THE MANAGEMENT OF FRACTURES, DISLOCATIONS, AND SPRAINS

THE MANAGEMENT OF
FRACTURES, DISLOCATIONS, AND SPRAINS

BY

JOHN ALBERT KEY, B.S., M.D.

ST. LOUIS, MO.

Clinical Professor of Orthopedic Surgery, Washington University School of Medicine;
Associate Surgeon, Barnes, Children's, and Jewish Hospitals

AND

H. EARLE CONWELL, M.D., F.A.C.S.

BIRMINGHAM, ALA.

Associate Professor of Orthopaedic Surgery, University of Alabama School of Medicine;
Consulting Orthopaedic Surgeon to the Tennessee Coal, Iron and Railroad Company and the
American Cast Iron Pipe Company; Member of the Committee on Fractures and
Traumatic Surgery of the American Academy of Orthopaedic Surgeons and Member
of the Fracture Committee of the American College of Surgeons. Associate
Surgical Director of the Crippled Children's Hospital, Attending
Orthopaedic Surgeon to St. Vincent's Hospital, South
Highlands Hospital, Jefferson-Hillman Hospital,
Children's Hospital and Baptist Hospitals,
Birmingham, Alabama

FOURTH EDITION

ST. LOUIS
THE C. V. MOSBY COMPANY
1946

Reprinted January, 1947

Printed in the
United States of America

Press of
The C. V. Mosby Company
St. Louis

DEDICATED TO

ELEANOR LAURENSON KEY
AND
BELLE ANDRUS CONWELL

PREFACE TO FOURTH EDITION

Partly as a result of lessons learned from the treatment of injuries incident to the war and partly as a result of the natural progress of the science of medicine, many new methods of treating injuries of the bones and joints have been introduced. We have incorporated what we consider the more valuable of these in this edition and have deleted methods which we consider obsolete. The principal changes have been made in the sections on the spine, the hip and on compound fractures. We have also omitted many of the less valuable illustrations and have added about two hundred new ones.

PREFACE TO THIRD EDITION

Recent advances in the treatment of fractures and dislocations have made it advisable to revise this book. In this edition the most extensive changes have been made in the sections devoted to fractures of the spine, humerus, hip, and foot. The chapter on Compound Fractures has been rewritten, largely as a result of the introduction of the sulfonamides in the treatment of these injuries, and a new section on war injuries has been added. Dr. James Barrett Brown has revised his chapter on Fractures of the Jaws and Face, and Dr. Edgar F. Fincher has revised the chapter on Skull Fractures and Brain Trauma.

PREFACE TO SECOND EDITION

In this edition we have incorporated those additions and changes in our methods of diagnosing and treating fractures which since the publication of the first edition we have found beneficial and which we believe to be sufficiently important and well tested to warrant publication in a textbook.

The most extensive changes are those in the treatment of fractures of the spine and the hip. However, every chapter has been carefully reviewed and many changes with numerous substitutions have been made.

Dr. Edgar F. Fincher, who was Dr. Dowman's associate, has kindly revised Dr. Dowman's chapter on Skull Fractures and Brain Trauma. Dr. James Barrett Brown has revised his own chapter on Fractures of the Face and Jaws. We gratefully acknowledge contributions of other surgeons.

J. A. K.
H. E. C.

PREFACE TO FIRST EDITION

This book is written for the student, the general practitioner, and the surgeon. Its purpose is to furnish a practical working guide in the management of fractures, dislocations, and sprains; and since the treatment of so many injuries of this type is influenced by the Workmen's Compensation Laws, a chapter on this subject is included.

The forms of treatment described are those which we have used and have found reliable and practicable. We make little claim to originality in the methods selected; we have used the work of other surgeons whenever this seemed desirable and have endeavored to give them due credit for procedures which they originated. We have, however, used many methods in common practice in various clinics without attempting to trace them to their sources.

There are types of fractures in which injury to the soft tissues is of more importance than the fracture itself. In such cases the treatment of these complications has been described. In the chapters on specific lesions, the after-treatment has been described in detail, and the restoration of function in the shortest space of time has been emphasized.

The reduction of some fractures is a relatively simple matter and may be successfully carried out by the general practitioner, who, however, should continually bear in mind that complicated fractures in the same region may tax the skill of the most experienced surgeon. Complications that may arise have been set forth in this book, with detailed information on how to treat them.

The automobile and the machinery age in industry have brought a new era, greatly influencing the occurrence, diagnosis, and treatment of fractures. The physician in the smallest town may suddenly be called to the aid of a patient suffering a severe fracture. He should know how to give the best form of emergency treatment, how to transport the patient to a hospital with the least possible additional injury should hospitalization be necessary. For this reason a special chapter on Emergency Treatment has been included.

It is not our belief that the time will come in medical practice when all fracture cases will be treated by specialists, but it is our opinion that every general practitioner should be able to recognize the possible occurrence of complications and deformities in certain fractures. In order to safeguard himself and give his patient the best possible care, he should procure the opinion and the aid of a specialist when necessary.

Since the possibility of damage suits in fracture cases is a constant cause of apprehension, a chapter on Medicolegal Aspects in Fracture Cases is included.

We believe that fractures of the skull and face require the attention of specialists. We have, therefore, requested specialists in these fields to write the chapters. The late Dr. Charles E. Dowman wrote the chapter on Fractures of the Skull and Brain Trauma shortly before his untimely death. The proof has been read by his associate, Dr. Edgar F. Fincher, but the text has not been changed. This chapter is a fitting memento to Dr. Dowman's great work in this field of surgery, and is a contribution of great value to the literature of fractures and neurological surgery. Dr. James Barrett Brown, of St. Louis, associate of Dr. Vilray P. Blair, has written the chapter on Fractures of the Jaws and Related Bones of the Face.

We wish to express our thanks to Dr. Lloyd Noland, Chief Surgeon for the Tennessee Coal, Iron and Railroad Company, and the Employees' Hospital, Birmingham, Alabama, for his cooperation and stimulus. We also desire to thank the past and present members of the Radiological Department and other services of the Employees' Hospital for their cooperation, and the various surgeons who furnished us with illustrations or with specific methods which we have incorporated in the book, for which due credit has been given. We thank Mr. James Whatley, the X-ray Technician of the Employees' Hospital, and Mr. R. H. Webb, of Birmingham, whose interest and energy are largely responsible for the quality of the photographs which are reproduced here, and Miss Lucille Weems, of St. Louis, who did the secretarial work involved and compiled the index.

J. A. K.
H. E. C.

CONTENTS

PART I

PRINCIPLES AND GENERAL ASPECTS

CHAPTER I

CHAPTER II

CHAPTER III

CHAPTER IV

CHAPTER V

CHAPTER VI

PART II

DIAGNOSIS AND TREATMENT OF SPECIFIC INJURIES

CHAPTER XI

CHAPTER XII

CHAPTER XIII

CHAPTER XIV

CHAPTER XV

CHAPTER XVI

CHAPTER XVII

CHAPTER XVIII

CHAPTER XIX

CHAPTER XX

CHAPTER XXI

CHAPTER XXII

CHAPTER XXIII

CHAPTER XXIV

CHAPTER XXV

CHAPTER XXVI

CHAPTER XXVII

THE MANAGEMENT OF FRACTURES, DISLOCATIONS, AND SPRAINS

THE MANAGEMENT OF FRACTURES, DISLOCATIONS, AND SPRAINS

PART I
PRINCIPLES AND GENERAL ASPECTS

CHAPTER I
GENERAL CONSIDERATIONS

FRACTURE EQUIPMENT

One of the principal reasons for the poor results so frequently seen in the treatment of fractures and one of the reasons why so many men who see an occasional fracture dislike to treat it is that adequate fracture treatment cannot be carried out efficiently and successfully without apparatus, and at the present time in the majority of general hospitals in this country there is a real lack of the necessary apparatus for the proper handling of fracture cases.

In certain hospitals in which an important member of the staff treats a large number of fractures, there is an adequate armamentarium; but unless this is true when a patient with a fracture comes into the hospital there is a scurrying about of internes, a fruitless search here and there for the required splint with finally the announcement that what is really needed is not to be had, and the surgeon after much waste of time will have to make out with something which may be rigged up to serve the purpose. For this reason we believe that every general hospital which accepts acute fracture cases for treatment should have a well-lighted splint room of ample size and that this room should be in a convenient location, that it should be kept locked at all times when it is not in use, and that some member of the hospital resident staff should be responsible for the condition of this splint room; the apparatus should be taken from the splint room only on requisition and should be signed for and returned to the room when it is no longer required for the treatment of a patient.

In addition to the splint room a hospital should have a fracture table in the operating room and should have an efficient system for the maintenance at all times of an adequate supply of plaster-of-Paris bandages.

In order to further this idea that if a surgeon is to do good fracture work it is necessary that he be supplied with good tools, we have listed (p. 22) the apparatus which we believe should be present in the splint room of a general hospital of from one hundred to two hundred beds which accepts acute fracture cases for treatment. In industrial hospitals where a larger proportion of cases are fracture cases, the amount of apparatus should be larger. In hospitals where an important member of the staff treats a large number of fracture cases the person responsible for the treatment will, of course, modify the list of apparatus according to his personal tastes. We have simply endeavored to make a skeleton outline which may be modified at will, but we believe that if the superintendent of every general hospital could be persuaded to invest a few hundred dollars in fracture equipment and inaugurate a system by which this equipment will not be lost or misplaced and will be readily available when needed, the results obtained will amply justify the expenditure. In addition to the equipment mentioned below the hospital should have on hand an adequate number of suitable fracture beds (Fig. 4).

Equipment to Be Kept in Splint Room

1. Overhead frame for treating fractures of the leg and femur in adults by suspension and traction (Army Balkan frame or its equivalent) (Figs. 1, 2, 3, 4, and 5)—4.

2. Round wood or metal bars (Trapeze bars)—6.

3. Overhead frame for treating fractures of the femur in children by suspension and traction (Conwell's frame or its equivalent) (Fig. 976)—2.

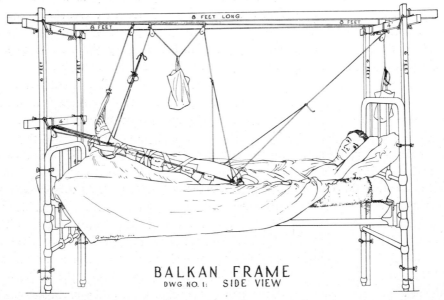

Fig. 1.—Balkan frame (United States Army pattern) for use in treating fractures of the lower extremity by traction. (Skeletal or adhesive.) (Courtesy Major General N. T. Kirk, Surgeon General, U. S. Army.)

4. Lateral traction frame for treating fractures of the upper extremity by traction and suspension (Conwell's lateral traction frame or its equivalent) (Fig. 7)—2.

5. Bradford frames for adults with extra covers—2.

6. Bradford frames for children with extra covers—2.

7. Adjustable canvas hammocks for pelvis with spreader (clean)—2.

8. Wooden or metal upright frames with pulley attachment for Buck's extension—4.

9. Braided rope, size ⅛ and ¼ inch—3 rolls each.

10. Awning pulleys for ¼ and ⅛ inch rope—2 doz. each.

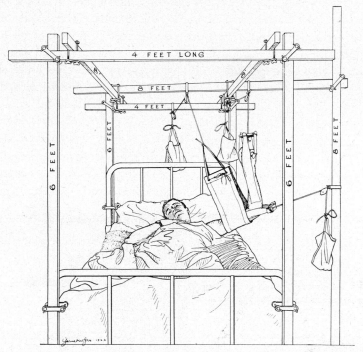

Fig. 2.—Balkan frame (United States Army pattern) as used in fractures of the humerus.
(Courtesy Major General N. T. Kirk, Surgeon General, U. S. Army.)

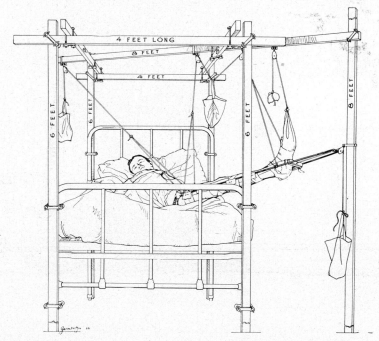

Fig. 3.—Balkan frame (United States Army pattern) showing thigh in abduction. (Courtesy
Major General N. T. Kirk, Surgeon General, U. S. Army.)

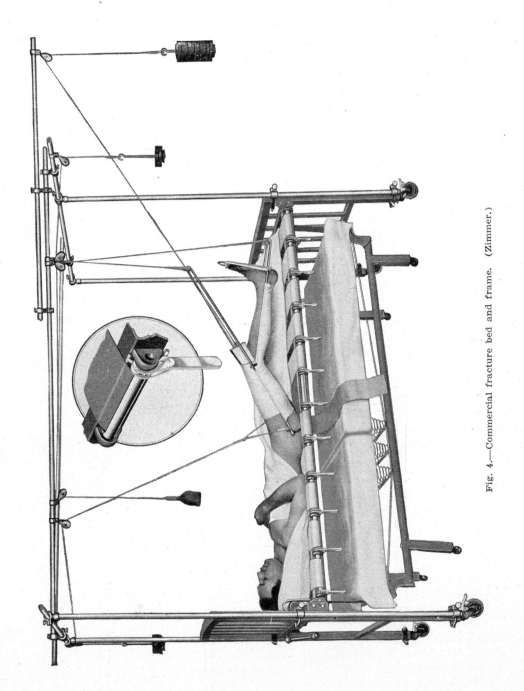

Fig. 4.—Commercial fracture bed and frame.   (Zimmer.)

11. Lower extremity Thomas splints, hinged or standard type and of various sizes—12. Pearson attachment for Thomas splints—4.

12. Foot supports for Thomas splints—12.

13. Hodgen splints—3.

14. Upper extremity Thomas splints—2.

15. Muslin or canvas strips 4 and 6 inches wide and 18 to 24 inches long—2 doz. each.

16. Safety pins for fastening the muslin strips in the splints as slings or for other purposes—6 doz.

17. Zinc oxide adhesive, 12 inches by 10 yards—3 rolls.

18. Spreaders (square wood blocks with hole in middle) (Fig. 73)—12.

19. Gauze and muslin bandages 2, 3, and 4 inches wide and 5 yards long—1 doz. each.

20. Elastic bandages (stockinet) 3, 4, and 6 inches wide and 5 yards long—6 of each.

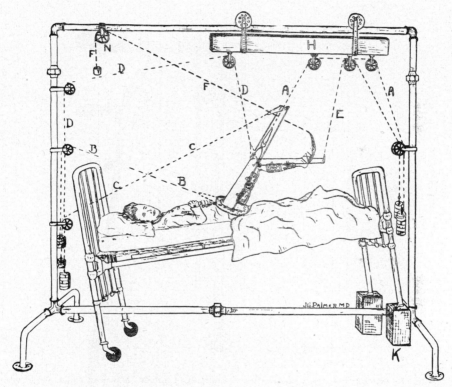

Fig. 5.—One type of overhead frame for treatment of fractures of the femur by suspension and traction. (Skeletal or adhesive.) (Conwell: Surg. Gynec. Obst., January, 1925.)

21. Cabot posterior wire splints—4.

22. Straight flat board splints either of pine or some other soft wood, ¼ inch thick and 3, 4, and 6 inches wide and 3 feet long—1 doz. each.

23. Sheet cotton rolls 3 and 6 inches in width—2 doz. each.

24. Jones' metal cock-up wrist splint or its equivalent—3.

25. Jones' humerus splints (Fig. 9)—2 right and 2 left or 2 reversible.

26. Metal abduction splints for the upper extremity—2.

27. Clavicular cross splints, small, medium, and large sizes—2 each.

28. Triangular slings for children and adults—12 each size.

29. Scale weights or window sash weights 1-, 2-, and 5-pound sizes amounting to 400 or 500 pounds. In case scale weights are used, pieces of heavy wire or iron rods bent properly for the reception of these weights—12.

30. Blocks for elevating foot of bed, 14 inches—6 pairs.

31. Fracture boards to be placed between the mattress and spring 1 inch thick and length and width of bed—6.

32. Sandbags 1, 2, and 3 feet long—4 each.

33. Plaster cutters, spreader, and knives (sharp).

34. Roll of webbing strap and buckles.

35. Pulley apparatus for foot of bed (Buck's extension) (Fig. 6).

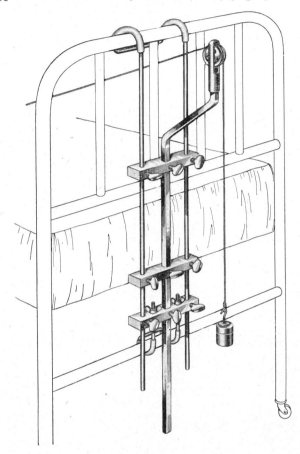

Fig. 6.—Buck's extension apparatus. (Courtesy Zimmer Manufacturing Co.)

Equipment to Be Kept in the Operating Room

1. Fracture table, a Bell, Hawley or Albee table or some other type permitting traction to the upper and lower extremities and the application of plaster spicas to upper and lower extremities with the patient in recumbency.

2. Apparatus for applying skeletal traction to upper and lower extremities. (Preferably some form of wire traction apparatus.)

3. An adequate set of bone instruments. These should be selected by a competent fracture surgeon.

4. An adequate supply of plaster-of-Paris bandages, sheet cotton, felt, and stockinet with suitable vessels for soaking the plaster bandages.

5. Plaster shears, spreader, and knives.

6. Heavy iron wire for making banjo splints for finger and toe traction.

7. Roll of webbing strap and buckles.

8. Tourniquets (two flat heavy rubber and one Campbell or its equivalent.

9. Electric band saw and accessories.

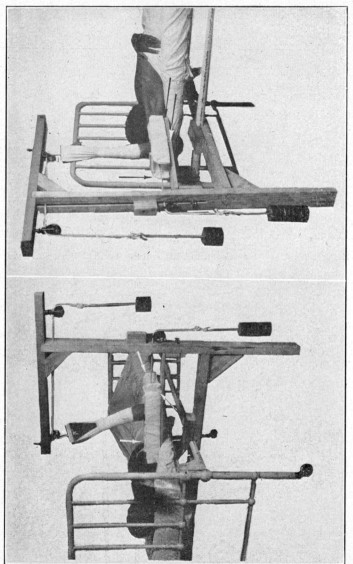

Fig. 7.—Lateral traction frame for treatment of fractures of the upper extremity by suspension and traction. (Conwell: South. Med. Jour., 1927.)

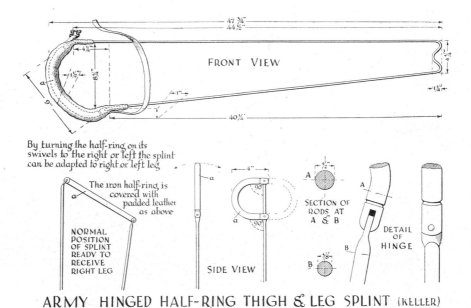

ARMY HINGED HALF-RING THIGH & LEG SPLINT (KELLER)

Fig. 8.—Keller hinged half-ring thigh and leg splint. (United States Army splint.)

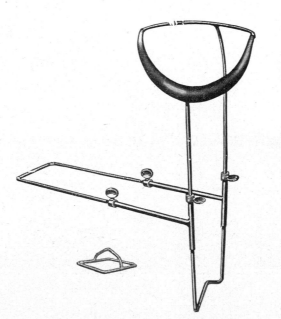

Fig. 9.—Jones humerus splint. (Zimmer reversible.)

Emergency Room

If the splints and other apparatus are kept in the splint room, there is no necessity for any special fracture equipment in the emergency room unless it is the practice of the given hospital to apply plaster-of-Paris casts here. Where this practice prevails, plaster equipment should be kept on hand in the emergency room.

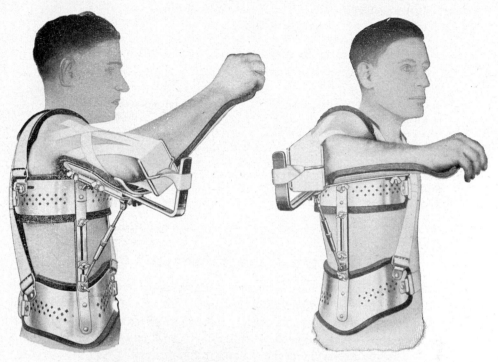

Fig. 10.—Abduction shoulder and arm splint. Two views. (Zimmer.)

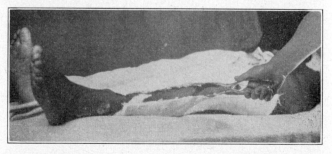

Fig. 11.—Use of Hoke's plaster spreader.

Equipment to Be Kept in the Office

In many instances physicians and surgeons who do much of their practice in their office and who do not take many of their fracture cases to hospitals find it advisable to keep a supply of splints on hand at the office. For this reason we are including the following list for the doctor's office and the doctor's automobile. This is the list recommended by the Cooperative Committee on Fractures of the American Medical Association and is taken from their report.

Splints to Be Kept in the Doctor's Automobile

1 Thomas leg splint
1 Thomas arm splint
½ dozen basswood splints
 Enough sheet wadding or cotton
  (padding)

1 tourniquet
1 can of ether
Bandages
Adhesive tape

Splints to Be Kept in the Doctor's Office

2 Thomas leg splints
1 Thomas arm splint
1 dozen splint boards of basswood ⅛ by
 3 by 24 inches
2 dozen plaster-of-Paris bandages wrapped
 in paper napkins, kept in an air-
 tight tin box in a dry place
2 dozen sheet wadding rolls 4 inches wide,
 5 yards long, of nonabsorbent cotton
1 yard of saddler's felt, ½ inch thick
½ dozen wire gauze rolls, 4 inches by 2
 yards; chicken wire, ¼ inch mesh

1 dozen iron wire rods, ⅛ inch, 1 yard
 long
1 roll of copper wire, 16 gauge
3 rolls of zinc oxide adhesive plaster 5
 yards long and 2 inches wide
6 sandbags made of heavy canvas 9 by 1
 or 2 inches
 Rubber tubing, ½ inch; several long
  pieces for a tourniquet
2 dozen webbing straps and buckles, 2 feet
 long
2 dozen 1- to 3-inch roller bandages

PLASTER-OF-PARIS TECHNIC

In this book we have used plaster of Paris more extensively than is usually recommended in textbooks on fractures. This is done because there are several advantages in using plaster of Paris in the treatment of fractures, and we believe that every surgeon who handles very many fractures should become skilled in its use. One of the principal advantages is that a plaster-of-Paris cast or splint, if properly applied, fits the patient more accurately and is more comfortable than any other form of apparatus with which we are familiar. Furthermore, when once the plaster has hardened and it is determined that the condition of the limb is satisfactory, the plaster requires very little attention on the part of the surgeon until the time comes for its removal, while splints fastened either with bandages, straps, or adhesive require frequent inspections, adjustments, and reapplications. Plaster of Paris is always available in hospitals equipped for its use, while the proper splint for a given case is frequently not available even in a large hospital.

Plaster of Paris

In this country practically all plaster-of-Paris casts are applied by means of bandages while in France many surgeons use attelles or pieces of crinoline cut to a definite pattern and impregnated with plaster cream. We shall not discuss attelles in this book. The first requisite in plaster-of-Paris bandages is good plaster of Paris. This is gypsum or calcium sulphate which is crushed and converted into an amorphous anhydride by heating. The heat causes it to lose 93 per cent of its original water of crystallization, and when it is again mixed with water a chemical union takes place which is called recrystallization or setting. In setting, the plaster becomes hard in whatever form it may be at the time and expands very slightly. Once it is set it retains its original shape indefinitely. Good plaster of Paris should set in about seven minutes. Higher grades of dental plaster may set more quickly. If quicker setting is desired in ordinary plaster of Paris, this can be obtained by adding salt to the water in which the plaster is soaked.

Plaster of Paris can be purchased in tins of various sizes or in barrels. Unless large amounts are used, it is better to purchase it in tins and keep the tin covered, for when exposed to moist air it tends to take up water slowly and crystallize.

The bandage material used is crinoline, which is book muslin sized with starch and not with glue. The meshes of this muslin should not be finer than from twenty to twenty-four to the inch.

At the present time excellent plaster bandages and splints can be purchased ready for use.

Making Plaster-of-Paris Bandages

The crinoline should be torn into lengths of from four to five yards and into widths of from two to eight inches as desired. After the strips have been torn, they should be folded lengthwise and the loose threads removed from the edges with a pin: otherwise these threads tend to pull out and tangle and prevent uniform unrolling of the bandage. The crinoline is now ready for the application of the plaster and the rolling into a bandage. This may be done by hand or by machine, as many plaster bandage machines have been devised from time to time and new ones are constantly appearing on the market. It has been our experience, however, that the best and most uniform bandages are those made by hand and that no machine yet devised is foolproof. The difficulty with making bandages by machine is that the person who makes them expects the machine to control the amount of plaster and tension with which the bandage is rolled and this does not occur.

In order to make the bandage by hand several pounds of plaster are poured out on a flat table and crinoline bandage is laid out on the table near the plaster. A handful of the plaster is then laid on the bandage and with a wooden paddle or with the hand this is pushed along over the bandage and the excess is removed while the bandage is drawn toward the person making it (Fig. 12). During this process the meshes of the bandage become impregnated with the plaster. As it is pulled in, it is rolled loosely, care being taken not to shake out the plaster which is in the meshes of the crinoline. If the bandage is rolled tightly, it will be found that when it is immersed in water the outside of the bandage will become saturated while the center will remain dry and when it is used the center will have to be thrown away. As the bandages are rolled, they should be wrapped in a tissue paper napkin, stored in a tin box, and kept in a dry place, for if they are kept a long time exposed to the outside air, the plaster tends to crystallize and deteriorate in quality.

Hospitals in which fractures are treated should keep a good supply of various widths of plaster-of-Paris bandages on hand, since these may be needed at any time and making them is a slow process.

Excellent plaster-of-Paris bandages and splints are now made in quantity in this country and are available. Many hospitals find it cheaper and more satisfactory to use this material. An ample supply should be kept on hand.

Soaking and Handling Plaster-of-Paris Bandages

As a rule when the plaster-of-Paris cast is applied, a nurse or orderly soaks and hands the bandage to the surgeon. The bandage should be soaked in a pail filled with lukewarm water. If quick setting is desired, a tablespoonful of salt should be added to the water. It is to be remembered that when a large plaster-of-Paris cast is required, such as a spica, and fifteen or twenty bandages are to be used, the ordinary pail does not contain enough water. After a certain number of bandages have been soaked in it, usually about eight or ten, the water left in the pail becomes saturated with plaster; consequently, when a large cast is to be applied two or more pails of water should be at hand to avoid the delay and inconvenience of emptying and refilling a pail during the application of a cast. Once a cast is started, it should be completed rapidly and without interruption; otherwise part of the plaster will set before the remainder has been applied and an unsatisfactory cast may result.

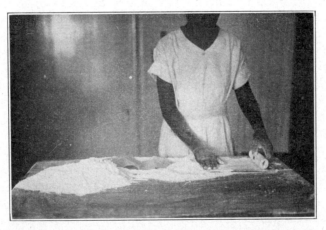

Fig. 12.—Method of rolling plaster-of-Paris bandage.

When the pails of water are ready and placed in a convenient position, the bandages are removed one at a time from the tin box containing them; a hole is punched in the tissue paper napkin around them at either end and the bandage is placed in the water and set on end to allow the contained air to escape. When bubbles cease to come from it, it is saturated with water and should be picked up gently without shaking and grasped at either end and slowly squeezed by pushing the ends together. By grasping at the ends one prevents the plaster from being squeezed out of the bandage. The tightness with which it should be squeezed varies with different surgeons. Some like bandages quite wet and some quite dry. Most of us prefer not to have them drip all over when they are being used, but we do like them thoroughly saturated with water.

Just before removing one bandage from the pail another should be inserted. If two surgeons are working on the cast, two bandages should be put in the water at the same time, but rarely should more than two be put in at once, because if the bandages are left in the water too long the plaster sets and the bandage must be discarded. It should be remembered that the setting is a chemical process and occurs just as quickly when the bandage is submerged in water as it does in the outside air. As the bandage is removed from the water and squeezed the person handling the bandage should remove the tissue paper, if this has not already been done, find the end of the bandage, and unroll it a little way in order to save the surgeon's time when applying it.

Application of Plaster-of-Paris Bandages

1. **Preparation of the Patient.**—The skin should be clean. If necessary it should be scrubbed with soap and water and then dried and washed with alcohol. It should next be protected by a small amount of padding unless the surgeon is adept in the use of the skin-tight plaster which has been popularized by Boehler, of Vienna. If a Boehler plaster is being used, no padding is necessary and the plaster of Paris is rolled directly on the skin. In Boehler's plaster the hair is not shaved, as hair on the skin plays an important part in making the plaster adhere. In this country we usually protect the skin with stockinet or sheet cotton and protect the bony prominences with saddler's felt.

We use the nonpadded plaster cast or skin-tight plaster in special instances, but not as a routine dressing. In applying a nonpadded plaster splint or cast the splint should be spread as smoothly as possible on the skin and the plaster bandage should be pulled snugly and evenly as it is rolled around the extremity. It is important that the nonpadded cast be as thin as is consistent with strength.

One of the secrets of applying a plaster-of-Paris cast is enough padding, but not too much. In other words it is just as bad technic to over-pad a part and then place a loose plaster-of-Paris cast around it as it is to neglect the padding and produce pressure sores as a result, because if too much padding is used it soon becomes compressed, the part moves around in the plaster, and fixation is inadequate. Not only this, but a loosely fitting plaster cast is less comfortable and may even result in pressure sores because of the movement of the limb in the case.

The stockinet can be purchased in rolls of widths of from two inches up to strips wide enough to cover the body of an obese patient. The stockinet is easier to apply than the sheet cotton and makes a neater cast. It has the disadvantage that it does not fit so evenly as the sheet cotton. When the stockinet is applied to the lower extremity for instance, a wider piece is required for the thigh than is necessary for the foot and leg; when it is pulled up into the groin, the edge tends to cut in; for this reason it should be split at the top.

In most instances we apply stockinet over the ends of the extremities, but depend upon sheet cotton for the greater part of the padding. This sheet cotton is torn into strips of from two to eight inches wide and is rolled into bandages of from four to five yards in length. It is nonabsorbable material and is applied as an ordinary bandage would be. It should be pulled snugly around the limb and applied in a thin layer, usually two or three layers of sheet cotton covering most of the limb.

After the sheet cotton has been applied, the bony prominences should be protected by pieces of felt. In a spica of the lower extremity a wide strip of felt is placed over the sacrum and extends up the spine, small triangular pieces are put over each anterior superior spine, and a long strip is put under the heel and up the tendo achillis. In some instances it is wise to put a piece of felt over the head of the fibula in order to guard against pressure on the peroneal nerve. In the upper extremity the ulna and the inner epicondyle of the humerus are the main points that need protection. We place a strip along the shaft of the ulna and extend it down to cover the styloid process and cover the epicondyle of the humerus and the olecranon.

Bandages should not be placed in water until the preliminary padding of the patient is complete. Strips of felt should be put on last, since it is desirable that they be next to the plaster; otherwise they may become loose and move around in the cast.

2. **Application of the Cast.**—The plaster-of-Paris bandage should be applied smoothly with an even tension. It should be tight enough so that it sets snugly to the patient, but care should be taken that when it is tightened, there is an even pressure across the full width of the plaster bandage to avoid cutting in at some point and causing a pressure sore, since these tension bands tend to remain as long as the cast stays on. A plaster-of-Paris bandage should be applied just as is adhesive; it should lie where it naturally falls and should never be twisted. In changing the direction of the bandage the plaster is reversed; it is pulled off the limb for a short distance, folded on itself, and started in the desired direction. The inside of the cast should be smooth.

If these rules are followed, a plaster-of-Paris bandage can be applied snugly with very little padding, no trouble need be expected from pressure sores, and it will rarely be necessary to bivalve the plaster afterward on account of swelling or pain.

It is important that the patient's limb be maintained in the original position until the plaster sets, as movements may cause either breaking of the plaster cast or a wrinkle in its surface which will result in a pressure sore later. Particularly to be warned against is the habit of supporting the limb by means of muslin or gauze slings from an overhead support, applying plaster over these slings, and then cutting them loose after the plaster has set. We have seen very extensive pressure sores result from this method. The assistant who holds the limb must avoid keeping his hands in one place and making indentations in the plaster, since these indentations tend to remain and may cause pressure sores and sloughing after the plaster has set.

The setting of the plaster takes only a few minutes and the patient may then be placed in bed. The cast should be left uncovered in order that it may dry out as much as possible; if the plaster remains wet too long a poor quality cast may result, breaking and necessitating reapplication of the cast. In order to hasten the drying process, we usually place an electric baker over the cast as soon as the patient returns to the ward.

The Skin-Tight Plaster.—Largely due to the writings of Dr. Boehler, the skin-tight plaster cast has been widely used during the past few years. Personally, we rarely apply such a plaster on fresh fractures, but use it more as a convalescent splint for the extremities, especially where we wish to apply a walking iron and have the patient use the extremity with the support of the plaster. It may be applied with plaster-of-Paris molds, which in turn are encircled with a thin plaster-of-Paris bandage, or it may be applied with the bandage. In applying a skin-tight plaster the skin should be clean, but should not be shaved as the hairs help the plaster to stick to the skin. It is important that good plaster-of-Paris bandages be used and that they contain sufficient plaster of Paris, but not an excess, which would tend to form lumps in the bandage or mold. It is also important in applying a plaster that the bandage or mold be quite wet in order that it may fit the skin closely with a minimum of wrinkles. In rolling the bandage on the limb it is important that it be applied snugly but not pulled sufficiently tight to cut into the skin at any point. Finally, the plaster-of-Paris cast should be made as thin as is consistent with the required strength. There is no special difficulty in applying a skin-tight plaster for anyone who is proficient in the use of plaster of Paris over the usual small amount of padding. We do not advise it in fresh fractures which may be expected to swell.

Reinforcements in Plaster-of-Paris Casts

Reinforcements are frequently used and are often advisable in the application of plaster-of-Paris casts, since by their use the cast can be made lighter. These are made of plaster-of-Paris bandage of the desired width

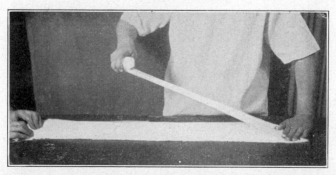

Fig. 13.—Method of constructing a plaster mold. A plaster bandage is simply unrolled on a flat surface to make a splint. This can be made on one or more thicknesses of padding (sheet cotton).

and length, simply rolled out on a table or other flat surface and folded on itself until a flat strip is obtained (Fig. 13). This is applied to the wet plaster dressing and incorporated in the cast. Reinforcements are particularly useful over the hip and shoulder; without them spica casts, even when properly applied, are apt to be broken. We do not incorporate iron or wooden reinforcements in the cast; they are bunglesome, interfere with the removal of the cast, and are not necessary if the cast is properly applied. In addition to the strips for reinforcement we frequently begin a plaster-of-Paris cast of the leg or arm with a plaster-of-Paris mold, made as described later, which is padded lightly with sheet cotton and fitted to the extremity. The advantages of this are that one obtains a certain amount of immediate immobilization and that it is easier to hold the limb while the cast is being applied than if the mold is not used.

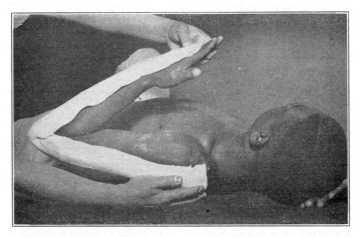

Fig. 14.—Plaster-of-Paris mold applied to the upper extremity for immobilization at the elbow with flexion of forearm at the elbow.

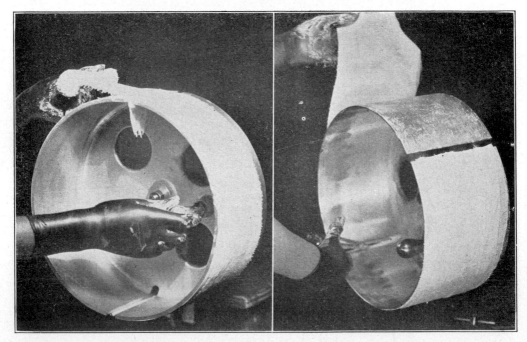

Fig. 15.—M. O. Henry's roller for making plaster reinforcements.

Plaster-of-Paris Molds.—Instead of applying a circular cast around the limb we frequently use a plaster-of-Paris mold for the arm, forearm, and shoulder and occasionally for the foot and leg in fractures in which there is relatively little danger of displacement and in others in which we desire simple immobilization. These molds are easily made by laying three or four layers of sheet cotton of the desired width and length on a table, applying ten to fifteen layers of plaster-of-Paris bandage over the sheet cotton, then laying this wet strip of plaster on the limb with the sheet cotton next to the skin, and bandaging it quickly and snugly with a gauze bandage (Fig. 14). The mold may be left on in this way, or as soon as the plaster sets the bandage can be cut and the mold slipped off, its edges trimmed and a neat plaster splint made. The splint should be as light as possible, but strong enough to support the extremity in the desired position. The chief difficulty in making these molds is that they may be made too thick so that the plaster begins to set before it is applied to the skin or to the limb; as a result it wrinkles or cracks and is uncomfortable and inefficient.

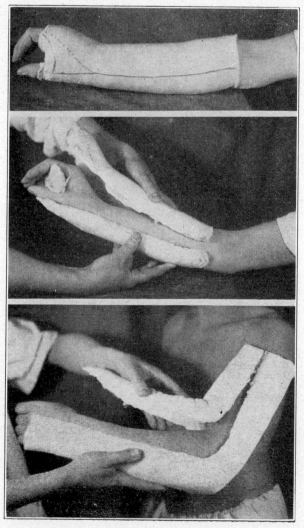

Fig. 16.—Plaster cast applied to the hand and forearm for immobilization of the wrist in the cock-up position (the optimum functional position at the wrist).

Fig. 17.—Same as preceding, bivalved for physiotherapy, or other treatment or inspection.

Fig. 18.—Plaster-of-Paris cast applied to the arm, elbow, and the forearm and bivalved for physiotherapy, or other treatment or inspection.

Splitting and Bivalving Plaster-of-Paris Casts.—Most textbooks and many surgeons in their writings advise that after a circular plaster-of-Paris cast is applied to the extremity it should be split or bivalved in order to allow for swelling and to prevent pressure sores. As a matter of fact, we rarely split our circular plaster casts until we are ready to take them off; but if we expect an extremity to swell to an unusual degree, we keep the patient in the hospital and have the limb elevated and the fingers or toes exposed in order that they may be inspected. If we find a marked impairment of the circulation we not only split the plaster on both sides, but we remove the upper portion and, what is equally as important, split the sheet cotton and inspect the leg. Then we strap the two halves of the cast together with adhesive. It should be remembered that it does little good to split the plaster if the circulation is impeded by a tight binding of sheet cotton or other material beneath the cast, and for this reason one should be particularly careful not to apply gauze or other bandages of unyielding material beneath the plaster cast.

We believe that most of the difficulties so much discussed and the dangers to the circulation after application of circular plaster casts are due not to the fact that the cast has not been split after it has been put on, but to the fact that the cast has been improperly applied in the first place. Of course, if a surgeon does not know how to apply a plaster-of-Paris cast properly, he should always split it as soon as it has set. However, plaster casts are frequently bivalved for physiotherapy or inspection of a part and are then strapped on. (Figs. 16, 17, and 18.)

DEFINITIONS

A **fracture** is the breaking of the continuity of a bone or of a cartilage.

An **epiphyseal separation** is a fracture in which the line of the fracture lies wholly or partly in the epiphyseal line.

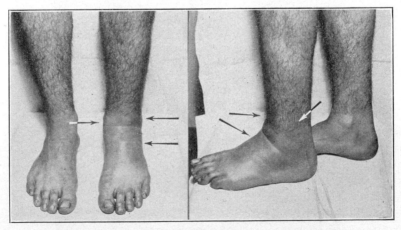

Fig. 19.—Severe sprain of the left ankle. X-rays negative.

A **dislocation** is the complete and persistent displacement of the articular surface of one of the bones entering into the formation of a joint from that of its fellow.

A **subluxation** is an incomplete dislocation in which the normal relationship of the articular surfaces is disturbed but in which they are partly in contact.

A **sprain** is a temporary subluxation in which the articular surfaces have returned to their normal positions and in which there has resulted more or less damage to the ligaments, tendons, and muscles around the joint.

A **sprain fracture** is a sprain in which a small portion of one of the bones, usually a ligamentous insertion, has been pulled off.

ETIOLOGY OF FRACTURES

The causes of fractures may be divided into predisposing or indirect, and exciting or direct causes. The predisposing causes may be divided into external and physical or physiologic.

External predisposing causes are those which are incidental to the occupations and modes of life of individuals with resultant variations in their exposure to injury. For instance, fractures are more frequent in the male and in the second, third, and fourth decades because during this period of life the individual is more active and exposed to injury. Under physical or natural predisposing causes we include the liability of certain bones to fracture because of their exposed positions, shape, osseous structure or function as levers. The bones of the extremities most frequently fractured are the (1) phalanges, (2) metacarpals, (3) clavicle, (4) radius, (5) humerus, (6) fibula and (7) tibia.

Age is a predisposing cause both because of its influence on the habits of the individual and because the structure of the various bones changes with age. In senility there is in many persons a rather marked osteoporosis which affects especially the upper end of the femur and humerus and the lower end of the radius, and makes these bones especially susceptible to fracture after relatively slight violence.

Direct or Exciting Causes

These may be divided into external violence and muscular action. Most fractures are the result of external violence, which may be either direct or indirect.

A fracture by direct violence is one in which the bone is broken immediately beneath the point of impact. These fractures are always accompanied by injury to the overlying soft tissues and are often compound. Examples are fractures due to blows or to falls in which the fracture occurs at the point of impact with the ground.

Fractures by indirect violence are those in which the fracturing force is transmitted through one or more bones and the fracture occurs at a distance from the site of the impact. Examples are fractures of the clavicle or humerus from falls upon the hands or of the spine or bones of the leg from falls upon the feet. The fracture is frequently due to leverage, as in a fracture of the lower end of the humerus in a hyperextension injury due to a fall upon the hand.

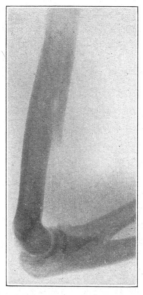

Fig. 20.—Spiral fracture of the humerus due to muscular violence. This fracture occurred in an eighteen-year-old boy, pitching a ball, just before his arm passed forward of the midline of the body. Treated by traction for 18 days; then a plaster cast for three weeks. Good result.

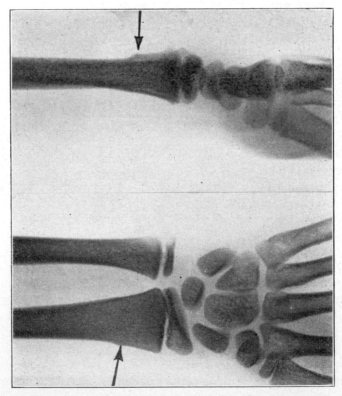

Fig. 21.—Typical infraction or torsion fracture of the radius. Treated by immobilization in a plaster cast to the forearm and wrist for four weeks.

In fractures from indirect violence the tissues are injured by the displacement of the fragments. These fractures are not often compound, and when they are compound the compounding is from within; that is, by the ends of the fragments being forced through the skin.

Fractures by muscular action are rare, but they do occasionally occur without the aid of any external violence. The fracture may be the result of violent contraction of muscles causing an abrupt strain on the bone or of sudden cessation of a muscular movement. For instance, a man may break an arm while throwing a ball (Fig. 20) or a patella while running. On the other hand, the fracture may result from contraction of a group of muscles against resistance in such a manner that great leverage is placed upon the bone, as occasionally occurs in a spiral fracture of the humerus when a woman is wringing out clothes, or when a rib is fractured from laughing.

March fractures are noted as the most frequent fracture in recruits under infantry training. They occur after or during a long march and are most frequent in the middle metatarsals, but may affect any of the bones of the lower extremity. They appear to be due to fatigue of the bone, much as metal may break after long-continued vibration or strain. (Fig. 24.)

CLASSIFICATION OF FRACTURES

1. **Dependent upon whether or not the fracture communicates with the outside air,** fractures are classified as **compound** and **simple.** Simple fractures are those in which there is no wound extending from the surface to the bone injury. It is to be noted that the term simple as used here has no reference to the treatment and that a simple fracture may be very difficult to treat satisfactorily. Compound fractures are those in which there is an open wound extending through the skin and down to the bone injury. A primary compound fracture is one in which the wound occurs at the time of the fracture, either from external violence or from within by the forcing of the end of a fragment through the skin. A secondary compound fracture is one in which a simple fracture has been rendered compound either by a surgical operation or by the sloughing of tissues over the site of the fracture. Primary compound fractures are always contaminated with bacteria and often become infected.

2. **Dependent Upon the Degree of the Fracture.**—Fractures are classified as **complete** and **incomplete,** dependent upon whether or not the continuity of the bone has been completely interrupted. A subperiosteal fracture is one in which there is no obvious displacement of the fragments and in which the periosteum is assumed to be intact. It may be complete or incomplete as regards the bone. A **greenstick fracture** is an incomplete fracture of the shaft of a long bone in which the cortex is broken on the convexity of the curve in the broken bone while the bone on the concave surface is bent and the bone is usually split longitudinally in either direction from the site of the fracture. Thus the fracture line resembles that which occurs when a green stick is broken. (Fig. 25B.) An **infraction type of fracture** is the opposite of a greenstick fracture; that is, it is one in which the cortex is broken and crushed on the concavity of the curve, while the cortex on the convexity remains intact. (Fig. 25A.) These fractures are practically limited to the bones of children, which

are considerably more flexible than are those of adults. Other types of incomplete fractures are **fissures** and **depressions**. **Sprain fractures** and **separations of an apophysis** are usually classed as incomplete fractures, but they are really

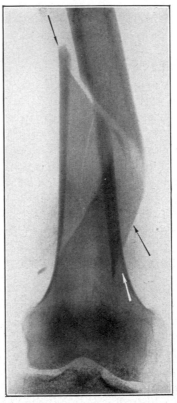

Fig. 22.—A spiral fracture, lower and middle third of femur. Treated by skeletal traction through lower end of femur with good result.

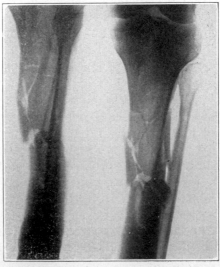

Fig. 23.—Compound comminuted fracture of the middle and upper thirds of the tibia due to direct violence. Treated by débridement and skeletal traction through tibia and later circular plaster cast with good result.

complete fractures of the part of the bone involved. A **complex simple fracture** is a fracture not compound, with or without laceration of the tissues, but with tissues severely traumatized. **Occult fracture** or **march fracture** is one which gives clinical signs of its presence yet which with excellent roentgen-ray technique cannot be demonstrated before reparative changes have taken place. (Hammond and O'Connor.)

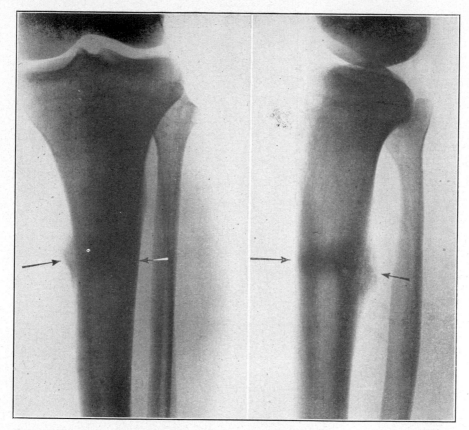

Fig. 24.—March fracture of the tibia. Treated by immobilization in a walking plaster. (Courtesy Major Hugh Smith.)

3. **Dependent Upon the Direction and Character of the Line of Fracture.**—Fractures are classified as longitudinal, transverse, oblique, spiral (Fig. 22), and V-, T-, stellate or Y-shaped. **Comminuted fractures** are those in which there is not only a break in the continuity of the bone, but the bone is broken into three or more fragments (Fig. 23). An **impacted fracture** is one in which one fragment has been driven into the other fragment and **remains** embedded there. Impacted fractures tend to occur at points where the ends of the two fragments are of different density, where the dense cortical bone of the shaft merges into the cancellous bone, as at the lower end of the radius, the upper end of the femur, and the upper end of the humerus. In such fractures the dense cortex is driven into the cancellous structure. Interlocking of fragments may occur without true impaction.

4. **Dependent Upon the Portion of the Bone Involved.**—In descriptions of fractures the site of the fracture is usually stated as fracture of the shaft

or lower end of the humerus, or fracture through the neck, or intertrochanteric or supracondylar fracture of the femur. If the fracture line lies entirely within a joint cavity, it is called an intraarticular fracture, while if it involves both intraarticular and extraarticular portions of the bone, it is called a true articular fracture.

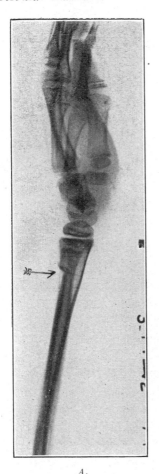
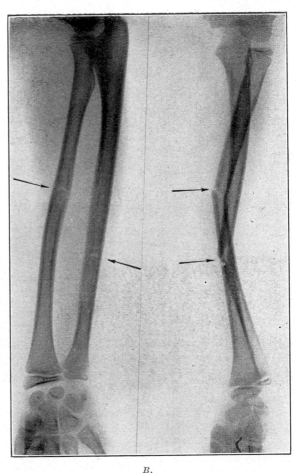

A. B.

Fig. 25.—A. Infarction fracture of the radius. B. Greenstick fracture of both bones or forearm in a child. Reduced by manipulation and immobilized in a plaster cast.

EPIPHYSEAL SEPARATIONS

Epiphyseal separations are fractures in which the fracture line lies wholly or partly within the epiphyseal line and the epiphysis may be wholly or partly separated from the shaft. Not infrequently in an epiphyseal separation a portion of the cortex of the shaft is split off with the epiphysis. Epiphyseal separations are most frequent in the lower end of the tibia, lower end of the radius, and upper end of the humerus.

Due to the fact that all of the epiphyses have united by the twenty-fifth year and that most of them have united before the age of twenty, epiphyseal separations practically do not occur after twenty years of age and are very rare after fifteen years of age. Most of the cases occur between the ages of

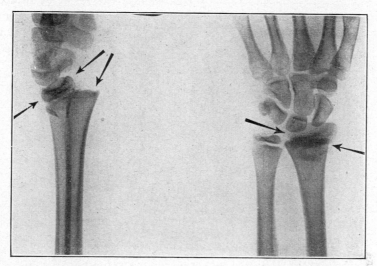

Fig. 26.—Showing the usual displacement in an epiphyseal separation of lower end of radius. Reduced by manipulation and immobilized in a plaster cast.

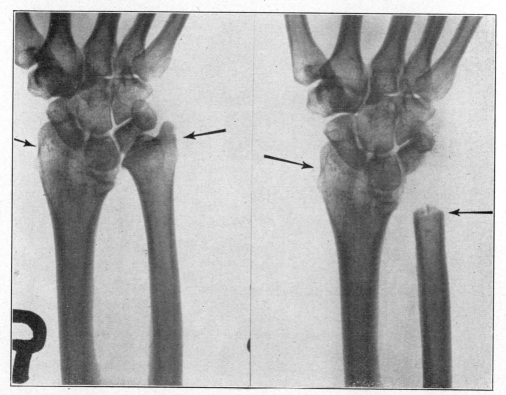

Fig. 27.—Epiphyseal arrest of the lower end of the radius following an injury in childhood. Treated by excision of the distal portion of the ulna with considerable improvement. (Darrach's operation).

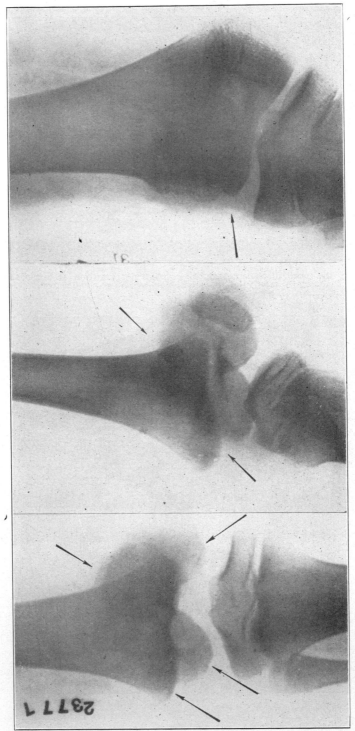

Fig. 28.—Partial epiphyseal arrest with valgus deformity following epiphyseal separation of the distal end of the femur despite good reduction. Treated by osteotomy.

six and twelve at a time when the epiphyses are rather large and the epiphyseal cartilage is relatively soft, this being the period of active growth.

The differential diagnosis between an epiphyseal separation and a fracture can in many instances be made only by the x-ray; but in a fracture near a joint in a young person in which the line of acute point tenderness lies at about the level of the epiphyseal line of the involved bone, an epiphyseal separation should be suspected. The symptoms are identical with those of a fracture except that if the fragments be moved upon one another a soft cartilaginous crepitus is obtained in place of the harsh bony crepitus of a true fracture.

In the treatment of an epiphyseal separation it is advisable that anatomic reduction be obtained where possible. Otherwise, deformity may occur as a result of abnormal growth at the site of the separation. It is also important that the surgeon warn the parents of the patient to the effect that occasionally after an epiphyseal separation there may result a disturbance of growth in the bone with resultant shortening, or even abnormal lengthening in rare instances. Fortunately, these growth disturbances are rare; but when they do occur, they are very serious and may demand operative interference and result in deformity despite the operative treatment. Consequently, the surgeon should not fail to let the parents know that such disturbances do occur and may occur in any given case despite proper treatment.

SYMPTOMS OF FRACTURES

The symptoms of fractures may be divided into objective and subjective. Subjective symptoms are those which are felt by the patient and knowledge of which the surgeon obtains from the patient. Objective symptoms are those which can be seen or felt by the surgeon himself. The subjective symptoms are the history of the accident, loss of function, pain and tenderness. The objective symptoms are surgical shock, deformity, swelling and ecchymosis, crepitus, abnormal mobility, and x-ray findings.

Subjective Symptoms

History.—The history should include a history of the accident and a history of any previous fractures or deformities which the patient may have suffered and which may have altered the form of the limb or which might lead the surgeon to suspect the presence of a pathologic fracture. In obtaining the history of the accident the surgeon should endeavor to ascertain as accurately as possible the degree of the traumatizing force and the manner and direction in which it was applied as well as whether there was direct trauma or only a twisting or muscular force produced. He should also find out whether or not the patient was rational at the time of the injury and whether or not the patient actually felt the bone break.

Pain.—Pain at the time of the injury and afterward, both spontaneous and upon movement of the fractured limb, is a constant accompaniment of fracture; but the degree of pain varies considerably in different fractures and in different persons with similar fractures. Not only should the surgeon learn as accurately as possible the character and location of the pain which the patient suffers while the extremity is at rest, but during the physical examination he should also endeavor to elicit pain at the site of the lesion by certain manipulations, since this pain may be of considerable aid in the diagnosis of obscure fractures.

In certain fractures without obvious displacement localized pain at the site of the fracture may be elicited by making axial pressure on the distal fragment or by making cross strain, such as when the bones of the leg or forearm are squeezed together, or by slight bending or twisting of the lower fragment while the upper is immobilized. For the purpose of diagnosis such localized pain need not be severe, but merely enough to indicate that when strain is put upon the given bone the pain occurs at a certain point.

Tenderness.—The amount of tenderness varies greatly in different persons and also varies directly with the amount of injury to the soft parts and with the time elapsing after the injury. Some patients complain of tenderness at any point along the limb, in which case it is more a question of apprehension than of true tenderness. If fractures are not seen until some hours after the injury and if there is considerable swelling and damage to the soft parts, there may be tenderness over a wide area.

An important point in the diagnosis of a fracture is what is called fracture tenderness or point tenderness. This is a narrow line of acute tenderness directly over the site of the injury. Point tenderness is difficult to elicit in bones which are covered by thick layers of soft tissue, as in the femur, but it is comparatively easy to elicit in superficial bones.

In order to elicit point tenderness the surgeon must handle the limb very gently and begin at some point distal to the site of the suspected fracture and with the tip of the finger gently press on the skin, gradually approaching the site of the fracture. When pressure is made directly over the site of the fracture, the patient will complain of acute tenderness. The surgeon should then begin at the other end of the limb and approach the fracture from the other direction. If true point tenderness has been located, the points of acute tenderness will tend to coincide.

Loss of Function also varies in different fractures and in different persons with the same fracture. The surgeon should first obtain a rough idea of the degree of loss of function from the history, and he should then corroborate the patient's statements by having the patient attempt to carry out certain movements. These should first be carried out without resistance, and then if this can be done, they should be carried out against resistance. In incomplete or impacted fractures the loss of function may be relatively slight; there are cases on record of patients who have walked on an impacted fracture of the upper end of the femur. Likewise we have seen patients walking with fractures of the shaft of the fibula.

Objective Symptoms

Constitutional Symptoms of Fractures.—All fractures are accompanied by more or less nervous shock to the patient and the degree of this varies with the person and with the severity of the injury. In the average simple fracture, shock is not present to any marked degree, but in a patient who has had a severe compound fracture of a large bone with extensive damage to soft tissues and severe hemorrhage, surgical shock may be the dominant feature and may demand immediate treatment before it is possible to attempt treatment of the fracture.

In a patient with a simple fracture who exhibits symptoms of severe surgical shock and in whom the fracture does not seem of sufficient gravity to account for the shock a careful search should be made for visceral injuries as otherwise these might be overlooked. The constitutional symptoms after an injury are apt to be more serious in older patients than in younger ones. During the first few days after the fracture, either simple or compound, many patients tend to run a temperature and a mild leucocytosis. This is apparently due to the resorption of the extravasated blood, but at times the temperature may reach 103° F. or even more and lead the surgeon to suspect some infection; in such instances the decision is a very delicate one as to whether or not a compound fracture which has been debrided and sutured should be reopened.

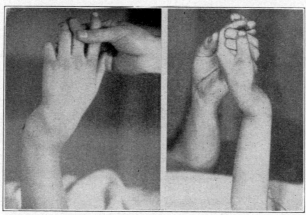

Fig. 29.   Fig. 30.

Fig. 29.—Marked radial deviation in a recent fracture of the lower third of both bones of the forearm.

Fig. 30.—Marked silver fork deformity is fracture of the lower third of both bones of the forearm.

Deformity.—Deformity signifies a change in the shape or position of the limb which is not due to swelling in the soft tissues, but is due to alterations in the bony structures. This deformity may be a shortening of the limb, a deviation from the normal alignment, an abnormal torsion of the limb, a separation of the fragments, or an abnormal posture of the limb. It is dependent upon displacement of the fragments and cannot be present unless the fragments are displaced. (Figs. 29, 30, 31, 32 and 33.)

The search for deformity should be the first step in the physical examination in a case in which a fracture is suspected. In order to detect a deformity, the injured limb and its fellow on the opposite side should be placed in the same relative positions and should then be compared by inspection, palpation, and measurements. In many instances in complete fractures with considerable displacement, the deformity is obvious at a glance. In others with very

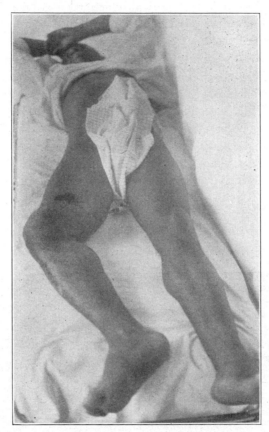

Fig. 31.—Deformity in a fracture of the lower third of the femur. This is a compound fracture (puncture wound).

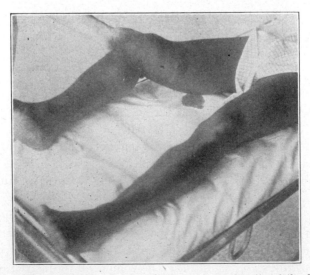

Fig. 32.—Same as preceding showing false motion at the site of the fracture.

slight displacement, the deformity is very difficult to determine, and the limb must be not only carefully inspected, but also measured and palpated.

In interpreting the results obtained by inspection, measurement, and palpation one must take into consideration any deformity which may have existed in the limb previous to the given injury and must also take into consideration the fact that slight asymmetry is not infrequently present in normal persons. This asymmetry is particularly common as regards the length of the lower extremity and in many normal persons one lower extremity as measured from the anterior superior spine to the tip of the internal malleolus is from one-fourth to one-half inch shorter than its fellow on the opposite side. Not only is this true, but there are cases reported in which there was a difference of from two to two and one-half inches in the length of the lower extremities in persons who were normal in other respects and who had received no injury.

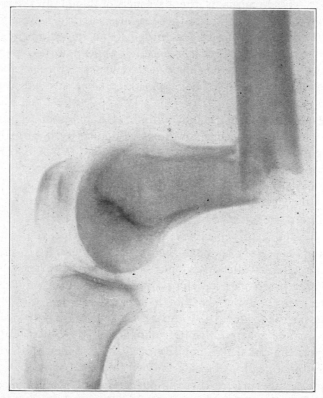

Fig. 33.—X-ray of the previous case. The deformity, however, is seldom this marked. Treatment: Skeletal traction in condyles of the femur five weeks, adhesive traction to the thigh three weeks, posterior molded plaster splint to the leg and thigh two weeks, and a walking caliper six weeks. Good results in seven and one-half months after injury.

In incomplete and in impacted fractures the deformity, if present, is persistent and cannot be corrected without either breaking up the impaction or bending the intact portion of the bone, in the case of an incomplete fracture.

Swelling.—The presence of considerable swelling or of a large amount of subcutaneous fat may obscure deformities which would be obvious in a normal slender limb or such swelling may cause a deformity to appear more marked than it really is.

Swelling in the vicinity of a fracture is the result of extravasation of blood and serum into the tissues and in severe fractures it may be so great as to be the dominant feature of the injury and demand immediate attention. This is especially true of fractures near the elbow. In addition to the swelling there may be a variable amount of thickening of the limb, the result of shortening of the muscles. The swelling comes on rapidly after the injury and tends to increase gradually over a period of several hours. In cases with extensive swelling large blebs filled with a yellowish brown serum may appear on the surface a day or two after the injury. In fractures which communicate with joints the synovial cavity becomes filled with blood and the joint presents the picture of an acute traumatic synovitis. In compound fractures the swelling is not a prominent feature, as the blood escapes through the wound.

Ecchymosis.—Ecchymosis is the presence of blood in the subcutaneous tissues and leads to discoloration in these tissues. It is almost always present after a fracture, but it is not to be regarded as an important symptom in an acute fracture because the ecchymosis may not appear until two or three days after the injury. In fractures in deep-seated bones the ecchymosis may not appear for several days, and it may appear at some site far removed from the site of the fracture.

Abnormal Mobility is motion in a limb at a point or in a direction in which it does not normally occur, and next to deformity is probably the most important single sign in the diagnosis of fractures. When it can be demonstrated in a bone, it is a pathognomonic sign of a fracture which is located at a point approximately the center of the abnormal motion. In the case of a joint it may be the sign of ruptured ligaments or of a fracture.

In seeking to demonstrate abnormal mobility in a limb the manipulations should be slowly and gently performed and the movement should be carried no further than is necessary to make the diagnosis definite. In most instances this can be done without causing further damage to the soft tissues and without inflicting very much pain on the patient.

In fractures through the shaft of a long bone either of the leg or arm all that is necessary is to grasp the upper fragment and gently raise the distal portion of the limb or gently move it from side to side. In fractures near the ends of the bones the abnormal mobility is, of course, more difficult to detect and in many instances cannot be satisfactorily demonstrated.

In certain fractures where there is overriding of the fragments the limb can be telescoped by applying slow gentle traction and then pushing upward very gently on the limb and carefully noting any change in its length. In other instances abnormal mobility in the direction of rotation may be detected by grasping the trochanter of the femur and rotating the thigh or by palpating the head of the radius while the forearm is being rotated. In the forearm and leg abnormal mobility of one bone when the other is intact can be demonstrated by placing the fingers over the seat of the fracture and either squeezing the bones together or grasping one fragment of the suspected bone and moving it from side to side.

Where an apophysis has been torn off, as in a fracture of the tuberosity of the humerus or of the femur, it is often possible to grasp the separated fragment and move it in an abnormal manner. The normal elasticity of the ribs and of the fibula may give one the impression of abnormal mobility when this does not really exist.

Crepitus.—In fractures crepitus is the grating sound or sensation produced by the friction of one fragment moving on the other. The crepitus of a fracture is a harsh grating sensation and is to be distinguished from the soft crepitus which occurs in arthritic joints and also from the soft cartilaginous crepitus which occurs in epiphyseal separations. When true bone crepitus is obtained, it is pathognomonic of fracture and for this reason is usually considered a most important diagnostic point, but crepitus is not as frequently sought for at the present time and is not considered of as great importance as it was before the day of the x-ray. In order to produce crepitus, the ends of the fragments must be placed in contact and must be moved upon one another. As a result many patients have been subjected to violent and useless manipulations in an attempt to elicit crepitus when the fracture could have been diagnosed without it. However, if the ends of the fragments are in contact, crepitus may be felt or even heard when the surgeon gently moves the limb in endeavoring to demonstrate false motion.

THE X-RAY IN THE DIAGNOSIS AND TREATMENT OF FRACTURES AND DISLOCATIONS OF THE EXTREMITIES

There is no question but that since the advent of the x-ray our knowledge of fractures has been greatly extended and the methods of treatment have been greatly improved. On the other hand, it is also true that since the advent of the x-ray the ability of surgeons to diagnose and treat fractures without the use of this method has been lessened.

Consequently, we wish to go on record to the effect that it is possible to make an approximately accurate diagnosis of most fractures without the use of the x-ray and that it is also possible to treat many fractures in quite a satisfactory manner without the use of the x-ray. We make this statement largely because many awards for damages are constantly being made in the courts on the basis that the attending surgeon did not take sufficient x-ray pictures either before or after treatment. We regard the x-ray as an aid to diagnosis and as a means of clearing up points about the injury which we have not been able to discover by means of a careful history and physical examination. If one looks at the x-ray in this manner, it is invaluable as an aid in the treatment. It is also important to note that the x-ray is not to be used as the sole guide in following the progress of a fracture under treatment. Clinical observation is not to be neglected.

On the other hand, we do not feel that any surgeon should be placed in the position where it is imperative to obtain x-rays in every case of suspected bone injury which comes under his care, and according to the courts this is the state of affairs at the present time. In many instances the patient cannot afford an x-ray picture or he must be transported for a considerable distance in order to obtain one, and there are many cases in which a satisfactory diagnosis can be made without difficulty and where correct treatment can and should be instituted immediately without resorting to x-ray.

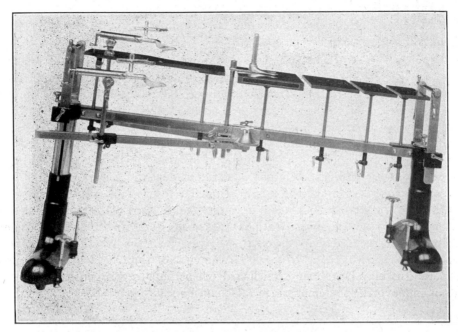

Fig. 34.—Bell fracture table with overhead frame removed.

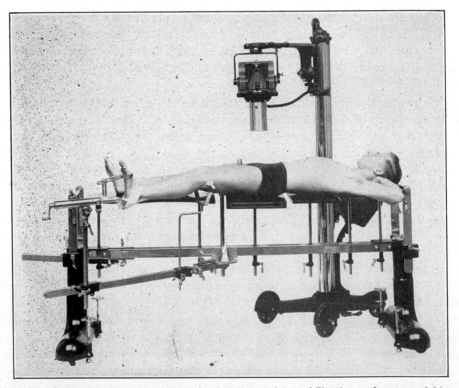

Fig. 35.—Same, showing arrangement for traction and immobilization and x-rays of hip.

The function of the x-ray in diagnosis is largely to elucidate the details of fractures which cannot be obtained by the history and physical examination and also to reveal certain fractures without displacement or small fractures in the vicinity of joints which it would be impossible to diagnose without it.

We do not mean to give the impression that we do not personally obtain x-rays on most of our fractures; we do. However, when it is not convenient or is impracticable we do not hesitate to treat a fracture without an x-ray. But if at any time during the treatment we are uncertain of our diagnosis or of the position of the fragments, we insist upon having an x-ray picture in order to clear up the questionable points.

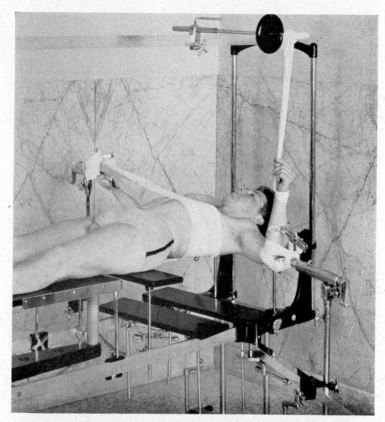

Fig. 36.—For traction to the upper extremity.

In addition to the use of the x-ray in the original diagnosis we feel that it is even more important to use it as a check on the results of treatment. This is not only true of fractures which have been treated by manipulative reduction followed by immobilization, but is also true of fractures which are treated by traction. In many of these, x-rays taken from time to time will enable the surgeon to regulate his traction so as to obtain the best possible result.

The x-ray pictures should be obtained in two planes at right angles to one another, and even in fractures of the hip and shoulder this is now possible. In injuries of the elbow, especially in children, and of the carpal bones it is often advisable to obtain x-rays of the opposite normal elbow or wrist for comparison.

In certain fractures oblique or other unusual views may be necessary to show the fracture. In others a fracture not seen in an x-ray taken shortly after the injury may be evident in an x-ray taken two weeks later after rarefaction of the adjacent fractured surfaces has occurred.

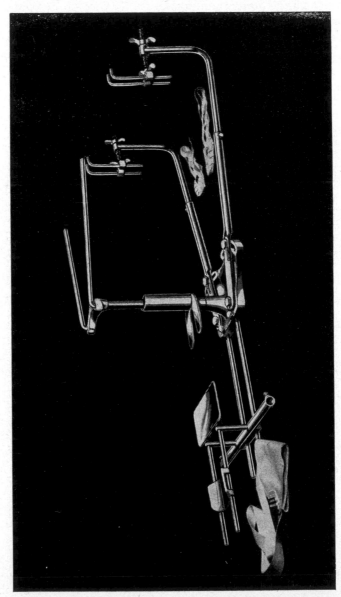

Fig. 37.—Zimmer portable fracture table.

Finally, it is to be noted that we have occasionally been sorry that we did not obtain an x-ray immediately in certain instances, but have never regretted having obtained one. Consequently, the surgeon should insist upon having an x-ray when there is the slightest doubt in his own mind as to the diagnosis, and he should never ignore a patient's request for an x-ray, even when he is quite satisfied that it is not necessary, because none of us is infallible.

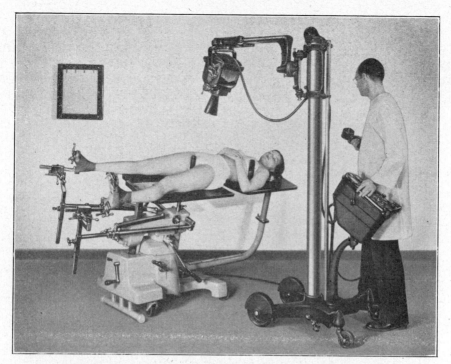

Fig. 38.—Albee-Comper orthopedic table. (Courtesy American Sterilizing Co.)

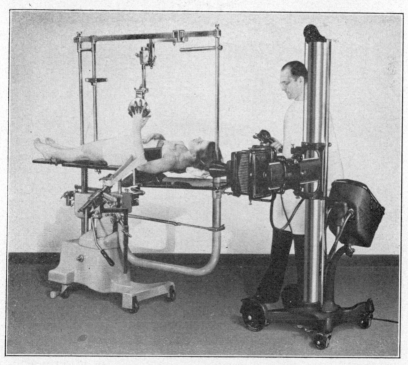

Fig. 39.—Albee-Comper orthopedic table. (Courtesy American Sterilizing Co.)

Reduction Under the Fluoroscope

Many surgeons are in the habit of reducing practically all of their fractures with the aid of the fluoroscope, while other surgeons treat identical fractures by manipulation and reduction without the aid of the fluoroscope and obtain practically identical results.   This is a matter of choice for the

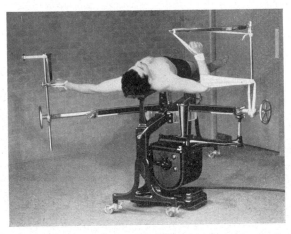

Fig. 40.—The Hawley-Scanlan-Morris table as used for a fracture of the right humerus. (Courtesy Scanlan-Morris Co.)

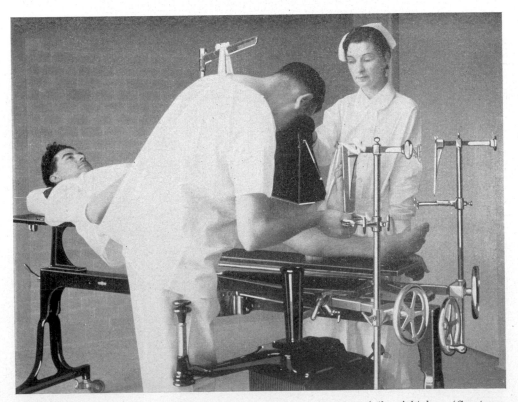

Fig. 41.—The Hawley-Scanlan-Morris table as used for a fracture of the right leg. (Courtesy Scanlan-Morris Co.)

individual surgeon. Personally, we rarely use the fluoroscope because we feel that we are able to work better in the light and thus see the condition of the soft parts during the manipulative procedure while we are able by inspection, measurement, and palpation to obtain sufficiently accurate knowledge of the position of the fragments for the purpose. Furthermore, reduction under the fluoroscope has some objectionable features in that the anesthetist cannot see the patient and the operator's attention is focused upon securing anatomic apposition of the fragments while he may neglect the more important factors of alignment and damage to the soft parts. We wish especially to warn surgeons against violent manipulations under the fluoroscope, since these may result in severe injuries to the soft tissues.

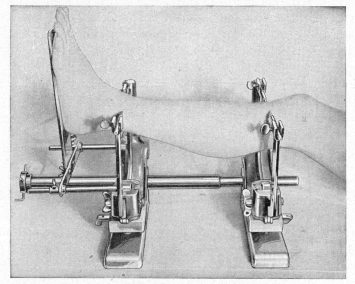

Fig. 42.—Mechanical reduction apparatus illustrating tibia and fibula reduction. (Courtesy Zimmer Manufacturing Co.)

There is also the danger of x-ray burns to the surgeon's hands if he does a considerable amount of fracture work and habitually manipulates his fractures under the fluoroscope. This may not seem to be worthy of notice, but the hands and deaths of many of our older surgeons bear witness that it is a very real danger.

We do not mean to detract from the value of the fluoroscope in the manipulation of fractures. We simply wish to emphasize the fact that the successful treatment of fractures is dependent upon the ability of the surgeon and not upon the method which he uses. In certain instances we use the fluoroscope to check the results of our manipulation before we immobilize the extremity in a cast or splint.

The Albee-Comper orthopedic table (Figs. 38 and 39), the Hawley-Scanlan-Morris table (Figs. 40 and 41), and the Bell table (Figs. 34, 35, and 36) are very useful aids in the reduction of fractures. Even with these, however, we are inclined to use the mechanical traction for reduction and then check the result with the fluoroscope. A postoperative film should be taken for a record of the case.

CHAPTER II

REPAIR OF FRACTURES

When a bone is broken there is a variable amount of rupture of blood vessels in the vicinity and a variable amount of damage to the soft tissues, not only within the bone itself and of the periosteum, but also of the muscles and connective tissues around the bone. In fractures by direct violence this soft tissue damage is partly due to the fracturing force, and in all fractures it is due to tearing of the tissues and to direct traumatism by the ends of the fragments. The rupture of blood vessels both within and around the bone leads to an extravasation of blood in the vicinity. This blood eventually clots and the fibrin clot contracts. Thus the ends of the bone are surrounded by a blood clot. As in any other portion of the body this blood clot tends to become organized by the ingrowth of young blood vessels and fibroblasts (granulation tissue), and concomitant with the ingrowth of granulation tissue there is an ingrowth of wandering phagocytic cells (macrophages) which tend to remove the extravasated red cells and débris. Under ordinary conditions a blood clot may be completely absorbed or may be replaced by scar tissue which varies in extent. The scar tissue is the result of the maturation of the granulation tissue which invaded the clot. Just what factors determine whether or not this primary granulation tissue will undergo involution and disappear or will form adult collagenic connective tissue and lay down a scar has not yet been determined.

The difference between the healing of a fracture and the disappearance of a blood clot in the subcutaneous tissues of the body lies in the fact that in the case of a fracture the normal tendency is for the granulation tissue to form callus and for this callus to be replaced by bone. This difference seems to be dependent upon the presence of bone in the hematoma.

When we make the statement that this difference is dependent upon the presence of bone in the hematoma, we include the mineral in the bone matrix and the osteogenic cells or osteoblasts which normally cover the surface and line the spaces in this bone. Which of these two elements; that is, the inorganic salts or the osteogenic cells, is the more important and whether or not either of these can be dispensed with, is at the present time a moot question, the answer to which has been attempted by many investigators who have devised hundreds of experiments in attempts to prove their theories. This book is not the place to digest this voluminous literature, nor is it the place to attempt to prove any given theory. We shall give the facts as we have observed them in clinical cases and in laboratory experiments.

When a bone is broken, the ends of the bone do not heal in the strict sense of the word; that is, there is no tendency for actual growth to take place from the end of a bone fragment, but under favorable conditions the continuity of the bone becomes reestablished by the soldering together of the ends of the fragments by new tissue which is laid down around and between them (Figs. 43 to 49). Whenever a bone is broken the living cells in the bone which are imprisoned in the lacunae adjacent to the fractured surface die (Figs. 43 and 44), and even if these cells lived, they would be unable to multiply and produce new bone because of their isolation in the lacunae. This is also true of cartilage. Whenever cartilage is cut, the cells adjacent to the cut surface die,

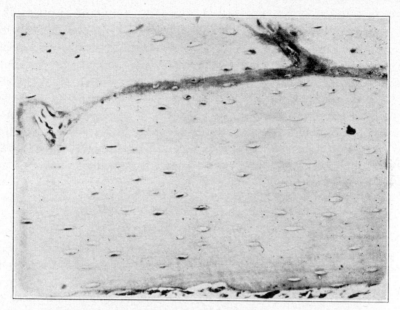

Fig. 43.—Photomicrograph of rib fracture in rabbit (three days), showing junction of living and dead bone. Empty lacunae on the right. (From Dr. A. W. Ham: J. Bone & Joint Surg., October, 1930.)

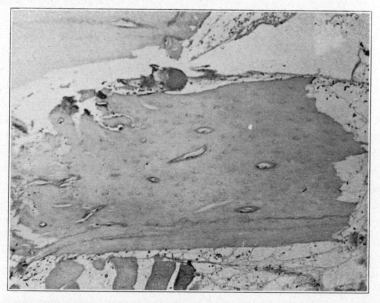

Fig. 44.—Photomicrograph of a completely detached fragment of bone in an experimental fracture three days after the injury, showing the death of the fragment as evidenced by empty lacunae. (Courtesy Dr. A. W. Ham.)

and repair cannot take place from these cells but must take place by the ingrowth of other tissue which binds the surfaces together.

In the case of a fracture, then, we have first the hematoma in which the blood clots and becomes organized. The difference between this and an ordinary blood clot is that from the sixth to the tenth day after the injury the fibrin clot begins to undergo a change into a tissue which is called callus. The characteristics of callus which distinguish it from other forms of granulation tissue are that it contains areas of cartilage and areas of calcification and ossification.

In the beginning the bone laid down in callus is formed in connective tissue and not in cartilage (Figs. 48 and 49). The amount of cartilage varies considerably and seems to be due to an attempt on the part of nature to immobilize the fragments by the formation of a temporary semirigid tissue. This statement is based on the observation that the amount of cartilage varies inversely with the amount of movement permitted at the site of the fracture. In other words, the more perfectly the fracture is reduced and immobilized, the less the amount of cartilage produced.

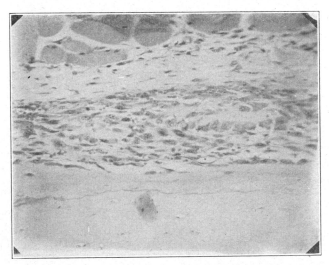

Fig. 45.—Photomicrograph of an experimental fracture (four days) showing proliferation of osteogenic cells beneath the periosteum near the fracture line. (Courtesy Dr. A. W. Ham.)

The invasion of the clot by connective tissue takes place from all sides; that is, from the surrounding tissues and from the periosteum and from the medullary canal. If the fragments are separated, the cartilage is formed in the space between the fragments and at various points in the organized hematoma. These islands of cartilage are apparently due to metaplasia of the ingrowing connective tissue cells. These cells swell, assume a mature or senile appearance, and the surrounding semifluid or gelatinous intercellular material tends to solidify and become cartilaginous in character. This is not true cartilage, but is better called chondroid tissue. These islets may coalesce so that the fracture is surrounded by a large mass of this tissue. This temporary healing of the fracture by a mass of chondroid tissue or cartilaginous callus serves to immobilize the fragments to a considerable degree.

In addition to cartilage in the callus as previously stated, there is a variable amount of calcification and ossification. This calcification is due to the deposition of lime salts in the matrix of the callus. Why and how these mineral salts are deposited here is not known. The ossification is apparently the

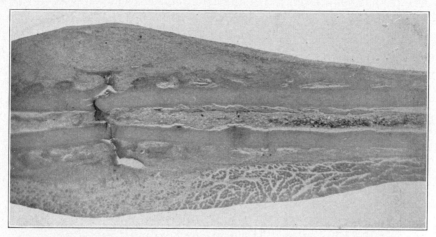

Fig. 46.—Photomicrograph of an experimental fracture of twenty-one days, showing spindle-like callus bridging gap in bone with new bone formation around the ends of both fragments. (Courtesy Dr. A. W. Ham.)

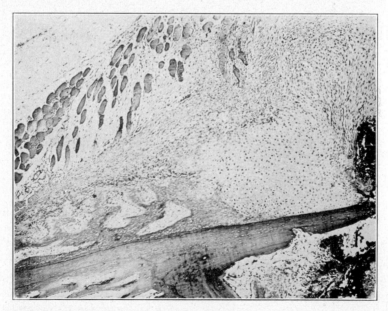

Fig. 47.—Photomicrograph of a twenty-one-day experimental fracture, showing end of fragment with empty lacunae and surrounded by new bone and callus. (Courtesy Dr. A. W. Ham.)

result of metaplasia of connective tissue cells in the mass of granulation tissue which has replaced the original hematoma. For some as yet unknown reason calcium salts are laid down in this connective tissue matrix or gelatinous mass which is inhabited by cells. These calcium salts surround the connective tissue cells and as they become imprisoned in the mass of calcium salts, they take on the appearance of bone cells and form true bone. This bone, however, differs from normal bone in that it is irregular in its structure and in that it is a type of cancellous or spongy bone in which the trabeculae are unusually coarse.

We have, then, at this stage the two bone ends surrounded by and imprisoned in a mass of callus which consists of connective tissue, cartilage, and coarse cancellous bone (Figs. 46 and 47). The bone and cartilage are formed in islands throughout the callus and these islands may coalesce to form large areas of either bone or chondroid tissue. The ends of the fragments play a purely passive rôle and act simply as dead pieces of bone, which they really are.

We have not yet considered the formation of the definite bone which is to be the ultimate factor in the healing process.

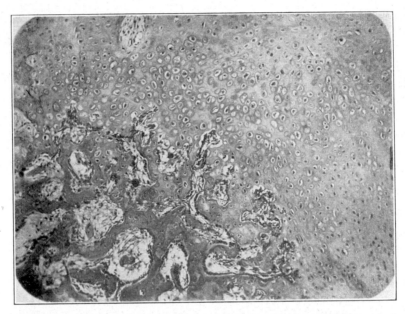

Fig. 48.—High power photomicrograph of callus, showing invasion and replacement of cartilage by new bone. (Courtesy Dr. A. W. Ham.)

Simultaneously with the formation of the callus there is a beginning formation of true bone. This usually begins beneath the periosteum around the fragments and at some distance from the site of the fracture (Fig. 45). This true bone is in the beginning cancellous in character and consists of fine trabeculae. It begins at the sixth to the tenth day and gradually grows down toward the ends of the fragments to invade and replace the callus.

In other words, a fracture is temporarily healed by callus and then this callus is invaded and replaced by the ultimate bone which, as stated above, usually begins at the junction of the stripped-up periosteum and the shafts and grows toward the bone defect.

Simultaneously with this invasion of the callus by the ultimate bone which is to heal the fracture, there is a tendency to resorption of excess callus around the site of the fracture. Eventually in the course of several weeks the true bone growing from beneath the periosteum of each fragment meets and fuses across the defect. This bone is first spongy in character. As time goes on this bone becomes transformed into dense cortical bone and an attempt is made by nature to restore the normal form of the original bone. If anatomic reduction has been obtained a new medullary canal is formed and the cortex gradually assumes its normal contour and thickness.

In the beginning and for several years after the accident, the site of the fracture is marked by a zone in which the cortex is somewhat thicker and in which the cortical bone is more dense than normal. In case anatomic reduction has not been obtained, nature reconstructs a bone which will meet the demands of function. Consequently, in such instances, the ultimate result is a new bone, the structure of which is so planned that it meets the demands of function in the most efficient mechanical manner and with the utilization of the least possible bone material. This is in accordance with Wolfe's law to the effect that a change in mechanical strains and stresses which a bone is called upon to bear is followed by a change in the structure of bone, so that ultimately the form and structure will be adapted to the demands made upon it. While Wolfe's law tends to be true at all ages, it is to be noted that the bones of young persons are more adaptable and that a deformity which would be corrected spontaneously in a child may persist indefinitely in an adult.

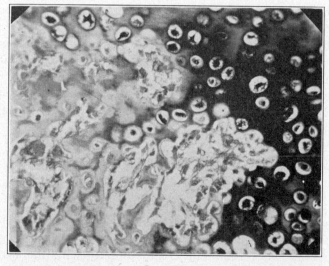

Fig. 49.—High power photomicrograph of seventeen-day experimental fracture, showing invasion of cartilage by bone. (Courtesy Dr. A. W. Ham.)

We mentioned in the beginning that it is a moot question whether or not the inorganic salts or the osteoblasts are the important factor. Those who believe that the inorganic salts are the important factor point out the fact that if a strip of periosteum which contains bone cells is transplanted to the soft tissues it does not form bone except under very exceptional circumstances, and the fact that along with the death of the ends of the fragments and also the death of all exposed surfaces of separated pieces of bone which occur in comminuted fractures, there is a tendency to absorption and rarefaction of these fragments.

According to this theory the ends of the bones and all separated bone fragments in the vicinity of the fracture act as a local calcium depot and supply not only the stimulus to the formation of bone from callus and to the growth of permanent bone to heal the fracture, but also supply the calcium salts which are necessary for this purpose. If this theory is carried to its ultimate conclusion, the content of the blood in calcium and phosphorus has nothing to do with the healing of fractures as all of the necessary calcium is supplied locally. This, of course, is not true as is evidenced by the fact that fractures in a case of severe active rickets tend to heal by osteoid tissue instead of bone. It is also obvious from a study of serial x-rays taken of fractures in which considerable callus has been laid down that the amount of bone formed is considerably more than that which could have been supplied by resorption from the fragments in the vicinity.

On the other hand, clinical and experimental evidence indicates that the presence of a local calcium depot is a definite factor in the healing of fractures.

If the osteoblastic theory is accepted in its purest form, we must assume that the osteoblast is a specific cell which has the power, and whose function it is, to form bone, this bone being deposited in the vicinity of and under the influence of the given cell and being formed of calcium and phosphorus which are withdrawn from the surrounding tissue fluids and eventually from the blood stream. Under this theory a local calcium depot is of no importance.

The truth of the matter appears to lie between the two: that is, in the first place, the osteoblast is not a specific cell, but any fibroblast can, under certain stimuli, become an osteoblast and may cause bone to be laid down in its vicinity. Just what these stimuli are we do not at present know. In the second place a local calcium depot tends to start the formation of bone in its vicinity and possibly tends to act as a stimulus for the transformation of fibroblasts into osteoblasts.

FACTORS TENDING TO CAUSE NONUNION

From what has just been said, whether or not a broken bone heals by bony union depends upon the following factors:

1. **Juxtaposition of the Bone Fragments.**—This is a simple mechanical problem, as the ability of the organism to form callus and bridge a gap is limited. The exact limitations of this ability vary directly with the size of the bone and, to a certain extent, in different persons—that is, in larger bones a larger fibrin clot is formed and as a result wider gaps can be bridged. On the other hand, if the gap to be bridged is wider than the callus or if the distance is greater than can be traversed by the bone which grows out from beneath the fragments, nonunion will result.

2. **Immobilization.**—Under ordinary conditions we believe that since fractures are healed by formation of new bone around the bone ends, it is important that the immobilization be as nearly absolute as possible. Every movement between the fragments results in an injury to and breaking down or tearing apart of part of the callus. It is true that callus is of such a nature that it heals rapidly and that it responds to injury incident to motion by the pro-

duction of more callus so that within certain limits the more motion there is between fragments the more callus will be formed and in a certain sense the firmer the primary union will be. However, if this motion or lack of immobilization is carried too far, it will tend to result in eventual involution of the callus and the formation of fibrous tissue and result in fibrous union.

3. **Interposition of the Soft Parts.**—If a layer of muscle or fascia be interposed between the fragments, the new bone growing from around either fragment may not be able to penetrate this layer of living tissue and nonunion may occur. (Figs. 50, 51, and 52.)

4. **Mineral Metabolism.**—Normally the blood contains from $9\frac{1}{2}$ to $12\frac{1}{2}$ mg. of calcium and from $3\frac{1}{2}$ to $4\frac{1}{2}$ mg. of phosphorus per 100 c.c. of serum. It is believed by many that the presence of a normal amount of calcium in the blood is necessary for the laying down of bone, and McCollum has stated that if the product of the calcium and phosphorus in the blood falls below 30 mg. per 100 c.c. of serum, ossification will not occur. However, our observations and those of other investigators have shown that it is extremely rare to find abnormally low calcium or phosphorus in patients with fractures and also that the calcium and phosphorus content of the blood of patients who develop nonunion is practically always normal. Furthermore, the bones of patients with severe rickets and osteomalacia tend to heal rapidly, but tend to calcify slowly and the poor union seen in these cases is different from the type of nonunion which occurs after fractures in normal persons.

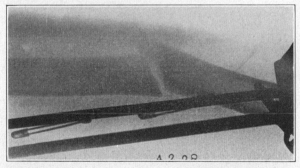

Fig. 50.—Nonunion of fracture of the femur due to interposition of soft parts between the fragments. Treated by open reduction, excision of bone ends, and bone graft. Good results.

5. **Extensive Damage to the Soft Tissue in the Vicinity.**—Compound fractures heal more slowly than do simple fractures, largely because the blood escapes and the hematoma is not formed in the normal manner. Not only this, but in fractures with extensive damage to the soft parts with destruction of blood vessels and ischemic necrosis of large areas in the surrounding tissue, repair is inadequate or fibrosis occurs or it is impossible for the invading granulating tissue to bridge the gap by the time calcification normally occurs in the callus. As a matter of fact most cases of nonunion may be traced either to extensive damage to local tissues or to incomplete reduction and immobilization.

6. **Infection.**—Infection by pyogenic organisms in some way stimulates the formation of bone as is seen in osteomyelitis, both in the form of an in-

volucrum around the dead shaft and also in the tendency of infected bone to become eburnated due to the laying down of calcium in the walls of the haversian canals with eventual occlusion of these canals. Infection, however, tends to cause nonunion in acute fractures because it tends to cause rapid autolysis of the fibrin clot and thus remove the framework which supports the ingrowing granulation tissue which is later to become callus. This is the result of the digestive action of the leucocytes which are accumulated as a result of the infection. On the other hand, chronic infection tends to cause eburnation of the bone and eburnated bone has a delayed power of healing, since the healing is dependent upon the growth of soft tissue from the fragments and in eburnated bone the soft tissue is practically nonexistent.

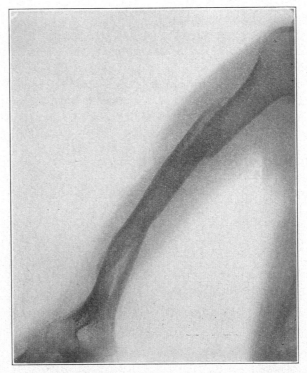

Fig. 51.—Nonunion of the humerus at junction of middle and upper thirds caused by interposition of soft parts. There was a small abscess on the distal end of the upper fragment in which diphtheroid bacilli were obtained in pure culture. This was a rare infection of a simple fracture.

7. Poor Blood Supply and Presence of Synovial Fluid.—Certain fractures are notoriously liable to result in nonunion. The chiefest of these are the fractures through the neck of the femur and the fractures through the carpal scaphoid. Next in order come fractures through the junction of the middle and lower thirds of the humerus or tibia. The importance of the presence of synovial fluid in the first two types is debatable, since other intraarticular fractures in which reduction and immobilization are carried out can be healed in the normal manner. On the other hand, there is no question but that if reduction is unsatisfactory and if immobilization is not obtained, the synovial fluid will tend to cause the fractured surfaces to become covered by a layer of fibrin and eventually by a layer of connective tissue, and nonunion will result. In either instance, however, if the fragments are jammed together, the synovial fluid is excluded and cannot be a factor.

Then there is the question of blood supply. The blood supply to the proximal fragment in fractures through the neck of the femur is unusually poor. The same is true of the blood supply to the carpal scaphoid and to the junction of the middle and lower thirds of the tibia. Another factor is of even more importance; in none of these areas are the bones surrounded by soft tissue of such a character as to make possible the formation and organization of an adequate hematoma and fibrin clot; as a result there is no preliminary framework which can be transformed into callus and later into bone.

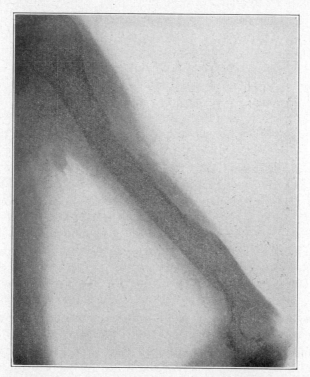

Fig. 52.—Same case as preceding, after excising the abscess, remodeling ends of fragments, perforating them with numerous holes, and tying them together with chromic catgut. Union in nine weeks after operation. Subsequent course uneventful after cut step operation.

8. **Unknown Factors.**—Most men who have treated and seen large numbers of fractures will admit that very rarely they encounter a fracture which is properly reduced and properly immobilized and which, in an otherwise normal person, either does not unite in the usual time or goes on to eventual nonunion. This is most marked in the case of so-called congenital or birth fractures in which even with a beautifully executed autogenous grafting followed by adequate immobilization union often fails to occur. It is true that these cases will be a very small proportion of the fractures which one sees; nevertheless they should be mentioned.

CLINICAL DELAYED UNION AND NONUNION

The term "delayed union" is applied to fractures which have not united after the lapse of the usual amount of time for the given fracture and the term "nonunion" is applied to those fractures in which not only has union not occurred after the usual lapse of time, but in which there is no probability that union will occur at any time without surgical intervention. Many authors reserve the term "nonunion" for those fractures which, after a year from the time of the injury, have not united. We prefer, however, to use this term for fractures in which clinical and x-ray evidence indicates that union will not occur regardless of the length of time which has elapsed.

In a consideration of delayed union it is to be remembered that the larger the bone the longer the time required for union; while fairly firm union may be expected in a finger within three or four weeks, the shaft of the femur will require from two to three months for the same degree of union to take place. The bones of children unite more quickly than do those of adults. It is often stated that the bones of the aged do not unite as rapidly or as certainly as do those of younger adults, but our experience has been that once the bones have obtained their normal growth, age has relatively little effect if the general condition of the patient is good. A possible exception is fractures through the neck of the femur. Cancellous bone unites more rapidly than does compact bone.

It also should be noted that delayed union may result in eventual healing or in true nonunion. The nonunion may be due to fibrous union between the fragments and a failure of the fibrous tissue to calcify. It may be due to the development of pseudarthrosis in which case there is free movement at the site of the fracture and the bone ends tend to become rounded and adapted to one another and a joint space which contains synovial fluid develops. In such instances the rounded ends of the bones are smooth and eburnated, but are not covered by cartilage. In other instances hyaline cartilage is interposed between the fragments; this may persist indefinitely and calcification not occur.

Especial mention should be made of nonunion occurring in young children, since in these cases the various types of bone grafting operations are usually doomed to failure. These cases most often occur at the junction of the middle and lower thirds of the leg and are frequently the result of fractures present at birth or occurring shortly after birth. In some instances the fibula remains intact while the tibia develops nonunion. In these so-called birth fractures the tendency of the bones not to unite is due to a local congenital defect in the bone structure.

Syphilis is often regarded as a cause of nonunion and many surgeons believe that the first thing to do when confronted with a case of delayed or nonunion is to get a blood Wassermann and then give antiluetic treatment regardless of the Wassermann. Personally we believe that syphilis rarely causes nonunion. We have seen fractures heal in the usual way in patients with syphilis, and have even seen a fracture of the leg unite in a patient who had a Charcot ankle on the same side. It is conceivable that a fracture through a bone at the site of a large gumma might fail to unite, unless proper antiluetic treatment is instituted. In pathologic fractures due to neoplasms union may be prevented by extensive growth of the tumor. We have seen such cases, but even these pathologic fractures generally tend to unite in the usual way, unless the tumor is osteolytic in character.

Another type of nonunion is one in which there is no connection between the fragments. This occurs in instances in which the ends of the fragments are widely separated and in intraarticular fractures, such as those of the neck of the femur in which there may be no fibrous connection between the fragments. Tables I and II summarize a study made by Henderson* in a series of 259 cases

TABLE I

Males	220
Females	39
Between the ages of 20 and 49 years, per cent	81
Originally compound, per cent	35
Originally simple, per cent	65

TREATMENT	PER CENT
Bone grafts	56.3
Plastic	23.2
Removal of sequestrums	13.5
Metal	**4.0**
Manipulations	3.0

	DELAYED UNION	NONUNION	TOTAL
Humerus	10	35	45
Ulna	4	6	10
Radius	2	20	22
Radius and ulna	17	14	31
Tibia	52	40	92
Shaft of femur	11	20	31
Hip	––	28	28
Total	96	163	259

in which he attempted to determine the distribution and cause of nonunion. It is interesting that in his series devitalization of the tissues incident to severe injury seems to be the most frequent cause of delayed union and nonunion.

Treatment of Delayed Union and Nonunion

In considering the treatment of delayed and nonunion it is important to determine as nearly as possible the probability as to whether or not union will occur under conservative treatment and to determine the cause of nonunion. If delayed union is due to inadequate immobilization or to inadequate reduction or to infection, union may occur after the cause has been removed. If, on the other hand, the fragments have been placed in good position, if adequate immobilization has been carried out, and if there is no infection and union has not occurred after the usual lapse of time, one should seriously consider the possibility of nonunion. Signs of definite nonunion as shown in the x-ray are eburnation of the ends of the fragments or absorption of the ends of the fragments, so that they become rarefied and pencil-like in character.

In certain instances of delayed union prolonged immobilization may result in a cure and this is especially true if this can be combined with function, as

*Henderson, M. S.: J. A. M. A. 86: 81, 1926.

TABLE II

	SEVERE INJURY ASSOCIATED WITH COMPOUND FRACTURE		SEVERE INJURY ASSOCIATED WITH SIMPLE FRACTURE		INADEQUATE FIXATION		POOR REDUCTION MALPOSITION		METAL		INDETERMINATE	
	NON-UNION	DELAYED UNION	NON-UNION	DELAYED UNION	NON-UNION	DELAYED UNION	NON-UNION	DELAYED UNION	NON-UNION	DELAYED UNION	NON-UNION	DELAYED UNION
Humerus	15	2	5	2	9	2	—	—	2	1	4	—
Ulna	—	—	2	3	3	1	—	—	—	—	1	—
Radius	4	5	8	1	—	1	6	—	2	—	—	—
Radius and Ulna	5	7	5	9	—	—	2	2	—	1	2	1
Tibia	21	1	6	10	4	—	—	15	3	1	6	—
Femur	2		3	2	—	—	8	7	1	1	6	19
Total	47	15	29	27	16	4	16	24	8	3	19	20
	62		56		20		40		11		39	
	118				60							

in the application of a walking plaster-of-Paris cast to the leg for a fracture of the tibia and fibula. This will sometimes result in eventual union.

The type of operation to be selected depends a good deal upon the conditions present at the site of the fracture. In the shaft of a long bone for instance, in which the fragments are in contact and in a satisfactory position

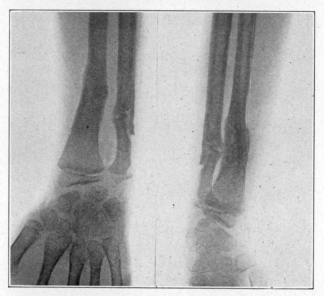

Fig. 53.—Inlay grafts in position for treatment of nonunion of both bones of the forearm three months after operation. Eventually firm union was obtained.

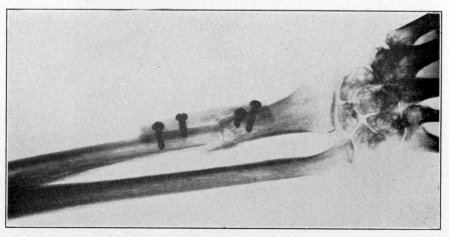

Fig. 54.—Fracture of the radius with nonunion; treated by bone graft and fixed with metal screws.

and are fairly firmly united by a short bridge of fibrous tissue or fibrocartilage, the multiple drilling operation is useful. This is particularly true in oblique fractures of the tibia with delayed union. The object of the operation is to traverse the fracture line with a number of drill holes (six to twelve or more, depending upon the area of bone involved). The drilling is frequently done subcutaneously through small stab wounds in the skin. However, several years

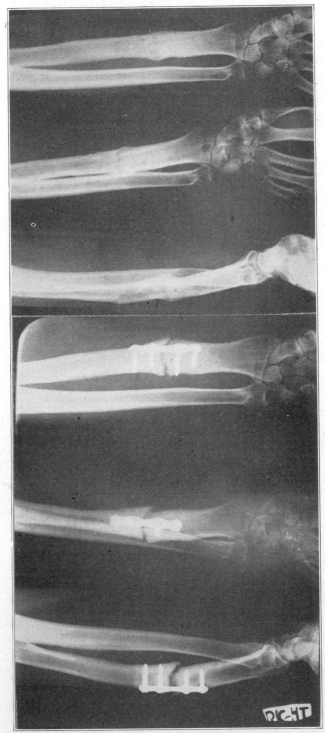

Fig. 55.—Old plated fracture of the radius, eighteen months' duration, with nonunion. Prompt union after inlay graft. Final result, slight limitation of rotation. (Courtesy Dr. Joseph Lembeck.)

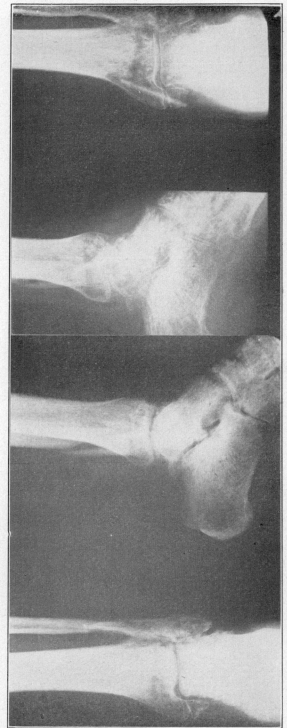

Fig. 56.—Old bimalleolar fracture with nonunion of the internal malleolus. Treated by open reduction, freshening of the surfaces, and a bone peg from the proximal third of the same tibia. Good result.

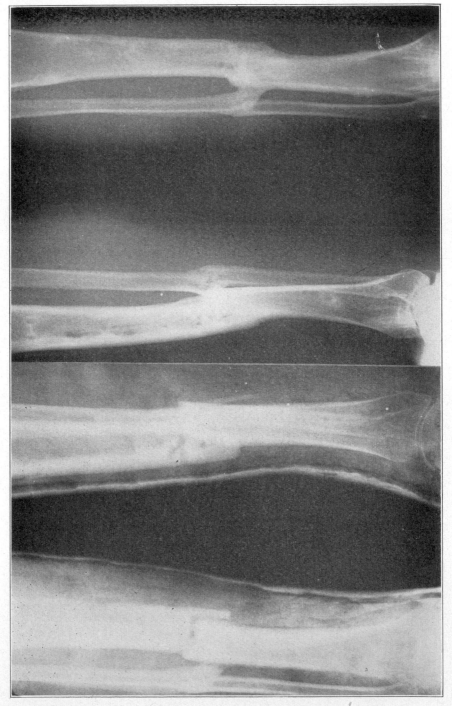

Fig. 57.—Fracture of tibia and fibula with nonunion, eight months' duration. Treated by multiple drilling and free graft. Immediately postoperative and eleven months after grafting operation. Primary treatment was by multiple pin fixation.

ago a patient subjected to the subcutaneous drilling by one of us (J. A. K.) developed a severe infection. After a rather stormy course chronic osteomyelitis developed and this required a saucerization operation and the removal of a large sequestrum before a cure was effected. Consequently, we now expose the bone in the usual way and make the drill holes under direct vision. The wound is then sprinkled with sulfonamide powder and closed and immobilized in a cast. We believe that this is a safer procedure than is the subcutaneous method. (Fig. 62.)

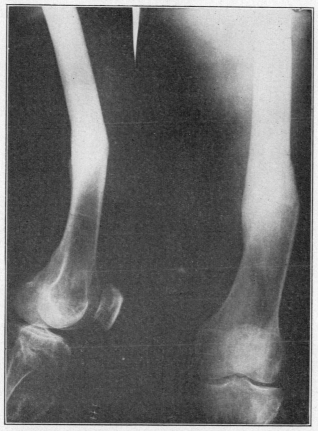

Fig. 58.—Fracture of femur in the same leg as shown in Fig. 57. Treated by traction in a Boehler frame with nonunion of the leg. Satisfactory union of femur.

If the bone ends are separated by soft tissue, if they are not firmly bound together, or if there is a defect, we advise the step cut operation or a bone graft. Where a small amount of shortening is permissible the step cut operation is useful. The bone ends are cut and overlapped and fixed with chromic catgut, kangaroo tendon, or wire through drill holes in each fragment (not around both fragments), or with a transfixing (Sherman) metal screw.

In every case the scar tissue and cartilage between the fragments and the eburnated bone should be removed, the marrow canal should be opened, the periosteum should be stripped up and later replaced, and either the ends of the fragments should be placed in contact and held in contact by suture or other

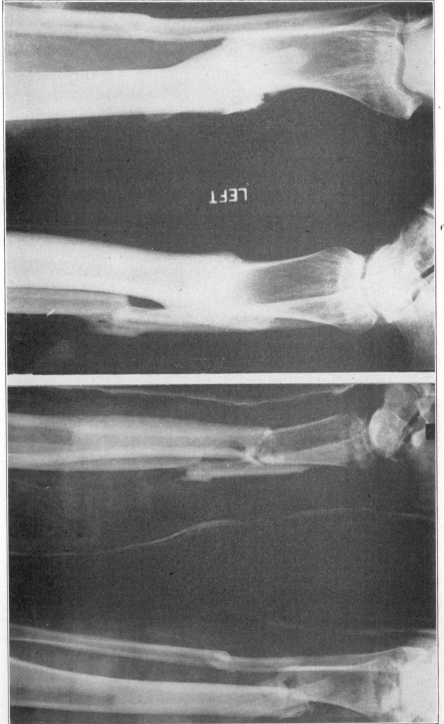

Fig. 59.—Same case as shown in Figs. 57 and 58. X-ray shows free bone graft of tibia, the proximal fragment of which has slipped mesially. Permitted to unite without attempt to correct the displacement. Resumed work as a switchman one year later.

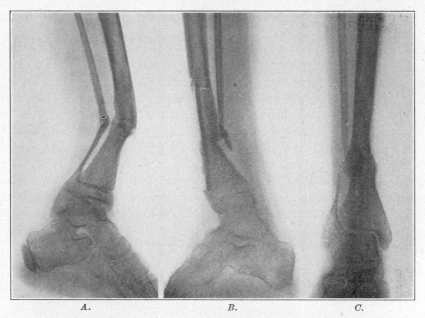

A.   B.   C.

Fig. 60.—*A.* So-called congenital or birth fractures with nonunion in a girl eleven years old.

B. Same as preceding, three years later, with inlay graft in place. A graft three years previous had united and then was absorbed a year later.

C. Same as preceding, six months later. Union apparently obtained.

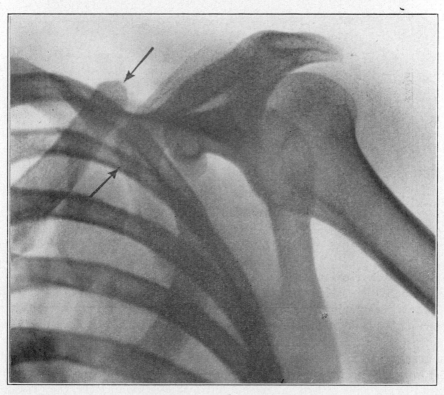

Fig. 61.—Nonunion of the clavicle, fifteen years' duration. Only limited loss of power of the arm at the shoulder joint.

mechanical means, or if a defect exists this should be bridged by an autogenous graft.

The type of graft to be used in cases in which there is a definite defect depends a good deal upon the choice and experience of the operator. Personally we usually use a large onlay or inlay graft (Figs. 53, 54, and 60*A, B,* and *C*). The inlay is cut slightly wider than the gutter and driven in. If the graft is cut too small and lies loose in the gutter, either a new one is cut or it is tied in with chromic catgut passed through drill holes in the bone. Intramedullary pegs are easy to insert and afford excellent insurance against displacement, but we rarely use them because we wish to keep the blood supply in the marrow cavity intact if possible. Henderson recommends the use of a large diamond-shaped graft, the points of which are inserted into the medullary canals of the fragments. Campbell uses an onlay graft which is firmly screw pegged onto both fragments and bridges the gap. Delagenier used osteoperiosteal grafts and many surgeons have used bone chips.

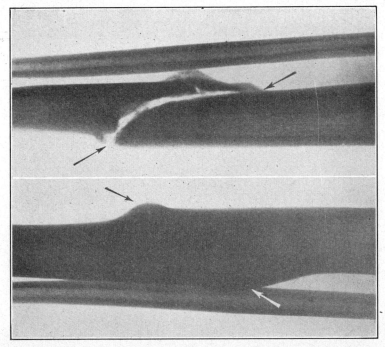

Fig. 62.—Old fracture of tibia with delayed union. At the bottom the result is shown four months after bone drilling with firm union. Synostosis is not present.

In all elective operations on clean bone a twenty-four-hour preparation of the skin should be carried out and strict asepsis should be observed. We do not use Lane's technic for reasons mentioned under the operative treatment of fractures. We believe that the autogenous graft is better than either beef bone or ivory pegs if a defect is to be bridged. We believe that in addition to the main graft osteoperiosteal strips and loose bone chips should be packed into the defect until the dead spaces are filled. We also believe that small holes should be bored in the ends of both fragments until, to a certain extent, they resemble cancellous bone.

After the operation is completed we immobilize the limb in a plaster-of-Paris cast over a considerable period of time and check the result by x-ray and clinical examination. It has been our experience that beautifully executed operations have sometimes resulted in failure and other operations with which we were quite dissatisfied at the time and in which everything went wrong, have resulted in rapid union.

During the past five years one of us (J. A. K.) has been using a large autogenous graft which is firmly fixed to each fragment by Sherman's self-tapping steel screws. In addition, the site of the fracture is bridged by several thin osteoperiosteal grafts, and if there is a defect between the fragments, this is filled with autogenous bone chips. The large slab from the tibia is used in the same manner as is a bone plate. It is fixed by one long and two short screws in each fragment when it is applied to a large bone and by two short screws in each fragment when it is applied to a small bone. In the relatively small series in which this method has been used, union has occurred in every instance and the metal screws have not caused trouble, even when used in nonunion resulting from compound fractures which had been infected. However, stainless steel or vitallium screws should be used if available. If the metal screws cause trouble, they can be removed after union is obtained. Sulfonamide powder is sprinkled in the wound before it is closed.

More recently he has been using the free onlay graft, as recommended by Phemister. This is easily applied and can be taken from the same leg (Key: Ann. Surg., 118: 665, 1944). Where the fragments are freely movable he uses dual bone plates supplemented by Paul Steele's barrel stave grafts or LeRoy Abbott's iliac grafts.

CHAPTER III

PRINCIPLES OF TREATMENT OF FRACTURES

When a bone is broken the object of treatment is to obtain union of the fragments in a good functional position, restoration of movements in the joints, and power in the muscles of the limb in the shortest possible time. Union is usually most rapidly and surely obtained if the broken ends are placed in contact and immobilized until they are quite firmly united by callus. Since union is the first consideration in the treatment, we believe that our efforts to secure union in good functional position should dominate the treatment and that our efforts to maintain movement in the neighboring joints and power in the muscles of the limb should be of secondary consideration. There is at the present time a wave of physiotherapy sweeping the country. We believe that in many instances this has done more harm than good because it has led surgeons to neglect the first principle in fracture treatment; that is, to obtain union of the bones in good functional position. We believe that the muscles and joints should be exercised whenever and wherever possible, so long as this does not jeopardize the obtaining of union in good functional position.

In simple fractures with displacement our first aim is to get the bones into good functional position: that is, to reduce the displacement. In simple fractures without displacement all that is necessary is to immobilize the fracture until union has occurred.

Anatomic and Functional Reduction.—Reduction is said to be anatomic when the displaced fragments are replaced in their normal position, and is said to be functional when the displaced fragments are placed in a position in which, if union occurs, the function of the limb will not be impaired regardless of whether or not the fragments are in their normal position. For instance, in a transverse fracture of the shaft of the femur, if the bone ends are placed in contact so that as much as one-fourth of their surfaces overlap, we are assured of full length and if the normal alignment of the shaft of the bone is maintained, we are assured of function when and if union occurs, and our experience has led us to believe that in these transverse fractures union occurs more rapidly and more surely after an incomplete, but good, functional reduction than after an accurate anatomic replacement.

In the case of joint fractures, and this is especially true in fractures involving weight-bearing joints, the terms "functional" and "anatomic" reductions are almost synonymous. That is, if normal function is to be restored to the part, an anatomic reduction must be secured and displaced fragments must be replaced in approximately their original positions in order that the contour of the joint surfaces be restored. This may require open operation. Otherwise a traumatic arthritis with a variable amount of impairment of function is to be expected.

Emergency Treatment of Fractures.—Most fractures occur some distance from a hospital, and for this reason more or less emergency treatment is indicated and necessary. Some form of splinting is usually necessary in severe

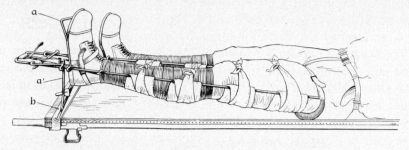

Fig. 63.—Emergency immobilization of fracture of thigh or leg for transportation. (United States Army Splint Manual.) (Courtesy Major General N. T. Kirk, Surgeon General, U. S. Army.)

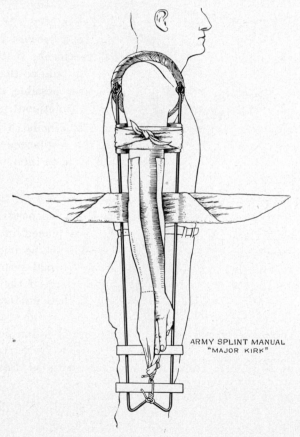

Fig. 64.—Emergency immobilization fractures of arm for transportation. (Courtesy Major General Kirk, Surgeon General, U. S. Army.)

fractures since transportation of the patient without splinting not only leads to great pain, but also to increase of surgical shock and may even be a cause of death. For this reason the principles of splinting the wounded on the field of battle was adopted in the various armies during the World War (Fig.

63).   However, in civil practice this is rarely practicable, since the Thomas splints for the arm and leg, which are probably the most satisfactory and efficient transportation splints yet devised, are rarely available.   Consequently the emergency treatment must be adapted to the circumstances as well as to the injury.   This is discussed in Chapter IV.

The emergency attention required by compound fractures is discussed under the heading Compound Fractures.

The object of emergency treatment should be to get the patient to a hospital or other place where definitive treatment is to be applied with as little pain and manipulation of the fracture as possible and to do this as quickly as possible.

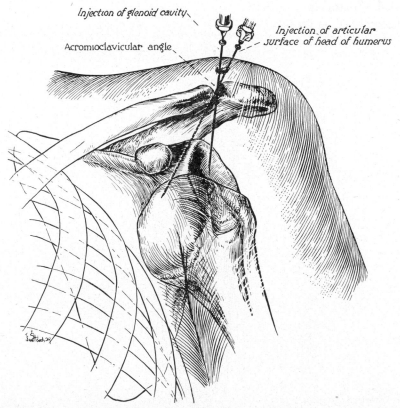

Fig. 65.—Drawing illustrating method of obtaining local anesthesia for the reduction of a traumatic dislocation at the shoulder.   (Figs. 65-71 from Rice: Minn. Med., September, 1929.)

Time Element in the Treatment of Fractures.—When the patient arrives at a hospital with a fresh fracture, this patient should be considered a surgical emergency and definitive treatment should be started just as soon as possible after admission.

Every hour that elapses after the injury usually adds to the swelling, and in the case of overriding adds to the shortening and to the muscle spasm which must be overcome if reduction is to be obtained.   Not only this, but the swelling incident to the extravasation of blood in the soft tissues renders reduction much more difficult and in many instances makes it necessary to postpone reduction and the application of a plaster cast for a week or ten days; whereas, in many instances, if the patient had been seen and treated immediately, the reduction could have been accomplished with relative ease and the patient could have been made comfortable within a few hours after the injury.

Anesthesia in the Treatment of Fractures.—When the patient arrives at the hospital and the surgeon takes charge, one of the first things for him to decide is whether or not the patient should have an anesthetic. It has been our experience that the surgeon is apt to err on the side of leniency in this phase of treatment and in order to spare the patient a general or local anesthetic will often be content with a mediocre result. We believe that where any manipulation or change in position of the fragments is indicated, it is advisable to administer an anesthetic in order that relaxation may be secured and the surgeon may be free to do what he sets out to do.

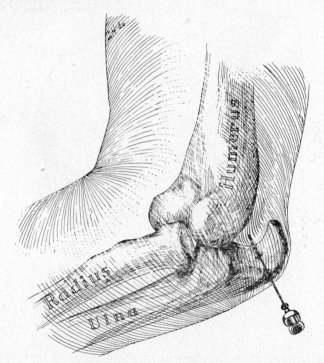

Fig. 66.—Insertion of needle in obtaining local anesthesia for reduction of dislocation at the elbow. (Courtesy Dr. C. O. Rice.)

Choice of a Local or General Anesthetic depends a good deal upon the surgeon's ability to use local anesthesia and upon his experience with this method as well as upon the availability of a skilled anesthetist.

General Anesthesia.—In fractures requiring merely a short manipulation and the application of a splint or plaster-of-Paris cast, gas oxygen anesthesia is usually to be preferred, while in fractures of the femur requiring complete muscle relaxation and a long anesthetic for the application of a plaster-of-Paris spica, ether is our choice. In some hospitals ethylene or cyclopropane is used and these are safe and reliable but inflammable. Many surgeons are now using spinal anesthesia for all fractures of the lower extremities. It is successful and safe when administered by some one who is skilled in its use, but for the most part nitrous oxide and oxygen or ether or ethylene will continue to be the method of choice. We are now using pentothal sodium intravenously in an increasing number of cases and find it very satisfactory.

Local Anesthesia.—Local anesthesia has certain advantages in that it is possible for the patient to cooperate with the surgeon and this is especially true in fractures of the humerus where it is desirable to apply a shoulder spica and plaster jacket for immobilization. It also has the advantage that the patient is not troubled with postanesthetic nausea and cuts down the risk of

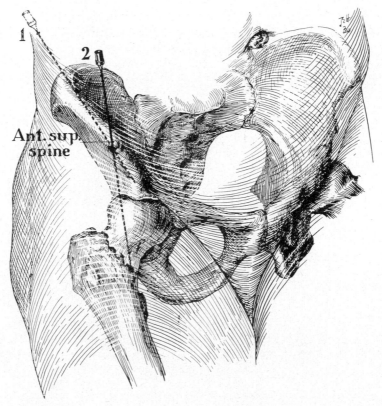

Fig. 67.—Insertion of the needle for obtaining anesthesia in intertrochanteric fracture of the femur. (Courtesy Dr. C. O. Rice.)

pneumonia after the reduction. Further advantages of local anesthesia are that relief of pain aids in combating surgical shock, and after the fracture is reduced and immobilized in a cast or splint, an x-ray can be made; and if the reduction is not satisfactory it can be repeated before the effect of the local anesthetic wears off. There are three methods of administering local anesthesia. One is by the nerve block or plexus block method which requires considerable skill and practice on the part of the surgeon. A second, the regional anesthesia, requires no especial skill but demands the use of a rather large amount of the anesthetic. The third is the injection of novocaine solution directly into the hematoma around the ends of the fractured bones.

This last method has been used for years and has lately been popularized by Boehler of Vienna. Its success is dependent upon the fact that when a fracture occurs the ends of the bones are surrounded by a hematoma and if the anesthetizing solution is injected into this hematoma, it will quickly permeate the surrounding tissues and will produce sufficient anesthesia to allay muscle spasm and render reduction painless. (Figs. 65-71.)

Circumferential Injection of Radius

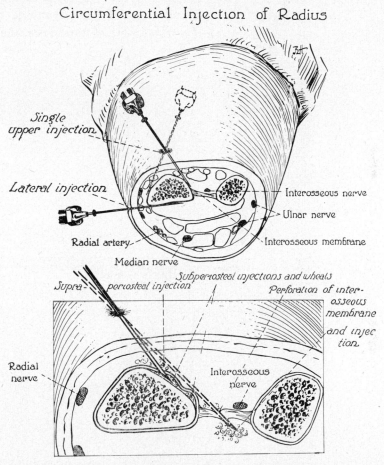

Fig. 68.—Insertions of needles for obtaining anesthesia of the shaft of the radius. (Courtesy Dr. C. O. Rice.)

The objection usually offered is that by introducing a needle into the hematoma the surgeon converts a simple into a compound fracture. However, if a small needle is used and if the skin over the site of the injection is painted with strong tincture of iodine, we believe that the danger of carrying infection into the area of the fracture is so slight that it is negligible. In order that this type of anesthesia be successful, the fracture should be seen early; that is, within the first twenty-four hours after the injury. Otherwise, the blood in the hematoma will have coagulated and it will be difficult to obtain satisfactory anesthesia. When two bones have been broken, as in the leg or forearm, both bones should be injected with a relatively strong (1 or 2 per cent)

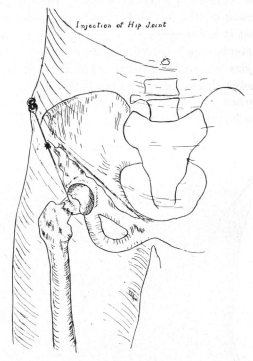

Fig. 69.—Insertion of needle for obtaining local anesthesia in fractures through the neck of the femur. (Courtesy Dr. C. O. Rice.)

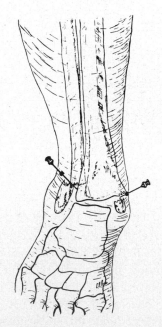

Fig. 70.—Points of insertion of the needle for obtaining anesthesia in fractures of both malleoli. (Courtesy Dr. C. O. Rice.)

solution of novocaine and the injection should be made in such a manner that every part of the fracture will be reached. For instance, in a fracture of the radius near the wrist it is necessary to inject on the dorsum and on the volar surface as well as laterally and mesially. The amount of novocaine to be used depends upon the size of the bone and varies from 10 to 30 or more cubic centimeters. The point is, use no more than is necessary, but use enough. It is remarkable how, when anesthesia is obtained, the muscle spasm tends to relax and the fracture can be manipulated at will.

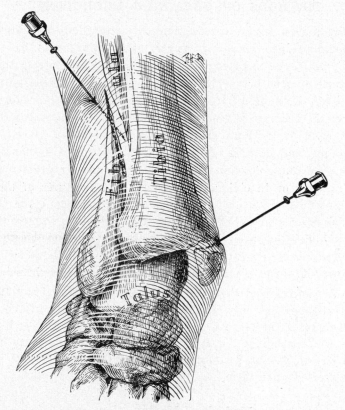

Fig. 71.—Points of insertion of the needle for obtaining local anesthesia in fractures of the fibula and of the internal malleolus. (Courtesy Dr. C. O. Rice.)

There is no special trick about the administration of local anesthesia in this manner except that it must be put into the hematoma. In a fresh simple fracture the long slender needle should be thrust down to a position as close as possible to the end of one of the fragments. Then the plunger should be withdrawn and if the needle is in the hematoma blood can be drawn up into the syringe.

In impacted fractures there is no hematoma between the fragments, and multiple subperiosteal injections must be made around the fractured area.

Spinal Anesthesia.—In some clinics spinal anesthesia is used in the treatment of fractures of the lower extremities. We would warn against its use in patients where shock is present or may be expected to occur.

Intravenous Anesthesia.—The newer intravenous anesthetics (pentothal sodium and evipal) are being used more and more extensively in the treatment of fractures. They have the advantage that general anesthesia is induced in a very short time and that consciousness returns promptly and that the patient is not sick afterward. In the hands of one skilled in their administration the anesthesia can be prolonged by repeated administration of small amounts of the anesthetic, and the method is relatively safe.

METHODS OF OBTAINING REDUCTION

The methods used to obtain reduction can be divided into closed manipulation, traction, and open operation. Other things being equal, closed manipulation is to be preferred in cases where the fracture lies close to the end of a long bone, such as fractures of the lower end of the radius and fractures about the ankle. Reduction by closed manipulation is also preferable in instances where the fracture is transverse and where one may expect to obtain stable engagement of the bone ends after they have been placed in contact with one another, and in cases of bones which are quite superficial, as in the fingers and in the tibia. Treatment by traction is usually preferred in severe compound fractures or in oblique and comminuted fractures of the shafts of long bones, especially of the femur and of the humerus where the bone is covered by a thick layer of muscles and where it is difficult or impossible to maintain reduction once it has been obtained. However, the choice between manipulation and traction treatment of a given fracture admits of wide leeway, depending upon the surgeon's skill in manipulating a limb, or in using traction.

It is to be emphasized that the term ''skill in using traction'' is used broadly and includes not only the ability to apply it properly, but also the interest on the part of the surgeon which will cause him to inspect it frequently and keep it efficient. Traction is dynamic energy and must be guided and varied from day to day as the positions of the fragments change in response to the forces exerted upon them.

Methods of Manipulation

Methods of manipulation vary with the training and methods of different surgeons and with the position and type of fracture. For instance, in a fracture through the shaft of a long bone one surgeon will prefer to obtain engagement of the fragments by means of direct traction in the long axis of the bone, traction being made in line with the position assumed by the upper fragment and being made while the joints at either end of the injured bone are in a neutral position; that is, semiflexed. By this method the sleeve of muscles and periosteum around the fragments may be depended upon to cause the bone ends to fall in place and engage one another when sufficient traction is applied to the limb to pull them by one another. Reduction is satisfactory if, with the traction relaxed, the normal length of the limb is maintained and is quite stable to upward pressure on the distal fragment. Various mechanical aids are used to supply traction and counter-traction. (Fig. 72.)

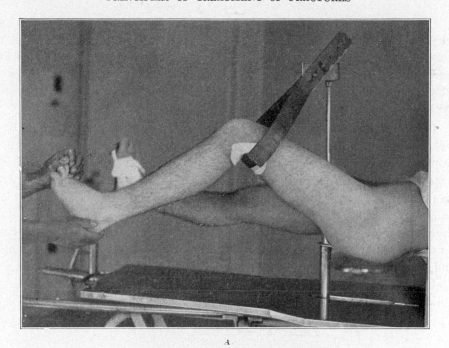

A.

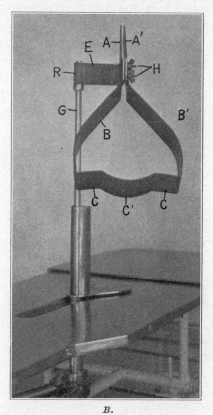

B.

Fig. 72.—Apparatus used by Conwell for supporting the knee and obtaining traction on the leg with the muscles relaxed for the reduction of fractures of both bones of the leg. (Two views.) (J. Bone and Joint Surg., July, 1931.)

Other surgeons depend upon angulation for engagement of the bone ends and place the joints in a neutral position—that is, semiflexed—and bend the limb at the site of the fracture until the bone ends are engaged. Then the limb is straightened, thus obtaining normal length. In fractures around the wrist and ankle the manipulation used is a combination of traction, leverage, and direct pressure on the fragments.

Before attempting the manipulation of a fracture the surgeon should, in most instances, obtain an x-ray, and his manipulation should be guided by the position of the fragments and by the pull of the various muscles and ligaments attached to the bone ends. Some surgeons prefer to manipulate all fractures under a fluoroscope. Others never use a fluoroscope even when it is available. A good deal depends upon the skill of the surgeon. With a fluoroscope the bone ends are visible, but the soft parts are not. Surgeons who do not use a fluoroscope are less likely to damage the soft tissues. On the other hand, they are less likely to obtain anatomic reduction. The results seem to be about the same and depend largely upon the skill of the surgeon in the application of the method which he uses.

Reduction by Direct Leverage

Dr. J. E. M. Thomson (Jour. Bone & Joint Surg., 1935) has shown that in certain fractures, especially those of one or of both bones of the forearm or leg in which manipulations have failed, it is possible to stick a thin steel rod or lever through a small incision in the skin, direct its end so that it lies between the ends of the bones and, under fluoroscopic control, lever them together much in the manner that one would use a small bone skid in an open operation. The operation is done under aseptic conditions and the fluoroscope is used only during the actual reduction. We have used this method successfully on a few fresh fractures and on a fracture of the radius (middle third, three weeks old) and on a fracture of the second metacarpal two weeks old. An ordinary small Steinmann pin was used as the subcutaneous lever or skid.

Reduction by Traction

Traction may be applied to the skin by means of adhesive tape (Figs. 73-76), moleskin adhesive, or various types of glue and muslin bandages; or

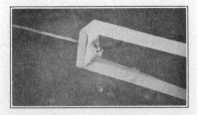

Fig. 73.—Spreader made of square wooden block with hole in the middle for use in applying traction to the extremities with adhesive tape.

it may be applied to the bone by means of the Kirschner wire or clamps or ice tongs or pins which pass through the bone distal to the fracture (Figs. 77-81).

Certain fractures of the femur, especially supracondylar fracture and compound fractures, or fractures in limbs in which the skin has been so damaged that it is impossible to apply adequate adhesive traction, must be treated by skeletal traction. The various methods of applying adhesive and skeletal traction are taken up under the bones for which they are indicated.

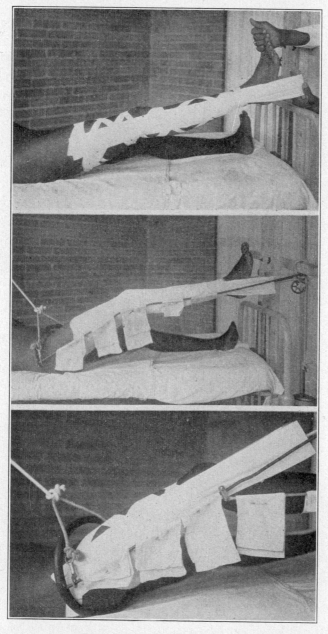

Fig. 74.—Method of applying adhesive to the lower extremity for traction.

Fig. 75.—Same as preceding. The adhesive has been covered by a firm gauze bandage and the leg is supported in a Thomas splint with Conwell's overhead pelvic-femur frame.

Fig. 76.—Method of applying adhesive traction to the thigh in fractures of the hip or upper portion of the femur. Supported in a Thomas splint and Pearson knee flexion support. The adhesive should be covered by a firm gauze bandage.

Skeletal traction has the advantages that it is more efficient, more weight can be used, and it is more comfortable to the patient if it is applied correctly. On the other hand, it has the disadvantage that occasionally, even under the best of conditions the bone will become infected either from the pin wound or from the wound around the clamps. During recent years the introduction of stainless steel wire and pins has greatly cut down the incidence of infection because these pins do not corrode and the pin wounds remain clean if they are clean in the beginning and if the skin is not pulled against the pin.

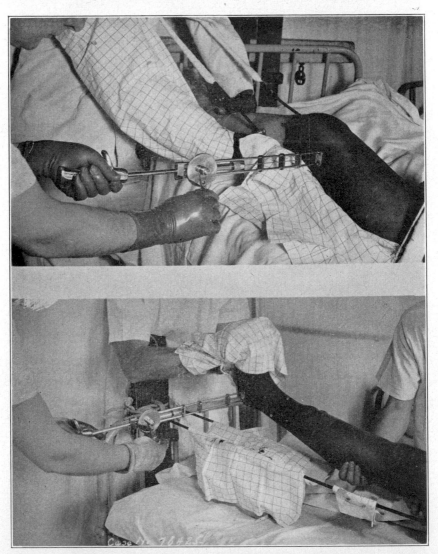

Fig. 77.—Application of Kirschner wire to femur (above) and os calcis (below).

The danger of infection has been further reduced by the recent introduction of stainless steel wire which is drilled through the bone making a very small skin wound. Other things being equal, it appears that danger to infection varies directly with the size of the pin or wire through the bone. . Consequently, the fine stainless steel wire passed through the bone and pulled taut by the traction apparatus is the safest method of applying skeletal traction. The only disadvantages are that the application of the wire requires a special drill and guide and the application of the traction requires a special clamp.

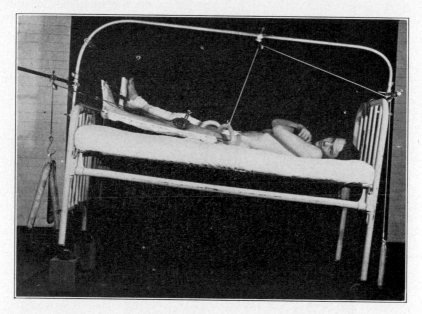

Fig. 78.—Traction clamp as used at the Shriners' Hospital for Crippled Children, St. Louis Unit. The gas pipe frame is one devised by Dr. A. O. Adams.

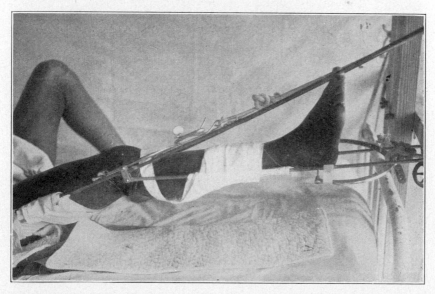

Fig. 79.—Patient with skeletal traction to both the femur and os calcis for fracture of the femur and both bones of the leg; ice tongs used for the femur and pin through the os calcis. Thomas splint and Pearson knee flexion with Conwell's overhead pelvic-femur frame is used.

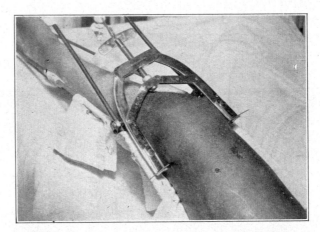

Fig. 80.—Wire traction to femur.   (Zimmer clamp.)

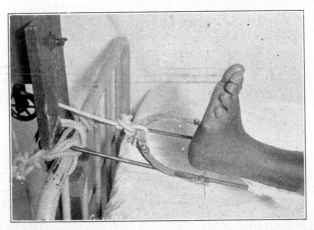

Fig. 81.—Wire traction to os calcis.   (DePuy clamp.)

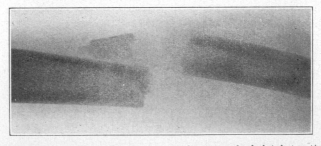

Fig. 82.—A fault sometimes encountered in the use of skeletal traction and one occasionally seen with adhesive traction. Too much traction has been applied and the bones have been pulled past one another. Unless this is corrected very soon after it occurs, it will lead either to delayed union or nonunion, since even when the traction is released, callus or soft tissue will be interposed between the fragments and it may be impossible to get them together again without open operation.

Mechanical Traction Reduction and Fixation Apparatus

The work on leg lengthening by Abbott and Crego and others showed that, by means of pins or taut wires through the fragments of a bone and the use of a screw traction apparatus, it is possible to lengthen a bone and control the position of the fragments. The same principle has now been applied to the treatment of fractures and several more or less complex and expensive reduction machines or automatic splints are now on the market.

These automatic splints or screw traction reducing machines are successful and we believe relatively safe in the hands of those who are skilled in their use, but we believe that their use requires considerable skill. It is a mistake to expect the splint to do the work unless it is used with intelligence and skill. In using such machines it is usually necessary to follow the position of the fragments with the x-ray and one should remember that it is possible to pull and hold the bone ends too far apart and thus court delayed union.

After the fracture is reduced the position is maintained by the special fixation apparatus which is attached to the pins or by incorporating the pins in the plaster which encases the limb. We have had very little experience with this method, but have each treated too many cases of delayed or nonunion with or without infection of the multiple pin holes or extensive infection of the bone and adjacent joints to extend this experience.

Immobilization

Immobilization is secured by recumbency, by bandages or slings, by traction, by splints, and by plaster-of-Paris casts. The character of immobilization depends a good deal upon the type of fracture and the tendency to displacement of the fragments either by muscle pull or by gravity, and also upon the choice of the surgeon. In fractures of the spine or pelvis, for instance, without displacement, simply placing the patient recumbent on a Bradford frame will often afford adequate immobilization.

In fractures of the clavicle or lower end of the humerus sufficient immobilization may be obtained by bandages and adhesive tape. The same is true in certain fractures about the ankle without displacement. In fractures with a tendency to displacement immobilization must be obtained by traction or splints and where traction is used, especially in the femur and bones of the leg, splints are necessary to support the limb and to prevent posterior angulation of the fragments. The same is true to a less degree in fractures of the shaft of the humerus. The choice as to whether a given fracture should be immobilized in a splint or plaster cast depends upon the availability of a suitable splint and upon the ability of the surgeon to use plaster of Paris.

We prefer plaster of Paris to the average splint with the exception of the Thomas or Hodgen splint for the lower extremity. Other surgeons who do not use plaster of Paris and are not adequately trained in its use will keep on hand a large supply of splints and use these in preference. It is our experience that most fractures can be adequately treated by plaster-of-Paris casts, that the patients are more comfortable in casts than in splints, and that the casts require less attention after they have been applied.

The former objection to plaster of Paris that it could not be used with traction has been met by the Hoke traction apparatus which is illustrated in fractures of the femur and of the humerus and which admits of adequate traction while the limb is encased in plaster (Figs. 84 and 85). It should not be used, however, by one who does not understand the application of plaster of Paris and who is not skilled in its use.

The following table of soft tissue injury devised by one of us (H. E. C.) is helpful in determining the type of immobilization to use in the treatment of fractures of the extremities:

One plus are cases in which there is a simple fracture with slight soft structure injury without comminution of the bone.

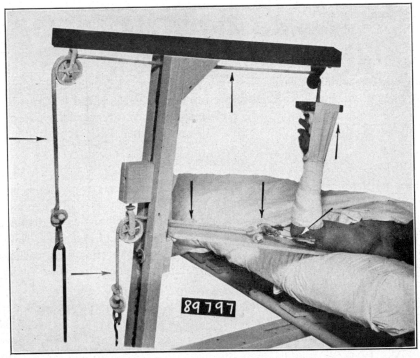

Fig. 83.—Skeletal traction to arm for fractured humerus. Kirschner wire in olecranon.

One and five-tenths plus are cases in which there is a simple fracture, usually not comminuted, with a moderate soft structure injury and slight intramuscular hemorrhage.

Two plus are compound or simple fractures in which there is a slight punctured wound of the leg, with or without a comminution of bone and with moderate soft structure injury and intramuscular hemorrhage.

The above three groups make up the largest part of all fractures.

Two and five-tenths plus are cases in which there is or is not a slight laceration through the skin and fascia, but with a severe soft structure injury and intramuscular hemorrhage with or without a comminution of the bone, which may or may not be compounded.

Three plus are cases in which there is one or more large lacerations extending through the skin and fascia and part of the muscle, with severe soft structure injury involvement, and marked intramuscular hemorrhage, with a compound wound of the bone and bone usually comminuted.

Three and five-tenths plus are cases in which there is a deep laceration through skin and fascia and muscle exposing the bone, with a severe soft structure injury and marked intramuscular hemorrhage with a compound wound of bone, the latter usually comminuted, with or without injury to the nerves.

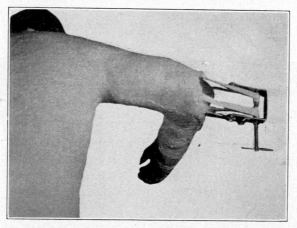

Fig. 84.—Hoke's traction apparatus as applied for fractures of the upper portion of the humerus.

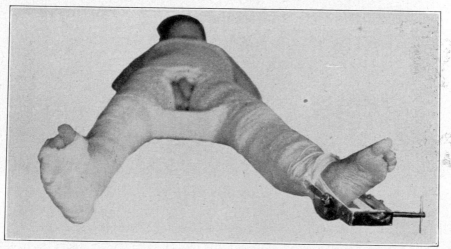

Fig. 85.—Hoke's traction apparatus as applied for fracture of the shaft of the femur. Well leg counter traction.

Four plus are fractured extremities with irreparable injury to soft structures, nerves, loss of blood supply, with or without compound comminution of the bone, demanding amputation.

The following applies generally to all extremities provided the fractures or fracture is in good position or can be reduced or held in position without possibility of a displacement.

In the one plus injury type the case can generally be treated in a circular plaster cast without bivalving.

In the one and five-tenths plus injury type the case can generally be treated in circular plaster cast with or without bivalving.

In the two plus injury type generally the case can be treated with a circular plaster cast with a window in the cast over the punctured wound, or it may be necessary to bivalve the cast besides the window.

In the two and five-tenths plus injury type we have the borderline case in which it is questionable whether extension or a circular cast should be used. Generally speaking if no comminution of the bone is present and no marked or severe laceration through the skin and fascia, the case can be treated with a

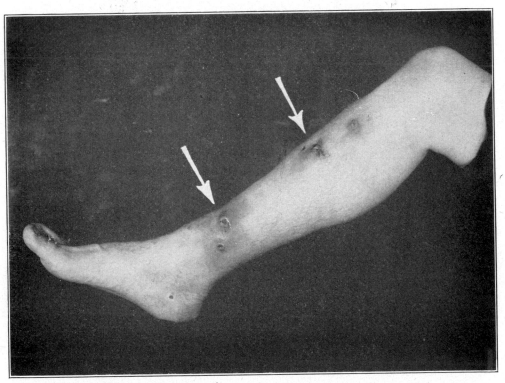

Fig. 86.—Infection of pin holes after external skeletal fixation. Union was obtained by multiple ring sequestra, and infection required multiple saucerization and chemotherapy.

circular plaster cast with bivalving of the cast immediately after the cast sets. In those cases in which there is comminution of the bone with severe lacerations of the skin and fascia and severe soft structure injury, traction should be used.

In the other types of injury, that is, three plus and three and five-tenths plus, traction, with wire or pin or adhesive, should be used. The traction, however, should be removed as early as possible and a circular cast applied to the extremity. Generally speaking the cast can be applied when overlapping of the fragments has been reduced, when sufficient callus formation has taken place to prevent malposition, and after all compound wounds have practically healed.

The other (J.A.K.) has no rules, but he believes that the more severe the soft tissue injury, the greater is the demand for immobilization and treats as large a percentage of his fractures as possible by immobilization in plaster casts. When necessary this is supplemented by internal or external skeletal fixation or traction. In certain fractures a cast is not necessary.

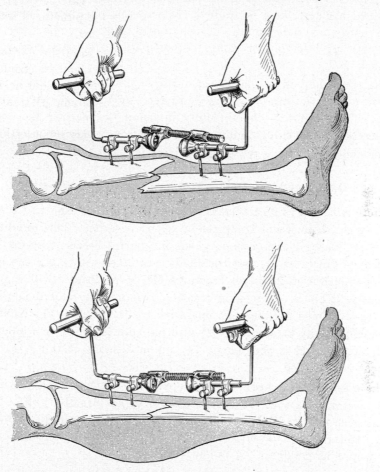

Fig. 87.—Fracture reduction apparatus. (Courtesy Zimmer Manufacturing Co.)

External Skeletal Fixation

By external skeletal fixation we mean the fixing of the fragments by one or more pins or wires which are inserted into the bone and extend out through the skin. There are three types in general use.

In the simplest type the fracture is reduced generally by open operation and the fragments are fixed by one or more stainless steel wires drilled through the two fragments and crossing the fracture site. One of us (J.A.K.) uses this type frequently for the proximal third of the humerus, the condyles of the humerus, the internal malleolus, and in other areas in order to avoid leaving metal in the wound. The projecting wire is cut off about 1 inch from the skin and then bent 90 degrees in order to prevent them from drifting into the tissues.

This is a reasonably safe procedure, as the wire is thrust through intact skin and the only strain on the wire is at the fracture site. The wires are pulled out as soon as they are no longer needed (about 4 weeks).

The second method is the reduction of the fracture by traction with from 2 to 4 pins or wires transfixing the extremity and the bone. While traction is maintained a plaster cast is applied, the wires or pins being incorporated in the cast and thus maintaining the position of the fragments. We have seen many cases of infection or nonunion, or both, after this method, and we rarely use it.

The third method is the use of multiple pins or half pins in one of the so-called automatic splints (Stader, Roger Anderson, Zimmer, Haines and others). On account of the difficulty in using the method successfully and the dangers of delayed or nonunion and infection, we do not use this method.

For oblique fractures the beaded wires of Thomson and Ferciot are useful.

Open Operation in the Treatment of Simple Fractures

There will always be a certain number of surgeons who will treat a large percentage of their recent fractures by open operation. This number will, we believe, gradually decrease as surgeons in general become more skilled in the treatment of fractures by closed methods. In other words, the frequency with which open operation in simple fractures will be performed will vary inversely with the skill of the surgeon in treating fractures by closed methods. The advantages claimed for the open operative treatment are: (1) Anatomical reduction can usually be secured; (2) internal splintage can be applied; (3) the convalescent period is shortened; (4) union is more certain; (5) the after-treatment is simplified.

The disadvantages are: (1) The operation converts a simple into a compound fracture and there is always danger of an infection; (2) after reduction has been obtained it must be, in most instances, maintained by adequate external splintage; (3) as little nonabsorbable foreign material should be left in the wound as possible; (4) union is slower.

The local implantation of sulfonamide powder in the wound has lessened the danger of infection and the use of vitallium or enduro stainless steel has largely overcome the objection to leaving foreign material in the wound. Consequently, open operations for the treatment of fractures can now be done with greater safety than at any time in the past.

The advantages of the closed treatment are: (1) There is practically no danger of infection and the patient's life is less endangered than by an operation; (2) union is more certain and is obtained more quickly after an adequate closed reduction than after open operation; (3) no foreign material is left in the wound; (4) the period of hospitalization is often shortened; (5) special operative skill is not necessary on the part of the surgeon.

There are certain fractures, however, in which open operation is necessary if the maximum restoration of function is to be obtained. These are largely fractures involving joints and fractures in which small pieces of the ends of the bone are separated and in which it is impossible to control these fragments by manipulation or by traction as well as fractures of the shafts of bones in which muscle or other tissue is caught between the fragments and in which it is found to be impossible to bring the fragments into direct contact or in which proper approximation has not been obtained after a fair attempt at the closed method has been tried (Figs. 88 and 89). We do not recommend repeated violent attempts at closed reduction. It is less traumatizing to perform an open reduction.

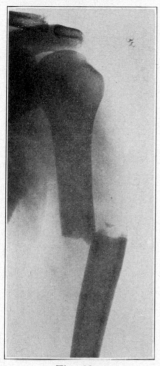

Fig. 88.

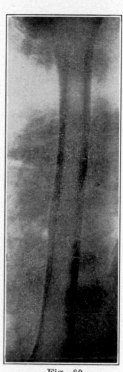

Fig. 89.

Fig. 88.—A simple transverse fracture of the humerus. Repeated attempts at manipulative reduction were unsuccessful as a result of interposition of soft tissues.

Fig. 89.—Same as preceding after open reduction. The ends were held together by kangaroo tendon and the arm was immobilized in a plaster-of-Paris spica. Firm union and complete restoration of function three months after operation. This is the simplest form of internal fixation and in most instances after operative reduction can be depended upon to immobilize the fragments sufficiently if adequate postoperative external fixation is employed.

Operative Treatment of Fractures

As stated above the choice between the operative and conservative or closed treatment varies greatly among different surgeons. When operative treatment is decided upon the first thing to be considered is the time most advisable for the operation. In simple fractures in which operation is deemed necessary, the operation is best performed immediately if the state of the skin over the wound permits; that is, if there are no abrasions or lacerations which may lead to infections, because just as in the closed method the operation will be much easier if it is done before the tissues have become infiltrated with blood and the fracture site surrounded by a partially organized exudate. On the other hand, if the operation cannot be done immediately; that is, within a few hours after the injury, it is best to postpone it for about five to seven days or until the swelling has largely subsided and the tissues have regained their vitality, since operating upon a fracture three or four days old always lays open a wide area of devitalized tissues and partially organized hematoma in which resistance to infection is relatively low.

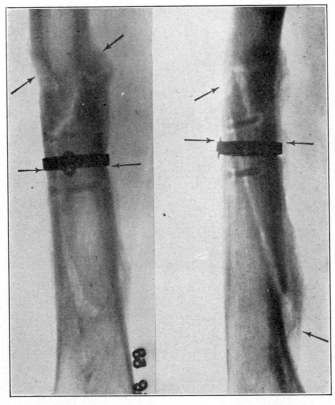

Fig. 90.—Parham band as applied for oblique fractures of the femur. We seldom use this form of internal fixation, since we believe that it leads to permanent weakening of the bone. The band should be removed when sufficient callus has formed. The bone has refractured one inch above the band.

Preparation for Operation.—If the operation can be done immediately the skin should be shaved, scrubbed with soap and water, then washed thoroughly with alcohol and ether and painted with full strength tincture of iodine or other skin antiseptic. The incision should be made in such a manner as to approach the bone by the shortest route possible without damaging important structures. After the incision is made through the skin, the skin should be protected by skin towels applied with clips with the limb completely covered so that no skin is exposed and so draped that it can be freely manipulated and traction applied when necessary. With a clean knife the wound should then be carried down to the bone and the fracture exposed. If the injury involves the joint, this should be opened freely and any loose fragments of bone removed or replaced. The fracture should then be reduced either by traction or leverage or direct pressure.

Internal Fixation.—After the fracture is reduced and the fragments are replaced, it is necessary that they remain in position. This brings up the question of internal fixation and there are a great many different types and materials used. Most of these will be ignored, but a few will be mentioned. The degree of internal fixation necessary varies inversely with the skill with which the fractured limb is handled and with the efficiency with which it is immobilized after the operation. In most instances it is possible to engage the bone

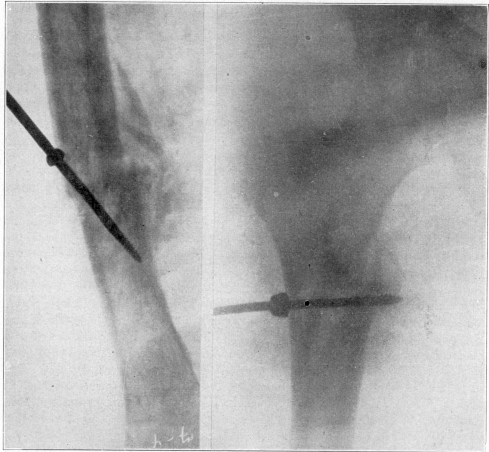

Fig. 91.   Fig. 92.

Fig. 91.—Removable screw with nut as used by Dr. W. B. Carrell for the fixation of difficult fractures. After the screw is applied, the limb is encased in a plaster-of-Paris cast with the screw projecting through the skin and incorporated in the cast. (Carrell and Girard: J. A. M. A., February, 1931.)

Fig. 92.—Same as preceding as applied for subtrochanteric fractures of the femur.

ends quite firmly so that there is relatively little tendency for them to slip by one another either with or without remodeling the bone ends and to hold them together with a piece of chromic catgut or stainless steel wire which is passed through small drill holes in each fragment. We now routinely use stainless steel wire which is passed through rather than around the fragments, and do not remove them after union is obtained, unless they cause trouble.

Formerly, we used chromic catgut, but now we use stainless steel wire and believe that if it is put in sterile and tight it causes less immediate reaction than catgut and will be tolerated indefinitely. The twisted ends of the wire are carefully pressed down against the bone so that they will not irritate the overlying soft tissues.

We do not use or advise encircling wires or bands for the fixation of oblique fractures, but prefer sutures or screws passed through drill holes in each fragment. When they are used they should be removed after union is obtained, since the encircling wire or band may lead to a fracture some years later. Carrell has recently devised a very clever removable screw for such cases. It is left projecting through the skin and plaster and is removed after union is fairly solid. We have not used it, but believe it to be useful in certain fractures. (Figs. 91 and 92.) The same is true of the beaded Kirschner wires devised by Thomson.

Some surgeons prefer to use bone or ivory, or metal plates. If bone plates are used, they should be fastened with beef bone screws or pegs if the surgeon wishes to avoid the use of metal in the wound. Or one may use a bone or ivory inlay of the type used by Magnuson which is set in a groove in the cortex and fixed by small bone or ivory pegs. The popular method, however, for internal fixation of the shafts of the long bones is by means of metal plates. (Figs. 93 and 94.)

The steel bone plate for the internal fixation of fractures is popular because if it is properly applied it is mechanically right and affords the maximum internal fixation with a minimum of foreign material. Through the efforts of the Fracture Committee of the American College of Surgeons the vanadium steel bone plates and self-tapping screws designed by Dr. W. O'Neil Sherman of Pittsburgh have been accepted as standard by the United States Bureau of Standards and in the future it should be possible to obtain plates and screws of uniform sizes and quality. These plates and screws are now made of enduro stainless steel or of vitallium. Since these materials are practically inert in the body and cause very little reaction, they can be used much more freely than could the older plates and screws and their adoption has greatly broadened the field of internal fixation of bone, just as has the local implantation of sulfonamide powder broadened the field of the open reduction of fractures.

One of us (J.A.K.) is now using dual plates of stainless steel in selected cases. These serve as clamps and afford very firm fixation. (Fig. 96.)

The Local Implantation of Sulfonamide Powder in Clean Operative Wounds.—In several publications one of us (J. A. K.) has demonstrated that sulfanilamide, sulfathiazole, or mixtures of these drugs can be implanted in clean operative wounds and that the presence of the drug in the wound does not interfere with the normal healing of the wound or the union of the fracture. A clinical experience of over 300 consecutive operations in which the powder was implanted in the wounds has proved that its local use leads to a decrease in the incidence of postoperative infection and is not toxic to the patient.

The powder is sprinkled lightly over the surface of the wound just before it is closed. It is slowly dissolved by the serum which collects in the wound and is then absorbed and excreted. While the drug is present in the wound (about forty-eight hours), it inhibits the growth of any bacteria with which it comes in contact. These bacteria are then eliminated by the normal defense mechanisms of the body. Sulfanilamide is more effective against streptococci and sulfathiazole is more effective against staphylococci and the organisms of gas gangrene. We now wash the wound with a saturated solution of the drug in normal salt solution.

When used in clean operative wounds the drug should be sterilized because it is not bactericidal. This can be done by autoclaving it at 18 pounds pressure for twenty minutes.

When infection is feared after operations on bone, we now inject from 10,000 to 20,000 units of penicillin intramuscularly after the operation and the dose of 10,000 to 20,000 units intramuscularly is repeated at 3-hour or 4-hour intervals for a few days, until the danger of infection has passed. This is especially indicated in instances where the bone has been infected in the past or where the operation has been unusually long and difficult.

Technic of Open Reduction and Application of a Sherman Bone Plate.— The first requisite for applying a bone plate is satisfactory plates, screws and instruments. These should be obtained and inspected before the patient is prepared for the operation. In addition to a dissecting set and the usual bone instruments, there are required (1) towel clips (two dozen for a large operation); (2) Sherman bone plates and self-tapping screws of approximately the correct sizes; (3) drill of the correct size ($\frac{3}{32}$ inch, No. 32 Brown-Sharp drill, hand or motor driven); (4) self-centering and holding screw driver; (5) bone skid; (6) bone-holding forceps; (7) clamp to hold the plate and bone ends while applying screws (Lowman or Lambotte); and (8) caliper for measuring the diameter of the bone in order to determine the proper length of the screws to be used.

The operation is best done immediately or from seven to ten days after the injury. After a twenty-four-hour preparation of the skin, the patient is anesthetized and the skin over the operative field is washed with alcohol and ether and painted with strong tincture of iodine. The excess iodine is then removed with alcohol and the extremity is so draped that it can be manipulated if desired without breaking the aseptic technic.

The surgeon and his assistants should take care that their gloved hands do not at any time come in contact with the patient's skin, even after it is painted with iodine.

A generous longitudinal incision is made through the skin and subcutaneous tissue over the site of the fracture. (The incision should be a little longer than necessary.) The knife and forceps used are discarded and skin towels are clipped to the edges of the incision in such a manner that no skin is left exposed.

With a clean knife the incision is carried down to the bone (avoiding important structures) and the fractured ends are exposed, seized with bone-holding forceps, gently curetted, and the displacement reduced either by means of a skid and traction or angulation and traction. (If a Berg clamp is available, it facilitates the reduction.) In a simple fracture a hair line anatomic reduction should be obtained.

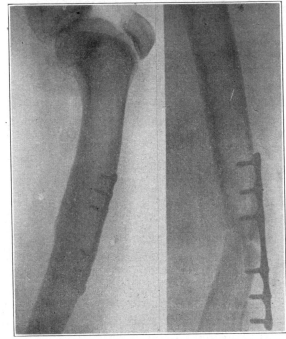

A.   B.

Fig. 93.—A. Metal bone plate as usually applied for fracture of the femur. More efficient fixation would have been obtained had the middle screw in each fragment extended through to the opposite cortex of the femur.

B. Metal bone plate as applied for fracture of the femur in which the screws have pulled out from one end of the plate. The plate, of course, in this instance is merely a foreign body in the thigh.

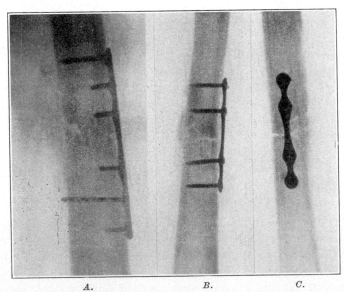

A.   B.   C.

Fig. 94.—A. Sherman steel bone plate properly applied to a fracture of the shaft of the femur. (Courtesy Dr. W. O'Neill Sherman.)

B. Sherman steel bone plate properly applied to a fracture of the shaft of the femur. (Courtesy Dr. W. O'Neill Sherman.)

C. Same as preceding, lateral view.

A suitable bone plate is selected and laid across the site of the fracture and the bone plate and bone ends are grasped firmly in the bone-holding forceps. With the plate in place, drill holes are made in the bone for the self-tapping screws. At least one of these holes in each fragment should penetrate both cortices. The diameter of the shaft is measured with the caliper and self-tapping screws of the correct length selected and driven home. Then the bone clamp is removed and the remaining screw holes are drilled and the screws driven home. (Figs. 93 and 94.)

Sulfonamide powder is now sprinkled over the surface of the wound, the muscle is sutured over the plate, and the wound is closed in layers without drainage. Care is taken to support the limb and not to manipulate it or put undue strain on the fracture site until it is supported by some form of external fixation (either a splint or a plaster-of-Paris cast).

Plates close to the skin, as on the subcutaneous surfaces of the tibia, should be removed after union is obtained, but plates covered by a thick layer of soft tissue, as on the shaft of the femur, are usually left in.

Short fragments near the articular surface when displaced can be replaced in their normal positions and fixed either by means of a small nail or screw or ivory screw or peg. A very convenient and cheap method is pinning the bones together with a bone knitting needle, using a drill slightly smaller than the knitting needle. The projecting part of the bone peg can be cut off with a pair of bone forceps. Very rarely where an articular surface is split is it advisable to screw or bolt two halves together by means of a transfixing screw or bolt. These larger pieces of metal should be removed after union has been obtained.

After the fracture is reduced and fixed by whatever means the surgeon chooses, the assistant who is holding the limb should secure a comfortable position in order to hold the limb securely while the wound is being closed. A plaster cast or splint is applied, since no type of internal splintage can be depended upon to hold the shaft of a long bone if it is subjected to very much strain. Not only must the limb be supported carefully, but the surgeon should check the alignment before the final external fixation is applied, since it is useless to operate upon and reduce a fracture if it is going to be immobilized in a poor functional position.

Rigid Internal Fixation and Balanced Traction.—For several years Dr. Wm. Darrach and Dr. Clay Ray Murray at the Presbyterian Hospital in New York City have advocated and used the principles of rigid internal fixation and balanced traction in the treatment of fractures of the long bones. The rigid internal fixation is obtained by fixation in two planes. The stainless steel plate is applied in the usual manner, and this is reenforced by a long oblique screw which traverses the fracture line at right angles to the screws holding the plate or by a second plate. The limb is then suspended in balanced traction and active exercise is begun a few days after the operation. Their results are good, but the method is not one which can be recommended for general use.

Lane Technic.—Many surgeons use the Lane technic routinely in open operations for fracture. By this we mean the nontouch technic in which nothing that has been touched by the hands of the operator or of his assistants

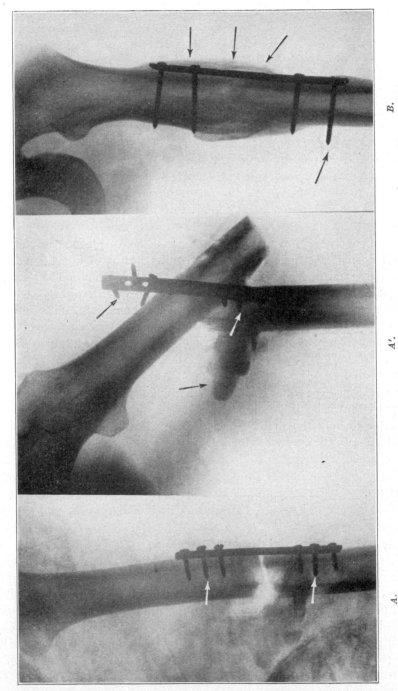

B.

A'.

A.

Fig. 95.—*A'.* Displacement after inadequate internal fixation with a bone plate (*A*) and external fixation with a cast.

B. Internal fixation of a fracture through the junction of the upper and middle thirds of the femur by vitallium bone plate and screws. Note the callus formation over lower screws, the screws having been inserted too far into the femur. Patient, however, had no disability from this. Good functional result. Internal fixation screw should not protrude beyond the distal cortex of the bone. We prefer six screws at this site.

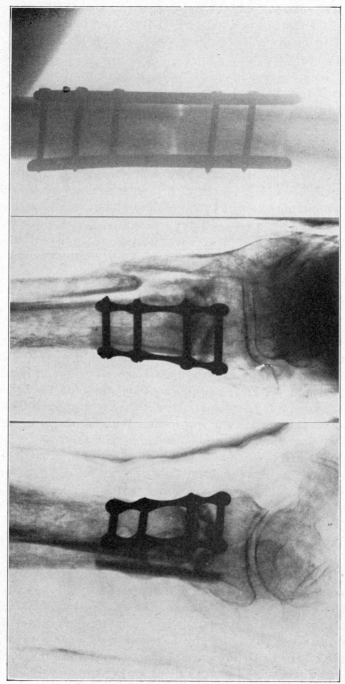

Fig. 96.—Dual plates supplemented by iliac grafts for old fracture of the femur with nonunion and for old supramalleolar fractures with nonunion supplemented by free graft. Both fractures united promptly after the operations.

enters the wound. All sponging is done with sponges on clamps, all needles are threaded by instruments, sutures are tied by instruments, and if the technic is properly carried out, the operator's and assistants' gloves at the end of the operation should be as clean and free from blood as they were at the beginning. In many instances, however, the technic is carried out in a more or less half-hearted manner.

Neither of the authors of this book use or recommend the Lane technic. We believe that if the surgeon scrubs his hands thoroughly, uses heavy rubber gloves which do not have holes in them, does not touch the skin with the gloved hand, and changes the gloves if they become torn, he will not infect the wound with his hands. There is absolutely no question but that for the average surgeon, use of the Lane technic greatly prolongs the operation and leads to the devitalization of tissues because of their long exposure to the outside air. The longer the operation the greater the chance for infection. We do not hesitate to put our hands into the wound whenever it is deemed advisable; but we do so only when there is a definite reason. We believe it is much more important to handle tissues gently, making adequate sharp dissection to expose the bone ends and do as little tearing and bruising of the tissues and stripping up of the periosteum as possible.

PHYSIOTHERAPY IN THE TREATMENT OF INJURIES OF BONES AND JOINTS

During and after the World War physiotherapy was used very extensively in the treatment of the various disabilities which followed wounds both with and without fractures, and in the base hospitals of the different armies a large personnel and elaborate equipment were provided for this purpose. Following this a tremendous wave of physiotherapy swept this country and has not only affected the medical profession, but has even impressed the laity. The result has been the establishment of physiotherapy departments in various hospitals and the purchase of various forms of apparatus by physicians and surgeons all over the country. We believe that this has been carried to the extreme and wish to emphasize the fact that in physiotherapy just as in most other forms of treatment, the therapeutic value of the method is largely dependent upon the skill with which it is administered.

We further wish to emphasize the fact that in the average fracture, if the bones are replaced in a good functional position and immobilized over a sufficient period of time, normal union will occur, and if the soft parts are not extensively damaged, normal function will return. This, however, is not true of joint fractures and the complications which arise in these injuries are mentioned under traumatic arthritis. It is well, however, to say here that in a great many instances physiotherapy has been used over periods of many months in futile efforts to restore normal function in joints the mechanics of which have been disorganized as a result of an injury.

We have not seen any adequate analysis of a series of fractures in which it has been shown to our satisfaction that by the extensive use of physiotherapeutic methods the period of disability has been shortened and the permanent result improved to such an extent that the result was worth the effort expended. Until this has been shown we shall continue to adopt a middle ground and shall particularly warn the average surgeon against the principles of early massage and mobilization as practiced and advocated by Lucas Championniere. His great dictum was "movement is life." We believe that a better dictum would be that "the healing of a fracture occurs more rapidly and more surely when rest is maintained." According to his method a minimum of splintage is used and very gentle, slow, rhythmic massage is begun on the day after the injury and is repeated and continued one or more times a day thereafter. He also began limited movements immediately after the injury and the range of movement was gradually increased. In certain fractures this method when applied by one skilled in its use is undoubtedly a successful one and is capable of producing excellent results. The average surgeon who treats fractures, however, is not a physiotherapist and furthermore we have no acceptable evidence that the results after intensive physiotherapy are any better than can be obtained by more conservative methods, and we have also seen fractures in which after an excellent reduction, displacement recurred as a result of too early and injudicious use of massage and movement. We endeavor to so apply our immobilization that the limb can be exercised or even used while the fracture is healing, but this must be done without danger of moving the fragments, and we do not bivalve our casts for heat, massage and passive movement of joints until the fragments are quite firmly united. The first dictum of the physical therapist should be "to do no harm."

The physiotherapeutic agents which have been proved to be of value in the treatments of fractures are:

1. Rest.
2. Movement (active and passive).
3. Heat.
4. Massage.
5. Ultraviolet light.

Rest.—Rest is placed first in this list because we believe that it is the most important, and should be used not only in the beginning of the treatment, but also, in joint fractures, from time to time during the convalescence whenever the joint becomes stiff and sore during a regime of active or passive movement. We have seen immobilization for a brief period in a plaster-of-Paris cast or splint result in marked improvement in joints which had been manipulated, heated, massaged, and exercised over a period of months without improvement.

Movement.—Movement is most important in the restoration, not only of motion to a joint, but also of tone and power to the muscles. It is to be remembered, however, that union of the fractured bone in good position is even more important than movement, that union must not be jeopardized by too early attempts to restore function, and that the rule should be to obtain union in good functional position first and restore function later.

The time at which active and passive movements can safely and profitably be begun depends largely upon the type and location of the fracture and the age and constitution of the patient. For instance, in children we are never concerned about the restoration of normal movement in a joint unless there has been some irreparable damage to the articular surfaces or to the soft tissues. We frequently see children whose joints have been immobilized over periods of six months or a year without permanent limitation of motion. On the other hand, in adults beyond middle life, and especially in those of the plethoric type or in those who are known to be afflicted with the arthritic diathesis, immobilization over a period of a few weeks may result in long continued and occasionally permanent limitation of motion in certain joints. For this reason in adults we endeavor to have our patients voluntarily put all of the joints of the extremity through the full range of movement at least twice a day when this can be done without any detrimental effect upon the treatment of the fracture. This is particularly true in fractures of the upper extremity in which stiffness of the hand is apt to follow immobilization. In fractures of the lower extremity if the limb is immobilized in good position, permanent limitation of movement does not, as a rule, occur.

The exercises should be begun as soon as possible after the injury, usually on the second or third day, and the patient should increase them gradually, but should not carry them to the point where they cause more than very slight pain. After union has occurred and between this period and the time when the limb is sufficiently strong for weight-bearing or other function, the active exercises should be encouraged and increased in order that by the time the patient is ready for the resumption of function, not only will considerable motion have been restored to the joints, but considerable power to the muscles. These exercises will, of course, vary with the patient and with the fractures, and they must be figured out by the surgeon for the individual case and so arranged that they do not disturb the position of the fragments until union has occurred.

Passive Movement.—Passive movement is not, as a rule, of great benefit in the restoration of motion to joints. We wish here to distinguish passive movement from assisted active movements. In certain instances in which the muscles are very weak the patient is able to carry out active movement if the effects of gravity or friction are removed from the part. In these movements, however, no appreciable force in the direction of movement is exerted by the physiotherapist. By passive movement we mean a forcible attempt to flex or extend a limb. Such attempts usually result not only in irritation of the involved joint, but in resistance by involuntary contraction of the muscles.

Manipulation Under an Anesthetic is occasionally resorted to in an effort to break up adhesions around or in a joint and to increase the range of motion in certain cases where apparently no other form of treatment can be expected to obtain the desired result. Before resorting to this, it is necessary first that the fracture be sufficiently healed that refracture will not occur; second, that too great a degree of atrophy not be present in the bones, otherwise, the bones may be fractured or the articular surfaces may be crushed and permanently damaged or fat embolism may occur; third, that slow, steady traction combined with active movements and function have been tried out over a period of weeks during which time careful observation of the joint has been maintained and that these measures have failed to restore function.

We mention the above precautions because we wish to emphasize the fact that *brisement forcé* is a dangerous procedure, really more dangerous than an open operation, and the patient and the surgeon should realize this before the manipulation is undertaken. One of us (J. A. K.) refractured an olecranon four months after the injury when attempting to regain flexion in the elbow, and in another case pulled off the condyles of the femur when manipulating the knee. The knee is illustrated in Figs. 97 and 98. There was fibrous ankylosis of about nine months' duration and the patient had been walking without support for about three months. The atrophy in this femur was not marked, yet it was fractured at approximately the epiphyseal line in a woman twenty-six years old and the force used was not excessive.

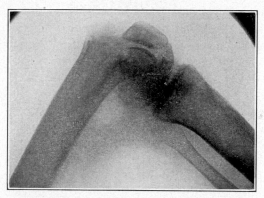

Fig. 97.—Fracture of the lower end of the femur in a woman twenty-four years of age, produced by manipulating the knee for the correction of fibrous ankylosis in a position of full extension. This patient had been walking on the leg for three months and bone atrophy was not marked.

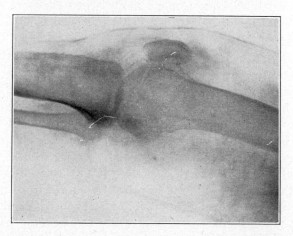

Fig. 98.—Same as preceding after correction and immobilization in a plaster cast.

Observing the precautions mentioned above, manipulation under an anesthetic or *brisement forcé* may be practiced with considerable benefit to the patient. This is particularly true of shoulders, elbows and knees. Stiff and contracted fingers, on the other hand, are much more satisfactorily treated by gradual stretching or, in certain instances, doing a capsulotomy and later traction, since manipulation of these small joints is apt to be followed by an acute irritation with an increase in the disability.

Heat.—It is difficult to evaluate the effect of heat in injuries. To many patients heat is grateful; they are made more comfortable; consequently, they believe that it is doing them a lot of good and the psychic effect is beneficial. So far as we know the principal effects of heat in fractures are (1) to cause dilatation of the blood vessels in the area and thus increase the circulation, and (2) to relieve pain. The mechanism by which heat relieves pain has not yet been determined. In regard to its effect upon circulation, local heat undoubtedly causes vascular dilatation, and it is said that it has a very marked decongestive action which tends to reduce the swelling in a part. Of this we are by no means certain. Heat is also used to maintain normal temperature in an extremity in which the circulation is impaired and thus acts as a preventive agent in surgical shock and impending gangrene.

The heat used for the relief of pain is usually applied locally over the injured area and the two most effective methods are diathermy or inductotherapy (sedative dosage), by which heat is produced in the tissues by means of an electric current, and infrared light. If these are not available, dry heat may be applied by means of a hot water bottle, an electric light, an electric pad, a hot iron or other object. It is important in the use of local heat to avoid burning the patient. In most cases moist heat seems to be more efficient than dry heat. It may be applied by means of hot soaks, poultices, or stupes.

When heat is used for its decongestive action it is important that the heat penetrate deeply into the tissues and for this reason either diathermy in sedative doses or the infrared lamp is more efficient than are other sources.

It is fairly well established that stiffened joints and muscles tend to loosen up temporarily and move more freely when they are heated. Consequently, exercises of hands or feet are often preceded by hot soaks or bakes.

Contrast Baths.—The alternate heating and cooling of a part tends to alternately dilate and contract the blood vessels; consequently, a very valuable form of physiotherapy for restoring the vascular tone in stiffened hands and feet that are cold, swollen, and cyanotic is contrast baths. The extremity is first plunged into water as hot as the patient can stand it and is held there two minutes; it is then plunged into cold water and held there one minute. These alternate hot and cold soaks should be kept up for about thirty minutes two or three times a day.

In heat used to combat surgical shock the heat should be applied to the entire body and should be sufficient to raise the temperature to normal. This can be done by means of heated blankets or electric bakes or hot water bottles, care being taken in the last instance not to burn the patient. For the prevention of impending gangrene, heat is best applied by means of electric bakes.

Massage.—Massage is of use principally as a preparation for active muscular exercises and joint movements. It should be begun lightly, should not cause pain to the patient, should be slow and rhythmic in character, and the stroking should be in the longitudinal direction of the limb from the distal end toward the body. As the massage is continued it can be more vigorous. Massage, if persisted in with sufficient vigor and over long enough time, may be of distinct benefit in decreasing the swelling in a limb. It is also helpful in increasing the circulation in a part where this is impaired.

The chief benefits claimed from massage, however, are that it restores power in paralyzed or weakened muscles and that it increases the range of movement in stiffened joints. This is not true. Power in weakened and paralyzed muscles can be restored only by active contractions of these muscles, and the exercises are most efficient when voluntarily performed by the patient. The contractions, however, can be brought about by stimulation of the given muscle by an electric current. It is doubtful whether electric stimulation is of much permanent value in the treatment of paralyzed muscles.

In the treatment of fractures we believe it is very important that the massage not be undertaken until quite firm union has been obtained. Motion of the fragments may result in delayed or even prevention of union. The chief value of massage in the treatment of fractures is the stimulating effect as a preliminary to active exercise of the limb; it is most efficient if the limb is first heated.

Ultraviolet Light.—Ultraviolet light is frequently advocated in fractures as a means of preventing nonunion. Most cases of nonunion, however, are not the result of any derangement of the calcium metabolism, but are the result of some local condition, and, of course, this cannot be affected by ultraviolet light. As a matter of fact it has not yet been proved that it is possible by any means at our command, either chemical or physical, to hasten the normal process of union in a fractured bone. If the patient is in a general run-down condition or if the patient has rickets or osteomalacia, ultraviolet either from the sun or some other source is a valuable adjunct in the treatment, but it should be understood that its effect is general, not local.

CHAPTER IV

FIRST AID IN FRACTURES AND AUTOMOBILE INJURIES

A large percentage of fractures occur at points some distance from a hospital. This is especially true of those injuries caused by automobile accidents which are ever becoming more frequent. As a result physicians who do not ordinarily treat traumatic injuries are frequently called upon to render first aid to injured individuals where little or no equipment is available.

Since the World War the usefulness of the Thomas arm and leg splints for the emergency treatment and transportation of fractures of the extremities has been stressed, but it is most unusual to find such a splint when one is called upon to render first aid. If such splints are available they should be used where indicated as is noted in the special part of this book. (Fig. 99.) Ordinarily the only materials available are boards, bandages, cloth and padding. These can be procured practically everywhere and with them the resourceful physician can immobilize the average fracture sufficiently to enable the patient to be transported to a hospital without danger of adding to the gravity of his injuries.

EXAMINATION

A rapid general physical examination is necessary, the purpose of which is not to arrive at an exact and complete diagnosis, but to determine whether the patient is seriously and perhaps fatally injured or whether the injuries are trivial. As a rule, this will not necessitate removal of all of the patient's clothes. Major fractures of the extremities which will require immobilization for transportation are usually obvious, and determination of the details of the fracture can be deferred until the patient is so situated that definite treatment can be begun.

EMERGENCY TREATMENT

If the patient is severely and dangerously injured, the emergency treatment has for its object the conservation of life. If in shock the patient should be given enough morphine to relieve the pain and should be kept warm and moved as little as possible. If open wounds are present, they should be covered with sterile dressings, but no attempt should be made to cleanse them. (See section on compound fractures.) If the patient is bleeding, the hemorrhage should be stopped either with a tourniquet or a tight compress, depending upon the location and the severity of the hemorrhage. If a tourniquet is used and it is necessary to leave it on more than one hour, the tourniquet should be loosened for a few minutes and then tightened again at the end of the first hour and at intervals of from twenty to thirty minutes thereafter. This is done to avoid gangrene.

It is much better to cover severely injured patients with blankets, allowing them to lie on the ground until they can be splinted and moved in an ambulance to the nearest hospital. The tendency is to dump them into the first available automobile and rush them to the nearest doctor's office or drug store where the superficial wounds are carefully cleansed and dressed while the patient is dying of shock.

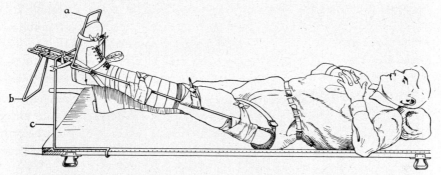

Fig. 99.—Immobilization of fracture of femur for transportation. (Courtesy Major General N. T. Kirk, Surgeon General, U. S. Army.)

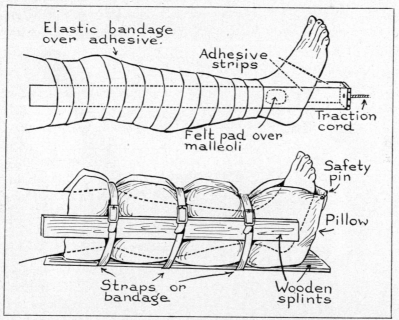

Adapted from United States Naval Medical Bulletin

Fig. 100.—Correct application of Buck's extension and pillow splint, the latter for emergency treatment, for fractures of the leg and ankle. (Courtesy Dr. J. W. Toumey.)

EMERGENCY SPLINTING OF FRACTURES

Major fractures in which there is a tendency for the fragments to move should be splinted before the patient is transported because the movement of the fragments causes great pain, damages the neighboring soft tissues, increases the hemorrhage and shock and may even result in the death of the

patient. It was for this reason that the practice of splinting the wounded on
the field was adopted by the various armies during the World War. And it
is said that the routine application of the Thomas splint on the field reduced
the mortality from 80 per cent to 20 per cent in gunshot fractures of the
femur. Since a Thomas splint is rarely available we shall describe methods

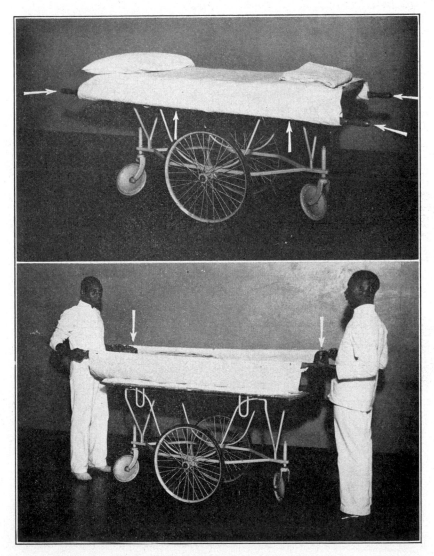

Fig. 101.—A stretcher which permits transfer of patient with relatively little movement.

of immobilizing major fractures by means of simple board splints. These
splints afford sufficient immobilization for emergency transport, but are not
suitable for the definitive treatment of fractures. In the illustrations padding
is omitted, but all of them should be padded with blankets, quilts, sheets,
clothing, cotton or whatever is available. It is to be noted that the splints immobilize the joints above and below the fracture.

Severe Fractures of the Spine or Pelvis

The ladder splint as illustrated in Figs. 102 and 103 is efficient and the materials for its construction can usually be procured. It consists of two long boards which are fastened together by three cross pieces. If hammer and

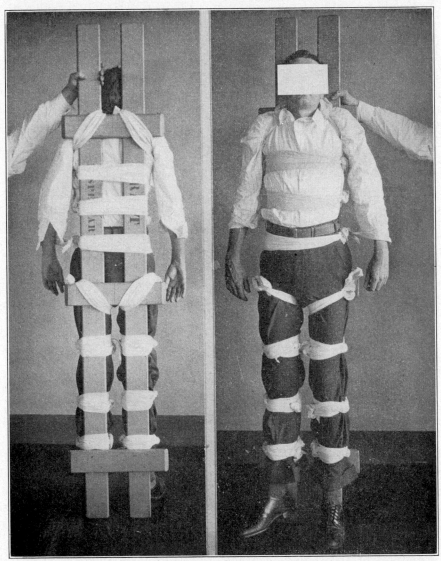

Fig. 102.   Fig. 103.

Fig. 102.—Ladder splint as used for the emergency immobilization of fractures of the spine or pelvis and for visceral injuries.

Fig. 103.—Same as preceding seen from the front.

nails are not available the cross pieces can be tied on. The splint is padded if material is available and the patient is bound to it as shown in the illustrations. It also serves as a litter and is useful for patients with visceral injuries. Lacking such a splint the patient should be transported and lifted face down to avoid further flexion of the spine. If the patient is very uncomfortable in this position, he may lie on the side or back, but the site of the fracture should be supported when he is lifted.

Fractures of the Upper Extremity

In simple fractures of the clavicle and minor injuries in the region of the shoulder all that is necessary is to place the arm in a snug triangular sling as illustrated in Fig. 112. In more severe injuries in the region of the shoulder the dressing illustrated in Fig. 107 is useful. It consists of: (1) a pad in the axilla (indicated by the pointer); (2) a scarf or band binding the elbow to the shoulder; (3) a band binding the arm to the chest (this should not be too tight as it may compress the brachial vessels); and (4) a sling to support the forearm and hand.

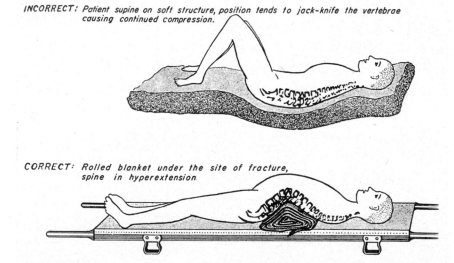

Fig. 104.—Method of transporting patient with fracture of the spine while hyperextension is being maintained. (Courtesy U. S. Army Medical Museum and Major General N. T. Kirk, Surgeon General, U. S. Army.)

Fractures of the lower half of the shaft of the humerus, elbow fractures, and fractures of the bones of the forearm in the upper third can be immobilized in board splints as illustrated in Figs. 108 and 109. Either a single long or two overlapping short boards can be used. Further immobilization can be secured by binding the arm to the side. The splint on the mesial surface should not extend too high in the axilla.

Fractures of the forearm in the lower two-thirds and fractures at the wrist can be immobilized in dorsal and volar board splints as illustrated in Fig. 110, and the forearm supported in a triangular sling (Figs. 111 and 112). The splints should extend beyond the elbow in order to prevent rotation of the forearm.

Fractures of the Lower Extremity

In fractures of the hip, shaft of the femur and knee it is necessary to immobilize the lower extremity and the trunk and in fractures of the leg it is

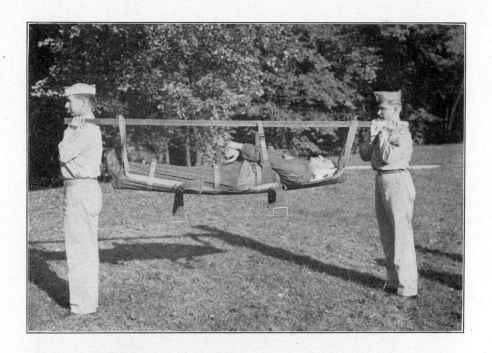

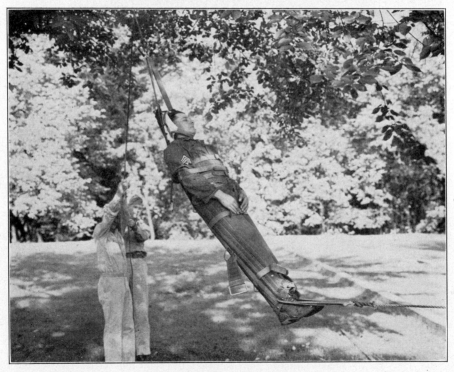

Figs. 105 and 106.—The Navy aeroplane litter, Neal Robertson model. (Courtesy Lieutenant Colonel A. R. Shands, United States Army.)

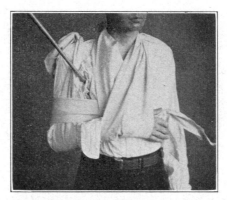

Fig. 107.—Emergency dressing for severe injuries in the region of the shoulder. The pointer indicates a pad in the axilla.

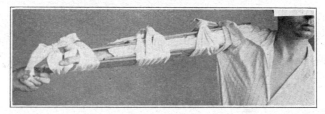

Fig. 108.—Board splints as used in emergency immobilization of fractures of the shaft of the humerus, elbow fractures, and fractures of the upper third of the forearm.

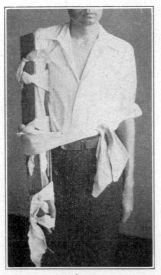

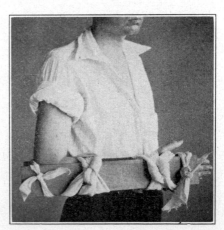

Fig. 109.   Fig. 110.

Fig. 109.—Same as preceding with arm bound to the side.

Fig. 110.—Board splint as used in the emergency immobilization of fractures of the forearm and wrist.

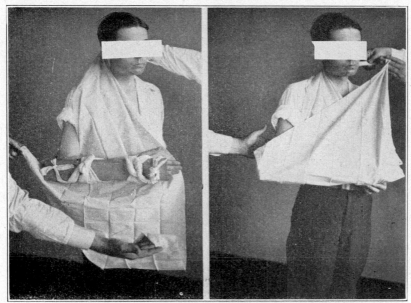

Fig. 111   Fig. 112.

Fig. 111.—Same as preceding with triangular sling being applied.

Fig. 112.—Same as preceding. The sling is folded and ready to be tied at the back of the neck.

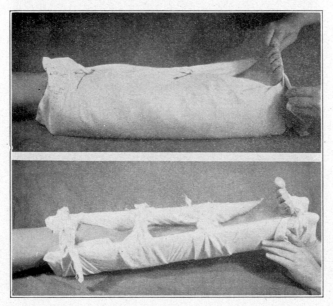

Fig. 113.—Pillow splint for temporary dressing of fractures of the leg. The pillow can be reinforced by straight boards under the leg and on the sides.

Fig. 114.—Lateral board splints for temporary dressing of fractures of the leg. Note that both knee and ankle are fixed.

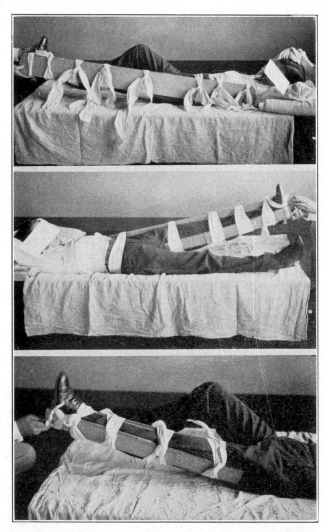

Fig. 115.—Long board splints for the emergency immobilization of fractures of the hip, shaft of the femur, and knee joint.

Fig. 116.—Same as preceding seen from the inner side. Note that the foot is bound to the splint to prevent rotation.

Fig. 117.—Lateral board splints as used in the emergency treatment of fractures below the knee. Note that the knee is immobilized.

necessary to immobilize the thigh and foot. A certain amount of immobilization can be secured by binding the two lower extremities together, but in fractures of the hip, thigh and knee it is advisable to apply boards as illustrated in Figs. 115 and 116. Note that the board on the outer side extends to the axilla and that rotation is prevented by tying the foot to the splint.

WIRE LADDER SPLINT

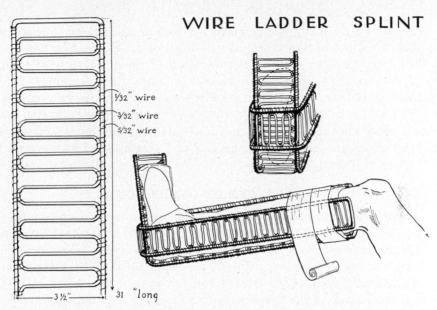

Fig. 118.—Use of wire ladder splint as emergency immobilization for fractures of the ankle. (Courtesy U. S. Army Medical Museum and Major General N. T. Kirk, Surgeon General, U. S. Army.)

In fractures below the knee it is not necessary to include the trunk, but it is desirable to include the thigh, and the shorter boards can be applied as shown in Fig. 117. If a pillow is available a very efficient and comfortable pillow splint can be applied. (Fig. 113.)

CHAPTER V

COMPLICATIONS OF FRACTURES

Fractures are usually accompanied by more or less injury to surrounding soft parts, and in addition there may be injuries or lesions in other parts of the body. In the strict sense of the word, all of these injuries are complications of the fracture, but we usually reserve the term ''complications'' for those conditions which are of sufficient gravity to demand treatment and to affect the prognosis in the given case. In certain instances the complication may be of more importance than the fracture itself, and the diagnosis and treatment of a fracture should include the diagnosis and treatment of any complication that may exist at the time of the injury or that may arise during the treatment.

1. FRACTURES OF OTHER BONES

Many fractures are caused by severe violence to the whole organism; this is especially true of those injuries resulting from falls or automobile accidents, and it is not unusual for more than one bone to be broken. For instance, we recently treated a man for a fracture of the femur incurred by being struck by an automobile. Several days later, when the patient was more rational, he complained of pain in the opposite heel, and physical examination and x-ray disclosed a fracture of the os calcis without displacement. This fracture had not been noted at the original examination. Other instances of this kind have occurred in our practice, as they doubtless have in the practice of other surgeons. When a patient comes under one's care for a fracture, a careful history should be obtained, and if the fracture is the result of violence, such as a fall or being struck by an automobile, or the result of a crushing injury, the patient should be subjected to a careful physical examination in order to rule out fractures in other parts of the body.

2. INJURIES TO THE OVERLYING SOFT PARTS

When the skin is broken and direct communication is established between the fracture and the outside air, we are dealing with a compound fracture, and these injuries are considered under that heading, but in fractures due to direct violence, the overlying soft parts are always crushed and may be devitalized over a wide area. Although the skin may not be broken at the time of the original injury, cinders, dirt or other contaminated foreign material may enter the skin and later the skin may slough over a wide area and either cause a simple fracture to become compound or considerably complicate the treatment and prolong the convalescence. In certain severe fractures, especially in those around the elbow and around the ankle joint, the swelling may be so great as to be a dominant factor in the injury and result in the formation of large blebs on the skin, thus rendering manipulation difficult and injudicious and greatly complicating the treatment.

3. INFECTION

The question of infection in compound fractures is taken up under that heading and in that section are discussed infection by gas bacillus, tetanus, and the pyogenic organisms. Very rarely simple fractures may become infected either by the later compounding of the fracture from necrosis of the overlying soft parts or in very rare instances by the metastatic implantation of bacteria in the fractured area (Figs. 51 and 52). One of us (J. A. K.) operated upon a patient with nonunion in a fracture at the junction of the middle and upper third of the humerus. The operation was performed about five months after the injury. At the operation a small abscess containing about 2 c.c. of thick white pus was found around the end of the upper fragment. A pure culture of rather large diphtheroid organisms was obtained from this pus. The wall of the abscess was excised and after the ends of the fragments had been remodeled, they were sutured with catgut and the wound was closed leaving a rubber tissue drain which was removed at the end of forty-eight hours. The convalescence was uneventful and union occurred in the normal way. The successful result in this case was due to the low virulence of the organisms. However, even in the presence of definite osteomyelitis and a fracture we believe that one should attempt to obtain union and hope to cure the osteomyelitis by some later operative procedure.

4. INJURIES TO MUSCLES

The muscles and tendons in the vicinity of the fracture may be injured or even severed by the fracturing force in fractures due to direct violence and by the displacement of the fragments in those due to indirect violence. In addition to the direct injury suffered at the time of the accident, the muscles in the area are usually infiltrated with blood and their function is disturbed over a considerable period. In cases which are necessarily subjected to prolonged immobilization, the muscles undergo atrophy of disuse. This atrophy tends to disappear with the restoration of function, but in senile patients and in patients in whom motion of the affected joints is not restored, the atrophy may be unusually prolonged or may be permanent.

Another type of injury to a muscle is one in which a muscle or tendon is caught in the callus or scar tissue incident to the healing of a fracture or to the wounds in the soft parts. These troublesome adhesions are more frequent in compound fractures than in simple fractures, but in simple fractures of the middle third of the femur the quadriceps may become adherent to the shaft and demand operative interference in order that motion in the knee may be restored.

Volkmann's Ischemic Contracture is the most severe form of muscle contracture with which we have to deal. The involved muscles become transformed into a mass of scar tissue, and according to the investigations of Brooks, the change is the result of an acute obstruction of the venous return from the involved muscles, while the arterial supply remains intact. Since the great majority of the cases occur in fractures of the elbow, this condition is discussed in detail in that section.

Rupture of Muscles and Tendons.—Occasionally tendons or muscles are ruptured by muscular violence (Fig. 119). Such accidents are not as a rule accompanied by a fracture, and the lesion should be repaired by open operation.

Myositis Ossificans is a condition in which the muscle becomes replaced by bone. The ossification may be so extensive as to involve a large part of the muscle, not only interfering with the function of the given muscle or muscles, but also blocking motion in the neighboring joint. Since this condition occurs most frequently in fractures and dislocations at the elbow joint it also is described in that section. (Fig. 120.)

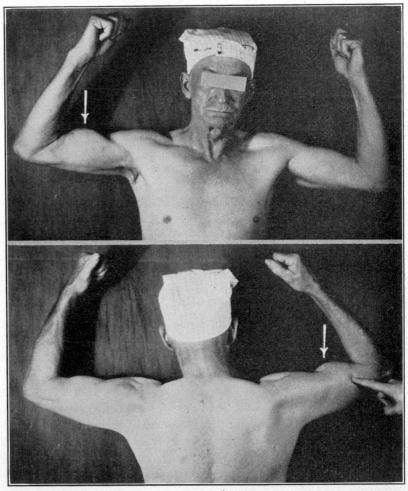

Fig. 119.—Rupture of the long head of the right biceps muscle. Treated by suture of the tendon to the short head.

Ossifying Hematoma.—This is the laying down of bone in a hematoma in a muscle or beneath the periosteum. It is usually caused by a contusion. With relative rest to the part, the abnormal bone tends to be resorbed over a period of months. If a troublesome mass persists, it may be excised (Fig. 121).

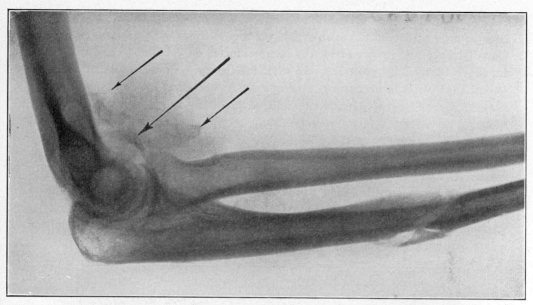

Fig. 120.—Myositis ossificans of elbow following fracture of ulna and dislocation of the head of the radius followed by manipulation. Treatment was rest and diathermy with improvement.

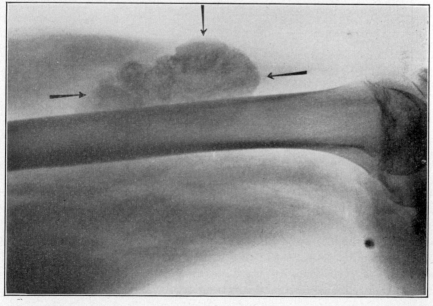

Fig. 121.—Ossifying hematoma three months after a contusion. Treated by relative rest and diathermy with gradual decrease in size.

5. INJURIES OF IMPORTANT BLOOD VESSELS

Because the walls of the blood vessels are unusually tough, these structures can be subjected to considerable trauma without serious damage. Occasionally, however, in fractures, the large arteries or veins may be torn, punctured or injured by pressure. If such an injury occurs and is of such an extent that blood is permitted to escape from the vessel into the surrounding tissues, there is a rapid extravasation of blood in the area; if the injured vessel is an artery, a false aneurysm may be produced and this may pulsate. With the false aneurysm the pulse in the artery distal to the point of injury is absent and the extremity tends to be cold and anemic; gangrene may occur. Occasionally the artery is crushed and may become thrombosed without the development of a false aneurysm. In such cases there is loss of pulse and loss of circulation in the distal portion of the extremity. Very rarely a traumatic aneurysm or an arteriovenous fistula or aneurysm may develop as a late complication of a fracture.

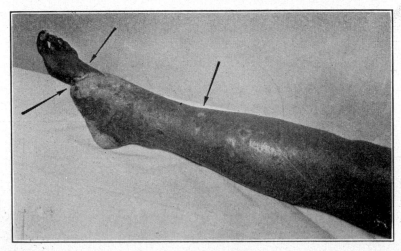

Fig. 122.—Dry gangrene of the foot following a compound fracture of the middle third of the leg with injury to the arteries.

When a large vein is injured, there is also an extravasation of blood into the tissues and an extensive hematoma is formed. The rapidity with which the hematoma develops depends upon the size of the vein. Such hematomas do not pulsate, but they may become very extensive and threaten gangrene of the extremity, which is apt to be swollen, cyanotic, and cold. A late complication, occasionally seen, especially in fractures of the pelvis and of the upper thigh, is thrombosis of the iliac or femoral veins with the development of edema and swelling in the extremity.

6. INJURIES TO NERVES

Injuries to important motor and sensory nerves are rather frequent and serious complications of fractures, especially of those in the arm and around the elbow, and occasionally in fractures of the lower extremity. Of course,

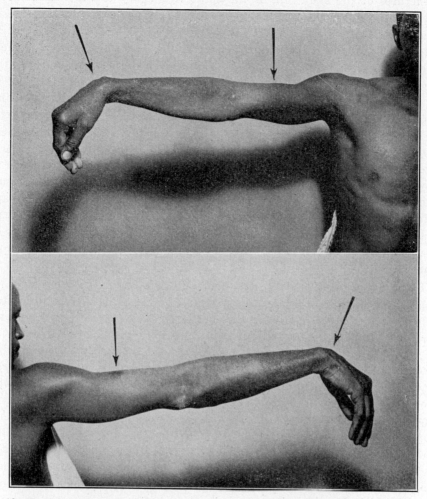

Fig. 123.—Radial nerve paralysis following a contusion on the outer side of the right arm. Cleared up in about six weeks with rest and support to the paralyzed muscles.

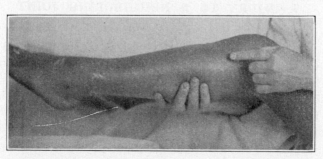

Fig. 124.—Peroneal nerve paralysis, the result of a blow at the point indicated by the finger. This is a typical picture seen after sciatic nerve paralysis in fractures of the femur, severe pelvic fractures, and peroneal paralysis in injuries around the upper end of the fibula. Recovery after conservative treatment with immobilization of the foot in a position of dorsiflexion.

in fractures of the skull and of the spine the injury to the central nervous system is the dominant feature and is discussed under fracture of those regions. In the case of peripheral nerves, the nerve may be contused (Fig. 124), stretched or torn or cut across either by the fracturing force or by the displaced bone at the time of the injury or during manipulation under an anesthetic. Later the nerve may be caught in the callus and compressed, or it may be compressed by the dressing or plaster cast or the splint used in the treatment. This last type is especially true in fractures of the lower extremity. Here the sciatic may be compressed by a band of plaster when the cast is applied with the thigh supported by a sling, or the peroneal nerve where it curves around the upper end of the fibula may be compressed either by a sling or by the plaster cast. Later still the presence of a deformity may result in irritation from stretching and friction of the nerve. This is especially apt to occur in fractures of the elbow which have healed with a valgus deformity. In these cases the ulnar nerve may become irritated or paralyzed years after the injury. The nerves most frequently injured are the radial, peroneal, ulnar, median, circumflex, and sciatic, in the order mentioned.

Since nerve injuries are so frequent and important, the original physical examination should include a rough neurologic examination in order to determine whether or not motor or sensory paralysis is present. If the paralysis is not noted until after the treatment of the fracture has been started, a question may arise in the mind of the surgeon and often of the patient, as to whether or not the paralysis is the result of the treatment. If paralysis is found, an effort should be made to determine whether or not it is complete. Severence of a nerve is unusual except in gunshot or cutting injuries. The symptoms of nerve injury are tingling, pain, numbness or loss of sensation along the sensory distribution and paralysis in the motor distribution on the involved nerve. In the case of partial or complete nerve injury, the paralyzed muscles should be supported and conservative treatment should be adopted. If some return of function is not noted within four weeks, exploration of the nerve should be considered.

7. INJURY TO A NEIGHBORING JOINT

Joint injuries as complications of fractures fall into two groups—those in which the fracture line communicates with the joint (Fig. 125) and those in which it does not. Either type of joint injury may result in a traumatic arthritis. The first type, in which the fracture line involves the joint, is taken up under the fractures of the various regions. But it is well to emphasize the fact here that joint fractures demand anatomic reduction with restoration of the normal contour of the articular surfaces, otherwise a variable amount of permanent disability may be expected. This is especially true of weight-bearing joints.

The second type is one in which the surfaces of the joint are contused as a result of the trauma which caused the fracture. This occurs especially in fractures due to indirect violence, as when a patient falls upon the hand and suffers a fracture at the wrist, forearm, elbow, humerus, or clavicle.

With any of these injuries the shoulder joint may be contused and may be the site of prolonged disability. Likewise, in fractures of the femur, the knee may be injured. The injury in these cases seems to be a contusion of the cartilaginous surface. In other instances the injury is in the nature of a sprain and is the result of leverage acting at the time of the fracture. Occasionally fractures are complicated by dislocations at a neighboring joint, the most frequent being a fracture of the upper end of the humerus with dislocation at the shoulder. These injuries are described in the chapters devoted to the regions in which they occur.

Even in joints that are not definitely injured at the time of the fracture, restoration of function may be delayed over a considerable period. This is especially true in the knee, where prolonged stiffness may follow the immobilization incident to a fracture at the hip or of the femur and at the ankle where in a fracture of the leg or ankle or foot immobilization of the ankle in a position of plantar flexion either of necessity or through carelessness has resulted in a shortening of the heel cord. In most cases this stiffness is gradually eliminated. For instance, it may be accepted as true that in young people a normal joint will withstand prolonged immobilization without injury. On the other hand, in persons beyond middle life prolonged immobilization may result in prolonged and even some permanent loss of movement in the joint.

As a rule, however, unless the joint has been immobilized in a position of deformity as in a case of the foot with immobilization in plantar flexion, complete restoration of function will gradually be accomplished, although this may require a period of several months or even one or two years. Restoration of function will occur with normal use and graded exercises and, as far as we can determine, cannot be materially hastened by other forms of physiotherapy. Hot baths and massage may hasten the restoration of motion.

8. TRAUMATIC ARTHRITIS

Traumatic arthritis may be defined as a low grade inflammatory condition which develops in a joint after an injury and is characterized by limitation of motion, pain and disability in the involved joint and may be accompanied by a variable amount of swelling. It differs from the normal disability following prolonged immobilization in that the symptoms do not tend to clear up with use, but are often made worse by attempts to exercise the joint and are usually relieved by rest. It also differs in that the disability may tend to progress rather than decrease as time passes.

Most cases of traumatic arthritis are the result of definite mechanical disorganization of the joint, fractures into joints which have been imperfectly reduced, or loose bodies in joints, such as joint mice or torn and displaced semilunar cartilages. The most common sites are the knee joint after fractures of one or both condyles of the tibia; the ankle joint after fractures of one or both malleoli; the subastragaloid joint after fractures of the os calcis; the hip joint after fractures of the neck of the femur; the shoulder joint after fractures of the upper end of the humerus or of the glenoid; and the elbow joint after fractures of the head of the radius.

In addition to those cases which are due to disorganization of the mechanics of the joint as a result of disturbance of the contour of the bearing surfaces we have occasional cases in which without a definite fracture of the bone there has been a severe contusion of the joint cartilage which has initiated a degeneration of the cartilage and which results in progressive arthritic changes in the joint.*   Other cases are the result of faulty weight-bearing caused by bony deformity, so that use brings about repeated mild injury to the joint surface or prolonged abnormal strain.   It is worthy of note that traumatic arthritis is most frequently seen in those patients who are of the heavy, or plethoric, type and who are beyond middle life.

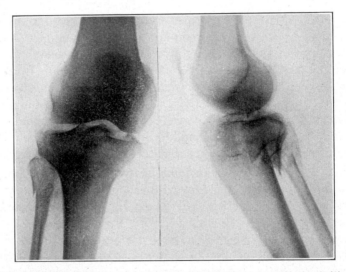

Fig. 125.—Type of fracture which tends to develop traumatic arthritis. Treated by manipulation, then followed by traction and active motion for four weeks. Weight-bearing in eight weeks. Result, flexion limited to 90 degrees, some pain after unusual amount of walking and in damp weather.

In considering the treatment of traumatic arthritis, the first thing to determine is why the arthritis has developed.   If the arthritis is the result of a condition which can be corrected by a surgical procedure, this should be attempted.   If, on the other hand, the fracture has united with the fragments in good position and the contours of the involved joint are practically normal, surgery can do little good.   Consequently no operation short of removing the joint and performing an arthrodesis should be considered.   The surgical treatment of the disability incident to fractures in various regions which result in chronic progressive arthritis in the involved joint is considered in the special part of this book.

In addition to the surgical treatment the surgeon should consider whether or not a given joint should be treated by physiotherapy or should be given rest.   In our experience this decision is a very difficult one and frequently can be decided only by trial and error.   In a weight-bearing joint the amount of weight-bearing should be restricted.   The patient should avoid

*Key, J. A.: Traumatic Arthritis and Mechanical Factors in Hypertrophic Arthritis, J. Lab. and Clin. Med. 15: 11-45, 1930.

those activities which result in prolonged pain or make the symptoms worse from day to day. At the same time mild exercises should be given and heat and massage may be employed. In certain instances in which the joint has been irritated by strenuous efforts to hurry the convalescence, the joint should be immobilized in a plaster-of-Paris cast. The surgeon and the patient will be surprised when the cast is removed at the end of a few weeks to find considerable more motion in the joint than was present when the cast was put on. The general health should be built up. In these patients we insist upon a diet high in vitamin content; we give them concentrated vitamins and see that the bowels move freely at least once a day.

In the case of weight-bearing joints, proper shoes should be worn and the joint should be protected from strain either by means of a splint or an elastic bandage or adhesive strapping, and the amount of protection can be reduced gradually as the patient's condition improves. Most cases eventually reach a point where fair function is obtained, but it is rare to find complete restoration of function.

9. ACUTE TRAUMATIC BONE ATROPHY (SUDECK)

Whenever an extremity is immobilized, there is a tendency for bone atrophy to occur. This is natural and should be expected in all fractures. In occasional cases, however, the atrophy is profound in degree and occurs with great rapidity. This curious condition is sometimes called Sudeck's atrophy because it was first described by him, or it may be called acute traumatic bone atrophy. It is a rapidly progressing osteoporosis which involves the bones of the extremity following an injury and is especially evident in the bones distal to the injured area. (Fig. 126.)

A remarkable thing about this type of atrophy is that it may be very severe following a trivial injury such as a sprain or contusion and also that it may occur in limbs which have not been immobilized. The cause is unknown, and Sudeck regarded it as a reflex neurotrophic phenomenon. It has never been produced experimentally and is not of frequent occurrence in clinical practice. When it does occur, however, it is a most troublesome condition.

Acute traumatic bone atrophy occurs most frequently in the bones of the hands and feet. It is characterized by persistent pain, stiffness and disability and is recognized by the facts that after an injury the extremity remains cold, tender and cyanotic and the joints are stiff and painful. The surgeon is at a loss to explain the failure of restoration of function. This condition may persist over a period of months and be very resistant to all forms of treatment. In the few cases that have come under our care, we have found restoration to normal is best accomplished by putting the patient on a high calcium and high vitamin diet with daily doses of cod liver oil and subjecting the involved extremity to contrast baths twice daily, and using diathermy, rest, and graded exercises. Exercises of the involved extremity should be begun very gradually; as the condition improves they should be carried out against resistance. Full weight-bearing in case the atrophy occurs in the lower extremity should be discouraged until improvement is well under way. Boehler reports prompt relief of acute atrophy of the tarsal bones by having these patients walk in a skin-tight plaster with a walking iron.

It is important that the swelling be reduced and controlled as early as possible. An elastic bandage may be adequate or a plaster cast may be necessary. Deep x-ray therapy and nerve block with novocain or periarterial sympathectomy have been recommended.

One of us (J. A. K.) believes that the condition is caused by the unusual swelling which has occurred after the injury and has persisted. Every effort should be made to prevent the swelling or to reduce it if it occurs.

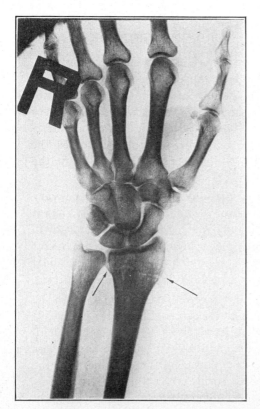
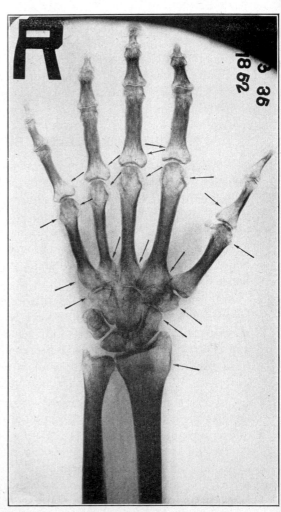

Fig. 126.—A minor fracture of the lower end of the radius. At the right is shown healing of fracture, but acute bone atrophy of hand and wrist.

FAT EMBOLISM

Fat embolism is a rare complication of fractures, demonstrated from time to time in postmortem material. While the occurrence of fat embolism is generally accepted, the mechanism has not been satisfactorily explained.

The current belief is that in extensive fractures of long bones and in crushing injuries of cancellous bone such as sometimes occur when very atrophic bones are manipulated, a variable amount of fat is forced out of the marrow cavity and enters the veins. The difficulty with this theory is that one would expect an amount of pressure necessary to cause mobilization of the fat to result in collapse of all open veins in the vicinity. However, if the pressure is great enough to tear off the vein from its attachment to the bony wall, then the mobilized fat could be forced into the canal in the bone and out into the vein at its point of exit.

Another theory is that the fat is absorbed by the lymphatics and dumped into the blood stream in unusually large amounts. The third explanation is that some chemical change occurs in the blood or in the fat which is normally present in the blood as an emulsion of chylomicrons and causes demulsification with the result that the chylomicrons form globules of fat which block the capillaries in various organs and especially those of the lungs. At autopsies the lungs are apt to show large amounts of fat in the capillaries and occasionally the capillaries in the brain, kidney, and other organs may be blocked by fat. Whether or not the fat found in these capillaries is the cause of death is still a moot question.

The symptoms arise only when a vital region of the brain is blocked or when many capillaries in the lungs are blocked and thus throw a large portion of the organs out of function. In the usual case the symptoms do not appear immediately after the injury, but come on after a period of from several hours to three days. The symptoms may be either pulmonary or cerebral in type, depending upon whether the fat collects in the lungs or in the brain.

In the pulmonary type there are signs of pulmonary edema with coarse râles in the chest, but normal resonance on percussion. There are also rapid breathing and rapid pulse with pallor which is later followed by cyanosis. In the cerebral type there may be delirium with pupillary changes, twitching, and coma. In either type the temperature may be normal, subnormal or elevated and there may be a combination of the two types, both pulmonary and cerebral.

The chief conditions from which fat embolism is to be differentiated are surgical shock, pulmonary embolism, and pneumonia. The time element is an important factor in the differentiation of the first three of these four conditions. In surgical shock the symptoms usually occur immediately after the accident, while in fat embolism the symptoms usually do not occur before twelve or more hours after. In pulmonary embolism due to thrombosis the symptoms usually appear between the tenth and the twentieth day following the accident, while in fat embolism they usually appear during the first three days. Pneumonia can usually be differentiated by the impaired resonance and signs of an acute infection. The only treatment is rest and sedatives. A good many cases of the cerebral type recover after a period of delirium or even of coma which may last for several days.

PULMONARY COMPLICATIONS AFTER FRACTURES

Pneumonia and embolism are the two types of pulmonary complications met with after fractures. Embolism is relatively rare, but may occur after fractures as after any other surgical procedure and is due to the dislodgment of the clot in a thrombosed vein and the passage of the clot through the right side of the heart and into the lungs where it blocks the pulmonary artery to a variable degree. In cases with small emboli only branches of the artery are blocked and the result is a localized infarct in the lungs accompanied by pain in the chest and usually by a pleural friction rub. With large emboli the entire artery may be blocked and the patient may die almost instantly.

Pneumonia after fractures occurs most frequently in aged and debilitated patients, and especially in those the nature of whose injury necessitates immobilization in bed in recumbency. It is so frequent in fractures of the hip in old persons that it is the chief cause of death in this injury, where the mortality is about 15 per cent. The most frequent type of pneumonia is a bilateral hypostatic congestion of the posterior portions of the lungs which gradually increases and terminates in a widespread bronchopneumonia with moderate fever and progressive weakness. The best prophylaxis against this type of pneumonia is treatment of the fracture so that the patient will be turned on the face in a plaster cast about four times a day. If it is treated by traction insist that the patient sit up in bed for a good part of the time. This pneumonia often terminates fatally; the progress of the condition is favored by prolonged recumbency.

In other aged patients there may result generalized bronchitis without marked hypostatic congestion; this may terminate in a widespread bronchopneumonia. More rarely there may occur a rapid and severe lobar pneumonia which progresses to a crisis and may terminate either fatally or in recovery, just as does lobar pneumonia in patients who have not had a fracture.

DELIRIUM

Alcoholic Delirium is an occasional complication of fractures in patients whose nervous systems have been damaged by the excessive use of alcohol. When this occurs it takes on the characteristics of delirium tremens.

Traumatic Delirium occasionally occurs in elderly patients or in those who have been under prolonged mental distress. It is similar to delirium after other operative conditions and is characterized by a low muttering, febrile state in which events of the past are recalled and remain uppermost in the patient's mind.

MALUNION OF FRACTURES

Malunion in the case of a fracture may be defined as a condition in which the fragments become united by bone, but in which the union is of such a nature that there is impairment of function or in which the cosmetic result is poor. (Figs. 127 to 133.) In the case of a fracture of a long bone, malunion may be the result of shortening due to overriding of the fragments or to loss of substance, or it may be due to faulty alignment resulting in abnor-

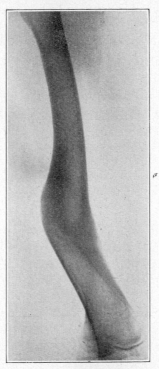

Fig. 127.—Malunion in fracture of the femur. (Shriners' Hospital case, Courtesy Dr. Crego.) The deformity and two inches shortening were corrected by plastic osteotomy and lengthening of the femur.

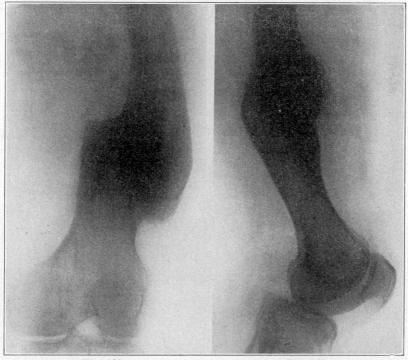

Fig. 128.   Fig. 129.

Fig. 128.—Malunion after an old fracture of the femur. There is also a traumatic arthritis in the knee joint. No treatment, as patient was too old and general physical condition was poor.

Fig. 129.—Same as preceding, lateral view.

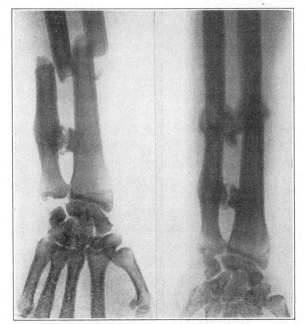
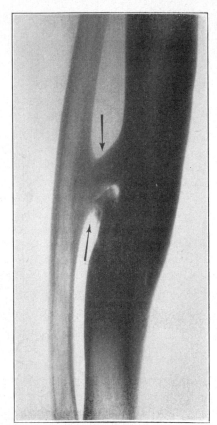

Fig. 130.   Fig. 131.   Fig. 132.

Fig. 130.—Synostosis six years after fracture of radius and ulna. There is a recent fracture above the synostosis.

Fig. 131.—Same as preceding, three months after reduction. A new synostosis is forming. Result: loss of rotation of forearm. Open operation done later. Cross union removed from both areas with good function.

Fig. 132.—Synostosis of the tibia and fibula following a fracture. Pain when walking necessitated removal of the synostosis.

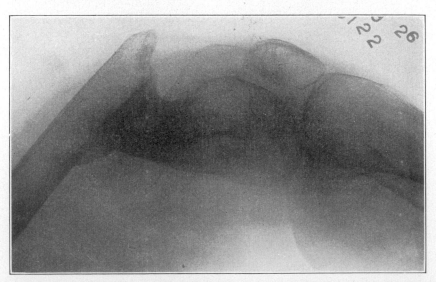

Fig. 133.—Malunion after an old supracondylar fracture of the femur with posterior displacement of lower fragment. Treatment refused.

mal angulation of the bone, or to union with the fragments in an abnormal position as regards rotation. In fractures of bones which are subcutaneous in position, a lateral displacement may result in union with a visible deformity which might be regarded as a malunion. In fractures into and in the vicinity of joints, union of the fragments may occur in such a manner that the motions of the joints are either blocked by projecting pieces of bone, or the joint surfaces may be deformed so that it is no longer possible for the movements of the joint to be carried out in the normal manner. In the forearm after fractures of one or of both bones, the radius and ulna may be united to one another by callus (synostosis), or angulation may occur in one or both bones, so that rotation of the forearm is limited or entirely prevented. The various types of malunion are taken up under the particular bones in which they are likely to occur.

The treatment of malunion depends a good deal upon the amount of disability and deformity which it causes. If the disability is great enough to warrant surgical interference, the bones can be separated by surgical operation or by manipulation and the malunion can in most instances be corrected. In certain fractures involving joints, as was stated elsewhere, it is frequently impossible to obtain a normal joint and sometimes it is impossible to obtain a joint which is stable and free from pain, and in such instances either an arthroplasty or an arthrodesis is to be considered.

PRESSURE SORES AND BED SORES

Pressure sores are the result of localized and long-continued pressure and are especially apt to occur under plaster-of-Paris casts which have been improperly applied. As a rule, they are not the result of insufficient padding, but are the result of improper holding of the extremity while the cast is applied or of improper application of the bandage. Sometimes a pressure sore results from a deep indentation in the plaster made by the assistant's hand while it supports the extremity.

At other times it is the result of a deep groove cut into the extremity by a bandage which acts as a sling to support the thigh. We have seen one such case in which during the application of the spica the thigh was supported by a bandage suspended from the upright on the Hawley table. In this case a pressure sore occurred which was so severe that the slough completely severed the sciatic nerve. In other instances pressure sores are due to the drawing of the plaster too tightly around the limb in some localized area or to the surgeon's twisting the plaster bandage during its application. It should be remembered that plaster of Paris "stays where it sets" until the cast is broken or removed.

In addition to the pressure sores incident to plaster casts, we have also seen them result from splints and slings. This is particularly true in debilitated persons in whom the heel rests in a sling while the rest of the leg remains unsupported. We have seen cases in which the entire posterior portion of the heel sloughed out so that the os calcis was exposed.

Another type is that in which the splint is bent rather sharply at the knee and in which traction is applied to the splint in such a manner that a tight sling is pulled around the leg below the knee. In such an instance we have seen a pressure sore over the upper end of the fibula with paralysis of the peroneal nerve.

In other cases the pressure sores develop over the malleoli where traction straps have not been separated by a spreader beyond the foot. We have also seen them around the elbow and wrist after both plaster cast and traction or splint treatment. In the forearm they are particularly to be guarded against after the application of anterior and posterior splints which may easily be applied too tightly or which may be applied loosely and become too tight as a result of later swelling of the part or of displacement of the fragments.

Pressure sores over the sacrum and posterior superior spines are usually the result of poor nursing care. This is especially true in patients who are treated in plaster-of-Paris casts, since practically no one ever applies a plaster spica without ample padding of these regions, but if the plaster is permitted to become soaked with urine and if the patient is permitted to lie in one position day after day, pressure sores are bound to result. This is particularly true in old and debilitated patients.

The difference between a pressure sore and a bed sore is that the pressure sore is usually the result of defective treatment and is usually due to the apparatus applied in an effort to immobilize the fracture, while a bed sore is the result of pressure incident to the patient's position in bed. Bed sores are likely to occur on the sacrum, elbows, shoulder blades, and heels, while pressure sores may occur over any bony points or even over soft tissues if they are subjected to prolonged abnormal pressure. Both types are especially apt to occur in debilitated patients, and bed sores are especially to be feared in patients with extensive paralysis, as is discussed under injuries to the spinal cord.

In preventing bed and pressure sores the skin should be kept dry and clean and rubbed with alcohol and powdered with talcum at least twice each day. The treatment is removal of the cause as soon as the pain and redness are discovered. As a rule when a patient complains of localized pain after the application of a cast there is apt to be undue pressure at the point or if the patient complains of more pain after the fracture has been reduced than before there is some fault in the reduction.

If the condition has progressed to such a degree that sloughing of the tissues has occurred, it is necessary, of course, to remove the slough before healing can result. The major portions of the slough can be excised with sharp scissors and the wound can then be packed with gauze soaked in Dakin's solution, the pack being changed about every four hours. In this way the necrotic tissue tends to disappear and the base becomes covered by clean granulation tissue. When this occurs, the edges of the pressure sores should be protected either by strapping with adhesive or with some ointment, and, as a rule, if the patient's general condition is good, the pressure sores will slowly heal.

CHAPTER VI

PATHOLOGIC FRACTURES

Pathologic fractures are those which occur in bones that have been weakened by some disease or abnormal condition. They are frequently called "spontaneous fractures," but are not really spontaneous, since they are always the result of some form of force, although this force may be far less than would be necessary to cause a similar fracture in normal bone.

Depending upon the cause of the deficiency in the bone, pathologic fractures may be divided into two groups: (1) those due to local bone changes; and (2) those due to conditions which affect the entire skeleton.

1. PATHOLOGIC FRACTURES DUE TO LOCAL BONE CHANGES

1. Bone Atrophy of Disuse

Whenever the functional demands on a bone are diminished, there is a tendency to resorption of the calcium salts in this bone, and in the case of a growing child, there is also a tendency for the bone to increase in size and in length less rapidly than normally. Consequently, we may have a condition of eccentric or concentric atrophy in the bone of the extremity. This is especially true after the extremities have been immobilized for a long period in plaster-of-Paris casts, and when such a patient gets up after a fracture, he is more susceptible to other fractures than is the normal individual.

In addition to the rather acute bone atrophy incident to treatment or immobilization after a fracture, there is a chronic bone atrophy that is always present in limbs which are extensively paralyzed and which as a result of the paralysis have not been used for weight-bearing. Fractures in such limbs often take on the characteristics of pathologic fractures in that they may result from relatively slight violence and may be accompanied by relatively little pain.

2. Inflammatory Processes in Bone

Any acute or chronic inflammation which results in the destruction of bone may cause such extensive weakening of the bone that a pathologic fracture may occur (Fig. 134), but the usual cause of pathologic fractures in inflammatory processes is osteomyelitis, and in the majority of instances the fracture occurs after the bone has been operated upon for the cure of the disease and in such a manner that a large portion of the shaft has been removed. This is especially true of the so-called extensive saucerization operation in which all of the shaft except a thin pencil of cortex on one side is removed. In such cases the limb should be handled with care and should be adequately splinted. This is especially true in adults; a fracture in such diseased bone may lead to nonunion. This occurs despite the fact that one

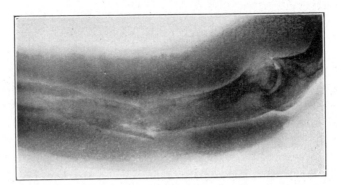

Fig. 134.—Double pathologic fracture of the humerus due to osteomyelitis.

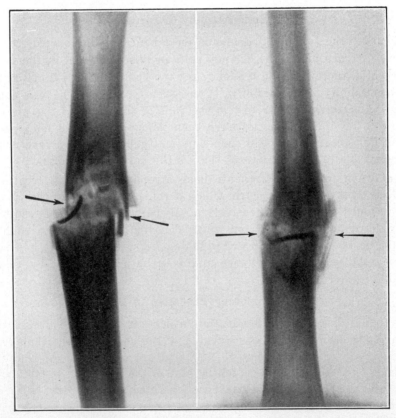

Fig. 135.—Benign bone cyst which healed after fracture. No bone grafting necessary. Treated by plaster cast fixation. Good results.

of the characteristics of osteomyelitis is that the disease is accompanied by new bone formation.

Another type of fracture occurring in osteomyelitis is a fracture through the dense eburnated bone. This bone is extremely hard and capable of sustaining great pressure, but it is brittle, and as a result may be broken by relatively slight force.

3. Neoplasms

Benign or malignant tumors may arise in the bone or metastatic malignant tumors may occur; any of these may result in a pathologic fracture. In young persons the most frequent cause of pathologic fractures from benign tumor formation is a bone cyst (Figs. 135, 136 and 137), which may occur in the

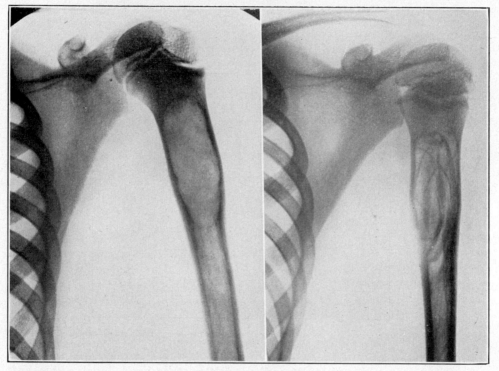

Fig. 136.—A similar fracture in which the cyst did not heal after the fracture. Excised and packed with bone shavings.

shaft of a long bone and by its gradual enlargement and expansion cause a progressive thinning of the cortex. Frequently, in fact in about one-third of the cases, the first sign of the bone cyst is a fracture which results from some trivial injury. Multiple, and occasionally solitary, bone cysts are associated with parathyroid adenomas and are apparently due to the hypercalcemia (Fig. 143).

In older persons metastatic carcinoma is a relatively frequent cause of pathologic fractures. When a pathologic fracture occurs in an older person, the surgeon should suspect the possibility of such a tumor immediately and rule it out by x-ray. (Figs. 141 and 142.)

Benign tumors of bone rarely cause pathologic fractures, largely due to the fact that most of these tumors are productive rather than destructive in character and result in considerable new bone formation. Another reason is that they tend to occur near the ends of long bones rather than in the shaft. For instance, a giant cell tumor occurring in the end of a long bone may result in marked destruction of the bone and yet even in this lesion a pathologic fracture is rarely seen.

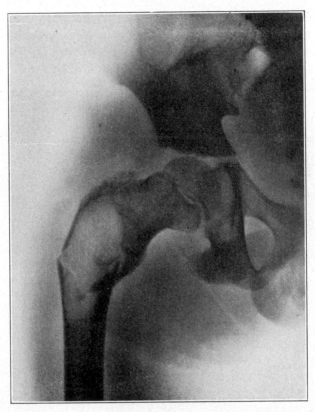

Fig. 137.—Pathologic fracture of the femur through a solitary bone cyst. Treated by closed reduction and abduction plaster cast with good results.

Osteogenic and periosteal sarcoma on the other hand, involve the shaft, but as a rule the progress of the tumor is so rapid and it invades the soft tissues to such an extent that the patient is either bedridden or succumbs to the disease before a pathologic fracture occurs. (Figs. 144, 145, 146, 147, and 148.)

Irradiation

Large amounts of deep x-ray therapy may so damage the bones that they may break spontaneously or as a result of slight violence. This is most frequently seen after deep x-ray treatment for cancer of the uterus. Roentgenologists should endeavor to so direct the rays that the hip is spared. (Fig. 138.) One of us (J. A. K.) also has seen aseptic necrosis of the head of the femur from the same cause.

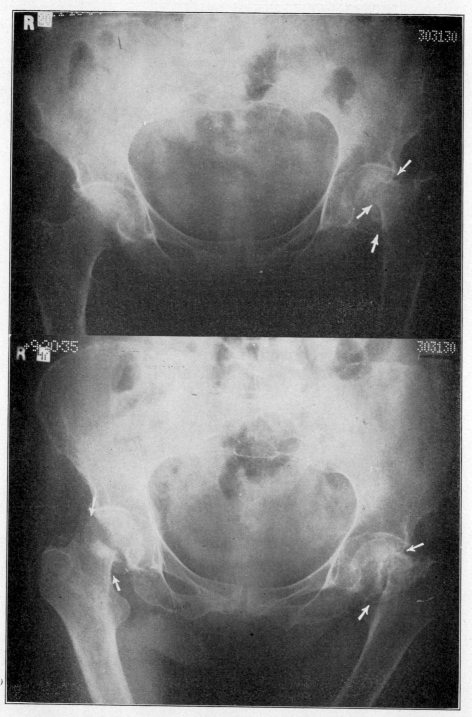

Fig. 138.—Pathological fracture of the first and then of the other hip following deep x-ray therapy for cancer of the uterus. These fractures did not unite. (Courtesy Dr. Carl E. Badgley.)

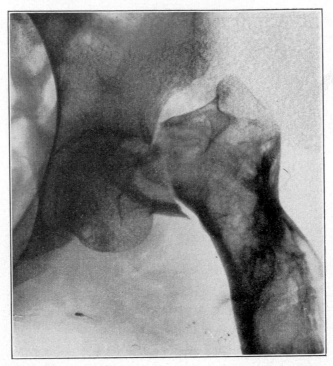

Fig. 139.—Pathologic fracture of the neck of the femur resulting from localized osteitis fibrosa with cystic formation in the femur. Nonunion. Whitman reconstruction later. (Courtesy Dr. J. Edgar Stewart.)

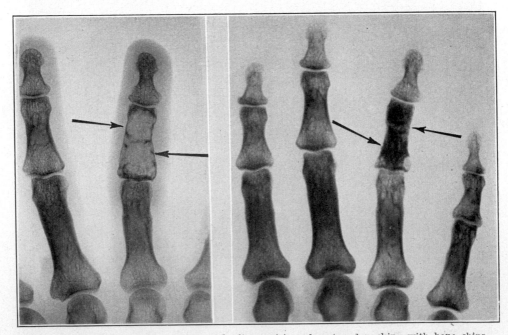

Fig. 140.—Cyst of phalanx before and after excision of cyst and packing with bone chips.

II. PATHOLOGIC FRACTURES DUE TO GENERAL CONDITIONS

1. Osteogenesis Imperfecta or Osteopsathyrosis

The general terms "osteogenesis imperfecta" and "osteopsathyrosis" are used to designate a condition in which there is a generalized hypoplasia of the skeleton and in which the bones of the affected individuals are not sufficiently strong to bear the wear and tear of normal existence. In these persons fractures occur from trivial accidents, and, depending upon the degree of hypoplasia, may be very numerous and occur at frequent intervals.

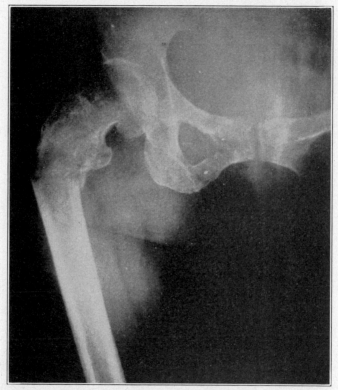

Fig. 141.—Pathologic fracture of the femur due to metastatic carcinoma of breast. (Courtesy Drs. Chas. Heacock and J. S. Speed, Memphis.)

So far as has been determined, the calcium and phosphorus metabolism of these patients is normal and the fragility of the bones is the result of a defect in development rather than of the inability of the patient to assimilate calcium and phosphorus and to form bone. In a paper by Key* these have been classified into osteogenesis imperfecta, idiopathic osteopsathyrosis, and hereditary hypoplasia of mesenchyme, or brittle bones and blue sclera. All of these three types are characterized by abnormal fragility of the bone; many of the individuals also exhibit an abnormal transparency of the white collogenic connective tissue, and the sclera have a blue tint, the depth of the blue varying in different individuals.

*Key: Arch. Surg., 1926.

In the cases classed as osteogenesis imperfecta the fractures are present at birth or are noted soon after birth and frequently in lifting the infant the arms or legs may be broken. A hundred or more fractures may occur in a single individual and practically all of these patients die in early infancy.

In the cases classed as idiopathic osteopsathyrosis the fractures do not as a rule occur until after the patient begins to walk and are usually the result of minor injuries. These cases may also have the blue sclera and their bones are abnormally slender and brittle.

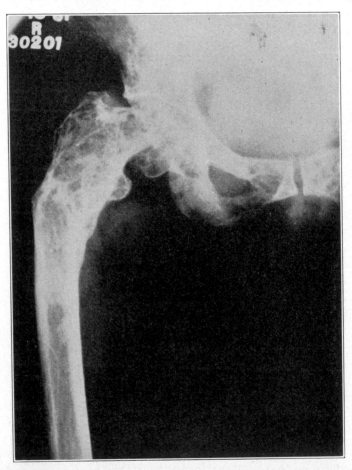

Fig. 142.—Same as preceding, twelve months later. The fracture has united despite the progressive destruction in the upper end of the femur and pelvis. (Courtesy Drs. Chas. Heacock and J. S. Speed, Memphis.)

Hereditary hypoplasia of the mesenchyme is identical with osteopsathyrosis except that it is transmitted as a dominant hereditary factor and the affected individuals have a tendency to develop deafness in early adult life. It should be borne in mind that if a patient affected with brittle bones and blue sclera gives birth to children, approximately half of the children will inherit the condition and they in turn will transmit it to their children, but nonaffected children do not transmit the condition.

2. Rickets

Rickets is a condition in which the individual is unable to calcify the bone formed, and in severe cases there is also a progressive rarefaction of the bones which leads to softening and bending with the development of deformities; but occasionally in very severe cases the rarefaction may be so great that pathologic fractures occur.

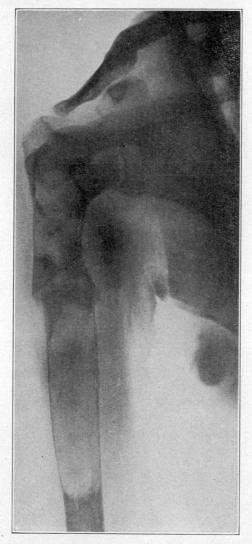

Fig. 143.—Pathologic fracture of the humerus due to a large bone cyst in a patient with a parathyroid adenoma and hypercalcemia. Fracture after the parathyroid tumor was removed. This fracture healed in spite of the extensive destruction of bone.

3. Osteomalacia

Osteomalacia is a condition similar to rickets in that there is a generalized osteoporosis. It is most frequent in pregnant women, and most of the cases can be traced to an inadequate supply of calcium in the diet. In very severe cases the osteoporosis may reach such a degree that pathologic fractures may occur.

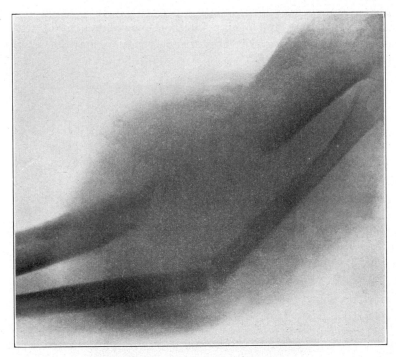

Fig. 144.—Pathologic fracture of both bones of the leg due to a large sarcoma. This fracture did not unite.

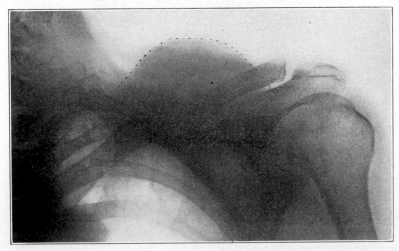

Fig. 145.—Pathologic fracture of the clavicle in a primary sarcoma. This fracture did not unite.

4. Senile Atrophy

In many old individuals there is a rather marked generalized osteoporosis, and in addition to the osteoporosis, the bones are often unusually brittle. The condition affects especially the upper end of the femur, the upper end of the humerus, the lower end of the radius and the bodies of the vertebrae. Fractures in these locations are apt to occur in senile individuals after relatively slight violence. These are not true pathologic fractures.

5. Osteitis Deformans, or Paget's Disease

Osteitis deformans, or Paget's disease, is accompanied by a fibrotic change in some of the bones, particularly in the tibia and femur; as a result these bones are frequently deformed and their structure may be so weakened that they are fractured by relatively slight violence.

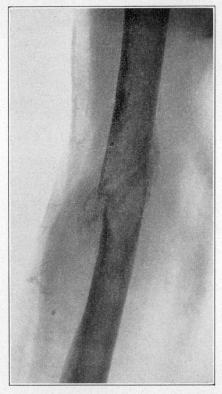

Fig. 146.—Pathologic fracture of the humerus in the same case as preceding. This is probably a metastatic tumor. (Sarcoma.) The fracture did not unite.

6. Syphilis

Since tertiary syphilis frequently attacks the skeleton, it is popularly regarded as one of the principal causes of pathologic fractures and of delayed or nonunion after fractures. As a matter of fact, syphilis may almost be disregarded as the cause of either of these. It is, of course, possible that a large gumma may so weaken a bone that a fracture will occur with relatively slight violence, as in the clavicle.

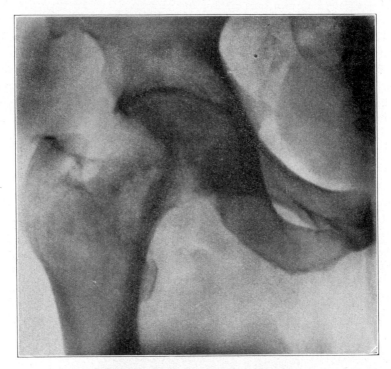

Fig. 147.—Sarcoma upper end of femur.

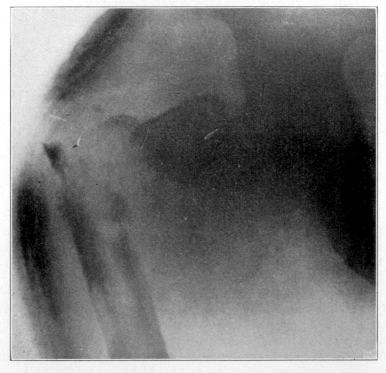

Fig. 148.—Same as preceding, two months later. This did not heal.

Congenital syphilis, however, in infants may result in a spontaneous separation of the epiphyses, the so-called pseudoparalysis of Parrot. These epiphyseal separations may occur spontaneously and can be recognized by the typical syphilitic lesions of the epiphyseal line as seen in the x-ray picture.

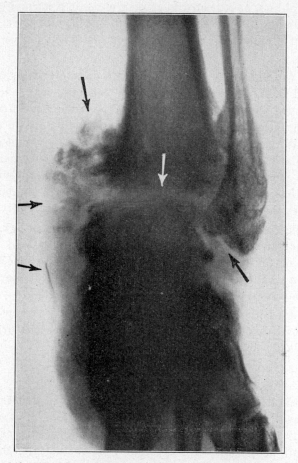

Fig. 149.—Charcot's ankle with fracture of the internal malleolus.

7. Diseases of the Nervous System

Tabes dorsalis and syringomyelia may result in trophic changes in the bones, particularly in the articular surfaces which lead to progressive erosion of these surfaces and a total destruction of the joint (Charcot joint). At the same time there is as a rule more or less rarefaction of the bones of the involved extremity, but we believe that is due to disuse rather than to the nervous disease. We have seen fractures in limbs affected with Charcot joint heal in the usual way and have not seen true extraarticular pathologic fractures which we could trace to disease of the nervous system.

DIAGNOSIS OF PATHOLOGIC FRACTURES

If the surgeon or the patient knows that there is disease or abnormal weakness in the bone, the diagnosis of pathologic fracture can, as a rule, be made with relative ease. On the other hand, if there is no known pathology present, the diagnosis of a pathologic fracture is often not made until the x-ray picture discloses the abnormality in the bone. However, if, in obtaining the history, the surgeon finds that the fracture occurred as a result of a trivial injury which would not be expected to cause a break in a normal bone, he should suspect the possibility of a pathologic fracture and should have x-ray pictures made in an effort to determine whether or not some destructive disease of the bone is present.

In addition to the history there are certain characteristics in the physical examination and in the subsequent course which may lead one to suspect a pathologic fracture even in the absence of a positive x-ray finding. One of these is that the patient, as a rule, suffers relatively little pain after the fracture and there is relatively little swelling or evidence of damage to the soft parts. The displacement of the fragments is, as a rule, less than usual and is dependent upon muscle action rather than upon external violence. Likewise, muscle spasm is less marked than one usually finds after a similar fracture and in many instances the fractured limb can be handled with relatively little pain.

In pathologic fractures the result of a neoplasm the presence of a visible or palpable tumor at or near the site of the fracture may lead one to suspect the true nature of the condition. Likewise, in certain instances where union does not occur an x-ray may reveal a neoplasm at the site of the fracture. The final diagnosis should be obtained from the x-ray photograph.

It is important both for the surgeon and the patient to know when a pathologic fracture is present because such a fracture may be the first evidence of some fatal neoplastic disease.

Prognosis of Pathologic Fractures

The prognosis depends upon the condition which caused the weakness in the bone. In cases due to bone cysts, for instance, not only do the fractures usually heal, but the bone cyst may disappear after the fracture. In cases due to malignant neoplasms, either primary or metastatic, the tendency is for the fracture not to heal because by the time the bone has been sufficiently involved to result in a pathologic fracture the local tumor has advanced to such a degree that it seriously interferes with the normal process of bone union. Consequently, in these patients when involvement of bone is known to be present efforts should be made by rest or supporting splints or braces to prevent the occurrence of a fracture as not only may the fractures fail to heal, but they cause the patients much discomfort and pain.

In inflammatory diseases such as osteomyelitis, the prognosis depends a good deal upon the type of bone which is broken and the amount of periosteal reaction which one may expect later. If the fragments become displaced, union may fail to occur and some of these cases eventually come to amputation.

In rickets, of course, the prognosis is good, since the rickets can be cured by a suitable diet and cod liver oil or ultraviolet rays from sunlight or artificial sources; the same is usually true of osteomalacia and of simple bone atrophy.

In Paget's disease union is apt to be slow but may be expected to occur. In osteogenesis imperfecta the fractures, as a rule, unite even more rapidly than do those through normal bone. However, we have seen bone so fragile that refractures are frequent and occasionally in these bones long delayed union is encountered.

TREATMENT OF PATHOLOGIC FRACTURES

The treatment is that of the fracture as described in the special sections of this book—that is, reduction and immobilization. Union may be expected in most cases. In the case of a giant cell tumor or other benign tumor it may be necessary to excise the tumor, while in the case of a bone cyst as the fracture heals the cyst tends to disappear and no operation is indicated. In malignant tumors operation is, as a rule, useless because in primary tumors, by the time the pathologic fracture has occurred, the tumor has metastasized to the lungs, and in metastatic tumors removal of a metastasis is futile.

In rickets and osteomalacia cod liver oil or ultraviolet light and high calcium diet are indicated, while in Paget's disease and osteogenesis imperfecta no treatment has yet been shown to have any effect upon either condition.

CHAPTER VII

COMPOUND FRACTURES AND WAR WOUNDS

A fracture or dislocation is said to be compound when communication is established between the site of the fracture or inside of the joint and the outside air. The open wound leading down to the fracture may have been caused by external violence or it may have been caused by internal violence. In the latter type the rupture in the skin is made by the end of one of the fragments. Lacerations near a simple fracture may be misleading. In case of doubt as to whether or not a wound communicates with a fracture, it is well to remember that in compound fractures with small wounds dark venous blood flows from the wound and can be forced out by pressing gently on the tissues and minute droplets of fat from the bone marrow can usually be seen in this blood.

From the standpoint of treatment the difference between a compound and a simple fracture is that a compound fracture is contaminated with bacteria which may be assumed to be pathogenic. This contamination occurs at the time of the injury and persists until such time as the organisms begin to grow in the tissues. From this time on the wound is infected.

Roughly, we may assume that a compound fracture becomes infected within from six to twelve hours after the injury. Consequently, injuries seen within the first six hours may be considered contaminated and those seen after the first twelve hours should be considered infected, while those seen between six and twelve hours after the injury are borderline cases and require surgical judgment if proper treatment is to be instituted. There are, of course, instances with virulent infections in which the infection starts within six hours after the injury, but these are unusual. Not only is the wound infected, but there is provided an ideal culture medium for the growth of pyogenic organisms because as a result of the injury causing the fracture there is always considerable damage and devitalization of the soft tissues and interruption of blood supply.

THE TREATMENT OF COMPOUND FRACTURES

The treatment of compound fractures includes the treatment of the patient at the scene of the accident, the transportation of the patient to a hospital or to some other point at which the injury will receive definitive treatment, and the treatment at the hospital. The last includes the treatment of the wound, the reduction and immobilization of the fragments in a position which will result in satisfactory function when and if union occurs, and whatever after treatment may be indicated.

1. **Treatment at the Scene of the Accident.**—This will depend upon the type of injury and also upon where the accident occurs and upon the facilities available for administering such treatment. If the patient is not very severely injured, if there are no general symptoms, if the patient has to be transported only a relatively short distance before the injury can receive definitive treatment, and if this transportation can be carried out without further injuring the patient,

no special treatment is necessary at the scene of the accident. However, a compound fracture is a surgical emergency, and the patient should be transported to a hospital as soon as possible in order that treatment of the fracture may be instituted.

If the patient is seriously injured, it is advisable that certain measures be taken at the scene of the accident in order to prevent further injury to the patient and prevent the development of shock. Other things being equal, it may be said that the more severe the injury, the less the patient should be handled. In other words, the severely injured patient should be left on the side of the road and made as comfortable as possible until an ambulance arrives, instead of being transported some distance and placed in bed until he can be lifted again from the bed into some conveyance and taken to a hospital. Given a case of a man who has suffered a severe compound fracture of the leg or thigh in a highway accident, for instance, it is better that he be handled very little and that the extremity simply be straightened and that he be covered and kept warm and made as comfortable as possible where he is and an ambulance sent for, rather than that he be carried into the nearest house where he will appear to be more comfortable once he is placed in bed. Handling of the patient necessarily causes pain and increases the amount of injury to the soft tissues and tends to increase the amount of shock.

If the patient is bleeding and the bleeding is considerable in amount, it is very important that this bleeding be stopped as soon as possible by pressure or by an improvised tourniquet, if this can be applied.

In a compound fracture it is also important that the wound be exposed and a clean dressing applied to the wound at the earliest possible moment. This dressing not only lessens the bleeding but also protects the wound from further contamination. If possible this dressing should include chemotherapy in the wound; sulfanilamide or sulfathiazole, or preferably a mixture of the two in powdered form should be sprinkled liberally in the wound. For this reason these drugs should be made available in emergency dressing stations in industrial plants and also carried in ambulances which are sent out for the specific purpose of picking up the injured person. The placing of the chemical in the wound at this time can do no harm and will tend to decrease the rate of the development of infection, and while it may not be necessary if the patient is going to be operated upon immediately, one can never be sure but that for some reason treatment will be delayed several hours, in which event the presence of the sulfanilamide or sulfathiazole will greatly lessen the tendency to the development of infection and will make the surgeon's work much more apt to be successful.

It is especially important that severely injured persons be kept warm and dry and that they be given fluids by mouth. Likewise, unless they are suffering from brain or intra-abdominal injuries, they should be given a hypodermic of morphine or other opiate as soon as possible after the accident and before they are transported to the hospital.

Splinting.—The question arises as to what fractures should be splinted and how. At the present time there is a campaign on to the effect that all fractures should be splinted where they lie before transportation is attempted. This, of course, can be carried to absurdity, and much valuable time may be lost or further injury may be done by an unskilled person who attempts to splint fractures before the patient is carried to the hospital. On the other hand, patients with severe fractures who are going to be transported long distances should be splinted before they are started on their journey because splinting not only tends to lessen the pain, but also tends to prevent further damage to the soft tissues which may be incurred if the patient is transported without splintage, and tends to prevent the development of surgical shock.

In Chapter IV there is illustrated a series of emergency splints which are suitable for both the upper and lower extremities and the spine. The splints are shown without padding and the figures are self-explanatory. These or similar splints can be improvised at the scene of the accident if splints are needed and if commercial splints are not available (and they usually are not available). It is to be understood, however, that the application of these splints is not necessary in every case. It is important that a patient with a fractured femur or a fracture of both bones of the leg be splinted if possible before he is transported for any considerable distance. Likewise, severe fractures of the upper extremity should be splinted if transportation over a considerable distance is anticipated. In many instances it is sufficient merely to place the extremity on a pillow or to bind the arm to the chest or to bind the lower extremity to its fellow.

It is important in fractures of the femur that the lower extremity be immobilized on the pelvis and prevented from rotating. For this purpose a Thomas hip splint is advisable, if this is available. However, it is rarely available at the scene of the accident, unless the accident occurs in an industrial plant with a well-equipped first aid station. However, by means of a long board similar to that illustrated in Fig. 115, adequate fixation even without adequate traction can be improvised, and the patient can be made relatively comfortable and safe for transport in an ambulance. In moving any broken extremity manual traction should be made on the extremity before it is lifted.

2. **Transportation.**—The manner of transportation will depend upon what is available and on the nature and severity of the injury. If the patient is injured in the spine, pelvis, or thigh, an ambulance is especially desirable. If he is injured in the lower leg and both bones are broken, an ambulance is also desirable. Injuries of the upper extremity, on the other hand, usually can be transported in an automobile and the patients are just about as comfortable as though they were in an ambulance, and valuable time is not lost in waiting for an ambulance.

The patient should be taken to a hospital where he can receive adequate treatment and not necessarily taken to the nearest hospital where perhaps the gravity of the situation and the importance of the time element are not appreciated and where he may be placed in a bed to await the convenience of a surgeon. It is much more satisfactory to transport the patient a few miles farther in order that he may receive appropriate treatment, despite the fact that the time interval is of great importance, as not infrequently patients are rushed to the hospital only to be placed in bed and left for several hours before anything much is done for them.

3. **Treatment at the Hospital**: *Admission.*—The patient suffering from a traumatic injury should be admitted as expeditiously as possible and red tape should be cut to a minimum. Immediately after admission he should be examined

by a physician and this physician's first duty is to estimate the general condition of the patient and decide whether or not he is severely injured and whether or not he is in a state of shock or of impending shock.

In compound fractures the time element is of great importance because the treatment of the wound is instituted in order to prevent the development of infection. The method of procedure at the hospital will depend upon the facilities provided.

In the case of a severely injured patient the first physician who sees him determines whether or not this patient is bleeding. If the patient is bleeding at an alarming rate, the first duty of the physician is to stop the hemorrhage if possible. In the hospital this usually can be done by the application of clamps or by a tourniquet or by a pressure bandage. After the bleeding has been stopped, the physical examination and history can be proceeded with. If the patient is not bleeding, the emergency dressing need not be removed until the patient is placed on the operating table.

The Examination.—The examination begins with a brief history of the accident and a notation of all of the regions in which the patient complains of pain and disability, because he may be suffering from multiple injuries, and it is embarrassing to find one or more unrecognized and untreated fractures several days after the more obvious lesion has been attended to. It should also include a notation of the number of hours which have elapsed since the injury because this is an important factor in determining the method of treatment of a compound fracture.

The patient is then subjected to a brief physical examination. This includes the heart, lungs, abdomen, and extremities. The injured part is examined more carefully, and a tentative diagnosis is made. The temperature, pulse rate, and blood pressure are recorded and an estimate is made of the patient's general condition. If indicated a hypodermic of morphine or other opiate is administered at this time. This will not only tend to lessen the pain, but it is also an important factor in preventing or treating surgical shock. As a rule, satisfactory dressings or splints are not removed until the definitive treatment of the fracture is started. The examination should include satisfactory roentgenograms of the injured part unless the patient is in shock. If surgical shock of considerable gravity is present, it may be advisable to defer the x-ray examination until after the patient has reacted favorably to the treatment of the shock. If severe shock is not present, the patient may be taken directly to the operating room from the x-ray room. Treatment of mild shock can be started in the operating room and continued during the operation.

Chemotherapy.—As stated above, at the earliest opportunity a liberal amount of sulfanilamide or sulfathiazole powder or microcrystals should be sprinkled in the wound and a dressing applied. This may be done at the time of the emergency dressing or at the first hospital dressing if the wound is dressed before the patient is taken to the operating room. The local themotherapy slows, but may not prevent the development of infection in the wound.

Penicillin, 25,000 units intramuscularly or intravenously, should be administered as soon after admission to the hospital as possible and from 10,000 to 25,000 units should be administered every two to three hours after that until danger of infection has passed. If penicillin is not available, sulfathiazole or sulfadiazine should be given in full doses. If oral administration is contra-indicated, the drug can be given intravenously as the sodium salt. The systemic sulfonamide therapy should also be continued until the danger of infection has passed.

The larger doses of penicillin or sulfonamide are given to the patients with large grossly contaminated wounds or with severe infection. The administration of both penicillin and a sulfonamide may be practiced in patients with severe infection.

Treatment of Patients in Shock.—Traumatic shock is indicated by unusual pallor and sweating, a cold clammy skin, pinched facies, dilated pupils, shallow respiration, a rapid thready pulse, subnormal temperature, and a low blood pressure. If the shock is chiefly due to hemorrhage, restlessness and air hunger may be present. Shock, on the other hand, should be differentiated from fainting, which may superficially resemble it, but from which the patient quickly recovers when placed in a recumbent position.

It is a moot question as to whether the surgical shock or the injury should receive the primary treatment in the case of a severely injured patient who enters the hospital in a condition of shock. Some hold that immediate treatment of the injury is the most efficient method of treating the shock. On the other hand, we believe that if the shock is at all serious this should receive the first attention and that the delay of an hour or a few hours in treating the injury will not greatly enhance the danger of infection. This is particularly true since we have available penicillin and the sulfonamide drugs which lengthen the time during which débridement and suture of the wound can be practiced with safety.

The patient in shock should immediately be put in a quiet room in a warm dry bed with heated blankets both under him and over him, and he should be surrounded by hot water bottles, particular care being taken not to burn the patient with the hot water bottles, as patients in shock are burned easily. The foot of the bed should be elevated so that the patient is in the shock position, and he should be given a full dose of morphine. He should be given fluids by mouth, if he can take them, and usually he should be given fluids intravenously as soon as possible. If plasma is available, a plasma transfusion can be given immediately. On the other hand, if plasma is not available, 5 per cent glucose can be given intravenously (an adult receives 1000 c.c.). Blood should be taken for matching and a suitable donor obtained; the patient should be given a transfusion of 500 c.c. of whole blood if he does not react promptly to the above measures. If the condition is grave, oxygen can be administered and this will help combat the anoxemia. Fractures of the extremities should be immobilized with sand bags or splints, if this has not been done before the patient entered the hospital.

If the hospital is equipped with a blood bank, whole blood is used instead of plasma and it is now considered good practice to give much more blood than was the custom in the past. One thousand or even 2000 c.c. may be given to patients who are exsanguinated and the transfusions of whole blood are repeated at one- or two-day intervals, until the patient's blood volume is restored and the hematocrit reading approaches normal. It is to be noted that plasma does not replace whole blood. In patients who have lost much blood it is used as an emergency measure to restore blood volume until whole blood can be supplied.

We have, then, as treatment of the shock patient, relief of pain by morphine, rest to the injured part, restoration of body heat by hot blankets and external heat, rest of the patient by recumbency in the shock position and isolation, the administration of fluids or blood to restore the blood volume and increase the blood pressure, and, in severe cases, the administration of oxygen to combat the anoxemia.

As soon as the patient reacts favorably to the shock treatment, specific treatment of the fracture can be undertaken. This includes x-rays because the patient in shock should not be transported to the x-ray room before he is treated for the shock.

ANTITETANIC SERUM AND GAS GANGRENE ANTITOXIN

Any compound fracture may be contaminated with tetanus or gas infection, and this is much more easily prevented than cured. Consequently, a combined prophylactic dose of antitetanic serum (1,500 U. S. P. units) and gas gangrene serum should be given subcutaneously and recorded immediately after admission; otherwise, in the press of duties incident to treating the fracture it may be forgotten. The large dose should be used in severely contaminated wounds and should be repeated at seven-day intervals until three doses have been given. If anaphylaxis is feared, the serum should be given in graded doses at thirty-minute intervals beginning with 0.5 c.c. In severe injuries the polyvalent gas gangrene antitoxin should be administered as a prophylactic measure.

Treatment of the Wound and the Fracture.—If a compound fracture is present, not only must the fracture be treated but usually it is advisable to débride the wound. This means an emergency operation.

What compound fractures should be débrided? This is a question to which the answer will vary with the individual surgeon. The fracture may be compounded from without—that is, by the fracturing force, in which case the overlying tissues have been crushed and more or less devitalized and foreign material including clothing and dirt may have been carried into the wound—or the fracture may have been compounded from within, particularly where the injury is due to indirect violence and the wound in the skin may have been produced by the end of one fragment sticking through the skin. In such instances the fracture is relatively clean, unless the end of the bone has been contaminated, usually by coming in contact with the ground or pavement.

In the past it has been our custom to débride all compound fractures in which the compound wound was caused by external violence—that is, fractures compounded from without, except those due to bullet wounds traveling at high speed—and not to débride those fractures which were compounded from within unless the bone appeared to be contaminated or unless there was good reason to believe that the bone had been contaminated and then pulled back into the tissues. However, with more experience in the use of the sulfonamide drugs implanted locally in the wound we have changed this point of view and now débride all compound fractures, except those caused by high-speed bullet wounds. These are not débrided because the bone is comminuted and such fractures tend to do better if treated as simple fractures, except that the wound is painted with an antiseptic and the patient is given sulfathiazole by mouth.

Since the local and systemic use of the sulfonamide drugs and/or penicillin has permitted us to operate upon bones with greatly increased safety, there is no reason why fractures which are compounded from within should not receive the benefits of operative treatment and also receive the further guarantee against infection which can be obtained by implanting sulfonamide drugs into the wound.

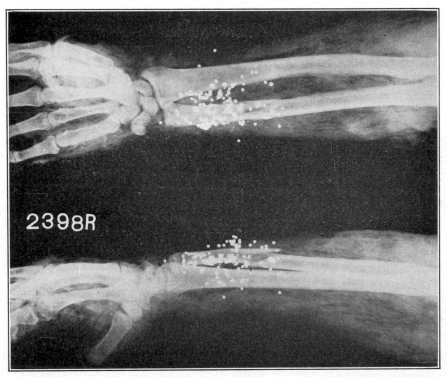

Fig. 150.—Gas gangrene of the forearm showing gas bubbles in the tissues following a shotgun wound. Treated by free incision and gas bacillus serum with good results. (Courtesy Dr. James J. Clark, Atlanta, Ga.)

If the patient is suffering from a compound fracture and is not in shock, he is taken to the operating room as soon after he has been admitted to the hospital as is practical to do so. He should first be taken to the x-ray room or a portable machine used and x-rays of the injury should be obtained. These should then be sent to the operating room. If he is in severe shock, this should be treated first and he is not moved to the operating room until he begins to react favorably to the shock treatment. In the operating room if the patient's general condition is satisfactory, he should be given a general anesthetic of pentothal sodium, or an inhalation anesthesia or local anesthesia may be used, depending upon the choice of the anesthetist and the surgeon.

The patient should be placed upon the operating table without removing his emergency dressing or splint, if this has been applied. If he is in a serious condition, the general anesthetic should not be started until the operating room and team are ready, because it is advisable not to prolong the anesthesia any longer than necessary.

Before proceeding with the preparation of the skin for the operation, a tourniquet may or may not be applied. Its use has the following advantages: (1) It conserves the blood supply of the patient; and (2) it enables the surgeon to work in a relatively bloodless field and he has a better view of the damaged tissues and is able to remove foreign material more thoroughly and to work more quickly. However, the tourniquet is removed at the end of the débridement and before the sulfonamide drugs are implanted in the wound and before an attempt is made to suture the wound, because it is important to stop all important bleeding points before the wound is sutured and in completing the débridement the presence of bleeding from the cut muscle is of aid in determining whether or not the tissue is viable. In applying the tourniquet the limb should be handled as gently as possible and, if one is available, a pneumatic tourniquet should be used. Never leave the tourniquet on too long.

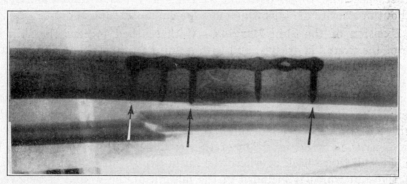

Fig. 151.—Compound fracture of the tibia. Treated immediately by débridement, internal fixation with a metal bone plate, and local sulfanilamide in wound. Uneventful recovery.

On the operating table the skin is prepared as for a clean surgical operation, an adequate field around the wound being cleaned and sterilized either by the dry or by the wet method. In using the dry method the wound is covered with a clean dry dressing, and the skin is washed with benzene or ether and shaved as close to the margins of the wound as possible. The skin, not the wound, is then painted with a skin antiseptic—tincture of iodine, merthiolate, metaphen, mercresin, or whatever antiseptic the surgeon prefers.

In using the wet method the skin wound is covered with a clean dry dressing and the surrounding skin is washed thoroughly with soap and water and shaved, the shaved area extending up as close to the wound edges as possible and covering sufficient area to allow an adequate operative field. After the limb is shaved and washed with soap and water it is then washed with benzene or alcohol or ether and after this has dried or evaporated the skin, not the wound, is painted with whatever skin antiseptic the surgeon prefers, as mentioned above in the dry method. This preparation of the skin and of the operative field must be performed or supervised by the surgeon with sterile gloves, unless he is fortunate enough to have a well-trained assistant who can be depended upon to carry out the procedure with care and gentleness. If the wound contains dirt or grease, it is washed with soap and water. The surgeon now dons a clean gown and gloves.

If a tourniquet is to be used, it should be applied before the preparation of the skin is started. Having been prepared, the limb is now pulled straight, supported on sand bags or by traction, and draped with sterile sheets and towels so that an adequate area is exposed for the operation.

DÉBRIDEMENT

The operation of débridement or cleansing of the wound is now proceeded with. The nature of this operation varies among individual surgeons. Some surgeons believe that it should include a block removal of all of the surface of the wound which is exposed, and this is rarely practical. Others merely enlarge the wound and pack it open, removing any gross foreign bodies which may be found in the wound.

The following outline of the operation is one which will be successful in most cases and one which does not sacrifice any tissue unnecessarily. It is carried out in a series of steps which may be enumerated as follows:

1. **Excision of the Skin Margins.**—With toothed forceps the skin at the margin of the wound is grasped and with a knife a thin strip of skin is cut away entirely around the wound. This strip is rarely over one-fourth of an inch wide. It includes the skin and any subcutaneous tissue which may be adherent to the skin, but no effort is made to carry this incision into the depths of the wound. If possible the margin of the wound is excised in one piece. However, usually the knife slips into the wound and the strip is divided at some point. When this happens the further excision of the wound margin is carried out, beginning a short distance back of where the knife slipped in so that all of that portion of the skin which is included in the margin of the wound is removed. At the same time if there is an adjacent area in which the skin is grossly devitalized by contusion so that it is perforated in small areas and ground down or crushed so that it is paper thin, this area is also excised, because if it is left it will slough and tend to cause infection. However, no skin should be removed unnecessarily, especially if the wound is to be closed, because it is important that the wound be sutured with as little tension as possible, and this cannot be done if a wide excision of the wound margins is practiced.

If more than one wound is present, the skin of each wound is excised in succession at this stage of the operation. The knife and forceps used in this maneuver are then discarded because they are grossly contaminated, but it is not necessary for the surgeon to change gloves as they have not touched the contaminated tissue.

2. **Enlargement of the Wound.**—The wound is enlarged by incisions up and down in the long axis of the extremity and the margins are retracted and its depths are inspected. The degree of enlargement will depend upon the size and depth of the wound and the damage to the underlying tissues. The longitudinal incisions are not made any longer than necessary. While it is true that wounds heal from side to side and not from end to end, it is also true that, other things being equal, small wounds cause less pain and heal with less complications

than do large wounds. As the wound is enlarged, blood vessels which are seen or are bleeding if the tourniquet is not on are clamped either before or immediately after they are divided, care being taken that as little blood is lost as possible. The larger vessels are ligated. The wound should be enlarged sufficiently to permit exploration of the entire damaged area when the edges of the wound are retracted.

3. **Débridement of the Wound Proper.**—It is now possible to inspect the depth of the wound and estimate the damage to the deeper structures. The surfaces are carefully sponged. Any foreign material or foreign bodies which are seen are removed. Not infrequently the skin and fascia are stripped up and separated in layers and form deep pockets which should be explored. It is usual to excise a thin layer of the superficial fat and of the fascia which may be exposed around the margins of the wound and of the exposed muscle which forms part of the walls of the wound. Likewise, severely damaged muscle which does not contract when pinched or does not bleed if the tourniquet is not applied is excised. However, no wide excision of undamaged muscle should be done if this can be avoided. Not infrequently masses of areolar tissue will contain small foreign bodies or dirt. It is advisable to excise such areolar tissue rather than to attempt to pick out the small bits of foreign material. If shreds of periosteum are torn off and contaminated, these are excised. Vessels which bleed after the clamps are removed should be ligated with fine silk or catgut.

At the end of this stage of the operation the wound should be relatively clean and contain no visible foreign bodies or unexplored pockets. All grossly damaged and devitalized tissues have been excised with a sharp knife. The wound should contain only living muscle and connective tissue, nerves and blood vessels, tendons, and bone and periosteum, if all of these structures are exposed in the wound. During this stage of the operation it may be necessary to manipulate the extremity, because not infrequently the wound extends around the bone or the bone may be entirely lifted up from its bed and foreign bodies may have lodged behind it. The entire wound should be inspected. If muscles or tendons or nerves are cut or severed and their ends are macerated or grossly contaminated, these ends should be excised with a sharp knife at this stage, care being taken to sacrifice no more of the structure than is necessary to insure the removal of devitalized or contaminated tissue.

4. **Treatment of Bone.**—In some instances the fragments of the bone are grossly contaminated—that is, the bone may have been forced out of the wound and driven into the dirt—and such bone cannot be cleaned as dirt and other foreign material have been forced into the bone spaces. This is particularly true of cancellous bone and such areas of grossly contaminated bone should be excised with heavy bone-cutting forceps or rongeurs and no attempt should be made to scrub them clean. Loose fragments of bone which have been completely detached from their periosteal attachments and are devoid of circulation should, as a rule, be removed. Occasionally, they may be left for support or to prevent a loss of substance which will necessitate shortening of the extremity. However, as a rule, it is advisable to remove them, because when they are left they usually remain as inert foreign bodies and, even though no infection may occur, they do relatively little, if any, good. This is particularly true of fragments

which include the entire thickness of the cortex as such fragments show little tendency to unite and do not act like a bone graft which is firmly fixed to the bone which it is supposed to aid in uniting.

Very rarely in an epiphyseal separation the end of the shaft has been forced out of the wound and grossly contaminated by being driven into the dirt or forcibly coming in contact with some other foreign substance. This epiphyseal surface or end can be forcibly scrubbed with soap and water rather than excised and can then be reduced and healing may be expected to occur without deformity and without infection.

If a joint is involved, the margins of the wound in the synovial lining are excised and the wound is enlarged and the joint cavity is explored carefully for foreign material and loose pieces of bone and cartilage, and contused and lacerated cartilage is excised.

The débridement is now complete. The skin edges have been excised, all visible foreign material has been removed from the wound and all grossly contaminated and devitalized tissues have been excised, and bleeding vessels have been ligated. In other words, the toilet of the wound is complete from the standpoint of mechanical excision.

5. **Irrigation of the Wound.**—It is now advisable to irrigate the wound with warm normal salt solution. This does not mean a prolonged irrigation, using several gallons of salt solution. However, it usually takes a gallon or more of saline solution to cleanse the average compound wound properly. The solution is placed in the irrigating can held by an assistant and to this is attached a rubber tube without a glass nozzle. The force of the flow is controlled by raising or lowering the height of the can and by squeezing the tip of the rubber tube so that the salt solution can be squirted into all portions of the wound. This will tend to float up loose tissue, especially areolar tissue, and may bring to light and remove foreign material which may have been missed during the preceding stage. After this irrigation is complete, the wound is sponged out and rendered relatively dry and is again inspected for the presence of any foreign bodies or devitalized tissue, and if such are found, they are removed.

6. **Repair of Deeper Structures.**—At this stage muscles, tendons, and nerves which are found to be cut or torn are repaired. If torn ends have been excised during the preceding stage of the operation, they are now carefully brought together and sutured with fine silk or catgut. Muscles are sutured very loosely, just enough suture material being used to hold the ends in contact. Nerves and tendons are carefully sutured with fine silk. It may be advisable in the case of both tendons and nerves to excise a small bit more from each end in order that accurate approximation of healthy tissues may be obtained.

7. **Reduction and Internal and Pin Fixation of the Fracture.**—By manipulation of the extremity or by manipulation of the ends of the fragments with bone-holding forceps the fracture is now reduced as accurately as possible. If the fracture is fairly stable, no internal fixation is advisable. If the fracture is a long oblique fracture or a comminuted fracture, it may be advisable to use some internal fixation. In certain instances of oblique fractures it may be advisable to reshape the ends of the fragments in order that they will be stable when placed in end-on contact.

In the past we have avoided the use of internal fixation wherever possible. However, during recent years with the use of vitallium and stainless steel, both of which are nonirritating, and also with the use of sulfonamide drugs which tend to lessen the tendency to the development of infection, it is now possible to use internal fixation in compound fractures with relative safety. Consequently, if plates, screws, or wires are indicated to hold the fragments together, there is no reason why they should not be used and applied at this stage of the procedure, and they will render the aftertreatment much more simple and tend to make it more successful. If internal fixation is used, it should be applied according to good mechanical principles, and plates, wires, and screws should serve the purpose for which they are placed in the bone. If internal fixation is not used an assistant should hold the limb after the fracture is reduced and is stable, being careful not to move it and thus cause the fragments to be displaced while the wound is being closed.

In certain instances, especially in comminuted or double fractures of the leg, one- or two-pin fixation may be more advisable than internal fixation or traction. At this stage of the operation the pins or wires may be driven or drilled through the proximal and distal fragments, if the operative field is extensive enough to permit this procedure without breaking the aseptic technique. The pins or wires are to be placed well away from the fracture wound. (H. E. C. prefers this technique in most instances.)

If a sufficient area of the limb is not exposed in the operative field to permit this, the pins or wires can be placed later after the wound is closed or packed open. They are to be incorporated in the cast which will immobilize the fragments.

8. **Final Inspection of the Wound and Control of Hemorrhage.**—If a tourniquet has been used, it is now removed. The wound is carefully inspected for bleeding points of any consequence and, if found, they are clamped, care being taken to include no excess tissue in the clamp, and they are ligated with fine silk or catgut.

9. **Chemotherapy of the Wound.**—Either sulfanilamide, sulfathiazole, or a mixture of the two drugs in powder form is now sprinkled over the surface of the wound, care being taken to place some of the drug in the depth of the wound and in pockets which may have been developed in fascial spaces in order that when it goes into solution in the fluid which will collect in the wound all parts of the wound will be exposed to a saturated solution of the drug which is used. The amount of the drug used varies directly with the size of the wound. In most instances from five to ten grams is sufficient, but fifteen or twenty grams can be used without causing toxic symptoms. Lately one of us (J.A.K.) has been washing the wound thoroughly with a saturated solution of the drug in normal saline.

When implanted in a wound, the drug is dissolved in the fluid which collects in the wound and is then absorbed and excreted. It does not appreciably interfere with the healing of the wound unless it is present in sufficient amount to form aggregates which are slowly absorbed and act as foreign bodies which keep the surfaces of the wound apart.

The sulfonamides inhibit the growth of susceptible bacteria and do not interfere with the normal defense mechanism of the body. Thus, in a compound fracture which has been débrided they prevent those bacteria which may have been left in the wound from multiplying and these can then be destroyed by the phagocytes. Of the two drugs in general use, sulfanilamide is effective against streptococci and is the more soluble. Sulfathiazole is more effective against staphylococci and the organisms which cause gas gangrene and because of its relatively slight solubility will remain in the wound longer (probably over forty-eight hours). We prefer a mixture of equal parts of sulfanilamide and sulfathiazole. Sulfadiazine can be used, but it is expensive and is not known to have any advantage over sulfathiazole when the drug is implanted in a wound.

The drugs can be sterilized by autoclaving, but if the sterile powder is not available we do not hesitate to implant the unsterilized powder in a compound fracture wound.

10. **Closure of the Wound.**—The question now arises as to whether or not the wound should be closed. Many surgeons believe that all compound fractures should be left open and that the limb should be immobilized and the wound permitted to heal by granulation. We believe that whenever possible the wound should be closed, and if the débridement has been adequate, most of these in civil life can be closed if operated upon within the first eight hours and many of them can be closed within the first twelve or twenty-four hours after the injury. Not only the time which has elapsed since the injury, but also the amount and character of the contamination and the amount of soft tissue damage and the mechanical conditions in the wound must be considered in determining whether the wound should be closed or packed open.

In military surgery under war conditions most compound fractures should be débrided, the wound sprinkled liberally with sulfanilamide or sulfathiazole powder, and packed open with vaseline gauze. A dry dressing should then be applied and the fracture immobilized in a plaster-of-Paris cast or splint; the surgeon who sutures a compound fracture should watch the patient until the danger of infection is past and under conditions of war this may not be possible.

In closing the wound no attempt is made to close it in layers as buried sutures are avoided when possible. The skin and underlying fat or superficial fascia are sutured in one layer with a continuous suture (H. E. C. prefers interrupted sutures) of silkworm gut, deknatel, or some other nonabsorbent material. Tension is avoided and, if necessary, tension incisions are made on either side of the wound in order to effect a satisfactory closure. Care is taken not to draw the sutures too tightly and the wound is closed without drainage. Sulfanilamide or sulfathiazole powder is then sprinkled over the sutured wound and a dry dressing is applied.

If, because of the lapse of too much time since the injury or for any other reason, it is deemed inadvisable to close the wound, interrupted sutures of silkworm gut may be placed in the wound to be tied a few days later, or it may be partially closed, or it may be packed loosely with petrolatum gauze and covered with a dry dressing, the sulfonamide powder having been placed in the wound as described above. If it is necessary to cut a flap or to make tension cuts in order to close the wound, the resulting defect may be covered immediately with a split skin graft which is sutured in place.

Delayed Suture.—In instances where immediate suture of the wound is not deemed advisable the chemotherapy is continued and the wound may be closed from four to ten days later. This secondary closure is done without excision and without bacteriological control. If the wound looks clean it can be closed.

Drainage.—In certain instances lateral or dependent drainage may seem advisable. This can be established by a stab wound and a rubber tissue drain which can be inserted before the wound is closed. The drain is removed two to four days later through a window in the cast.

Dressing.—If the wound has been closed, we usually sprinkle the suture line with sulfonamide powder and cover this with a single layer of petrolatum gauze; a dry gauze dressing is then placed over the wound and the limb is bandaged snugly with a gauze roll. This is covered with a thin layer of sheet cotton and a snugly fitting cast is applied. Wounds which are left open are treated in practically the same manner. Davis and Fortune apply a meticulous pressure dressing, using an Ace bandage under the cast and mechanic's cotton waste or sea sponges where indicated to combat postoperative edema.

IMMOBILIZATION

The fracture has been reduced before the wound was closed and it must now be immobilized by external fixation. This is true whether or not internal fixation was used and whether or not the wound was closed. The immobilization is necessary not only for the treatment of the fracture, but it is also one of the most important measures in combating the infection. It can be immobilized in splints with or without traction or in a plaster-of-Paris cast which may or may not be padded. We use a plaster cast in most instances and usually use very little padding. It is important that the cast be applied while satisfactory position of the fragments is maintained and that it include the joints above and below the fracture. If the fragments are not stable when reduced, we do not hesitate to tranfix each end of the bone with a stainless steel pin or wire and to incorporate this in the cast in order to maintain length of the limb, or we may use a pin or wire in the distal fragment and apply traction.

AFTERTREATMENT

The aftertreatment includes chemotherapy, supportive treatment, if indicated, leaving the wound and the fracture alone, watching the patient for evidence of infection, and opening the wound and treating the infection if it occurs.

Chemotherapy.—As soon as the patient is sufficiently recovered from the anesthetic he should be given penicillin or sulfonamide in full doses (1 gram by mouth every four hours). This should be continued for from four to seven days until the danger of infection is past.

Supportive Treatment.—The patient may need transfusions or intravenous fluids and these should be given as indicated.

Leaving the Wound Alone.—The wound should not be dressed or the fracture disturbed for three or four or more weeks, unless there is some reason for doing so. Sutures may be left in for four weeks or more, or even until the fracture has united. If the wound is packed open, the cast may be changed or a window cut in the cast at the end of three or four weeks and the vaseline gauze removed and fresh petrolatum gauze placed in the wound. Then the cast is reapplied.

Evidence of Infection.—As a rule the first evidence of infection is pain and with the development of gas gangrene this may be excruciating. The pain is accompanied by an elevation of the temperature and a disproportionate increase in the pulse rate. The toes or fingers may become swollen and cyanotic. The leucocyte count is elevated and the wounds are red, hot, and edematous.

Treatment of Infection.—If infection supervenes, the wound should be opened widely if it has been sutured, or the petrolatum gauze should be removed if it has been treated by the open method, and thorough drainage assured. Immobilization and chemotherapy should be continued. Also, supportive treatment should be intensified as indicated. If gas gangrene is present, this should be treated as indicated below and this should dominate the picture.

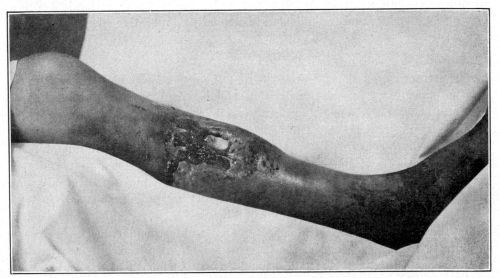

Fig. 152.—Old osteomyelitis of the tibia with sequestrum following compound fracture. Healed after saucerization operation.

TREATMENT OF INFECTED COMPOUND FRACTURES

Compound fractures which are compounded from without and which are seen twelve hours or more after the injury may be considered infected and consequently the surgeon must attempt to evaluate the gravity of the infection and regulate his treatment accordingly. The degree of infection varies directly with the virulence of the infecting organisms and with the length of time that has elapsed since the accident, and with the amount of damage to the soft tissues in the vicinity of the wound. The first consideration is to determine whether or not gas gangrene is present or imminent and whether or not severe pyogenic infection is present or imminent.

In cases in which there is severe damage to the soft parts with relatively little drainage through the skin even without infection, there will be marked swelling of the limb and discoloration in the subcutaneous tissues. A glance at the wound will usually disclose serum or even frank pus, and a smear from this material when stained and examined usually reveals bacteria, either staphylococcus or streptococcus or a number of different organisms. One should be particularly impressed by the presence of large short thick bacilli in the exudate from the wound as these are apt to be the organisms of gas gangrene. On the other hand they may be relatively harmless saprophytes.

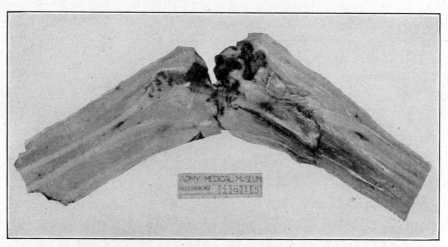

Fig. 153.—Amputated specimen from infected gunshot fracture of the knee. (Courtesy U. S. Army Medical Museum.)

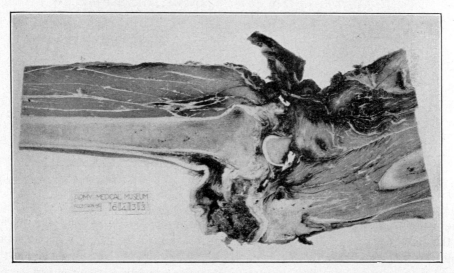

154.—Amputated specimen from infected gunshot fracture of the lower portion of the thigh involving the knee. (Courtesy U. S. Army Medical Museum.)

Diagnosis of Gas Gangrene.—The diagnosis of gas gangrene is not a simple matter in its early stages, as any infected wound in the presence of a compound fracture with saprophytic organisms and devitalized tissues may give rise to a foul or even fecal odor. Likewise, the severe pain, rapid pulse, moderate elevation in temperature, and general appearance of an extremely ill patient may result from staphylococcus or streptococcus infection as well as from gas bacillus.

Gas gangrene should be suspected, of course, when the wound has a foul odor, when dark pus exudes from it, when the surrounding skin is tense or marble-like in appearance and copper colored, when the patient's pulse rises disproportionately to the increase in temperature, and when the patient appears unusually sick and has an icteric color. If smears from the pus show short thick bacilli in large numbers, the diagnosis should be considered sufficiently established to warrant surgical intervention for gas gangrene. The crucial point, however, in the diagnosis is the presence of gas in the wound or tissues or both, and if this is carefully looked for, it can usually be detected. It should be remembered, however, that gas may be present in the wound or tissues without gas gangrene. This is due to the physical characteristics of the wound so that air is drawn in and pocketed there and may result from dead spaces between the

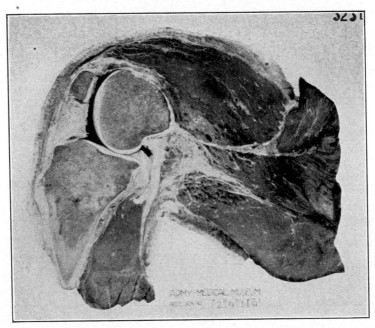

Fig. 155.—Amputated specimen of gas gangrene in the muscle. (Courtesy U. S. Army Medical Museum.)

fragments or in the tissues which communicate with the outside air. Also, air in the tissues may be found occasionally in chest injuries where it has escaped from the lungs and through a pneumothorax. The presence of air or gas in the tissue may be determined by palpation if a fine crackling crepitus can be obtained. In large amounts between muscle planes it can also be identified in the x-ray picture, but the diagnosis should be made long before the gas is sufficient in amount to show in the x-ray. (Figs. 165, 166, 167 and 168.)

In a compound fracture in the presence of gas gangrene, if the area around the wound be gently palpated, a few small gas bubbles can be pressed out. This may also occur if the fragments be gently moved so that changes in pressure inside the wound occur. This gas will have a faint fetid odor and not necessarily a foul fecal odor.

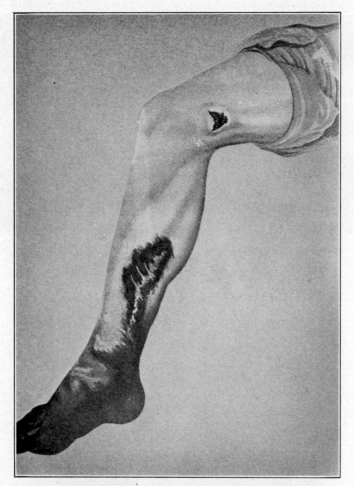

Fig. 156.—Gas gangrene of leg and foot following a gunshot laceration of the femoral artery. (Courtesy U. S. Army Medical Museum.)

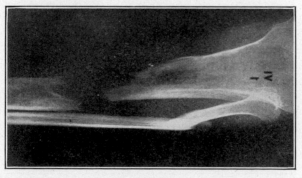

Fig. 157.—Old infected gunshot wound of the leg with loss of substance and nonunion. (Courtesy U. S. Army Medical Museum.)

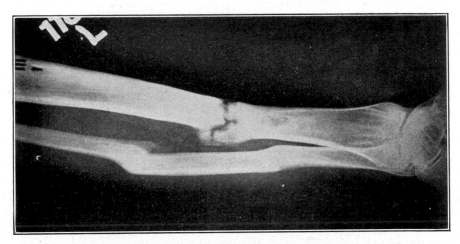

Fig. 158.—Old infected gunshot wound of the leg with nonunion. (Courtesy U. S. Army Medical Museum.)

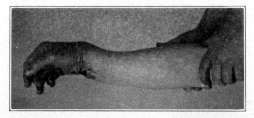

Fig. 159.—Compound fracture of both bones of the forearm due to indirect violence with protrusion of the upper fragments through the skin. Treated by débridement although compounded from within, because the ends of the fragments were soiled. Good result.

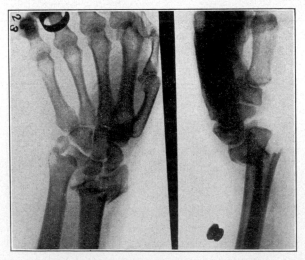

Fig. 160.—Roentgenograms of preceding case.

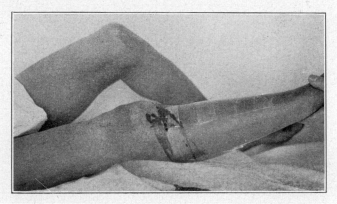

Fig. 161.—Compound comminuted fracture both bones of the leg (puncture wound). Treated by skeletal traction, after débridement, for three weeks; then a circular cast for four weeks. Weight bearing with metal brace ten weeks. Good result.

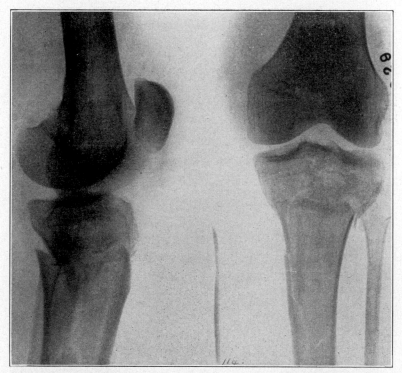

Fig. 162.—X-ray picture of preceding case.

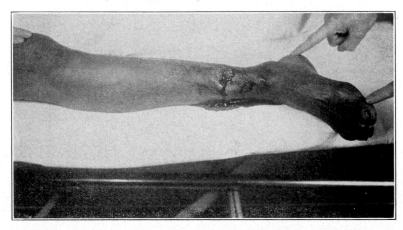

Fig. 163.—Compound comminuted fracture of tibia and fibula. Treated by débridement and a Kirschner wire through the lower fourth of the tibia. The wound was closed with one Dakin tube in fascia. Dakin's irrigation and later with a circular plaster cast. Good result.

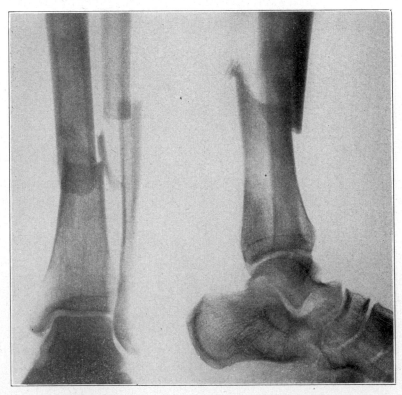

Fig. 164.—X-ray pictures of the preceding case.

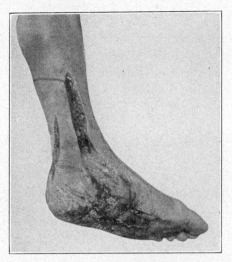

Fig. 165.—Moderately advanced gas gangrene in compound comminuted fracture of the os calcis with gangrenous areas around ankle and plantar surface of the foot. These have been incised. Bronzing of the skin above the incisions. Treated by amputation about four inches below the knee. Dakin's solution to stump and antigas bacillus serum. Recovery. (Courtesy Dr. J. O. Dieterle, Milwaukee.)

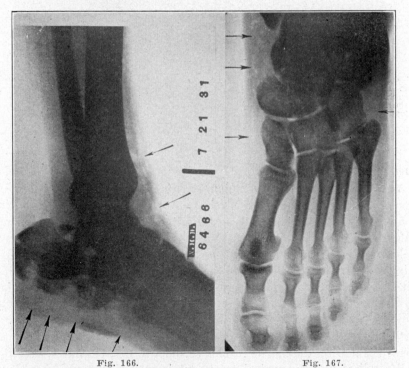

Fig. 166.   Fig. 167.

Figs. 166 and 167.—Roentgenograms of preceding showing the fracture and gas in the tissues. (Courtesy Dr. Dieterle.)

If the surgeon is uncertain about the presence of gas in the wound, the limb should be immobilized, the wound covered with a dressing and left for an hour. The surgeon should then return, re-examine the wound by gentle palpation and, if necessary, manipulation. In the presence of gas gangrene infection more gas will have accumulated in the wound during the interval, and it will be possible to express it and confirm the diagnosis. Cultures should be made, but surgical intervention should not be delayed.

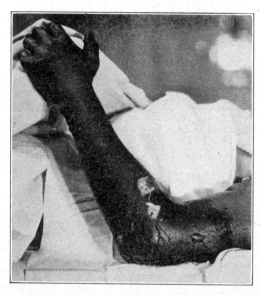

Fig. 168.—Advanced gas gangrene of lower arm, forearm, and hand, following a compound fracture at the elbow. The line of demarcation can be seen in the middle third of the arm. Treated by shoulder joint amputation and antigas bacillus serum. Recovery. (Courtesy Major General N. T. Kirk, Surgeon General, United States Army.)

TREATMENT OF GAS GANGRENE

Chemotherapy.—The dosage of penicillin or of sulfathiazole, or of both, should be increased as soon as gas gangrene is suspected. The penicillin may be given in doses of 25,000 units every two or three hours or by continuous intravenous drip. If sulfathiazole or sulfadiazine is used, the patient may be given the drug by mouth or intravenously as the sodium salt. He is given an initial dose of 2 to 4 grams and 1 gram every three hours. The chemotherapy is continued after the operation and penicillin (250 units per c.c. of salt solution) or sulfathiazole may be implanted in the wound. When penicillin is used locally, it is advantageous to include a small rubber tube in the dressing and to instill the penicillin solution into the wound two or more times a day.

Antitoxin.—The patient should be given full doses of the polyvalent antitoxin which is now on the market. This serum will not, of course, save the patient's life unless proper surgical treatment is carried out and should not be depended upon to do so. It should always be used because it apparently does no harm and may make the difference in the patient's resistance between survival and death after the operation. It is our practice to give a full dose of the serum immediately after the diagnosis is made; then, to proceed as soon as possible with the surgical treatment and repeat the serum after the operation until the patient reacts favorably or dies. The usual initial dose is from 10,000 to 20,000 units of the antitoxin given intravenously or intramuscularly and this is repeated at six-hour intervals until 100,000 units have been given or the patient reacts favorably or dies. Sulfathiazole should be given in full doses, and the patient should be transfused when this is indicated.

Surgical Treatment.—The surgical treatment is wide incision and excision of all infected and devitalized tissue. With massive gas gangrene this may necessitate amputation, and this should be high enough to include all infected and devitalized tissues. Too often amputation is done at the site of election in the leg for a gas gangrene in the foot and ankle and the extremity is later re-amputated in the thigh only to have the patient die of the infection. On the other hand, the surgeon should not sacrifice a knee and upper half of the leg needlessly. In other words, he should, if possible, determine how high the gangrene has extended and should save as much of the extremity as possible, but his first consideration should be the life of the patient.

In certain instances where the infection is localized in the wound or in the subcutaneous tissues, wide incision and local excision and drainage after sprinkling sulfathiazole powder in the wound are sufficient. More often muscle will be involved, and the devitalized muscle is brownish in color, does not bleed when cut or contract when pinched with forceps. Such muscles should be exposed generously by longitudinal incision combined with transverse incisions in the deep fascia and widely excised, leaving only healthy, red, bleeding, contractile muscle, and the wound sprinkled generously with sulfathiazole powder and left wide open and packed lightly with dry gauze. At times it is necessary to remove entire groups of muscles, such as the anterior tibial and the extensors of the toes. After operation sulfathiazole or penicillin is continued in full doses and the polyvalent antitoxin is continued, and the patient is watched closely for the appearance of the infection in other parts of the extremity.

Where the main blood vessels of the extremity are hopelessly damaged or the massive gangrene involving the distal portion of the extremity is present, amputation is necessary. The circular or guillotine type of amputation is usually advised. This has the disadvantage that reamputation is usually necessary if the patient survives. We now recognize the fact that most of the infection is in the muscles and that the subcutaneous tissues are not extensively involved. Consequently, we recommend the usual anterior and posterior flaps of skin and subcutaneous tissue, but excise the muscle well above the level where it is devitalized. If, when the distal portion of the limb is removed and hemostasis is obtained, it is found that certain muscles in the stump are involved by the infection, the stump may be incised longitudinally and these muscles excised at a higher level, if this is indicated. The stump is sprinkled generously with sulfathiazole powder and is packed lightly with dry gauze and bandaged loosely. The skin flaps may be tacked together over the gauze with a few sutures.

If the infection continues up the limb, wide incision of the stump with excision of involved muscle or reamputation at a higher level is indicated.

X-Ray Treatment.—A good deal has been written about the x-ray treatment of gas gangrene, but this is based on clinical observations and is not sup-

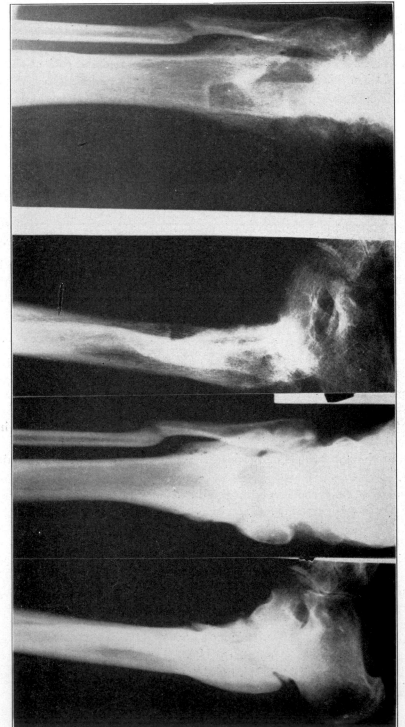

Fig. 169.—Severe compound fracture dislocation at the ankle with infection, three years' duration. Treated by sequestrectomy and arthrodesis with bone graft. Patient returned to work as a brakeman.

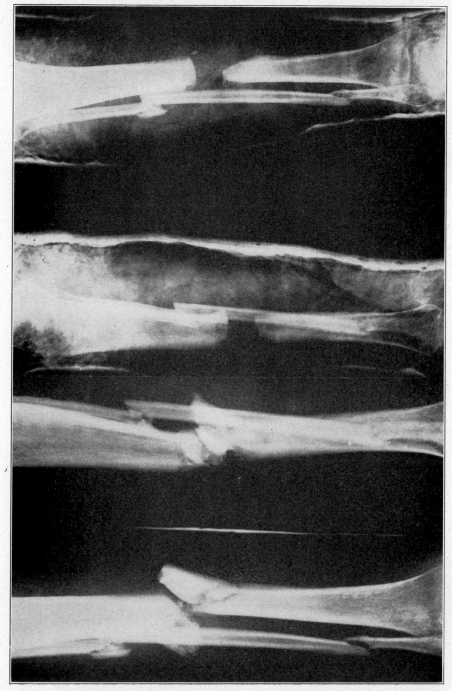

Fig. 170.—Severe fracture of the leg with infection. Treated by excision of infected area with closure and chemotherapy.

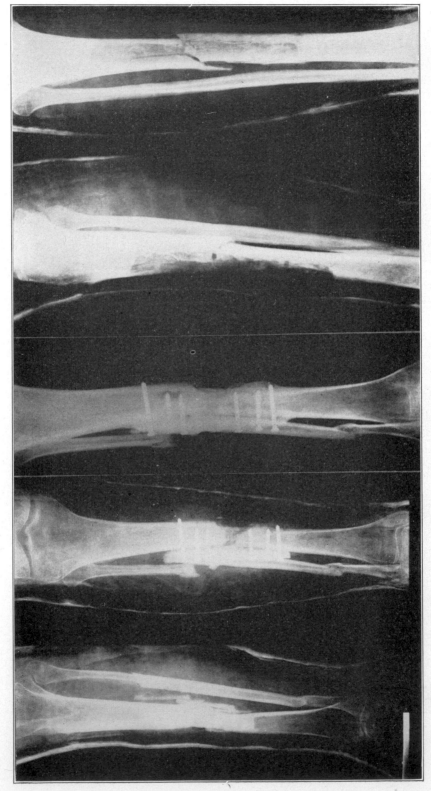

Fig. 171.—Same case as shown in Fig. 170, four months later. Treated by osteotomy and shortening of the tibia; a large bone graft was fixed to both fragments with stainless steel screws. This united promptly, but a fracture at the graft site in the opposite leg occurred from a fall and this united slowly. Eventual good result.

ported by experimental evidence. We do not know whether or not it is of value, but see no objection to using the deep x-ray therapy as adjuvant treatment provided the surgical treatment, chemotherapy, and antitoxin administration are carried out as described above and the patient can be given the treatment without subjecting him to a great deal of pain. A portable x-ray machine is advisable and the advised dose is small (100 roentgen units twice a day for two or three days).

THE TREATMENT OF INFECTED COMPOUND FRACTURES WITHOUT GAS GANGRENE

These are wounds in which the bacteria have begun to invade the tissues and from six to twenty-four hours or more may have elapsed since the injury. The infection is usually mixed and, in addition to staphylococci and streptococci, various saprophytic bacteria may be present. The infection may be relatively mild or it may be a rapidly progressing fulminating infection. The patient may be in good general condition, or he may be moribund. If his general condition is not good, this may be due to the severity of his injuries or to the infection.

From the above it is evident that these patients present problems similar to those discussed above in the section on the treatment of compound fractures plus those directly due to the infection and that clinical judgment is even more important than surgical skill in their treatment.

If shock from the injury dominates the picture, supportive treatment of the patient is the first consideration and this may include transfusion and rest. If toxicity from the infection is the most important feature, this demands intensive chemotherapy, adequate drainage, and immobilization of the infected tissues.

The treatment is carried out along the lines discussed above, except that in the presence of an acute fulminating infection chemotherapy is started immediately; it is advisable to administer penicillin in full doses or sulfathiazole (2 to 4 grams of sodium sulfathiazole) intravenously in order that an adequate blood concentration of the drug may be obtained as quickly as possible, and that the operation of débridement is replaced by one for drainage; even this may not be necessary, because the wound may be wide open and drainage may be adequate. Local chemotherapy is useful, but is not effective against bacteria which have deeply invaded the tissues. Immobilization must not be neglected, because this is one of the most effective measures in combating the infection. The limb and the patient should be moved as little as possible.

The Operation.—If the wound is obviously infected, the operation is for drainage and is not a débridement. The wound is enlarged in the long axis of the limb, and the deep fascia is cut transversely, if necessary, in order to expose the depths of the wound. Bleeding vessels are clamped and ligated with fine catgut. Foreign bodies and loose pieces of bone are removed. Necrotic tissues are excised, but no effort is made to excise the walls of the wound. The wound may be flushed with normal salt solution or wiped out with gauze. The fracture is then reduced, but no internal fixation is applied. No attempt is made to repair muscles, tendons, or nerves. After the wound is dry, it is sprinkled liberally with sulfathiazole or with a mixture of sulfanilamide and sulfathiazole and is packed loosely with petrolatum gauze, and a dry dressing is placed over the wound or a solution of penicillin (250 units per c.c.) may be instilled into the wound two or more times a day.

The fracture is then immobilized in a plaster-of-Paris cast, and if transfixion pins or wires are necessary for the maintenance of position of the fragments, these may be used but are placed as far from the infected area as possible.

In a borderline case in which the wound is not obviously infected a débridement may be carried out, as described in the preceding section, if the general condition of the patient permits, but the wound is not closed. It is sprinkled liberally with the sulfonamide powder, packed open, and immobilized in a cast.

Aftertreatment.—Penicillin in large doses or chemotherapy (1 gram of sulfathiazole by mouth every four hours) is continued until the infection is well controlled. Supportive treatment and rest are used as indicated.

The wound is not inspected or dressed until the odor of the discharge from the wound renders a change of the cast advisable, unless there is evidence of continued invasion of the tissues by the infection. This is indicated by pain, fever, increased pulse rate, toxemia, and progressive anemia.

At each change of plaster the skin around the wound is smeared with zinc oxide ointment in order to combat scalding and local skin infection.

TREATMENT OF OLD INFECTED COMPOUND FRACTURES

Old infected compound fractures are those in which osteomyelitis has occurred. This differs from the ordinary hematogenous osteomyelitis, however, in that the infection in the bone tends to be limited to the vicinity of the fracture. (Figs. 172, 173, 174 and 175.) The treatment of these cases is usually operative, but it is important that the operation be done at the proper time and that it be so planned as to remove all infected bone and result in union in good functional position. When union is present, it is advisable not to interrupt the continuity of the bone if possible, because the presence of a fresh fracture not only greatly complicates the aftertreatment but may result in nonunion. For this reason we do not believe in subperiosteal resections in the treatment of these cases. This is especially true in adults where the power of osteogenesis is considerably less than in children.

As a rule these patients are ready for a definite operative attempt to eliminate the infected bone in from three to six months after the injury, whether or not sequestration of dead bone has occurred. In some instances the dead bone will be sequestrated and simple removal of the sequestra will result in permanent healing of the infected wound. In others, and these are the majority, whether or not sequestra are present, there will be a variable amount of infected and dead bone enclosed in the callus, and it will be necessary to perform an operation such as we ordinarily plan for the attempt to cure osteomyelitis. That is, we approach the bone by a long longitudinal incision between muscle planes, being careful to avoid important blood vessels and nerves, expose the bone subperiosteally and excise a wide saucerized area, beginning with what in the surgeon's judgment will be sufficient to remove all of the infected bone. This saucerization process is continued upward and downward on the shaft until all of the infected area is removed. The wound is then packed open with petrolatum gauze, and a plaster cast is applied according to the Orr method.

In the operation we remove as little of the cortex as is consistent with an adequate saucerization. Since the mature bone of adults regenerates slowly or not at all, it is advisable not to so weaken the bone that its function will be seriously impaired. The removal of too much cortical bone is to invite a pathological fracture. The wound is then sprinkled generously with sulfathiazole powder, packed with petrolatum gauze, the gauze being well impregnated with petrolatum, and is left open. A gauze dressing is then applied, the limb is wrapped with sheet cotton, and a plaster cast is applied. This cast is left on for from three to six weeks and the drainage from the wound is allowed to accumulate in the dressing beneath the plaster. At the end of this time the plaster is removed, the petrolatum gauze will have been partly pushed out by the healing

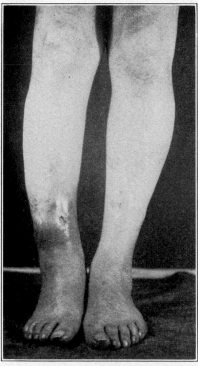

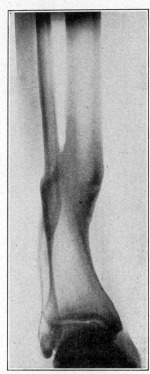

Fig. 172.

Fig. 173.

Fig. 172.—Old compound fracture at the junction of the middle and lower thirds of the right leg with deformity, poor alignment and chronic infection.
Fig. 173.—X-ray picture of preceding case.

of the tissue beneath, the wound is simply wiped out, and the limb is washed with soap and water and then thoroughly washed with alcohol. The wound is again sprinkled with sulfathiazole powder, repacked with petrolatum gauze, and a plaster cast is reapplied. This cast is left on as long as possible and is removed only when the odor causes it to be too unpleasant or secretions cause the cast to soften. If necessary a third or fourth cast is applied in the same manner. If the operation is successful—that is, if all of the infected bone has been removed—the wound may be expected to heal by granulations from the bottom and to remain healed.

This Orr method has an advantage over the Carrell-Dakin method as used formerly, in that the patient can be placed in a cast and sent home; the painful dressing is eliminated; the aftertreatment is greatly simplified; and we believe that the results are better. The principal objection to the Orr method is the odor. This is lessened by implanting the sulfonamide drugs at each dressing.

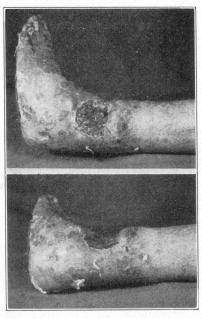

Fig. 174.—Old compound infected fracture of lower end of the left tibia and fibula. Eventual healing with fair function.

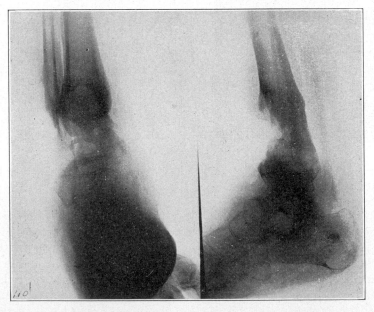

Fig. 175.—Roentgenograms of preceding case.

The Chemotherapeutic Method.—An even more satisfactory technic is one described by Drs. Frank Dickson and Rex Diveley. We have used it with success in a high percentage of the cases in which it was tried. It is as follows: Two days before the operation the patient is started on sulfathiazole by mouth (1 gram every four to six hours) or penicillin (1000 units every three hours).

The skin of the operative field is prepared as for a clean surgical operation.

The walls of the sinus tract and wound are excised back to healthy tissue, care being taken to remove all infected granulation tissue.

Sequestra are removed.

The cavity in the bone is saucerized or the ends excised if nonunion is present. The object is to remove all necrotic or infected bone.

Hemostasis is obtained and the wound inspected for any infected tissue. The entire wound surface is sprinkled with sulfathiazole powder.

The wound is closed without drainage. We use a deep skin suture of silkworm gut and avoid the use of buried sutures.

The limb is immobilized in a plaster-of-Paris cast.

Sulfathiazole by mouth or penicillin intramuscularly is continued for from five to seven days after the operation.

We have on several occasions performed the above operation on old ununited infected compound fractures and within two or three months have reopened the wound, placed a large onlay bone graft across the fracture, and fixed it with metal screws. The ends of the fragments were drilled, and bone chips and cancellous bone were placed around the fracture line. The entire wound was then sprinkled with sulfathiazole and closed. All healed by primary intention, and the fractures united in those in which sufficient time had elapsed.

This operation is suitable for chronic infections and not for acute infection or a chronic infection in which there is an acute flare-up.

GUNSHOT FRACTURES

Gunshot fractures are compound fractures by force from without and are either penetrating or perforating wounds, and as such are all potentially infected wounds. For this reason many of these wounds demand operation and débridement. Experience has shown, however, that gunshot wounds when inflicted by high velocity bullets from rifles or pistols may be treated expectantly just as can compound fractures which are compounded from within, because the high velocity sterilizes the bullet, and it does not carry clothing or other foreign material into the wound. In the penetrating wounds the bullet tends to remain in the tissues as an inert foreign body and should be let alone. (Figs. 176, 177, 178, 179, and 180.) We practically never probe for or operate to remove a bullet. In gunshot wounds which demand operation the operation is performed to prevent or combat infection and not to remove a now harmless bullet. Fractures from shrapnel, shell fragments, hand grenades, etc., are caused by projectiles which are low in velocity, irregular in shape, and larger in size than are the high velocity bullets, and these wounds demand immediate operation and débridement just as do grossly contaminated compound fractures.

The operative treatment of a gunshot wound requiring an operation demands a large longitudinal incision which is laid open to the depth of the wound or, if it is a perforating wound, demands a longitudinal incision on either side of the limb.   The track of the missile is lined by devitalized tissue, and this must be excised by sharp dissection, it being remembered that the track may be irregular because of the contraction of muscles after the infliction of the wound.   Foreign bodies are removed and bone fragments are treated just as in other compound injuries, the viable fragments being left in situ. The wound may be left open or closed, depending upon the time which has elapsed since the injury, just as in the case with other compound fractures.

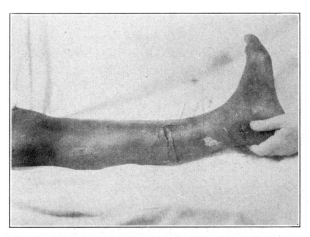

Fig. 176.—Comminuted gunshot fracture of both bones of the left leg, treated by traction with skeletal traction without débridement.   Primary healing, with good functional result.

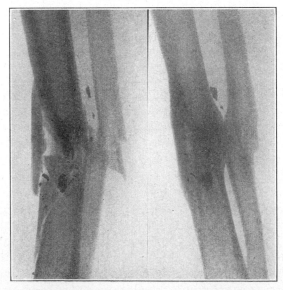

Fig. 177.—Roentgenogram of preceding case.

Bullet wounds may be simple, perforating wounds in the bone as from high velocity bullets, or may be relatively simple fractures in case of spent bullets, or the bones may be extensively shattered, the fragments being driven far into the tissues and the bullet broken into fragments which are also scattered through the tissues.   The bullets should not be probed for, since the bullet itself can usually be tolerated by the tissues. The wound should either be left entirely alone and treated as a simple fracture after the skin wounds have been painted with iodine and dressed with dry sterile dressing, or it should be widely opened and adequate débridement performed.

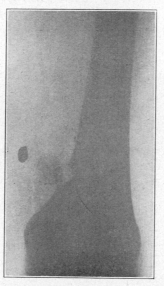

Fig. 178.—Gunshot wound of the femur with an incomplete fracture. Note the fragments of the bullet in the soft tissues. Treated by posterior wire splint to leg and thigh with antiseptic dressing to the skin and simple bandage for twelve days, with good results. Weight-bearing without support one month.

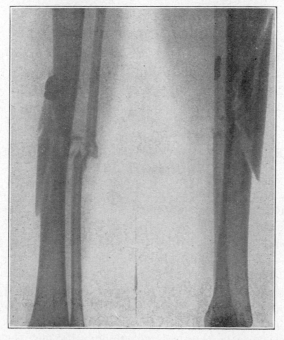

Fig. 179.—Compound fracture of both bones of the leg. Treated by traction with wire through lower fourth of the tibia without débridement. Circular plaster cast later. Good result.

A special type of injury in civil life is a compound fracture due to a shot-gun fired at close range. This injury produces a large gaping wound; shot are scattered widely through the tissues; there is a great deal of destruction of the soft tissues; and it is not unusual that some of the wadding from shotgun shells is carried into the wound and buried in the tissues, and this wadding may contain spores of tetanus or of organisms which produce gas gangrene. Such wounds must be thoroughly débrided, and the patient should be given tetanus antitoxin and treated with chemotherapy just as in other compound fractures.

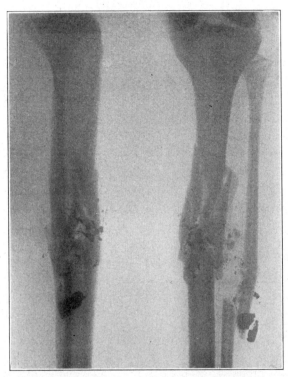

Fig. 180.—Severe gunshot wound with extensive shattering. Treated by skeletal traction for three weeks without débridement, then plaster cast. Walking without supports twelve weeks. Good result.

THE TREATMENT OF COMPOUND FRACTURES AND WOUNDS IN WAR

Compound fractures in civil life are considered in the preceding section, but present conditions make it advisable to include in this book a brief consideration of wounds and compound fractures which are suffered in times of war and as a result of military activities. The treatment of such cases must be modified on account of several factors, among which are the following: (1) There are the difficulties in transportation which may increase the time between the inception of the wound and the surgical treatment; (2) large numbers of wounds may have to be handled by relatively few men in a relatively short time; (3) it may be necessary for the surgeon to work with a reduced armamentarium because of the demands of mobility and the possible failure of supplies; (4) surgical technic must be simplified and speeded up or streamlined. A meticulous time-consuming operation may be admirable in civil life, but it slows up the work in the machinery of an evacuation hospital during a push; and (5) usually wounds must be packed open and the limbs immobilized, because the patient will be evacuated as soon as he is ready to travel, and the surgeon cannot watch the patient for evidence of infection.

In this chapter we shall consider briefly the treatment of the wounded man from the time of his wound until he has received his final treatment. We shall not attempt to follow any prescribed military plan, but shall merely consider the first aid in the field, the treatment at the field dressing station or regimental aid post, the treatment in the field hospital, and the treatment in the base hospital. What is said of the soldier in battle is also true of civilians who are injured in the bombing of cities.

First Aid Treatment.—It is assumed that each soldier will carry with him a first aid kit and that in addition to a dressing and bandage this will contain about 5 grams of sulfanilamide or sulfathiazole or preferably a mixture of the two drugs. When a man is wounded, if he is close to his dressing station and can get there under his own power, he naturally will go to the dressing station without preliminary treatment. However, if he has suffered a severe wound and is not able to get to the dressing station, he must be picked up and carried there and will probably have to remain in the field for some time before he is picked up. It is now recognized that it is poor economy to send stretcher bearers and surgeons over the top with advancing troops. They must follow the troops and wait until there is a lull in the battle or it may be necessary to collect the wounded during the night. In a war of movement many of the wounded will be left behind, and this is true whether the army is advancing or retreating. Consequently, first aid dressings should be applied after the sulfanilamide powder is poured into the wound. It is also advisable if the soldier is supplied with tablets of sulfathiazole or sulfanilamide that he swallow 2 grams of the drug immediately.

If he has suffered a compound fracture of the femur or of the leg, it is advisable that he be splinted in the field. This is especially true if he has to be carried for a very long distance to the first aid station. It is also advisable that all casualties with fractures of the lower extremities, as well as wounds of the abdomen and chest, be moved on stretchers.

Upon arrival at the first aid station a rough estimate of the severity of the wound is made. The dressing is examined, and if necessary more sulfonamide powder is poured into the wound and a dry dressing is applied. If hemorrhage is sufficient to be of consequence, it is stopped by means of pressure bandages, if possible, or a tourniquet, if this is necessary. The patient should be kept warm and dry and given a hot drink and he should be given morphine and tetanus antitoxin. All fractures of the long bones and wounds of the joints are splinted, if possible, before the patient is put in an ambulance and sent back to the field hospital. If the patient is in a state of surgical shock or of impending shock and if he is seriously injured, every effort should be made to get him back to the field hospital with as little delay as possible.

Treatment at the Field Hospital.—On arrival at the field hospital the patient is subjected to a brief examination and is classified and the subsequent treatment is outlined. It is the duty of the examining physician to decide whether or not the patient is in a condition of shock and whether or not he is fit for operative treatment and whether or not this is indicated. Slightly wounded patients may be treated in the dressing station or may need no immediate treatment, this having been administered at the field dressing station. If the patient is in a state of severe shock, he should not be sent to the operating room immediately, but he should be given appropriate treatment for shock, as noted in preceding sections, and, if indicated, he should then be taken to the operating room as soon as he has reacted sufficiently from the shock to permit operative treatment.

It is to be noted that soldiers wounded in battle may be exhausted mentally and physically and debilitated by cold and exposure before they are wounded. Consequently, shock is more apt to be present than in a group of similar injuries in civil life. In addition there is another type of shock caused by the blast of high explosives, and this must be looked for, especially in bomb casualties.

Likewise, virulent infections are more apt to be present in the wounds of soldiers in battle, because they may not have had an opportunity to bathe for some time and their clothes may be dirty. This is especially true of lower extremity and buttocks wounds.

This sorting out of the wounded *(tirage)* requires considerable surgical judgment and should not be entrusted to an inexperienced medical officer, as the decisions made in the receiving room at a time when large numbers of wounded are being brought to a field hospital may make considerable difference not only in the mortality of the patient, but also in the effectiveness of the surgical teams who are working in the hospital. In addition to determining the general condition of the patient and whether or not operative treatment or shock treatment is indicated or necessary, he should also check for the presence of a tourniquet and determine how long it has been on and he should determine whether or not the patient has had tetanus antitoxin and, if this has not been administered, it should be administered. If the patients are suitable for operation, they are then sent directly to the operating room as fast as the operating room can take care of them or sent to the x-ray room where they are x-rayed or fluoroscoped for the presence of foreign bodies and fractures, and if such are present, their position is noted on the skin in two planes and they are then sent directly to the operating room. Care is taken to move severely injured patients as little as possible and the splints and dressings are not removed until the patient is on the operating table and usually not until he is under the anesthetic.

Chemotherapy.—Systemic and local chemotherapy with penicillin and the sulfonamides is used intensively, as described in the preceding section on compound fractures.

The Anesthetic.—This will depend a good deal upon the choice of the surgeon in charge of the particular hospital. In the past, ether has been the most generally used anesthetic. However, it is possible that in the presence of war intravenous anesthesia with pentothal sodium or some similar preparation will be used. Not only can this be transported easily, but in the hands of one skilled in its use it is relatively safe, and when it is used, considerable time can be saved between operations as the patient goes to sleep almost instantly and awakens very quickly after the anesthetic is stopped.

On the operating table the dressings applied at the field dressing station are removed, and the type of treatment is then decided. Certain wounds caused by high velocity bullets, such as machine gun bullets and rifle bullets, as a rule do not need to be débrided. In such wounds the margins of the wound should be excised under local or general anesthesia after the skin has been painted with a skin antiseptic. Sulfonamide powder should be implanted in the wound, and it should be covered with petrolatum gauze and a dry dressing and the fracture, if present, should be reduced and immobilized just as though it were a simple fracture.

On the other hand, large wounds from shell fragments, bombs, hand grenades and other projectiles which are traveling at relatively slow speed and which consist of large or irregular fragments nearly always carry infectious material with them into the tissues. These irregular missiles frequently damage the tissues widely and sometimes carry a portion of the patient's clothing into the tissues. All such wounds demand débridement or incision and drainage, depending upon whether they are in the contaminated or infected stage. The presence or absence of missiles in the tissues and the condition of the bone will have been determined and noted at the x-ray examination, and this knowledge will have been conveyed to the operating surgeon so that he has a rough idea of what he will encounter.

What has been said above about the necessity of débridement or drainage of all wounds due to shell or bomb fragments must be modified because many of the modern air bombs break into small fragments which travel at high velocity and cause wounds similar to those of rifle or machine gun bullets and these need not be débrided.

In patients with multiple wounds the number of wounds may be so great that débridement or even superficial excision of all wounds is not practical. This is especially true in instances where a patient has been sprayed with small fragments from a high explosive bomb. Such a patient may contain many small foreign bodies. These foreign bodies will probably do no harm and no attempt should be made to remove those which are buried in the tissues. Common sense should be the guide in treating patients with multiple injuries, and the surgeon should consider the patient as a whole rather than concentrate his attention on one or two specific injuries.

Preparation of the Skin.—Either scrubbing with soap and water followed by alcohol and ether and a skin antiseptic (one of the mercurial tinctures, such as merthiolate, mercresin, or metaphen, or weak tincture of iodine) or the dry method of painting the skin antiseptic on the unwashed skin, either with or without shaving, may be used. In times of stress when large numbers of wounded are to be treated, it is obvious that the wet method which is time consuming will not be used, nor will the limbs be shaved, but will simply be painted thoroughly with whatever skin antiseptic is at hand and is being used in that particular hospital.

The Operation of Débridement.—The limb is then straightened and draped and traction is made to steady the limb. The skin edges are excised, usually removing not more than one-fourth of an inch of the skin around the margins of the wound. If the skin adjacent to the wound is burned deeply, this charred area is excised. If there are a wound of entry and a wound of exit, the skin edges from both wounds are excised at this stage. Usually the wound of exit will be larger than the wound of entry. The knife and forceps used in excising the skin edges are then discarded.

Enlargement and Exploration of the Wound.—It is nearly always necessary to enlarge the wound in order that its depth may be adequately explored. For this reason incisions are made at its upper and lower borders in the long axis of the limb, and these are extended as far as is necessary to permit examination of the deeper structures. The primary incision for enlargement of the wound extends through the skin and the superficial and deep fascia to the muscle. Blood vessels of consequence are clamped where they are encountered, but only the larger vessels are tied off, usually with 0 plain catgut or finer catgut, if this is available. The wound edges are now retracted gently, the traumatized and devitalized margins of the subcutaneous tissue and fascia around the wound are excised, and this is then retracted and the deep fascia is incised transversely to expose the underlying muscles. Any foreign bodies encountered are removed as they are seen. The devitalized margins of the muscles which are more or less macerated and discolored are excised until only healthy muscle is left in the wound. Muscle which does not bleed or which does not retract when pinched is excised with a sharp knife or with scissors. If necessary the enlargement of the wound through the fascia is carried down through the muscle in order to explore the depths of the wound and to determine the condition of the bone, but when possible this is done through intermuscular planes.

Treatment of the Bone.—Fragments of bone which are completely detached, or so nearly detached from the surrounding soft tissue that their blood supply appears to be inadequate, are removed. Large fragments which have a periosteal attachment and blood supply deemed sufficient to keep the bone viable are usually left in situ, because it is important to avoid complete loss of continuity of the bone if this can be preserved with safety. The ends of the bone which are grossly soiled are excised with rongeurs or bone-cutting forceps. The ends of the bone are then lifted up and a further search is made for foreign bodies and also any devitalized tissue found in the depths of the wound is excised. It is desirable to remove all foreign bodies, but it is not absolutely necessary and the surgeon should not devote a great deal of time to searching for small foreign bodies which may be buried in the tissues adjacent to the wound. Likewise, he should not extend the wound widely through healthy tissue in order to remove a missile which may have fractured the bone and then traveled some distance through healthy tissue before coming to rest. The important thing is to excise devitalized tissues, remove foreign bodies from the wound proper, and pack the wound open. This was true in the last world war and is even more true today when we have strong reinforcements in the form of penicillin and sulfonamides in our war against infection.

The wound of entrance is now enlarged slightly and this, too, is explored, but not to the extent that the larger wound of exit is explored. Its margins are excised, and fascial and muscle walls are excised in order that as little devitalized tissue be left as possible. If a tourniquet has been used, it is now removed. The wound is now dried as thoroughly as possible. The hemostats are removed, and bleeding points which persist are tied with fine catgut. The wound is irrigated thoroughly with normal saline and is then sprinkled generously with one of the sulfonamides.

Chemotherapy.—The sulfonamide used may be either sulfathiazole, sulfadiazine, sulfanilamide, or a mixture of sulfanilamide and sulfathiazole. We prefer the mixture of equal parts of sulfanilamide and sulfathiazole. The sulfanilamide is more soluble and will be present in the wounds in a higher concentration and should penetrate the surrounding tissues more deeply. Consequently, it should be more effective against streptococci. Sulfathiazole, on the other hand, will remain in the wound longer and is more effective against staphylococci and the bacteria which cause gas gangrene. The status of sulfadiazine and its effect when implanted locally have not yet been determined. However, it is even less soluble than is sulfathiazole. Any of these chemicals can be used in the wound and will not interfere with the healing of the wound, nor will the amount used be toxic to the patient or to the tissues. This is especially true in wounds which are left open and packed with vaseline gauze and from which a considerable portion of the implanted drug will be drained out with the secretions from the wound. Penicillin (250 units per c.c.) may be used locally and instilled two or more times daily through a small rubber tube incorporated in the dressing and led out through the cast. In such wounds an excess amount of the drug should be implanted. It is possible that gramicidin (derived from soil bacilli) or penicillin (from molds) may be effective when implanted locally in wounds. If so, they can be used instead of or in combination with the sulfonamides.

Treatment of Nerves, Blood Vessels and Tendons.—Nerves, blood vessels, and tendons which are severed by the bullet or projectile, or are almost severed, should have the devitalized ends excised, care being taken not to remove any more tissue than is necessary. The severed ends may then be left to retract, and this is the safer procedure from the standpoint of sepsis, or they may be brought together with one or two strands of fine, plain catgut, as this may make subsequent repair more easy or unnecessary in the case of muscles and tendons and tends to contribute to the ultimate restoration of function of the extremity. Whether or not these tissues are brought together will depend upon the judgment of the surgeon and on the condition of the wound. If the wound is relatively fresh and the tissues are in good condition, they can be brought together with impunity, especially if one of the sulfonamide compounds is implanted in the wound. On the other hand, in a wound ten or twelve hours old which contains considerable devitalized tissue, it is probably wiser not to attempt to repair any nerves, tendons, or muscles.

Reduction of the Fracture.—The fracture is now reduced, usually by direct traction and manipulation, and the ends of the bones are opposed under direct vision. In certain instances it may be advisable to reshape the ends of the fragments in order to make the reduction more stable. In many instances, however, the fracture will be comminuted, and the ends of the bone will be oblique and stable reduction of the fragments will not be possible. The question arises as to whether or not one should use internal fixation.

In civilian life internal fixation is advised in compound fractures which have been operated upon before bacteria have invaded the tissues and which have been adequately débrided because the use of stainless steel or vitallium plates, screws, and wires and the sulfonamides render this relatively safe. In war injuries, on the other hand, internal fixation is not advised except under unusual conditions. However, it is permissible to transfix each fragment with a stainless steel pin or wire of sufficient length to project out from the side of the limb for about two inches and this can be incorporated in the plaster-of-Paris cast and will maintain length and aid in maintaining the position of the fragments. If it is decided that transfixion and immobilization by the two-pin method are to be used, this can be done at this time. The pins or wires are drilled or driven through the bone well away from the wound or may be placed through other bones in the extremity if necessary. If the fracture is being operated upon on a fracture table or fracture machine in which the limb is held by transfixion with pins and the fracture reduced, these pins are incorporated in the plaster-of-Paris cast.

After the pins are in place, the wound is again inspected, again rendered dry, and more sulfonamide powder is sprinkled in the wound, if this is thought to be indicated. The wound is then packed relatively loosely with petrolatum gauze and a dry sterile dressing is placed over the wound and a plaster-of-Paris cast is applied. This cast may be of the skin-tight variety or it may be applied over a moderate amount of cotton sheet wadding or other padding, depending upon the choice of the surgeon. If the surgeon is skilled in using plaster-of-Paris and can apply a skin-tight plaster with reasonable skill, this affords more complete immobilization. On the other hand, if he is not skillful in the use of this type of plaster, the patient may suffer considerable discomfort from pressure aside from the discomfort incident to his wound, and it is advisable to use some padding. It is important to remember that the cast should immobilize the joints above and below the injury; that is, for an ankle fracture the knee joint should be immobilized and for a fracture involving the knee joint or thigh the patient should be immobilized in a plaster-of-Paris spica cast.

It is advisable to draw a rough outline of the fracture and note the date of the operation on the damp cast.

Treatment of Wounds of Joints.—If the wound involves the joint, this should be opened widely at the time of the incision of the skin and fascia, and the joint should be thoroughly explored. Loose fragments of bone and any foreign material present in the joint should be removed. Any soiled bone exposed in the wound should be excised. The joint may or may not be irrigated with salt solution, depending upon the choice of the surgeon. In most instances we advise thorough washing out of the joint cavity with normal saline. The wound should then be dried and the joint cavity sprinkled liberally with one of the sulfonamide drugs, and the wound should be treated just as described above in the case of fractures not involving joints. The petrolatum gauze packing should extend down to the joint cavity. In some instances the synovial membrane can be closed with fine catgut. In wounds which are not very recent or which are in questionable condition, the joint should be left open. As a rule, no attempt should be made to suture the capsule or ligaments exposed in the wounds and severed. The joint should be immobilized in a plaster-of-Paris cast as described above.

Treatment of Wounds in Which Infection Is Present.—In the preceding section we considered wounds which were not definitely infected. These wounds may be five or six hours old, or they may be fifteen or twenty or more hours old. The presence or absence of infection in such wounds depends upon the general condition of the patient, the nature and severity of the wound, the type of organisms which were implanted in the wound at the time of the injury, and whether or not one of the sulfonamide compounds was placed in the wound shortly after the injury, as well as upon the elapsed time.

Whether or not the wound is infected can be determined by the surgeon when he examines the wound after the dressing has been removed. If the tissues are red, hot, and edematous and if pus is present in the wound, there is no question but that infection is present. In such instances and in instances where the wound is not relatively clean, the operation is not one of débridement, but the treatment is drainage followed by chemotherapy and immobilization. Unless they are necrotic or burned, the wound edges are not excised after the skin has been painted with a skin antiseptic, as described in preceding paragraphs. The wound is enlarged in the long axis of the limb by incisions through the fascia, and the deep fascia is cut transversely and the depths of the wound are gently explored. All visible foreign material is removed. Obviously necrotic tissue is excised, but no attempt is made to remove all damaged or infected tissue. Deep pockets of the wound are opened. The granulating margins or walls of the wound are not excised as these are nature's attempt to form a barrier against the spread of the infection. Loose particles of bone are removed, and the wound is then washed out thoroughly with normal saline and sprinkled generously with one of the sulfonamide compounds and packed loosely with petrolatum gauze. The skin around the wound is covered with petrolatum gauze or zinc oxide ointment because the purulent discharge from the wound will tend to macerate the skin and cause blistering and burning pain. A rather voluminous dressing is placed over the petrolatum packing, and the limb is then encased in a plaster-of-Paris cast. This is usually a cast over padding. Transfixion pins and fixation incorporated in the cast may or may not be used. If the pins can be placed in parts of the limb not involved in the infection, they may be driven or drilled through the bone without danger of spreading the infection and the added immobilization which they afford more than compensates for the slight increase in this danger. If the main blood vessels of the limb are occluded or destroyed, amputation is necessary.

Treatment at the Base Hospital.—Most of the above patients will be evacuated to the base hospital before the original plaster cast which was placed on the limb at the time of the operation for débridement and reduction of the fracture has been removed. Under favorable conditions these patients should be kept in the evacuation hospital until the danger of a spreading infection is over and it is relatively safe to send them back to the base. The time involved will vary with the seriousness of the wound, the general condition of the patient, and whether or not the wound was infected when it was operated upon and the virulence of the infection. On the other hand, military necessity may demand immediate evacuation, and the patient may reach the base hospital a day or so after operation.

In the great majority of instances in which the wound has been operated upon while it was in a state of contamination rather than infection, the convalescence will be uninterrupted. The pain will not be excessive and the patient will not have more than two degrees of fever, and his general condition will continue to improve rather than deteriorate. The presence of infection is suggested by an increase in temperature, increase in the pulse rate, and above all by a throbbing pain in the limb, and when this occurs, it calls for inspection of the tissues around the wound. This entails the cutting of a large window in the cast or removal of the cast. If the tissues are found to be tense, red, and tender, it is advisable to remove the packing and to explore the wound and it may be necessary to provide more adequate drainage or in certain instances where there is a fulminating infection to operate for gas gangrene or to amputate, as noted in a preceding section on the treatment of gas gangrene.

At the base hospital the original dressing and plaster-of-Paris cast are not disturbed until about three weeks or longer after the operation, unless there is some reason for doing so. It is to be noted that inspection of the wound exposes the wound to contamination with virulent bacteria and to the danger of a loss in the position of the fragments. It is now believed that secondary or cross infection of wounds in the wards of military hospitals is an important cause of the prolonged disability which is so frequent in these patients. Usually the reason for the early application of a new cast is that the cast is soiled and has a bad odor. This is especially true in the case of wounds which were infected. Wounds which are not infected tend to heal slowly beneath the petrolatum gauze dressing without much discharge or odor.

At the end of three weeks, or about that time, the original dressing should be removed, and as a rule in the case of fractures, especially those with transfixion pins, this can be done through a window in the cast and will not necessitate a change of cast which will disturb the position of the fragments. After the window is cut in the cast, the dressing and petrolatum gauze are removed and the surface of the wound is wiped gently with a dry sponge. It is then sprinkled liberally with sulfonamide powder, packed with petrolatum gauze and covered with a dry dressing. This is bound firmly to the leg, either with or without replacement of the window. The local pressure tends to prevent local edema with bulging of the tissues through the window in the plaster and aids rather than interferes with healing. This dressing is repeated at weekly, or longer, intervals when indicated until the wound is healed. The cast is changed when this is necessary.

The subsequent course of these patients in the base hospital does not differ greatly from that of similar patients in civilian life, except that they are not worried about hospital bills and time lost from work.

Also in Army hospitals transfusions of whole blood are used more freely in convalescent compound fractures and the restoration of the patient's blood to an approximately normal condition is accomplished more quickly.

Early Secondary Suture.—As was noted in the preceding section on compound fractures, it is often possible to suture the débrided wound during the period from the fourth to the tenth day after the débridement without excising the wound. This is similar to the excision and secondary suture of soft tissue wounds as practiced during and after the last war. It is now done early and without bacteriological control and with the aid of chemotherapy. It is done on wounds which look clean clinically, but are not necessarily sterile on culture. The use of this method on compound fractures is more limited than in soft tissue wounds, but it is successful in selected cases and even may be combined with internal fixation in fractures where external fixation or traction is not satisfactory. The screws or plates may be applied through the wound or through a separate incision and the increased immobilization lessens the danger of infection and thus counterbalances the increased danger caused by leaving the metal in the tissues. These wounds should be sutured and drained for a few days after the operation. The rubber tissue drain may be inserted through a separate stab incision. The early secondary suture of a compound fracture without or with internal fixation should be followed by adequate external fixation and chemotherapy.

CHAPTER VIII

DISLOCATIONS

Compared to fractures, dislocations are relatively rare injuries; they occur only about one-tenth as frequently as do fractures. It is also of interest to note that about 85 per cent of all dislocations occur in the upper extremity and about 50 per cent occur at the shoulder joint.

Causes.—The predisposing causes are instability of the joint and exposure of the joint to injury. This is particularly illustrated in the shoulder in which the large head of the humerus fits into the small glenoid and is held in place largely by the tone of the surrounding muscles. This joint also occupies an exposed position where it is frequently subjected to trauma, both directly on the shoulder and indirectly by means of leverage of the upper extremity.

The determining cause is usually external violence which is in most instances applied in an indirect manner; that is, through leverage exerted on the distal portion of the extremity. In addition to primary dislocations we occasionally see recurrent or habitual dislocations. Most of these cases occur at the shoulder joint and the subject is treated in that section.

PATHOLOGY OF RECENT DISLOCATIONS

In a traumatic dislocation the articular surface of one of the bones entering into a joint is violently pushed or pulled away from its fellow and forced through the joint capsule and into the surrounding tissues where it comes to rest and is fixed by muscle spasm. It is obvious that not only must the capsule of the joint be ruptured to permit the passage of the articular surface of the dislocated bone, but also the ligaments of the joint must be ruptured to a variable degree and many of the muscles which control the joint are either stretched or torn. The degree of displacement and the extent of damage to the soft tissues vary directly with the severity of the dislocating force and with the size of the joint.

In addition to the damage to the capsule, ligaments, and muscles, fractures of the articular surfaces or of the bones in the vicinity may occur, and blood vessels and nerves in the vicinity may be torn or stretched or contused. The damage to the soft tissues and the extravasated blood cause swelling just as in fractures.

The progress of the displaced bone is eventually arrested by the untorn ligaments or muscles which are attached to it and by the soft parts which lie in its path. In cases of very severe violence, the end of the bone may be forced through the skin and a compound dislocation result. The primary displacement, as in fractures, is caused by the fracturing force, and eventual displacement is the result of tension of untorn ligaments and muscles, of gravity, and of the fracturing force.

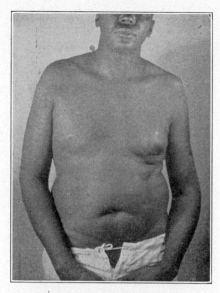

Fig. 181.—Anterior dislocation of the shoulder, subcoracoid. Note the typical posture of the upper extremity and the deformity of the shoulder. Treated by manipulative reduction, immobilization by strapping arm and forearm to the body with adhesive for three weeks. Good result.

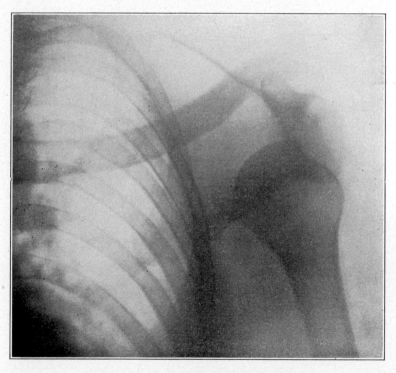

Fig. 182.—Roentgenogram of preceding.

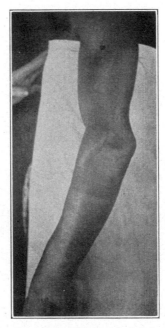

Fig. 183.—Posterior dislocation at the elbow with typical deformity. Treated by reduction and immobilization in moderate flexion for three weeks. Good result.

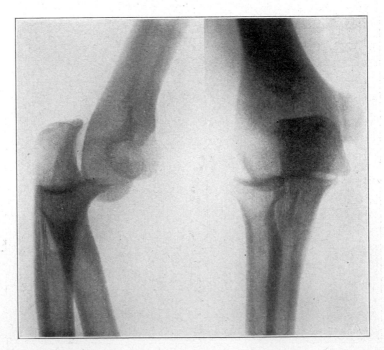

Fig. 184.—Roentgenogram of preceding case.

COMPLICATIONS OF DISLOCATIONS

In addition to the possible fracture of the involved bone or bones, complications of dislocations are practically the same as are those of fractures and are considered under the section on Complications of Fractures. It is important to mention old unreduced dislocations which are considered under the section on Injuries of the Shoulder.

REPAIR OF DISLOCATIONS

If the dislocation is reduced without excessive trauma and if the joint is immobilized, the extravasated blood will be absorbed and the tear in the capsule will heal by the formation of granulation tissue and a scar as does any other fibrous tissue. Eventually this scar will be covered by a layer of cells corresponding to those lining the rest of the joint. The ligaments and tendons also tend to heal by scar tissue, but if the immobilization be continued over too long a period, the ligaments and capsule tend to become shortened and considerable difficulty may be experienced in restoring normal motion in the joint.

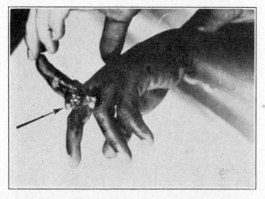

Fig. 185.—Compound fracture dislocation of the finger treated by débridement under local anesthetic, primary suture, and immobilization on a tongue depressor for fourteen days. Good result in nine weeks. No tendons were cut in this instance.

Tears in the muscles will heal and muscles which are torn off from their insertions also tend to heal by scar tissue. Any fractures incident to the dislocation heal in the normal manner if the fragments are approximated. In cases in which there has been extensive stripping up of the periosteum at the time of the dislocation, considerable new bone formation may occur during the process of healing and this may be so extensive as to interfere with movements of the joint. This is especially to be feared after severe dislocations at the elbow.

SIGNS AND SYMPTOMS OF DISLOCATIONS

The signs and symptoms of dislocations are similar to those of fractures. There is a history of an injury; if one is able to obtain an accurate description of just how the injury occurred, one is frequently able to predict the type of lesion which is to be found on physical examination. Particularly should one ask whether this is the first dislocation or whether there have been others at the same joint.

With the dislocation there is severe pain which may be described as sickening or nauseating in character. It may subside gradually after the injury, but tends to persist for an indefinite time until the dislocation is reduced. There may be paralysis or a tingling of the nerves. Loss of function may be present,

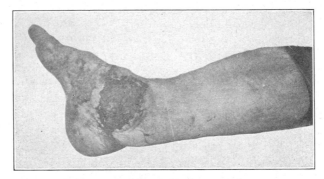

Fig. 186.—Compound fracture dislocation at the right ankle. Treated by open reduction, débridement with primary suture and immobilization in plaster-of-Paris cast for seven weeks. Walking with metal ankle support, ten weeks; no support, fourteen weeks. Good results.

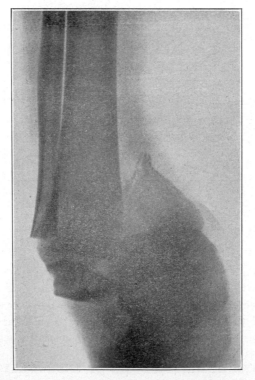

Fig. 187.—Roentgenogram of the preceding case.

and, as in a fracture, it may vary greatly in degree in different individuals even with the same lesion, and one occasionally sees a dislocation which has been present for some time in which considerable power and movement are present in the affected limb.

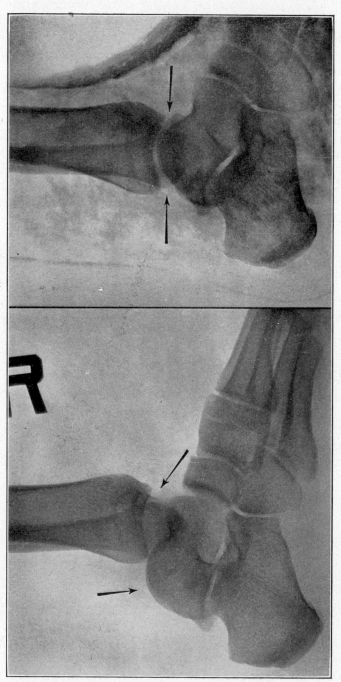

Fig. 188.—Posterior dislocation at the ankle before and after closed reduction.

Objective Symptoms

Deformity.—The pathognomonic signs of a dislocation are the identification of the articular end of the displaced bone in an abnormal position and the demonstration of its absence from its normal position. This can usually be accomplished by inspection and palpation. (Figs. 181, 182, 183, and 184.) In addition to the deformity due to the displacement of the articular end of the bone, there is also a deformity of the limb as a whole which is characteristic of the given dislocation. This fixation of the limb in an abnormal attitude is one of the most important points in the differential diagnosis between a dislocation and a fracture. Whereas in a fracture the limb can be moved freely and even false motion may be obtained, in a dislocation it will be found that the limb is fixed in some abnormal posture. There may be shortening or apparent lengthening of the limb, and if its axis be projected toward the dislocated joint, the axis will be found to run in an abnormal direction and not to pass through the articulation.

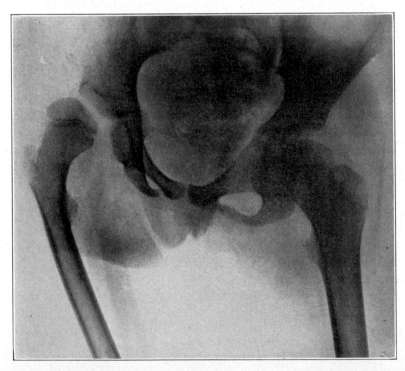

Fig. 189.—Pathologic subluxation of the right hip, the result of poliomyelitis at an earlier period. Note the coxa vara, atrophy of the femur and of the right side of the pelvis.

In dislocations which are the result of severe injuries with extensive tearing of the ligaments and muscles, the characteristic posture may be absent because the structures which maintain it have been torn; in such a case the picture is more that of a fracture than of a dislocation. It is also characteristic of a dislocation that once the dislocation is reduced, there is little tendency for it to recur, whereas in a fracture the opposite is true. In compound dislocations the articular surface of one or both bones may be exposed. (Figs. 185, 186, and 187.)

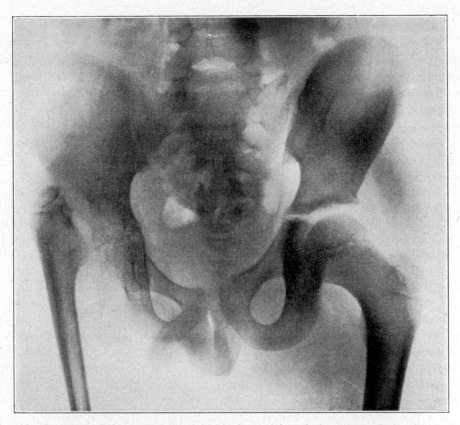

Fig. 190.—Pathologic dislocation of the right hip due to tuberculosis with wandering acetabulum.

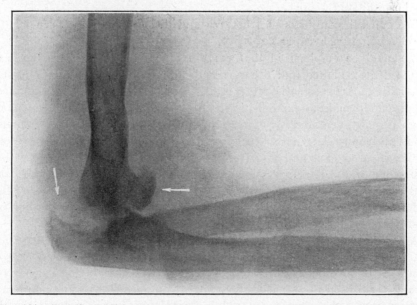

Fig. 191.—Pathologic dislocation of the elbow due to previous pyogenic infection.

PATHOLOGIC DISLOCATIONS

A dislocation is said to be pathologic when it is not the result of severe external violence. The dislocation may occur spontaneously from the distention of the capsule by fluid as in an acute arthritis, or it may be the result of muscular action or of some slight injury.

The Causes of Pathologic Dislocations.—1. Distention of the capsule by fluid as in acute arthritis. 2. Extensive muscular paralysis as in poliomyelitis. 3. Erosion of the bones due to infectious disease, neoplasms, or a neurotrophic arthropathy (Charcot joint). (Figs. 188, 189 and 190.)

DIAGNOSIS OF FRACTURES AND DISLOCATIONS

The diagnosis of the various types of fractures and dislocations is given in detail in the special part of the book and should be looked for there, as only some general principles will be mentioned here. Probably the most important point in the diagnosis is that the surgeon who examines the patient after an injury bear in mind the fact that his responsibility does not end with the diagnosis of any particular fracture or dislocation, but that it is his duty to determine as soon as possible the nature and extent of all the injuries which the patient may have suffered. At the present time when so many fractures and dislocations are the result of automobile accidents, frequently multiple lesions are present, and there is always the possibility that the surgeon in examining the patient may direct his entire attention to some major injury as, for instance, a fracture of the femur, and fail to recognize some other injury, perhaps a fracture of one of the metatarsal bones of the foot, which may be called to his attention some days later by the patient or by some other member of the hospital staff.

The general symptoms of fractures and dislocations have been mentioned in the preceding paragraphs.

It should be emphasized that certain fractures and dislocations can be recognized at a glance and others can be diagnosed only after painstaking x-ray studies. After as satisfactory a history as possible has been obtained, the surgeon should make a careful physical examination of the injured part and a rough physical examination of the entire body, unless it is quite obvious that there is no injury elsewhere. In examining the limb the clothing is removed from the injured part and also from the opposite limb in order that the two may be compared. The surgeon then inspects the limb carefully from various angles and notes the presence of any visible deformity; the results of this inspection are checked by various measurements to determine whether or not shortening or other deformities exist.

After the inspection and measurements are completed, the injured area is palpated with gentleness in order that as little pain as possible be caused the patient. It is possible to palpate the extremity without moving it to any great degree. In addition to palpation for general tenderness and for point or fracture tenderness, the surgeon should in certain instances palpate deeply for the deformity. It is well to remember that in cases with extensive swelling, if slow steady pressure be made in the swollen area, the edema over a bony prominence can be pushed aside into the surrounding tissues and with relatively little pain to the patient it will then be possible to palpate bony prominences and arrive at a diagnosis. In most instances the rough diagnosis can be made by inspection and palpation.

In certain instances it is advisable to manipulate the limb and attempt to demonstrate abnormal mobility or crepitus or at least to elicit pain at the site of the injury. If abnormal mobility or crepitus or pain are not elicited after gentle manipulations, and if more severe manipulations cause pain, the surgeon should not attempt to complete his diagnosis by physical examination, but should obtain an x-ray picture in order to determine the exact nature of the lesion.

It is also very important that an x-ray picture be obtained when the history and symptoms point to a fracture which the surgeon is unable to demonstrate by physical examination; otherwise certain fractures without much displacement will be missed.

In the examination of compound fractures it is important not to contaminate the wound any more than is necessary during the examination. A significant point in the diagnosis of a compound fracture in the presence of a laceration of the skin is that if the bone is broken and if the break in the bone communicates with the external wound, the external wound will bleed more freely than will a similar wound not connected with a fracture. One is often able to see small fat globules, which come from the bone marrow, floating in the blood in the wound.

CHAPTER IX

THE WORKMEN'S COMPENSATION LAW AFFECTING FRACTURE CASES

It is now recognized that an employer has a certain amount of responsibility for his workmen, and most of the states have workmen's compensation laws. Employers operating under these laws are required to carry compensation insurance or to carry their own insurance and post a suitable bond for the protection of their employees. As a result of this general adoption of workmen's compensation, a large percentage of the traumatic and industrial surgery is practiced under the rules laid down by the laws in the various states. Consequently, surgeons who are interested in this type of work should familiarize themselves with the laws under which they practice. In this chapter we shall give a brief general discussion of the system.

HISTORY OF WORKMEN'S COMPENSATION*

"The present compensation statutes were born of an evolution of the law respecting an employer's liability to an employee for injuries sustained while at work. In its earliest development this branch of the law was classified under what was known as Master and Servant liability. While the term Master and Servant continued in general use, and even today is not uncommon, later practice used the term Employers' Liability when referring to this branch of the law. Today in practically every state the law defining the workmen's rights, however, and the employers' liability for injury or death, is governed by workmen's compensation statutes.

"A brief review of the history and effect of master and servant law and employers' liability statutes seems necessary for an intelligent appreciation and understanding of the present laws.

"In its earliest development our industry was, of course, quite primitive and simple. The 'master,' more often than not, worked alongside or in close supervision over his 'servants.' The means employed to complete a given task were also free from complexities; only the ordinary tools and implements were used and these were all manually employed or operated. In this state of development of our industry the master, in the event of injury, was held liable for damages to the servant only in the event that the master had been negligent in some regard, which negligence had proximately caused the injury. Even in cases where the master's negligence may have proximately caused the injury there were, nevertheless, certain effective defenses which might be interposed to a claim for damages. One of these was that of 'contributory negligence.' If it could be shown that the servant had also been guilty of negligence which proximately contributed to his injury, then there could be

---

*Mr. W. H. Beatty, of Birmingham, Alabama, has kindly contributed these paragraphs on History of Workmen's Compensation to this chapter.

no recovery. Another defense, effectively interposed to injury claims, was that of 'assumption of risk.' There are risks inherent in almost every employment. Could it be shown that the servants' injuries resulted from such a risk, there could be no recovery, since in undertaking the employment the servant was held to have assumed the risk of injury from these inherent hazards. Yet a third defense was available to the master; this is what is known as the 'fellow servant rule.' If the master could show that the servant's injury resulted from the negligence of some fellow servant of the injured man, then there could be no recovery. So, in the early development of industry, it resulted that a man could rarely receive payment for injuries sustained while at work. The master's denial of negligence or the interposition of some one or all of the defenses enumerated presented barriers almost impossible to overcome save in the most flagrant cases.

"As industry became more widespread and complex following the industrial revolution, wherein it might be said that industry passed from the tool age into the machine age, injuries to workmen mounted fearfully. In situations where risks of employment existed that could not be foreseen even by the employer or master it was a harsh rule that denied recovery to a workman because he was held to have assumed a risk of which he did not know or could not reasonably have suspected. Also, in situations where numerous employees were engaged in a given enterprise, one might be injured by the negligence of a fellow employee whom he had never seen or with whom he never came in contact; hence, the harshness of a rule which precluded recovery because of the negligence of a 'fellow servant' became apparent. These rules, viz., 'assumption of risk,' 'fellow servant' doctrine, 'contributory negligence,' had developed under the old English Common Law. They were not rules declared by specific legislative enactments, but which had grown up from judicial precedent; that is, from a line of decisions by the Courts rendered as specific cases were presented for a decision. It might be said that they resulted from custom quite like the familiar laws of the highway, such as the custom of approaching vehicles to drive to the right, or to the left in some countries, arise from long-established custom.

"As the harshness of these old common law doctrines became apparent, when applied to later day circumstances and conditions, the legislatures of our various states modified their effect somewhat in a series of enactments known as 'Employers Liability Statutes.' Even under these modifying statutes, however, there could be no recovery for injuries unless it could be shown that the employer or some one for whose acts he was *legally* responsible had been guilty of some negligent act or omission which proximately caused the workmen's injury. Negligence on the part of the employer remained the primary basis for recovery under the Employers Liability Acts as it had been prerequisite to recovery under the old common law rules.

"However, even the most remedial of the Employers Liability Statutes were found to be inadequate as industry expanded. Accidents, resulting in grievous injury or death, were found to be inevitable in a highly developed industrial community. An employee and his dependents suffered just as greatly whether the injury resulted from a negligent act of the employer or not. If there could be no recovery from the employer, the employee and his dependents, during the period of disability, were cast upon the charity of relatives, friends, or the public for their sustenance. Out of this realization of the utter inadequacy of the existing laws, the theory underlying the workmen's compensation laws was evolved.

"The workmen's compensation laws indemnify the workman for injuries sustained which arise out of and in the course of his employment, irrespective of whether the injuries resulted from any negligent act or omission of the employer. Also the defenses of contributory negligence, assumption of risk, and fellow servant rules were abolished. Recovery is denied where the accident occurs in line and scope of one's employment only in the case of willful misconduct or some unlawful act on the part of the injured employee. The Compensation Statutes attempt to substitute for the old laws a system based upon a higher conception of man's obligation to his fellow men. The payment for injuries is regarded as a legitimate item in the cost of production to be charged to the industry and liquidated in steps ending with consumption by the public. The burden, therefore, in theory is ultimately cast upon the community generally.

"Under the former laws it will be appreciated, employers had no great concern, from a purely economic viewpoint, in the severity of the injuries or their proper treatment by the medical profession. Of greater concern was his escape from any liability whatever by the interposition of the various defenses to the employee's action. With the advent of the Workmen's Compensation Law this aspect of industrial accidents was radically changed. When the law declared every accidental injury to be compensable, it became of vital economic importance to the employer to see that the injured man received proper medical and surgical treatment to the end that the severity of the disability and hence, the economic loss, might be minimized. Employers, therefore, sought the most skilled physicians and surgeons to treat their employees. Also, physical examinations of applicants for employment were demanded and in some instances periodical physical examination of employees was demanded in order to safeguard against economic loss which might result from the employment or continued service of the physically unfit.

"While the general theory underlying all compensation laws is the same in all states, they vary greatly in their specific provisions. The practitioner should secure a copy of the Acts of the State of his residence and devote a few hours to study of its particular provisions."

WHAT IS WORKMEN'S COMPENSATION?

The compensation paid an injured employee is not to be construed as payment of damages for injuries suffered while at work, but is a continuation of wages during time lost as a result of an accident while at work, or in the case of a permanent disability, is compensation for the reduction in earning power. In other words, an employer is not punished because a workman mashes his finger; but if a workman mashes his finger while at work, it is the duty of the employer to furnish medical attention and to see that the workman does not suffer undue financial loss as a result of the accident. This is true even when the accident was due to negligence on the part of the injured workman, provided the negligence did not amount to willful violation of reasonable rules of the employer, or the violation of some statutory rule, or constitute willful misconduct.

The compensation is paid weekly during the period of temporary total and partial disability and is usually paid in a lump sum at the time of settlement in case of total or partial permanent disability. The maximum amount of weekly compensation varies from twelve to twenty-five dollars in the different states and is usually figured as a designated percentage, usually from one-half to two-thirds of the weekly wage, but not to exceed the maximum as stated under the law.

Temporary partial disability is usually compensated for by the payment of from one-half to two-thirds of the difference between what the workman earned before the injury and what he is able to earn by diligent effort, but the amount paid is not to exceed the maximum as provided under the law.

Permanent total or partial disability is paid for on the basis of specific schedules for the total loss of a part of the body. These schedules vary in different states. As will be mentioned below, in the great majority of cases the permanent disability is not complete and the percentage of loss must be decided by the state workmen's compensation board or other tribunal designated by statute which administers the law and decides questions where a difference of opinion arises between the workman and the employer. In Table III* there is given a condensed list of the number of weeks for which compensation for specified injuries is payable in the several states.

NOTIFICATION OF ACCIDENT

When a workman is injured while at work he should notify his employer or his representative and it then becomes the duty of the employer to provide medical attention. It frequently happens, however, that the workman fails to do this and later selects and consults his own physician. In such an instance the physician should send the employer a complete report of the accident if he expects the employer to pay for his services. If compensation is to be paid to the workman, the employer must be notified within a certain time (five to thirty days in the various states). If the employer has been notified, a claim for compensation must be made within a certain time (six months to two years); otherwise it is outlawed. However, decisions in practically all states have held that if the employer has actual knowledge of the accidental injury to the employee, the giving of notice by the injured employee is not required as a condition precedent to his right to compensation payments or medical benefits.

CHOICE OF PHYSICIAN

The laws in the various states differ on this point and the physician should familiarize himself with the law in the state in which he practices. The law may provide that the physician be selected by the employer or by the employee at the expense of either one or the other. It may also grant authority to either the employer or the employee to change physicians.

In states where the employee is authorized to select the physician, difficulty sometimes arises, because when the physician sends in his report of the accident to the employer, the patient is then ordered to discontinue the previous treatment and to report to a physician or to any one of a panel of physicians furnished by the employer or by his insurance company. In such an instance the employee's physician should withdraw from the case.

PHYSICIAN'S RECORDS IN COMPENSATION CASES

Since physicians are notoriously careless about keeping accurate records and especially on patients who are seen outside a hospital, it is in order that this chapter include a word of warning on this subject. Ordinarily clinical office records are kept to enable the physician to study and follow his patients and to enable the physician to make his charges for the services rendered. In compensation cases the physician should bear in mind the fact that every such case is a potential subject for dispute before the industrial compensation board and that at some future time he may be called upon to testify as to (1) the extent and nature of the patient's injuries; (2) whether or not they could have resulted from the accident as claimed by the patient; (3) the treatment rendered the patient; (4) the progress made by the patient while under treatment; and (5) the end-result and the amount of permanent disability which has resulted from the accident. In addition, he is usually called upon by the employer or his carrier for a preliminary and a final report; in cases of prolonged disability he may be asked for reports on the progress of the patient.

Consequently, the physician's record should include a brief account of the accident, the chief symptoms, the subjective and objective findings and the diagnosis as made at the first examination, the treatment rendered with dates, important changes in the patient's condition and the final diagnosis and the end-result. Such a record need not be voluminous, but is a great help when called upon some months later.

Too great an emphasis cannot be laid upon the necessity of keeping accurate and detailed records of treatments given the patient in cases where the circumstances of the injury are such that controversy over its nature and extent may subsequently arise. The physician or surgeon who has not kept accurate records usually makes a most pitiable spectacle when called to court as a witness and is taken over by adverse counsel for rigid cross examination. The uncertainty of his answers casts a good deal of reflection even upon his professional fitness. On the other hand, when the medical or surgical witness has his accurate and full records to refresh his memory he can then testify confidently and positively and usually is able to leave the stand after a most favorable and indelible impression upon the court, jury and spectators.

The fracture record as recommended by the American College of Surgeons (Figs. 192 and 193) meets all requirements, but is more elaborate than the average surgeon will keep.

THE X-RAY IN COMPENSATION CASES

The roentgenograms are part of the physician's record and should be preserved by him. Due to the fact that disputes may arise as to the extent and nature of the injury, the physician should be more liberal in ordering x-ray pictures in compensation cases than in ordinary civil practice. In ordinary practice he should order x-ray pictures when he is in doubt as to the diagnosis and when the x-ray may help him in the treatment, but in compensation cases he should in many instances order x-ray pictures as a matter of record even when he is quite sure of the diagnosis and when the x-ray will not help him in the treatment.

ESTIMATION OF DISABILITY

As will be seen from Table III the workmen's compensation laws of the various states provide a specific compensation for the total loss of a specific portion of an extremity, but make no provision for partial loss or impairment of the function of a given member. As in the great majority of instances there is a partial loss of or an impairment in the function of the injured part, it is necessary for compensation commissions to determine what this loss or impairment amounts to in order that the compensation allowed may be fair to the workman and to the employer.

In the determination of the end-result it should be remembered that in many fractures, and this is especially true of joint fractures, it is at least a year after the injury before the end-result is obtained and in occasional fractures such as those of the hip in the elderly, the final result may not be obtained until several years after the injury. With this in mind the surgeon should hesitate to rate a patient as permanently or partially disabled a few months after the injury because in our experience many patients, especially those with joint injuries, continue to improve slowly and almost imperceptibly over a period of several months. This improvement occurs without physiotherapy and without active treatment, but as a result of the normal use of the part by the patient.

For this reason all workmen's compensation acts and all accident insurance policies should include provision for temporary partial disability; otherwise the surgeon who is treating a case is faced with the problem of classifying a patient as totally disabled during a considerable period of his convalescence when the man would be much better off if he were working at some lighter work, or of cutting him off entirely from his compensation. Not infrequently we see patients who loaf along for several months doing no work because they cannot return to their regular occupations and consequently are not permitted to do any work without losing their compensation entirely. This method is expensive both to the insurance company and to the workman, and tends to encourage the type of case where a cure is accomplished by an early settlement.

Attempts to reduce permanent partial disability in injuries of the extremities to a percentage basis are usually based upon loss of motion in the various joints. If such a system is used the loss of motion should be accu-

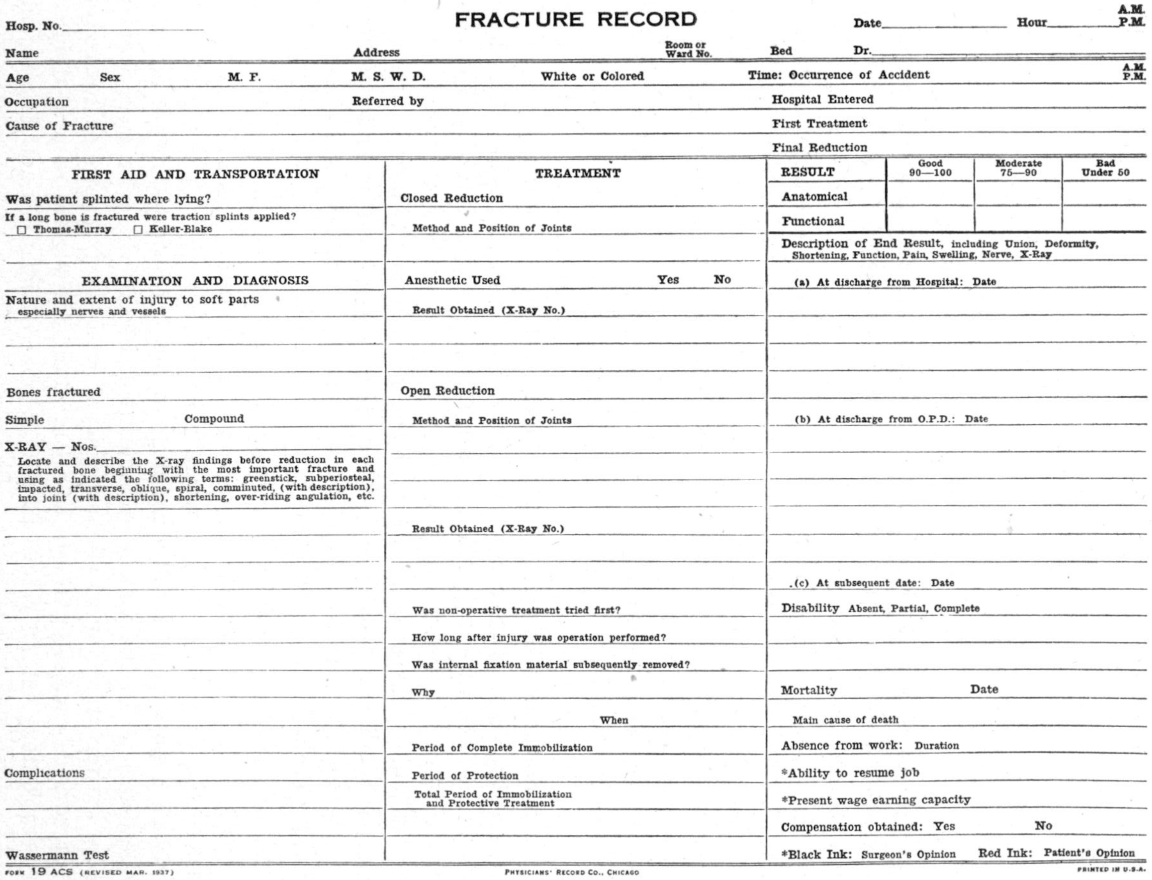

FRACTURE RECORD

Hosp. No. _____   Date _____   Hour _____ A.M. P.M.

Name _____   Address _____   M. S. W. D.   White or Colored   Room or Ward No.   Bed _____   Dr. _____

Age   Sex   M. F.   Occupation   Referred by _____   Time: Occurrence of Accident _____ A.M. P.M.

Cause of Fracture

Hospital Entered

First Treatment

Final Reduction

FIRST AID AND TRANSPORTATION

Was patient splinted where lying?

If a long bone is fractured were traction splints applied?
□ Thomas-Murray   □ Keller-Blake

TREATMENT

Closed Reduction

Method and Position of Joints

Anesthetic Used   Yes   No

Result Obtained (X-Ray No.)

EXAMINATION AND DIAGNOSIS

Nature and extent of injury to soft parts especially nerves and vessels

Open Reduction

Method and Position of Joints

Bones fractured

Simple   Compound

Result Obtained (X-Ray No.)

X-RAY — Nos.
Locate and describe the X-ray findings before reduction in each fractured bone beginning with the most important fracture and using as indicated the following terms: greenstick, subperiosteal, impacted, transverse, oblique, spiral, comminuted, (with description), into joint (with description), shortening, over-riding angulation, etc.

Was non-operative treatment tried first?

How long after injury was operation performed?

Was internal fixation material subsequently removed?

Why   When

Period of Complete Immobilization

Complications

Period of Protection

Total Period of Immobilization and Protective Treatment

Wassermann Test

RESULT	Good 90—100	Moderate 75—90	Bad Under 50
Anatomical			
Functional			

Description of End Result, including Union, Deformity, Shortening, Function, Pain, Swelling, Nerve, X-Ray

(a) At discharge from Hospital: Date

(b) At discharge from O.P.D.: Date

(c) At subsequent date: Date

Disability Absent, Partial, Complete

Mortality   Date

Main cause of death

Absence from work: Duration

*Ability to resume job

*Present wage earning capacity

Compensation obtained: Yes   No

*Black Ink: Surgeon's Opinion   Red Ink: Patient's Opinion

Form 19 ACS (Revised Mar. 1937)

Physicians' Record Co., Chicago

Printed in U.S.A.

Fig. 192.—Fracture record as recommended by the American College of Surgeons.

Family History

Past History

Present Injury

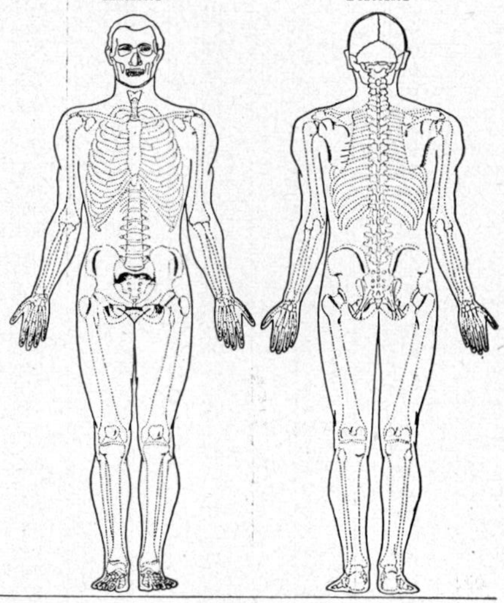

(Details of Treatment, Operation, etc.)

Anterior

Posterior

FORM 19 ACS (REVISED MAR. 1937)

Fig. 193.—Same, reverse side.

TABLE III.—NUMBER OF WEEKS FOR WHICH COMPENSATION IS PAYABLE FOR SPECIFIED INJURIES IN THE SEVERAL STATES

STATE	PERMANENT TOTAL DISABILITY	LOSS OF: ARM AT SHOULDER	HAND	THUMB	INDEX FINGER	MIDDLE FINGER	RING FINGER	LITTLE FINGER	LEG AT HIP	FOOT	GREAT TOE	OTHER TOES	SIGHT OF ONE EYE	HEARING, ONE EAR	HEARING, BOTH EARS
Alabama	550	200	150	60	45	30	20	15	175	125	30	10	100	--	150
Arizona	Life	260	217	65	39	30	22	17	217	173	30	11	108	87	260
Arkansas	450	200	150	60	35	30	20	15	175	125	30	10	100	40	150
Colorado	Life	208	104	50	26	18	11	13	208	104	26	11	104	35	139
Connecticut	520	225	175	60	38	30	25	20	208	156	38	13	208	52	156
Delaware	475	194	158	60	35	30	20	15	194	135	30	10	113		
District of Columbia	*	280	212	51	28	18	17	7	248	173	26	8	140	52	200
Florida	350	200	150	60	35	35	20	15	175	125	30	10	100	40	150
Georgia	350	200	150	30	35	30	20	15	175	125	30	10	100	--	150
Hawaii	312	312	244	60	46	30	25	15	288	205	38	16	128	60	312
Idaho	Life	240	200	70	40	40	30	20	180	125	30	12	120	35	115
Illinois	Life	225	170	70	40	35	25	20	190	135	35	12	120	50	125
Indiana	500	250	200	60	40	35	30	20	200	150	60	10-30	150	--	200
Iowa	400	225	150	40	30	25	20	15	200	125	25	15	100	50	150
Kansas	416	210	150	60	37	30	20	15	200	125	30	10	110	25	100
Kentucky	416	200	150	60	45	30	20	15	200	125	30	10	100		
Louisiana	400	200	150	50	30	20	20	20	175	125	20	10	100		
Maine	500	150	125	50	30	25	18	15	150	125	25	10	100		
Maryland	To $6000*	200	150	50	30	25	20	15	175	150	25	10	100	50	100
Massachusetts	*	75	75	40	20	12	12	12	50	50	12	12	50		
Michigan	500	200	150	60	35	30	20	15	175	125	30	10	100		
Minnesota	To $10,000*	200	175	60	35	30	20	15	200	150	30	10	100	52	156
Missouri	Life	232	175	60	45	35	35	22	207	150	40	14	108	44	168
Montana	500	200	150	60	30	30	20	12	200	125	30	12	100	20	120
Nebraska	Life	225	175	60	35	30	20	15	215	150	30	10	125	50	100
Nevada	Life	260	217	65	39	30	22	17	217	173	30	11	108	87	260
New Hampshire	300	170	140	40	25	20	15	10	170	120	20	8	100	42	170
New Jersey	400-Life	230	175	65	40	30	20	15	175	125	30	10	100	40	160
New Mexico	550	180	110	50	25	20	15	12	180	100	30	12	110	35	135
New York	Life	312	244	75	46	30	25	15	288	205	38	16	160	60	150
North Carolina	400	200	150	60	35	30	20	15	175	125	30	10	100	70	150
North Dakota	To $15,000*	234	195	45	29¼	24¾	15¾	13½	234	136½	19½	7½	100	29¼	156
Ohio	Life	215	165	60	35	30	20	15	190	140	30	10	125		
Oklahoma	500	250	200	60	35	30	20	15	175	150	30	10	100	--	To $3000
Pennsylvania	500	215	175	60	35	30	20	15	215	150	--	--	125	--	150
Puerto Rico	340	300	200	50	35	25	25	15	250	160	25	15	125	25	200
Rhode Island	1000	100	80	50	36	26	20	18	100	80	30	10	80		
South Carolina	500	200	150	60	35	30	20	15	175	125	30	10	100	70	150
South Dakota	To $3000*	200	150	50	35	30	20	15	160	125	30	10	100		
Tennessee	550	200	150	60	35	30	20	15	175	125	30	10	100	--	150
Texas	401	200	150	60	45	30	21	15	200	125	30	10	100	--	150
U. S. (Longshoremen)	*	280	212	51	28	18	17	7	248	173	26	8	140	52	200
Utah	Life	200	150	60	30	30	20	12	180	125	30	12	100		
Vermont	260	170	140	40	25	20	15	10	170	120	20	8	100	42½	170
Virginia	500	200	150	60	35	30	20	15	175	125	30	10	100	50	
West Virginia	Life	240	200	80	40	28	20	20	240	140	40	16	132		
Wisconsin	Life	500	333⅓	125	50	40	30	30	500	250	83⅓	25	250	50	333⅓
Maximum	Life	500	333⅓	125	50	40	35	30	500	250	83⅓	30	250	87	333⅓
Minimum	260	75	75	30	20	12	11	7	50	50	12	7½	50	20	100

*During disability.

From *Accidental Injuries* by Henry H. Kessler (Lea and Febiger, Philadelphia, 1941).

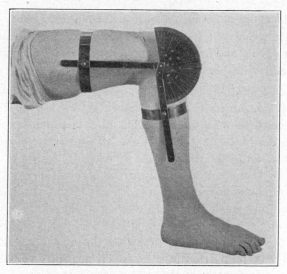

Fig. 194.—Conwell's goniometer as used in measuring range of motion at the knee joint. (Geo. P. Pilling & Son Co., Philadelphia.)

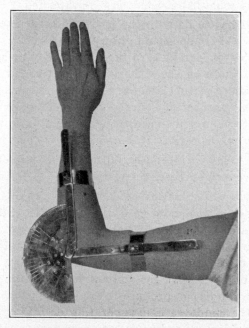

Fig. 195.—Conwell's goniometer as used in measuring the range of motion at the elbow.

rately determined by a goniometer (Figs. 194 and 195). Our objection to such a schedule is that it is based almost entirely upon limitation of motion and does not take into consideration other factors such as the cosmetic result, anatomic result, economic result, and functional result, nor does it consider disabilities due to spine injuries which we all know are the bugbear of industrial surgeons, and which, even with a negative x-ray, are frequently and rightly awarded the maximum of temporary total disability by the workmen's compensation board.

In most states there is no compensation for a poor cosmetic result. However, in many instances in the treatment of fractures, for instance in the treatment of fracture of the clavicle in a female, the cosmetic result is one of the most important considerations.

In regard to the anatomic result, the most important consideration is that normal alignment of the limb be maintained. The second is that approximately normal length be maintained. The third is that normal apposition of the fragments be maintained. All of these, of course, presume that the fracture unites by bone and that there is no permanent injury to the soft tissues which may add to the disability. Anatomic apposition of fragments is of relatively little importance in fractures of the femur and of the humerus end of the fibula and frequently in fractures of the tibia, since it makes no difference in the end-result whether the bones are end on or whether there is 50 per cent or even less apposition, provided the alignment is good and firm union is obtained. In joint fractures, however, accurate reduction is of great importance, since it is necessary that the normal contour of the joint be restored and that the ligaments heal, especially in weight-bearing joints; otherwise permanent functional impairment may be expected.

Economic result has to do with the patient's return to his original occupation. If not, is he able to do some lighter type of work? If he has returned to his original occupation, can he earn the same salary as before and turn out the same volume of work in the same length of time or does he require a longer period for doing the same amount of work? Does he earn as much per day working the same number of hours as he did before or does he earn more or less? If forced to change his occupation, is he able to perform some type of work in which he can as readily obtain regular work as he did before?

The functional result is the most difficult of all to estimate, since it involves both objective and subjective factors.

The principal subjective factors are—does the patient have pain or is he comfortable, and does he tire more easily than before? Information on these points must be obtained from the patient. Where there is doubt as to the patient's veracity, we believe that it is up to the compensation board to accept the patient's statements unless the insurance company or employer can produce evidence to prove that the patient has performed work which he states he is unable to do or can produce reliable medical testimony which will tend to show that the employee is exaggerating or faking his symptoms. In other words, pain and lack of endurance are very real causes of disability and must be taken into consideration even in the presence of joints with a normal range of movement and in the presence of very minor objective findings. We have frequently seen patients who were not subjects of compensation after a fracture of one condyle of the tibia or of an injury to the shoulder with no positive x-ray findings who suffered prolonged disability of a high degree in the involved extremity.

Another important factor in estimating functional disability is power in the involved muscles. It makes little difference to the patient whether or not the joints have the normal range of movement if there is insufficient muscle power present to render these movements useful. In the lower extremity a patient may be able to walk normally without a limp, but he may be totally unable to carry a weight of fifty or one hundred pounds over any considerable distance. Such a man has real disability.

The range of movement in the involved joints is at the present time the consideration of prime importance in the rating of most disabilities. We believe that the importance of this is considerably overrated. As a matter of fact, we not infrequently advise ankylosis of a joint which is unstable or painful in order to eliminate pain and instability and restore function in an extremity by rendering this joint stiff.

This is particularly true of the subastragaloid joint after fractures of the os calcis and of the shoulder joint after fractures at the upper end of the humerus and occasionally of the knee and wrist joints. In addition to freedom from pain, power in the muscles and range of movement in the joints, the patient must be able to control and coordinate the movements.

Finally, the possibility of lessening the permanent disability by operative intervention must be considered. For instance, a workman with a torn and displaced semilunar cartilage in the knee may be restored to full earning capacity if the offending cartilage is removed, but he may suffer considerable permanent disability if it is not removed. If the workman refuses to submit to the operation, this should be taken into consideration in making the award. The same is true of a nonunion which may be cured by a successful operation. In many instances reconstructive surgery offers the probability of restoration of function to a very considerable degree. If expert treatment is available and if the employer is willing to furnish such treatment, it is up to the employee to submit to the treatment and to cooperate in the efforts directed toward his ultimate rehabilitation.

From what has been said above, it is obvious that the estimation of the patient's disability after an injury is a very complicated procedure, one which it is practically impossible to reduce to a mathematical basis, and one which will always require the most delicate judgment of an impartial and experienced observer who draws his conclusions from observations and history which he believes to be reliable, and that such an estimate should not be given without a careful history and physical examination.

CHAPTER X

MEDICOLEGAL ASPECTS OF FRACTURE CASES

With the transfer of a large percentage of accident cases to the jurisdiction of the workmen's compensation boards there was a decrease in the number of lawsuits against employers. Partly as a result of this and partly as a result of the depression, actions against physicians for malpractice have become increasingly frequent. It is advisable, therefore, for every physician to have some definite knowledge concerning his rights and responsibilities before the law under which he practices. A very large percentage of the actions for malpractice are brought by patients who have been treated for fractures. This is probably due to the fact that the results obtained in the treatment of fractures are usually obvious and speak for themselves, and it is the tendency of the patient and of his lawyer to decide that what they believe to be a poor result is caused by improper treatment and to make this decision without due consideration of the gravity of the lesion that the patient had in the beginning. Consequently, we believe that a modern book on fractures should include a brief chapter on the medicolegal aspects of these conditions. It is not intended to make this a textbook on medical jurisprudence, but merely to point out some of the salient features of the subject as applied to fractures.

RELATION OF DOCTOR TO PATIENT

In the beginning it is advisable to define briefly the relationship and duty of the doctor to the patient. When a doctor is consulted by a patient the doctor is a free agent and may or may not undertake to treat the patient. If, however, he chooses to accept the patient then a definite contract is expressed or implied, and in the practice of medicine it is almost always implied. This contract begins at the time that the doctor accepts the patient for treatment and it ends when the doctor is discharged by the patient or when the doctor discharges the patient, either because he does not choose to treat him any longer or because he is no longer in need of treatment. It is to be noted, however, that if the patient is in need of further treatment, the doctor cannot quit the case until he has given ample opportunity to the patient to obtain further medical treatment if this is needed. In other words, after the implied contract begins, the patient is a free agent and can terminate it at any time, but the doctor must continue to treat the patient and can terminate the contract only after due notice. If the doctor merely drops the case without giving the patient notice, then the case is considered to have been abandoned by the doctor; if the patient suffers injury as a result of this abandonment, the doctor may be held liable for the injury.

THE DOCTOR'S DUTY TO THE PATIENT

In a decision in the Pike case the New York Court of Appeals laid down the law as follows: "A physician and surgeon, by taking charge of a case, impliedly represents that he possesses, and the law places upon him the duty of possessing, that reasonable degree of learning and skill that is ordinarily possessed by physicians and surgeons in the locality where he practices, and which is ordinarily regarded by those conversant with the employment as necessary to qualify him to engage in the business of practicing medicine and surgery. Upon consenting to treat a patient, it becomes his duty to use reasonable care and diligence in the exercise of his skill and the application of his learning to accomplish the purpose for which he was employed. He is under the further obligation to use his best judgment in exercising his skill and applying his knowledge." This decision was rendered thirty-seven years ago and is still extensively quoted. The court further emphasized that the physician must keep abreast of the times and that he must not depart from methods in general use.

In the above statement the word *reasonable* as applied to the degree of learning and skill and the word *ordinarily* as applied to the learning and skill of physicians in the locality where he practices are important. It is thus evident that the law does not demand that a doctor possess a high degree of skill, but it is presumed that a doctor in a city will possess a higher degree of skill than will one who practices in a rural community. Likewise, the word *reasonable* is applied to the care and diligence which the physician should exert in the exercise of his skill and in the application of his learning. It is, therefore, not obligatory that he exert extreme care and diligence. As regards judgment, it is demanded that the physician use his best judgment. In regard to keeping abreast with the times, it is further demanded that the physician familiarize himself with the important and accepted developments in medical science. On the other hand, the law requires him to use approved methods in general use. The purpose of this last requirement is to protect the patient from being used by the doctor as an experimental animal. On the other hand, it is obvious that if a physician never uses anything except approved methods in general use, the science of clinical medicine cannot advance. Consequently, this last provision should be modified to the extent that a physician may use methods of his own devising or new methods devised by others which offer a reasonable hope of benefiting the patient and which apparently will not result in any harm to the patient.

It is further to be noted that the doctor is responsible for the acts of his assistants, nurses and internes if they are in his direct employ. On the other hand, he is not responsible for the acts of assistants, nurses and internes who are not paid by him, but are employees of a hospital or of some other institution. If the doctor sends another physician to substitute for him on a case, he is not responsible for the acts of the substitute, because it is assumed that the substitute acts not as an agent, but as a principal. Where two or more doctors treat the same patient one is not responsible for the negligent acts of the other unless he in some way participates in them or unless he observes or should have observed wrongful acts by the other physician and should have stopped or prevented them.

OPERATIONS WITHOUT CONSENT

"The courts hold that every human being has a right to determine what shall be done with his own body; and a surgeon who performs an operation without his patient's consent commits an assault for which he is liable in damages. . . . . . . This is true except in cases of emergency where the patient is unconscious and where it is necessary to operate before consent can be obtained." The rule which permits a surgeon to operate without his consent where the life or limb of a patient is in danger applies even in the case of a minor. On the other hand, if the operation is not a bona fide emergency the surgeon should not operate upon a minor without the consent of the parents or of whoever is legally responsible for the child. In cases of emergency it is, of course, wise to obtain a consultation before operating upon either an adult or a minor in order that the surgeon may produce evidence if necessary that the emergency really existed. The most frequent violations of the above rule are in cases where the patient is under an anesthetic for one operation and the surgeon then discovers some other condition which should be treated and proceeds to perform the indicated operation. Under such circumstances the surgeon should not proceed to the second operation without the patient's consent unless it is absolutely necessary and failure to do so would endanger the patient's life.

X-RAYS

In the section on the Use of the X-ray in the Diagnosis of Fractures we have made the statement that a large percentage of fractures can be adequately diagnosed and even treated without the aid of an x-ray and that satisfactory results may be obtained in such cases. On the other hand, the x-ray is now a well-recognized diagnostic method and where its use is indicated and is neglected and a bad result ensues the doctor may be held liable for not having used it. This means that the x-ray should be used in all doubtful cases, and if the physician wishes to be absolutely on the safe side, he should accept no fracture case for treatment unless the patient will agree to have x-ray pictures made before treatment is instituted and at intervals until the final result is attained. This interpretation of the law, however, puts an undue financial burden on the patient and we do not think that it is just. In other words, we think that the physician should be permitted to use his own judgment as to whether or not x-ray pictures are necessary in a given case. If he errs in judgment he cannot be held liable if he has used his own best judgment.

THE MEDICAL WITNESS

Not infrequently the surgeon who has treated fractures, dislocations and sprains will be called as a medical witness to testify before a court or commission. He will be called to inform the court or jury as to the nature and extent of the patient's injuries and disabilities. Before reporting to court in answer to subpoena, the doctor should review carefully the hospital charts and the x-rays and thoroughly refresh himself on the case. Should the doctor delay this review of the case until he has reached court or possibly placed upon the witness stand and continually have to refer to the charts and pictures before attempting to answer questions, he must expect to be thoroughly embarrassed by his hesitant answers and the close cross questioning of counsel. The doctor who presumes to be examined as a witness, yet who must constantly refer to his records to answer the simplest questions makes a sorry spectacle of himself and leaves a bad impression, not only as to his capacity as a witness, but also as to his professional fitness. Only a few minutes' review of the charts and pictures before reporting to the court will enable the medical witness to testify resolutely and confidently and without hesitancy. He will thus be of the greatest assistance to the court, commission or jury in their efforts to ascertain the truth concerning the patient's injuries and disabilities. Moreover, this ability to answer questions promptly and accurately cannot fail to impress those before whom the testimony is given.

DUTIES OF THE PATIENT TO THE PHYSICIAN

The patient is also a party to the implied contract and should obey the orders and follow the directions of his physician. If he fails to do so, he cannot hold the physician responsible for the consequences of his own disobedience or neglect. In other words, if the patient does not cooperate with his physician, he is guilty of contributory negligence. "It is further held that the patient must exercise ordinary prudence: that is, such prudence as could reasonably be expected from an ordinary prudent patient under similar circumstances." For instance, if a patient who is being treated for a fracture removes the splint or cast without the consent of the attending physician and the fragments become displaced and a poor result ensues, the physician is not responsible for the poor result.

THE ACTION FOR MALPRACTICE

An action for malpractice is based on the presumption that the physician has failed to perform one or more of the duties which evolved upon him as a result of his implied contract with the patient and that as a result of this the patient has suffered injury. Lawyers speak of it as "an action in tort." A tort is a civil wrong founded upon some breach of duty. In order to establish malpractice the plaintiff must prove that (1) he was actually treated by the physician; (2) that the physician departed from some duty owed by him to the patient; and (3) that that departure from duty caused the injury or bad result complained of. In regard to the relationship of the physician to the patient, this is rarely a question of dispute, but it should be emphasized that this relationship is not dependent upon the payment of a fee by the patient. The physician is just as responsible to his charity patients as he is to the patients who pay a regular fee.

In most malpractice cases it is claimed either that the doctor did not use care and diligence in his professional work or that he departed from approved methods in general use. The mere fact that the doctor is licensed to practice medicine establishes the fact that he possesses the requisite skill and it is very difficult to prove that he did not use his best judgment.

One weakness in most malpractice cases is that the plaintiff does not attempt to prove or finds it impossible to prove by expert testimony that the injury which he claims to have suffered was actually caused by negligence or malpractice on the part of his physician and that it could not have been caused by anything else. It is the tendency of the plaintiff to exhibit his poor result and expect it to speak for itself. The difficulty is that a poor result is not evidence of malpractice and the courts have held that a physician cannot guarantee the results of his treatment to a patient. In case of dispute the burden evolves on the plaintiff to prove that the proper and approved practice was not followed and that as a result of failure to follow the proper and approved practice the patient was injured. It is recognized that only other physicians are qualified to state what the proper and approved practice would be in a given case and that only other physicians are qualified to determine whether or not the result complained of is due to failure on the part of the physician to follow the approved method.

For these reasons it is evident that expert testimony is usually necessary to prove that malpractice really occurred. There are certain exceptions to the above rule and these are cases such as those in which a surgeon has operated upon the wrong limb or other part of the body; or in which the patient has been injured or burned while under treatment, as in the large number of cases in recent years in which patients have been injured by diathermy given by a doctor's assistant.

In addition to the suit for malpractice, which, as we have seen, is an action based upon the alleged negligence of the physician, there is a possibility that a suit may be brought upon the theory of a breach of contract; that is, the patient may claim that the doctor had contracted to cure and correct some condition and had failed to effect the cure or correct the condition. This type of action, however, is rare. Nevertheless, care should be taken never to guarantee or contract to effect a cure or remedy a disability. A doctor should only undertake to use his best judgment and professional skill and should a patient demand more, the doctor would do well to refuse treatment of the case.

DEFENSE IN MALPRACTICE SUITS

When faced with a suit for malpractice the physician should immediately notify his insurance company and follow their instructions or if he does not carry liability insurance he should employ a competent lawyer and enter a general denial of the charges. Especially should he deny that he had failed to use proper and approved methods and that anything which he has done or failed to do has resulted in causing the injury complained of.

In addition to the above there are certain other defenses: (1) One of these is that the matter has been considered previously and has been decided in the doctor's favor in a previous trial. In other words, if the doctor has sued and has recovered for his professional services, the judgment in his favor in that action is a bar to a later suit by the patient for malpractice. This is not true in every state. (2) Contributory Negligence: If it can be proved that negligence on the part of the patient or on the part of others who were acting for him caused or contributed to the injury complained of, then the doctor is not responsible. On the other hand, if both the patient and the physician have been negligent and the injuries due to the respective negligence of each can be separated, then the doctor is liable for the results of his own negligence. (3) The Statute of Limitation: Statutes of limitation are laws, the object of which is to prevent fraudulent and stale claims from springing up after long lapses of time and after the evidence appertaining to the facts has been obscured or lost. In other words, a suit for malpractice must be instituted within a certain time after the alleged injury; otherwise it is thrown out of court. This time varies from one to three years in the various states and the statute begins to run at the time that the injury or negligent act was committed. That is, it runs in favor of the physician rather than from the time of the consequential injury. For instance, if a needle is left in a wound and is discovered five years later, the statute of limitations may be used in defense, because it begins to run at the time of the operation rather than at the time of the discovery of the needle.

However, it is important to note that in the case of minors who are claiming malpractice, the statute of limitations does not begin to run until the minor becomes of age. This is especially important in epiphyseal injuries which may be followed by disturbance of growth. Such disturbances are not common, but they may occur even after perfect reduction and it should be generally recognized that they are not necessarily caused by improper treatment and are not a basis for action for malpractice.

AVOIDANCE OF MALPRACTICE SUITS

The little book *Courts and Doctors* by Lloyd Paul Stryker* contains an excellent chapter on avoiding being sued and states that "the best way to avoid a lawsuit is not to deserve one." Of course there will be instances in which a surgeon who treats fractures will be sued or threatened with a suit when he does not deserve one, because an unfortunate result may occur in spite of excellent treatment. However, in such instances the jury should render a verdict in favor of the defendant.

If the following suggestions are adhered to the number of malpractice suits in fracture cases should be materially reduced:

1. Examine the patient carefully and arrive at a satisfactory diagnosis.

2. Be sure that you have not overlooked a fracture in some other part of the body while concentrating on the most obvious injury.

3. If in doubt as to the diagnosis, procure a satisfactory roentgenogram before beginning treatment.

4. Having arrived at a satisfactory diagnosis decide whether you are qualified to treat the condition by methods which are accepted in modern surgical practice.

---

*The Macmillan Company, New York, 1932.

5. If you cannot arrive at a satisfactory diagnosis or if you do not feel qualified to treat the condition in a manner which will be to the best interest of the patient, ask for a consultant or refer the patient to an expert if one is available.

6. If you treat many fractures procure the necessary equipment.

7. Hospitalize the patient if necessary.

8. If a general anesthetic is necessary, procure the services of a skilled anesthetist if possible, and see that the patient has a general physical examination before the anesthetic is administered.

9. If the fracture is compound or if lacerations are present give anti-tetanic serum.

10. Keep adequate records.

11. If roentgenograms are indicated during the course of the treatment, insist that these be obtained.

12. If a plaster cast or constricting bandage has been applied to an extremity, inspect the limb within four to eight hours or obtain a reliable report upon the condition of the circulation in the limb, and if it is not satisfactory do not hesitate to loosen the constricting dressing.

13. If things are not going well ask for a consultant.

14. If the patient or his family wish a consultant do not object, but try to obtain the services of a man whose opinion you respect.

15. Do not abandon the patient; that is, do not discontinue your services without notifying the patient and giving him an opportunity to secure the services of another physician.

16. Strive for functional rather than anatomic results.

17. Do not use x-ray or diathermy unless you are qualified to do so.

18. If the patient insists upon leaving the hospital against advice, have him sign a statement to that effect.

19. Do not undertake operations upon bones or joints unless qualified and equipped to perform them satisfactorily.

20. In such operations be especially careful of your asepsis and be sure that no foreign body is unintentionally left in the wound.

21. If you treat many fractures keep informed as to the modern methods of treatment.

22. Be honest with your patient and his family and conservative in your prognosis. Do not make rash promises which you may not be able to fulfill.

23. Be charitable to your colleagues and do not be too quick to condemn the methods used or results obtained by another physician. Such criticism may lead to a malpractice suit and you may be called upon to prove statements which were thoughtlessly made and which the evidence may show to have been unjust or untrue.

PART II

DIAGNOSIS AND TREATMENT OF SPECIFIC INJURIES

CHAPTER XI

FRACTURES OF THE SKULL AND BRAIN TRAUMA

BY EDGAR F. FINCHER, M.D.
ATLANTA, GA.

In this chapter on fractures of the skull and the associated injuries of the intracranial structures, an attempt will be made to discuss this subject in a manner which will be most helpful to the general practitioner of medicine and surgery rather than those who specialize in neurologic surgery. In dealing with fractures of various bones of the body, the fracture *per se* usually assumes primary importance. This is particularly true of long bones of the skeletal system. Such complications as involvement of the surrounding structures naturally assume importance according to their character and degree. In dealing with fractures of the skull, the reverse is the situation, and a treatise on fractures of the skull resolves itself largely into a discussion of *brain trauma*. The character and degree of damage which may be done to the intracranial structures are of prime importance, and the fracture itself in many cases may claim only a radiological interest. It is absolutely essential to think of injuries to the head in terms of *brain damage*. It is, however, of interest and importance to know whether or not the bone encasing the brain be broken, and if so, the type and degree of fracture. Any practical discussion of injuries to the head must take these facts into consideration. Attention will be given entirely to acute head injuries with or without skull fractures and no attempt will be made to discuss the late posttraumatic sequelae such as headaches, vertigo, nervousness, mental or character changes, epilepsy, etc., which sometimes develop following injuries to the brain.

The attempt to rewrite this chapter proved to be a futile task. The original manuscript so well covered the subject from a practical standpoint that only a revision* seemed all that was necessary. Entire sentences, paragraphs and even pages appear as they were in the original edition. Minor changes have been made in the grouping of the various types of head injuries. Sketches emphasizing some of the discussion in the text have been added. Radiologic reproductions have been included, illustrating some of the experiences gained from the study of skull fractures as correlated with the underlying intracranial damages. The operative treatment of the surgical cases has not been changed. The medical treatment as outlined for some of the grouping has been altered in keeping with the advances made, since the last edition, in chemotherapy and in the treatment of shock.

*This chapter was originally written by the late Dr. Charles E. Dowman.

There has been no time in civilization in which the occurrence of various types of injury in civil life has been so prevalent as it is today. The advent of rapid methods of transportation, particularly the automobile and improved highways, is unquestionably responsible for this increased incidence of traumatic conditions. Among the thousands of lives lost each year as a result of automobile accidents, the proportion dying from head injuries is astounding. An even larger number of head injuries without loss of life occurs. Such accidents not infrequently happen in locations remote from recognized medical centers and almost every practicing physician is called upon to treat one or more such injuries every year. It is often impractical to transport these patients hundreds of miles to such centers, and the burden of properly diagnosing and treating such cases may fall upon the shoulders of the physician living in the vicinity of the accident. A classification of the various types of cranial and intracranial injuries will be offered and a method of treatment which experience has proved most efficacious in each of the various groups will be discussed. In order to aid in the proper classification of the various types of injury the clinical phenomena which may occur in each of the various groups will be discussed. It is to be remembered that such a classification is not always clinically easy. It is also realized that in any large series there are some cases which do not fit into any of the various groups suggested. From a practical standpoint, however, it is best for the average physician to have something concrete on which to rely. From a large experience with the management of head injuries a classification, and the methods of treatment as herein submitted, has been applicable to the greater majority of cases that suffer injuries to the head.

There are some general considerations of head injuries that command attention before taking up the details of the classification and treatment of these cases. It is hoped that a review of these considerations will serve to stimulate more interest and help make the solutions of these problems easier.

FRACTURES OF THE SKULL

The skull is an irregular sphere. Just as a football when kicked may change its shape momentarily, so the skull as the result of some sudden impact will change its shape momentarily. Whether or not the skull is fractured as the result of a blow depends largely upon whether or not its normal degree of elasticity has been exceeded. Should the force be of small mass and great velocity, such as may be produced by a hammer, there may result a circumscribed depressed fracture. Should, on the other hand, the force be of great mass and moderate velocity, such as the head striking the ground, as when an individual is thrown from a vehicle, linear fractures in various regions may result. Such linear fractures may radiate from the point of impact, or as frequently happens, they may be more or less remote from the area receiving the blow. When on the side opposite to the area struck, the fracture is spoken of as *contrecoup*. A favorite site for such remote fractures is the so-called "base" of the skull. Two factors may explain this. In the first place the bones forming the base of the skull are of irregular degrees of thickness and therefore of a relatively low degree of elasticity. In the second place the base of the skull is supported on the upper end of the spinal column. A blow on the vault may drive the base of the skull against the spinal column with such force as to cause a bursting fracture radiating from this point of support. Another type of basilar fracture may be produced by a blow on the chin in such a manner as to transmit the impulse against the floor of the middle fossa with sufficient force to cause a fracture in this location.

Fractures of the base of the skull have usually a graver prognosis than linear fractures of the vault of the skull. This is due to the fact that the brain stem is more liable to injury when the base of the skull is fractured. Fractures of the base of the skull may produce paralyses of one or more of the cranial nerves. The sixth cranial nerve is the most commonly involved in brain stem damage, resulting in an inability to turn the eye outward. As a unilateral phenomenon this nerve may be peripherally injured; if bilateral paralyses, the damage is usually the result of damage to the nuclei in the brain stem and is accompanied by other ocular nerve palsies. The seventh nerve which controls facial movements is very commonly associated with injuries about the mastoid region and there follows a peripheral type of facial paralysis. It is not uncommon that the eighth cranial nerve is affected in basilar fractures and this is particularly true where there is sufficient force to rupture the ear drum, causing auditory canal hemorrhage. Ofttimes an impairment in hearing, vertigo and tinnitus persist as residuals where the auditory nerve has been injured. Rather often, permanent dysfunction follows the injuries to cranial nerves incurred in fractures to the base of the skull.

Linear fractures may communicate with one or more of the various accessory sinuses of the skull. When such fractures are so located as to involve the frontal and sphenoidal sinuses or the cribriform plate of the ethmoid bone, the danger of infection which may lead to meningitis or to brain abscess cannot be overestimated. Fractures involving the petrous portion of the temporal bone are frequently associated with bleeding from the ear, and the danger of a subsequent meningitis or brain infection is likewise a complication which may be feared.

The penetrating fractures are but manifestations of the localized injuries caused by a force of small mass and great velocity. A depressed fracture may be associated with an overlying laceration of the scalp. Such fractures are spoken of as *compound fractures* of the skull. The correct treatment of such compound fractures is all-essential, in order to eliminate the possibility of a subsequent infection which may lead to more serious complications than a simple wound infection.

It is evident from the foregoing that the fracture of the skull is an important consideration in head injuries, even though the treatment and prognosis are prompted by the damage to the intracranial contents.

Roentgen Ray Examination.—An x-ray examination of the skull is always desirable provided the patient's condition be such as to permit the necessary manipulations without jeopardy of the patient's life or physical condition. If the skull is fractured, the location and type of fracture are a matter of clinical importance. A fracture, for example, which extends across the meningeal vessels will cause one to watch carefully for evidence of epidural hemorrhage. A fracture extending into one or more of the accessory bony sinuses should cause one to anticipate a possible complicating meningitis or pneumocephalus. In depressed fractures, the x-ray examination is of particular value in determining the location and extent of the bone pathology. A depressed fracture over the lateral sinus, for example, should prepare one for a troublesome sinus hemorrhage at the time of operation. The absence of evidence of fracture should never warrant the dismissal of the case as one of trivial character. It has been emphasized that grave brain injury may occur where the degree of elasticity of the encasing skull has not been exceeded sufficiently to cause a fracture.

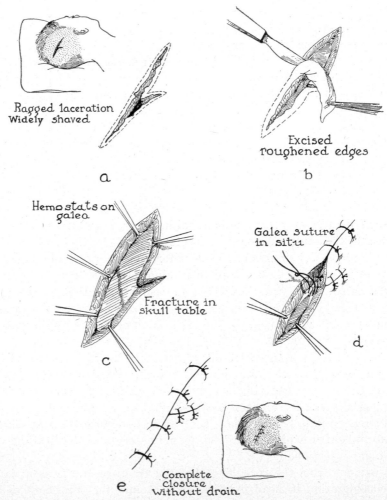

Ragged laceration
Widely shaved

a

Excised
roughened edges

b

Hemostats on
galea

Fracture in
skull table

c

Galea suture
in situ

d

Complete
closure
without drain

e

Fig. 196.—Suggestions for primary wound healing in scalp lacerations: Extensive shaving of the scalp about the wound; scrubbing of the wound and adjacent scalp briskly with sterile soap and water for not less than five minutes; selection of effective antiseptic preparations; sterile draping of the wound as meticulously as if it were an elective craniotomy; thorough débridement of all devitalized tissues; hemostasis by galea retraction; thorough inspection of the bone for any foreign debris or fracture damage; wound closure, without drainage, in two layers; removal of scalp sutures within forty-eight hours.

Proper technic should be insisted upon when an x-ray examination of the skull is made. The technical criteria of skull plates in cases of suspected fractures are much greater and more difficult than in cases where the long bones of the body have broken. Too many times the normal vascular or suture markings of the skull have been interpreted as fractures. These mistakes are usually the result of faulty technic. A flat lateral view of the skull is of little value. One should insist on true lateral stereoscopic films, preferably with first one side of the head to the plate and then the other. A single true antero-posterior position so as to show the foramen magnum as well as other basilar structures is sufficient, unless the frontal bone structures are suspected as being injured. Under such circumstances a true posteroanterior plate should be made. In about sixty per cent of adult skulls a calcified pineal shadow can be demonstrated on x-ray studies. In a true anteroposterior position this calcification normally occupies a midline position. A shift from this normal position is of pathologic significance and may be of great value in the presence of definite neurologic findings, whether there be a skull fracture or not. As was hinted in the beginning of this brief discussion, on roentgen ray examination the principal thing to be remembered is the patient's condition. There is no x-ray film that is more important than this consideration. A patient *in extremis* should not be moved for roentgen ray study; neither should any suspected case of brain injury be subjected to unwarranted risks simply for the sake of making such a laboratory examination.

INJURIES TO THE INTRACRANIAL STRUCTURES

The skull encases the brain with its membranes and blood vessels, and these structures lie snugly in their bony container. When there is a momentary alteration in the shape of the skull as the result of some sudden impact, the intra-cranial structures are simultaneously affected. Nature has provided certain fluid filled cavities within the brain called ventricles which act as a "water bed" for this delicate and highly organized structure. This provision of nature permits, within certain limits, the brain and associated structures to escape injury when the skull receives a blow of the usual limited intensity. Should, however, the force of impact exceed the so-called physiological limits, the intracranial structures will be "squeezed" (as it were) beyond the limit of normal range, with resulting lesions of varying degrees of severity and extent. These lesions may vary from scattered microscopic hemorrhages with rupture of nerve fibers to gross lacerations of the brain, torn blood vessels, and rup-tured membranes.

Martland[1] found small perivascular intracerebral hemorrhages in the brains of nine out of three hundred and nine persons who died from injuries to the head. These microscopic hemorrhages were in or near the corpora striata and were rarely or never in the cerebral cortex or in the cerebellum and brain stem. There were no fractures of the skull demonstrated in any of these nine cases. Martland suggests that the hemorrhages are the result of forces op-erating under the laws of hydrostatics. Such hemorrhages are explained by Cassasa[2] as due to sudden overfilling of the perivascular lymph spaces with cerebrospinal fluid, thus causing lacerations of the vessels by tearing the fine fibrillar attachment between the wall of the vessel and the brain tissue, in the Virchow-Robin's spaces. This is due to fluid from the surface of the brain being driven into the perivascular spaces. This explanation of "concussion" was further developed by Osnato and Giliverti.[3] Such hemorrhages may be followed by parenchymal changes which form a basis for postconcussion symptoms, such as headaches, vertigo, nervous and mental disorders, which are frequently referred to as "neuroses" because of the paucity of objective clinical signs. They propose the term "traumatic encephalitis" for such cases.

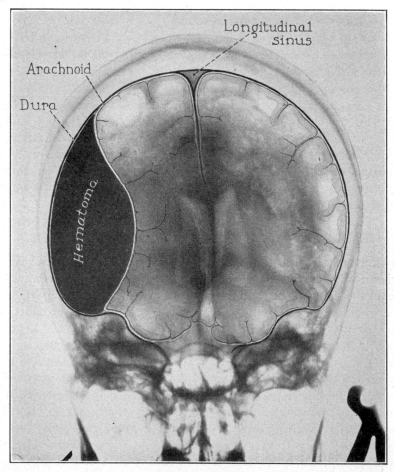

Fig. 197.—A composite ventriculographic sketch of the gross pathology of a chronic subdural hematoma. Such a condition as this may develop following a trivial head injury and the symptomatology be deferred many weeks or even months after the trauma.

The character of the applied force often modifies the pathologic findings. For example, in a circumscribed depressed fracture there may occur a localized area of brain contusion lying directly under the fractured area. A force of great mass and moderate velocity, on the other hand, may cause scattered and remote areas of contusion varying from lesions of microscopic proportions to gross lacerations. Such lesions may occur as the result of a severe blow even when the skull has not been fractured. The most common sites for such gross lacerations are the undersurfaces of the frontal lobes and the tips of the temporal lobes.

Gross hemorrhages may result from ruptured meningeal vessels, from the torn vessels of the pia arachnoid, and from ruptured subcortical vessels. There not infrequently occurs, as the result of an apparently trivial injury which may not have caused a fracture of the skull, a tear of one or more of the cortical veins at the site where they leave the cortex to enter one of the venous sinuses. Such veins are particularly numerous on both sides of the longitudinal sinus and along the posterior border of the occipital lobes near the lateral sinuses.

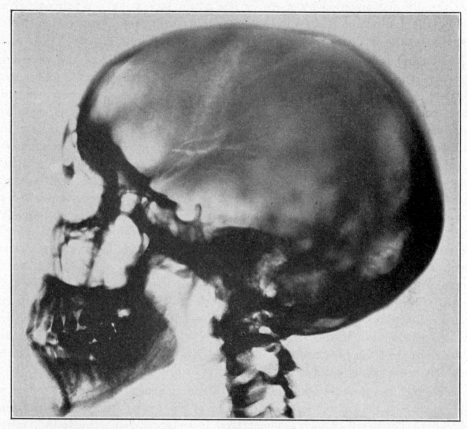

Fig. 198.—When there is a skull fracture across the bony groove of the middle meningeal artery, careful observation for the possibility of an extradural hemorrhage must be maintained.

A few such veins also leave the surface of the tip of the temporal lobe and enter the veins of the adjacent dura. When one or more such veins are torn there results a slow but progressive escape of venous blood into the subdural space. As the venous pressure is only slightly higher than the normal intracranial pressure, such hemorrhages do not become immediately gross enough to produce marked symptoms. For this reason the gravity of the condition does not always become manifest until the subdural hematoma has been organized into a membrane lying snugly under the dura and a second membrane lying over the brain cortex. Between these two layers the blood becomes liquefied and degenerated, to which may be added an exudation from the organized membrane. The gravity of the condition, therefore, does not manifest itself until the hematoma has reached a sufficient size to give rise to symptoms and signs of increased intracranial pressure. This may be many days or months after the accident. Such a condition is spoken of as "chronic subdural hematoma" and presents a well-recognized clinical entity.

When the intradural hemorrhage is arterial in nature, the clinical manifestations are of rapid onset and are of a more immediate grave nature than is the case where the hemorrhage is of venous origin. Such arterial hemorrhages are usually accompanied by more or less brain laceration. When occurring below the tentorium there develops a rapid medullary compression which usually results in death within a few minutes to an hour.

Hemorrhages of a less degree of severity may occur from the vessels of the pia arachnoid and remain confined largely to the subarachnoid space. Bagley[4] has called attention to the evidences of meningeal irritation resulting from such subarachnoid hemorrhages. When subarachnoid hemorrhages are very severe in extent and located principally in the interpeduncular cistern the blood may extend into the vaginal sheath of the optic nerves. Such an extension of blood may compress the central retinal vein as it crosses the sheath diagonally to enter the neighboring cavernous sinus. This causes a marked engorgement of the retinal veins with the formation of flamelike hemorrhages in the retina. It was Dowman's good fortune to see the occurrence of such flamelike hemorrhages within the retina during an ophthalmoscopic examination of a patient who had a very extensive subarachnoid hemorrhage of traumatic origin Such subarachnoid hemorrhages may be the cause of a subsequent optic atrophy. When located largely below the floor of the third ventricle, there may result subsequent lesions in this area which may give rise to posttraumatic diabetes insipidus. Fay[5] believes that subarachnoid hemorrhages cause injury to the pacchionian bodies, interfering with spinal fluid absorption, and are thus a cause of the pressure atrophy of the brain following trauma, which he has demonstrated by encephalography.

Bagley[6] has described a type of intracranial hemorrhage which occurs as the result of a tear of the vein of Galen or of the contributory or lesser veins of Galen. The result of such a hemorrhage is a marked hemorrhagic infiltration of these structures in the region of the internal capsule, with resulting hemi- or diplegias. At no time in such cases is there evidence of increased intracranial pressure.

Isolated subcortical hemorrhages may also occur as a result of trauma. A favorite site for such a subcortical hemorrhage is the temporal lobes. Such hemorrhages may result from an apparently trivial injury, the patient developing several days later symptoms of an alarming neurologic nature.

The large venous sinuses of the dura are not usually torn as the result of trauma unless there is a fracture directly over them. Sargent and Holmes during World War I described the compound depressed fracture as the result of a high explosive shell fragment across the vault of the skull with injury to the longitudinal sinus and resulting disturbance of the cortical centers for the movements of the legs. Depressed fractures in the occipital region are not infrequently accompanied by rupture of the lateral sinuses. Gross hemorrhages from the torn sinus, however, may not occur until the fragment has been removed at operation.

An extradural hemorrhage of grave clinical significance is that which results from rupture of the meningeal arteries. The hematoma which develops from such torn vessels lies between the skull and the dura and produces symptoms and neurologic manifestations when the hematoma has reached a sufficient size to cause pressure on the underlying brain. It is of interest to note that large extradural hemorrhages may also result from fractures which have extended across the large venous channels which lie in the diploe of the skull.

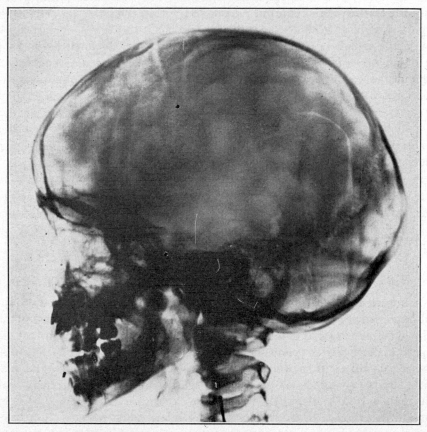

Fig. 199.—The scalp wound in this case was located in the center of the bony depression and was less than 2 cm. in length. Had it not been for the radiologic depiction of a circumscribed depression the bone damage would have escaped observation through the débrided wound.

Should the fracture extend through the outer plate of the skull, the blood may escape outward under the flap, giving rise to a scalp hematoma. If, on the other hand, the blood from torn diploetic channels cannot escape outward, it may escape between the inner surface of the skull and the dura and give rise to a compressing hematoma with symptoms similar to those caused by a rupture of the meningeal arteries. Such a venous extradural hemorrhage develops a little less rapidly than the meningeal arterial bleeding. The clinical picture of the diploetic blood escape might be compared to a slow motion picture of the arterial type. This is due to the fact again that the normal intracranial pressure is only slightly less than the normal venous pressure, so that signs of rising intracranial pressure and localizing neurologic developments are a little delayed as compared to the brisk arterial pressure alterations of cerebral physiology.

As the result of perivascular hemorrhages and gross lacerations of the brain there usually occurs an accumulation of fluid within the brain substance. Rand[7] made microscopic studies of the choroid plexus and the perivascular spaces within the brain in several cases that died from two to four hours after being injured. He demonstrated the presence of an abnormal quantity of fluid within the stroma of the choroid plexus and within the cuboidal cells covering the plexus, several globules of fluid having the appearance of just bursting through the cells into the lateral ventricles. He also demonstrated the presence of an excessive amount of fluid within the perivascular spaces of the brain substance. As the result of tears in the pia arachnoid there may occur an abnormal accumulation of fluid in the subdural space. This fluid probably escapes from the subarachnoid space through the ruptured arachnoid. When such fluid is present the underlying brain may be actually compressed. Naffziger[8] first called attention to this condition and emphasized the grave clinical picture which may thereby be produced.

Such intracranial lesions as may result from a blow on the head serve to illustrate the importance of looking upon cases of head injury in terms of intracranial damage. In each of the above-mentioned conditions the encasing skull may or may not be fractured, depending entirely upon whether or not the normal elasticity of the skull has been exceeded.

HISTORY, EXAMINATION, DIAGNOSIS AND TREATMENT

A knowledge of the nature of the accident and the progress of symptoms is all-important in order properly to estimate the nature and degree of injury to the skull and its contents. It is well to know whether the patient has in his past history any previous head injuries or whether there is any chronic illness or debility. It is well known that linear fractures in adults may be depicted on x-ray studies as late as five years after the original head trauma. More than once a bradycardia with a pre-existing hypertension has been interpreted as evidence of acutely increasing intracranial pressure. It has happened that a head injury patient upon regaining consciousness explains to the examiner that "the dilated pupil" condition was one developed following some childhood injury or disease. Thus it is evident that a careful history is just as important in acute head injuries as it is in any other diagnostic problem. A syphilitic or alcoholic background may materially influence one's prognostic acumen. If a patient is struck on the head by some instrument in the hands of another with sufficient force, a localized depressed fracture of the skull is to be expected. Such a type of injury is commonly accompanied by an overlying laceration of the scalp and an underlying contusion or laceration of the brain. The same pathology may be expected from smaller missiles. A blow on the temple by a baseball or a brick is a favorite cause of a rupture of the middle meningeal artery. In contrast to the damage from small objects, the skull and brain damage when the head is thrown against the side of an automobile or when the injury is the result of being thrown to the pavement, the bone damage is less likely to be circumscribed but more extensive. These later types of injuries are more prone to result in linear types of fractures. There is another factor in skull fractures and damages to the intracranial structures that must be taken into account. If the head is mobile or immobile at the time of the injury is important. Rather extensive bony damages may occur when the head is fixed and immobile without the interruption of consciousness, whereas if the trauma occurs to a mobile skull the damage to the intracranial structures may be extensive and remote from the site of head contact.

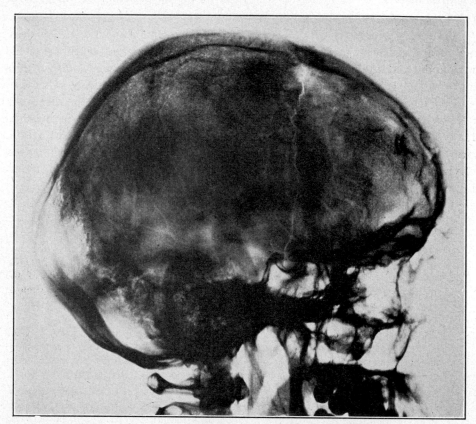

Fig. 200.—This patient had no subjective or objective neurologic symptoms of a head injury. The history of a blow on the vertex prompted the radiologic evidence of a lengthy linear fracture.

Details of the accident are not always available but often a few questions help in establishing something of the nature of the injury as well as subsequent clinical developments. Did the patient fall and strike his head or was he thrown against the ground or an irregular object? If so, what was the distance of the fall or what did he strike before reaching the ground? Did he fall from some stationary position or was he hurled from a moving vehicle? Was the patient rendered unconscious immediately? If so, was the unconsciousness temporary or continuous? Did unilateral paralysis or convulsions develop? Such questions are but examples of the importance of obtaining a careful history, as the proper estimate of the type and degree of injury often depends upon the type of the accident and the subsequent development of symptoms.

Examination

A complete neurologic examination requires the cooperation of the patient. For this reason such an examination is rarely possible in cases of acute trauma. It is of great importance, however, to make as complete a neurologic survey as circumstances will permit. It is well to have a system of examination in mind and to carry out this system as far as possible. A very useful system of examination that is applicable to a variable degree is as follows:

General.—Symmetry of the skull on palpation and inspection. The presence of any stiffness or rigidity of the neck. The presence of scalp abrasions or wounds, and the extent and character of each. The presence of Kernig's sign. Any bleeding from the ears or nose. It is well to note any other evidence of injury to the chest, abdomen, long bones, etc. Ofttimes the discovery of a clavicular fracture or a contused shoulder will lead one to a brachial plexus damage in preference to classing the monoplegia as of cerebral origin. After a careful general study noting the color, respirations, consciousness, activities of the patient's extremities, etc., neurologic observations are undertaken.

CRANIAL NERVES.

1. Ability to smell on each side. Noting any spinal fluid or bleeding from the nose.

2. Ophthalmoscopic and visual field findings.

3, 4, 6. A study of the pupils as to size, equality, and reaction to light and accommodation. The presence or absence of parallelism of the eyes, and the action of the various external ocular muscles. The history of diplopia and the demonstration of any ocular palsies on testing all eye movements. The presence of unilateral or bilateral enophthalmos or exophthalmos.

5. The perception of touch and pain sensations over the face and forehead, and the condition of the corneal reflex. The contraction of the masseter and temporal muscles, and the action of the pterygoid muscles as shown by the presence or absence of deviation of the jaw when the patient opens the mouth.

7. The presence of facial asymmetry and the action of the facial muscles in the performance of emotional and voluntary movements. When the patient is unconscious a unilateral facial paresis may be detected by the paralyzed cheek being "blown out" during expiration. The ability to taste over the anterior two-thirds of the tongue.

8. The history of otitis media and the presence of the discharge of pus, blood or cerebrospinal fluid from the ears. The degree of hearing as tested with watch tick and tuning fork and the relative degree of bone and air conduction. The history of tinnitus and vertigo; the presence or absence of nystagmus.

9. The disturbance of the ability to swallow. The presence of the gag reflex. The movements of the palate.

10. The history of vomiting. The blood pressure and the pulse rate.

11. The voluntary action of the sternocleidomastoid and trapezius muscles.

12. The deviation of the tongue when protruded. Fibrillations.

CEREBRUM.

A. FRONTAL LOBE: Mental changes, such as disturbances of memory and orientation, changes in disposition, indifference to sphincter control, etc. The history of drowsiness, the presence of motor aphasia.

B. TEMPORAL LOBE: Auditory aphasia, word or object blindness (angular gyrus), hallucinations of smell (uncinate gyrus), hemianopsia, the history of dreamy states and the history of hallucinations of vision. It is of particular importance to know whether the patient is right- or left-handed.

C. PRECENTRAL CONVOLUTIONS AND ALLIED TRACTS: The history of convulsions, general or localized, unilateral or bilateral paresis of movements, the strength of muscles, the presence of spasticity or flaccidity.

D. POSTCENTRAL CONVOLUTIONS AND ALLIED TRACTS: The appreciation of sensation to touch, pain, temperature changes, vibratory sense, and disturbances of the so-called psychotactile sensations (stereognostic sense, joint sense, sense of position, etc.), and the history of paresthesias.

E. OCCIPITAL LOBE: The history of visual hallucinations and the presence of visual fields defects. (Either confirmation test or perimetric studies.)

CEREBELLUM.

The history of staggering gait, tests for coordination (finger to nose, heel to knee, past-pointing, ataxic gait, Rombergism, etc.), the presence of nystagmus, the presence of hypotonia and hypermetria.

REFLEXES.

Superficial—Abdominal, cremasteric and plantar reflexes (Babinski, Gordon and Oppenheim). Deep—Arm (triceps, biceps and forearm), leg (patellar, and tendo achilles). Pathologic (Babinski, Gordon—ankle or patella clonus).

SPHINCTERS.

Vesical and rectal.

This more or less complete outline for a routine neurologic examination can be only partially followed in examining cases of acute injury to the brain. By having some such system in mind, however, many neurologic manifestations will be observed which otherwise might escape the examiner's attention. In order to estimate correctly the degree and type of intracranial lesions one must obtain as much detailed information as possible. For example, the presence of a unilateral facial paralysis may have great localizing significance; the presence of a unilateral spasticity of the extremities, a unilateral Babinski reflex, etc., are findings of great value in locating the area of greatest damage. Such findings can only be properly interpreted by falling back on our knowledge of the anatomy and physiology of the nervous system.

The correct diagnosis depends largely upon the utilization of every available means to gain as many facts as possible concerning the particular case under study. A correct interpretation of the various symptoms and findings is all-important in order to determine the nature and degree of intracranial damage which may be present. It is not only necessary that the presence or absence of brain damage be determined, but, in order to be in a position to determine the character of treatment which should be instituted a further differentiation of the type and degree of injury is all-essential. Many cases can be properly estimated when first examined. Other cases may have to be kept under careful observation for several hours before a correct interpretation can be made.

Symptomatology and Clinical Manifestations

In the presence of an extensive intracranial hemorrhage whether intra-dural or extradural, there may result an immediate increase in intracranial pressure due to the blood per se. Where there is contusion, either general or local, an edema ensues which likewise causes increased intracranial pressure. Tissues deprived of oxygen will take up fluid and swell. With the rupture of many vessels of varying sizes and with traumatic thrombosis of others a considerable bulk of brain tissue may be deprived of oxygen, resulting in an extensive edema.

Acute cerebral compression, whether due to intracranial hemorrhage or edema, may give rise to certain physiologic responses manifested by certain symptoms and findings. A clear understanding of the effects of cerebral compression is therefore necessary in order properly to interpret certain clinical phenomena which may occur in cases of cerebral trauma.

There are three vital centers situated in the medulla oblongata: namely, the vasomotor, the respiratory, and the cardioinhibitory centers. Experimentally these centers compensate in a classical manner (up to certain limits) in the presence of an increasing intracranial pressure. Clinically the reaction of these centers is not always as prompt as in experimental studies. In the experimental production of intracranial pressure there are not the added factors of cerebral contusion and lacerations so often present in clinical studies. With this difference in mind, however, it is still possible to explain satisfactorily certain reactions to compressing forces.

There are four stages of cerebral compression, as follows:

1. **Mental Dullness.**—The compressing agent may be compensated for by the displacement of some of the cerebrospinal fluid. It has been shown experimentally that about 6 per cent of the space occupied by the cerebrospinal fluid can be encroached upon without producing symptoms. Beyond this, even though the pressure be relatively mild, there may result headache and slight mental dullness.

2. **Irritability.**—As the intracranial pressure becomes more marked some of the cerebral veins become blanched and there develop such symptoms as increased headache, restlessness, irritability, vertigo, and excitement.

3. **Medullary Compensation.**—The circulation in the vessels supplying the medullary centers becomes interfered with as the intracranial pressure increases. Normally the blood pressure is considerably higher than the intracranial pressure. Howe[9] called attention to the fact that a moderate increase in spinal fluid pressure is balanced by a similar increase in venous and capillary pressure, a condition which continues the normal circulation. Under normal conditions the spinal fluid pressure is roughly equal to the venous pressure. The arterial pressure is six times the venous pressure. As the intracranial pressure increases, a point may be reached when there is a cessation of circulation of blood through the brain. The resulting anemia stimulates the medullary centers to react in a compensatory effort to restore the cerebral circulation. The increased activity of the vasomotor center causes a compensatory rise in the blood pressure to a degree sufficiently high to restore cerebral circulation. If

the cerebral compression continues, a point will again be reached when the brain becomes anemic. The medullary centers are again stimulated and the blood pressure ascends to an even higher level than before. This physiologic response of the medullary centers may continue until the centers become exhausted. This period of activity of the medullary centers is spoken of as the period of "medullary compensation." During this period the blood pressure increases, the pulse becomes slow and bounding and the respiration deep and stertorous.

4. **Medullary Exhaustion.**—As the intracranial pressure increases there results a cessation of the activity of the medullary centers. This period is spoken of as the period of "medullary exhaustion." During this stage the blood pressure falls, the pulse rate increases, respiration ceases, and death ensues.

Temperature.—During the first few hours following the accident the temperature may be subnormal. It should be remembered that during this time there is frequently an attending condition of traumatic shock. This subnormal temperature may be followed by a rise above the normal. As a rule the factor which determines the rise in temperature is the degree and location of brain damage. As a general rule the greater and more extensive the brain contusion the higher the temperature. As an exception to this rule should be mentioned a type of injury described by Bagley[6] in which there is a marked rise in temperature a few minutes after the accident. This hyperpyrexia continues throughout the course and may rise to 106 or 107° F. In Bagley's cases there was a corresponding increase in the pulse and respiratory rate. The lesions found at necropsy were limited to the structures anatomically related to the vein of Galen and its tributaries, and consisted of extravasations of blood into the corpus callosum, optic thalamus and internal capsule.

As a general rule an increasing temperature warrants a grave prognosis. Accompanied by an increasing degree of unconsciousness it may indicate an increasing intracranial pressure due to edema of the brain and subdural hemorrhage. An excessive amount of blood in the subarachnoid spaces may not only cause a rise in temperature but give rise to the signs of meningeal irritation which may simulate the picture of an infectious meningitis. Under such circumstances the daily withdrawal of bloody cerebrospinal fluid may cause the symptoms to subside. A delayed rise in temperature in those cases in which there has been a compound fracture or in which the fracture has extended into the sphenoid or frontal sinuses, or across the cribriform plate, should lead one to suspect the presence of a secondary meningeal infection. Another cause of a late elevation of temperature may be overdehydration, a condition which will be discussed when the treatment is considered.

Pulse Rate.—During the period of shock immediately following the accident the pulse rate may be increased. Should reaction take place the pulse rate may descend to normal. On the other hand, a definite bradycardia may be observed, the pulse rate descending as low as forty to fifty to the minute. Should this abnormal slowing of the pulse rate be accompanied by an increasing blood pressure it is safe to assume that it is caused by an increasing intracranial pressure. In the absence of other signs of increased intracranial pressure one is hardly justified in concluding that there is a material increase of intracranial pressure because the pulse rate is low, as not infrequently a slow pulse may be observed in minor degrees of brain injury. A slow pulse indicates that very close and constant observation should be made in order not to overlook a rapidly increasing intracranial pressure. A persistently rapid pulse is of grave prognostic significance, particularly when accompanied by a marked hyperpyrexia. In those cases in which there is only a moderate increase in temperature there is usually no corresponding rise in the pulse rate. The pulse rate in acute cerebral compression is usually slow and of full volume and increased tension.

Blood Pressure.—Experimentally it has been shown that as the intracranial pressure increases, an anemia of the medullary centers eventually ensues. The temporary anemia stimulates the vasomotor centers with the result that there occurs a compensatory rise in blood pressure. This physiologic response may likewise occur in clinical observations, but not always, as not infrequently there may have occurred contusions of such gravity and extent as to interfere materially with this normal physiologic response. Clinically, therefore, absence of increased blood pressure is not incompatible with increased intracranial tension, but on the other hand when there occurs a gradually increasing blood pressure with a corresponding decrease in the pulse rate, it is safe to conclude that there is increasing intracranial pressure. Immediately after the accident during the period of shock the blood pressure may be below normal. When the blood pressure continues to fall, especially when accompanied by a rising pulse rate, the prognosis is grave and indicates an exhaustion of the medullary centers.

Respiration.—During the period of shock immediately following the accident the respiration may be very shallow. As reaction takes place the breathing becomes deeper and if the intracranial pressure is increasing, it changes to a heavy stertorous character. As the pressure becomes greater, the respiratory rate may be slow and the rhythm becomes irregular. At times the respiration may assume the Cheyne-Stokes type. Just before death the breathing may again become shallow. When an increased pressure is exerted directly on the medulla (as in extensive hemorrhage into the posterior fossa) the respiratory rate may descend to from two to four per minute and there may occur simultaneously a marked cyanosis and pulmonary edema. After a complete respiratory failure as the result of medullary compression the heart may continue to beat for several minutes.

Pupils.—The sympathetic fibers which enter the cranial cavity with the internal carotid artery consist partly of those fibers which have to do with dilatation of the pupils. The area of entrance of these fibers into the cranial cavity is not infrequently the site of fracture. Injury to these fibers may stimulate or paralyze, thereby causing either dilatation or contraction of the pupil on the side of the injury. The third cranial nerve which contains the fibers causing pupillary contraction is rarely injured in its peripheral course, but the third nerve nucleus or its cerebral connections is subject to contusion just as any other area of the brain. Thus it is seen that any type of pupillary change may occur in cases of injury to the brain. It has been noted that most frequently when there are unequal pupils the larger pupil is on the side of greatest intracranial pressure. Rand[10] called attention to the presence of a dilated pupil with homolateral hemiplegia as indicating bilateral subdural hemorrhage. That the dilated pupil is not always on the same side as the lesion in cases of chronic subdural hematoma overlying the cerebral hemisphere is an exception to the rule. It is an established fact that dilated and nonreacting pupils indicate as a rule a grave prognosis. It must be kept in mind, however, that the significance of pupillary changes depends largely upon other signs and symptoms which may be present.

Eyegrounds.—A routine ophthalmoscopic examination should always be made in cases of head injury. Although the information obtained may not be as valuable as in cases of chronic increased intracranial pressure, there are certain changes of definite value in the eyegrounds which may take place in acute cases. There are seldom any noticeable changes within from four to six hours following the injury. After this time a definite fullness of the retinal veins may be noticed when the intracranial pressure is increasing. This may be accompanied by a hyperemia of the discs and at times by a beginning edema of the nasal half of the disc. After twenty-four hours there may occur a distinct choking of the discs provided the intracranial pressure is markedly increased. A more rapid development of a true papilloedema has occasionally been observed. When there has occurred an extensive subarachnoid hemorrhage the retinal veins may be tremendously engorged and large flame-like hemorrhages may occur. Should the ophthalmoscopic examination disclose large retinal hemorrhages in cases of brain injury, it is reasonable to assume that there has occurred an extensive subarachnoid hemorrhage. When a choking of the optic discs occurs a week or longer after a brain injury, particularly in cases that were not apparently seriously injured at the time of the accident, there is usually a marked subdural accumulation of fluid, a subdural hematoma, or a large subcortical hematoma. Such late changes in the discs are of sufficient importance to make necessary the periodic examination of the eyegrounds for several weeks following the accident.

An attempt to outline a classification into which every head injury case might be pigeonholed would be impractical and very lengthy. Some classification is necessary, not only for the instigation of proper treatment but for its prognostic value. The following grouping of cases has been found to be of practical value:

    I. Massive brain injury.
        These cases show clinical evidence of rapidly increasing intracranial pressure and may show:
            A. Rapid exhaustion of the medullary centers.
            B. Evidence of being within the period of medullary compensation.
    II. Definite brain injury. Exhibiting no findings of acutely increasing intracranial pressure.
    III. Depressed fracture of the skull. Simple or compound.
    IV. Linear fractures of the skull. Simple or compounded in which repeated examinations fail to show any evidence of brain damage.
    V. Middle meningeal hemorrhage.

VI. Miscellaneous head injuries.
    A. Concussion.
    B. Chronic subdural hematoma.
    C. Isolated subcortical hematoma.
    D. Tear of Galen vein or its tributaries.
    E. Traumatic pneumocephalus and cerebrospinal fluid drainage.

I. Massive Brain Injury

A. Evidencing Rapid Exhaustion of the Medullary Centers

Patients belonging to this class have sustained a fall or blow of such severity as to cause a massive brain injury. As a general rule they are profoundly unconscious; the pupils are dilated and do not react to light; there is heavy stertorous breathing which soon becomes irregular; the pulse may be either very slow and irregular or very rapid and almost imperceptible; the blood pressure, though possibly high soon after the accident, may descend rapidly; and there may be evidence of a rapidly occurring edema of the lungs. The roentgen ray may reveal one or more fractures of varying extent and location. Blood may be escaping from one or both ears and often from the nose and mouth. The extremities are more or less flaccid and both superficial and deep reflexes are usually abolished.

The brain in such cases is grossly lacerated and there is extensive intradural hemorrhage. Death occurs in from one to several hours, although such patients may occasionally live as long as twelve hours. In this group also belong those cases in which the subtentorial structures have been injured. Such cases have extensive hemorrhage in the posterior fossa which compresses the medulla. The medullary compression is evidenced by the slow and irregular respiration which ceases soon after the accident. After the respiration has stopped, the pulse which is slow and bounding may continue to beat for several minutes. Such patients rapidly become cyanotic and death occurs in from a few minutes to an hour after the accident.

Treatment.—As a general rule cases belonging to this type can be properly classified when first seen. No specific treatment is indicated in this class of patients. The best that can be done is to employ the usual methods for shock and to keep the patient under careful observation in the hope that the diagnosis of a hopeless massive injury to the brain may prove incorrect and permit the case eventually to be reclassified into a more hopeful group. There is no operation which will accomplish anything or any medication which will be of value. The nature of the injury is such as to preclude the possibility of recovery.

B. Cases of Rapidly Increasing Intracranial Pressure Which Are Well Within the Period of Medullary Compensation

The cases which belong to this group are usually rendered unconscious at the time of the accident and give evidence of increasing intracranial pressure. This is usually caused by a subdural hemorrhage. Contusions and lacerations of the temporal lobes and undersurfaces of the frontal lobes may be present. These lacerations may be unilateral or bilateral. The hemorrhage is from torn cortical arteries and veins—if from arteries the accumulation of blood is rapid, if from veins alone, the hemorrhage is much slower and may not accumulate rapidly enough to cause acutely increased intracranial pressure. There may occur a gradually rising blood pressure unless the brain injury is so great as to interfere materially with the expected physiologic responses to increasing intracranial pressure. The blood pressure should be recorded every fifteen minutes until the case is properly classified. The pulse rate may remain normal or become slow as the blood pressure rises. Should a spinal puncture be done, the fluid is found to be bloody and its pressure increased above the normal upper limit. The pupils are not infrequently unequal, the larger being as a rule on the side of greatest damage. Repeated eyeground examinations disclose an increasing fullness and tortuosity of the retinal veins. After six to twelve hours the physiologic cup may be filled up and an actual papilloedema may be observed. There may be a suppression of the superficial abdominal reflexes on the side opposite to that of the greatest pressure, and the contralateral deep reflexes may be hyperactive. Should the pressure increase with great rapidity, the deep reflexes may become abolished. As the pressure increases, the degree of unconsciousness becomes more and more profound and the respiration becomes slower and more stertorous. Even when the blood pressure remains low an increasing degree of unconsciousness, a rising temperature, venous engorgement of the retina, and increased spinal fluid pressure are evidences of an increasing intracranial pressure. The roentgen ray may or may not reveal the presence of a fracture of the skull.

Treatment.—It is in this group of cases that there are many divergent opinions in regard to the best method of treatment. The rapidly increasing intracranial pressure is usually caused by intracranial hemorrhage. A period may be reached when the intracranial pressure increases to a sufficient degree to stop the active hemorrhage. To permit a patient to lie for many days or weeks with marked increased intracranial pressure may lead to such organic changes within the brain itself as to give rise to many and various distressing posttraumatic neurologic manifestations. It is felt that patients belonging to this group should be given the benefit of a decompression operation as soon as it has been decided that there is a rapidly increasing intracranial pressure, provided the period of medullary compensation has not already been exceeded.

The operation of choice under such circumstances is a subtemporal decompression, either unilateral or bilateral according to the individual case. The side on which a unilateral decompression is done should be that which neurologically exhibits the greatest degree of intracranial damage. This is not always an easy matter to determine. As a general rule, the side which should be operated upon is that on which there is a dilated pupil, if such a finding be present. In rapidly increasing intracranial pressure there may be a sluggishness or absence of the contralateral abdominal reflexes. Should such a finding be associated with hyperactive deep reflexes on the same side as the sluggish abdominal reflexes, a clue as to the side which should be decompressed can thus be obtained. In cases belonging to this group the operator should always be prepared to follow the operation with a decompression on the opposite side, provided the condition found at the first operation is such as to lead one to suspect that the greatest damage is on the opposite side.

The technic of such an operation is that which was first described by Cushing, with certain modifications later developed by him. The operation can usually be done under local infiltration with one-half to one per cent novocain anesthesia. The incision of choice should begin about six centimeters above the ear and extend diagonally downward and forward to the zygoma, about one centimeter in front of the ear. In order to control the hemorrhage from the scalp the galea is caught with hemostatic forceps at distances of one centimeter apart and held in groups by means of rubber bands. The weight of the forceps will evert the edge of the scalp incision sufficiently to control all hemorrhage from this structure. An incision is then made through the aponeurosis overlying the temporal muscle in the direction of its fibers. The temporal muscle is then divided in the direction of its fibers and by means of a periosteal elevator separated from the bone overlying the temporal lobe. By means of decompression retractors the muscle is now elevated from the underlying bone. The skull is entered with a perforator and burr and the dura separated from the inner surface of the bone by means of a separator. With rongeurs the bone is removed for a diameter of from five to seven centimeters. Through such an incision it is well to remove as much bone as possible down under the thickest portion of the temporal muscle. In order to avoid injury to the underlying brain cortex in effecting the dural opening it should be picked up by means of a small dural hook and a small incision should be made, large enough to admit the end of a grooved director. This incision can then be extended in various directions by incising the dura against the groove of the director thus making several crucial incisions so as to obtain a dural opening corresponding to the size of the opening of the bone. The middle meningeal artery and its branches can be either ligated or clipped with silver clips as encountered. Not infrequently lacerations of the tip of the temporal lobe and the undersurfaces of the temporal lobe will be encountered. Should ruptured cortical vessels be brought into view, they should be either ligated or clipped. By retracting the brain gently by means of a brain spoon, the undersurface of the frontal lobe can be investigated. Not infrequently a large amount of blood will then escape from under the frontal lobe. This can be removed by means of cotton pledget or by suction. If there seems to be a continued bleeding from the structures deep under the frontal lobe and the bleeding vessels cannot be brought into view and clipped or ligated, a folded rubber tissue wick should be placed under the frontal lobe and allowed to escape at the lower angle of the wound. This should be removed at the end of twenty-four to forty-eight hours. The wound is now closed by means of several layers of fine interrupted silk sutures and suitable dressings are applied.

For several days following the operation it is sometimes well to do daily lumbar punctures, particularly if the cerebrospinal fluid is very bloody. These punctures should be made at intervals thereafter until the fluid becomes clear.

II. Definite Brain Injury

Exhibiting No Acutely Increasing Intracranial Pressure

Patients belonging to this group when first seen are usually in a semiconscious condition. The blood pressure as a rule is somewhat higher than normal but does not increase. The pulse rate is about normal and remains so. There may or may not be bleeding from one or both ears. The roentgen ray may or may not reveal linear fractures of varying degrees and locations. The spinal fluid contains blood but the spinal fluid pressure is not excessively high. The neurologic examination may or may not give findings indicating the presence of localized contusion. Repeated examinations of the eyegrounds fail to show the venous engorgement and tortuosity so characteristic of rapidly increasing pressure. After several hours of observation one feels safe in assuming that there has occurred definite brain damage with subarachnoid hemorrhage, although there is no rapidly increasing intracranial pressure.

Within a few days such patients are likely to show definite signs of increased intracranial pressure unless measures are employed to prevent such a complication. This delayed increase of intracranial pressure is due to an accumulation of fluid between the dura and the arachnoid. Why this fluid should be so located is an interesting question. A plausible explanation is that, at the time of the injury, there were definite contusions of the brain and small tears in the arachnoid through which the fluid from the subarachnoid space escaped into the subdural space. It is physiologically impossible for fluid to be absorbed from the subdural space, as the normal cerebrospinal fluid absorption takes place from the subarachnoid space. When fluid accumulates in the subdural space there is produced a definite increase of intracranial pressure.

Patients belonging to this particular group may have progressed satisfactorily for a few days, after which they become increasingly restless and complain of intense headache. The scalp veins become distended and a papilloedema develops. Should a lumbar puncture be done, the spinal fluid will be found to be under markedly increased pressure and of a yellowish tint. This is caused by blood pigments in the fluid, since such cases have more or less subarachnoid hemorrhage at the time the injury is sustained. The fluid which may be removed by lumbar puncture is that which has remained in the various subarachnoid cisterns and the ventricles. The fluid which has accumulated between the dura and arachnoid and which is causing the increased intracranial pressure cannot be removed by lumbar puncture, as the needle enters the subarachnoid space. The subdural fluid is usually of yellowish tint. It actually compresses the brain. When the dura is opened under such circumstances the fluid will spurt out to a height of several inches and the underlying brain is found to be compressed.

Treatment.—On account of this tendency to develop increased intracranial tension due to fluid accumulation the treatment of this particular class of cases is directed largely toward preventing such a complication.

Weed and McKibben[11] have shown experimentally that the pressure of the cerebrospinal fluid and the bulk of the brain can be reduced by intravenous injections of hypertonic sodium chloride solution. Foley and Putnam[12] demonstrated that giving hypertonic sodium chloride solutions by mouth likewise reduces cerebrospinal fluid and brain bulk, although the action is much slower than when the solution is given intravenously. With these findings in mind, the clinical application of hypertonic solutions in the treatment of certain types of head injury has been used in the author's clinic for many years.[13] Our earliest experience was with 30 per cent sodium chloride solution given intravenously in order to relieve an already existing edema of the brain following injury. Later, in an effort to prevent the accumulation of fluid with the resulting symptoms of increased pressure in certain types of head injury, saturated solutions of magnesium sulphate were given by mouth, and the more rapid action of sodium chloride solutions was reserved for those cases in which an edema already existed. During the past few years hypertonic solutions of sucrose (50 per cent solution) administered intravenously have been used in certain selected cases in order to accomplish the same results.

Hypertonic solutions of sodium chloride administered intravenously in order to combat edema of the brain is not an absolutely safe procedure. That the edema will be temporarily relieved has been proved both experimentally and clinically. Sodium chloride, however, is a dialyzable salt and will very readily go through cell membranes and become fixed tissue chloride. When a hypertonic sodium chloride solution is introduced into the blood stream, the blood is rendered hypertonic. An isotonic state is eventually attained by fluids being "drawn" from the various fluid filled cavities, tissues, etc., into the blood, and by an excretion of excessive sodium chloride through the kidneys and sweat glands. Some of the salt, however, on account of its dialyzable quality may be taken up by the cells of the various organs, so that the sodium chloride content of these cells may cause the cellular protoplasm to become in turn hypertonic. After the existing edema has been temporarily relieved by the intravenous injections of hypertonic sodium chloride solution there will come a time when the tissue cells, on account of the excessive amount of fixed cellular sodium chloride, will in turn begin to draw upon fluids of the circulating blood in an effort to become isotonic. This will give rise to a secondary edema which may be even greater than that which existed before the sodium chloride was administered.

There does not seem to be the same objection to the use of hypertonic solutions of magnesium sulphate given by mouth or by rectum, or to hypertonic solutions of sucrose given intravenously. When it is possible for the patient to swallow, one-half ounce of a saturated solution of magnesium sulphate without water may be given by mouth every 3 to 4 hours for the first twenty-four to forty-eight hours. Thereafter the time of administration may be lengthened to every six for a day or two, and then gradually decreased according to the condition of the patient. After seven to ten days the drug may be withdrawn entirely. Children should be given a smaller dose, estimated according to the age of the child. No plain water is allowed but the patient may be given a sufficient amount of fluids of a hypertonic nature in the form of sweetened lemonades, salty broths, etc. It is interesting to note that patients so treated are very rarely excessively purged. One or two watery stools daily is the rule. If water is allowed freely with the magnesium sulphate excessive purgation results. As such, no water is given by mouth thirty minutes before or after the administration of the saturated solution of magnesium sulphate. The total fluid intake for an adult on such a dehydration regime should be limited to forty to fifty ounces per twenty-four-hour periods.

If the patient is unable to take or retain the magnesium sulphate by mouth it may be given by rectum—three ounces dissolved in six ounces of water every twelve to twenty-four hours. When so administered the depletion of fluid in the cranial cavity seems to be as efficacious as when the drug is administered by mouth.

When magnesium sulphate cannot be satisfactorily administered either by mouth or by rectum, hypertonic solutions of glucose or sucrose (preferable) may be given intravenously. Twenty cubic centimeters of a 50 per cent solution of either may be given intravenously every four hours for a period of several days. The depleting effect seems to be just as effective as that obtained by the use of sodium chloride or magnesium sulphate solutions. Larger quantities of glucose in weaker concentrations may be used with equally as good effect. Two hundred to five hundred cubic centimeters of a 5 per cent glucose solution may be given intravenously once or twice daily with satisfactory depleting effects. The use of such solutions may have a distinct advantage over the other methods of hypertonic treatment, since the patient is given a reasonable amount of fluid and nourishment intravenously in addition to preventing the fluid accumulation in the cranial cavity. In administering such large quantities of glucose the urine should be examined for evidences of glycosuria and the treatment supplemented by the hypodermic administration of insulin in case it may seem necessary to aid in the proper catabolism of such excessive amounts of sugar. Cases are not infrequently observed in which a rise in temperature and marked restlessness develops, despite the administration of magnesium sulphate by mouth. In cases of this nature the intravenous administration of five hundred cubic centimeters of 2.5 per cent glucose solution seems to have a marked beneficial effect—the temperature descends and the restlessness is improved.

In those cases in which the hypertonic treatment is used, symptoms of overdepletion of intracranial fluid should be carefully watched for. Such symptoms are, usually, a marked increase in pulse rate, a rise in temperature, increased restlessness, and at times an increased degree of coma. When such symptoms arise overdepletion should be suspected. Under these circumstances the patient should be given five hundred to one thousand cubic centimeters of normal salt solution intravenously and the hypertonic treatment should be discontinued.

The use of the hypertonic treatment in this particular type of brain trauma will prevent the occurrence of the symptoms of increased intracranial pressure due to intracranial fluid accumulation. Patients falling into this particular group of cases constitute fully 50 per cent of all cases of head injury admitted to any large traumatic service. When treated along the lines suggested the mortality is reduced to nil. It is also believed that such treatment usually prevents the occurrence of posttraumatic neurologic manifestations in cases belonging to this large group. This is explained by the fact that the patients are not allowed to lie for days and weeks with a frankly increased intracranial pressure.

Patients belonging to this particular group may present definite evidence of increased intracranial pressure if first seen several days to several weeks following the injury, during which time no hypertonic treatment has been given. Examination of the eyegrounds under such conditions may reveal a marked papilloedema. The increased pressure is usually caused by a marked accumulation of fluid between the dura and the arachnoid. This fluid cannot be removed by repeated lumbar puncture as in such a procedure the needle drains the subarachnoid and not the subdural space. The treatment of choice under such circumstances is operation. This consists of a small incision in the temporal region and the opening of the skull with a perforator and burr. The dura is then incised, whereupon the subdural fluid will spurt out to a height of several inches. After the subdural fluid has been allowed to escape, the underlying brain is seen to be actually compressed and not increased in volume. A small rubber tissue wick may then be used for drainage and allowed to escape between two of the sutures used in closing the wound. After two or three days the drain can be removed. After such an operation some form of hypertonic treatment should be instituted for several days in order to prevent the reaccumulation of fluid.

Should a lumbar puncture be done in this particular group of cases and the cerebrospinal fluid found to be bloody, it may be well to supplement the treatment already outlined by doing a lumbar puncture at least every other day until the fluid becomes clear. It has been shown by Bagley[4] that blood in the subarachnoid spaces may cause symptoms of meningeal irritation. It is a logical procedure, therefore, to remove periodically the bloody subarachnoid fluid as long as there is evidence of blood being present. In this way the marked irritability so often observed in patients belonging to this group can very often be controlled. Repeated spinal puncture also aids in the prevention of increased intracranial pressure due to fluid accumulation. In the author's opinion to rely on lumbar punctures alone is not as beneficial as to combine lumbar puncture (when indicated) with the hypertonic treatment.

III. Depressed Fracture of the Skull, Simple or Compound

The diagnosis in this type of injury can in most cases be readily made. The injury is usually produced by a force of great velocity and of small mass. A blow on the head with a hammer or some other weapon may cause a localized depressed fracture. The penetrating wounds produced by bullets or shell fragments belong also to this group of cases. A fall during which the head strikes some sharp or irregular object not infrequently causes a depressed fracture. The overlying scalp may or may not be lacerated. The brain underlying the fracture may or may not be contused. When present, such contusion may be the result of the blow, or, as is most frequently the case, it may be caused by indriven bone fragments which actually tear through the dura.

The degree of contusion in cases of penetrating wounds depends largely upon the velocity of the bullet or shell fragment.

The symptoms and signs in this group of cases depend upon the extent and location of the injury. Naffziger[15] has pointed out the lack of serious symptoms from depressed fracture without brain contusion. As a rule the patient is not rendered unconscious except perhaps for a few minutes following the accident. If the injury be over a so-called silent area of the brain, there may be no neurologic manifestations. Under such circumstances the clinical or roentgen ray evidence of depressed fracture may be the only positive findings on examination. If, on the other hand, the injury be over areas of brain of known function, there may be findings indicating irritation or destruction of the involved centers. Examples of such manifestations would be the disturbance of the contralateral psychotactile sensations (astereognosis, disturbance of joint sense, etc.) in parietal lobe injuries, contralateral paresis in precentral injuries, auditory aphasia in temporal lobe injuries, etc.

Should the injury be of the vault of the skull with a tear of the underlying longitudinal sinus the clinical picture might be that described by Sargent and Holmes during World War I; namely, a bilateral spasticity of the legs due to contusion and hemorrhagic infiltration of the cortical leg centers.

These examples are mentioned to emphasize the importance of making as complete a neurologic examination as possible in all cases of suspected brain trauma. The roentgen ray examination is of particular value in cases belonging to this group. Such an examination will accurately locate the area of fracture and give a clue as to the degree of depression. A spinal puncture in this group of cases is not necessary, since the diagnosis can be made by inspection, palpation, and roentgen ray examination. The presence of blood in the spinal fluid may be of value in determining whether there is a subarachnoid hemorrhage as the result of a contusion underlying the fracture, and might aid in determining the character of treatment to be employed. As a rule, a spinal puncture is not indicated.

Treatment.—It is a matter of more or less dispute as to whether or not any particular treatment is indicated in the case of a small simple depressed fracture without evidence of lesion of the underlying brain. There are many such fractures which will never produce symptoms and there would be no particular necessity for elevating the depressed bone were one sure that there is no underlying brain contusion or hemorrhage and that the fracture is located over a so-called silent area of the brain. One cannot be sure, however, that there is no underlying damage. For this reason it is the author's opinion that except in very unusual instances such depressed areas should be investigated by means of operation, in order to correct as far as possible underlying damage if such be found to exist. By elevating the bony depression one also insures the patient against any latent cortical damages that might occur from the normal cerebral pulsations against a focal indenture.

As to large depressed fractures with evidence of underlying brain damage, there is no dispute in regard to the choice of operative treatment. This is particularly true when the overlying scalp has been lacerated. The method of treatment is in general similar to that employed for penetrating wounds of the brain in the American hospitals during World War I. The method is that which has the principle of débridement in mind.

In the case of a compound depressed fracture the incision should be so devised as to excise completely the edges of the contused and lacerated scalp. If the lacerations are of any appreciable size, in order to effect a satisfactory closure, a Y-shaped incision should be used, each incision converging with the others at the site of the laceration. When such an incision is made, there will be three flaps of scalp which can be reflected back from the underlying bone and sufficiently undermined to permit of a satisfactory closure without undue tension. When the bone is thus exposed the depressed area will be in its center. An opening is made at the border of the depression by means of a perforator and burr. Through this opening a stout elevator can be carefully inserted and the depressed fragments pried upward and removed. All fragments should be removed and placed in sterile salt solution. The exposed dura is now inspected. If it be torn, the opening in the dura should be enlarged to a sufficient extent to permit a careful inspection of the underlying brain. If no dural tear be present, the dura should be incised in such a manner as to expose the underlying brain. Torn cortical vessels should be ligated or clipped. If there be a softened area of contused brain, it should be removed. This can be accomplished either by excision or by suction. After the contused brain has been removed and all foreign bodies irrigated away, thorough washing with normal saline solution should be carried out. If there is no indication for leaving a decompression, the dura should be closed tightly with interrupted black silk sutures. If the dura can be closed tightly the bone defect should be obliterated by fitting in several of the removed bony fragments which have been preserved in some antiseptic solution. The scalp wound is then closed in two layers, using fine interrupted silk sutures. Drainage is not only unnecessary if all bleeding has been properly controlled, but the dangers of infection are minimized. The scalp stitches should be removed within forty-eight hours.

Occasionally cases of compound depressed fracture of the skull may come to operation too late to permit of primary wound closure after débridement. In such cases the brain has already become infected and a primary closure cannot be done safely. This may also be the case when the scalp lacerations are so extensive as to preclude the possibility of closure. After a removal of the contused brain, in driven bone fragments, etc., the dura is left wide open and the scalp closed loosely with interrupted through-and-through silk sutures and the development of a brain fungus is expected. The fungus is caused by the marked edema caused in turn by the infection. Chemotherapy as indicated by bacteriologic studies should be immediately instigated and a sufficient concentration of the chemical in the blood stream maintained, as determined by daily blood examinations and tests, until all evidence of edema and infection has disappeared. Epithelization by now will have been almost completed. The local application or the introduction of large quantities of these sulfonamide drugs into a potentially infected wound is not advocated at the present writing. When a traumatic brain fungus has developed it will not subside until the infection and edema have completely disappeared. It is these two factors which cause the fungus except in cases of subcortical abscess or hematoma. The slightest trauma of the surface of the fungus will increase the edema. For this reason the fungus should never be touched with gauze or chemicals. If, on the other hand, every precaution is taken to avoid manipulation or pressure on the fungus, and the surrounding scalp is kept thoroughly shaved and surgically clean, the edema will gradually subside and the protruding brain will drop back into the cranial cavity. The surface of the fungus will become smooth, and healthy granulations will form. When the surface of the exposed brain reaches the level of the scalp, epidermization of the raw surface will gradually take place; if not, pinch grafts may be applied.[16]

Daily dressings should be applied in the following manner: The surface of the fungus is syringed off with normal salt solution. No effort should be made to remove necrotic areas. The surrounding scalp is scrubbed with soap and water and shaved with a sterilized razor blade. The scalp is then cleansed with alcohol and dried with a sterile sponge. A large square of sterile gutta percha tissue is now placed over the fungus. If the rubber tissue has been in alcohol or bichloride solution it should be washed off with normal salt solution before being placed over the fungus. A sterile cotton "doughnut" of sufficient size to surround the fungus and protect it from all pressure is then applied. Numerous squares of sterile gauze are laid over the "doughnut" and the whole bandaged neatly to the head in such a manner as to avoid slipping. Wet crinoline bandages hold the dressing in a satisfactory manner. The time required for the fungus to subside and heal over depends upon its size and the degree of infection. As a rule about three to six weeks will suffice for a cure to be effected.

IV. Linear Fractures of the Skull, Simple or Compounded in Which Repeated Examinations Fail to Show Any Evidence of Brain Damage

Cases falling into this group have a relatively low degree of elasticity of the skull, permitting the skull to be fractured without damage to the intracranial contents. There is a history of a blow on the head which may be followed by momentary unconsciousness. After a few moments the patient may become mentally clear and neurologic examination fails to reveal any evidence of damage to the intracranial structures. The spinal fluid is clear and under normal pressure, and there is no particular alteration of the pulse, blood pressure or respiration. The picture presented is that which is usually described as concussion and would be so diagnosed if the roentgen ray examination did not reveal an actual fracture of the skull.

Patients falling into this group usually recover promptly without any neurologic manifestations. They may perhaps have sustained scattered perivascular hemorrhages of mild degree without gross lesions or subarachnoid hemorrhage. On account of this possibility they should be kept at rest and under close observation for at least a week or ten days.

Treatment.—It is felt that such patients should be kept under careful observation and at rest in bed for at least one week in order to be sure that they have been correctly diagnosed. During this period of observation it is well to have these patients on a modified dehydration regime, limiting their total fluid intake (adults 1200 c.c. per 24-hour period) and administering saturated magnesium sulphate by mouth. With such a regime the greater number of cases will escape any frank sequelae. Should repeated examinations fail to reveal evidence of intracranial damage, there is no indication for any operative treatment. Should symptoms and findings arise indicating an intracranial lesion, reclassification of the case would be necessary.

V. Middle Meningeal Hemorrhage

The history and findings in cases of rupture of the middle meningeal artery are usually typical. There is a history of a blow or a fall on the head which may or may not have produced a slight degree of temporary unconsciousness. The patient may recover sufficiently from the transient unconsciousness to appear almost normal. After a period of freedom from symptoms (which may vary from a few minutes to several hours) there begin to develop symptoms and findings contralateral to the side injured. The first finding of note is a contralateral weakness of the facial movements. This is followed by a spastic paresis of the contralateral hand and leg. On the other hand, there may first develop contralateral irritative phenomena such as convulsions of jacksonian type, followed by paralysis. As these symptoms and findings develop, the patient lapses into an unconsciousness which gradually or rapidly becomes more and more profound. The contralateral deep reflexes are exaggerated and the superficial reflexes on this side are usually suppressed. The blood pressure progressively increases and the pulse rate descends.

Such a picture indicates that there is something within the cranial cavity which is causing a rapidly increasing intracranial pressure in spite of the fact that at the time of the accident the patient was not rendered profoundly unconscious. Such a lesion is usually a rapidly increasing extradural hemorrhage due to rupture of the middle meningeal artery. Since the artery enters the skull through the foramen spinosum in the floor of the middle fossa and courses upward in the dura where it lies so closely approximated to the inner surface of the skull as to cause definite grooves in the bone, one can readily understand why the artery may be torn when there is a fracture in this region. Although a fracture is usually present, cases have been reported in which there was no roentgen ray evidence of such a lesion. The ruptured artery may be on the side opposite to that on which the blow was received— a true illustration of the so-called contrecoup injury. This is mentioned in order to emphasize the importance of making a neurologic examination rather than depending entirely on the superficial evidence of injury.

The so-called lucid interval is usually spoken of as that period which elapses between the primary and secondary unconsciousness. From a practical standpoint the lucid interval should be that period of time which elapses between the time of the accident and the development of neurologic manifestations. The results of treatment in this group of cases depend upon the diagnosis being made at the earliest possible moment. The slightest contralateral facial paresis may be the first evidence of a progressing pressure and should therefore have great diagnostic significance. Should the diagnosis be withheld until the patient becomes unconscious, the brain may have been so profoundly damaged by the increasing pressure as to prevent recovery, even though the pressure be relieved.

Treatment.—There is no dispute in regard to the absolute necessity for immediate operation in cases of middle meningeal hemorrhage. The operation is for the removal of the extradural blood clots and for the checking of continued hemorrhage. The method to be employed depends largely upon how well versed the operator is in accepted neurologic technic. The incision and the exposure of the bone underlying the temporal muscle are the same as that already described for the performance of a typical subtemporal decompression. As soon as the skull has been opened, the diagnosis can be verified or disproved by the presence or absence of an extradural blood clot. If no clot is found but the exposed dura seems to be under greatly increased tension, it should be incised in order to determine whether or not there is a subdural hemorrhage. If such be found, a subtemporal decompression can be done as already described. If, on the other hand, there is doubt in the operator's mind in regard to the side of the hemorrhage (in case no hemorrhage is found) an exposure on the opposite side should be made in a similar manner.

In case a clot be found when the skull is opened, the further procedure depends largely upon the skill of the operator. If he is not well versed in the technic of controlling a ruptured meningeal artery, he should temporarily abandon the subtemporal operation and ligate the external carotid artery through an incision along the anterior border of the sternocleidomastoid muscle. As the middle meningeal artery is one of the terminal branches of the external carotid artery, a continued bleeding from the torn vessel will be prevented as soon as the external carotid artery is ligated. The operator should then return to the subtemporal exposure and remove a sufficient amount of bone to permit the complete evacuation of the extradural clot. Whether or not this should be followed by opening the dura in order to give the patient a subtemporal decompression depends largely upon the probability of a subdural injury associated with the middle meningeal hemorrhage. An operator of experience in this type of injury can usually ligate or clip the ruptured meningeal artery without having to resort to ligation of the external carotid artery. After the extradural clot has been removed and the hemorrhage controlled, the wounds are closed in layers, preferably with fine silk sutures.

VI. Miscellaneous Head Injuries

A. Concussion

Concussion is a poorly defined term that has acquired publicity through the press and in the courtroom; it may imply mild or severe brain damage. The term should, however, apply only to those cases in which there is a transient lowering of cerebral activity with no evidence of any structural changes. An individual is knocked down, hit about the head or strikes the head, and is momentarily dazed or unconscious. This period of diminished cerebral function may be from a few seconds to a few minutes. Regaining consciousness, the patient may notice a dull unlocalized headache or localized scalp discomfort at the site of the injury. What has actually happened to the patient is that he has suffered a momentary cerebral anemia from the blow, not sufficient to produce any subsequent cerebral edema, but sufficient to interfere momentarily with circulation. The blow is not of sufficient force to cause a fracture, nor is the force great enough to result in any damage to any of the structures encased in the skull. If either of these latter are involved in a head injury, then the case must be classified other than one of concussion.

Treatment.—There are no specific efforts indicated in this type of injury. Should a spinal puncture be resorted to, to exclude any subarachnoid hemorrhage, the patient should remain in bed for twenty-four hours to minimize the possibility of a postpuncture headache. Careful observation for any error in classification is the only precaution in this group.

B. Chronic Subdural Hematoma

As the result of an apparently trivial injury, often not associated with a fracture of the skull, one or more of the cortical veins may be torn as they leave the cortex to enter one of the dural sinuses. As the result of such a venous injury blood escapes between the dura and the arachnoid. Such patients may not present any neurologic manifestations at the time of the injury. They usually complain of some persistent headache. The gravity of the condition may not be appreciated until a sufficient amount of intracranial pressure to produce symptoms has developed. Why these symptoms of increased pressure should so frequently be delayed for many weeks or months offers a fertile field for speculation. When such patients come to operation, there is found an organized membrane closely attached to the inner surface of the dura and rich in capillaries and spaces lined with mesothelial cells, also a second thinner and avascular organized membrane lying over the brain cortex but not attached to the arachnoid except at the point of rupture of the cortical vein. Between these two organized membranes is a large quantity of fluid containing the elements of degenerated blood and varying in color from a clear yellow to a greenish brown. Peet[17] describes such a condition in which the fluid was of yellowish color and occurred in babies of several months to several years of age. All gave a history of a difficult labor. It is quite possible that the symptoms of increased pressure do not occur until there is an actual exudation into the area between the organized membranes from the membranes themselves. The condition has been found to occur bilaterally in about one-third of the reported cases.

The symptoms of this condition of chronic subdural hematoma may be for many weeks or months simply a headache of gradually increasing intensity. In a series of forty-two cases gathered from the literature by Jelsma,[18] headache was the first symptom noted in all of the cases. As the intracranial pressure increases, mental changes may be noted. These changes may simulate those frequently found in lesions of the frontal lobe. A late symptom may be drowsiness which may eventually deepen into coma. Contralateral motor weakness or evidences of motor irritability may develop. The other symptoms and findings are usually those of increased intracranial pressure such as choked disc, vomiting, disturbance of vision, and very late in the disease, irregular respiration.[19, 20, 21, 22]

Treatment.—The treatment of chronic subdural hematoma should consist of a removal of the organized membranes and the fluid which is present between them. This should be done at the time the diagnosis is made. There are cases in which the diagnosis of chronic subdural hematoma may be suspected, but not verified until the patient is subjected to ventriculography or to exploration through a small trephine opening. As soon as the diagnosis is confirmed, operation is the only hope for a cure. Operative procedures until recent years were all carried out through an osteoplastic flap, evacuating the liquefied blood and resecting the organized membranes.

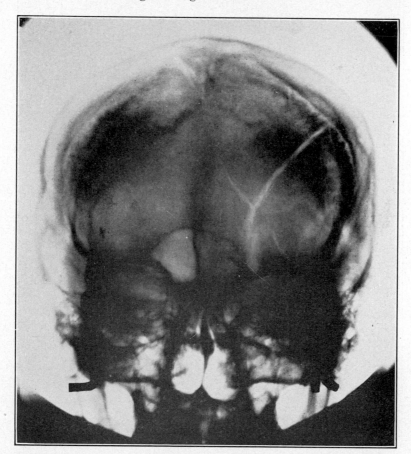

Fig. 201.—Most commonly there is an associated tear of the meninges in this type of fracture and infectious avenues are established.

In 1932 McKenzie[23] and in this same year Fleming and Jones[24] reported the treatment of cases by simple trephine drainage of the subdural clots. Not all cases are cured so simply, later requiring an osteoplastic flap before successfully relieving the patient. It is felt that if the trephine opening is enlarged to a diameter of at least one and one-half inches and as much of *both* membranes as possible through such an opening be removed, the likelihood of subsequent operations will be further minimized. By rupturing the inner membrane the expanding cerebrum helps prevent reaccumulations of blood, whereas, if only the liquefied blood is drained away, the remaining dead space invites a reformation of the clot. An enlarged trephine opening permits daily observation of the patient's progress. As long as free pulsations are visible one has no fears of any gross intracranial tension.

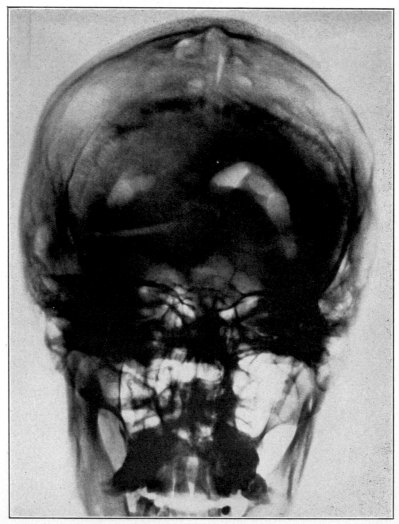

Fig. 202.—The introduction of air into the cranial cavity, either subdurally or into the ventricular cavities, more commonly results from fracture damages about the anterior base of the skull.

When an osteoplastic flap is necessary, a careful dissection of the adhered membrane from the dura must be accomplished. Meticulous hemostasis can be carried out with electrocoagulation. The removal of the inner membrane is more easily carried out than in removing the dural membrane. Care must be exercised not to tear the pial vessels so as to prevent subarachnoidal bleeding. This inner membrane strips away easily with cotton pledget dissection. Once the membranes are removed and complete hemostasis is effected, the bone flap is sutured in place and the scalp closed without drainage using interrupted silk sutures for the galea and the scalp.

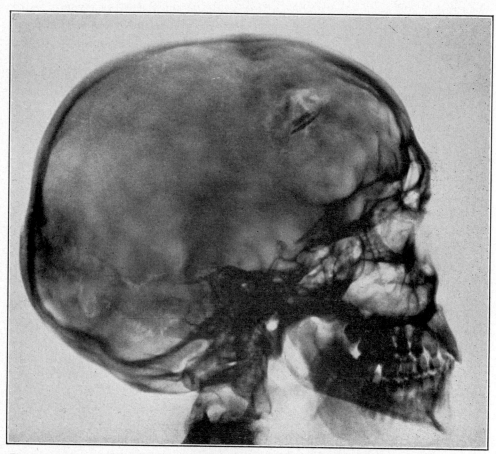

Fig. 203.—Such a fracture as this is most commonly the result of a force of small mass and great velocity. This was a simple depressed fracture.

C. Isolated Subcortical Hematoma

Isolated subcortical hemorrhages apparently following what may appear to have been a trivial head trauma are occasionally observed. The site of election for such an isolated hemorrhage is the temporal lobe. When seen several days or weeks after the history of trauma such patients present evidence of increased intracranial pressure and develop a contralateral facial weakness.

An illustration of such a case is as follows: A man, thirty years of age, on the night of January 1, 1929, was struck on the right side of the head with a bottle. He was rendered unconscious for three or four hours. The following day he returned to his home where he remained for several days apparently free from symptoms. On the sixth day after the accident he developed a condition of status epilepticus. The convulsions involved the left side more than the right. On examination there was a left facial weakness, a marked venous engorgement of the retinal veins, and a beginning bilateral papilloedema. Lumbar puncture was done and the spinal fluid was found to contain fresh blood. The right temporal region was explored by Dr. Dowman and a large subcortical hematoma of the temporal lobe with an apparent recent rupture through the overlying cortex was found and evacuated. The patient made an uneventful recovery.

Although the occurrence of such isolated temporal lobe hemorrhages may not be frequent, the condition should be kept in mind when unilateral symptoms suggesting temporal lobe involvement develop several days following an apparently trivial injury. Ventricular air studies will give accurate localization where neurologic symptoms and findings are misleading.

Treatment.—Isolated subcortical hemorrhages when properly diagnosed should be treated by means of operation. The object of the operation is to expose that part of the brain which is suspected of containing the hematoma, to verify the subcortical hemorrhage by means of puncture, and to incise the overlying cortex, and remove the clot. When the hemorrhage is in the temporal lobe this can be done by the usual subtemporal exploration already described. When in other portions of the brain the operation can best be done through a properly placed bone flap exploration. After removing the clot the cavity should be carefully inspected and if a bleeding vessel be found it should be clipped or ligated.

D. Tear of Galen Vein or Its Tributaries

This is a type of injury which does not present the clinical manifestations of any of the above-mentioned groups. Bagley[6] described the pathologic findings in several cases belonging to this group which came under his observation. He found an injury of the vein of Galen or of the contributory veins of Galen with an associated hemorrhagic infiltration in the region of the internal capsule and the central ganglia. On account of the marked hyperpyrexia in such cases Bagley thought perhaps the heat-regulating mechanism might be represented in this portion of the midbrain.

Patients belonging to this group are rendered profoundly unconscious. The pulse rate is rapid, the respirations are rapid, and the temperature is greatly elevated. The neurologic examination reveals evidence of unilateral or bilateral pyramidal tract involvement. There is no evidence of increased intracranial pressure. The spinal fluid is bloody and under decreased pressure. The patient may live as long as a week or ten days without regaining consciousness. An occasional case of this type may recover,[25] although death is the usual result. Should such a patient be operated upon on account of hemiplegia, the brain is found to be under decreased rather than increased pressure and actually falls away from the dura when this structure is opened.

Treatment.—Other than general measures, particularly those employed for the reduction of fever, there is no specific type of treatment indicated in this group of cases. The spinal fluid usually contains blood and as long as such patients are living the removal of the bloody spinal fluid by daily lumbar puncture may be done. There is no indication for hypertonic treatment, since these cases do not develop increased intracranial pressure. A mistake which is not infrequently made is that of misinterpreting an existing hemiplegia as being caused by a large extradural or subdural hemorrhage. Such a misinterpretation may lead one to perform an unnecessary subtemporal exploration. When such an operation is done in cases belonging to this group no blood clot is found, and (as already mentioned) when the dura is opened, the brain actually falls away from this structure.

E. Pneumocephalus and Cerebrospinal Rhinorrhea

The importance of traumatic pneumocephalus presenting a problem in head trauma has been emphasized by Rand.[26] It has been known for many years[29] that following a fracture of the skull when the fracture communicates with one of the bony sinuses, air may escape from the sinus under the subaponeurotic layer of the scalp. That air may also escape into the cranial cavity as a complication of such a type of fracture was first demonstrated in roentgenograms by Leuckette[28] in 1913. In 1884 Chirrari[29] reported a case of air within the cranial cavity complicating a chronic inflammation of the ethmoid cells. Rand reviewed the literature on this subject and reported eight cases of traumatic pneumocephalus, emphasizing the importance of recognizing the condition and suggesting an appropriate treatment.

The most common site for the development of pneumocephalus is the frontal region. The dura underlying the frontal sinuses is very thin and tightly adhered to the skull. A fracture of the inner wall of the frontal sinus can therefore be easily complicated by a tear of the underlying dura. Talking, sneezing, or straining will increase the air pressure within the sinus and if a fracture be present, this air may be forced into the cranial cavity. The condition is practically identical with that which may permit the outflow of cerebrospinal fluid in cerebrospinal rhinorrhea.

Rand emphasizes the importance of carefully watching for the possible development of pneumocephalus in any case of fracture of the skull communicating with an accessory nasal sinus. Complications may appear immediately after the injury or more often several weeks later. The presence of cerebrospinal rhinorrhea should cause one to suspect the possible development of pneumocephalus. When the condition develops, the symptoms depend largely upon the amount of air and the rapidity of its entrance into the cranial cavity. The symptoms of increased intracranial pressure appear; namely, headache, nausea, and vomiting. Drowsiness and stupor which even progress to coma may develop. Mental symptoms such as disorientation, disturbance of memory, and illusions may occur. Although not constantly present, a papilloedema may be observed on ophthalmoscopic examination. Convulsions of a jacksonian type have been observed. The signs and symptoms characteristic of a rapid developing meningitis such as chills and fever, stiffness of the neck, and a positive Kernig's sign are usually present. The roentgen ray examination will reveal the presence of air which may be located in the frontal region of the cranial cavity or in one or both ventricles.[29, 30, 31]

Treatment.—The treatment of traumatic pneumocephalus is by means of operation. Dandy[29] in 1926 suggested a practical method of treating this condition by releasing the entrapped air, searching out the dural defect and closing this defect by suture or by a fascial transplant. His method of approach varied according to the type of fracture and position of the dural tear. Two procedures were suggested: (1) simple exposure of the fracture near the supraorbital ridge and repairing of the dural defect which lay directly beneath, or (2) an extensive frontal bone flap, searching for the dural defect along the posterior wall of the frontal sinus or in the region of the ethmoid cells, and closure of the same. The same type of operation should be done in cases of persistent cerebrospinal rhinorrhea, as cases of this nature may later develop a meningitis unless this condition is corrected.

GENERAL MEASURES

Treatment Which May Be Applicable at Times in Any Particular Type of Head Injury

The reason for utilizing a classification of head injuries is to instigate proper treatment as soon as possible. The employment of operative measures depends entirely upon the individual case under consideration. In general, an operation is not indicated unless there is something to be removed. If, for example, there is a rapidly increasing intracranial pressure due to extra- or intradural hemorrhage and the patient is well within the period of compensation, an operation for the removal of the accumulated blood should be performed. If there be indriven bone fragments and localized areas of contused brain, the bone fragments and the softened contused brain should be removed. If there be a late development of increased intracranial pressure due to subdural fluid or blood, the fluid or blood should be removed. On the other hand, there are many cases of brain injury which can be handled without operation, provided there is nothing present which should be removed by operation. There are certain general measures which are more or less applicable to all cases regardless of the group to which they belong. Such measures are those which are employed during the period of shock, for the control of hyperpyrexia, for restlessness, general irritability, etc.

Shock.—Many patients who have sustained a head trauma when first seen are in a condition of profound shock. Under such circumstances, measures for the relief of shock should be first instituted before subjecting the patient to any of the various methods of treatment already discussed. It is of prime importance to differentiate between shock and the condition of marked increased intracranial pressure of rapid onset. In the former condition the respiration and pulse are usually very rapid and shallow, temperature subnormal, skin clammy, and the patient may be covered with profuse perspiration. In marked increased intracranial pressure the respirations are usually much slower and more stertorous than in a condition of shock. It is also of great importance to determine whether the shock is the result of an excessive loss of blood or purely traumatic in character. When due to loss of blood some method for restoring blood volume should be instituted. If transfusion is not possible the intravenous administration of 250 to 500 c.c. of blood plasma may be used. If neither blood nor blood plasma can be obtained, the patient can be given 500 to 1,000 c.c. of 2½ per cent glucose in normal saline solution, intravenously. Whether the shock is due to loss of blood or traumatic in nature the patient should be warmed by the means of warm blankets and hot water bottles. Stimulants such as caffeine sodium benzoate (grains viiss.), camphorated oil (minims xxx), or adrenalin (minims v to x), may be given hypodermically. If the patient is extremely restless sodium luminal (grains ii to iv) may be given hypodermically. It is well to avoid the use of morphia, immediately after an injury of this nature, on account of masking important symptoms and findings which may aid in a correct diagnosis of the type of injury sustained. Indicated operative measures should be postponed until the patient has recovered from the condition of shock.

Hyperpyrexia.—When hyperpyrexia occurs in cases of head injury, measures should be employed to reduce the temperature. An ice bag to the head, cold sponges, and cold colonic irrigations will usually reduce temperatures of moderate degree. Should these measures fail to bring down the temperature, the extremities should be wrapped in cloths which have been saturated with ice water. Many times the hyperpyrexia is secondary to faulty peripheral circulation and brisk massage of the extremities with a roughened towel will be as effective as hydrotherapeutic efforts. Excessive degrees of temperature may be due to subarachnoid hemorrhage. Under such circumstances the bloody cerebrospinal fluid should be removed as much as possible by means of lumbar puncture. Not infrequently the intravenous administration of five hundred cubic centimeters of 5 to 10 per cent glucose solution will have a marked beneficial effect in lowering the temperature when a hyperpyrexia exists. In cases receiving hypertonic treatment, the sudden rise in temperature may indicate an overdepletion of body fluids. Under such circumstances the administration of 500 to 1,000 c.c. of normal salt solution subcutaneously will usually correct the condition. If the condition of overdepletion persists despite the subcutaneous administration of normal salt solution, 500 to 1,000 c.c. administered intravenously very slowly may be resorted to.

Restlessness and General Irritability.—Restlessness and general irritability is not an infrequent condition in cases of brain injury. When these symptoms are present, two to four grains of sodium luminal may be given intramuscularly. If the restlessness is not thus controlled, forty to sixty grains of sodium bromide or one-half ounce of paraldehyde in four ounces of water may be given, by rectum, once or twice daily. As a general rule it is well to withhold the use of opium, not only for the reason mentioned above, but the use of morphine is known to elevate the spinal fluid pressure. Everyone is familiar with its constrictor effects on the pupils of the eyes and the depressant effect it has on respiration. Despite all sedative treatment there are some patients with marked restlessness and irritability who have to be restrained by the use of a strait jacket. It is probably the wiser part of judgment to resort to guarded doses of morphine before increasing the patient's irritability with this torturous method of restraint. The use of the strait jacket should be reserved for those cases which cannot be otherwise controlled.

Various other therapeutic measures which may be necessary in cases of brain injury differ little from such general measures as used in other types of injury. The same care of the bladder, bowels, etc., applies here as in other cases. An overdistended bladder may sometimes be the cause of extreme restlessness. Under such circumstances catheterization should be resorted to. Not infrequently in spite of the use of large quantities of magnesium sulphate given in saturated form without water the bowels will have to be evacuated by means of enemas.

In case of bleeding from the ear, the canal should be swabbed with a non-irritating antiseptic and a sterile cotton pledget placed in the ear and removed when saturated with blood. Irrigation of the ear should be avoided as such a method of treatment tends to carry an infection which might extend to the meninges. Should a blood clot form within the external auditory canal it should be removed through a speculum.

Spinal Puncture.—The advisability of performing a spinal puncture in cases of head injury is a matter of great dispute among various neurologic surgeons. It is a well-recognized fact that spinal puncture is not a safe procedure in cases of chronic increase of intracranial pressure caused by brain tumor. Under such circumstances there is grave danger of promoting a medullary herniation into the foramen magnum by releasing the pressure within the spinal canal. When such herniation occurs, the patient may die of respiratory failure. It is a matter of dispute whether the same danger is present in cases of acute intracranial pressure due to trauma. Some fatalities following spinal puncture in brain trauma have been observed, and such observers advise strongly against the procedure. There are other neurologic surgeons who consider spinal puncture of such great value as to adopt it as a routine measure. There are two conditions in which it seems wise to perform spinal puncture. In the first place, there are many cases of head injury in which it is difficult to say definitely that the brain has been injured. Under such circumstances the presence or absence of blood in the spinal fluid is of great diagnostic value. This can be decided definitely only by doing a spinal puncture. When the puncture is done, the cerebrospinal fluid pressure can also be determined, thereby giving information of great value. An accurate estimate of the spinal fluid pressure can be made only from manometric observation. In the second place, blood in the subarachnoid space may act as a great irritant. This has been emphasized particularly by Bagley.[4] The withdrawal of the bloody cerebrospinal fluid by repeated punctures is therefore a measure of definite therapeutic value.

A reasonable position to assume, therefore, in regard to spinal puncture is as follows: In cases of unquestioned brain damage, and particularly in those cases in which the major injury seems to concern the structures in the posterior fossa, lumbar puncture is not only unnecessary, but may be dangerous. On the other hand, in those cases in which there is some doubt as to the presence of brain contusion, spinal puncture is indicated as an aid to a correct diagnosis. When blood is found to be present, it indicates that there have been injuries sufficiently near the surfaces of the brain to permit blood to escape into the cerebrospinal fluid spaces. Furthermore, if during the course of the illness there develop symptoms of brain irritation, spinal puncture is indicated therapeutically in order to withdraw the bloody fluid or it may give an accurate estimate of the intracranial tension which may have developed slowly enough to not allow acute manifestations.

PROGNOSIS

The mortality in cases of injury to the brain with or without fracture depends largely upon the character of the intracranial lesion. This is, of course, provided the cases have been properly classified and the proper type of treatment employed to meet the individual case. The mortality in any large series of cases, properly treated, depends upon the number of patients falling into the class of so-called massive brain injury with evidence of rapid exhaustion of the medullary centers. As a general rule approximately 20 per cent of all types of head injuries fall into this group. Such cases die in spite of any type of treatment which has been employed. Most cases in which there has been a midbrain lesion, such as described by Bagley, die regardless of any form of therapy. Fortunately, these cases constitute a very small percentage of the injuries encountered. The results in cases of middle meningeal hemorrhage depend upon the early recognition of the condition. If the diagnosis is not made until the patient has relapsed into the secondary stage of profound unconsciousness, death usually results even though the blood clot be removed. Therefore, it is highly important in this particular group of cases to resort to operation just as soon as unilateral neurologic manifestations appear. Under such circumstances the mortality in this group should be nil.

The morbidity in cases of intracranial trauma depends upon several factors. If, for example, there be a depressed fracture with marked brain contusion of the cortical motor centers, a certain amount of residual mono- or hemiplegia is to be expected. Contusions of the temporal lobe may leave the patient with a residual auditory aphasia or visual field defect; destruction of certain areas of the occipital lobe may result in the patient having a homonymous hemianopsia, etc. On the other hand, extensive and widely scattered contusions of the brain may so interfere with various associated nerve pathways as to result in such mental disturbances as forgetfulness, change in disposition, errors in judgment, etc. It is the author's opinion that many posttraumatic neurologic manifestations can be prevented by instigating the proper treatment at the time of injury. There may be permanent damage to nerve cells and fibers as the result of circulatory disturbances in patients who are permitted to lie for days and weeks with a marked increased intracranial pressure. This damage leads to posttraumatic manifestations which would not occur had measures been employed to prevent the intracranial structures from being subjected to such long periods of increased intracranial tension. In general it may be said that the more accurately the individual cases be diagnosed and classified in order to institute the type of treatment which may seem indicated in each particular case, just so the posttraumatic manifestations will be lessened.

REFERENCES

1. Martland, H. H.: Punch Drunk, J. A. M. A. 91: 1103, October 13, 1928. Editorial, J. A. M. A., January 26, 1929.
2. Cassasa, C. B.: Multiple Traumatic Cerebral Hemorrhages, Proc. N. Y. Path. Soc. 24: 101, January-May, 1924.
3. Osnato, Michael and Giliverti, Vincent: Post Concussion Neurosis. Traumatic Encephalitis, Arch. Neurol. and Psych. 18: 181, August, 1927.
4. Bagley, Chas. Jr.: Blood in the Cerebrospinal Fluid. Resultant Functional and Organic Alterations in the Central Nervous System, Arch. Surg. 17: 18, July, 1928.

5. Fay, Temple: Generalized Pressure Atrophy of the Brain, Secondary to Traumatic and Pathologic Involvement of Pacchuonian Bodies, J. A. M. A. 94: 245, January 25, 1930.
6. Bagley, Chas. Jr.: The Grouping and Treatment of Acute Cerebral Trauma, Arch. Surg. 18: 1079, April, 1929.
7. Rand, Carl: Before American Medical Association, Section on Nervous and Mental Diseases, June 27, 1930.
8. Naffziger, H. C.: Subdural Fluid Accumulations Following Head Injuries, J. A. M. A. 82: 1751, May 31, 1924.
9. Howe, H. S.: Physiologic Mechanism for the Maintenance of Intracranial Pressure, Arch. Neurol. and Psych. 20: 1048, November, 1928.
10. Rand, Carl: The Significance of a Dilated Pupil on the Homolateral Hemiplegic Side in Cases of Intracranial Hemorrhage Following Head Injuries: Report of Seven Cases, Arch. Surg. 18: 1176, April, 1929.
11. Weed and McKibben: Pressure Changes in the Cerebrospinal Fluid Following Intravenous Injections of Solutions of Various Concentrations, Am. J. Physiol. 48: 212, 1919-1920.
12. Foley and Putnam: The Effects of Salt Ingestion on Cerebrospinal Fluid Pressure and Brain Volume, Am. J. Physiol. 53: 464, 1920-1921.
13. Dowman, Chas. E.: Management of Head Injuries with Real or Potential Brain Damage, J. A. M. A., December 30, 1922.
14. Fay, Temple: The Treatment of Acute and Chronic Cases of Cerebral Trauma by Method of Dehydration, Ann. Surg. 101: No. 1, 76, January, 1935.
15. Naffziger, H. C.: Effects of Depressed Fractures, Surg., Gynec. and Obst. 51: 17, July, 1930.
16. Dowman, Chas. E.: The Treatment of Brain Fungus, Trans. South. Surg. Assn. 41: 170, 1928.
17. Peet, Max: Symptoms, Diagnosis and Treatment of Acute Cranial and Intracranial Injuries, N. Y. State J. Med. 28: 555, May 15, 1928.
18. Jelsma, Franklin: Chronic Subdural Hematoma: Summary and Analysis of Forty-Two Cases Collected From the Literature; With Report of Two Additional Cases, Arch. Surg. 21: 128, July, 1930.
19. Putnam, Tracy, and Cushing, Harvey: Chronic Subdural Hematoma, Arch. Surg. 11: 329, September, 1925.
20. Rand, Carl: Chronic Subdural Hematoma, Arch. Surg. 14: 1136, June, 1927.
21. Griswold and Jelsma: Chronic Subdural Hematoma, Arch. Surg. 15: 45, July, 1926.
22. Holmes: Chronic Subdural Hemorrhage, Arch. Neurol. and Psych. 20: 162, July, 1928.
23. McKenzie, H. G.: A Clinical and Surgical Study of Nine Cases of Chronic Subdural Hematoma, Canadian M. A. J. 26: 534, 1932.
24. Fleming, H. W., and Jones, O. W., Jr.: Chronic Subdural Hematoma. Simple Drainage as a Method of Treatment, Surg., Gynec. and Obst. 54: 81, January, 1932.
25. Bagley, Chas., Jr.: The Grouping and Treatment of Acute Cerebral Trauma, Arch. Surg. 18: 1079, April, 1929.
26. Rand, Carl W.: Traumatic Pneumocephalus, Report of Eight Cases, Arch. Surg. 20: 935, June, 1930.
27. Wernher: Pneumatocele Cranii, Deutsch. Ztschr. f. Chir. 3: 381, 1873.
28. Leuckette, W. H.: Air in the Ventricles of the Brain Following a Fracture of the Skull. Report of a Case, Surg., Gynec. and Obst. 17: 237, 1913.
29. Chirrari, H.: Ueber Einen Fall von Luftansammlung in den Ventricel des menschlichen Gehirns, Prag. Viertelyahrs, schr. f. Heilk. 5: 383, 1884.
30. Dandy, Walter E.: Pneumocephalus, Arch. Surg. 12: 949, July, 1926.
31. Allen, T. P.: Arch. Neurol. and Psych. 20: 1390, December, 1928.
32. Lewis: Traumatic Pneumocephalus, Brain 51: 228, 1928.

CHAPTER XII

FRACTURES OF THE JAWS AND RELATED BONES OF THE FACE*

By James Barrett Brown, M.D., St. Louis, Mo.

FRACTURES OF THE LOWER JAW

The lower jaw is in an exposed position; it is relatively poorly protected by soft tissues and in some cases it appears to be relatively brittle. External violence applied directly to the jaw in fights, sports, falls, and traffic accidents accounts for most fractures. Fractures occur most frequently near the mental foramen or the angle, and, if both sides are broken, usually near the mental foramen on one side and near the angle on the other.

Fractures through the symphysis, ramus, and condyle occur less frequently. The force that breaks a condyle is necessarily transmitted from another part of the jaw and the most frequent cause is a fall or a blow on the chin. This type of injury may also jam the condyle backward or upward and splinter the bony ear canal or even the floor of the middle fossa. This is perhaps the only way in which a skull fracture may directly complicate a lower jaw fracture, whereas in upper jaw fractures brain injury is frequently present and fracture of the cranial bones must be looked for carefully.

Fractures may occur in areas weakened by pathologic processes such as osteomyelitis, benign cysts and tumors, and malignant growths inherent in the jaw itself or secondary involvement as from a carcinoma of the buccal mucosa. They may also occur during the extraction of teeth, most frequently in removing difficult third molars. (Figs. 204-208.)

Displacement

The immediate displacement of the fragments is dependent on the direction of the force, but the attached muscles soon modify the deformity according to their direction of contraction. A knowledge of the action of these muscles will help one to find where the fragments are and then to replace and maintain them correctly. With this information and rather simple equipment, the surgeon may accomplish excellent results in most instances, without resorting to a study of all the numerous forms of apparatus that have been recorded.

It is well to remember that the direction of the fracture line itself may govern the displacement and also that irregular lines or fragments may be a help or a hindrance in correctly aligning the fracture; for example, if the obliquity of the fracture line as shown in Fig. 210 were from below upward

---

*Many of the principles involved are included in the legends of the illustrations and may be followed as part of the text.

and backward, the posterior fragment might be held down in position, while if it were in the opposite direction, some direct aim would have to be made at holding the fragment down.

In fractures of the condyle and its neck it is frequently stated that the external pterygoid muscle pulls the small fragment forward so that the remaining large fragment cannot be reduced on this small fragment. This in turn calls for open reduction of or excision of the small fragment if it undergoes necrosis or if ankylosis occurs. We have found, however, that the condyle is more often separated with a small part of the posterior border of the ramus attached to it and this luckily tends to hold the condyle in a position close enough to normal so that fixation of the jaw in correct occlusion usually suffices.

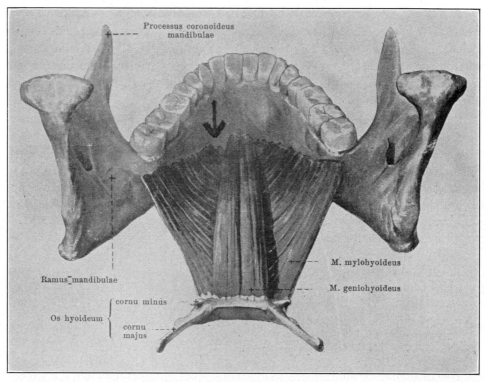

Fig. 204.—Opening muscles of jaw. The muscle groups attached to the front part of the jaw are the depressors, and, accordingly, tend to pull fragments down in the direction of the arrow. The digastrics on the outer side have the same action. The displacement is somewhat guided by the direction of the fracture lines, but is directly affected by the movement of the hyoid bone on swallowing, and one of the most troublesome lower jaw fractures to maintain in position may be a simple appearing one near the symphysis. In the posterior part of the jaw the closing muscles are attached and tend to pull the fragments upward. See Figs. 205 and 206. (From Spalteholz.)

The coronoid process is very infrequently broken, but it may be pulled high in the zygomatic fossa by the temporal muscle.

Voluntary movement of the jaw and swallowing always influence displacement and cause pain.

Diagnosis

If displacement, abnormal movement, loss of normal occlusion of the teeth, pain on movement, and hemorrhage from around one or more teeth is present, the diagnosis of fracture is clear, and there is little use trying to elicit crepitus. It is not always easy to determine where or in how many places a jaw is broken, however; and a careful examination should always be made, noting the points of tenderness, and having x-rays of the entire jaw including both condyles.

Displacement may not occur in fractures of the ramus and condyle, and occasionally even in the body, and here the x-ray must be depended on.

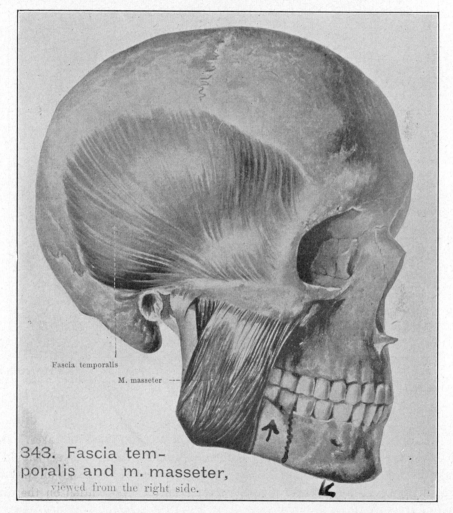

Fig. 205.—Closing muscles of jaw. The main closing muscles—the masseter, the temporal and internal pterygoid—all pull the posterior fragment upward. The masseter also pulls it outward so that its end may lodge in the upper buccal fornix. This deformity, if not corrected early, gives the most frequent and most troublesome displacement of lower jaw fragments with which to deal. (From Spalteholz.)

Dislocation occurs much less frequently than fracture. It results in deviation rather than displacement and there is no abnormal movement or crepitus. Loosening of teeth or avulsion of the alveolar process may simulate complete fracture, but there is no false motion through the entire thickness of the jaw.

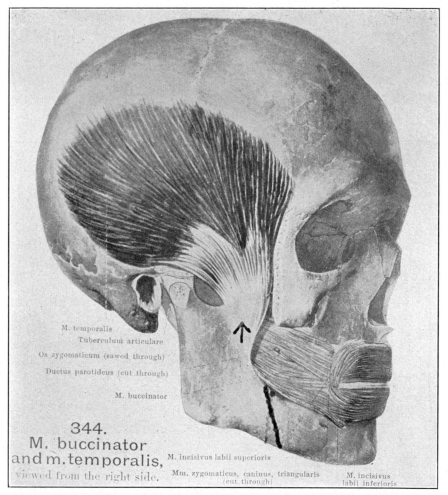

Fig. 206.—The temporal is a powerful closing muscle that elevates the posterior fragment. If the coronoid itself is fractured, this muscle may pull it high in the fossa out of reach. (From Spalteholz.)

X-ray Diagnosis

X-ray diagnosis should be relied upon in all questionable cases. Complete views of both sides, including both condyles and the symphysis should always be taken, because one or more fractures may be missed on physical examination. X-ray pictures give the most accurate information on the direction of fracture lines, the involvement of tooth roots in the fracture lines, the injuries and general condition of the teeth themselves, and the position of fragments after reduction.

Treatment of Uncomplicated Cases With Teeth Present

Fixation with bandages, or the use of a molded chin cup with a rubber sling over the head or attached to a plaster cap will give some support and probably some comfort to the patient during transportation or until firmer fixation can be made. This may be used overnight or until the stomach is empty and possible effects of alcohol have cleared up. The bandage should be put on so that the jaw is in a sling from the top of the head, and no turns should go around the front of the chin, since these may tend to increase displacement. The teeth should be brought into occlusion as nearly as possible, supported there, and the bandage applied with a gauze or sponge pad under the chin. A two-inch elastic bandage is perhaps the most comfortable. (Fig. 209.)

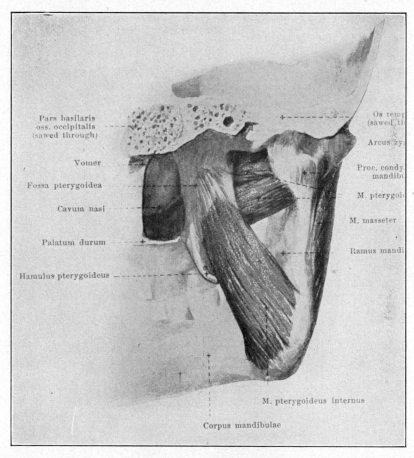

Fig. 207.—The internal pterygoid elevates and pulls inward the posterior fragment. The masseter and temporal together, however, usually pull the fragment upward and outside of the anterior fragment. (From Spalteholz.)

If there is any tendency to displacement, bandaging and even the use of long strips of adhesive plaster will only occasionally suffice to hold the jaws in occlusion during the period of healing. In some instances there is little tendency to displacement and rest is all that is required. This is usually the type in which credit is given for bandage fixation, and the bandage does give some sense of support.

Fixation by Interdental Wiring.—The objects of treatment are to align the fragments, to bring the entire lower jaw into a position so that the occlusion of the upper and lower teeth is the same as it was before the accident, and to hold the jaw in this position until it will maintain itself. This does not

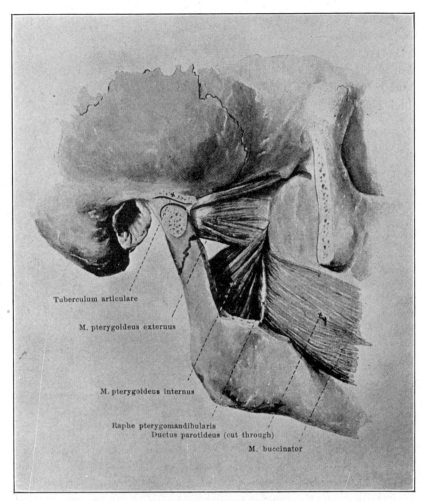

Tuberculum articulare

M. pterygoideus externus

M. pterygoideus internus

Raphe pterygomandibularis
Ductus parotideus (cut through)
M. buccinator

Fig. 208.—The external pterygoid may pull the condyle forward, but, as stated in the text, it most frequently breaks with a wedge or prolongation down the ramus so that it may be held in fairly good position.   (From Spalteholz.)

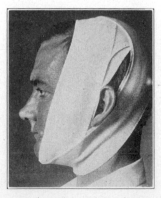

Fig. 209.—Bandage for supporting fractured jaw. The jaw is closed in as accurate occlusion as possible. A small pad is put under the chin and the bandage is applied so that the chin is literally slung from the top of the head. No turns go around in front of the chin.

necessarily mean normal correct occlusion, but normal occlusion for the individual patient. To try to improve on occlusion is not good practice, and one may gain information from the patient's own sensations as to what is his normal occlusion.

The best splint that can be employed by the surgeon is the upper jaw; and the best fixation is by means of wires fastened around appropriate teeth on both jaws and then fastened together. If there is any question in the surgeon's mind about correctly aligning the teeth, the ideas of a dental or oral surgeon should be obtained on this point. (Figs. 210 to 217.)

There will be found in the literature an endless number of ideas for mechanically fixing the jaws, many of them advocating complicated dental splints, but it is thought that even a discussion of them in a general text of this type is unnecessary. If these devices are to be used, they of course have to be applied by their own advocates. The majority of uncomplicated fractures of the lower jaw will undoubtedly do best if fixed directly to the upper jaw, the position of rest, which is with the lower jaw open slightly, being disregarded.

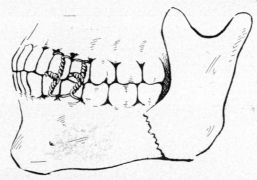

Fig. 210.—Diagram of wire fixation. The bicuspids are preferably used as they have good interdental spaces and good necks for the wires to lock around. The ends of the wires are cut off cleanly and turned toward the teeth to protect the mucosa. No wax covering is needed if this is done smoothly. Note retention of third molar in fracture line to prevent elevation of posterior fragment. (This is essentially the Gilmer method.)

Method of Wiring.—The patient should be able to cooperate, free from the effects of alcohol, and the stomach empty. A preoperative sedative is desirable but not necessary. A gentle effort at reduction of the fracture should be made, and, if there is too much discomfort, block anesthesia of the mandibular nerves, local infiltration from the outside about the fracture or deep block anesthesia of the third division of the fifth nerve should be done. It is not a safe procedure to wire jaws closed under general anesthesia unless some arrangement is made for separating them if there should be respiratory difficulty in waking from the anesthesia. Local anesthesia may be necessary for applying the upper wires. (Figs. 227, 228, 229.)

At the time of reduction, a studied effort should be made to determine what is normal occlusion for the patient, and his ideas of sensation should be closely followed if there is any question. With this accomplished the teeth upon which to apply the wires are next determined. If the bicuspids are present, they are the ideal ones to use, the molars next, and the cuspid and incisors last as they can hardly be counted on to retain wires because of their shape.

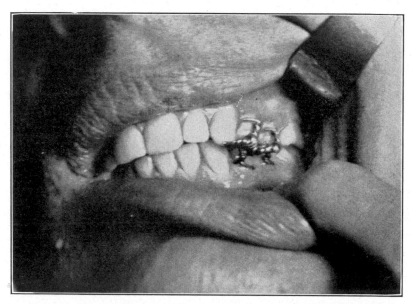

Fig. 211.—Interdental fixation of all eight bicuspids for fracture through angle. This patient was treated twelve hours after injury in a soccer game. The last molar was left in place to hold the posterior fragment down; external drainage was done. The patient worked after the fourth day entirely through the period of fixation of three weeks. The last molar was easily removed about two weeks later, and the jaw has remained solid with normal opening and occlusion.

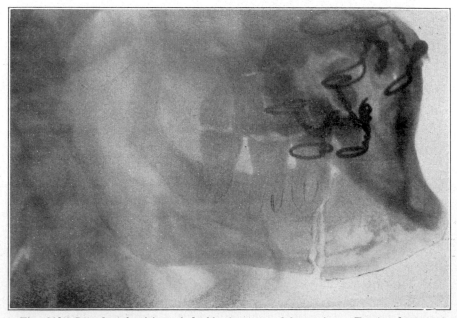

Fig. 212.—Interdental wiring of double fracture of lower jaw. Fractured at angle on opposite side as shown in Fig. 213. Note accurate occlusion obtained, the firmness of fixation apparent from the wires, and the placing of one wire on a molar in the posterior fragment. Shows definite need of retention of teeth close to fracture line for utilization in fixation. Also definite need of external drainage because of being compounded into the mouth and because of loose, small fragments in the fracture line.

If the fracture is behind the bicuspids and tends to displace, it is well to use one of the molars; in other words, try to place one wire on the posterior fragment if possible. Where there is marked abnormality of occlusion, there may be difficulty in getting any set of wires that will remain firm throughout the period of fixation. (Figs. 210-213.)

Various types of wire may be found satisfactory: No. 24 or 26 plain iron wire cut in about 16-inch lengths and the strands kept good and straight.

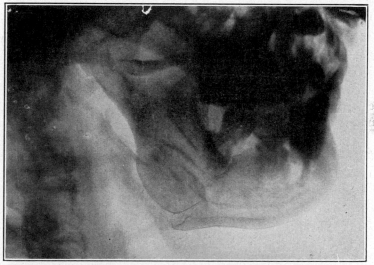

A.

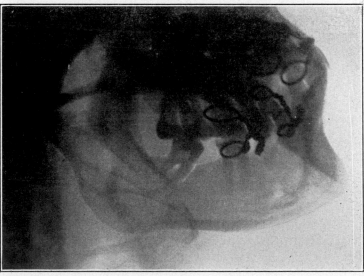

B.

Fig. 213.—Retention of tooth in fracture line for support of posterior fragment. *A.* Fracture near angle through socket of third molar. Fracture definitely compounded into the mouth and external drainage indicated for this reason. This third molar should definitely be retained during the period of fixation, to hold down in place the posterior fragment. *B.* Shows preceding fracture reduced and the jaws wired in normal occlusion. The third molar holds the posterior fragment down in place during the period of fixation. It can be gently lifted from its socket seven to fourteen days after the wires are removed and union is solid enough to withstand the manipulation.

Other kinds used are No. 24 Angle's brass ligature wire, nickeled silver wire, and stainless steel wire. The iron wire discolors the teeth temporarily, but is strong, cheap, and is easily available. Plain silver wire is not strong enough.

A separate wire is put around each tooth, preferably on two teeth on each side, above and below. The wire loop is made to drop firmly in place around the neck of the tooth by a final tug gently on one end. It is tightened firmly in place with the hands; the turns of all wires should be made the same way.

The long ends of the wires are brought outside the mouth and the patient's eyes are protected by hanging a surgical clamp on each wire.

When all eight wires are on, the jaw is reset into what has been determined the best position. An assistant stands at the head and cups his hands under the chin and, if possible, the patient flexes his head to relieve the tension of the opening muscles. The wires are then fastened together firmly with the fingers (not twisted with forceps) bringing the wires directly from one bicuspid to its opposite. This is about the only change from the original Gilmer method of wiring in which the wires were crossed from before backward. This does not permit of opening the mouth for inspection, but in a long series this has not been necessary, and other methods give less firm fixation. Even with this method the wires will stretch and loosen some and give some play in a few days' time so that they may have to be carefully tightened if too much play of the fragment develops.

If accurate reduction and firm fixation are obtained, the patient will be comfortable within from five to ten minutes, and the long ends may be cut off. The short sharp ends are then turned in neatly so that the buccal mucous membrane is protected, and there is no need for a protective covering of wax or cotton. There may be minor adjustments necessary from time to time for these ends, but the use of a gum covering only makes more pockets for débris.

For cutting the wire small, pointed, electrician's wire-cutters are far more satisfactory than any surgical tool, and are almost indispensable when finally removing the wires. About the only other instruments necessary are small clamps and a small retractor for the cheek. (Fig. 211.)

Interdental Fixation That Permits Opening the Jaws.—If a method of wiring is desired so that the mouth can be opened, that of Ivy (Figs. 214-217) is excellent; or that of wiring short bars to two or three teeth and then ligating between them, as advocated by J. A. Brown, may be used.

Disposal of Teeth in the Fracture Line.—If a jaw is broken through alongside a tooth or directly into its socket, this is considered a compound fracture and especially liable to infection because of contamination from the mouth. This classifies all such fractures as compound fractures. Although frequently recommended there is one serious drawback to the routine removal of teeth from fracture lines because these very teeth may give valuable aid in fixation, and, in the case of fractures through the molar region and angle, may be indispensable in holding down the posterior fragment. (Figs. 210 and 212.) Even if one of these last teeth were quite loose in its socket, great help may be had by retaining it during the period of fixation. Also, near the symphy-

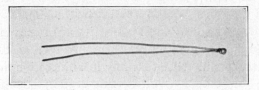

Fig. 214.—Ivy method of interdental wiring. Eyelet twisted in strand of wire. (From Ivy and Curtis: Fractures of the Jaws.)

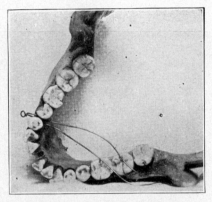

Fig. 215.—Ends of eyelet wire inserted between premolars.

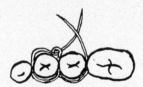

Fig. 216.—Eyelet wire passed around the teeth, with one end through the eyelet ready to be twisted.

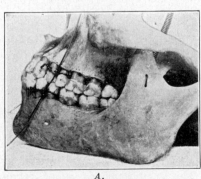

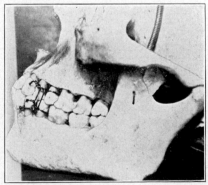

A.   B.

Fig. 217.—A. Ends of upper and lower eyelet wires twisted and tie-wire passed through eyelets. B. Upper and lower teeth drawn into occlusion, ends of tie-wire twisted and cut off short.

sis, the retention of teeth during the healing period is important, because if they are removed the space tends to be filled by tilting of the fragments.

About ten to fourteen days after the wires are removed and it is seen that the jaw will maintain its continuity, these involved teeth may be carefully lifted from their sockets in order that any local infection may have a chance to clear up and the jaw become solid in this region. Care must of course be taken to prevent refracturing the jaw. Patients who do not report for these extractions almost invariably have trouble from infection around these teeth later on.

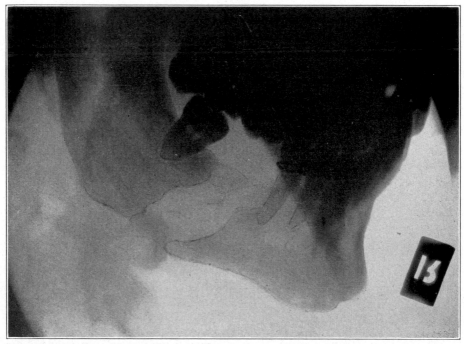

Fig. 218.—Loss of substance from infection. Shows area of loss where a low grade infection persisted over a long period without external drainage. The third molar has fortunately been present to hold the posterior fragment down in place.

External Drainage.—As mentioned under the last heading, we think that any fracture that goes through the jaw in the region of a tooth should be considered compounded; and certainly so, those with displacement sufficient to tear the gum fringes visibly. If these fractures are seen and wired in the first forty-eight hours, it has been a rule to establish external drainage through the skin clear up to the fracture line. If a patient is seen after this period and no infection has developed, and the wiring can be done without too much manipulation, external drainage may be omitted, but careful watch should be kept for any sign of its necessity. The occurrence of small fragments between the main ones is further indication for drainage.

The external incision need be only 1.5 cm. long. It is placed under the jaw, usually in the general direction of the inframandibular branch of the seventh nerve. This crosses over the body about the midpoint along with the facial artery and so incisions behind this point are especially likely to cut it. The knife should go just through the skin, and deep separation to the bone be made with forceps or scissors. These wounds usually heal with little scar, and may prevent serious infection with prolonged or permanent swelling of the side of the face. This is a surgical procedure that offers dependent drainage of an almost assuredly infected field (Fig. 218).

This rule is not as important if chemotherapy is employed locally and generally (see page 325).

Removal of Wires, General Results, X-ray Findings.—Single fractures should be kept fixed three to five weeks. At the end of this time there will usually be some play between the teeth and the patient will have a good idea about the solidity of the fragments. If there is infection still present, fixation may be prolonged. Double fractures are usually fixed from six to eight weeks.

The wires are removed carefully after cutting them apart and cutting each loop around the teeth, with the sharp, strong wire-cutters.

If a tooth in the fracture line has been saved for fixation, there will frequently be some springiness in the union, but this should become solid after the tooth is finally removed. Only very infrequent cases will need to be resplinted.

Occlusion should be normal but one of the involved teeth may be loose and throw it off a little or it may be necessary to have an annoying cusp of some tooth cut down.

Persistent swelling of the face about the fracture line may occur and especially if abscess formation has occurred from lack of, or inadequate, drainage (Fig. 218).

Persistent infection and discharge either internal or external usually means a low grade osteomyelitis, or a small fragment that nature is trying to throw off.

Anesthesia of the lip and teeth may be permanent if the mandibular nerve has been cut across by the fragments.

X-ray pictures should be taken toward the end of, or just after, the period of fixation. If the teeth have maintained normal occlusion and function is good, the position of the fragments will necessarily be good though perhaps not perfect. Valuable information is also given concerning the condition of the tooth roots close to fracture lines.

Persistence of Fracture Line on X-Rays.—An important point in late x-ray findings in lower (and also upper) jaw fractures is that the fracture line may be solid objectively and subjectively, and still show plainly on the plate as though there were little or no union. This has been frequently observed, but as yet we have no satisfactory explanation of the phenomenon (Figs. 219 and 220).

Fixation With Dental Splints and Wire Arches.—There are many satisfactory dental appliances for splinting fractured jaws, but most of them require the skill of a dental surgeon, and it would be impossible to include here all the individual ideas that have been recorded.

A simple procedure is to ligate a metal bar around the buccal surface of several teeth. If this doesn't suffice, a similar bar can be put on the upper teeth and the two fastened together. (Fig. 222.)

Risdon has suggested that the arch be formed by using regular fracture wires on the posterior teeth on both sides and then bringing them around in

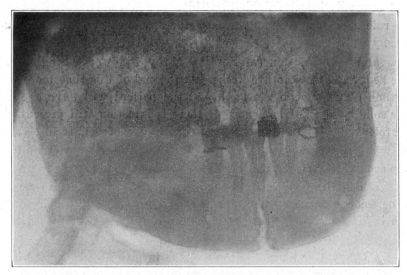

Fig. 219.—Symphysis fracture; persistence of fracture line on x-ray. Shows lack of calcification throughout fracture line in patient who had a solid functioning jaw when the wires were removed just after this x-ray picture was taken. More density may develop when the teeth in the fracture line are removed, but in some instances the fracture line remains evident indefinitely.

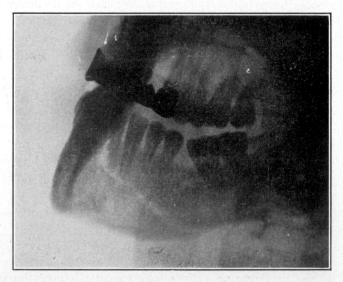

Fig. 220.—Persistence of fracture line on x-ray. Fracture beginning at symphysis and extending obliquely back to molar region. This type may be slow in becoming solid if held with interdental wires because of rocking of the fragments on swallowing, and it may be necessary to use a band splint around the teeth.

Shows persistence of fracture line visibility almost one year later although union is solid objectively and subjectively. The reason for lack of calcium deposit in some lower jaw fractures is not clear. There may be only a fibrous union that is solid enough to appear functionally bony. Prolonged infection or delayed union from poor fixation may be contributing causes but this lack of calcium may be found at times in cases where healing has progressed normally. This is an important medicolegal point.

front and fastening them together.   Smaller individual wires then are used to fasten this arch to the teeth.   (Figs. 221 and 223.)

Elastic Traction in Treating Jaw Fractures.—Although it is found by most surgeons that immediate firm fixation of jaw fractures gives the best results, there are some instances in which elastic traction from one jaw to

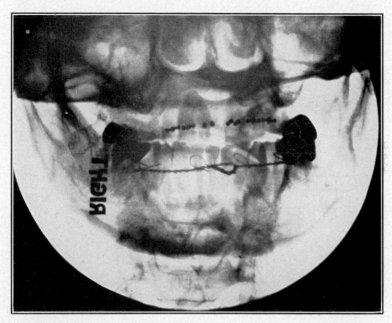

Fig. 221.—Simplest type of anterior splint with simple wires from posterior teeth fastened in front and to separate teeth and held to the upper denture with elastic bands.   Chin vertex bandage is used for support.

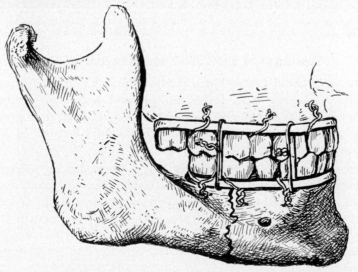

Fig. 222.—Use of anterior band splint or buccal arch with or without elastic traction. Shows general method of ligating a heavy wire or a one-half round band to the buccal surface.   This may be used alone for fixation of some symphysis fractures, but it usually is best to fasten to an upper bar as shown.   This general method can be used for elastic traction also.   If one fragment is depressed out of line, a separate bar is ligated to its teeth and then orthodontic rubber bands are used from this bar to the upper in any desirable direction.

the other may be indicated. If a patient is seen some days or weeks after the injury and the fracture line is not solid but the jaw is out of position, then, instead of breaking up what union has already been obtained, the orthodontic principle of elastic traction may be applied as outlined in Figs. 221 and 222.

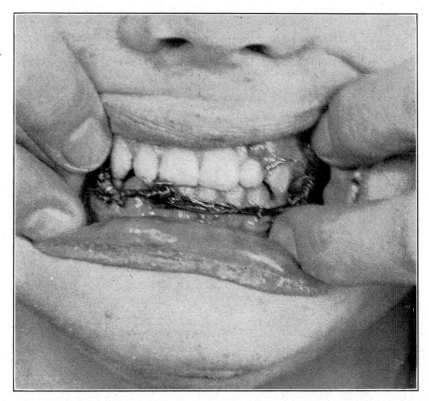

Fig. 223.—Buccal arch fixed to upper jaw. Photo of buccal arch used in a very difficult symphysis fracture complicated by multiple fractures in the upper jaw.

Treatment of Individual and Complicated Cases

Where a fractured jaw is but a part of the injury it can usually be supported with bandaging until full diagnosis and necessary treatment is afforded other parts. Full x-ray studies of the skull and cervical spine may frequently be indicated and the entire situation should be well in hand before attempts are made at fixation of the jaw.

Fractures Compounded Externally.—The fragments are cared for as described above if teeth are available for fixation. The soft parts should be approximated accurately, but external dependent drainage can be provided for through the wound if it is situated properly. There is frequently a drawing in of these scars to the bone and secondary suture may be necessary. Figs. 224 and 225 illustrate the result occasionally seen of closing a wound of external compounding without drainage or fixation of the fracture.

Fractures With Depressed Fragments and Need of Circumferential Wiring.—Where a block of the full thickness has been broken out and has been pulled down into the neck, it may be necessary to encircle this fragment with wire to pull it up in place and fix it. Double strands of No. 24 silver wire are used and passed through the floor of the mouth on the inside of the fragment with a large needle. This comes out through a wound (or stab wound) under the jaw and is passed back into the mouth on the outside of the jaw. If teeth are present, the loops are twisted together after one has been brought through an interdental space. This gives a good hold on the fragment, and it may be manipulated into position and fastened to wires on upper teeth or to what-

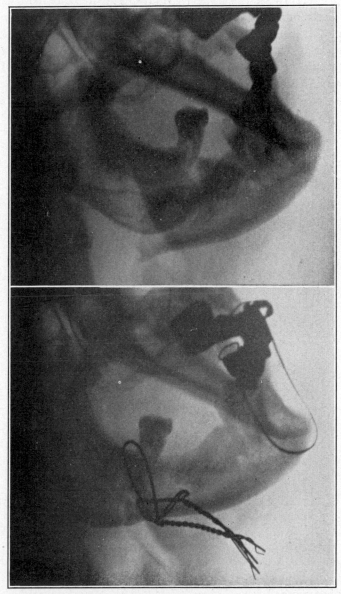

Fig. 224.—Direct bone wiring: circumferential wiring. Compound fracture sustained in fall on plowshare. External wound closed, no drainage established, and nothing done to replace jaw fragments, giving good chance for development of osteomyelitis. Marked displacement and comminution of fragments. Open reduction with direct and circumferential wiring necessary. Circumferential wire also placed around symphysis and anchored above to interdental wire.

ever fixation is employed. Ivy recommends the use of an antral trocar and cannula to pass through the tissues and then passes the wire through the cannula (Figs. 224 to 226).

Compound, Comminuted Fractures result from crushing injuries, explosions and gunshot wounds. There may be badly fragmented and sloughed soft tissues containing dirt and foreign bodies. Here again the main object of treatment should be carried out and that is alignment of the lower jaw so that it occludes properly with the upper. Widespread débridement of bone fragments with little or no replacement or fixation followed by a laborious débridement and closure of the soft parts cannot be too severely condemned. It would be better to save detached bone fragments than to throw away viable ones, and it would be better to pack the soft tissues open than to fail to align the bone fragments. Periosteum if recognized should never be sacrificed. Each of these cases presents special problems, but a general plan of care may be outlined.

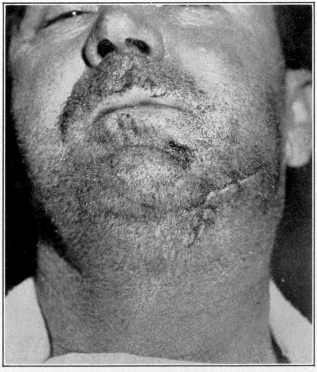

Fig. 225.—External wound of patient, shown in Fig. 224. It has been roughly but tightly closed and the jaw fragments left unfixed and not drained. Wound opened to afford drainage when wires were applied as shown in Fig. 224.

Some type of anesthesia is necessary. Deep block of the third division is ideal; general anesthesia of any type including rectal is to be avoided unless tracheotomy is arranged for. (Figs. 227 to 229.)

A careful search should be made of the wound, and dirt, foreign bodies, and accessible bullets removed. Frank sloughs and completely detached bone fragments should be removed and viable bone fragments replaced. It may be necessary to drill the fragments for fixation with silver wire or tendon, or circumferential wires may be used. When the very best possible plan for bone replacement is worked out, then the soft tissue replacement may be done. Known points are searched for and closed and the remaining areas are closed with these key points as guides. Dependent drainage up to the bone must be adequate. If the floor of the mouth is torn open, it is not closed tightly, but preferably is packed with iodoform gauze. (Figs. 224 to 226.)

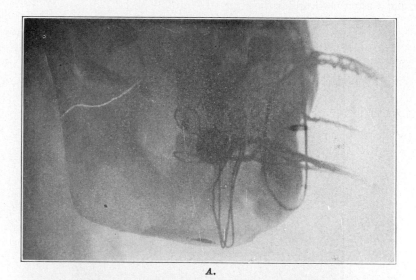

A.

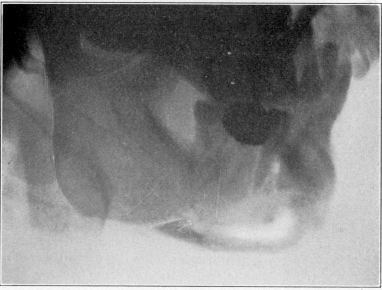

B.

Fig. 226.—Circumferential wiring. Compound comminuted fracture. *A* and *B*. Shows circumferential wires in place to hold up in position block separations of several pieces. Five distinct fracture lines were made out, one of them being just below the neck of the condyle as shown. The long fragment along the lower border was retained throughout the period of fixation but did not survive and was removed through the drainage incision after the wires were removed.

If fixation to the upper jaw is impossible, the metal band wired to the teeth may be used. The jaws may be closed as accurately as possible and supported with a well-padded chin and elastic bandage, or by a plaster cap and sling down under the chin. (Fig. 251.)

If the patient is edentulous and his dental plate is available, the fragments may be fitted into it and fastened to it with circumferential wires all the way around plate and jaw. This plate may in turn be fastened to the upper and a sling used under the chin. (Figs. 230 and 231.)

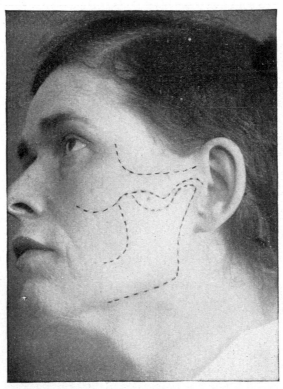

Fig. 227.—Deep injection fifth nerve branches. Showing bony landmarks roughly located by palpation. The lower border of the zygoma is determined first and then the condyle by having the patient open or protrude the mandible. It is almost always definitely felt as it slides forward on the articular tubercle (eminence). The point of insertion of the needle is 2.0 to 2.5 cm. in front of the tragus just below the lower border of the zygoma. From here it passes between the coronoid process and the condyle of the mandible (sigmoid fossa) and just anterior to the articular tubercle. Occasionally it may be necessary to have the mouth held open so that the space between the zygoma and the mandible may be increased. (From Brown, J. B.: Surg., Gynec. & Obst., 1931.)

The after-care of these patients is tedious and discouraging, especially when bone fragments keep separating. Drainage must be kept up and some fixation maintained frequently as long as twelve weeks. It is these cases that suffer full thickness loss with resultant narrowing of the jaw, but if separation of the fragments can be maintained, sepsis controlled and any surrounding periosteum preserved, regeneration and solidity may occur.

Fractures With Loss of Substance.—In these cases if any teeth remain in any fragments, wiring them in position is to be done, even though there may be a definite gap in the bone. A dental splint especially constructed should be used, but if this is not available, a metal bar fastened around the buccal surface of the teeth may be used.

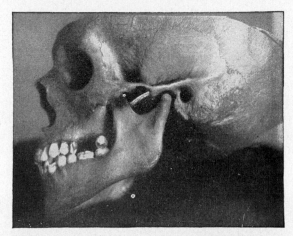

Fig. 228.—Deep injection fifth nerve branches. Showing approximate relation of needle and bony landmarks. Needle represented by a straw held in place with short modelling clay. On its course inward to the pterygoid plate the needle passes through the parotid gland, the masseter, temporal, and external pterygoid muscles. It may also encounter the transverse facial, internal maxillary, middle meningeal, and masseteric arteries. So far we have not seen any untoward results from the passage of the needle through these structures, although we have had several brisk hemorrhages through the needle.

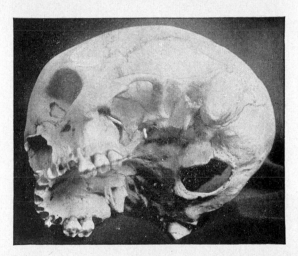

Fig. 229.—Deep injection fifth nerve branches. Showing the deep course of the needle. After gently striking the pterygoid plate, by short withdrawals and reinsertions, the point of the needle is carried up to the undersurface of the great wing of the sphenoid, which is about at a right angle to the pterygoid plate. From now on this undersurface of the greater wing is equally as important as a landmark as the pterygoid plate itself.

To inject the third division the needle is carried backward by short withdrawals and reinsertions against the pterygoid plate being held up against the sphenoid wing. When the posterior border of the plate is reached, the needle slips off and the patient usually experiences momentarily severe pain. The fluid is injected here. It is not absolutely essential to get the pain of a direct "hit" of the nerve before injecting the fluid. If it is not thought that a direct "hit" has been obtained, an extra amount of fluid may be deposited and a longer time should be allowed for the development of anesthesia. (Ten minutes may be necessary.) It is important to remember the rule of not going posteriorly or deep more than 0.5 to 1.0 cm. from the edge of the plate. Damage may be done to the internal carotid artery, the middle meningeal artery, or the Eustachian tube. The pharyngeal mucosa may even be punctured and fluid gotten into the throat. (This might also happen if enough were deposited in the Eustachian tube.)

It is also possible to go entirely through the foramen ovale and inject the ganglion directly. This has not been done so far, nor have attempts been made to inject the first division, because it is thought that the probable paralysis of other nerves and the puncture of the dura might not justify the procedure.

To inject the second division, the needle is carried forward to the sphenomaxillary fossa and the fluid deposited here. Straws are placed to show the third division emerging from the foramen ovale and the second division coursing across the sphenomaxillary fossa. (From Brown: Surg., Gynec. & Obst., 1931.)

If any viable slivers or periosteum have been left in the defect, good regeneration may be the result, but the general result is a narrowing of the jaw, that will require bone grafting if function is impossible. (Fig. 232.)

Fracture of Both Upper and Lower Jaws.—These usually require dental splints though here again the metal bar ligated around the buccal surface of the teeth may suffice for the lower jaw. If there is not much displacement of the upper jaw, the regular interdental fixation may be done and then if there is a tendency for a dragging down of the upper jaw a plaster cap with sling under the chin may be applied for support. Occlusion is probably best insured this way. The open bite splint of Gunning, or its modifications, may be employed

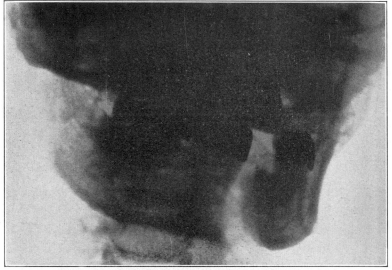

A.

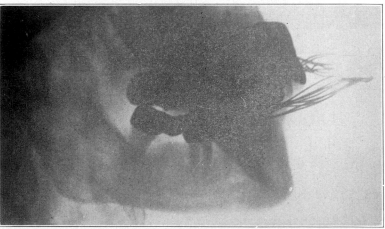

B.

Fig. 230.—Automobile door handle injury; use of dental plate for fixation. Patient caught in the mouth by handle on a passing automobile, dragged several feet, with fracture and extensive lacerations.

A and *B.* Wide separation of fragments in partly edentulous jaw. X-ray shows lower jaw with interdental wires fastened to an upper dental plate. The plate was held up in place by firm fixation of jaws with plaster cap and sling down under chin.

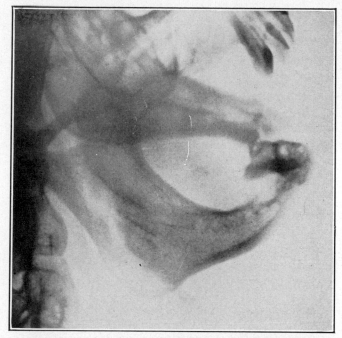

A.

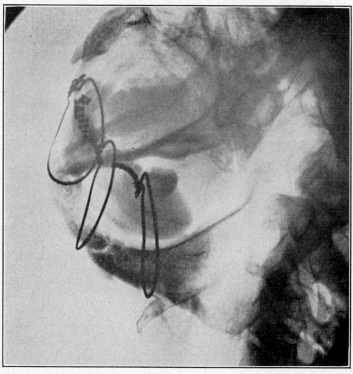

B.

Fig. 231.—Use of lower dental plate for splint. Fracture in edentulous jaw. Use of lower dental plate and circumferential wires for fixation of fracture in molar region. Left film used in *A* to show fracture on right side.

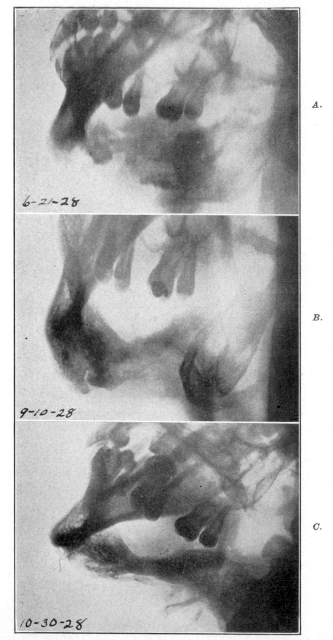

A.

B.

C.

Fig. 232.—Loss of substance from infection; osteomyelitis. *A.* Widespread osteomyelitis following fracture during extraction of an acutely infected tooth, with full thickness loss of substance. External dependent drainage was maintained for some weeks and the dead fragments allowed to separate themselves after which they were removed from the area. The jaw tended to collapse toward the midline, but the large fragment with teeth in it was wired to the upper jaw in its correct occlusion.

B. Three months later shows new bone growing across gap, no sequestra visible.

C. Shows complete regeneration of bone through the area that gave normal function and occlusion in the rest of the jaw.

but these do not give as good assurance of correct occlusion. They may be used for a time and then before the fragments are solid, normal occlusion may be established and maintained for the rest of the fixation period by inter-dental wiring. (Fig. 251.)

Fractures of Edentulous Jaws. Direct Bone Wiring.—These cases are not considered compound in the mouth unless there is definite evidence, and exter-nal drainage is guided accordingly. If there is little or no displacement, rest may be sufficient. If plates are available, to have these in place and a suppor-tive bandage under the chin may increase comfort. If there is displacement and the fragments can be fitted into the plates, fixation may be obtained in this way or it may be necessary to put circumferential wires around the plate and jaw. (Figs. 230 and 231.)

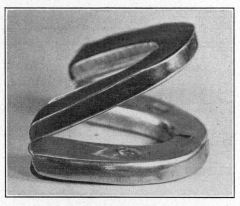

Fig. 233.—Open-bite splint, supplied by the Detroit Dental Mfg. Co., that can be used oc-casionally. The tray is filled with dental compound which is softened, the splint introduced, and the jaws brought together in it. Dr. S. L. Ledbetter of Birmingham, Ala., has made a personal report of the earlier use of this principle with only the dental wax.

If there is much obliquity of the fracture line one or two circumferential wires directly around the bone plus a supportive bandage may suffice (Fig. 234).

If displacement is marked, open reduction, drilling and direct wiring of the fragments may be necessary. It is frequently necessary to have some change made in the fitting of the dental plate after healing is complete.

Fractures of Ramus and Condyle and Coronoid.—As mentioned previously fractures through the neck of the condyle are not as apt to displace badly as is commonly believed and interdental wiring in occlusion will usually suffice. The same thing applies to fractures of the ramus itself. (Figs. 235 and 237.)

If the condyle does tip clear out of line, necrosis or ankylosis may result and resection become necessary. The advisability of immediately excising these displaced condyles is not clear because good function may result even in these cases following a period of fixation in occlusion. Operative methods have been advocated for pushing condyles down into place with certain designed in-struments both from within the mouth and from the outside. Fractures with dislocation may require only fixation but if there is complete displacement, open reduction with or without direct wiring or resection may be necessary.

For condyle resection see "Dislocation and Ankylosis of Jaw."

The coronoid is only infrequently fractured. There may be a complicating fracture of the zygomatic process that requires elevation or there may be a trismus that requires physiotherapy, dilating the jaws and blocking them open for from ten to fourteen days. There should be no effect on occlusion from this fracture. The temporal muscle may pull the fragment high up in the fossa (Fig. 238).

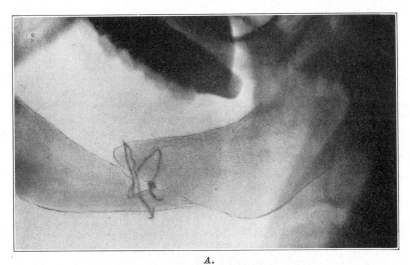

A.

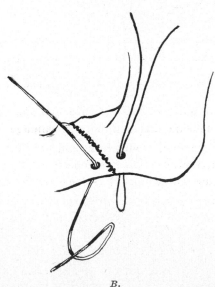

B.

Fig. 234.—Direct wiring of jaw. *A.* Wires through and around edentulous fragments. If the fragments are oblique as shown here, it may not be necessary to drill holes for the wires.

B. Method of drilling and fixing fragments. A wire loop has been passed through the hole in the posterior fragment to receive the silver wire or Kangaroo tendon used for fixation.

Fractures in Children and Infants.—Children with teeth may have interdental wiring done, using light wire, or some form of dental splint may be applied. Fractures in infants are luckily infrequent. If there is uncontrollable displacement, it may be necessary to do direct bone wiring.

Very occasionally an infected second dentition unerupted tooth may become infected and cause persistent drainage until it is removed from the jaw.

Pathologic Fractures.—If these result from benign processes, fixation in occlusion should be done and an attempt made to remove the offending cyst or tumor without destroying the periosteum. If such a growth is removed first and the danger of fracture is recognized because of the reduced volume of bone, interdental wiring is frequently resorted to for protection against fracture.

If a malignant process accounts for the fracture, the immediate treatment should be of the process and in this instance little thought is given to the occlusion unless it is possible to wire one side of the jaw in occlusion.

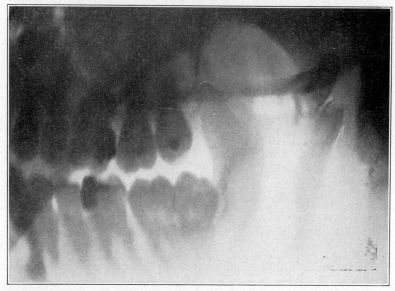

Fig. 235.—Fracture of condyle. The neck of the condyle has been fractured and pulled forward somewhat by the external pterygoid muscle. The original force drove this condyle backward, to impinge on the auditory canal and cause bleeding from it. Treatment by wiring the jaws in normal occlusion was successful and the condyle apparently retained its vitality. Opposite condyle broken also, but not displaced as much.

Infected Fractures. Osteomyelitis.—If there is communication with the mouth, contamination about the fracture site is certain, and frequently a mild infection develops. If drainage is inadequate there may be widespread soft tissue infection with abscess formation and some loss of bone if the infection continues over a long period. This type of infection seldom goes on to the wide bloc necrosis that may be associated with dental infection; but conversely those instances of widespread bone necrosis that are associated with extraction of acutely infected teeth may develop fractures. These should be cared for as other fractures with special effort at maintaining soft tissue drainage, preserving the periosteum, and allowing necrosed bone to separate itself from surrounding live bone before attempting to remove it. This conservative treatment in regard to dead fragments gives the quickest and least complicated healing, position may be the most accurately maintained and the efforts at regeneration are best insured. (Figs. 218 and 232.)

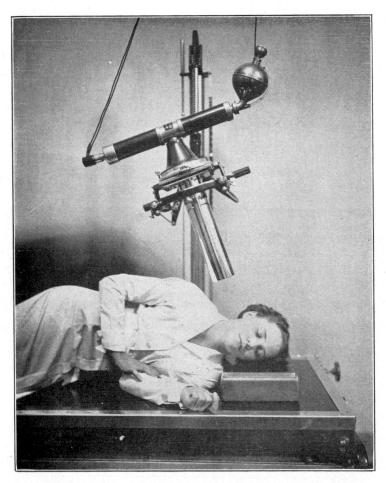

Fig. 236.—Position for radiograph of condyle and associated region in the ramus. Kilovoltage, 60; milliamperage, 20; distance, 28 inches; time, three-fourths of a second. (Courtesy Dr. Sherwood Moore, Mallinckrodt Institute of Radiology, Washington University School of Medicine.)

Late Treatment of Malunion and Nonunion; Bone Grafts; Loss of Substance

Elevation of Posterior Fragment.—Union in bad position or failure of union occurs most often with a posterior fragment elevated; it also occurs following comminuted or infected fractures with or without loss of substance. The main signs are external deformity with flattening and loss of the angle, or a narrowing of the jaw. Inside there is loss of occlusion, narrowing of the floor of the mouth, and the posterior fragment may be so elevated that it prevents the mouth from closing completely.

It will be found that some patients prefer to accept the deformity if they are able to get adequate nourishment and keep on with work. (Fig. 239.)

Some form of open operation is usually necessary for the alignment of the fragments and frequently fixation with dental splints is necessary.

For opening old fracture lines an elevator or Gigli saw is usually used. If the fragments can be aligned, direct bone wiring may be possible.

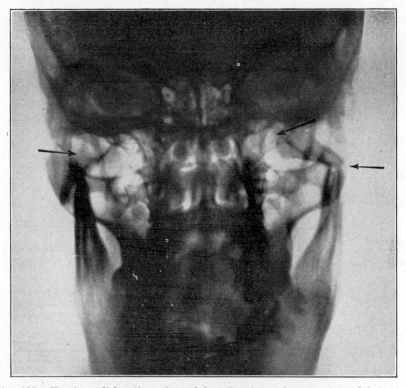

Fig. 237.—Fracture dislocation of condyle. Fracture of neck of condyle with medial dislocation of head. This is an excellent x-ray although this view does not show the more usual lesser displacements of this area. Good result reported by Conwell from open reduction and direct wiring in this patient.

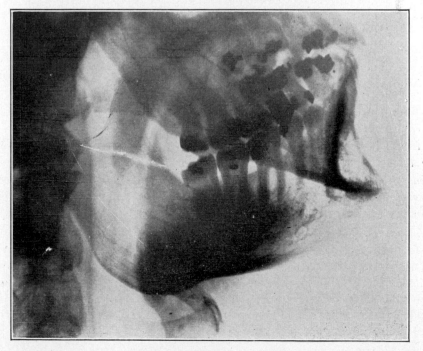

Fig. 238.—Fracture of coronoid process. Fracture of coronoid from a lateral blow that also crushed the zygoma down and in.

For restoration of bad deformities the plan should be to free and return the fragment to as close its normal position as possible and if necessary fill in any defects or splint any necessary areas with bone grafts.

The elevated posterior fragments may be gradually reduced by the method recommended by Ivy and Curtis* in which an elastic pull is fastened in a drill hole through the angle and to a fixed point held at the back of the neck by a plaster cap. The internal wire method, described later, is applicable if the fragment can be reduced, Fig. 240. If it cannot be reduced, a screw right through into the angle should suffice for traction instead of an open operation to get a wire in.

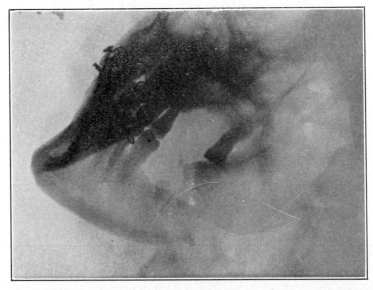

Fig. 239.—Elevation of posterior fragment with malunion following fixation with no attempt at reduction of posterior fragment. Only treatment in this case was to extract the upper third molar which was encroaching on the elevated fragment. Union was strong, but there was some external deformity.

Bone Grafts.—For any bone graft, adequate means of fixation must be provided; if there are teeth in both fragments, interdental wiring may suffice, but frequently dental splints will be necessary. There must be complete freedom from infection, and there must be no entry into the mouth cavity. If, during the course of an operation, it is found that the oral mucosa has been broken through, the application of the graft should be delayed until there is again perfect healing.

For nonunion with small or no loss of bone we have found the rib graft satisfactory. The fragments are aligned and freshened back 1 to 2 cm. A piece of a rib is removed with its periosteum on the outer surface; this is split in two, and the medullary surface placed across the fragments. It is held in place with silk mattress sutures over it which catch the periosteum and surrounding soft tissues. The wound is closed in firm layers and a firm dressing using damp marine sponges is applied.

*Ivy and Curtis: Surg., Gynec. & Obst. 52: 849, 1931.

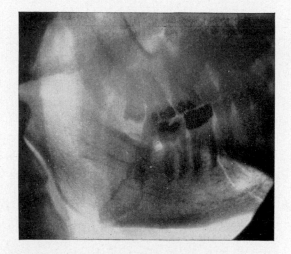

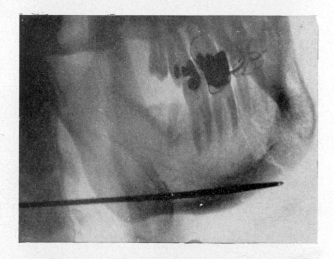

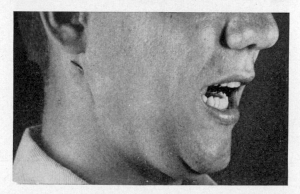

Fig. 240.—Fracture at angle with elevation of posterior fragment and loss of mandibular nerve sensation. Fixation with single internal wire put in from behind and below the nerve canal. Avoidance of open reduction or elastic traction reduction of posterior fragment. Interdental wiring was done because of second fracture in body. At bottom, mouth open, with wire in place. (From Brown, J. B., and McDowell, F.: Surg., Gynec. & Obst., 1942.)

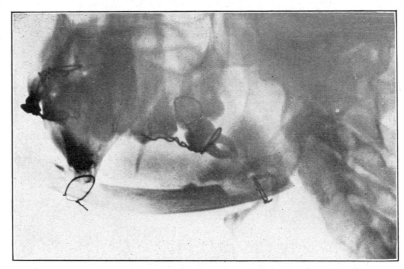

Fig. 241.—Massive bone graft. Huge rib graft used successfully to bridge gap in jaw.
Held with wire to give support to the posterior fragment and help hold it down in place during
period of fixation. Wires removed later.

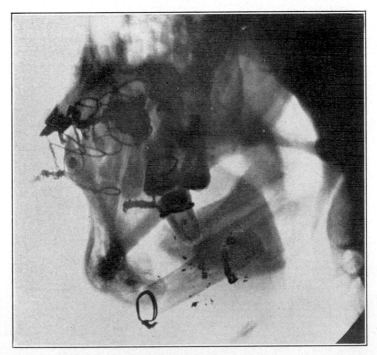

Fig. 242.—Bone graft for loss of substance. Rib graft used to bridge eleven-year-old
gunshot loss in lower jaw. Full fixation of graft fragments obtained by wiring graft in
place. Interdental wiring done also.

As mentioned before, anesthetic complications must be guarded against if the jaws
have been wired together under general anesthesia. In this patient, a curved rubber breathing tube (McGill tube) was left through the nostril so that its opening rested in a correct
position for free respiration, for five days.

Other types of free grafts employed are osteoperiosteal and cortical grafts (usually taken from the tibia).

The pedicle graft described by Cole utilizes a piece of the jaw itself and leaves attached a pedicle of platysma muscle from below to insure vitality. The fragments are aligned, a piece is removed from the lower border of one (usually the anterior) and a block is cut from the other, but leaving the platysma attached. This piece is carried across the defect and fixed to both fragments.*

For replacement of any length of bone, heavier grafts from the tibia or ilium or of the full thickness of the rib are used. The fragments usually have to be separated at preliminary operations and frequently held in position with dental splints, or the dental splints may be attached to the teeth and arrangements made for locking them in place when the fragments are separated. If good fixation of the fragments has been provided for, the graft may be held in place with fixation to the soft tissues or with absorbable material through drill holes in the fragments.

In large defects where there are no teeth to use or other methods of splinting available, it is possible firmly to fix the graft to the fragments so that it actually acts as a splint also and itself holds the fragments in position immediately as it is supposed to do eventually. To obtain this firm fixation of the fragments and graft it is best to rely on wire to hold the graft in place. One drill hole in each end of the graft and one in each fragment usually suffice and either stainless steel or silver wire can be used.

It is, of course, necessary to fix the lower to the upper jaw, either by interdental wiring or by the use of dental plates and bandaging (Figs. 241 and 242).

Direct Wiring of Jaw Fragments and Fate of Wires.—A separate heading is made of this subject to call attention to the fact that wires put through the jaw bone, either in direct approximation of fragments or in holding bone grafts in place, usually have to be removed before there is permanent final healing, and this can be done whenever solidity seems adequate—usually after three months (Figs. 224, 225, 234, 241, and 242).

FRACTURES OF THE TEETH AND ALVEOLAR PROCESSES

The alveolar processes may be broken away carrying the contained teeth with them. The diagnosis is easily made usually, but thorough study should be made for any possible complete fractures. Single teeth may be loosened without block separation of the alveolar processes and single roots may be broken. For the block separation of an alveolus, replacement and circumferential wiring with silver wire directly around the fragment and remainder of the jaw usually offers the simplest relief. Wiring to adjacent teeth on either side rarely suffices. The use of the metal bar ligated to the teeth all the way around the arch or interdental wiring with the teeth in occlusion may be necessary. The ultimate fate of these bony fragments is usually good, although the teeth are frequently so damaged that they may have to be extracted later.

---

*Cole and Bubb: Brit. M. J., Jan. 18, 1919, pp. 67-70.

In badly comminuted fractures of the teeth and their supporting alveoli it is best to get completely detached fragments out early as they form foreign bodies and when caught under the mucosa delay healing unnecessarily.

Loosened teeth should be supported with light wire fixation to adjacent ones if simple rest will not suffice. The replacement of teeth that have completely left their sockets is not an accepted procedure although they have been reported as successfully regrafted, and the main consideration of this procedure should be for upper front teeth. If one would survive, the next consideration should be the advisability of a root resection and canal filling.

If roots are broken across, there is little hope for viability. If there are not subjective symptoms early and the tooth becomes solid, it might be left in place but there is usually trouble or discomfort later that necessitates extraction.

Feeding During Treatment

It is never necessary to remove teeth to feed these patients. The use of a stomach tube, passed through the nose, would be preferable to the removal of sound front teeth.

Many patients already have one or more teeth missing, there is usually some space behind the last molars, and occlusion is seldom so accurate that fluids cannot be got between the jaws.

The diet will necessarily have to be liquid or very soft. After a few days an enterprising patient will be looking after his own diet satisfactorily.

The following basic diet has a fairly normal balance of protein (71), fat (102) and carbohydrate (362), and supplies about 2,600 calories.

		Calories
Eggs	6	450
Milk	1½ pt.	480
Cream 20%	½ pt.	480
Strained tomatoes or other vegetables	½ pt.	36
Sugar, Karo or glucose	10 oz.	1200
Salt	1 teaspoonful	
		2646

This diet may be mixed together and fed through a tube, or the ingredients may be made into any combinations desired. Coffee, tea, ice cream, fruit juices and any flavoring may be added at will.

As other articles of diet are taken such as cereals and ground meat, the total caloric value of the above may be cut down accordingly.

FRACTURES OF THE UPPER JAW

General Considerations

The upper jaw presents a complicated problem for consideration when dealing with injuries about the face for the following reasons:

1. Both sides must be taken into account because of the transverse involvement in many instances. (Figs. 250, 253, 255, 256, 262.)

2. Skull fracture and brain injury are such frequent complications that the possibility must always be considered. (Figs. 248, 252, 263.)

3. All of the associated bones of the face may be involved and these include the maxilla, zygoma, zygomatic arch of the temporal, nasal, ethmoid, frontal, palate and both the bony and cartilaginous nasal septums (Fig. 255).

4. The presence of the sinuses and fracture lines through them enhances the chance of infection. (Figs. 250, 253, 262.)

5. The nasal passages may be occluded and require early restoration. (Figs. 248, 255, 261.)

6. Displacement of the eyeball may occur with resultant diplopia. (Figs. 255, 256.)

7. Blindness may result from direct section of the nerve by one of the thin fragments of bone, or by intraocular injury. There may also be direct injury of the external ocular muscles or their nerves. (Figs. 248, 252, 263.)

8. The lacrimal duct may be occluded. (Fig. 263.)

9. The associated injuries of the soft parts may be so great as to delay or hinder attention to the bone displacement. (Fig. 252.)

10. Because of the possible permanent changing of the features, both from soft tissue injury and from bony displacement, it is necessary to include consideration of this point in carrying out treatment in addition to the consideration of function. (Figs. 255, 261.)

Heavy blunt crushing blows are usually the cause of fractures of the upper jaw, such as a heavy impact of another's head or knee in sports, the kick of a horse, or a jam against a steering wheel or other part of a car in a traffic accident. As stated above, any other of the facial bones may be involved, and in fact many fractures of the maxilla are from indirect violence, which has been first received by the zygoma (malar or yoke bone), the prominent bone of the cheek.

The extent of the fracture may vary from a simple alveolar avulsion to a complete transverse separation of all the facial bones from the skull so that they hang in a soft tissue sling. (Fig. 250.)

The bony orbit may be broken through and displaced so that the action of the extrinsic ocular muscles is interfered with and diplopia may result.

Blindness may result from direct injury to the globe, intraocular hemorrhage, or occasionally by direct injury to the optic nerve. In one severe case the globe was not grossly injured, but the nerve was found cut in two and the remaining distal end turned around and pointing forward. (Figs. 252, 263.)

When the nasal sinuses are involved in the fracture line, the question of infection and drainage arises. This depends to a great extent upon the condition of the nose and sinuses before the accident, and the underlying principles of treatment are restoration of contour and maintenance of drainage.

If the lacrimal duct is torn or blocked a dacrocystitis may develop that finally may require excision of the sac. This is never done primarily. (Fig. 263.)

Displacement and Diagnosis.—The displacement is due to the original violence, and where there has been a complete transverse separation of bone gravity may cause a dropping of all the tissues of the face. If a violent force is transmitted directly from the front, the maxillae may be spread laterally by a wedge of the frontal processes and nasal bones; even the medial walls of the orbit may be displaced laterally.   If the force is driven upward, the nasal fossae and antra may be impinged upon by the palate and alveolar processes.

Most commonly the cheek bone receives the blow.   This bone is so wedged that the separation of its suture lines or fracture close to them plus fractures of the zygomatic process of the temporal bone and of the orbital border of the maxillae is the most common occurrence.   Examination of the bony

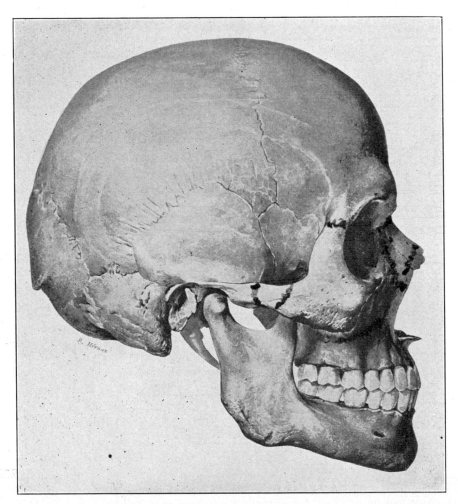

Fig. 243.—(*See opposite page for legend.*)

structure about this region will show that fracture in more than one area would be the rule.   The force may be transmitted entirely across the face causing a complete transverse fracture.   This fracture may occur at any level, but on the opposite side usually causes separation at or near the maxillo-zygomatic suture line.   It is with these transverse facial fractures that basal fractures and damage to the eyes is most apt to occur.   Any of these fractures may be impacted in place, but most of them sag downward and, by taking hold of the upper teeth, the whole face can be made to move on the

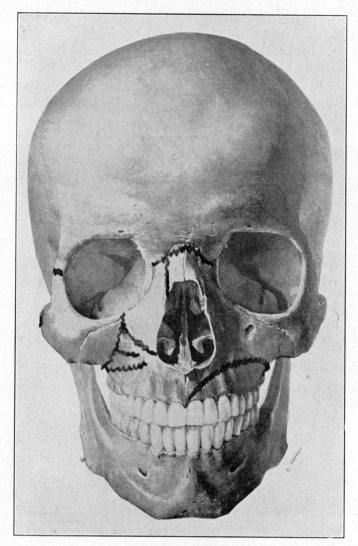

Fig. 244.

Figs. 243 and 244.—The usual sites of separation in the upper jaw are roughly shown, inked in. The zygoma itself usually separates from its suture lines with the zygomatic process of the temporal, the frontal, and the maxilla, and is crushed down onto the antrum which crumples under it. The body of this bone is only infrequently fractured. The zygomatic arch which is part of the temporal bone is either crumpled in by a sharp blow from the side, or collapsed backward by a blow from the front transmitted through the zygoma.

The maxillary fracture may be an avulsion of the alveolus with its teeth or a comminuted fracture entirely around the antrum. The frontal process may be completely detached as shown along the right side of the nose and such a fragment may be very hard to locate and hold in correct position.

Fractures that carry across the face are usually at the highest level (inked in at the glabella), but may also be down lower just above the alveolus.

The separation may extend into the frontal and ethmoid sinuses, through the lacrimal bone to occlude the lacrimal duct, deep in the orbit, and through the bones of the palate to cut through the soft tissues.

The nasal bones may be separated from any attachment and are frequently shattered into small pieces along with the frontal processes that support them so that they may flatten out close to the level of the cheeks. (From Spalteholz.)

cranium. The face elongates so that it has been said to resemble a horse face. There may be severe facial lacerations and comminution of bone, but complete fractures may occur with only external contusion.

Emphysema may occur about the nose and face, and the tissues may even be seen to dilate with each respiration.

There can be little difficulty in knowing that fracture has occurred in the extensive cases. The location of all the ramifications, however, may not be possible.

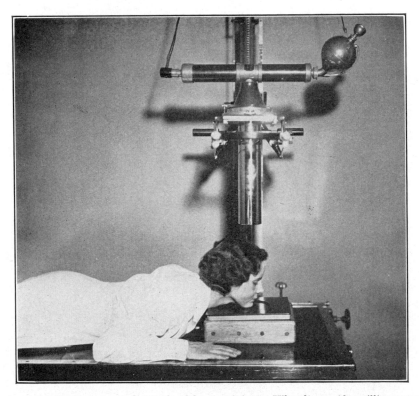

Fig. 245.—Position for radiograph of bones of face. Kilovoltage, 68; milliamperage, 20; distance, 28 inches; time, 3 seconds; screens. (Courtesy Dr. Sherwood Moore, Mallinckrodt Institute of Radiology, Washington University School of Medicine.)

Movement, loss of normal occlusion, palpable disruption of contour about the orbit, and local tenderness should all be looked for. Slight depressions of the zygoma, zygomatic process, or the orbital border may easily be overlooked or obscured by swelling. Trismus may result from impingement about the coronoid process of the lower jaw by a comminuted fracture of the zygomatic arch.

X-Ray Findings.—Demonstrating the regions of the maxillary bones and locating fractures may be very difficult. Good ideas may be obtained of the position of the heavier ridges of bone, such as the orbital borders, frontal processes of the maxilla and the whole zygomatic arch; and, since these are the main guides for the restoration of contour, attention should be centered on them, and an adequate number of views taken. (Figs. 245, 246.)

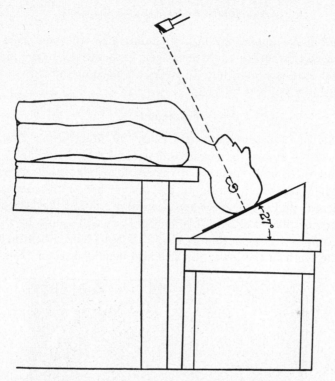

Fig. 246.—Radiography of zygoma. Table with twelve-inch square top about three-fourths the height of radiographic table and an angle table about 10 inches wide with an angle of 27 degrees.

The patient is placed in supine position with head extended over end of table and hyper-flexed so that the vertex of the head rests firmly on the angle board which has been previously placed atop the smaller table. The central x-ray beam is directed in the center of the infra-mandibular area. The patient's head is so placed that there is no rotation to either right or left (Conwell).

Sixty-two Kv. 100 ma. seconds at 30 inches distance using double intensifying screens. This method may be somewhat difficult in acute injuries and in the patients frequently seen with neck injuries also.

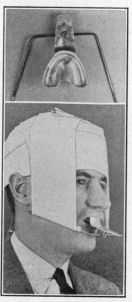

Fig. 247.—Simple type of splint for elevating dental arch and face. Made by Dr. J. A. Brown for use in patient shown in Fig. 230. The tray is filled with dental compound before it is used and is held with a simple elastic sling from the top of the head.

Every extensive upper jaw injury should have the benefit of a complete skull series study, whether there has been evidence of brain injury or not. Upon slightest evidence of injury to the cervical spine an x-ray study of this region should also be done.

Treatment

Treatment of Fracture Through Body of Maxilla on One Side.—The fragment should be aligned in correct occlusion and held in place. A metal bar ligated around the buccal surfaces of the teeth may be used. Firmer fixation can be had by interdental wiring to the lower jaw or, if edentulous, by inserting the dental plates in correct occlusion and holding the mouth closed with a chin bandage or plaster sling. This fracture usually occurs by the lower jaw striking the upper teeth so that a block of bone and its attached teeth is loosened. The teeth in the lower jaw are also usually broken (Fig. 255).

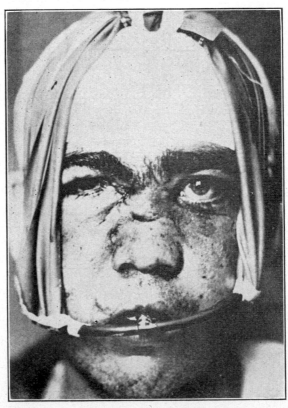

Fig. 248.—Cast splint in place and elevation of face effected by simple overhead rubber dam pull.

Treatment of Transverse Fractures Through the Dental Arch and Through the Orbit.—If it is thought that a plaster cap and sling or a rubber sling from the vertex around the chin will support the fragment, interdental wiring with the teeth in correct occlusion should be done and the support applied. This is the simplest type of fixation.

If the fragment cannot be got into position at one sitting, or if there is contraindication to interdental wiring, some type of dental splint fixation to the upper dental arch should be applied. A satisfactory method is as follows: An impression is taken of the upper arch, and either a cast or vulcanite tray is made from it; to this tray is attached a bar that comes out of the mouth and to this a second bar that extends around in front of both cheeks. This splint is put in place and held with rubber dam pulled over the top of the head. In a short time the fragment will be elevated into position and it is maintained there from one to three weeks. This splint can be taken loose and cleaned. The occlusion of the lower jaw should be closely watched, since there is likely to be some tilting of the upper fragment if pressure is uneven

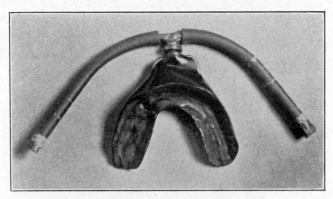

Fig. 249.—Simple type of dental splint that will usually suffice. Care must be taken that it does not tip from before backward or from side to side, and, in most instances, after the bones are elevated, interdental wiring should be done to insure normal occlusion.

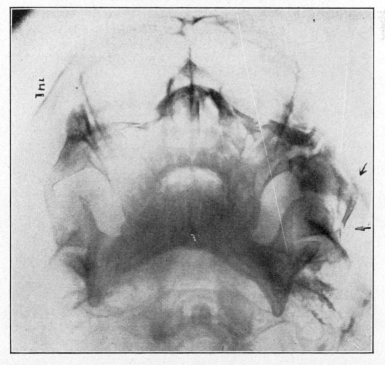

Fig. 250.—Shows one view of patient with badly comminuted fractures with complete separation and elongation of the face. The orbital borders are well shown here as is also the crumpled-up zygomatic process. The frontal processes of the maxilla have also been detached and flattened out.

from side to side, or from before backward. As soon as elevation is complete and fixation has begun, the jaws may be wired in occlusion and held with support from the vertex. This last step may not be necessary, but helps greatly if there has been difficulty in preserving the position of occlusion with the dental splint alone. (Figs. 247, 248, 249, 250.)

Other types of fixation are open bite splint in one or two pieces and in emergencies even impression trays may be used. One type of fixation depends on a head band from which rods are brought down, and the dental splint is

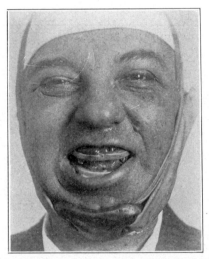

Fig. 251.—Method of supporting complete transverse fracture of face and multiple fracture of lower jaw with an adjustable open bite splint. (Detroit Dental Mfg. Co.) The insides of the trays are inlaid with dental compound, and a dental compound cup under the chin is held with rubber dam over the head.

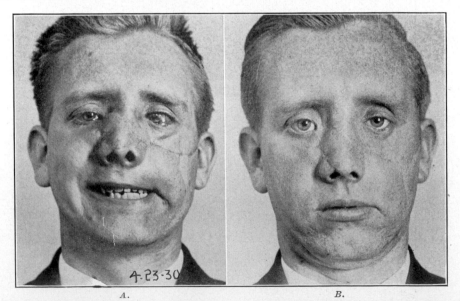

A.   B.

Fig. 252.—A, Patient with blindness in left eye, complete transverse and multiple facial fractures with almost total loss of the left upper jaw. B, Restoration of occlusion, nasal position, and of the cheek prominence with a free costal cartilage transplant. The right inner canthus is still somewhat displaced, as evidenced by the sharp curve of the tarsal border.

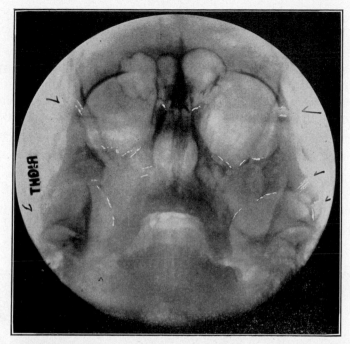

Fig. 253.—Multiple comminutions of the facial bones, some of the areas having been scratched in for clearness. Note arrows indicating separation of the zygomatic-frontal suture lines on both sides, and the crumpling of the zygomatic arches, and the comminution about the orbital borders and antrum.

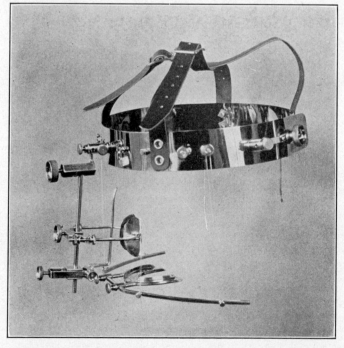

Fig. 254.—Apparatus designed by Dr. C. L. Straith for supporting bad facial fractures. The dental tray supports the alveolar arch and the apparatus just above it supports the nose, having adjustments for lifting it forward and for compressing it from the sides. Ball and socket joints give a wide range of adjustment.

fastened to these. Innumerable mechanical variations have been described, one of the best of which is that designed by Straith, of Detroit, which has an accessory arrangement for supporting nasal fractures. (Figs. 251, 254.)

Federspiel puts on an arch wire and then attaches another wire to this in the molar region and passes this wire through the cheek quite high up in the fornix. This wire is then firmly attached to a plaster-of-Paris head cap, and the fragment is drawn up into position and held there.

Treatment of Fracture of the Orbital Border, Zygoma and Zygomatic Arch.—A blow on the zygoma or directly on the orbital border may depress the border so much that diplopia may result as the globe follows the orbital floor downward. This one result of displacement makes replacement imperative.

It is possible to raise some orbital borders from the outside with hooks or special clamps on the order of towel clips that engage the fragment through the overlying soft parts.

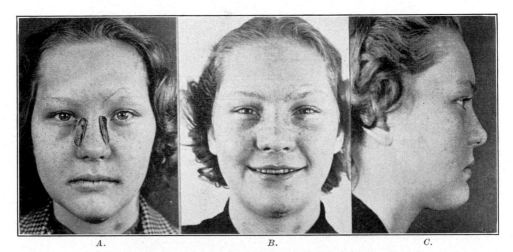

A.　　　　*B.*　　　　*C.*

Fig. 255.—Restoration of contour after complete facial fractures. *A.* Patient shown four weeks after accident in which there were multiple comminuted fractures of practically all the bones of the face: (1) Both orbital borders were down with wide separation of the inner canthi. (2) The nose was completely loose and shattered and, with swelling, it was just on a level with the cheeks. (3) Both zygomas were down and (4) both antrums were comminuted. (5) The upper alveolus was broken through in two places on the left and the palate process had cut entirely through the covering of the hard palate. (6) The right frontal process was completely free and could not be locked against any fragment at the time of operation. (7) Fracture lines were visible into the frontal sinus, but none were seen farther back in the skull. (8) The lower jaw was broken through the symphysis. The lead plates on the sides of the nose support a mattress suture of fine silver wire which is the entire support of the nose, and has insured normal narrowness, prominence of the dorsum and, most important of all, correct position and direction of the inner canthi.

B. Restoration of contour after complete facial fractures. Patient shown twenty-five days later with practically normal expression. The canthi are in good position and the occlusion is normal. The lower arch splint, as shown in Fig. 223, is still in place.

At operation, done one week after the accident, under hyoscine and block anesthesia: (1) The airway was established through both nostrils and maintained with rubber tubes. (2) The orbital borders were raised through the antra and held with iodoform packs; at this point it was found that the right frontal process could not be controlled by any intra-antral manipulation. (3) The dorsum of the nose was elevated and, although shattered into multiple small fragments, it was held with the sling of silver wire from side to side as shown in *A.* These wires were put through on large cutting needles. (4) The canthi were re-placed at the same time the nose was molded and held with the same fixation. (5) The upper alveolus was folded into position by pressure on the teeth and direct wiring of teeth across fracture lines. (6) A buccal arch wire was put around the lower jaw and (7) interdental fixation was done with the teeth in normal occlusion. (8) The symphysis fracture was drained externally through a wound already present.

C. Restoration of contour after complete facial fractures. The most prominent feature of the profile is the dorsum of the nose and here it has been restored to practically normal position. There is no loss of vision or diplopia, occlusion is normal and, aside from the loss of teeth in the fracture line, no further restoration need be done. (Patient referred by Dr. Robert Schlueter, Dr. Henry Thym, and Dr. C. G. Jungk, St. Louis.)

Where external elevation does not suffice, outline may be restored by reduction with a steel sound or forcep introduced through the buccal fornix into the antrum. The displaced orbital border is carried into position and molding is helped by external palpation along the border. If there is not too much comminution the fragments may stay in place, but an iodoform gauze pack is usually carried high up and placed firmly to act as an internal splint. The end is brought through the buccal fornix wound and the whole pack is removed in seven to ten days. During this time the area is gently cleaned with fluids through a small tube that is left in alongside the pack. This hole that is made into the antrum rarely fails to close after the pack and tube are removed. The antrum is usually crushed by the orbital border coming down and this fracture line may be palpated or located with a needle through the mucosa. When it is found, the mucosa is opened over it and the antrum easily entered. (Description continued in Figs. 255 to 258.)

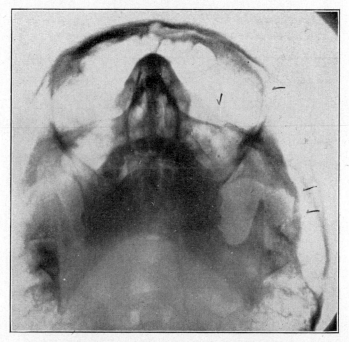

Fig. 256.—X-ray to show mainly depression of orbital border, but accompanied by the usual separation at the frontal attachment and two fractures through the zygomatic arch.

If there is bulk displacement of the whole side of the face and tendency for recurrence of the deformity, open reduction and wiring of the fragments may be necessary.

If diplopia does not occur and there is only slight external deformity that the patient is not concerned about, no special attempt need be made at elevation.

Many methods have been offered for elevating a depressed zygomatic arch: (1) towel clips and hooks to pull it in position from the outside; (2) heavy sound-like instruments to elevate it from the inside of the mouth by application high up outside the coronoid process; (3) open reduction by inserting a sound through the scalp of the temporal region, down along the temporal muscle toward the coronoid and then elevating the fragment from here (Gillies).

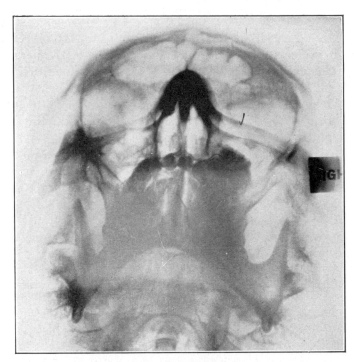

Fig. 257.—Accurate replacement of depressed orbital border. Same patient as shown in Fig. 256. Entry to the antrum was made through an incision in the buccal fornix mucosa and then through the fracture of the antral wall. The orbital border was carried up into place and packed with one inch iodoform gauze. A small rubber tube was also left in the antrum for irrigation and the application of mild antiseptics. The iodoform gauze is shown in place seventeen days later just before it was removed.

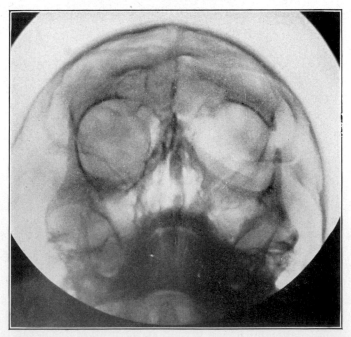

Fig. 258.—Shows late result of fracture of zygoma without replacement. The wide separation from the frontal, the distortion of the orbit, and the crumpled zygomatic process can be plainly seen. Diplopia will nearly always result with displacement as marked as this, and this patient had learned to disregard the vision of this eye. In respect to diplopia, it is important to determine whether it is due to bony displacement carrying the globe out of alignment, or to paralysis of one or more extrinsic ocular muscles. It is evident that replacing depressed bone or otherwise elevating the globe would not correct a true muscle paralysis.

Simple depressions of the zygomatic arch are, however, rather infrequent. To have this injury alone a blow is necessary directly from the side and applied directly to the arch itself. If there is no trismus and no appreciable deformity, little need be done except perhaps a simple external elevation with a hook. If this does not suffice the other procedures may be tried. (Fig. 260.)

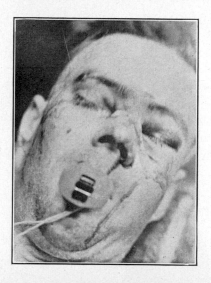

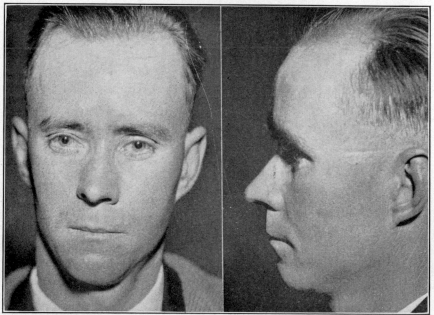

Fig. 259.—Comminuted fractures of facial and frontal bones. X-ray shown in Fig. 262. This patient was seen soon after a fourteen-foot fall in which he struck directly across the face. Immediate replacement of the markedly comminuted fragments was done, rubber tubes were left in the frontal sinuses (these tubes were not irrigated), and the fragments of the nose were held up and in place with through-and-through wires as shown in Fig. 255. The final results show good restoration of the nasal bridge and, more important, good situation and direction of the internal canthi. These patients should be watched for evidence of sinus blockage, and it was suspected at one time later in this patient but he did not return for treatment. (Patient referred by Dr. Glover Copher.)

Many fractures of the zygomatic arch are out-bowings, rather than depressions, a sort of a crumpling-up having occurred as a result of a blow on the zygoma itself where it has been driven backward.

The reduction of this displacement is usually effected by external pressure and this may be combined with open reduction through the antrum of the depressed zygoma itself.

Treatment of Complicated Cases.—There may be extreme laceration, contusion, comminution of bone and presence of foreign bodies. Hemorrhage may be severe and the airway obstructed. The general and neurologic care of the patient may first require some hours.

Emphysema is best controlled by cleaning out a free airway and if necessary packing the nostrils. Hemorrhage may require this pack plus one in the posterior nares. Tracheotomy may be necessary, although a simple rubber tube placed through the mouth may suffice and make the patient comfortable until the difficulties can be controlled. (Figs. 255, 259, 260.)

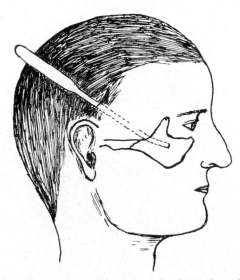

Fig. 260.—Gillies' method of elevation of depressed malar bone through temporal skin incision. (From Gillies, H. D., Kilner, T. P., and Stone, D.: Brit. J. Surg., 1927.)

For cleaning up the individual case with torn soft tissues, careful débridement, removal of foreign bodies, alignment and fixation of fragments and closure of soft parts should be carried out. No considerable portion of bone should be sacrificed. Fragments will live with surprisingly little attachment and they should be replaced along with any known periosteum even if the contour is maintained by but a shell of bone. As in the lower jaw, this bone replacement should not be sacrificed in favor of soft tissue restoration.

The nasal airway should be restored if possible, preferably by carefully sorting out the passage through with normal lining pieced out as accurately as possible and then inserting a large rubber tube through the inferior meatus. These injuries may show extensive crumpling and displacement of the turbinates and medial wall of the antrum so that parts may have to be excised later to insure an airway. (Fig. 255.)

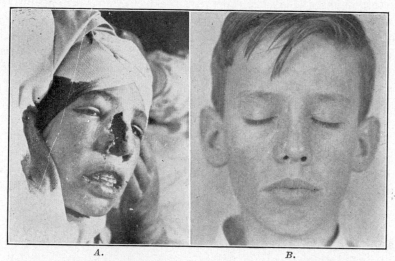

A.   B.

Fig. 261.—A, Extensive soft tissue tearing combined with comminution of facial bones. There is wide separation of soft tissues and bone to a depth of five centimeters, the inner canthus being badly displaced. The patient was seen immediately and allowed complete fixation and repair to be done under block anesthesia. The most important features here are to set in the inner canthus and maintain it, to hold the frontal process of the maxilla and the nasal bones in place and to close the soft tissues accurately.

The final result is shown in B with good position and direction of the canthus and a linear scar on the nose; the nostril is somewhat small due to an actual loss of tissue at the alar border. Closure of this type of soft tissue laceration without replacing and holding the bones would almost certainly necessitate further operation. (Patient referred by Dr. E. O. Breckenridge.)

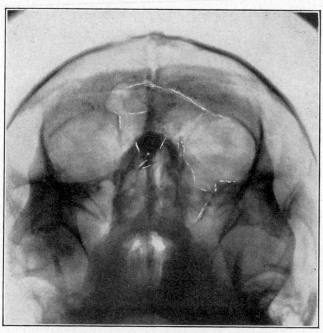

Fig. 262.—X-ray of compound injury to the facial and frontal bones; a few of the many fracture lines have been scratched in. Same patient as shown in Fig. 259.

Infection in cases seen some time after the accident require adequate drainage usually including opening of previously sutured wounds. Gentle irrigation or mechanical swabbing and a general regime of cleanliness cover the available measures. Forceful irrigating should not be done for fear of carrying infection through some possible channel to the meninges. If packing is to be done it should be lightly with iodoform gauze and changed frequently.

Involvement of the sinuses presents no further complications than those already mentioned except that drainage of the sinuses themselves may have to be maintained, and the final outcome cared for after there has been some progress in bone fixation. If it is definitely known that the frontal or ethmoidal sinuses have been involved, especial care must be taken to maintain drainage and to curb activities that might carry infection higher up. (Figs. 259, 261.)

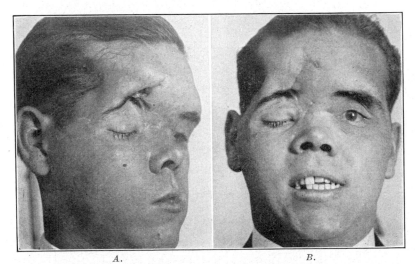

A.   B.

Fig. 263.—*A.* Compound facial injury with loss of one eye, lacrimal duct blockage on other side and midline separation through maxilla and palate. Patient seen eleven months after accident; the right eye has been lost, the right frontal and parietal bones and the nasal supports have been crushed in. The right frontal sinus drains externally and the left naso-lacrimal sac is obstructed and keeps the remaining left eye so covered with pus that vision is impaired.

B. The right frontal sinus has been obliterated and the eyebrow moved downward. The left lacrimal sac has been removed at the same time as the most important step in getting the patient back to work. The mouth is open to show the total lack of occlusion from the depressed dental arch on the right. See Fig. 223.

Late Complications.—Loss of substance or unrestored displacement may have to be cared for by cartilage or soft tissue transplants to restore contour. Late open reduction of depressed orbits with drilling and wiring of the fragments may be required and care should be taken that the masseter attachment to the zygomatic arch does not displace the fragments again.

Wide lacerations through the face may result in cut branches of the seventh nerve and resultant sagging of the features. (Figs. 252, 263.)

The infraorbital nerve occasionally forms a painful neuroma if it has been damaged and excision of it at its exit through the infraorbital foramen may be necessary. The resultant anesthesia of the lip is usually very disagreeable.

The teeth may or may not survive; if there has been a complete transverse fracture through the body of the maxilla, there is usually continued discomfort in the teeth, although many patients seem to accept the fact philosophically.

Bony union of any fracture of the maxillary bones is questionable.   It does not often occur, and of course the amount of infection, comminution and loss of substance will determine the final solidity even of the fibrous type. Many patients with complete transverse fractures even though occlusion and function seem normal, are conscious of some false movement on chewing, and

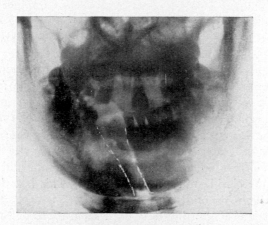

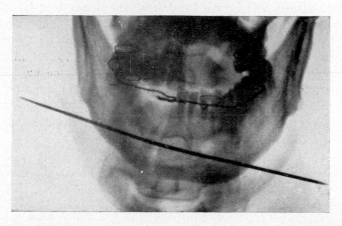

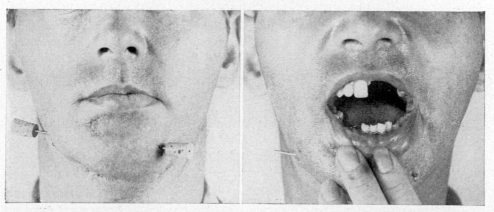

Fig. 264.—Bad comminution at symphysis with only small points of bone in contact, left condyle and many teeth broken. Fixation at symphysis with one internal wire and a second plane of fixation obtained with an anterior wire arch. Jaws wired together because of the condyle fracture opened after four weeks with internal wire still in place. (From Brown, J. B., and McDowell, F.: Surg., Gynec. & Obst., 1942.)

in some the movement may even be felt by the examiner. The advisability of attempting free bone grafts on these patients is as questionable as the original chance for bony union is.

INTERNAL WIRE FIXATION FOR FRACTURES OF JAW*

"In some fractures of the lower jaw, in which interdental wiring cannot be done, a wire—of the Kirschner type—drilled across the fracture line may be an easy and satisfactory method of treatment.

"*The indication* for this internal fixation may be present when the opportune early time for interdental fixation has passed and the fragments have become displaced, with compounding into the mouth, infection, and local sloughing. It also may be considered in edentulous jaws; when there is much comminution and accompanying injury, as in gunshot and war injuries; when many teeth have been loosened or broken; in displaced symphysis fractures; and in fractures at the angle in which the posterior fragment is pulled out and up into the upper buccal fornix by the closing muscles (Fig. 240). This last deformity is one of the worst to contend with, and, if left uncorrected, may result in non-union of the fragments. It is also of value in certain separations of the upper jaw.

"The internal wire will insure fixation in one plane—that is, the fragments cannot slip up or down past each other. However, they might rotate, in or out, or they might pull apart and, therefore, *the addition of an anterior wire dental arch* will give a second plane of fixation that will prevent rotation and will jam the fragments in impaction so that separation will not occur. If there is a condyle fracture to deal with also, or if normal occlusion cannot be maintained, then there can be the *further addition of interdental fixation to the upper jaw.*

"Multiple internal wires can be used for multiple fractures, or to give the second plane of fixation if desirable.

"*Avoidance of the nerve canal* is advisable even though the nerve may have been cut in two by displacement of the fragments. The same is true of any good teeth and this can usually be done by staying below the canal. When a second wire is placed above the lower one, there is more chance of damage of the nerve and teeth.

"An electric power drill is practically necessary, as the hand drill may not give enough speed for easy penetration of the bone. Regular Kirschner wires may be used, but stainless steel wires, recommended by Dr. C. H. Crego in leg lengthening, are cheaper and can be obtained in suitable lengths of thickness from .05 inch to .08 inch, a three-sided point being put on them.[1] Bicycle spokes also are used.

"Local or deep block anesthesia is usually employed. The fragments are alined with the hands, or an open reduction may be necessary, an elevator being used between the fragments. It is important that reduction be accurate, as only slight adjustment is possible after the wire is in.

"A puncture incision is made to get the wire in against the bone, and the wire and drill are lined up accurately. Then, perhaps most important of all,

---

*This section is taken directly from "Internal Wire Fixation for Fractures of Jaw," by James Barrett Brown, M.D., and Frank McDowell, M.D.: Surg., Gynec. & Obst. 74: 227, 1942.

[1]This wire is 18-8 stainless steel. The smallest size to give the necessary stiffness is preferable.

the fragments have to be held in accurate position with the hands while the wire is drilled into place. (Little mention need be made of the necessity of care with the drill and wire, and for avoidance of injury to the hands that are holding the fragments.) The wire usually is drilled on through the bone and a small opening is made to let it through the skin on other side. Secondary internal wires may be needed occasionally.

"The anterior arch wire is applied by putting No. 26 stainless steel wires on posterior teeth on each side, twisting the strands tightly for 2 inches, then twisting them together in midline and holding them with individual No. 28 wires around separate teeth. Any other type of arch appliance may be used, but this one requires no added equipment and is usually satisfactory.

"This is the wire that should suffice for the second and final plane of fixation and should impact the fragments together over the internal wire

"*Interdental fixation* is done as mentioned, if there is some final adjustment of occlusion to be secured or if the condyles also have been fractured. The jaws may be fastened directly together or by any effective method of elastic traction.

"*In edentulous jaws,* when dental plates wired or bandaged in place with the mouth closed will not suffice, a single internal wire may be effective as the jaws are usually small from atrophy anyway. This plan for edentulous jaws seems much less trouble for the patient and surgeon than attempting any rigid fixation within the mouth with screws down into the bone and nerve canal.

"*Pressure dressings,* of soft cotton mechanic's waste, are applied to give support to the soft tissues and prevent, as far as possible, hematomas, hemorrhage, and swelling, and also to lend further support to the bone fragments.

"The jaw seems solid immediately and the patient experiences the usual comfort of a set fracture. The ends of the wire are covered and the patients do not object much to discomfort. In some instances, the wires may be cut short enough to be covered by the skin, but it is probable that they all should be removed finally. Just one or two days are required in the hospital, and some patients can open the jaws and take soft foods almost immediately.

"*The removal of the wires* can be done easily after 3 to 5 weeks, depending upon the progress. There may be some irritation around the wires but no serious osteomyelitis should develop.

"This plan was thought to be new, but articles on the subject were found by Ipsen and Sobye in Denmark and Meade in Ireland, and these men seem to have been the only ones to have reported it.

"In the voluminous literature from the last war and since then, there has been a multiplicity of dental splints, often with emphasis on some contrivance of little fundamental bearing. If this simple direct method of internal wire fixation by drilling a wire across the fragments will help avoid the use of complicated dental splints, overhead plaster-cap traction for elevated posterior fragments, and wide open reductions, it will be worthwhile."

CHEMOTHERAPY IN COMPOUND FACIAL INJURIES AND JAW FRACTURES

Wounds of the mouth, jaw, and neck, with their marked tendency to infection, make a field of great importance for the use of penicillin and the sulfonamides. They are used systemically and locally in all wounds and right in the fracture line, if they can be gotten in, so that external drainage is not as necessary as formerly. Chemotherapy is continued in full doses for eight to ten days after the accident.

FRACTURE OF THE NASAL BONES

The nasal bones are broken oftener than any other bones of the face (perhaps oftener than any other bone in the body). Fracture of the nasal bones themselves is not so frequent as separation of their suture line from the frontal processes of the maxilla, or separation of the lateral cartilages from the nasal bones themselves. The frontal processes of the maxilla may also be separated from the body of the maxilla and be classed as a nasal fracture. It is this type that frequently accompanies extensive fractures of the facial bones and displacement inward is almost sure to occlude the airway.

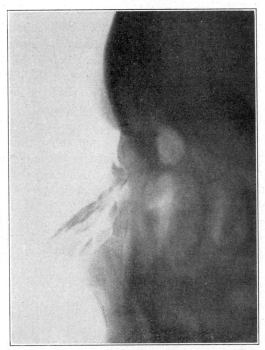

Fig. 265.—Comminuted fracture of nasal bones. (Conwell.)

Displacement.—A blow direct from the front is apt to comminute and crush down the nasal bones themselves and perhaps break or deform the septum. From the side the nasal bone or frontal process is broken in, or the lateral cartilage is separated from the bone. This last displacement may almost correct itself, but other fractures usually stay where the force has placed them.

Diagnosis.—Following a blow on the nose if there has been hemorrhage from the inside some type of fracture or separation has occurred that has been great enough to cut the nasal mucosa. This is an important point because by the time the patient is seen there may be so much external swelling that little can be made out about external deformity. If there is not frank displacement, careful palpation should be done, feeling for any slight clicks or grating of bone fragments. The nasal passages should be carefully cleaned out (cocainized if necessary) and careful inspection of the mucosa should be made. Gross occlusion of the passages may be present and dilation by the speculum may elicit a click and some pain. If this is not present, but there has been bleeding, the tear in the mucosa can nearly always be found. This gives an idea of the site of the separation, and the septum and its mucosa should be carefully gone over. If there is no tear there may be a submucous hematoma (which should be opened). As much information as possible should be obtained from the patient about the condition of the inside of his nose and the septum and also about the external contour. It should be remembered that very few noses are perfectly straight, but unfortunately few patients seem to know this and until the injury have paid little attention to the exact contour of their noses, but just suppose it to be perfectly straight and in the midline.

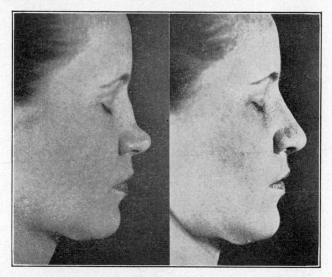

Fig. 266.—Correction of old depressed nasal fracture with costal cartilage transplant. This operation is thought to be necessary frequently because of the similarity of the deformity to that of a loss of structure from syphilis.

X-ray Diagnosis.—X-ray pictures may help some for records and to determine the degree of comminution. Their most accurate information is given in cases of fracture of the frontal process of the maxilla but this shows best on a posteroanterior or vertico-submental view. X-ray pictures of children's noses are usually worthless. (Fig. 265.)

Treatment of Uncomplicated Cases.—Most simple fractures can be set (under cocainization) with a Kelly forceps inside the nostril to raise the fragment into position. Frequently a distinct click will be heard and felt both by the operator and the patient as the fragments approach their normal positions. External molding with the fingers may help if there is wide displacement. The replaced fragments frequently will remain in position without support but narrow iodoform gauze may be packed high up in the nostril to be retained as a splint. This is changed in forty-eight hours or left out if fixation is firm. (The use of packs in nasal fractures is questioned frequently because of danger of blocking infection toward a possible basal fracture. This is an excellent caution in extensive cases, but is not applicable to the average simple nasal injury.)

A light metal splint may be used over the nose and cold compresses are valuable if used one to three hours a day.

Firm fixation is usually counted on in ten days and during this time the air passage should be watched and, if there is any tendency to redisplacement, it should be corrected.

The nose should be kept clean and oil drops used regularly.

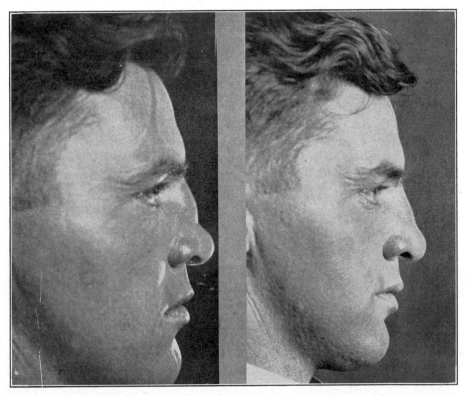

Fig. 267.—Correction of early nasal fracture deformity by replacement of bone and cartilage. This fracture was treated after some weeks by loosening and replacing the deformed lateral cartilages and by removing some of the dorsal bony hump and transplanting it lower down.

Complicated Cases.—Severe comminution and displacement with soft tissue laceration requires careful sorting and replacement of parts; packing should be light and, if there is question of fracture higher up, rubber tubing might be used through the meati, or the packing changed at least every twenty-four hours. A simple method of restoring narrowness when the nose has been flattened out is to put a through and through silkworm-gut stitch from side to side under the fragments and through the septum and tie them over perforated lead plates on the side of the nose, pulling them up carefully so that necrosis will not occur. (Figs. 223, 261.)

There are as many nasal splints advocated as there are jaw splints; one type is a mold to go over the nose, to be held in place by adhesive or straps; this does not appear adequate for a depressed fracture. Another is an internal support (or external mold) held by a headband.

Late Complications.—There may be loss of substance that leaves a depressed bridge, and, if a natural appearance is desired, a transplant of costal cartilage may be necessary. (Fig. 266.)

There is occasionally a periostitis that proliferates along the bony dorsum so much as to make a definite humped deformity. This is removed with the chisel preferably inserted through an incision just inside the ala and up under the skin of the dorsum which has been raised. (Figs. 267 and 268.)

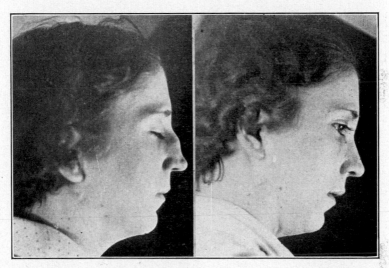

Fig. 268.—Osteoplastic operation for correction of fourteen-year-old nasal fracture deformity. Patient shown to illustrate the deformity that may result from fracture in childhood; corrected in one operation and nose held in its new position with the wire sling shown in Fig. 255. (Patient referred by Dr. Sumner L. Koch.)

Continued bony displacement with deviation to one side may need complete freeing of the bony nose and replacement in midline. This is done with saws or chisels carried along the maxilla at the point of reflection of the frontal processes, beginning inside the nose. It may also be necessary to free the septum from the palate and if one side is a great deal higher than the other it may be necessary to remove a triangle of bone from this side before the nose is moved to the center. (Fig. 269.)

When the nose is mobilized, it is swung into a little overcorrection and held there either with the external splint and packing, as a broken nose, or with a wire looped around the lower angle of the detached bone, or through the septum with a lead plate to prevent cutting, and brought on out into the buccal fornix and wired to a tooth, as in Fig. 270.

Septum Deviation.—The nasal spine in old cases may be firmly united on one side of the midline and carries with it the septum so as to produce asymmetry and possibly interference with breathing. The displaced nasal spine may be detached with a chisel and held over in position with a wire anchored to a tooth as is shown in Fig. 270.

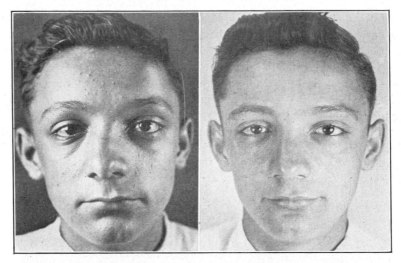

Fig. 269.—Progressive deformity result of fracture in childhood. This nose had deviated so far to the right that, in the correction, it was necessary to remove a triangle of bone from the left side and then swing it to the left after sectioning the frontal process on the right. The position was maintained by a wire anchored to a molar tooth on the left side with the loop of the wire caught around the lower angle of the loosened frontal process on the right side. See Fig. 270.

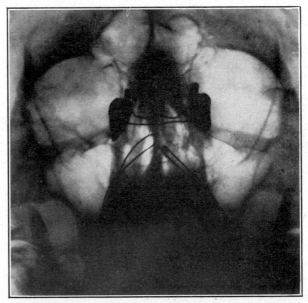

Fig. 270.—Wire through the septum and buccal fornix, fastened to another one around a tooth to hold the nose after mobilization from a deviated position.

If the cartilaginous septum itself is deviated at its tip into one nostril, it may be loosened along its lower attachment and sectioned from above downward where it bends over and then pushed over into the midline and held with mattress sutures through the columella and its own edge. Some excess mucosa may be excised from the prominent side. Resection of parts of the septum may be necessary later if breathing is impaired. Whether these offending parts of the septum are the direct result of the trauma or whether they are old deviations made more noticeable is not always clear. (Fig. 271.)

Fractures in Infants and Children.—Gross fractures are to be cared for much the same as outlined above. The instance difficult to deal with is that in which the child has fallen on the nose, but does not present any apparent deformity except swelling. Many of these injuries really are fractures with a pinching in or a mashing down of the nasal septum. It is possible that this condition, if allowed to remain uncorrected, may account for some of the unexplained bad deformities of the nose seen later in life. (Figs. 268, 269.)

For this reason it is perhaps good practice in all cases of fracture in infants or children to give an anesthetic and gently elevate any possible depression with a forceps high up in the nostril. This is a simple procedure, and its application may seem a bit questionable, but it is not so much so as allowing a depression to remain and having the patient suffer extreme nasal deformity as he grows up.

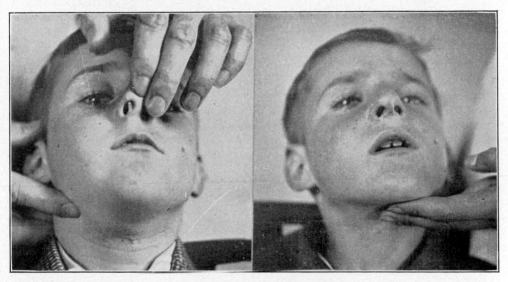

Fig. 271.—Displacement of nasal spine and septum. Following an injury the lower end of the septum presents directly into the right nostril. It was replaced by loosening it below and cutting through it at the bend and then fixing it in its new central position with mattress sutures through the septum and columella. If the bony nasal spine is also displaced, it is freed with a chisel and held over with a wire to a tooth as the nose is in Figs. 269 and 271. (Patient referred by Dr. T. K. Brown.)

DISLOCATION OF THE LOWER JAW

The joint is made up of the condyle, the glenoid fossa and the articular tubercle of the temporal bone, the meniscus, the capsular and three other ligaments. There is a wide range of motion in the joint and the articular surface of the temporal bone is several times greater than that of the condyle. General laxity of joint capsules, chronic subluxation, and bad occlusion of the teeth are predisposing causes, and most cases occur in women. In many cases of fracture of the condyle there is also a dislocation.

Forward Dislocation is the most frequent type and there is no fracture necessary for its production. As the mouth opens, or the chin is protruded, the condyle rides forward on the articular tubercle; if it slips forward over the crest anterior dislocation results. Causes are chronic subluxation, blows on the jaw or chin with the mouth open, and blows on the ramus. Some spontaneous cases occur presumably from overactivity of the external pterygoid muscle which draws the condyle forward, followed by contracture of the masseter. (Fig. 272.)

Displacement and Symptoms.—The jaw is held forward with the mouth open. Chewing is impossible, and swallowing and talking are difficult at first. The condyle may be felt and seen on the x-ray to be in front of the tubercle. The chin deviates to the opposite side in unilateral dislocation; this finding is the opposite in fracture and ankylosis when deviation is toward the affected side. Hysterical opening of the mouth may be confusing, but may be differentiated by x-ray or under anesthesia (local or general).

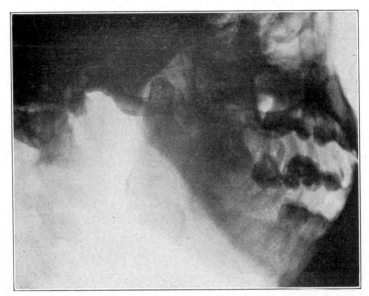

Fig. 272.—One side of a double anterior dislocation that had been unreduced six weeks and for which double open reduction was necessary.

Treatment of Forward Dislocation.—If seen soon after dislocation, complete relaxation under anesthesia itself may effect reduction. If not, traction and manipulation may be employed by grasping the jaw with both hands, thumbs inside the mouth on the molars (being ready to get them out of the way if the jaw should snap shut) and the fingers outside on the body of the jaw. Gentle depression of the molars and then backward pressure on the whole jaw should carry the condyle down to the level of the articular eminence and then allow it to drop into the joint. First one side and then the other may be done by pulling downward, outward and backward on the jaw by holding it firmly in the molar area inside and out. The backward pull is not important because the condyle will slip in the fossa if the head can be gotten well up on the eminence. General anesthesia is best, but block anesthesia of the third divisions has been satisfactory.

If this does not suffice as in cases that have been displaced some time, more traction may be secured by Gilmer's method. A stout flat stick 2 feet long in put into the mouth, the end resting on the posterior molars, and the upper molars acting as a fulcrum. The teeth are protected with rubber or gauze and a good amount of pressure can be exerted to depress the condyle just below the eminence. Obstacles to reduction are tenseness of the muscles and ligaments, and infiltration of the surrounding tissues if displaced very long. Bony block of the coronoid under the zygoma has been described, but is very infrequent.

Open reduction may have to be done. The joint is approached as outlined under ankylosis, and the condyle elevated back in place with a curved elevator. If both sides are done, the first wound should be left open until the other side is reduced. The jaw should be fixed shut in occlusion for from two to three weeks. Bandage or plaster cap and sling may suffice, but interdental wiring as for fracture gives the safest retention.

After-care should be protection of the joint: avoiding tough food, large bites of any kind, and subduing convulsive laughing or wide yawning.

Upward Dislocation.—A severe upward blow with the mouth open (most likely if many teeth were missing) might drive the condyle through the thin roof of the glenoid fossa into the middle cranial fossa. Movements would be impaired and the ramus apparently shortened.

Closed reduction should be attempted under anesthesia, or trephining above might be necessary. The usual case would not be far out of position and wiring the jaws in occlusion would suffice.

Backward Dislocation.—A backward blow on the chin with the jaw closed might drive the condyle against the tympanic plate of the glenoid and crush it into the auditory canal. This might frequently be complicated by fracture of the condyle itself. Dislocation clear in under the bony auditory canal has been reported. (Fig. 235.)

Treatment should be dragging the jaw forward into its correct occlusion and fixing it. If the canal has been deformed, its contour should be restored.

Outward Dislocation has been reported. It is almost necessarily complicated by fracture some place in the jaw. The condyle should be freed from the zygoma and gotten into the fossa and fixation in occlusion done along with whatever care is necessary for the fracture.

Medial Dislocation is almost always associated with fracture of the neck of the condyle or ramus; it is extremely rare, but may require open reduction. (Fig. 219.)

Unreduced Dislocations necessarily throw off occlusion, but the patient may develop surprising function. If open reduction fails, it may be necessary to resect the condyle.

Chronic or Recurrent Dislocation may tend to occur if not guarded against in some instances, the condyle slipping over and in front of the eminence at any time the mouth is thrown open. The first treatment should be voluntary rest and protection of the jaw, and the use of a supportive chin bandage a great part of the time. Next should be partial fixation of the jaw with dental bands and rubber or silk ligatures that may be removed at will. Such an appliance may be worn a number of months.

There are many operative procedures described for shortening or excising joint capsule ligaments and intraarticular cartilage.

Subluxation or "Cracking Jaw."—Due to some derangement of the joint mechanism and probably of the intraarticular cartilage, there may be a click on moving the jaw. This may be a loud audible noise and even temporary locking open may occur. The condition is mainly seen in persons with bad occlusion, so that all their lives they have unconsciously had to make some effort to get the jaws into occlusion. There may be a nervous element besides, in which the jaws are kept more or less constantly in motion. There may be recurrent pain for a long period, but many patients with loud audible "cracks" have no other discomfort. Dental manipulation is apparently a frequent starting point of the trouble when the mouth has been held open a long time or the joint traumatized during an extraction.

X-ray studies of this condition are somewhat disappointing. Although patients with marked symptoms may show marked excursion of the condyle beyond the eminence of the glenoid fossa, other patients without symptoms may show even more marked excursion. (Figs. 236, 273.)

Treatment is the same as for chronic dislocation and must be continued permanently in some cases. In bad attacks, firm fixation by interdental wiring may be done. Many operative procedures have been recommended by Annandale, Ashhurst, Blake, Brockenheimer, Darcissac, Dubecq, Monro, Morris, Summa and others so that they cannot all be referred to here.

Syndrome of the Mandibular Meniscus.—Dubecq* has given a concise review of the subject and from his study thinks that all names such as "snapping jaw," "cracking jaw," etc., should be discarded and the term "painful cracking of the jaw" substituted. He states that the triad of symptoms of pain, cracking and eventually blockage should justify recognition of the "syndrome of the mandibular meniscus." This triad of symptoms is not always present however as pain is frequently absent and there may be early blockage in cases due to trauma of orthodontic manipulation or tooth extraction. In Dubecq's description it is pointed out that the mandibular meniscus is an intraarticular fibrocartilage that is movable and that its main function is to deaden the blow of the condyle in the glenoid and against the auditory canal. It may be affected by disease or trauma, and may be worn through when the teeth are lost. In the dog the meniscus may be removed without producing symptoms and if traumatized in situ blockage of movement develops. This blockage finally disappears due to complete absorption. In the patients he has seen pain has been an almost constant finding, followed by cracking and only occasionally by blockage. He has divided the patients observed into 3 groups in relation to treatment: (1) Conservative without operation. (2) Alcohol injections of the joint, dental appliances to correct occlusion or limit opening, etc. (3)a. Operations on the glenoid or articular tubercle to block the opening, local bone grafts. b. Operations on the capsule for reefing it, operations on the meniscus for reefing it, and total removal of the meniscus. This last procedure was the most favored and was done 11 times out of 30 cases.

*Dubecq: Journal de Medicine de Bordeaux **114**: 125, 1937.

Pain Symptomatology of the Mandibular Joint.—This joint is quite complicated in itself in its anatomy and its movements and is in close association with other important anatomical structures. Much investigation has been done of its movement, and deafness has been reported from interference with the cartilaginous auditory canal and eustachian tube. Painful conditions about the ear and tongue have been traced to injury to the chorda tympani

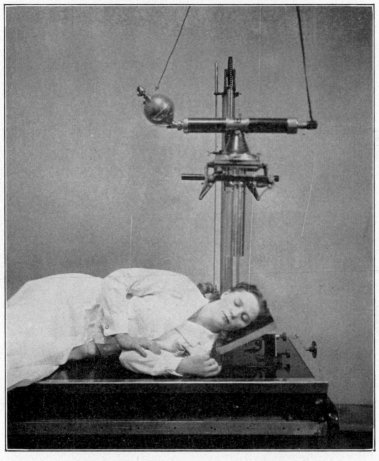

Fig. 273.—Temporomandibular joints. Should be taken with mouth opened and closed. Kilovoltage, 66; milliamperage, 20; distance, 28 inches; time, 3 seconds; angle board, 23°. (Courtesy Dr. Sherwood Moore, Mallinckrodt Institute of Radiology, Washington University School of Medicine.)

and auriculotemporal nerves by a condyle that has become misplaced or eroded or has not been held away from the glenoid because of lack of molar teeth. Many such patients have been relieved of symptoms by increasing the separation of the jaws in the molar region by the use of discs between any existing teeth or by building up old dentures or supplying new ones. Costen has recently summarized these investigations and added many of his own observations.*

---

*Arch. Otolaryng. 22: 556, 1935, and J. A. M. A. 107: July, 1936.

ANKYLOSIS

Bony ankylosis may result from a fracture of the condyle with resultant necrosis, dislocation, unreduced fracture dislocation, or from any type of infectious arthritis, and may be a complication of mastoid disease.

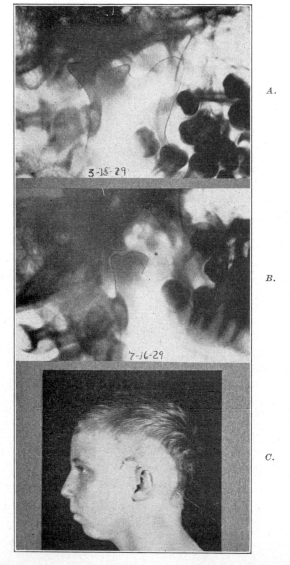

Fig. 274.—*A*. Solid bony ankylosis of six years' duration. At operation cortical bone appeared to be continuous from the ramus to the temporal bone.

B. Same joint four months after operation. Normal function of lower jaw except for somewhat limited opening.

C. Scar from incision two weeks after operation. The incision arches through the temporal region, goes down just in front of the crus of the helix, over the tragus and down just in front of the lobe. It is practically unnoticeable later and may be used for all approaches to the joint to replace those incisions placed farther out on the face.

Diagnosis.—The jaw deviates to the ankylosed side; this makes a flatness on the opposite side so that it looks more deformed than the affected side. There is usually some swelling about the joint and on carefully palpating both sides the lack of movement can usually be noted. The preangular notch along the lower border of the jaw is deepened on the ankylosed side. The mouth can be opened little or but very slightly and there is further deviation to the affected side. This is evidence against an anterior dislocation which throws the jaw toward the opposite side. It is also important to differentiate ankylosis due to scar bands inside the mouth. In long-standing cases no one in the patient's family may remember which side was originally involved, and accurate determination of the fixed side must be made.

Roentgenograms are helpful in determining the extent of bony fixation. (Fig. 274.)

Treatment.—Resection of the condyle with possibly the coronoid and some of the ramus itself may be necessary for a cure. Stretching or forcefully dilating the jaws apart will never suffice in real bony ankylosis and will usually do harm. Fascia transplanted into the space may be of help and also allow early movement and may cut down the amount of bone to be resected, thereby preventing retraction of the jaw.

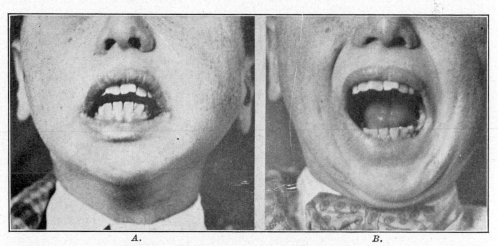

A.   *B.*

Fig. 275.—Bony ankylosis with relief by joint resection. *A.* Only slight opening is possible several years after mastoid disease. *B.* Shows patient fifteen days after operation with good opening and with some deviation to the resected side.

The skin incision is a flap from the temporal region down in front of the crus of the helix, over the tragus and down close to the lobe of the ear. This gives an almost unnoticeable scar. A fascial flap may be turned back, but this never is large enough to cover the bony raw surface and it retracts into almost nothing. These superficial flaps are retracted forward, but without too much traction on the seventh nerve fibers. (Figs. 274, 275.)

The fascia and masseter are cut and moved downward from the zygoma, and the joint is exposed. Removal of bone is done so that free movement is obtained. The operation is often a wide resection, more than an arthroplasty. Some authors recommend the removal of part of the zygoma, but this does not appear necessary. The bone is removed with rongeurs or chisels and if desired a wide drill may be used to start or to remove certain areas. There should preferably be a free space of at least 1 cm. from ramus to skull with the mouth closed.

When sufficient bone has been removed and movement gotten as free as possible, the fascial flap is carried down in the empty space over the cut ramus and the superficial wound is closed with drainage, or free fascia lata is used. Hemorrhage from the internal maxillary artery may occur, and if it does, it may have to be controlled with an iodoform pack which may be removed through the lower part of the wound several days later.

The jaws are carefully dilated to full opening with a mouth gag between the molars and finally are blocked open with a wood block wired between the molars. This may throw the jaw closer to the skull, but the advantage of the soft tissue stretching is important. The block is removed in from seven to fourteen days. If this block is omitted in children, active motion of the jaw is encouraged as soon as possible.

Anesthesia must be guarded because of danger of blocked respiration before the ankylosis is relieved.

Bilateral Ankylosis may occur and the only hope of function is operation on both sides. The worst joint should be treated first, and then if the mouth cannot be opened, the other side should be excised. This is a radical procedure and may be extremely shocking to the patient.

The jaw is forcefully dragged forward as far as possible, even past normal occlusion and wired firmly in position for from ten to fourteen weeks. Note that it is not to be blocked open, because to do so may result in the patient's inability to close the mouth later.

Good function usually results if enough bone has been excised. In double resections the jaw may drop back when the patient goes to sleep on his back and occlude the airway. Some suitable position in sleeping will be a matter of training.

Risdon of Toronto has proposed another procedure for ankylosis that he believes is superior to joint resection. The soft tissues are elevated from the external surface from beneath the angle upward, the masseter is taken loose from the border of the jaw, leaving a small part attacked. The ramus is drilled through in several places from before backward, about one-half way up, or high enough to avoid the maxillary nerve and artery. Complete section of the bone is then done and the masseter is split in two from below upward so that a broad flap may be carried through the separated bone ends and sutured to the internal pterygoid muscle on the inner side of the jaw. The remaining masseter is resutured to the stump on the bone and the wound is closed. The seventh nerve is not disturbed and neither is the ankylosed joint. A new false joint is produced and advantages are an easier and less shocking operation, and less subsequent retraction of the jaw. This procedure should be a great improvement over double resection when there is ankylosis on both sides.

CHAPTER XIII

INJURIES OF THE SPINE

SURGICAL ANATOMY

The spine is a flexible column composed of thirty-three bones called "vertebrae." The upper twenty-four of these are movable, or true, vertebrae and the lower nine, or false, vertebrae are fused to form two bones, the sacrum and the coccyx. The true vertebrae are divided into seven cervical, twelve dorsal, and five lumbar. In this section we are concerned with the true vertebrae, the sacrum and the coccyx being included in the section on the pelvis. (Fig. 276.)

The Individual Vertebrae.—Each vertebra consists of a body, a neural arch, and a number of processes. The body is a short thick section of cancellous bone covered by a thin sheath of cortical bone. Its upper and lower surfaces are flattened, while its borders are slightly concave from above downward. The bodies are piled one upon another to support the head and trunk.

The neural arch projects backward from the body as an osseous ring and in the articulated spine these arches form a flexible bony cylinder for the protection of the spinal cord. Each neural arch consists of two pedicles and two laminae. The pedicles are two short thick processes which project backward from the upper part of the posterolateral portions of the bodies. The laminae are broad, thin plates of bone which project backward and inward from the pedicles and fuse to complete the neural arch.

Processes.—The spinous process projects backward from the junction of the laminae and serves for the attachment of muscles and ligaments. The transverse processes project laterally from the junction of the pedicles and laminae and serve for the attachment of muscles and ligaments. The articular processes are four in number and spring from the junction of the pedicles and laminae. The superior articular processes face upward and backward and the inferior articular processes face downward and forward.

The First and Second Cervical Vertebrae differ radically from the other true vertebrae. The first, or atlas, has no body or spinous processes but consists of two lateral masses which are united by anterior and posterior arches. The lateral masses support the occiput and articulate below with the axis. The arches form a large ring for the inclusion of the odontoid process of the axis and the spinal medulla. The second or axis is remarkable in that its body is extended upward as the odontoid process which fits in the anterior portion of the ring of the atlas where it is held by the strong transverse ligament. Embryologically the odontoid process represents the body of the

---

In the revision of this chapter we have been helped by Dr. Arthur G. Davis, and he has contributed a decription of his gravity suspension method for the treatment of compression fractures of the spine and the section on cervical fractures and dislocations.

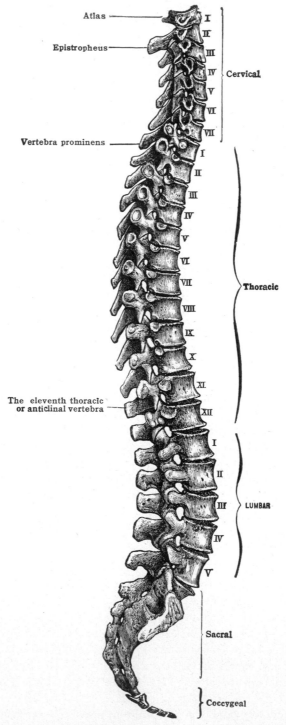

Atlas

Epistropheus

Vertebra prominens

The eleventh thoracic
or anticlinal vertebra

I
II Cervical
III
IV
V
VI
VII

I
II
III
IV
V
VI
VII
VIII
IX
X
XI
XII Thoracic

I
II
III LUMBAR
IV
V

Sacral

Coccygeal

Fig. 276.—The vertebral column, right lateral view. (From Morris: Human Anatomy. P. Blakiston's Son & Co.)

atlas. The axis also possesses a large bifid spinous process which is the first spinous process that can be palpated below the skull.

Articulations and Ligaments of the Spine.—The bodies of the vertebrae are held together by strong anterior and posterior common ligaments which extend from the occiput to the sacrum and by intervertebral discs which are interposed between the adjacent surfaces.   Each disc consists of a central, semifluid nucleus pulposus and a peripheral annulus fibrosus.   The semifluid center is maintained under pressure and the fibrous border is compressible. Thus the discs act as shock absorbers and permit bending of the bodies on one another.   (Fig. 277.)

The articular processes possess a surface of articular cartilage and form true joints with the processes of vertebrae above and below.

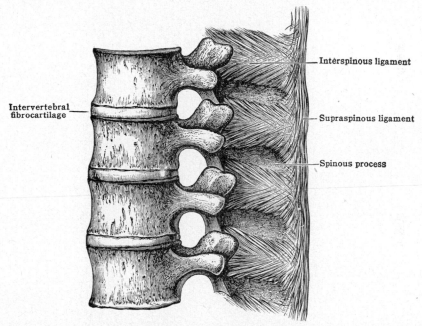

Intervertebral fibrocartilage

Interspinous ligament

Supraspinous ligament

Spinous process

Fig. 277.—The interspinous and supraspinous ligaments in the lumbar region. (From Morris: Human Anatomy. P. Blakiston's Son & Co.)

The ligamenta subflava unite the laminae of adjacent vertebrae, and the interspinous, supraspinous, and intertransverse ligaments unite the spinous and transverse processes of adjacent vertebrae.

Physiologic Curves.—Normally the spine is straight in the lateral plane and presents four curves in the anteroposterior plane.   These are cervical, dorsal, lumbar and sacrococcygeal curves.   The dorsal and sacrococcygeal are convex backward and are primary curves, while the cervical and lumbar are concave backward and are secondary curves.   (Fig. 276.)

Movements of the Spine.—The cervical region possesses the widest range of movement and the dorsal region is relatively fixed.

Nodding forward and backward of the head occurs at the occipitoatlantoid joints and rotation of the head occurs at the atlantoaxoid joint.   Lateral bending of the head occurs in the midportion of the cervical spine and flexion and extension of the head occur in the lower portion.

Due to the fact that it enters into the formation of the bony thorax, relatively little motion in flexion, extension or lateral bending is possible in the dorsal spine, but most of the rotation which occurs below the cervical region takes place here.

The lumbar spine admits of practically no rotation but allows a wide range of motion in flexion, extension, and lateral bending. Much of the motion occurs at the dorsolumbar and lumbosacral regions.

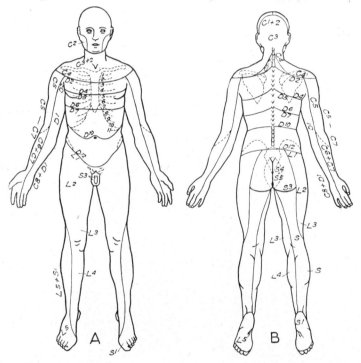

Fig. 278.—Sensory distribution of spinal nerves. Pain and temperature. (From Davis and Voris: Arch. Surg., January, 1930.)

Surface Landmarks.—The tips of the spinous processes can be palpated in the midline of the back. The bifid tip of the spinous process of the second cervical vertebra is the first one which can be palpated below the occiput. In the cervical and upper dorsal region the tip of the spinous processes lies opposite the body of the corresponding vertebra. The spinous process of the fourth lumbar vertebra lies at the level of the crest of the ilium.

The anterior surfaces of the bodies of the second and third cervical vertebrae can be palpated by inserting the finger into the posterior pharynx.

The Spinal Cord and Its Membranes.—The spinal cord is much shorter than the spinal column and in the adult its lower end lies at the level of the disc between the first and second lumbar vertebrae. Anterior and posterior nerve roots spring from the sides of the cord and pass outward and downward to emerge between the vertebrae as the spinal nerves. Due to the relative shortness of the cord the centers for the spinal nerves lie at a higher level than the vertebrae beneath which each emerges and by which it is designated and this disparity increases as the distance from the upper end of the cord increases. Chipault's rule for determining the relation of the segments to the spinous processes of the vertebrae is ''in the cervical region add one to the number of the vertebra, and this will give the segment opposite it. In the upper dorsal region add two, and from the sixth to the eleventh dorsal add three.'' The lower part of the eleventh dorsal spinous process and the space below it are opposite the lower three lumbar segments. The twelfth dorsal spinous process and the space below it are opposite the sacral segments.

The spinal cord presents two enlargements—the cervical for the upper limbs which comprises the lower four cervical and upper two dorsal segments and ends opposite the seventh cervical spine; and the lumbar for the lower limbs which lies opposite the three lower dorsal spines.

As the spinal nerves pass through the intervertebral foramina they lie close to the articular facets and are exposed to injury if these are fractured or dislocated. In the lumbar region of the canal the filum terminale of the cord and the roots of the lumbar and sacral nerves form a leash-like bundle called the ''cauda equina.'' Injuries in this region cause lesions of the nerve roots and not of the cord proper.

The cord is covered by three membranes: dura, arachnoid, and pia mater. The dura is a dense fibrous sheath which forms the outer covering and sends prolongations to invest the nerve roots as they enter the intervertebral foramina. It is attached to the walls of the vertebral canal at various points, but in most places is separated from the bone by a layer of fat and areolar tissue which contains the arteries to the cord and a rich plexus of veins.

The arachnoid is a delicate membrane which lines the dura and is attached to the cord by a multitude of thin web-like strands. The space between the dura and the cord which is crossed by these strands is called the ''subarachnoid space.'' It contains the cerebrospinal fluid. The pia is a thin membrane which is closely applied to the cord.

INJURIES OF THE SPINE—GENERAL CONSIDERATIONS

To the lay mind and, unfortunately, to many medical minds as well, a broken back or neck is a broken back or neck, and as such is a dreadful accident which results in sudden death or complete and permanent paralysis below the level of the lesion. This gloomy point of view is the heritage of pre-Roentgen days when only the severe fracture dislocations of the spine with extensive damage to the spinal cord were recognized as spine fractures. At the present time we know that more than half of the fractures of the spine are not accompanied by paralysis and that with adequate treatment most of these patients may be expected to recover and return to their former occupations.

It should be emphasized that fractures of the spine are not dangerous on account of the skeletal injury, but are dangerous to life only when associated with damage to the spinal cord or other visceral or skeletal injuries. On the other hand, it is also to be emphasized that the skeletal injury may cause prolonged disability if proper treatment is neglected. In this chapter we shall emphasize the treatment of the skeletal injury, because we believe that it is more important to recognize these minor spinal fractures and return these patients to their former occupations than it is to make careful neurologic studies of the hopelessly injured cases. For this reason we shall deal rather briefly with the neurologic findings in lesions at different levels of the cord and refer our readers to textbooks of neurology for information on that phase of the subject. To those who criticize this attitude our answer is that we determine the level and extent of the bony lesion by the x-ray and the presence of pressure on the cord by the Queckenstedt test.

We believe that fractures of the spine should be treated by reduction and immobilization until the lesion has healed and that pressure on the cord is most effectively relieved by early reduction and immobilization which tends to restore and maintain the normal diameter of the spinal canal. We recognize the fact that many cases of paralysis gradually clear up spontaneously, but that anatomic lesions of the cord may be permanent and that treatment may not affect them. We shall discuss the care of these paralyzed patients.

Spinal injuries will be considered under the following headings:

1. Compression Fractures of the Vertebral Bodies.
2. Fracture Dislocations of the Spine.
3. Luxation of the Cervical Spine.
4. Injuries of the Spinal Cord, Nerve Roots and Cauda Equina.
5. Isolated Fractures of the Transverse Processes.
6. Isolated Fractures of the Spinous Processes and Laminae.
7. Isolated Dislocations of the Vertebrae.
8. Jumped Process Complex.
9. Traumatic Lesions of the Atlas and Axis.
10. Traumatic Spondylolisthesis.
11. Traumatic Lesions of the Low Back (Lumbosacral and Sacroiliac Strains).
12. Injuries of the Sacrum and Coccyx are included in the section on the pelvis.

COMPRESSION FRACTURES OF THE SPINE

Incidence and Cause.—More than 50 per cent of all fractures of the spine are of the compression type. The majority of the cases are due to automobile accidents or falls, usually from a height in which the patient lands upon the feet or buttocks and in which the spine is hyperflexed or jackknifed by the superincumbent body weight. It is to be emphasized, however, that a compression fracture of the spine may result from an apparently trivial injury, such as occurs when a patient slips and suddenly sits down upon the floor. Other cases are due to the same mechanism in which a weight falls upon the patient's back, head, or shoulders from above, hyperflexing and crushing the spine. Rarely a compression fracture results from a fall or dive on the head or shoulders, and in these cases the cervical or upper dorsal vertebrae are usually involved, while in those due to falls upon the feet or buttocks or to crushing injuries, the fracture usually occurs in the dorsolumbar region.

Over 70 per cent of the cases of compression fractures occur at the dorso-lumbar region; that is, at the junction between the relatively fixed thoracic and the movable lumbar spine. In a series of one hundred and twenty-five fractured vertebral bodies, Wallace found that the first lumbar vertebra was broken thirty-three times and the second lumbar vertebra was broken nineteen times. The third, fourth, and fifth lumbar were broken seven, nine, and ten times, respectively. The other dorsal and cervical vertebrae were broken from one to six times with the exception of the first and second cervical and the first dorsal in which fractures did not occur in his series.

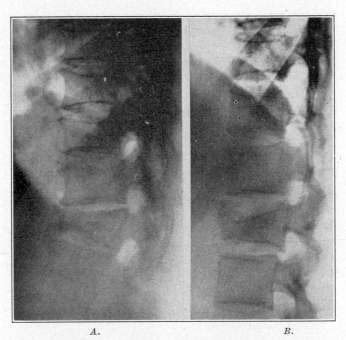

A.   B.

Fig. 279 A and B.—Anterior compression fracture of the third lumbar vertebra, lateral view. Before (A) and after reduction (B) on hyperextension frame. Body cast with recumbency in bed for two months; then body cast from axillae to hips for eight weeks, out of bed with this cast; then Taylor back brace for four months. Good results in ten months.

In Wallace's series there were one hundred and twenty-five compression fractures of the vertebral bodies in eighty-two cases and in Conwell's series there were one hundred twenty-six fractures in one hundred patients. Not infrequently two adjacent vertebrae are crushed and occasionally definite fractures of two or more vertebrae with one or more normal vertebrae between them may occur from a single accident. One of us has recently treated a patient who had five distinct vertebral fractures from an automobile accident. None of the vertebrae was severely crushed or displaced and there were no neurologic disturbances.

Pathology of Compression Fractures of the Spine.—As the force in hyperflexion is applied, the anterior portion of the body of one of the vertebrae tends to give way and is crushed by the body of the next vertebrae above (Figs. 279-285), the two bodies being folded together on the articular facets and pedicles which act like a hinge and are relatively stronger than the bodies of the vertebrae. As the cancellous bone is crushed, it may be spread apart or broadened, and loose fragments may be forced outward in any direction, usually forward or to either side, but occasionally backward into the spinal canal where they may impinge upon and compress the cord. With the compression of the vertebral body, the fragments may be impacted quite firmly so that considerable force is necessary to loosen the impaction and restore the normal height of the vertebral body. In addition to the fixation in hyperflexion by impaction of fragments there is also a variable amount of fixation in this position as a result of muscle spasm incident to the fracture.

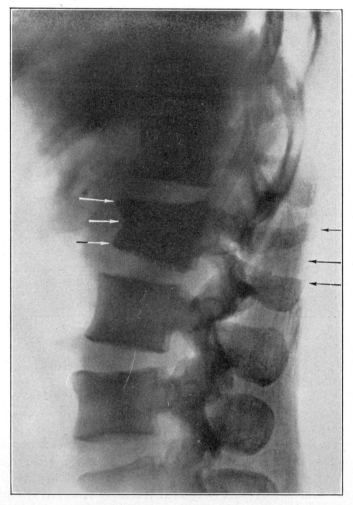

Fig. 280.—Compression fracture of the first lumbar vertebra before reduction with splitting of the spinous process.

There is also a variable amount of damage to the intervertebral discs in the vicinity of the fracture, and these may be torn and the contents of one or more of them may be forced out into the surrounding tissues and the disc flattened. The strong anterior common ligament which is continuous across the discs and vertebral bodies usually remains intact, although it may be stripped up from the anterior surface of the body of the fractured vertebra. The fact that this ligament remains intact enables us to correct the deformity in these fractures by hyperextension of the spine with little fear of damaging the cord by pulling the vertebrae apart.

Occasionally in very severe injuries when the force continues to act, the vertebra above is displaced forward or forward and to one side on the vertebra below. When this occurs there is a fracture of the posterior arch or of the articular facets and the spinal cord tends to be crushed between the posterior border of the body of the vertebra below and the posterior arch of the vertebra above the point of fracture. In rare instances there may be tearing of the interspinous ligaments or splitting of a spinous process with subluxation or even dislocation of the articular facets. The injuries to the spinal cord and nerve roots are considered under a separate heading.

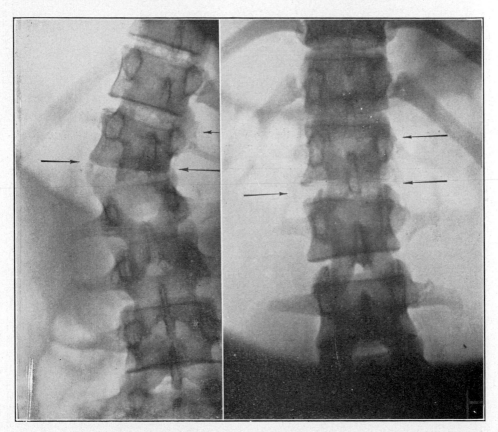

Fig. 281.—Compression fracture of the first lumbar vertebra with lateral angulation before and after treatment with traction on a hyperextension frame.

Diagnosis of Compression Fractures of the Spine.—The diagnosis of compression fractures of the spine is now made a great deal more frequently than it was a few years ago. This is largely due to the fact that surgeons are learning to suspect compression fractures after certain definite types of injury, and to take routine anteroposterior and especially lateral x-ray pictures of the spine in these suspected cases. In the past most of these cases went unrecog-

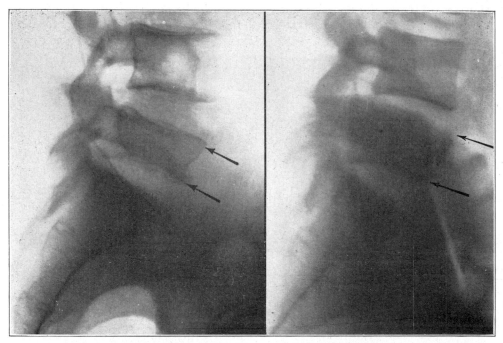

Fig. 282.—A compression of the fifth lumbar vertebra before and after reduction by hyper-extension.

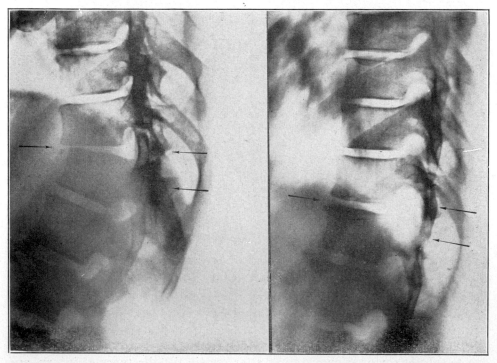

Fig. 283.—Slipping forward of the eleventh on the twelfth dorsal vertebra before and after reduction by hyperextension.

nized, and the only cases that were diagnosed fracture of the spine were those that presented obvious deformity or marked cord symptoms. However, even at this time many mild cases of compression fractures are missed by physicians and surgeons, and as a result these patients receive inadequate treatment and may suffer prolonged or sometimes permanent disability.

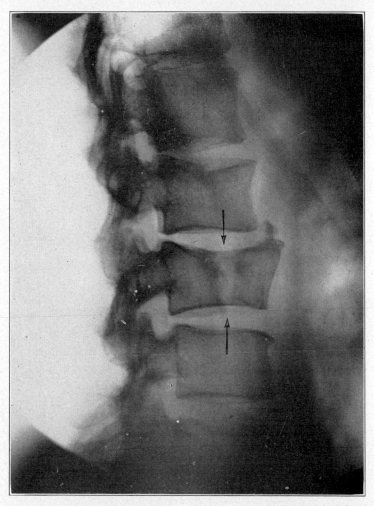

Fig. 284.—An unusual compression fracture of the third lumbar vertebra with anterior and posterior fragments. (Courtesy Dr. Jim Mason.)

Osgood has very aptly stated that the key that opens the door of diagnosis is suspicion and that one should never fail to suspect a compression fracture of the spine after an accident that may have caused sudden hyperflexion of the spine. Once suspicion is aroused, the diagnosis is usually easy, because at the present time x-ray pictures are practically always available. The point to be emphasized is that after a fall or hyperflexion injury, a patient may get up and walk and even return to work in the presence of a compression fracture of one or more vertebrae, and that a mild compression fracture may exist with no deformity which can be demonstrated by physical examination. In such cases unless one is suspicious because of the hyperflexion or compression injury the diagnosis is apt to be missed and the case dismissed as a contusion or strapped with adhesive and treated as a low back strain.

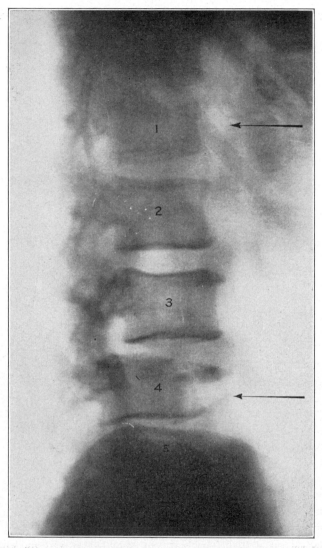

Fig. 285.—Crushed compressed fracture of the first and fourth lumbar vertebrae, lateral view with dislocation of the fourth lumbar. Total transverse lesion of cord at level of first lumbar. Cord was severed as shown by laminectomy, treated by fixation in a body cast for six months. Lower extremities paralyzed. Died three years after injury. (This case shows the importance of looking for fractures at different levels, following injuries to the spine.)

The diagnosis then depends largely upon the history. In the examination of back injuries the surgeon should endeavor to obtain an accurate history of the mechanism of the injury. A history of a compression or hyperflexion injury followed by localized pain in the back makes it imperative for the surgeon to rule out fracture of the spine whether or not girdle pains or motor or sensory paralysis are present. This can be done only by x-ray pictures (especially lateral views) and these should be made in every suspicious case.

The pain may be a dull ache or burning in character and may be localized in the back or in the abdomen or it may be distributed along the nerves emerging at the site of the fracture (girdle pains). It is usually aggravated by movement, and most patients with a fresh fracture of the spine prefer to lie on the side with the knees drawn up, but some patients are able to sit up or even walk with very little pain.

Physical Examination.—The most constant and reliable sign which can be elicited by physical examination is tenderness over the spinous process of the broken vertebra. This tenderness is nearly always present in fresh compression fractures and is distinct from the tenderness along the side of the spines over the muscles and articulations, which can be elicited after contusion and sprains of the back. We have, however, seen mild cases of compression fractures in which no tenderness could be demonstrated.

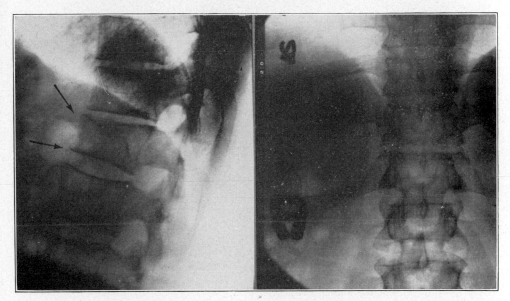

Fig. 286.—A mild compression fracture of the twelfth dorsal vertebra.

Next to tenderness, the most constant physical finding is muscle spasm over the involved area. This, however, is present in sprains or strains and is also difficult to demonstrate in injuries of the dorsal spine. Consequently it is not of great importance in the diagnosis of spine fractures as differentiated from other back conditions. In some patients there is marked rigidity of the abdominal muscles and the surgeon may suspect a visceral injury.

A knuckling of the spine—that is, the presence of a kyphos or unusual prominence of one or more spinous processes—is almost pathognomonic of compression fracture if it occurs after injury. (Figs. 287, 288, and 289.) Of course, one must rule out previously existing deformity, but in the lumbar region considerable compression must occur before the knuckling can be demonstrated. Consequently the absence of a visible or palpable deformity does not rule out a compression fracture.

Every case of suspected spine fracture should be subjected to a neurologic examination in order to rule out injury to the spinal cord or nerve roots. If the patient can move the arms and legs freely and the deep reflexes are normal, and if there are no obvious sensory disturbances, there is probably no injury to the spinal cord or nerve roots and the surgeon's attention can be concentrated on the skeletal injury. If paralysis is present its limits should be determined and reduction of the deformity performed immediately in order to relieve pressure on the cord as will be mentioned in the Section on "Injuries to the Cord."

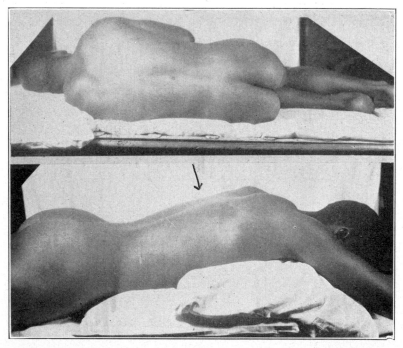

Fig. 287.—Usual attitude assumed by a patient with a fracture of the spine. This patient has a fresh fracture of the ninth thoracic vertebra.

Fig. 288.—Same as preceding. An arrow points to the slight deformity (kyphosis) at the ninth thoracic vertebra.

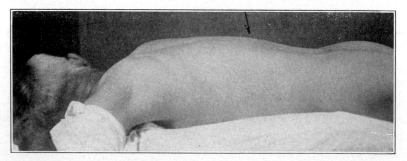

Fig. 289.—Anterior compression fracture of the twelfth thoracic vertebra. Note the moderate kyphosis.

When neurologic symptoms are present they, of course, lead the surgeon to suspect a fracture, but in very rare instances concussion of the cord may occur from trauma and paralysis result with no demonstrable fracture.

The X-Ray.—Every case of spine injury in which one is even suspicious of fracture should be subjected to both anteroposterior and lateral x-ray views of the involved area and in selected cases oblique views should be made in order to demonstrate obscure lesions of the posterior arch. Even the best x-ray technic may fail to reveal all of the lesions present, or a lesion may be obscured by the recoil factor. Compression fractures of the body and fractures of the spinous processes are best shown in the lateral x-ray pictures.

Treatment of Compression Fractures of the Spine

In this section we shall consider only the treatment of the injury to the spine proper. The treatment of any lesion of the spinal cord or nerve roots which may be present is considered under "Injuries of the Spinal Cord and Nerve Roots."

In the past, fractures of the spine have been treated by simple immobilization in a plaster cast in whatever position the fragments happened to be when the diagnosis was made. In 1923 Wallace* published his method of gradual correction of the deformity by the use of a special frame which was placed over the bed and which could be elevated. The patient is placed on the frame in such a position that the upper end of the frame coincides with the level of the fracture and his feet are strapped to the bottom of the frame. Then the frame is gradually elevated, thus permitting the head and trunk of the patient to fall backward and gradually hyperextend the spine and correct the deformity. In Wallace's paper most of his cases were old cases and he did not emphasize the correction of fresh fractures. Consequently most of these cases continued to be treated by simple immobilization until 1929, when A. G. Davis published his method of manipulative correction of the deformity in spine fractures. The dramatic method of Davis attracted much more attention and led to the general recognition of the fact that these deformities can and should be corrected, and the method was soon followed by various types of frames for the gradual correction of the deformities, because many surgeons felt and still feel that the manipulative method is dangerous. At present the most popular method is immediate hyperextension, usually with the patient supported on a loose canvas hammock, and immediate immobilization in a hyperextension plaster jacket.

Treatment of Compression Fractures of the Spine in Which There Is Little or No Deformity

In these cases all that is necessary is to immobilize the spine in a position of hyperextension. In young vigorous patients in good general health this can be done by applying a plaster-of-Paris jacket in a position of hyperextension as described below. However, many patients cannot tolerate this immediately and must be given a preliminary period of rest in bed or it may be necessary to apply the hyperextension gradually.

The simplest method of accomplishing this is to place the patient upon a hospital bed which is so constructed that it can be broken and elevated under the patient's knees. The patient's head is placed at the foot of the bed (wrong end to) or the head and foot pieces are reversed. This will place the break in the

---

*Wallace: J. Bone and Joint Surg. 5: 28, 1923.

springs at about the dorsolumbar region. The bed is then cranked up to secure the desired amount of hyperextension, and this may be increased or decreased at will. It is to be noted that some patients cannot tolerate much or even any hyperextension until several days after the accident. Elevating the head of the bed renders the patient's head and chest more horizontal and makes the hyperextension more tolerable.

As soon as it is judged that the patient can tolerate the hyperextension jacket, this is applied. This may be the day of the injury, or in obese females the cast may be omitted entirely and the patient may remain in hyperextension in bed for from four to eight weeks and then be fitted with a high back brace with shoulder straps (Fig. 298) and gotten up.

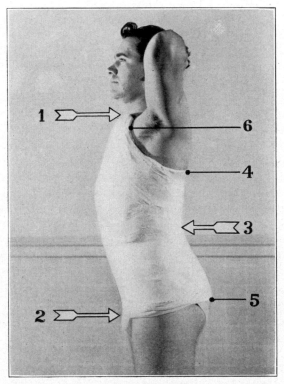

Fig. 290.—Typical hyperextension ambulatory jacket. *1, 2, 3,* indicate three-point pressure thrusts; *1, 2, 4, 5,* levels anterior and posterior necessary to control canting backward of torso; *6,* space between sternum and jacket can be padded with felt, increasing backward thrust. (Courtesy Dr. Arthur G. Davis.)

Lacking a bed which can be elevated a fracture board can be placed beneath the mattress on an ordinary bed and the desired amount of hyperextension secured by placing a roll of blankets beneath the mattress. In many hospitals convex or adjustable Bradford frames are used for this purpose, but we find that our patients are more comfortable in beds.

The advantage of the plaster jacket is that the patient can turn over in bed or lie on the face and that the patient may be up and about as soon as the acute pain and tenderness have subsided. We formerly kept these patients recumbent for from eight to twelve weeks, but now with a well-fitting plaster jacket which holds the spine in hyperextension, we often get them up in a few days after the accident and not only let them go home, but often permit them to carry on their regular business.

In old or debilitated patients and in obese women who are relatively inactive, one of us (J. A. K.) makes no attempt to correct minor compressions of the lumbar and lower thoracic spine or even rather marked compressions of the middle and upper thoracic spine. He simply keeps them in a bed with a firm mattress and a fracture board under the mattress for about four weeks and then gets them up gradually with a high Taylor type back brace or a light hyperextension plastic jacket. He has not noted that the failure to correct these deformities has resulted in any pain or disability. In patients with minor compressions the period in bed may be only a few days.

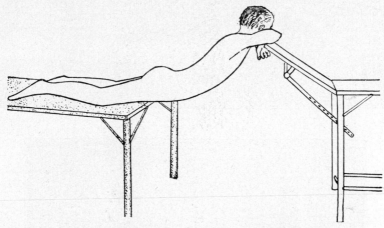

Fig. 291.—Reduction of compressed vertebra by hyperextension in its simplest form. (Courtesy Dr. Watson Jones: J. Bone & Joint Surg., 1934.)

Supports for Application of Plaster Cast in Fractures of the Spine.—For the application of a plaster cast the patient must be supported in a position of hyperextension and the support must be so arranged that the major portion of the trunk is exposed to permit the application of a plaster jacket which will maintain the position of hyperextension and thus relieve the pressure on the body of the fractured vertebrae. In order to do this, the cast must get a firm grip on the pelvis, fit snugly against the upper part of the front of the chest and against the back at the level of the fracture. There are thus provided three points of pressure: pressure forward at the level of the fracture and pressure backward at the front of the chest and the symphysis pubis and anterior superior spines of the ilia. As a result, with the patient in the upright position, the weight above the site of the fracture is shifted from the bodies of the vertebrae to the articular facets. Consequently, if adequate hyperextension has been achieved and if the plaster jacket fits properly, the patient may sit up or walk without danger of causing collapse of the body of the fractured vertebrae. This being true, the prolonged recumbency in plaster shells or on hyperextension frames is rarely necessary and many patients with compression fractures of the spine may now leave the hospital in a relatively short time and frequently they may attend to their regular business during the prolonged convalescence.

The plaster jacket may be applied with the patient lying prone or lying on the back. If the patient lies prone it is necessary to have the body weight partly supported by a canvas or muslin hammock which can be slackened in order to obtain the desired hyperextension. Watson Jones (Jour. Bone and Joint Surg., 1934), in his simplest form of hyperextension (Fig. 291), suspends the patient between two tables, one higher than the other, the lower table supporting the lower extremities as high as the groins and the higher table supporting the head and upper extremities.

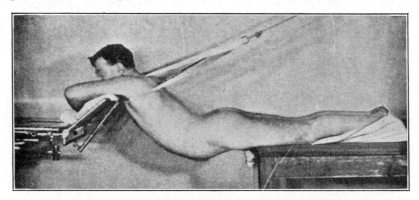

A.

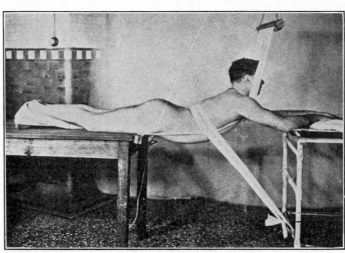

B.

Fig. 292.—Watson Jones' method of obtaining hyperextension and reduction of compression fractures of the spine. A, for lower dorsal and lumbar; and B, for middorsal fractures. (J. Bone & Joint Surg., 1934.)

We have used various types of hammocks, a simple one being a strip of canvas stretched on a rectangular gas pipe frame which has a ratchet at one end so that the hammock can be tightened or loosened at will. Boards placed crosswise on the frame under the canvas at the level of the mid thigh and chin provide fixed points of support, and as the hammock is slackened the trunk sags and the spine hyperextends. The head end of the hammock should be split in order that the canvas may fit closely to the shoulders and upper chest. Of late years various appliances have been fitted to fracture tables in order that hammocks may be attached to these. If a Bell table is

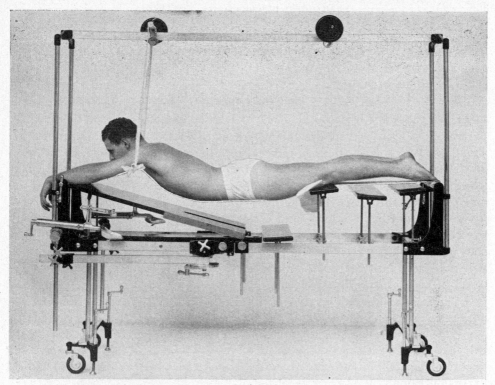

A.

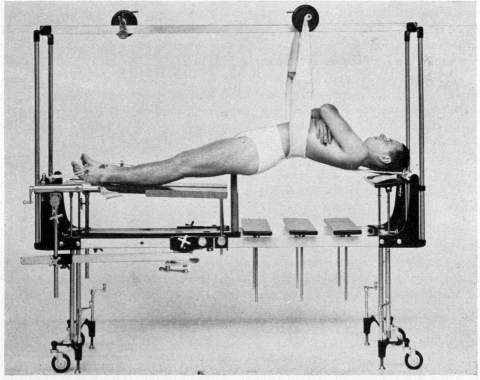

B.

Fig. 293.—Hyperextension of the spine and immobilization as obtained on the Bell table. Two methods. (Courtesy Mr. G. H. Chick, Oakland, Calif.)

available it may be used as illustrated in Fig. 293. It should be emphasized that when the hammock is used its upper end should be split in order that the hammock may approximate the chest and that the plaster jacket may get a firm grip around the upper thoracic region.

For the application of a plaster jacket with the spine in hyperextension while the patient is lying on his back, it is to be emphasized that the Hawley, or any other type of fracture table with a pelvic rest and a support for the shoulders, is not efficient as it is necessary to support the spine at the level of the fracture. A popular method of doing this is by means of the Goldthwait irons. These are two softly tempered steel bars which are strong enough to maintain a part of the body weight and are supported at each end by steel standards. We have used these irons on the Hawley table by resting one end on the pelvic support and the other end on the upper end of the table. The irons are kept from turning by having the lower end fitted with studs which project into the holes in the pelvic support and the upper ends are fitted in notches in a flat steel bar.

The irons are bowed upward to obtain the desired hyperextension and the patient is laid upon them. After the plaster cast has set, the irons are pulled out of the cast. The Goldthwait irons have the advantage that the plaster can be molded well around the front of the chest and pelvis. They have the disadvantages that they cannot be accurately adjusted and that the hyperextension cannot be sharply localized.

The above disadvantages are met by the automobile jack fitted with a removable pad as used by Ryerson and O'Donohue or a long strip of flexible steel, as used by James Bost. If a Bell table is available any desired amount of hyperextension can be obtained gradually by means of a canvas sling under the site of the fracture, as illustrated in Fig. 293.

The methods described above are suitable for lumbar or low dorsal fractures, but not for middle or high dorsal or cervical fractures. For the middle dorsal fractures Watson Jones uses the ventral hammock, but fixes the spine just below the level of the fracture by drawing a strong bandage over this area and tying it to the foot of the table in front of the patient (Fig. 292).

For the reduction of fractures in the cervical region a narrow strip of board is nailed to a table and padded and the patient lies on his back with the projecting end of the board at the level of the fracture and the head and neck are hyperextended over this end while the cast is applied to include the head, neck and upper trunk. (Fig. 336.) We use a long, thin metal slab instead of the board.

The plaster jacket is applied snugly over a thin layer of sheet cotton or a single layer of stockinet with a felt pad over each anterior superior spine of the ilium and a vertical strip of felt to protect the spinous processes from pressure.

When the patient is in position, either on a hammock or on the iron supports and the padding has been applied, the plaster-of-Paris bandages are rolled on in a circular manner, pulling them fairly tight and avoiding wrinkles until a jacket about a sixth of an inch thick has been made. This is allowed to set and the patient is taken off, either by cutting the hammock or lifting up on the irons, and placed in bed. In case the hammock has been used, it is withdrawn from the front of the cast, and in case the irons have been used they are withdrawn from the back of the cast. A small pillow is placed beneath the patient's back in order to prevent sagging of the cast while it is hardening. It is then trimmed to permit flexion of the thighs and movement of the arms and a large window is cut out over the abdomen.

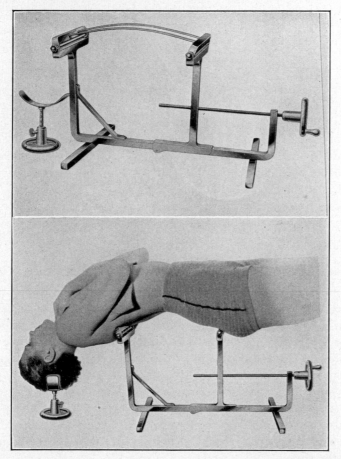

Fig 294.—The Johnson hyperextension back frame. (Courtesy Dupuy Manufacturing Company.)

Convalescent Treatment of Compression Fractures of the Spine

As soon as the plaster has hardened and the patient is comfortable, he may sit up or walk about at will. It is to be remembered, however, that a well-fitting plaster jacket which maintains the spine in the area of the fracture in a position of hyperextension is a sine qua non for the ambulant treatment of fractures of the spine.

In practice we wait one to four weeks, depending on the severity of the fracture, and then let the patient be up at intervals and the ambulant period is gradually lengthened until he is permitted to be out of bed at will.

In addition we prescribe certain exercises which are intended to strengthen the muscles of the back, abdomen, and lower extremities. We do not expect to make gymnasts out of our patients simply because they have broken their backs, but try to maintain their musculature in as good condition as it was before the accident.

Consequently, the exercises are graded to suit the individual, and the amount of exercise taken is increased as the patient's muscles become stronger. The two simplest ones which are given to all patients are the following:

1. Hyperextension of Hips: Lie on the face. Cross the hands behind the back and raise one leg and the head slowly as high as possible, keeping the knee straight and the chin in. Lower slowly and relax. Repeat with the other leg.

2. Straight Leg Raising: Lie on the back, pull both feet up, turn them in, curl the toes and raise one leg slowly as high as possible, keeping the knees straight. Lower slowly and relax.

In the beginning these are done three or four times, three times a day; then the number is gradually increased and other exercises are added as the patient improves. All exercises are done slowly and with full muscular power.

Renal calculi are a frequent complication of the convalescent fractured spine (8 per cent of Conwell's series).

The plaster jacket is worn for from four to eight weeks, and the patient is then fitted with a high Taylor back brace with shoulder straps which is worn for from two to four months, or longer, and then gradually discarded.

Treatment of Compression Fractures of the Spine in Which Deformity Is Present

We have seen compression fractures of the spine heal with deformity and the patients return to their original occupations and remain symptom-free for years. This is probably because a considerable percentage of these patients develop physiologic fusion at the site of the fracture. This is especially true of the severely injured spines.

On the other hand, we have seen these patients complain of pain and disability over a period of years. This may occur even with physiologic fusion and in these cases the pain tends to be localized just below the injured area where the faulty mechanics lead to the development of a localized hypertrophic arthritis of the spine.

Consequently, we believe that if a deformity is present, an attempt should be made to correct it. This can usually be done by hyperextension with or without traction. In former editions we described the original methods of Davis and some of the methods of correction by gradual hyperextension on an adjustable frame, because they illustrate the principles of correction and are useful in certain patients where it is not practical to correct the deformity immediately and apply a plaster jacket. But since the introduction of the ambulant treatment in hyperextension jackets, we rarely use either of the above methods, but try to obtain immediate correction of the deformity and apply a plaster jacket in hyperextension.

Transportation of the Patient.—Since the injury is due to hyperflexion and it is possible to cause further damage by further flexion, it is advised to transport and lift these patients in the prone posture—that is, horizontal and face down. However, it is much more important that they be handled gently, and care should be taken that a couple of orderlies or other uninformed individuals do not pick up a patient with a severe fracture of the spine with a heave and a jerk and severely wrench the fractured area and possibly do irreparable harm to the spinal cord. In our experience these patients can be lifted face down or face up and transported either way or on the side, provided the trunk is lifted as one piece and the fractured area supported when they are lifted.

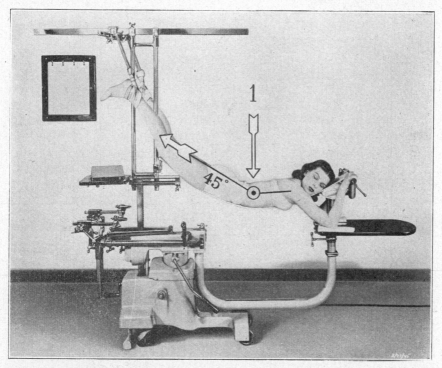

Fig. 295.—Typical foot suspension with Comper-Albee table. *1*, indicates thrust induced by levering the lower section of spine against the fixed thoracic section. *2*, Note 45-degree or ideal angle of suspension. Component of leverage thus safeguarded by the component of horizontal traction. (Courtesy Dr. Arthur G. Davis and American Sterilizer Co.)

The Gravity Suspension Method of Davis* is based upon the fact that the anterior common ligament practically always remains intact and that the strength of this ligament is such that hyperextension may be applied to the spine without danger of pulling the fractured vertebrae apart and thus causing further damage to the spinal cord. The firm attachment and relative invulnerability of the intervertebral discs, together with the firm incorporation of the annulus fibrosus with the anterior common ligament and epiphyseal plates insure restoration of the circumference and of the general contour of the vertebral body by the manipulation.

The method consists of actually restoring the contour of the body of the vertebra by obtaining the limit of hyperextension and of maintaining this position with adequate fixation. In cases in which the fragments are impacted,

*J. Bone & Joint Surg., 1929. The description of this method is contributed by Dr. Arthur G. Davis.

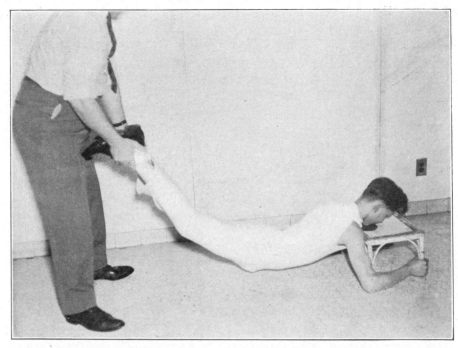

Fig. 296.—In the absence of apparatus of any kind, the simple raising of the feet as in the game of wheelbarrow may be used. A plaster jacket can be applied with as much efficiency as with special apparatus. (Courtesy Dr. Arthur G. Davis.)

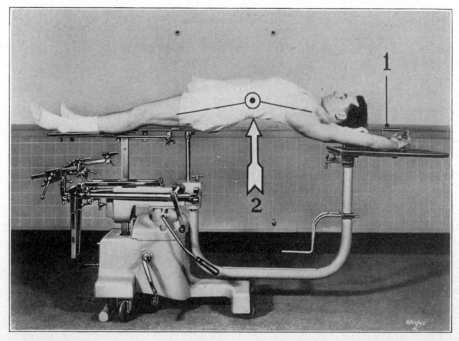

Fig. 297.—Hyperextension with adjustable Goldthwait irons on Comper-Albee table. *1*, Crank to adjust arc of curvature. *2*, Indicates thrust. (Courtesy Dr. Arthur G. Davis and American Sterilizer Co.)

it may be necessary to manipulate the region of the fracture while the spine is held in a position of hyperextension, thus causing disimpaction with a general restoration of contour. As the spine is hyperextended leverage is exerted through the pedicles and posterior arches which tend to act on the impacted body and pull the fragments apart to a point where the anterior common ligament is taut and the width, depth, and height of the body are restored.

Davis wishes to correct an erroneous impression created by the use of the word *manipulative* correction or reduction. The word manipulation was never intended to convey the necessity of the use of force. The method from the beginning never used more force than that involved in gravity suspension of the feet, except in cases when x-ray afterward showed incomplete restoration of the anterior vertical height. In such cases gentle pressure forward on both sides of the kyphos by "measured thrusts" was used to disimpact. Davis stressed from the beginning that no more than *gentle* manipulation is ever necessary. While foot suspension or any other type of hyperextension involves manipulation in the generic sense of the word, "gravity suspension" is a more specific and more accurately descriptive term. Gravity suspension implies avoidance of force. The force involved is no more than that involved in the child's game of wheelbarrow. Foot suspension apparatus does exactly what one does in this game and nothing more (Fig. 296).

Treatment of Uncomplicated Crush Fractures From the Tenth Thoracic to the Fifth Lumbar Vertebrae

Since this section of the spinal column sustains 75 per cent of the compression fractures, the following sequence of steps is outlined. Experience with some two hundred and fifty cases shows an almost universal return to former occupation with symptomless spines and completely uneventful convalescence, regardless of the degree of collapse of the centrum.

1. Provision for a suspension hammock and overhead block and tackle as illustrated in Fig. 295.

2. Without anesthesia and usually without opiates, the patient is then rolled into the prone position on the hammock and asked to hold himself from sliding by grasping the head end of the apparatus.

3. The feet are then simply elevated. This is done in a few seconds and the line controlling the block and tackle is secured in place.

4. The position is then scrutinized:

   A. The angle of inclination of the lower extremities should be about 45 degrees with the torso. Less elevation exerts too little traction on the anterior common ligament. More vertical suspension of the feet may dangerously compress the posterior arch.

   B. During suspension of the feet the projecting spinous process or kyphos may be observed to disappear.

   C. It will be noted at this point that the conformation of the spine is that of a hockey stick.

5. A plaster jacket is then applied. The jacket must conform to the requirements shown in Fig. 290.

6. Ordinarily fifteen to twenty minutes are sufficient for the plaster to harden. The feet are lowered and the patient is rolled simultaneously onto his side and the canvas hammock is withdrawn. The form of the jacket is carefully preserved for the rest of the day with the jacket exposed to air for evaporation.

7. By evening the patient is allowed to roll about the bed on his side, supine or prone, but with instructions not to sit up.

8. The next day a check x-ray picture is taken to show the degree of restoration of vertical height. Ordinarily such vertical height will be completely restored. If not, however, the jacket should be removed and another attempt at foot suspension with greater hyperextension is made. A forward thrust is made with the thumbs at a point 2″ lateral to the midline. Such thrusts should be gentle.

It has been the author's experience that it is rarely necessary to resort to this manipulation, since quite universally the x-ray picture taken the day after reduction shows complete restoration of anterior vertical height.

9. Present practice allows the dependable patient to leave the hospital in a day or two to spend six weeks recumbent at home, free to change about in bed but forbidden to sit up.

10. After a lapse of six weeks the patient is again checked by x-ray, the plaster jacket is trimmed enough for sitting purposes and to give arm room and, unless the patient has lost considerable weight, he is instructed to be up and about. Felt pads may be introduced between jacket and skin surface to produce greater hyperextension (backward thrust), Fig. 290, or the jacket is changed.

11. The object of ambulatory activity at this time is to induce perpendicular trabeculations in callus. The vibrational influence of walking serves to induce the necessary trabeculations for unrestricted weight bearing. It is not only important to start walking at this time, but it is considered definitely harmful to keep the patient recumbent because, as is well known, structural trabeculations are the direct result of imposed strain. At six weeks the callus must be considered as amorphous. After he has been up and about for an additional six weeks, the amorphous callus then becomes structurally strong enough as evidenced by massive clinical experience so that compression does not recur.

Gradual Correction of the Deformity.—Unless there is some contraindication to immediate correction of the deformity, such as multiple rib fractures, fracture of the femur or an unconscious patient, we rarely attempt to correct the deformity of the body of the vertebra gradually by hyperextension in bed. In the hands of J. A. K. it has been painful and inefficient.

The deformity may be corrected gradually by means of the frame of Wallace or by means of the extension frame of Rogers or Herzmark, or Conwell, or by means of a plaster jacket which has been applied in the position of maximum extension and then wedged. All of these methods aim at the gradual correction of the deformity by hyperextending the spine and letting the patient's body weight effect the correction. All frames are excellent, and are based upon the same idea concerning reduction. The Rogers* frame can be adjusted for a fracture at any level. It consists of a rectangular frame of spring steel bands one and one-half inches wide by three-sixteenths inch thick. Canvas is stretched across this as on a Bradford frame and the patient is placed upon it with a crossbar or yoke supporting the frame at the level of the fracture. With the ends of the frame fixed, the crossbar can be raised by means of a screw apparatus, thus obtaining the hyperextension, or with the crossbar fixed, the ends of the frame can be lowered and the hyperextension can be obtained in this manner.

The Herzmark† frame is simply a Bradford frame which is hinged about the junction of the middle and upper thirds and has a turnbuckle rod beneath it and attached to each end in such a manner that by tightening the turnbuckle the convexity of the frame is increased. It is somewhat more easily made than

---

*Rogers: Surg., Gynec. and Obst. 5: 101, 1930.
†Herzmark: J. Bone & Joint Surg. 11: 794, 1929.

the Rogers frame and has the advantage that the upper end can be elevated to any desired point, thus keeping the patient's head and thorax level while the extension is being made.

Treatment on these frames should be started with the patient in a comfortable position; that is, as a rule, with the frame slightly concave and with the site of the fracture opposite the hinge in the frame. The hyperextension may be made gradually, and usually at the end of fifteen to twenty minutes full correction of the deformity is obtained, and this correction should be controlled by lateral x-ray pictures taken while the patient is on the frame in a position of hyperextension. At the limit of extension the patient feels tension in the abdominal muscles and physical examination will disclose a disappearance of the abnormal prominence of the spines at the site of the fracture. In resistant cases we apply head and foot traction and combine the traction and hyperextension methods. Narcotics may be necessary during the rapid correction or the patient may be left recumbent for a few days and the correction carried out very gradually over a period of days.

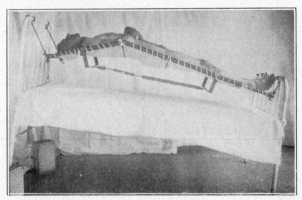

Fig. 297A.—Photograph showing patient on Conwell's modified Herzmark Bradford frame for gradual correction of compressed fractures of the spinal vertebrae. Any amount of convexity of the frame can be accomplished with the aid of the turnbuckle, thereby bringing about any desired hyperextension of the spine. The hyperextension can be secured with any degree of rapidity. The convexity can be easily adjusted to the area of compression. Traction and countertraction are applied to the head and pelvis and the lower extremities if necessary. An anesthetic can be given but is seldom indicated.

After correction has been obtained, the patient may be shifted to an ordinary Bradford frame which is bent to the same degree of extension or may be left on the adjustable frame or may be placed in anterior and posterior plaster shells which are applied in extreme extension, the anterior shell being made with the patient on the frame and the posterior shell being made while the patient is in the anterior shell. After the patient has been placed in the shell, clear lateral x-ray pictures may be obtained by cutting windows in either side of the plaster opposite the site of the fracture.

In order to simplify the after-care, the patient may be shifted to the Goldthwait irons or a suspension hammock and a plaster jacket may be applied as soon as hyperextension is obtained.

It has been our experience that some patients do not tolerate the prolonged hyperextension on the frame and may suffer from abdominal distention and vomiting in addition to severe pain. These symptoms can usually be relieved by placing the patient on a bed with fracture boards under the mattress. After a few days' rest he can be given a dose of morphine and placed on Goldthwait irons or a suspension hammock and a plaster jacket applied in hyperextension. The front of the jacket should be cut out over the abdomen and lower chest in order to prevent recurrence of the abdominal symptoms.

The patient should remain recumbent in hyperextension either on a frame or in a plaster shell or jacket for a period of from six to eight weeks, depending upon the severity of the fracture. At the end of this time he may be permitted up either in a well-fitting plaster jacket or in a brace. (Fig. 298.)

COMPRESSION FRACTURES OF THE MIDTHORACIC REGION

The posterior curvature represented by the prominence of the back roughly corresponding to the area between the fourth and ninth thoracic vertebrae calls for a special adaptation of the hyperextension principle. In this case two levers of almost equal length are available to "pry apart" the upper and lower sections of the fractured body and to render the anterior longitudinal ligament taut.

Since the thrust in this case is against the convexity of a curve, the force required is considerably less than is necessary in gravity foot suspension. One therefore resorts to the Goldthwait irons with the patient supine as illustrated in Fig. 294. Some fracture and orthopedic tables are equipped with such irons, or the irons and standards can be made of strap iron properly tempered. If the malleable types are used, they should be prepared with the proper arc of curvature in advance and laid on the standards. In any case, the patient is rolled from prone to the supine position on the irons and it is ordinarily found that the patient is quite comfortable for the necessary length of time required to apply a jacket. There should be 2 inches of space between the irons because this distance apart is found most comfortable. If the irons are farther apart, they press on the ribs uncomfortably; if they are close together, they press on the spinous processes. The patient is either held in place on the irons by attendants or he holds himself by grasping the table edge. No anesthetic or opiate is necessary; in fact it is almost impossible to carry out this technique except in a fully conscious patient. The jacket is applied from the sternal notch to the pubis and ordinarily low enough to clear the shoulder blades. The plaster is applied over stockinet and sheet wadding with felt padding for the bony prominences. After the plaster has hardened sufficiently but while still green, the patient is tumbled, irons and all, off of the standards on to a stretcher and the irons are then withdrawn while the patient remains on his side. Some modeling may be necessary in the lumbar region to restore the conformation at this point temporarily distorted by the withdrawal of the irons. The cast is then allowed to dry thoroughly.

The x-ray check is made the following day; the bed and the ambulatory convalescence are all conducted in the same manner as for lumbar compression fractures.

"High Thoracic Fractures"

None of the standard texts deal with this problem and it *is* a problem.

The section of the spinal column from the middle of the curve of the thoracic region (prominence of the back) upward presents unusual problems. No completely satisfactory method of reducing these fractures exists. Because this section is relatively rigid and does not enter into spinal movements except in a negligible way, the restoration of vertical height need not be as complete as the demands imposed by the highly mobile cervical and thoraco-lumbar sections. X-rays taken at the time of the process of reduction frequently show complete reduction but the application of the Minerva jacket is difficult to do at the moment and it is impossible to maintain hyperextension otherwise for long periods because of the unbearable pressure. Figs. 306 and 307 illustrate especially arranged equipment for the immediate reduction and immediate application of the Minerva jacket. Apparatus closely simulating that illustrated in Figs. 306 and 307 may be improvised by using a canvas hammock attached to a gas pipe frame. The level of the fracture should be marked on the stockinet. The mark should clear the crossbar to avoid pressure on the involved spinous process.

It will be seen that just as in the reduction of the much commoner thoraco-lumbar fractures, gravity *only* acts upon the upper and lower sections of the spine levers. Due to the fact that the thoracic spine curves backward at this point, very little leverage is required. In this case the operator is hyperextending against a convexity rather than with a concavity as is the case in the lumbar spine. The author has experienced great difficulty even with the precise method and apparatus herewith depicted in maintaining full vertical height throughout convalescence. Some after results have not been entirely pain free due no doubt to a traumatic arthritis in the posterior spinal joints at the involved level. This painful aftermath is the inevitable result of wedging (in this case partial collapse following complete reduction due apparently to the impossibility of holding the reduction). We have therefore arrived at the conclusion that in cases where such wedging recurs and the check x-ray shows twenty-five per cent plus loss of anterior vertical height of the centrum, an immediate fusion should be done covering the two or more vertebrae involved and after two weeks of convalescence following operation, another Minerva jacket should be applied. Fusions in this area involve but very little loss of normal spinal range of motion. The duration of convalescence is approximately the same, whether or not a fusion seems necessary. The obvious advantage is the more certain promise of a painless spine. We do not believe that early fusion is indicated often in these cases, even though reduction is not perfect. Painful backs following fractures in this area are not frequent enough and severe enough to warrant early fusions. We have found that fusion is only necessary when pain continues after convalescence and this is unusual.

Immediate Correction of the Deformity and Immobilization in a Plaster Jacket.—This is now the method of choice in most fracture clinics because soon after the patient has been fitted with a hyperextension plaster jacket, the nursing care is simplified and the patient may be gotten up out of bed. Not only this, but the patient is more comfortable in a jacket than on a frame or in a plaster shell.

Since the deformity is the result of forcible compression and hyperflexion, it is usually readily corrected by hyperextension with or without traction.

If the patient is in a state of shock, he should be placed on a firm bed or hyperextension frame, and treatment for shock should be instituted. The fractured spine can then be reduced and immobilized as soon as he has reacted from the shock. As a rule no anesthetic is necessary.

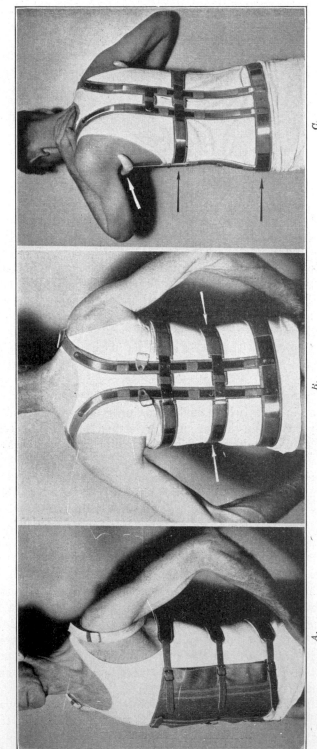

Fig. 298.—A and B. Taylor back brace as used in convalescent treatment of fractures of the spine. C. Same with axillary crutches.

The hyperextension may be obtained by any of the methods mentioned in the preceding section on the application of a hyperextension jacket. We have usually used a hammock which is lowered gradually. If necessary, gentle traction can be made on the extremities or gentle pressure can be made over the kyphos in order to complete the reduction.

As soon as the reduction is complete, the plaster cast is applied rapidly as described in the preceding section, except that a double layer of felt is placed over the kyphos. In severely compressed or comminuted fractures the cast is worn longer; that is, from four to six months or until the x-ray shows restoration of bone. Since we have learned to apply the plaster jackets properly, we not only get our patients up much earlier, but do not use a brace as much as we did in the past.

Prognosis in Compression Fractures of the Spine.—At this point we shall limit our discussion to the spine proper and shall ignore any cord or nerve lesions which may be present, since these are discussed under "Cord Injuries."

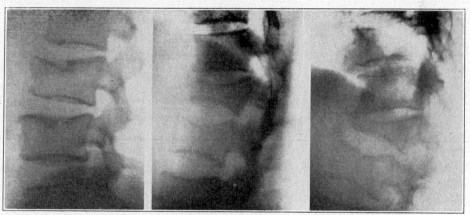

Fig. 299.   Fig. 300.   Fig. 301.

Fig. 299.—Compression fracture of third lumbar vertebra. Treated by hyperextension on frame for twelve weeks, then ambulatory body cast for eight weeks, and a Taylor back brace for four months.

Fig. 300.—Preceding case nine months following injury showing further compression or collapse. (Kümmell's disease.)

Fig. 301.—The same case eleven months following injury. Treated by Hibbs' fusion after the conservative methods had failed. Good results. This shows that a satisfactory reduction of the body does not always mean a good result and also that when the body alone is injured, delayed collapse may occur.

The body of the vertebra, being cancellous bone and having an abundant blood supply, tends to heal rapidly after a fracture and if the fragments are pulled apart the space between them tends to be filled with new bone. However, the callus tends to remain soft for a considerable time, and if it is subjected to full weight-bearing before it is hard, it will give way slowly, and the vertebral body will become flattened. This is true not only of the callus, but also of the adjacent cancellous bone which becomes rarefied after the injury. Consequently, we believe that if the vertebral body is protected long enough, it will eventually regain its normal solidity in whatever form it may be.

In addition to the vertebral body we must consider the intervertebral discs and the posterior arch. It is due to the injuries of these structures that physiologic fusion may develop. Physiologic fusion may be due to injury to the articular facets and laminae and may develop in the posterior arch, but it is usually due to injury to the intervertebral disc and develops between the involved vertebral bodies. In either case physiologic fusion tends to develop in the more severely injured spines and tends not to develop in the mild compression fractures. As a result a severe compression fracture may heal by fusion and the patient be free from symptoms while a mild compression fracture may heal without fusion and the patient may complain of some pain and disability over a period of years.

In compression fractures of the spine which have been adequately treated and permitted thoroughly to heal with or without physiologic fusion, but with little or no deformity we expect the patient to be able to return to his former occupation even though it involve heavy lifting, and to have no pain in the back as a result of the fracture. This eventuality, however, does not occur in a great many cases. One reason for this is that in the past a very small percentage of these cases have been adequately treated and as a result most of the cases with compression fracture with deformity have been permitted to heal with the deformity present. This has disorganized the mechanics of the back and has resulted in a stiff and painful back with the development of hypertrophic arthritis of the spine in the vicinity of the lesion. As a result many of these cases have suffered more or less prolonged disability. We have not been correcting these deformities long enough to be able to give a definite prognosis in the corrected cases, but the results so far obtained indicate that a much higher percentage of them will be able to return to their former occupations without symptoms.

Old Compression Fractures of the Spine.—As stated above many of these cases of old compression fractures have pain and disability months or years after the injury. Many of these are cases which were undiagnosed and received no treatment; others are cases which were inadequately treated; and still others are cases in which symptoms occur in spite of treatment. There is as yet no definite agreement as to the treatment of these cases. A conservative method of handling them is to place the patient recumbent in hyperextension on a frame in which the hyperextension can be gradually increased and after a period of from two to six weeks fit him with a plaster or celluloid jacket or high back brace which he should wear over a period of from a few months to a year. The object of the hyperextension is not to restore the normal contour of the fractured vertebra, as this is obviously impossible, but to correct the mechanics of the spine by the creation of secondary curves above and below the lesion.

About half of the cases of old fractures of the spine with pain show bony fusion of the fractured vertebra with the one above or below, and many of these show hypertrophic arthritis in the neighboring vertebrae. In the cases with bony fusion the pain tends to be localized just above or just below the point of fracture and is probably due to the faulty mechanics of the spine and the resultant abnormal strain in this area.

Some surgeons believe that these cases with pain demand spinal fusion in order to eliminate motion in the painful area. It should be remembered, however, that if fusion is to effect relief of the symptoms, it should fix that portion of the spine which is painful. Consequently, in cases of old fracture with ankylosis of the fractured vertebral bodies, the fusion should include the fractured vertebra and the ones above or below which are painful, and the fusion should be preceded by a period of rest in hyperextension in an effort to correct the abnormal mechanics of the spine. After the fusion the patient should be immobilized in a position of hyperextension until the fusion is solid; that is, over a period of from eight to twelve weeks. After the patient is up he should wear a high back brace or celluloid or plaster jacket over a period of at least six months until there is no longer any danger of breaking the fused area.

Whether conservative treatment or fusion in a given case is to be advised will have to be decided by the individual surgeon. Successes and failures have followed both forms of treatment.

Kümmell's Disease

Theoretically the condition described by Kümmell is one in which after a compression injury a vertebral body which at the time of the injury was not fractured or compressed, gradually gives way and collapses some months later, and the condition is supposed to be due to a rarefying osteitis which is caused by a disturbance of the circulation at the time of the injury. We now believe that most of these cases are the result of unrecognized compression fractures of the bodies of the vertebrae which may remain practically free from symptoms over a period of several months and then gradually collapse with resultant pain and disability.

The symptoms are those of pain and weakness in the back, usually with the development of a visible and palpable kyphos, the degree of deformity depending upon the amount of collapse of the vertebra. The x-ray shows the typical wedge-shaped vertebra and is differentiated from Pott's disease by the facts that the intervertebral disc is intact and there is no abscess. There may or may not be girdle pains or pains along the spinal nerves emerging at the site of the fracture, and in many cases it is difficult to obtain a history of the injury, and a neoplasm of the spine may be suspected. (Fig. 300.)

Treatment of Kümmell's Disease.—The patient should be fitted with a hyperextension plaster jacket as described under compression fractures of the spine or he may be put to bed with hyperextension either in a plaster shell or on an adjustable convex frame and an effort should be made to correct the deformity. We believe that many of these cases should be fused and that in most instances the fusion should include two vertebrae above and two below the site of the lesion.

Technic of Spinal Fusion.—The operation which we use is that of Hibbs and we supplement this by grafts removed from the tibia or ilium and placed along the sides of the broken-down spinous processes. If this operation is done properly, it is a serious and rather difficult procedure and should not be undertaken lightly by an inexperienced surgeon. The operation is expedited if the special instruments devised by Hibbs are used. It is performed as follows:

After a twenty-four-hour preparation of the skin of the back and leg, the patient is placed prone upon the table and anesthetized. Sandbags are placed under each shoulder in order to permit expansion of the chest. The patient is draped, leaving one foot free. Then by flexing the knee the tibia is exposed and through a longitudinal incision four or five long osteoperiosteal grafts and a considerable number of bone chips are cut from the tibia. These are wrapped in a blood-soaked piece of gauze and placed in a covered dish to prevent drying or the grafts may be removed from the ilium if this is to be used.

The leg wound is then closed by an assistant while the operator proceeds to expose the spine through an incision about seven inches long directly over the spinous processes. The tissue is removed from the tip of each spinous process with a sharp osteotome and knife. Then, by means of a periosteal elevator the periosteum and muscles are stripped from the spinous processes and reflected outward. The Hibbs' method is to begin at the top of the wound, strip about a third of one side of a spinous process and insert a gauze pack; then move down to the next process and strip about a third of that; and so on down the length of the wound leaving gauze packs in as each spinous process is exposed for a short distance. He does the same thing on the other side and then comes back to the first side and increases the amount of bone exposed. In this way the bleeding is controlled by the gauze packs and relatively little blood is lost. This is kept up until the desired number of spinous processes and laminae out to the articular facets have been exposed by subperiosteal dissection. The interspinous ligaments are then removed by sharp dissection. The cartilage of the articulations is removed by means of a very small sharp curette, and with a small curved chisel two slivers of bone are elevated from the base of each spine and lamina on each side. One of these slivers is turned up and the other one down so that they overlap with those from the laminae above and below. Then each spinous process is split longitudinally into three pieces. The upper piece is turned upward and the lower piece downward, thus overlapping with those of the spines above and below while the middle piece is left standing. Finally the osteoperiosteal grafts and bone chips are laid down along the side of the spines on top of the grafts from the laminae thus, to quote Forbes, "creating a veritable forest of bone." The muscle and periosteum are then pulled back with deep interrupted sutures of catgut, and fascia is sutured, and the skin is closed without drainage.

This is a serious operation and may result in considerable shock. It has been our impression that the shock is largely due to the cleaning out of the articulations. Consequently, we usually do the operation under local anesthesia, using 3 drops of adrenalin to the ounce of $\frac{1}{2}$ per cent novocaine, and do the articular facets last. The adrenalin lessens the bleeding and is used even when the operation is performed under general anesthesia. If the patient's condition is not good on the table, we do not fuse the articular facets. Firm fusion may be expected even without arthrodesis of the articular facets. It should be emphasized that this is the personal opinion of one of us (J. A. K.), because Dr. Hibbs believed that most of the failures after fusion operations are due to the fact that the operator did not properly remove the cartilage from the articular facets.

The patient should remain recumbent in bed with a fracture board under the mattress for from three to four weeks, when he is fitted with a high hyperextension plaster jacket or back brace and permitted to be up. The brace is worn about three months and then gradually discarded.

Treatment of Fracture Dislocations Without Paralysis

Fracture dislocations with or without paralysis present infinitely greater difficulty in regard to diagnosis, therapy and end result than does the compression type. While it is important ever to be watchful in the apparently simple compression type for involvement of the posterior arch, in the fracture dislocation type one must always allow for the limitations of roentgenography to exhibit details of the posterior arch which in this case is as certainly involved as though the fracture lines or dislocation were actually seen. *Diagnosis by inference* must be resorted to as in the "jumped process complex" referred to below.

Therapy is fraught with danger. The greatest danger is that the surgeon may produce injury or paralysis in a case of fracture dislocation without paralysis. The outstanding feature in the lateral projection is the very clearly defined crush of the body. This tends to blind the observer and he ordinarily looks no further. The lack of visual evidence of fault in the posterior arch will undoubtedly continue to create a false sense of security because of the apparent negative findings. Fracture dislocations constitute an exception to the rule of hyperextension so universal in the simple compression type. While hyperextension still remains the most constant factor in the mechanics of reduction, in cases such as the "jumped process complex," hyperextension type and avulsion type, any kind of hyperextension is not only contraindicated but is considered illogical and futile.

First Aid.—It is primarily because of the impossibility of diagnosing the dangerous type from the simple uncomplicated type when a case is first seen that special instructions for the handling of fractures of the spine should begin with the emergency service and specialized care start at the site of the injury. Fig. 302 and Fig. 303 depict the dangerous type of handling. Fig. 304 shows proper handling. All transfers in the hospital should also be guarded. Correct handling is illustrated in Fig. 305. When the patient is rolled on to the back, a pillow is first placed on the bed or stretcher opposite the fractured vertebra. The patient is rolled from prone to supine with a pillow under the fractured region. Whether for roentgenography or for any other reason, the patient should be rolled like a bundle, keeping the plane of the shoulder blades and the buttocks parallel.

Diagnosis.—The history of the nature of the accident may be helpful in determining the degree of force. Extreme hyperflexions result from collisions at high velocity, falls from a height, mine cave-ins or the falling of heavy objects on the shoulders or falls from a height in which the patient strikes foot first fracturing one or both os calces.

Pain, shock, ileus, bladder disturbance, internal organ rupture and associated fractures obviously are more likely in these cases. The treatment of such complications may for the moment outrate in importance the diagnostic study of the spinal lesion. As soon, however, as appropriate measures have been outlined, a preliminary survey x-ray examination is in order. The anteroposterior film will show very little of significance unless there is an element

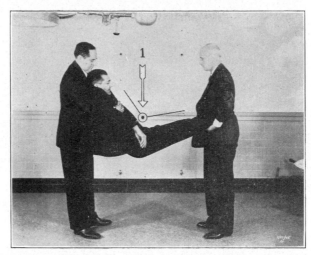

Fig. 302.—Damaging types of carry. Opens dislocations, increases compression fractures. (Courtesy Dr. Arthur G. Davis.)

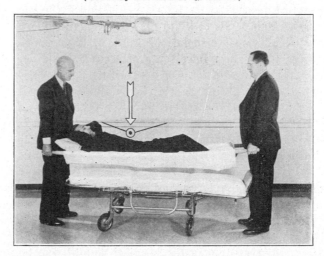

Fig. 303.—Damaging first aid. *1,* Ordinary attitude in recumbency increases angulation. (Courtesy Dr. Arthur G. Davis.)

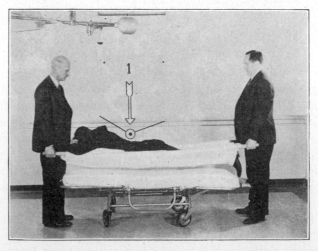

Fig. 304.—Correct first aid in prone position. *1,* Uses anterior longitudinal ligament as check strap. Actually tends to reduce compressions by tensing anterior ligament. (Courtesy Dr. Arthur G. Davis.)

of twist entering the mechanics of the injury. In the lateral view besides noting the immediately obvious compression, comparison of the posterior borders of the bodies is the best criterion to show the degree of dislocation, encroachment on the spinal canal and jackknifing. Further x-ray analyses are contained under the different following subheadings.

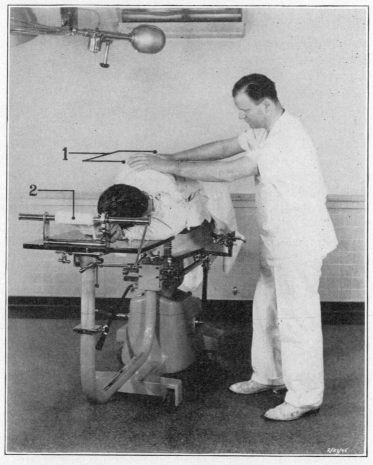

Fig. 305.—Method of hospital handling "rolling the bundle." *1*, Plane of shoulders and pelvis the same; *2*, adjustable hammock. (Courtesy Dr. Arthur G. Davis and American Sterilizer Co.)

Jumped Process Complex.—This type fracture dislocation represents a radical departure from the usual, both in diagnosis and treatment. It is thought that the mechanics producing this rarely occurring clinical entity represents a spiral twist of the torso along with the usual flexion "whiplash" effect. Figs. 306, 307, and 308 show the nature of the roentgenographic findings in such cases. A study of the anatomical specimen shown in Fig. 309 helps more clearly to visualize the actual status of the posterior arch. In approaching the diagnosis in any case of thoracolumbar fracture, the clinician should always have in mind the necessity of diagnosing by inference from observations made in the anteroposterior and lateral planes. With this approach in mind, certain points become immediately obvious. The correlation of a number of these points frequently will enable the surgeon to decide whether to employ manipulation or open operation. By observing all roentgenograms of spinal injuries in this light, the surgeon will safeguard himself against disasters owing to forceful manipulation. The use of hyperextension when hyperextension is not only positively contraindicated but also is positively illogical and futile will be avoided. On the other hand, the surgeon must inevitably arrive at the conclusion that open reduction with the possibility of fusion is the only logical indication. Fig. 308 shows an anteroposterior and a lateral roentgenogram made in the case of a fracture dislocation of the third lumbar vertebra. Neurological signs were normal. The following findings were noted in the anteroposterior projection:

1. Lateral angulation with its apex at the third interspace.

2. A wide interval between the spinous processes of the third and fourth lumbar vertebrae.

3. A rotation of the entire upper section of the spine as indicated by the defective alignment of the spinous processes of the upper section of the spine with those of the lower section.

4. An unequal compression of the two halves of the body of the vertebra. The patient was a slender boy; in a corpulent person such details would be still further obscured.

A lateral roentgenogram revealed the following additional findings:

1. Gross enlargement of the intervertebral foramen.

2. The appearance of one articular process being impaled on the one below.

3. The two different levels appearing in the centrum.

Wherever this apparently double shadow of the vertebral body appears, the dislocation of one articular process must be anticipated as the most logical cause of such asymmetrical compression.

An analysis of the anatomical specimen depicted in Fig. 309 shows why the angulation, rotation and disalignment of the spinous processes with large interspinous space all combine to make certain the diagnosis of a "jumped" articular process and demonstrates conclusively the impossibility and the illogic of attempting reduction of such a dislocation by manipulation. In the light of this analysis and Davis states that in view of the fact that eleven proved cases of this kind seen by him are a matter of record, it is clear that such cases for the most part in the past have eluded diagnosis. Since the means of identifying this type fracture dislocation has been established, a review of cases treated prior to this time indicates that some of them underwent spontaneous fusion with deformed and somewhat disabled spines. Some were relatively pain free on account of the fusion, others were fused and attained comfortable backs in spite of the deformity, others continued with permanently disabled backs due to painful radiation from the deformed area.

Hyperextension Fractures With Elements of Dislocation.—This type constitutes another outstanding exception to the rule of hyperextension reductions. Unusual conditions are required to disrupt the spinal column with this kind of force. Violence of this kind occasionally happens. Falling backward from a height, striking a projecting object directly against the back is an example. In this case the mechanics of injury are directly opposite from the usual hyperflexion "whiplash," the "whiplash" being in the opposite direction. In this case the upper and lower sections of the torso plus the gravitational velocity involved in falling objects combines to produce a fracture dislocation of the avulsion type. The hinge of movement in this case is the tip of the spinous process. This unusual conjuncture of mechanics has occurred, resulting in a transverse rupture of the anterior longitudinal ligament. The check strap effect of the ligament therefore is lost. Hyperextension obviously is not only ineffective but positively dangerous. The diagnosis of such hyperextension fractures may be immediately apparent from the lateral projection in which an open space appears between the upper and lower fragments of the

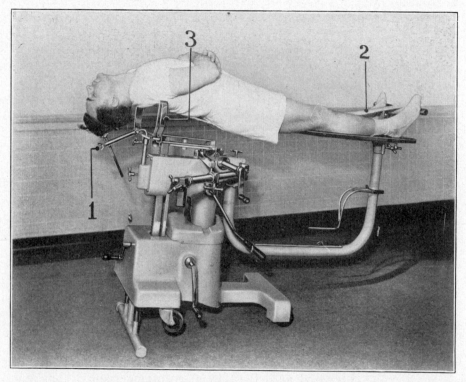

Fig. 306.—Setup for high thoracic and cervical cases. *1*, Adjustable headrest; *2*, adjustable hammock; *3*, handle of withdrawable crossbar. (Courtesy Dr. Arthur G. Davis and American Sterilizer Co.)

centrum and the vertical height of the body is *increased*. This appearance should give the surgeon pause and from this point on extreme caution must be brought to bear for fear of dire and immediate results of ill-advised treatment. Hyperextension in such cases may cause immediate paralysis. In this case the spontaneous recoil must also be allowed for. Such recoil obviously would be in flexion. The flexion in this case may serve to partially or completely reduce the avulsed centrum. In this case posterior projection of the upper posterior angle of the body into the spinal canal furnishes another mark of identification of this type. In this case, however, conclusive differentiation is impossible. Evidence of a contusion over a spinous process also will apprise the surgeon of the role of hyperextension in the causation of the injury. W. A. Rogers also speaks of involvement of the posterior vertical diameter in such cases and that this also constitutes another contraindication to hyperextension. Fortunately the chance of encountering a hyperextension fracture is remote. Head-on collisions, falls from a height, cave-ins, falling objects; all involve a hyperflexion since most attitudes at rest or at work finds the torso already in a flexed attitude. The chance, therefore, of encountering a hyperextension fracture is indeed remote.

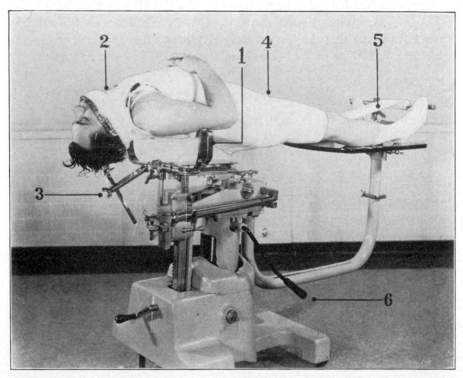

Fig. 307.—Minerva jacket application. *1*, Handle of withdrawable crossbar; *2*, note deep grooving beneath mandible; *3*, adjustable headrest; *4*, lower edge of jacket; *5*, adjustable hammock. (Courtesy Dr. Arthur G. Davis and American Sterilizer Co.)

The Avulsion Type.—This type is easily recognized if the avulsion persists and remains unaltered until the time of roentgenography. The appearance of increased anterior vertical height with an open space between the fragments and, in some cases, actual avulsion forward of the main fragments of the body, obviously implies that the anterior longitudinal ligament has undergone horizontal rupture. Such hyperextension avulsions usually involve a horizontal fracture line at the mid most portion of the anterior cortex where both anterior longitudinal ligament and cortex are weakest. Fortunately, such cases also are extremely rare and are easy to identify in the lateral projection. in such cases, however, it must be realized that the usual sheet anchor of the anterior longitudinal check strap has been lost and one has to depend in this case upon the intact ligaments of the posterior arch.

Treatment of Fracture Dislocations Without Paralysis.—From the above descriptions of unusual clinical types, it will be seen that the most important element in designing treatment is a careful differential diagnosis, depending

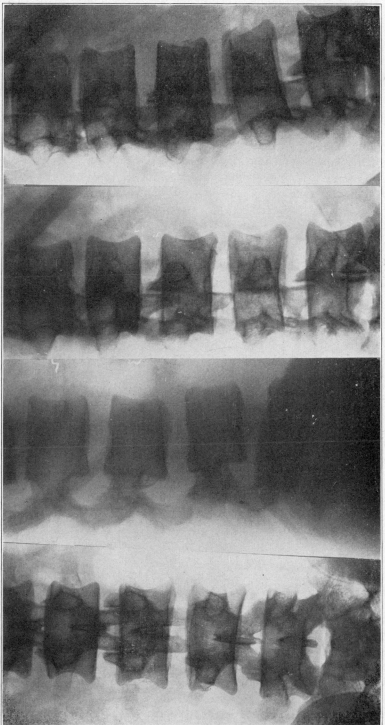

Fig. 308.—Jumped process complex, third on fourth lumbar. Bilateral dislocation. Asymmetrical compression. Irreducible by hyperextension. No paralysis. Operative reduction refused. Outcome unknown. (Courtesy Dr. Arthur G. Davis.)

primarily upon carefully detailed roentgenography frequently involving oblique views and upon scanning the x-ray films with a foreknowledge sufficient to forearm against disaster. Treatment must be highly individualized if the differential diagnosis eliminates the three special types just described and one has to deal with a simple fracture dislocation without paralysis. Hyperextension in the prone position, using foot suspension, seems by far the safest. If the formula outlined for compression fractures under the heading, "Foot Suspension," is elected, the element of horizontal traction contained in the 45 degree pull tends to safeguard all elements involved. The foot suspension is simply done more guardedly. If the prominence (kyphos) is carefully watched during the suspension and the degree of purely gravity suspension limited to the point where the deformity disappears and normal contours are restored and a three-point pressure jacket immediately applied, most cases will show a surprisingly normal appearance on the following day. The steps in the convalescence need not vary from those outlined for simple uncomplicated compression fractures.

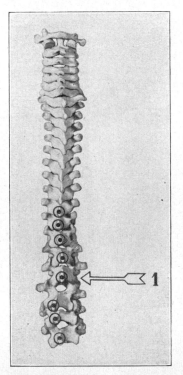

Fig. 309.—Demonstration of factors entering into diagnosis of jumped process complex. Note (1) lateral tilting of second; (2) different alignments of upper and lower series of spinous processes; (3) lateral angulation of two spinal segments; (4) rotation localized. (Courtesy Dr. Arthur G. Davis.)

Treatment of "Jumped Process Complex."—The patient is placed prone on an operating table which breaks in the middle. The posterior arch at the point of kyphos is exposed by the usual subperiosteal method as in fusion. The laminae and articular processes are exposed in detail. One articular process will then be found to be mounted in front of its subjacent partner. Evidence of fracture of the articular processes must be sought for. Ordinarily, however, the opposite joint will be found luxated but not completely dislocated. Provided the case is being operated upon within a few weeks of injury, the table is then broken so as to induce the necessary flexion to disengage the jumped processes. A bone forceps then grasps the spinous process of the dislocated vertebra or a blunt elevator may be used to pry the process into proper position. When the process has been cleared by thus eliminating the factor of rotation, the table is straightened. The articular processes will then be seen to engage in normal relationship.

At this point it will be remembered that there exists the factor of compression of the body. Therefore, with the operative wound still open, the patient is hyperextended by foot suspension and a lateral roentgenogram is taken to show the degree of vertical restoration of the body. If this shows unsatisfactory reduction, a fusion may be immediately considered and executed according to the technic previously described. In case the articular processes have been fractured, fusion ordinarily restricted to the two vertebrae involved should be done with or without the accompaniment of hyperextension as indicated.

Most of the cases encountered by Davis have been seen so long after the injury that the operative treatment just outlined could not be considered. When callus formation has occurred in a deformed and wedged centrum, it has been found by actual experience that this prohibits the possibility of reducing the dislocation factor. Such unreduced cases may or may not have painful symptoms. If such painful symptoms persist, a simple fusion of the area should be done.

Treatment of Hyperextension Fractures.—When from the history and the nature of the accident or by x-ray or other diagnostic measure such hyperextension fractures are identified, the first precaution is to avoid completely any attempt at hyperextension. It will be remembered that the posterior ligamentous investiture of the area is probably intact so that if the patient is placed either supine or prone upon the canvas sling and a three-point plaster jacket is applied, such cases ordinarily promise to go throughout the usual convalescence without incident. Check x-rays taken with the Bucky diaphragm the next day after the plaster is dry will help to determine whether anything more needs to be done or whether immediate fusion should be considered. Prediction at this point as to the nature of the end result is quite impossible. A few of such cases that have simply been jacketed have returned to their former occupation with relatively symptomless spines. Other cases having gone through the typical three or four months of convalescence have demonstrated that a return to ordinary work is impossible because of painful disability with the result that a fusion is required and another three months of convalescence is involved. Davis no longer hesitates to do an *initial* fusion in such questionable cases combined with a reasonable correction of gross deformity especially when he anticipates the probability of the eventual necessity of a fusion. The disuse atrophy and prolonged hospitalization involved in the ultraconservative approach seems, in view of the satisfactory end result experienced in fusions involving only the two involved vertebrae, to decide the question in favor of immediate fusion in questionable cases.

Avulsion Type of Fracture Dislocations.—Treatment in this type case should be largely concerned with the avoidance of catastrophe through hyperextension of any kind. The patient is placed supine on a canvas sling, the patient is asked to rock the pelvis forward and flex both thighs, the lumbar spine is thus flattened. Without any further ado a three-point pressure jacket is applied and the convalescence is conducted as outlined for simple uncomplicated compression fractures. The sheet anchor to all manipulative procedures is destroyed. Horizontal rupture of the anterior longitudinal ligament is proved. Again reasoning by inference decides that the posterior arch ligaments are probably intact. The defect in the centrum will probably fill in. The factors surrounding prognosis will decide the question one way or another as to further measures at the time in a similar manner as outlined under the heading of "Hyperextension Fractures," just cited.

POSTERIOR DISLOCATION OF LUMBAR VERTEBRAE

Occasionally as the result of direct hyperextension traumata of the low back, a posterior dislocation of the fourth or fifth lumbar vertebrae occurs and it is conceivable that they may occur higher up the lumbar area. Interpretation of the x-ray film must be especially guarded. It is well to remember that there is no standard anatomy in this lumbo-sacral area. If it is suspected from the first lateral roentgenogram that the disalignment at this point is sufficient to justify the diagnosis of posterior dislocation, a second lateral film should be taken with a cone in order to verify that the suspected dislocation actually exists. Special precaution should be taken to see that the plane of the pelvis is perpendicular to the plate, since small degrees of rotation induce artifacts. Oblique films should also be taken to show discrepancies in the intervertebral foramen, since if the dislocation actually exists, disruption of the posterior spinal joints or fracture at this point must be suspected.

Treatment

If such cases do not respond to conservative treatment such as hyperextension and the three-point pressure jacket or brace wearing, fusions are usually necessary and just as in the case of spondylolisthesis, the fusion ordinarily eliminates all painful disability and yields a quite limber spine with possibly some restriction of forward bending.

INJURIES OF THE SPINAL CORD AND NERVE ROOTS ASSOCIATED WITH INJURIES OF THE SPINE

As was stated above, spinal injuries present two distinct problems: (1) the injury to the vertebral column and (2) the injury to the spinal cord and nerve roots. We believe that the subject is simplified by considering these two problems separately. In the preceding pages we have discussed the diagnosis and treatment of the compression fractures of the vertebral column. This section will include the diagnosis and treatment of the injuries of the spinal cord and nerve roots.

Occurrence and Mechanism of Spinal Cord Injuries

The spinal cord is so well protected by its fluid bed and covering membranes and fits so loosely in its bony canal that in the majority of fractures and dislocations of the vertebra it escapes injury. However, in severe crush fractures or fracture dislocations, or dislocations or fractures of the laminae, the spinal cord is frequently crushed or lacerated and may be completely severed.

The most frequent mechanism is one in which with a fracture dislocation a vertebra is displaced forward upon the one below it and the spinal cord is crushed between the posterior border of the body of the inferior vertebra and the posterior arch of the one above. Occasionally the displacement is lateral and the same mechanism acts in the lateral plane. It is to be noted that the displacement may be temporary and that after crushing the cord the vertebra may snap back into approximately its normal position, so that the x-ray may reveal no apparent cause for the extensive cord lesion. Occasionally the cord may be stretched tightly over the kyphos or it may be compressed or penetrated by fragments of the body or posterior arch of the fractured vertebra.

Hemorrhage.—In addition to actual mechanical damage by displaced bone the cord may be injured by hemorrhage. All fractures are accompanied by hemorrhage and in fractures of the spine this hemorrhage may be extradural, subarachnoid, or intramedullary. Very rarely extradural hemorrhage may cause pressure on the cord from a large localized hematoma. Due to the large size of the subarachnoid space hemorrhage here practically never causes pressure on the cord as the blood usually settles below the level of the cord. Here the contracting clot occasionally irritates the cauda equina and symptoms of root pressure may develop as a late complication.

Intramedullary hemorrhage or hematomyelia is bleeding into the substance of the cord; this is always accompanied by injury to the adjacent nerve cells and fibers. The gray matter is much less resistant to damage by hemorrhage than the white and consequently suffers more. The symptoms vary with the location and extent of the bleeding and this varies from microscopic extravasations to relatively large hemorrhages involving several segments, or multiple hemorrhagic areas may be present. The symptoms may resemble those of syringomyelia and in the cervical region may result in diaphragmatic paralysis while hemorrhage in the lumbar enlargement may result in paralysis of the bladder and rectum.

Contusion and Edema of the Cord.—"Contusion of the cord is a crushing without physical solution of continuity" (Fraser). The experimental work of Allen has shown that the contusion is followed by edema of the substance of the cord and that this edema appears early and if it is not relieved it may lead to secondary softening and permanent loss of function, while if it is relieved by making a longitudinal incision in the cord within six hours after the injury, much of the permanent paralysis may be prevented.

It is to be noted that intramedullary hemorrhage (hematomyelia) and contusion of the cord with edema may occur in spinal injuries in which no fracture or dislocation can be demonstrated.

Diagnosis of Injuries of the Spinal Cord and Nerve Roots

From the practical point of view, what the surgeon wants to know is whether or not a cord injury is present and, if it is present, whether or not the lesion is a complete transverse lesion or a partial lesion, and in either instance it is important to know whether or not there is pressure on the cord. A careful neurologic examination will usually enable the surgeon to determine the level of the lesion from the extent of the motor and sensory paralysis, it being recalled as was pointed out in the section on Anatomy that the lesion in the cord is higher than the level of the sensory changes would indicate.

If there is marked motor and sensory paralysis it is, of course, obvious that there is a cord lesion. Minor lesions, however, may escape notice; consequently, when a patient with a fractured spine is first seen, the knee jerks, plantar reflexes, ankle jerks and abdominal reflexes should be tested. The patient should be asked to move the legs and arms in various directions in order to determine whether or not there is motor paralysis. Then a rough sensory examination to pin prick and deep pressure should be made. This should include the perineal region. If there are no abnormalities noted, there is in all probability no cord lesion. If there is motor paralysis or loss of sensation there is a lesion of the cord or of the nerve roots. The location of the fracture as determined by physical examination and x-ray and the location of the sensory level and motor paralysis as determined by a more careful neurologic examination will enable the surgeon to roughly estimate the extent of the paralysis.

Brown-Séquard's syndrome should be mentioned although it rarely occurs in fractures. It is a spastic paralysis on the side of the lesion in the cord, below the lesion, with exaggeration of the tendon reflexes and often hyperesthesia, while on the opposite side there is loss of touch, pain and temperature sense below the lesion. The typical Brown-Séquard's syndrome is due to a hemisection of the cord. Very rarely an atypical syndrome of this type may exist in unilateral injury to the cord.

Total Transverse Lesions of the Cord.—In the case of a total transverse lesion there is complete symmetrical motor and sensory paralysis below the level of the lesion. The paralysis is flaccid in type and the tendon reflexes are lost. The upper limit of the paralysis is quite sharply defined and is bordered by a narrow zone of hyperesthesia, the result of irritation of the posterior roots at the level of the fracture. There may be dilatation of the superficial blood vessels in the paralyzed parts with an increased temperature. There is also loss of control of the rectum and bladder with a tendency to priapism.

It is important to remember that the symptoms of a total transverse lesion of the cord, while usually due to a complete anatomic section, may be due to an incomplete anatomic lesion with physiologic block of the intact fibers, and that partial recovery may follow relief of pressure on the cord and immobilization. Furthermore, it is not possible by physical examination to differentiate the anatomic from the physiologic block. Consequently, these cases should be treated as though the lesion were physiologic until it has been proved otherwise.

Bladder and Rectal Disturbances.—Bladder and rectal disturbances not only occur in all complete cord lesions, but also occur in incomplete lesions in which the centers controlling the bladder and rectum are involved. These centers lie in the third and fourth sacral segments which are situated at the level of the first and second lumbar vertebrae. Consequently in fractures involving the first and second lumbar vertebra or in fractures below this in which the third and fourth sacral nerve roots are injured, there may be relaxation of the sphincters and incontinence of urine and feces. In lesions situated above these centers, if the afferent fibers in the posterior column or efferent fibers in the lateral columns are involved there is retention of urine and constipation.

Lesions of the Cauda Equina and of the Nerve Roots.—The nerve roots emerging at the level of the fracture may be involved in fractures at any level while in fractures below the second lumbar vertebra the cord is not affected as it normally ends here, but the lumbar and sacral nerve roots comprising the cauda equina may be injured either in the canal or at their points of exit. In these lesions of the cauda equina the lower the lesion the fewer the nerve roots that can be injured. These lesions of the nerve roots and of the cauda take the form of a peripheral nerve injury in the distribution of the affected root or roots with a complete severance. There is flaccid paralysis of the muscles, loss of reflexes, complete sensory paralysis and incontinence of the rectum and bladder. These lesions are not necessarily symmetrical as it is not necessary that both roots at a given level be involved.

In addition to the paralysis these lesions of nerve roots and of the cauda are frequently accompanied by severe lancinating pains radiating along the course of the involved nerve roots. These pains are due to irritation or contusion without complete severance of the given nerve roots.

Treatment of Fractures of the Spine With Paralysis

In these patients time is very important because the cord lesion may be due to pressure or edema and, as stated above, the spinal medulla does not tolerate long-continued pressure and a lesion which is physiologic may become anatomical after six hours.

Consequently, it is imperative that the pressure, if present, be reduced immediately. We believe that the most effective manner of relieving pressure and widening the spinal canal is to institute hyperextension at the site of the lesion. This may be combined with traction. It may be done by placing the patient on his back over pillows or a blanket roll or prone between similar support. It can be more effectively done by the gravity suspension method of Davis and a plaster cast applied immediately.

With severe paralysis the lesion of the cord is the most important factor in the treatment and should be treated first. The fracture of the spine and other fractures or lesions are relatively unimportant and can be treated later if the patient survives. There is little profit in surviving with a total transverse lesion of the cord.

As stated, hyperextension should be applied as an emergency procedure even before x-ray films and and a Queckenstedt test are made. The patient

should be handled very gently, as described under treatment of fracture dislocations of the spine.

X-ray pictures are then made and examined carefully for evidence of displacement of the lamina inward with pressure on the cord or of irregularities in
the line of the posterior margins of the bodies of the vertebrae. If the x-ray
films indicate a possibility of improving the condition of the spinal cord by
more hyperextension or by laminectomy and removal of displaced fragments
which are causing pressure on the cord, the indicated procedure is instituted
without delay.

The next procedure is a Queckenstedt test to determine by a lumbar puncture and a manometric reading whether or not there is a spinal block. If this
has been done before hyperextension was instituted it should be repeated, as
the hyperextension may have relieved the block.

Indications for Laminectomy in Injuries of the Spine

In a severely injured patient with fracture of the spine and evidence of
injury to the spinal cord, it is usually stated that complete motor and sensory
paralysis and abolition of all reflexes below the level of the lesion are evidences of a complete transverse section of the cord. In recent years, however, it has been shown that occasionally complete physiologic block of the
spinal cord may exist without anatomic block being present. This fact, together with the possibility that in cases which do not give evidence of complete block there may be pressure on the cord with the possibility of relieving
this pressure by operation and thus eliminating some of the paralysis, has led
many surgeons to become very radical in their treatment of these cases and
to operate on a great many people without in any way benefiting the patient.
This radical stand is encouraged, of course, by the patient and the patient's
family who are anxious that everything possible be done to save the patient
and to prevent permanent paralysis.

On the other hand, an equal number of conservative surgeons, after
analyzing the results obtained by laminectomy in these cases, have concluded
that it is rare indeed that laminectomy has any definite influence on the ultimate result, and they have almost entirely abandoned the operation in fractures of the spine, because it is a serious operation if performed on a patient
who is already seriously injured, and in addition to the general shock and
depression it results in further weakening the already broken back.

It has been shown that by a neurologic examination it is impossible to
determine whether or not the paralysis following a spine fracture is anatomic
or physiologic. Consequently a neurologic diagnosis of a complete transverse
lesion is not a contraindication to laminectomy. However, it is important for
the surgeon confronted with such a case to remember that laminectomy can
perform only one function and that is to relieve pressure on the spinal cord.
Whatever anatomic damage is present is permanent and laminectomy has no
effect on any anatomic lesion in the cord.

Pressure on the cord may be due to displacement of the vertebra with
narrowing of the vertebral canal, to pressure on, or penetration of, the cord by

displaced fragments of bone, to the accumulation of blood in the subdural or subarachnoid space, or to edema of or bleeding in the cord itself as a result of the injury.

The x-ray is, as a rule, of relatively little benefit in determining whether or not pressure is exerted upon the cord, because many cases are on record in which, in spite of considerable displacement, there was no marked cord damage and other cases are recorded in which, with no evidence of displacement and no evidence of narrowing of the intervertebral canal, there was a complete transverse lesion of the cord. This is frequently due to the fact that in the case of a fracture dislocation the vertebrae tend to spring back into place or into approximately their normal positions before the x-ray picture is taken. Consequently the temporary displacement is not shown. However, the x-ray may reveal a fracture of the posterior arch with displacement of a fragment into the spinal canal and this justifies immediate laminectomy.

During recent years the work of Coleman and Dowman have greatly simplified this difficult question as to whether or not operation is indicated. Recognizing the fact that the only possible benefit to be obtained from the operation is relief of pressure on the cord, these authors have used the Queckenstedt test in all spinal cord injuries and by means of this relatively simple procedure have been able to determine definitely whether or not pressure is present. The test is performed as follows:

Technic of the Queckenstedt Test.—With the patient lying upon the side, a lumbar puncture is performed in the ordinary way, care being taken to use sufficient novocaine at the site of the lumbar puncture to secure complete anesthesia of this area and prevent pain with resultant coughing or straining on the part of the patient.

After the lumbar puncture needle has been introduced an ordinary water manometer which, in its simpler form is a glass tube filled with water, is connected with the lumbar puncture needle and the level to which the fluid rises in the manometer is noted. Then after a stationary level has been reached, the internal jugular veins on both sides are compressed by pressure with the thumbs and fingers in the neck anterior to the sternomastoid muscle at the level of the angle of the jaw. If there is no pressure on the spinal cord and the subarachnoid space is free, there is a prompt rise of the fluid in the manometer and when the pressure on the jugular is released there is a prompt fall of the fluid to the normal level.

In case of a complete block of the subarachnoid space, there is no rise in the fluid in the manometer or a very slow, step-like, slight rise, and this higher level is maintained after the pressure is released. With a partial block there is a rather slow, step-like fall when the pressure is released, and the fluid does not fall quite to its former level. This change in the fluid level in the manometer is due to the fact that the intracranial pressure is increased by compressing the jugular veins, and this increase in intracranial pressure is transmitted to the subarachnoid fluid below the level of the lesion if the canal is open, and is not transmitted if the canal is occluded.

In performing the Queckenstedt test there are certain precautions which must be taken in interpreting this test, since any increase in intrathoracic or intraabdominal pressure may cause congestion in the cord below the block and result in an increase in intraspinal pressure even with a complete block of the subarachnoid space. Consequently, care must be taken that the patient does not cough or strain while the actual test is being made.

Coleman points out that occasionally there is a rise in the fluid level in the tube when the fingers are placed upon the neck preliminary to making pressure upon the jugular veins. This is due to a reflex straining of the patient at this time. It is also on this account that Dowman emphasized the fact that the lumbar puncture should be practically painless. Another point to be taken into consideration is that if only a few drops of fluid are obtained when the needle is introduced a block is probably present.

Delayed Cord Compression.—In addition to the cases which show compression of the cord at the time of admission and in which early operation is indicated, there are certain cases in which a Queckenstedt taken soon after the injury reveals no blocking of the subdural space, but in which, if this test be repeated twelve or twenty-four hours later, a gradually increasing occlusion of the space may be detected.

These are cases which enter the hospital with neurologic evidence of only a partial lesion of the cord and in which pain continues or increases, or in which a neurologic examination made twelve or fifteen hours later reveals an increase in the motor and sensory paralysis. In such cases the Queckenstedt test should be repeated at least every twelve hours, and if the later tests show evidence of a partial or complete block, laminectomy should be resorted to. The pressure on the cord may be due to hemorrhage outside the dura or into the cord or to progressive edema of the cord.

The question of edema of the cord without narrowing of the canal and without direct pressure on the cord is one of the most difficult problems presented by these cases. Allen has shown experimentally that with a uniform traumatism of the cord produced by dropping a weight upon it after the canal has been opened a complete and permanent paralysis may be produced and that this paralysis is probably the result of edema in the cord itself because if the dura be split and a longitudinal incision be made into the cord immediately after the compression, the animal will recover. He has further shown that this edema reaches its height in about four hours and that if the release of the pressure is delayed longer than six hours after the injury the operation does little or no good. For this reason surgery, if it is to be of benefit in cases due to edema, must be done immediately; otherwise it cannot prevent permanent paralysis.

It is conceivable that in very rare cases of this type the Queckenstedt test may be misleading. The same is true of very rare cases in which a small splinter of bone has punctured the dura and has lacerated or compressed the cord without causing complete block. Such spicules might not be visible in the x-ray and their removal might benefit the patient. However, we believe that these cases are so rare that they may be ignored and think that the safest procedure at the present time is for the surgeon to be guided by the Queckenstedt test and to operate when pressure is present and to refrain from operating when the Queckenstedt shows no evidence of pressure, regardless of the neurologic findings.

Technic of Laminectomy.—Preparatory for laminectomy the patient is placed prone upon the operating table, care being taken in compression fractures and fracture dislocations which have been reduced by manipulation not to move the patient any more than necessary. Sandbags are placed under his shoulders in order to permit free expansion of the chest. The operation can be done under local anesthesia. One of us (H. E. C.) uses local infiltration supplemented by sodium pentothal.

Especial care should be taken to make the center of the incision over the site of the fracture. This having been localized by the x-ray, the skin is prepared and an incision about seven inches long is made directly over the spinous processes, and is carried down to them, exposing six or seven spinous processes. When the superficial bleeding has been stopped, skin towels are adjusted to the edges of the wound and with a heavy knife and osteotome the fascia is dissected from the tips of the spinous processes beginning at the top of the wound and freeing one side of each process down the length of the wound and packing gauze sponges in to stop the bleeding. Then the other side is freed and packed. The periosteum and muscles are gradually freed from the spinous processes and laminae and pushed laterally, this part of the operation being done in stages, no attempt being made to free one entire process and lamina at one time. The subperiosteal dissection is carried down a short distance on the spinous process and then this portion of the wound is packed with gauze and the next spinous process is freed and so on, working down one side of the wound and then the other until the desired number of spinous processes and laminae are exposed.

The interspinous ligaments between the spines to be removed are then cut with a knife, and the spinous processes are excised with sharp bone-cutting forceps. After the spines have been removed, the laminae are removed piecemeal with rongeur forceps. Great care is taken in removing the laminae not to let the blade of the forceps slip into the spinal canal and further traumatize the cord.

When sufficient laminae have been removed to expose the traumatized area, the subsequent steps of the operation will depend upon whether the lesion is extra- or intradural. Any pieces of bone pressing upon the cord should, of course, be removed. The same is true of any extradural hematoma.

In many cases the laminectomy itself will have accomplished relief of pressure on the cord. On the other hand, if laminectomy is performed the dura should be opened by a longitudinal incision and the cord inspected. Any intradural clots should be removed and if the cord is tense and swollen the operation of cordotomy should be performed; that is, a longitudinal incision about an inch long should be made in the midline of the cord. This will permit the escape of fluid which may have accumulated in the cord, and the operation may prevent damage from edema.

The dura should be sutured loosely and the muscles drawn together with deep interrupted sutures of chromic catgut. The fascia should be sutured with interrupted sutures of chromic catgut and the skin closed in the usual way. Dr. Hibbs (personal communication) stated that when a laminectomy is performed for a fracture of the spine as complete a spinal fusion as possible should be performed before closing the wound. After the laminectomy the patient should be treated for the fracture as described above just as though no operation had been performed.

Care of Patients With Paralysis

The care of patients with paralysis may be considered under the following headings:

1. Correction of the deformity.
2. Immobilization of the fracture.
3. Prevention of bed sores.
4. General nutrition.
5. Care of the bladder and rectum.
6. Prevention of deformities.

Correction of the Deformity.—Since patients with paralysis do not stand immobilization in hyperextension on a frame of any sort, it is wise to correct the deformity immediately by hyperextension either by the Davis method or by traction and hyperextension with assistants.

Immobilization of the Fracture.—In case of paralysis patients are best immobilized in a hyperextension plaster jacket or a large plaster-of-Paris shell, especial care being taken to make the inside of the shell smooth and have it extend, as a rule, down to the groins. In this way the body weight is distributed over a wide area and localized pressure is prevented. The anterior shell should be made immediately and the patient should be turned on the abdomen and lie in the anterior shell approximately half of the time, beginning as soon as the shell is dry. If the Davis method of correction is used, a heavy plaster jacket reinforced by longitudinal strips may be applied while the patient is on the hammock and this can be bivalved in order to make the plaster shells. Or the two halves of the shell may be made separately with the patient lying prone in hyperextension and then the anterior shell is made on the patient while he is lying in the posterior shell.

Prevention of Bed Sores.—During the first few weeks after the cord lesion, the vasomotor control of the superficial vessels is lost as well as the sensation below the lesion, and the skin is very prone to develop pressure sores from abnormal or prolonged pressure at any one point. The nurse should turn the patient and inspect the skin carefully twice daily for beginning pressure sores. These are more easily prevented than cured and the premonitory symptoms of a pressure sore can be recognized as an area of redness. Such areas, when they appear, should be relieved of pressure either by cutting out the shell or having the patient turned on the other side.

The skin should be kept dry and warm, but bakes should not be used because the skin is very easily burned, nor should hot water bags be applied to any part of these patients as they may be seriously burned without knowing it. It is not advisable to apply any form of ointment to the skin, but it should be rubbed gently with alcohol twice daily and then powdered.

If bed sores are already present, or if they appear in spite of precautions, they must be treated and if possible permitted to heal. The essentials to be observed in healing a pressure sore are to relieve the area from pressure, remove the necrotic tissue, and protect the skin edges. Pressure is best relieved by a well-fitting plaster shell. The necrotic tissue may be removed by means of scissors and the sore packed with gauze saturated with Dakin's solution which should be changed about every four hours. When the necrotic material has separated and been removed, the area should be protected by cross strapping of adhesive just as is used in the treatment of burns. The adhesive keeps the area moist and protects the skin edges. This should be changed about every twenty-four hours. In most instances pressure sores will heal eventually if the patient survives and the above regime is carried out.

General Nutrition.—The patient should, if possible, be placed in cheerful surroundings, given a normal diet, and it is helpful if the bed can be moved out on the porch or out of doors during part of the day. Occupational therapy is of use to those patients who can use their hands and may be begun within the first two weeks after the accident. The muscles which are not paralyzed should be exercised daily.

Care of the Bladder and Rectum.—Most of the patients with severe paralysis who are not killed by the original injury and the shock following it, die from either bed sores or infection of the bladder and kidney, and a large percentage develop renal or bladder stones. For this reason many men advise against catheterizing these patients at all and strive for the development of an automatic bladder. The patients who have complete cord lesions have relaxed sphincters and develop the automatic bladder immediately; that is, they continue to dribble urine almost continuously. The patients with partial cord lesions develop distention and are unable to void. Distention is the cause of great pain, and it is impossible in private practice to carry these patients along for the time necessary for the development of an automatic bladder. Consequently our experience is that these patients must be catheterized at least twice a day. Catheterization should be done under the strictest aseptic precautions, and after the bladder has been emptied, it should be washed out with a weak antiseptic solution. Saturated solution of boracic acid or a weak silver nitrate solution is usually used.

Due to the loss of sensory nerve supply to the urinary tract these patients do not tolerate indwelling catheters well, and for this reason many surgeons prefer to perform a suprapubic cystotomy within a few days after the fracture and drain the bladder through this wound.

Since these patients develop constipation or incontinence, the lower bowel should be emptied by a daily enema. If this procedure is carried out, they get along with relatively little trouble.

Prevention of Deformity.—Incomplete cord lesions with spastic paralysis are apt to develop flexion contractures of the knees and hips and equinus deformities of the feet. These contractures can, to a certain extent, be prevented by plaster molds or braces which hold the extremities in the normal position, but if the muscle imbalance is at all pronounced and persists over a long time, deformities usually develop and will demand correction either by tendon lengthening or neurectomies of the stronger muscles.

Prognosis.—In complete transverse lesions the paralysis is permanent and there is no chance of any regeneration taking place. However, it is to be emphasized that it is not always possible to determine whether or not the complete paralysis is due to a physiologic or anatomical lesion, and some of these cases improve later with immobilization. Other things being equal, the lower the lesion the better the prognosis.

If the patients can be prevented from developing severe infections of the genitourinary tract and severe bed sores during the first four weeks after the time of the injury, many of them may live for years and pursue a rather active life, although confined to a bed or a wheel chair, since the skin later on becomes more resistant to pressure and the general condition improves.

Prognostic Value of the Reflexes.—The knee and ankle jerks are usually lost, even in relatively mild lesions, but their early reappearance is regarded as a favorable sign and is often followed by a considerable amount of recovery. The same is true of sphincter control. Its early reappearance points to a relatively mild lesion. The persistence of the plantar reflex or its early reappearance after having been lost, or a change from a flexor to an extensor type of response within the first week, is indicative of an incomplete lesion and of a more favorable prognosis.

It should be pointed out that in flaccid paralysis even with complete transverse lesion of the cord, there may occur a period of reflex activity a few weeks after the injury in which the deep reflexes are present or even exaggerated and in which movement of the limbs may occur as a result of peripheral stimulation. These are reflex movements and are not necessarily signs of recovery. They may be differentiated from the typical reflexes which reappear in incomplete lesions by the fact that these pseudoreflexes tend to spread to the other extremity or even more widely forming a mass reflex and affecting the abdominal wall and causing evacuation of the bladder. After a few months these pseudoreflexes tend to disappear and the patient returns to the original condition of complete paralysis.

Prognosis as to Life.—In the majority of cases with complete transverse lesions the prognosis is bad. In the Burrell series of 244 cases the mortality was 71 per cent, and in Gurdt's 277 cases there was a mortality of 80 per cent. With better after-care this can, of course, be lessened as was shown by the series reported by Wilson and Mixter in which the mortality was approximately 40 per cent. Many of the patients die from shock or other injuries received at the time of the accident. Those who survive the immediate injury, frequently die from infection of the bladder and kidneys or bed sores.

ISOLATED FRACTURES OF THE TRANSVERSE PROCESSES

These fractures were practically never recognized before the advent of the x-ray, but during recent years, since it has been the custom to take x-ray pictures of injured backs, it has been found that they are not infrequent.

Etiology of Isolated Fractures of the Transverse Processes.—Nearly all of the isolated fractures of the transverse processes occur in the lumbar region, but they occasionally occur in the cervical region. For the most part the injury is the result of direct trauma, as a blow or a weight falling upon the lumbar region while the spine is flexed. Very rarely they may be the result of muscular violence as in heavy lifting or straining. It is quite possible that many of the fractures are due to a combination of muscle action and direct trauma. When caused by muscle action, they are largely the result of contraction of the iliopsoas muscle, aided somewhat by the quadratus lumborum. The processes most frequently broken are those of the second, third, and fourth lumbar vertebrae, because these processes are more exposed to injury, since the transverse processes of the first lumbar are protected by the lower ribs and those of the fifth by wings of the ilia. Frequently two or three or more processes are fractured and occasionally the transverse processes on both sides are fractured. (Fig. 310.)

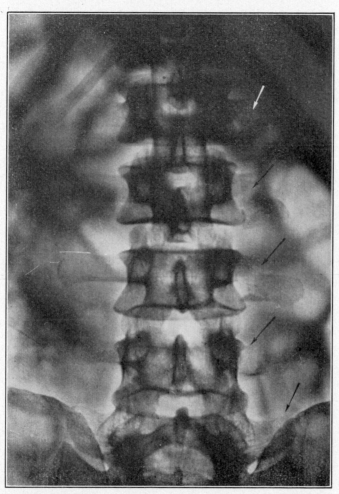

Fig. 310.—Fractures of the transverse processes of all lumbar vertebrae on the right side. Treated with a short plaster jacket. Union did not occur in vertebrae 1, 2, and 3, but the functional result was good.

Diagnosis of Isolated Fractures of the Transverse Processes.—There is a history of direct trauma to the back or of a fall from a height or of a sudden pain in the back during violent muscular exertion followed by pain and disability in the low back.

On physical examination the patient complains of pain in the low back which is localized in the region of the fractured transverse process, but may be widely distributed in the lumbar region, and there is tenderness which is most marked directly over the fracture or fractures. All movements of the back are painful and are limited by muscle spasm. When the patient is lying down, raising the leg on the affected side causes pain, which is especially pronounced if he attempts to flex the thigh against resistance. This is due to the pull on the iliopsoas muscle. Likewise, if the hip is passively hyperextended, pain is produced at the site of the fracture.

All of the above signs and symptoms may be present in an ordinary low back strain. The most important diagnostic point is the presence of acute tenderness over the broken transverse process. It should be pointed out that there may or may not be evidence of damage to the skin and subcutaneous tissues, even when the injury is the result of a direct trauma.

Finally, the diagnosis must be made by the x-ray, taken in the anteroposterior plane; this will show the fracture if it is present. In interpreting an x-ray picture of the transverse processes, it should be remembered that each of these normally has an epiphysis at the end which does not unite until after the twentieth year. Also, that occasionally the transverse processes are asymmetrical and that one of them may point in an abnormal direction. A third factor to be considered is that the first lumbar may present an anomalous rib which resembles a fracture of the transverse process. Finally the shadow of the psoas muscle may cause a line across a transverse process which resembles a fracture.

In a fresh fracture the line of the fracture as seen in the picture is usually irregular, sharply defined, and in many instances there is more or less separation of the loose distal fragment. As a matter of fact this may be displaced several centimeters. The fracture usually occurs about the middle of the shaft of the process.

Treatment of Isolated Fracture of the Transverse Processes

There is no especial reason why these fractures should cause prolonged disability, and the patient should not be told that he has a broken back, but should be told that he has a fracture of a small process of one of the vertebrae and that he will be all right again in a few weeks. This is urged because so many of these cases result in prolonged disability largely as a result of the mental attitude of the patient rather than of the fracture itself.

Many cases have been reported of fracture of the transverse processes in which the patients have continued their active occupations, not knowing they had suffered a fracture until some weeks later. As a rule, however, it is better to treat these patients in bed for the first two weeks, and sometimes longer when multiple fractures are present. During this period of rest in bed if the patient has considerable pain, it can be relieved by strapping with adhesive or by the application of a plaster-of-Paris jacket which is well fitted and extends from the axillae to the pelvis. The jacket should get a firm grip upon the pelvis and the shoulder straps may or may not be included to prevent twisting of the body in the cast. (Fig. 311.)

The cast should be worn for from two to five weeks, depending upon the severity of the fracture and the reaction of the patient. During this time the patient need not remain in bed unless he has considerable pain when sitting or walking. At the end of this time the cast should be removed and the patient may go without support or may wear a wide lumbar belt or corset or a high or low brace, the amount of support being determined by the pain. The surgeon should be cautioned against overtreating these patients; otherwise they get the idea that they are seriously injured and are apprehensive of resuming their normal occupations.

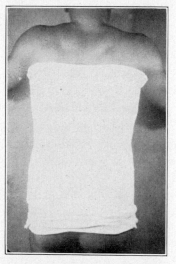

Fig. 311.—Type of short plaster jacket used in the treatment of fractures of the transverse process of the lumbar vertebra.

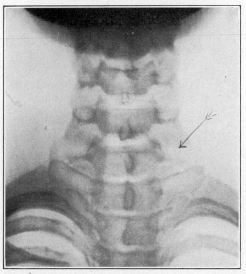

Fig. 312.—Fracture of the transverse process of the seventh cervical vertebra. Treated by immobilization in a Thomas collar with good results.

In fractures of the transverse processes of the cervical region (Fig. 312) sufficient immobilization and support can be obtained by means of a Thomas collar which is made out of pasteboard padded with sheet cotton and tied around the neck with a bandage. This should be worn for about four weeks. At the end of this time it can usually be dispensed with. In certain patients it is necessary to continue this support a few weeks longer.

Prognosis of Isolated Fractures of the Transverse Processes.—Most of these patients should be able to resume their normal occupations in from eight to ten weeks after the injury except in case of multiple fractures with severe contusion of the soft parts or low back strain. In these cases the disability may extend to four months or longer. Union usually occurs in cases with little or relatively slight separation and nonunion usually occurs in cases with wide separation, but we have never seen nonunion result in disability and have never found it necessary to operate for the removal of a transverse process which has failed to unite after a fracture.

ISOLATED FRACTURES OF THE SPINOUS PROCESSES AND LAMINAE

These are relatively rare injuries and are practically always due to direct violence, although occasional cases have been reported as the result of muscular violence. Most of the cases occur in the cervical region and are caused by blows or falls upon the back of the neck. The spinous process may be broken off, usually about the middle of its shaft, or one or both laminae may be fractured. When only one lamina is fractured, there is usually no displacement. When both laminae are broken, the separated portion of the arch of the vertebra may be driven inward and cause pressure on the spinal cord.

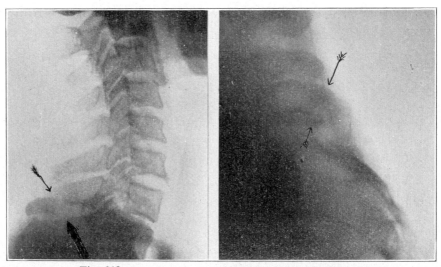

Fig. 313.   Fig. 314.

Fig. 313.—Fracture of the spinous process of the seventh cervical vertebra (shoveler's fracture). Thomas collar for three weeks, local heat. Good results in two months.

Fig. 314.—Fracture of the spinous process of the fifth lumbar vertebra. Treated by rest in bed for eighteen days; then out of bed for few hours each day for one week. Pain and tenderness for two months. No support except adhesive strapping. Good result.

Diagnosis of Isolated Fractures of the Spinous Processes and Laminae.— There is usually a history of direct trauma to the back of the neck followed by pain and disability with limitation of motion in the involved region of the spine. On physical examination there is acute localized tenderness over the fractured spinous processes and muscle spasm in the involved area. It may be possible by palpation to detect abnormal mobility of the spinous processes.

The final diagnosis depends upon the x-ray which, when taken in the lateral plane, will show the fracture (Figs. 313 and 314). As a rule there is little or no displacement as the attached muscles and ligaments tend to prevent displacement or to pull the broken fragment back into position if it is displaced by the fracturing force.

Treatment of Isolated Fractures of the Spinous Processes and Laminae

Just as is the case with fractures of the transverse processes these fractures of the spinous processes and laminae are not, as a rule, serious injuries and should not be overtreated. Since there is little or no displacement, union may be expected either with or without immobilization. However, in most instances it is advisable to immobilize the fractured area either in a plaster-of-Paris jacket or a well-fitting Thomas collar. Rest in bed after the first day or two is not necessary unless there are other injuries or unless the patient is very uncomfortable when up. The Thomas collar is made of pasteboard and padded with sheet cotton and is usually sufficient to keep the patient comfortable; it should be tried first. If this is not adequate, a plaster-of-Paris jacket, which takes its base of support from the pelvis and includes the neck and head, may be used.

The immobilization should be continued for from two to four weeks, depending upon the severity of the lesion and the reaction of the patient. It should be discontinued as soon as the patient is comfortable without it and no disability need be expected. If nonunion occurs and the patient continues to complain of pain and disability, the loose fragment should be excised. This can be done under local anesthesia.

Fractures of the laminae are best treated by rest in bed with or without a plaster jacket or shell, as may be deemed necessary, over a period of about four weeks. At the end of this time the patient is permitted up with a back brace or a jacket or Thomas collar which should be worn from two to four weeks longer.

In fractures of the laminae in which the fragments are displaced in such a manner that they cause pressure on the spinal cord and cause cord symptoms, immediate operation should be performed and the offending bone should be lifted off the cord. As a rule, this is a relatively simple procedure and it will not be found necessary to remove the spinous processes and laminae, although the surgeon should not hesitate to do this if any difficulty is experienced in keeping it away from the cord. After the operation these cases should be treated as described above; that is, immobilized in bed for from four to eight weeks, then got up with support which should be worn from two to four weeks or longer if necessary.

ISOLATED FRACTURES OF THE ARTICULAR FACETS

These are rare injuries which occasionally present in patients who have received a severe low back strain. They are not as a rule diagnosed until the strain has been present for some time and has failed to respond to the usual forms of treatment. Then the fracture of the articular facet may be seen in the anteroposterior x-rays, but if such an injury is suspected, it is best demonstrated by oblique x-rays as Ghormley and Kirklan have shown. The supine patient is rotated 32° to the right to show the right articular facets and 32° to the left to show the left articular facets. The tube is placed directly above the spine. When diagnosed late, these fractures usually demand fusion of the involved joints for permanent relief, but may respond to prolonged immobilization or support and this should be tried first.

RUPTURE AND HERNIATION OF THE INTERVERTEBRAL DISCS (SCHMORL'S NODES)

The extensive pathologic studies of Schmorl have drawn attention to the fact that the thin bony plate which separates the spongy bone of the vertebral body from the nucleus pulposus may give way and semifluid nucleus may

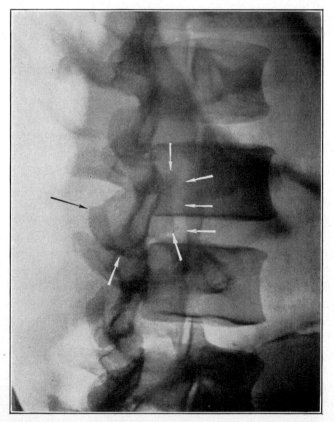

Fig. 315.—Right oblique view of lumbar spine to show fractures of inferior articular facets and pedicle of third lumbar vertebra. Other standard views were negative.

project or herniate into the vertebral body and be visible in the x-ray. Whether or not such lesions have any clinical significance is questionable. It is probable that the herniation into the bone causes no symptoms, but that in certain instances the collapse of the disc may cause irritation and pain sufficient to justify supporting the spine with a brace or corset or postural exercises until the symptoms are relieved.

The work of Barr and Mixter has shown that in the lumbosacral region this lesion is an important cause of low back pain and sciatica. The syndrome is considered at the end of this chapter under low back pain.

INJURIES OF THE CERVICAL SPINE*

The cervical section of the spinal column stands apart in a number of important respects. The cervical vertebrae are broad, shallow, with thick intervertebral discs and possess large range of motion. The functional anatomy as ordinarily described in standard textbooks of anatomy needs to be supplemented by evidence from roentgenograms of the normal to show the nature and range of motion in this area. A study of Figs. 316, 317 and 318 is necessary to arrive at a proper evaluation of the nature of the injury and a differentiation of the normal from the abnormal. In the three attitudes contained in Fig. 316 the fibers of the posterior articulations and the interspinous ligaments are most susceptible to hyperflexions of the "whiplash" type.

It will be remembered that nodding occurs largely at the occipito-atlantoid joint, that rotation occurs largely around the odontoid, or in other words, at the atlanto-axial joint. Other than these two highly specialized vertebrae, however, all of the cervical vertebrae participate in the act of flexion and extension. Two components of movement combine in a rocker motion, one component is between adjacent articular processes, the other between the bodies and involving shifting of the nucleus pulposus. Motion in one component inevitably involves motion in the other. All vertebrae participate in motions of extreme rotation or torsion. Movements of circumduction of the head are thus made possible as effectively as the ball and socket mechanism at the hip. When the accidental force carries the head and neck beyond the normal range, fractures, dislocations, fracture dislocations, luxations and/or intervertebral disc injuries are the result. Which one or combination of two or several of these occurs depends largely upon the degree of movement beyond the normal limit. With the exception of unilateral dislocations, practically all injuries occur as a result of hyperflexion. Starting with the fact that the great majority of injuries of the cervical spine are in the nature of a "whiplash" and accepting the meaning of the term "whiplash" as a hyperflexion followed by spontaneous extensor recoil, the nature of a great variety of injuries of this section of the spinal column becomes understandable. The common automobile head-on collision, the sudden stopping of public vehicles, falls from a height, diving accidents, blows striking the head, sudden throws of the head resulting from slipping or loss of footing; all result in the same mechanics of injury. An analysis of 134 consecutive cases in the author's experience shows the automobile head-on collision to be the most prolific cause. It must be remembered that the velocity of the car is also the velocity of the individual and his parts. Ordinarily the torso and the legs are braced at the moment of impact of the head-on collision. The extreme mobility of the cervical section of the spine permits the weight of the head to continue its forward momentum after the moment of impact. The degree, therefore, of hyperflexion

*With the exception of the section on the manipulative treatment of dislocations of the cervical vertebrae this section was contributed by Dr. Arthur G. Davis.

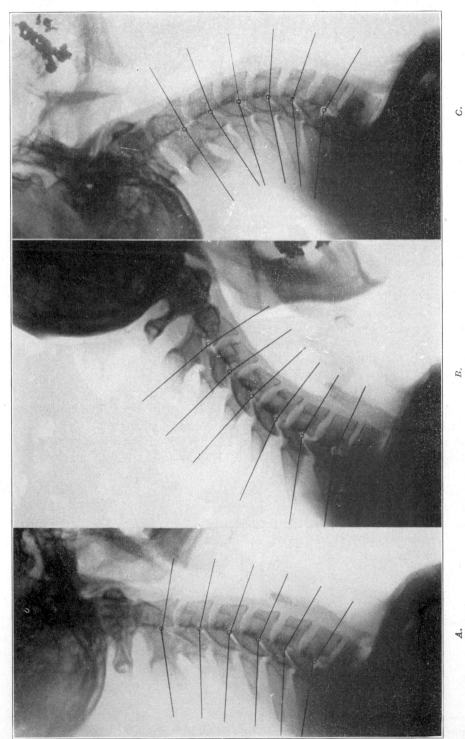

A.

B.

C.

Fig. 316.—Functional anatomy. For this purpose arbitrary points were selected on each vertebra and lines extended to visualize the movement. A is in relaxation with the eyes horizontal, position 1. Note that the posterior lines are nearly parallel, evenly spaced, and horizontal (in balance). B shows the "chin-chest" position and the degree of deviation of the lines is variable. The sixth and seventh vertebrae remain nearly horizontal. The greatest range is seen between the fourth and sixth. Note in C the convergence of the posterior lines is maximal between the third and sixth. In terms of the "whip lash" mechanism it will be seen that the sixth and seventh form the stock of the whip and the upper vertebrae the lash. The movement indicated by the anterior lines is best explained by the movement involved in the shift of the nucleus pulposus, the approximation of the anterior edges of the vertebrae in B being consistent with the convergence of the lines just as the divergence of the lines in C is accompanied by an approximation of the posterior edges of the body. (Courtesy Dr. Arthur G. Davis.)

"whiplash" is directly proportional to the speed at the moment of collision. Any degree of injury must, therefore, be anticipated from slight strain involving the tearing of a few fibers of the posterior articular ligaments, disc injury, complete dislocation to the fatal cases in which the cord is severed. Immediately following such a hyperflexion, the elastic extensor recoil mechanism provided by the static posterior musculature and the ligamentum flavum is the mechanism which serves to conceal the damage which has occurred since it effects a variable degree of reduction spontaneously. The individual types of lesions will therefore be described in sequence starting with those of less degree to those of intermediate and severe degrees closing with those exhibiting paralysis.

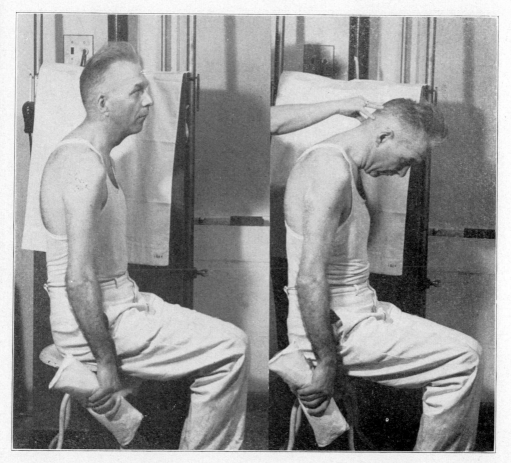

Fig. 317.   Fig. 318.

Fig. 317.—Sitting relaxed. Eyes horizontal. Sandbags in hands to depress shoulders. (Courtesy Dr. Arthur G. Davis.)
Fig. 318.—"Chin-chest" position. Flexion may be held voluntarily or with passive assistance. (Courtesy Dr. Arthur G. Davis.)

Luxation Type (Cervical Sprain).—Many patients present themselves to the physician with the complaint of pain in the neck with or without spasm with variable pain radiation with gradations from those of trivial annoyance to those exhibiting intractable causalgia. The question of injury, whether recent or remote, is frequently slurred over by the patient for the reason that painful symptoms do not develop until some time after, a good many times years after the injury occurs. Special questioning on this point usually brings out the history of a definite injury, one or several days before, or months or even years prior to the onset of disabling symptoms. The matter of a specific diagnosis is as much a matter of pain to the physician confronted with such a complaint as it is a matter of pain to the patient. The patient interprets the original fleeting symptoms as a sprain either not worthy of medical attention or as something merely requiring liniments, massage, manipulation or drugs. In this connection the word "sprain" is unfortunate since sprain implies something of very small degree but it should indicate to the physician a

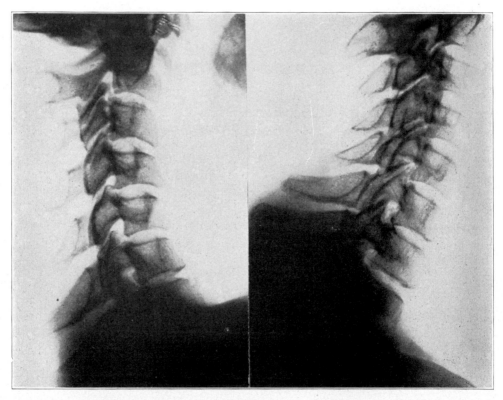

Fig. 319.—Luxation of the sixth and seventh cervical vertebrae. Disc lesion associated with fracture. Note the anterior projecting fragment of seventh vertebrae as well as the contacting exostoses of the posterior edges of sixth and seventh, the narrowing of the intervertebral space; also that no change is noted in the posterior articulations. Pain of a causalgia type radiated to the finger tips of the right hand. There was also paralysis of the serratus anterior. (Courtesy Dr. Arthur G. Davis.)

torn muscle, fascia, ligament or joint capsule. In the case of the ankle, the knee, the wrist or shoulder, the word "sprain" indicates a partial or complete ligamentous avulsion. In the case of these joints, however, there is accompanying swelling, point tenderness and ecchymosis. In the case of the cervical region there is no evidence of hematoma, ecchymosis and swelling although there may be some diffuse tenderness on pressure. The usual objective evidence is missing because of the several inches of soft parts interposed between the skin and the cervical joints. When partial or complete ligamentous avulsions surrounding other joints are neglected, the healing process is incomplete, leaving an elongated weak structure which with ordinary normal use continues to stretch. The cervical spine is no exception, in fact its extreme mobility renders it peculiarly susceptible to such progressive elongations of weakened ligaments or capsular tissues with or without the secondary involvement of the other components in the intervertebral joints.

Diagnosis of Luxation.—The key to the diagnosis of a luxation is the proper interpretation of the first lateral projection of the cervical spine. If the first x-ray plate taken with the patient in position 1, Fig. 317, i.e., sitting relaxed, the gaze focused on a point level with the eye and the cervical spine shows *straightness* throughout its length, it must be assumed that some kind of mechanical derangement has taken place since this is just as abnormal a finding as is bowing in the tibia. This occurrence of straightness of the cervical spine in a recently or remotely injured case has not received the attention it deserves. It provides the clue to these lesser degrees of injuries which heretofore have for the most part eluded specific diagnosis.

The spasm of the cervical musculature serves to avoid painful contact of the injured part, therefore the facets are not restored to their normal apposition. The natural result is that the patient automatically protects himself from pain. The entire cervical spine is held slightly forward to avoid such painful contact of the posterior articular processes. If such cases report immediately afterward and the lateral projection shows a straight cervical spine, obviously a picture should be taken in the "chin chest" position or position 2 (Fig. 318). Figs. 319, 320, 321 and 322 show typical examples of what is revealed by this simple procedure. A great many of such cases, however, have but fleeting symptoms which disappear in a few days and the individual resumes the normal use of his head and neck. In exactly the same manner as a neglected ankle sprain, such torn ligaments heal in the long and weakened position. Normal use thereafter continues to stretch the ligaments, accounting for the increasing disabling symptoms occurring from three months to years afterward. Such neglected cases present themselves with pain in the cervical region with variable pain radiation. The analysis of a consecutive series of 74 such cases from the point of view of their pain radiation reveals 7 different syndromes:

1. The occipital syndrome.
2. The third and fourth cervical root syndrome.
3. The fifth cervical root syndrome.
4. The sixth cervical root syndrome.
5. The seventh cervical root syndrome.
6. The precordial syndrome.
7. The syndrome of the long thoracic nerve.

In referring to the root numbers it will be remembered that the number of the root corresponds with the space above the vertebra of the same number. The occipital syndrome associated with lesions of the axis or atlas is recognized by pain radiating up one or both sides of the occipital region together with limitation in nodding, rotation and tilting of the head or "wry neck." The third and fourth cervical root syndrome is associated with muscle spasm

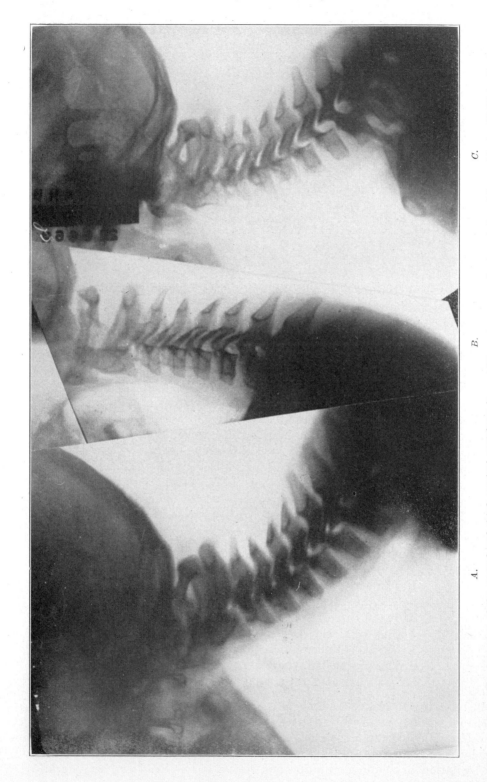

Fig. 320.—Luxation of the second and third cervical vertebrae in a child seven years of age. Automobile accident. Multiple fractures. Could not sit up, fell over each time from dizziness. Limited neck movements. Note the dislocation well forward at B, "chin-chest" position. Complete recovery in plaster collar. A, Standard lateral view; B, voluntary flexion ("chin-chest"; C, extension in Schanz collar. (Courtesy Dr. Arthur G. Davis.)

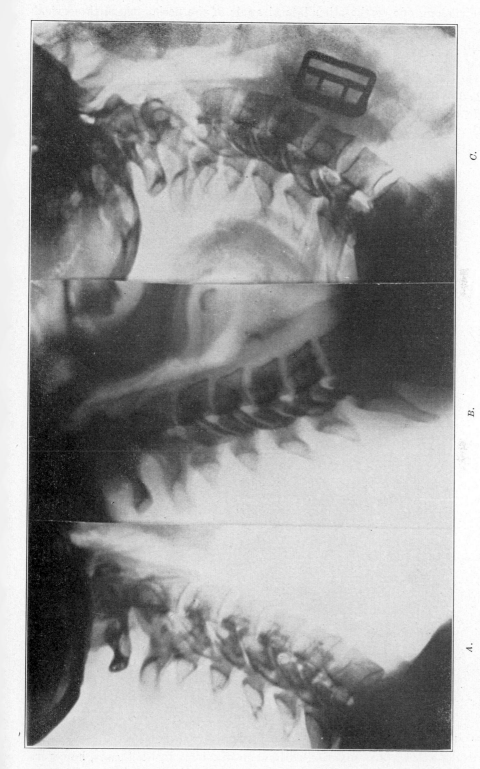

A.

B.

C.

Fig. 321.—Luxation of the fourth and fifth cervical vertebrae. Patient stumbled on a slippery floor. First seen ten days later. Bilateral shoulder girdle pain. *A*, Normal lateral view; *B*, chin-chest; *C*, hyperextension in plaster collar. Disappearance of symptoms immediately. Collar removed six weeks later. No recurrence. Note discrepancies at C 4-5 level posterior borders, anterior borders, and interspinous space in *B*. (Courtesy Dr. Arthur G. Davis.)

and pain along one or the other lateral angle of the neck. The fifth cervical root syndrome in which pain radiates over the shoulder region, the sixth to the radial side of the hand and the seventh to the radial side of the hand including the index and in some cases the middle finger. The syndrome of the long thoracic nerve has been seen twice in this series, both cases showed "winged" scapula, complete paralysis of the serratus anterior and roentgenographic evidence of injury at the seventh cervical level. The tearing of the long thoracic in its peripheral section is an equally logical explanation of these two cases. Both, however, showed cervical disc lesions at the seventh level.

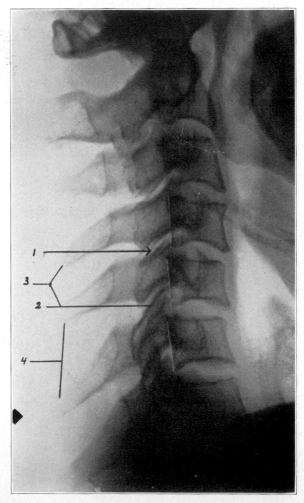

Fig. 322.—Luxation of the fifth and sixth cervical vertebrae. One-month-old luxation injury. The separation of the posterior margins of the articular processes between the fifth and sixth vertebrae is easily demonstrated with flexion. The wide separation as indicated in four as compared with three confirms this conclusion. The patient complained of pain over both shoulders which disappeared with the hyperextension collar. Complete recovery, six weeks. Symptomless nine months after. (Courtesy Dr. Arthur G. Davis.)

In the case of disc protrusion, the signs are considerably more definite than in the case of pure luxation without protrusion. In both cases, however, they cover the same areas. Mixter and Barr, McKenzie, Oppenheimer, Semmes and Murphy, Spurling, Stookey and Stuck have all pointed to syndromes associated with disc protrusion showing sharply delineated areas of sensory and motor change. Semmes, Oppenheimer and Nachlas point to the association of precordial pain with sensory changes involving the radial side of the hand while in other contributions the precordial pain of an anginoid type is not referred to. It is obviously important to eliminate the scalenus syndrome in all chronic cases involving pain radiation to the hand. In scalenus cases, cervical roentgenography is negative. Fig. 319 shows involvement of the seventh nerve root. Fig. 320 illustrates a typical case of fifth root radiation.

Differential Diagnosis.—With the clue to mechanical derangement established by the fact that the cervical spine exhibits a straight line in the lateral projection, differential diagnosis depends upon a proper correlation of x-ray findings with nerve pain radiation and, or motor changes. In disc lesions the biceps, triceps, and thenar eminence may undergo atrophy with a corresponding diminution of the triceps or biceps jerks. Semmes, Spurling and Oppenheimer have noted straightness of the cervical spine in disc lesions. Watson-Jones also makes note of taking films in the flexed position in "sprains" of the cervical spine. Oppenheimer notes lesions of the articular processes and encroachment on the intervertebral foramina due to spurs surrounding the intervertebral disc. The scalenus syndrome has been mentioned. This obviously is not associated with straightness or other changes of the cervical spine. Pure muscle ruptures are not ordinarily painful beyond the first two weeks.

A specific diagnosis therefore rests upon the correlation of positive x-ray findings corresponding to a definite level of root radiation as described. Spurling very recently has shown that disc protrusions can be shown with pantopaque. He also finds that compression downward of the head on the side of involvement produces pain in one of the root areas mentioned. Careful roentgenography in the sitting relaxed position with eyes horizontal and the "chin chest" position and bilateral oblique films to show the intervertebral foramina will frequently reveal a lesion of one or other of four kinds:

1. Luxation of the posterior facets.
2. Narrowing of the intervertebral space.
3. Lesions encroaching upon the intervertebral foramen.
4. Lesions combining any two or all three features.

One of us (J. A. K.) believes that practically all of these obscure lesions of the cervical spine: sprains, subluxations, or idiopathic pains in the neck are really lesions of the intervertebral discs in this area and that most of them respond to conservative treatment.

Diagnosis of the Obvious Group.—The immediately preceding paragraphs dealt with the diagnosis and outlined special means of detecting a group of lesions which from the point of view of diagnosis may well be referred to as "obscure." In contradistinction to this obscure group, the following group may be referred to as "obvious." Two degrees of injury are immediately separated by the severity of the accident. In the obscure group the victim of the accident can usually handle himself and usually does not require emergency measures. In the obvious case involving much greater degrees of force, immediate disability is the rule, the patient is unable to handle himself and emergency rescue is usually necessary. When paralytic signs or gross lesions immediately obvious in the x-ray film are present, the diagnostic problem is a simple one. The following injuries are those most frequently encountered:

1. Unilateral dislocation.
2. Bilateral dislocation.
3. Fracture dislocation.
4. Compression fracture.
5. Fracture dislocations with paralysis.
6. Fractures and dislocations of the atlas and axis.

Since regardless of the type of accident, the general rules regarding treatment and prognosis are the same, only the diagnostic features of each type will be mentioned at this point and the treatment and prognosis discussed, as a group. It will be seen that the all-important factor in differentiating the types is the preliminary survey x-ray. Next in importance comes the neurological examination.

Unilateral Dislocation.—Pure dislocations are limited to the cervical portion of the spinal column. There is a history of an injury or sudden twist of the neck followed immediately by pain and stiffness in the neck and fixation of the head in an abnormal attitude. In unilateral anterior dislocations the head is always rotated away from the side of the lesion so that the chin points to the opposite shoulder, and if the dislocation is complete, the head is inclined toward the side of the lesion, thus producing a type of torticollis similar to that caused by the contracture of the sternomastoid on the side of the lesion. When the dislocation is incomplete, the head is rotated so that the chin points to the side away from the lesion and is also inclined to the side away from the lesion, thus differing from a torticollis produced by a contracture of the sternomastoid on the side of the lesion. In any case the "wry neck" attitude is characteristic of unilateral dislocation.

The muscles on the side toward which the head is tilted are relaxed and those on the opposite side are taut. Attempts to straighten the head are resisted by an abrupt block and cause pain. In many instances there is also pain referred along the nerve root emerging on the side of the lesion or there may be paralysis of the peripheral nerve type in the distribution of this nerve root.

On palpation in an acute case, there is tenderness over the displaced articular facet, and it is usually possible to recognize the displacement of the transverse process by deep palpation in the side of the neck. There may also be sufficient deviation of the spinous process for it to be detected by palpation, and pressure on the spinous process of the dislocated vertebra causes pain.

The chief difficulty experienced in diagnosis is the occasional case of acute torticollis due to irritation of the sternomastoid. In these cases the history is an important differential point, since the torticollis comes on without history of accident, is rather gradual in onset, on physical examination the sternomastoid is contracted and there is no tenderness of the spinous processes or palpable displacement of the transverse processes.

The diagnosis should be confirmed by the x-ray, but it should be remembered that these dislocations are difficult to demonstrate in the x-ray picture and are best shown in views taken in slightly oblique lateral planes. In addition to the articular facets the bodies should be examined carefully as the body of the dislocated vertebra is displaced anteriorly a short distance and what is even more important, there is a tendency to a flattening out or even reversal of the normal anterior curve (cervical lordosis).

The unilateral cervical dislocation also involves "diagnosis by inference" as is described under the heading of "Jumped Process Complex." The offset of the spinous processes in the antero-posterior view, the enlargement of the intervertebral foramen in the oblique view and the laminagram are all helpful in arriving at a precise diagnosis.

Diagnosis of Simple Bilateral Dislocation of the Cervical Vertebra.—Since the articular processes of the dislocated vertebra are impaled on the pedicles of the subjacent vertebra, there is necessarily a complete avulsion of the capsule and ligaments of the posterior arch with the probability of a partial or complete avulsion of the posterior common ligaments with some of the fibers of the annulus fibrosis with variable disruption of the intervertebral disc.

In bilateral dislocations the head is usually displaced forward and the chin is fixed in the midline; that is, the patient is unable to rotate the head either to the right or to the left. The deformity of the spinous processes at the level of the dislocation can be palpated with relative ease, as the anterior displacement renders the spinous process of the next vertebra below unusually prominent. Deep palpation in the side of the neck will reveal the abnormal prominence and anterior displacement of the transverse processes of the dislocated vertebra. There is usually pain or paralysis in the distribution of the anterior root of the spinal nerve on both sides which emerge at the level of the dislocation. These bilateral cases may occur without cord symptoms but are more apt to exhibit symptoms of cord compression or damage than are the unilateral cases.

Lateral x-rays will rule out a fracture and reveal the anterior displacement of the body and of the articular facets and will show the flattening out or even reversal of the normal anterior cervical curvature.

INJURIES OF THE CERVICAL SPINE—DISLOCATIONS WITH PARALYSIS

Prior to the beginning of the use of x-ray for bone and joint diagnosis, medical literature records the occurrence of "whiplash" dislocations of the cervical spine sufficient to cause paralysis and sudden death, yet the extreme recoil has been so complete that no evidence of bone or joint injury or disalignment remains at autopsy. In such cases the spinal medulla is found pulpified, the dura usually intact, local hemorrhage, ligament avulsion, and the transverse medullary lesion being the only marks left to show the level of injury.

In approaching the diagnosis of cases showing complete or incomplete neurological signs, it is important to have the possibilities of lesser degrees of this "whiplash" mechanism in mind. Were it possible to record the degree of compression of the centrum, the degree of jackknifing or the extent of dislocation at the exact moment of extreme hyperflexion, a fuller appreciation of the possibilities of spinal cord, nerve root and posterior arch involvement would be the rule. However, by the time the patient is x-rayed, the element of spontaneous recoil of the extensor muscles and intelligent first aid care such as the hyperextension position, has served to reduce considerably the *extent* of the compression or dislocation.

The "rocker" action between adjacent vertebrae involved in all movements of the spine in the anteroposterior plane also must be borne in mind, since unless there is a complete fracture of the pedicles or articular processes sufficient to make two units out of a single bone, all movements of the interbody joints are accompanied by movement of the posterior joints to the point of complete dislocation. Except in rare instances, whether the case in hand be one of dislocation, fracture or fracture dislocation, the mechanism producing the injury is a hyperflexion beyond the normal range of motion. The center of action of the "rocker" is toward the anterior side of the intervertebral foramen up to the point of normal range. As the accidental force increases in intensity and therefore in range forward beyond the normal, the center of effort shifts to the anterior border of the body of the vertebra. If the bone yields, as it usually does in the case of a lumbar compression, a crush fracture is the usual result; if the capsular ligament of the posterior articulations yield, as they most often do in cervical "whiplash" events, a dislocation results. When greater degrees of force are experienced, the posterior common ligament is the next most common point of yield, permitting derangement of the intervertebral disc and nucleus pulposus. The case at hand should be regarded from the point of view of any conceivable degree or combination of yield of these three vulnerable structures.

From the obscure cases caused by the avulsion of a few fibers of the posterior joints in the cervical region to the hopelessly paralyzed where the section of spine and torso above the injury moves forward on the lower section, shearing the cord as it moves, the mechanics of injury is the same. With rare exceptions, the broad anterior central leaflet of the anterior longitudinal ligament remains intact. Were it not for this ligament, neither traction, hyperextension or other manipulative reductions would be possible without damage to the spinal meninges. In cases of fracture dislocations, both clinical and autopsy evidence demonstrate that the ligament may become separated from the cortex of the bodies, i.e., is lifted off, but nevertheless the ligament remains intact in the longitudinal axis, thus providing the necessary check strap to prevent overstretching. The dire consequences of reduction done *without* the agency of the anterior ligament are enough to stagger the imagination. The fact that the ligament does not contain elastic fibers is also of great importance since, if it did, root avulsion from traction or hyperextension would occur. As the evidence stands today, untoward results from hyperextension or manipulation are extremely rare. Cases in which such untoward results may be anticipated are mentioned elsewhere in this text.

COMPLETE PARALYSIS WITHOUT X-RAY EVIDENCE
OF ABNORMALITY

Starting with Kocher of Berne 50 years ago, cases appear now and again where a complete bilateral dislocation has occurred by the usual mechanics of complete hyperflexion and the recoil mechanism has been sufficient to reduce completely the dislocated vertebra, so that a lateral film shows no defect at the point of dislocation. If the spinal cord has undergone complete compression or severance at the level of the dislocation, such cases are obviously fatal. They may live for a variable length of time, even up to weeks. Intercurrent internal organ infection is the usual contributory cause of death. Autopsies show pulpified medullary substance at the level involved.

Fracture Dislocations With or Without Paralysis.—In this case combined roentgenographic and neurologic examinations aid in arriving at a decision for the kind of definitive treatment necessary to the case in hand. Just as in fracture dislocations of the thoracolumbar spine with paralysis or in cases with spinal subarachnoid block, the neurologic findings preclude the possibility of exact diagnosis as between transitory edema, contusion, compression or transection. Examination of the reflexes and for sensation and motion should be repeated following first aid and throughout the course of treatment in order to determine the status of the spinal cord. In partially paralyzed cases repetition of the complete neurologic examination should be made at frequent intervals in order to determine the question of increase or decrease of such signs. If it is felt that the patient is being adequately treated, yet the signs are increasing, such increase is probably due to hemorrhage within the medullary substance and may indicate the necessity of immediate incision of the posterior commissure. While it is true that in the majority of cases showing complete paralysis at a definite level, irreparable damage has been done, nevertheless the occasional patient with such complete signs recovers. It is this paradoxical clinical experience which demonstrates that conclusions regarding the status of the spinal cord are impossible to reach from the neurological evidence alone.

INJURIES OF THE CERVICAL SPINE

Fractures and Dislocations of the Atlas and Axis.—Because of their structural individuality these two vertebra must be considered in a separate group. Fracture of the odontoid process and dislocation of the atlas on the axis is regularly encountered. In the case of these two vertebrae, aside from the complaint of pain with occipital radiation and spasm with tilting of the head, one is entirely dependent upon roentgenography for diagnosis. Such special methods as the laminagraph and directing the rays through the foramen magnum may be necessary for detail.

The routine roentgenography necessary to exhibit odontoid fractures consists of the lateral view in the usual manner and an anteroposterior taken through the open mouth. The odontoid usually fractures near its base although not necessarily so. The figure indicates an oblique line of fracture. The base of the odontoid and the two components of the atlanto-axial articulation being at the same level, an anteroposterior view which shows these joints adequately also ordinarily shows the base of the odontoid. The anteroposterior detail is more important than the lateral since unless the odontoid fragment is displaced forward or backward no defect will ordinarily show in the lateral view. In positioning the head for x-ray photography in the anteroposterior plane, the mouth should be held wide open with a cork between the teeth to hold the spread and the line connecting the occipital protuberance with the lower margin of the teeth must be perpendicular to the plate. If the evidence is negative on the preliminary survey and symptoms persist, a second attempt using a number of the recent innovations available to the roentgenologist should be brought to bear. Oblique roentgenography and projections through the foramen magnum will occasionally reveal fractures of the lateral masses of these vertebrae.

Special precautions must be taken during all handling of the head until the odontoid is found free from involvement. After the standard anteroposterior and lateral survey films have been taken and found negative, further x-ray work at a 45 degree angle, with the head flexed, with the head extended, should be done. The patient should undertake his own movements under the direction of the roentgenologist because of the danger of manipulation or other handling. Numerous contributors have shown individual cases of unusual fractures of the atlas and axis by such carefully detailed roentgenography.

Treatment of Injuries of the Cervical Spine

While the different types of injuries of the cervical spine are separated for the purpose of diagnosis, for the purpose of treatment it seems more profitable to discuss them collectively. Whether the case be one of dislocation or simple compression fracture or fracture dislocation, with or without paralysis, the aim is to attain hyperextension. Whether the injury is of the "obscure" group or the "obvious," three important principles underlie all treatment:

1. The aim is to attain hyperextension and maintain it.
2. All treatment hinges upon the proper interpretation and use of the intact anterior longitudinal ligament.
3. The emergency care in all types of cervical injuries is of the utmost importance because of the possibility of damage through unintelligent handling.

The following routine is therefore outlined for the hospital emergency service:

1. Medical responsibility begins at the site of the accident. The ambulance personnel is instructed to place the head in immediate hyperextension with a blanket roll or other material under the neck and an attendant remains in charge of the head position throughout all transport directly to the hospital bed, never once allowing the head to be bent forward or lifted. (Fig. 323.)

2. After the patient is transferred to the hospital bed, a halter is applied to take over the hyperextension. Five pounds of weight is attached through a pulley and the head of the bed is elevated. (Fig. 324.)

3. Not until the patient is so established in hyperextension with traction is the preliminary x-ray survey permitted. A lateral picture is then taken and an anteroposterior, particularly to show the odontoid. An anteroposterior otherwise is mostly a deception.

4. Meanwhile a neurological examination is made. If there is no evidence of spinal cord involvement and the preliminary survey films are negative, the case is further investigated in the roentgenological department at leisure,

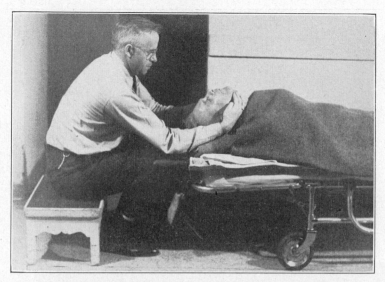

Fig. 323.—First aid for ambulance service in cervical spine injuries. (Courtesy Dr. Arthur G. Davis.)

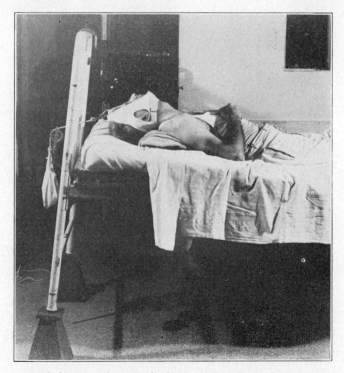

Fig. 324.—Temporary halter traction. Preliminary to roentgenography in cervical spine injuries. (Courtesy Dr. Arthur G. Davis.)

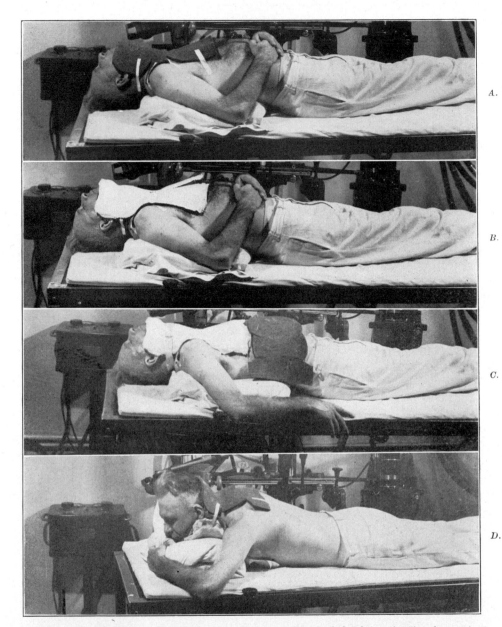

Fig. 325.—Application of plaster collar with or without skeletal traction in place. *A*, A layer of felt is cut and fashioned to fit between the jaw and the chest. *B*, Plaster slabs are laid in place while the jaw is being tilted back to attain the maximum space between the point of the mandible and the chest. This is allowed to harden. *C*, A strap and buckle or bandage is passed around the neck and the anterior half collar. The tongs are then removed and with the patient thus protected against forward flexion, he is rolled over face down. *D*, A short posterior plaster section is made in similar manner. The patient is allowed ambulatory to test out the comfortable fit of the collar. More padding may be required to remove uncomfortable pressure from the jaw or from the clavicles. After this is done a plaster bandage is passed around and around the neck and the two extensions to the chest. Of the various types of metal and leather collars, this type made in two halves is the most comfortable and satisfactory. (Courtesy Dr. Arthur G. Davis.)

using bilateral oblique films, repeating the odontoid films if necessary and taking films in the sitting position, position 1 and 2 mentioned above.

If the lateral projection in position 1 shows elimination of the normal forward curvature and all other evidence is negative, this of itself is sufficient to indicate the application of a hyperextension collar (Figs. 325 and 326), to be worn without interruption for a minimum of three weeks, three weeks being the time of sound repair of fibrous tissue. A great many cases of chronic disability involving both intervertebral disc and posterior spinal joints will thus be prevented.

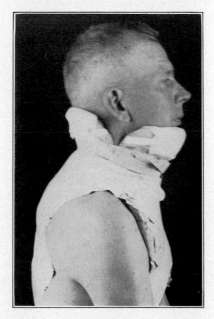

Fig. 326.—Same patient as shown in Fig. 325 in finished collar. (Courtesy Dr. Arthur G. Davis.)

Outline of Definitive Treatment

When the survey x-ray examination shows a gross lesion such as a crush fracture, unilateral or bilateral dislocation, fracture dislocation or fracture of the odontoid process:

1. Skeletal traction is almost invariably indicated. (Fig. 327.)

2. If there are neurological signs, skeletal traction also is indicated.

3. Provision should be made to raise or lower the pulley and weight traction and the amount changed to suit the case. Up to forty-five pounds of weight have been used over a considerable period of time. However, fifteen to twenty-five pounds with skeletal traction are ordinarily quite sufficient.

UNILATERAL OR BILATERAL DISLOCATIONS

In case of unilateral or bilateral dislocations or fracture dislocations, it is important to start traction in a straight line. Traction in flexion is dangerous because of avulsion of the posterior roots. Traction in extension is not effective because of the check strap effect of the anterior longitudinal ligament. Straight line traction therefore under x-ray control using as much weight as is necessary to disengage the articular processes is the rule. This procedure has been illustrated by Cone and Turner. (Fig. 328.)

This method seems by far the safest and simplest of the manipulative procedures. It recognizes that pulling in a *straight line* is without danger because of the check strap effect of the anterior longitudinal ligament. It also recognizes that once the facets are replaced, strong traction is contraindicated so the traction is reduced to a negligible amount or entirely removed. It has been my practice that when such pure dislocations are properly reduced, a plaster collar

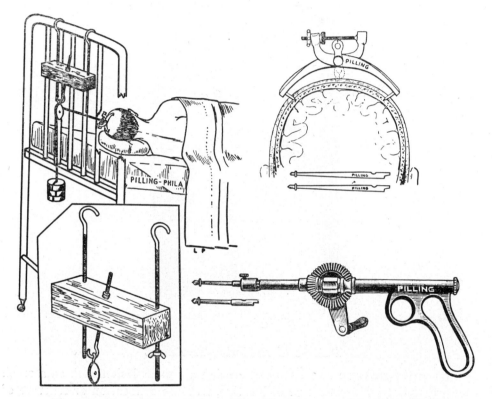

Fig. 327.—Crutchfield tongs in position. Showing ease of turning patient.

should be applied with the neck in hyperextension as soon as possible after the reduction has been accomplished. The skeletal traction is then immediately removed since it can serve no useful purpose. In fact, traction after complete reduction in hyperextension is definitely contraindicated. This is done in order to allow repair of the posterior ligaments in the short position, otherwise progressive luxation or recurrence of the dislocation may be experienced. There are numbers of cases on record that have gone through this experience. It is therefore important after the reduction has occurred not only to remove all traction but to immobilize the cervical spine in complete hyperextension in a rigid irremovable plaster collar for the necessary length of time for healing of the torn ligamentous tissues which is from three to four weeks.

In the rare case where dislocations are found irreducible by skeletal traction, one resorts to the Taylor or Walton technic. In spite of several attempts some dislocations or fracture dislocations remain irreducible. When all attempts at reduction fail, resort to operative approach is justifiable for the removal of an obstructing articular process with fusion. In some cases it will be necessary to fuse in the presence of deformity because the fusion of two or three cervical vertebrae does not materially restrict range of head or neck motions.

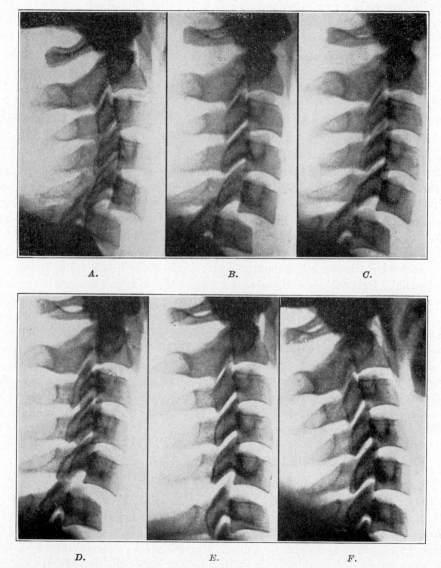

A.   B.   C.

D.   E.   F.

Fig. 328.—Reduction with skeletal traction under roentgenographic control, reproduced from the *Journal of Bone and Joint Surgery*, 1937, by courtesy of W. G. Turner. This method consists of gradual reduction by proper interpretation of the skeletal traction method. In cases of bilateral complete dislocations with or without subarachnoid block, skeletal traction is applied, using twenty-five pounds of weight, pulling in line with the vertebra above the dislocation. Lateral films are taken at ten-minute intervals, and it is found that after twenty minutes or more the processes are unlocked. At this time the head traction is lowered in order to induce hyperextension, thus replacing the jumped process. The traction is then reduced to eight pounds or less. In the case cited the author states the subarachnoid block was completely relieved.

PARTIAL OR COMPLETE PARALYSIS

If there is nerve involvement or complete paralysis with a definite level, a Queckenstedt test should be made. Traction can be easily maintained and the position remained unchanged with such skeletal traction guarding the injured region while the patient is turned on his side for the test. If there is a complete block, it is obviously important to attain complete restoration of the caliber of the spinal canal at the point of fracture or dislocation. Hyperextension more than any other one factor will bring this about. After a roentgenographic check has demonstrated full reduction and full hyperextension, with release of the block, there is obviously no indication for laminectomy. If the pressure readings still show block, laminectomy may be indicated. In spite of the well-known futility of laminectomy in such cases, if laminectomy is to be done, it should be done under local anesthesia and as quickly as possible. Allen has shown that spinal cord substance has the ability to recover from pressure up to five hours, but that if pressure is continued longer the condition is irreversible.

Where there is partial paralysis it is important to have repeated neurological examinations at short intervals to determine progress or not of the lesion. In cases showing progressive paralysis or where the roentgenogram shows the intraspinal projection of a bone fragment such as a fractured lamina, an emergency laminectomy is indicated. Clinical experience has shown that hyperextension is much more effective as a decompressor than is laminectomy. The projection of the posterior upper angle of the vertebral body into the spinal canal is the most frequent compressing medium. This deformation disappears with adequate hyperextension, releasing the block, by enlarging the spinal canal. Several cases showing an initial block have shown a restoration of pressure in the lumbar needle after hyperextension or manipulative reduction. Too often, however, laminectomy proves to be an antemortem exploration and the cord is found pulpified. A number of fatal cases in which complete reduction has been attained by hyperextension in which laminectomy was not done because of its apparent futility have shown pulpified cords on necropsy. Prediction in any case is impossible when the case of complete paralysis is first seen because of the fact that edema, contusion, hemorrhage and compression may temporarily produce complete signs and it is quite impossible to differentiate these entities.

FRACTURES OR DISLOCATIONS OF THE ATLAS AND AXIS

Fractures or dislocations of the first and second cervical with the exception of fractures of the odontoid defy classification as to treatment. Fractures in these vertebrae, however, obey the general rule as regards the immediate application of the Crutchfield tongs although they are frequently an exception to the rule of hyperextension. Experience has taught that the head may have to be lowered or raised depending upon the appearance of the odontoid in the lateral projection. As soon as the odontoid has become stable and the fragments correctly apposed, this position should be maintained either by the tongs or a plaster collar which may be fitted while the tongs are still in place. It is important to eliminate all motions in rotation, nodding or lateral tilting for several months.

Indication for Laminectomy

The indications for laminectomy in the cervical region do not depart essentially from the outline for other parts of the spine. There are, however, cases of partial or progressive paralysis in which despite skeletal traction and attempts at hyperextension, the spinal subarachnoid block persists. In a personal communication from W. G. Turner, two cases were operated under these conditions within the first few hours following injury and in both cases a projecting bar of the intervertebral disc was found to be the cause of the pressure. It is questionable whether these cases would have undergone recovery had they not been laminectomized promptly.

Anesthesia

General anesthesia is definitely contraindicated for all cervical spine manipulations, traction or even laminectomy. Traction in a straight line is practically without pain. Traction of itself ordinarily relieves pain and spasm. In paralyzed patients the area of laminectomy is already partially anesthetized by the paralysis and the hypersensitive area just above the level of injury can be completely anesthetized with 1 per cent procain. Local anesthesia for the introduction of tongs either in the outer table of the skull or in the zygomata or if wire loops or fish hooks are used, can all be executed with local anesthesia. From the experience of the author, the Crutchfield tongs is by far the easiest and surest method of skull traction. These ingenious tongs of high mechanical efficiency have greatly simplified all treatment of injuries of the cervical spine.

Convalescence

Here a single general rule may be said to cover the entire conduct of convalescence to the point of sound healing. Hyperextension is that rule. Nowhere is it more necessary to maintain complete hyperextension throughout convalescence than in the cervical spine. Whether the case be recumbent or ambulatory, whether a unilateral or bilateral dislocation or a compression fracture, whether a partial luxation or a suspected intervertebral disc lesion, whether the patient must look skyward or not to hold the extension, the rule holds. Removable braces are the least trustworthy; irremovable plaster casts the most dependable. Plaster collars when carefully made are also more comfortable than braces. In fashioning such plaster collars or Minerva jackets, the principal criterion is the separation of the jaw from the chest.

A number of cases appear in the literature where redislocations have occurred after complete reduction because of inadequate splintage. Recent ligamentous lesions should be protected for three to six weeks, complete dislocations for three months, compression fractures for three months, odontoid process fractures for three to five months. Where fracture dislocations are found to be irreducible and there are no paralytic signs, posterior fusion of two or three of the vertebrae in the involved region is quite sufficient to produce a fully functioning spine minus symptoms except slight limitation of mobility.

Different types of fixation will be required for the different types of cases. One may choose between a Thomas or cardboard collar, a bivalved plaster collar, a cuirass or a Minerva jacket. The author ordinarily uses the Thomas or card-board collar or brace only for greater comfort after the critical fibrous tissue or callus forming period is finished. The bivalved plaster collar is ordinarily used for unilateral or bilateral pure dislocations or luxations, the cuirass or Minerva jacket for fracture dislocations.

Recumbency or Ambulatory Convalescence

Cases of the pure luxation type without paralysis may be ambulatory from the beginning. Unilateral or bilateral dislocations unaccompanied by fracture may be ambulatory in adequate hyperextension from the time of complete reduction. Cases of fracture dislocation without paralysis should remain recumbent for a minimum of six weeks for the necessary bone differentiation and callus formation. Cases of odontoid fracture may be made ambulatory as soon as reduction is demonstrated to be 100 per cent and a proper Minerva jacket or cuirass has been applied. A check x-ray should be taken after the patient has become ambulatory in order to see that the fragments have not changed position.

Prognosis

In a consecutive series of 61 hospital admissions of serious accidents to the cervical spine, 11 patients died. All but 2 of the fatal cases were autopsied and showed irreparable pulpifaction of the spinal cord. The remainder of the serious injuries have for the most part fully recovered. Several cases showing complete neurological signs at a definite level experienced complete or almost complete recovery with hyperextension only. None of these cases were lami-nectomized. Of the 61 hospital admissions of serious injuries to the cervical spine, 50 have for the most part fully recovered. Thirty-five of the patients complained of arm or hand signs. In the luxation type of injury, if the inter-vertebral disc is also involved with protrusion to the point of atrophy and diminution of reflexes in the affected arm, it is impossible to prognosticate the outcome, there being no general agreement as yet as to the proper treatment for such combined lesions. Further investigation and end result studies are necessary to decide the type therapy and prognosis in these cases. In general, however, it may be said that due to recent advances in anatomical interpreta-tion, roentgenological, neurological and orthopedic technic, a more favorable prognosis in all types of injury of the cervical spine is possible except those with complete neurological signs.

Manipulative Treatment of Simple Unilateral and Bilateral Dislocations of the Cervical Vertebra

The surgeon may elect to treat these lesions by immediate reduction by manipulation. In the unilateral cases this is most satisfactorily done by the method of Walton while in the bilateral cases the Taylor* method is probably the safer, but the method of Walton† can be used and is recommended by Langworthy, while Brookes‡ uses Taylor's method.

*Taylor, A. S.: Ann. Surg. 90: 321, 1929.
†Walton, G. L.: Nerv. & Ment. Dis. 20: 609, 1893.
‡Brookes, Theodore P.: Surg., Gynec. & Obst. 57: 772-782, 1933.

In Walton's method the object is to unlock the articular process by bending the head forward and to the side away from the lesion and at the same time slightly increase the rotation in the direction of the deformity (away from the lesion); then to reduce the dislocation by rotating the head in the opposite direction (toward the lesion). (Figs. 331, 332, 333.)

In Taylor's method the dislocation is reduced by slow, steady traction with the cervical spine in a position of slight flexion. (Figs. 334 and 335.)

In all fresh dislocations and fracture dislocations the patient should be handled with extreme care because one of the most important considerations is to protect the spinal cord from further damage, and unguarded movements or manipulations on the part of the patient or surgeon may result in severe damage to the cord or even death. For this reason the patient should be placed immediately on a stretcher or hard bed without a pillow under the head, but with sandbags or hard pillows on either side of the head and should be moved with great care. X-ray pictures should be taken and, when possible, without moving the patient from the stretcher or bed. But here traction on the head and countertraction on the shoulders are necessary if a view of the lower cervical vertebrae is to be obtained. With the patient sitting up and leaning slightly forward with the shoulders drooped, a six-foot exposure will often give a good lateral view of the entire cervical spine.

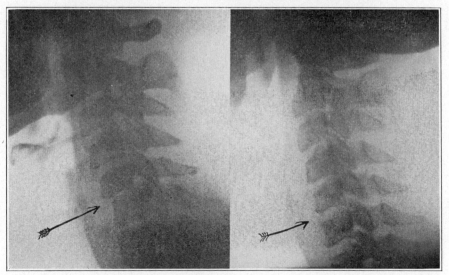

Fig. 329.   Fig. 330.

Fig. 329.—Bilateral dislocation of the fifth cervical vertebra, lateral view.

Fig. 330.—Same as preceding after reduction by Taylor's traction method. Cast extending from chin, neck, and occiput to pelvis for two months, then metal brace for four months.

Anesthesia in Cervical Dislocations.—The question of anesthesia must be decided by the surgeon and in part by the method used for the reduction. If the Taylor method is used, reduction can in most cases be accomplished without any anesthetic other than a dose of morphine. If Walton's method is used, the manipulation may be very painful and an anesthetic may be necessary, especially if the dislocation has been present for some days. In recent cases the manipulation may be tried without anesthesia and if unsuccessful a general anesthetic may be given by inhalation or pentothal. Boehler uses novocaine injected between the spinous processes and laterally in the region of the displaced articular facets and applies traction up to seventy-five pounds.

Before the operation the patient should be placed on an orthopedic table in a position for the immediate application of a plaster-of-Paris cast with the cervical spine in hyperextension. It may be necessary for the cast to include the head and extend down to the pelvis, and materials should be at hand for making a plaster jacket as well as for taking lateral x-ray plates in order to verify the reduction.

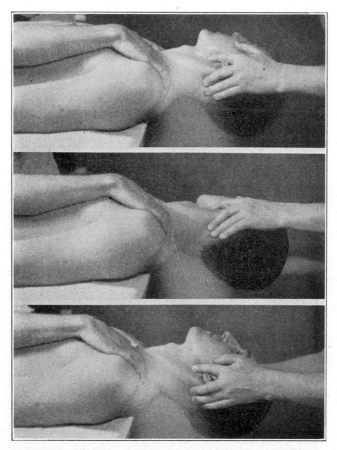

Fig. 331.—Walton's method in the reduction of dislocation of the cervical vertebra on the left side. With moderate traction and flexion the deformity is increased by rotating the head to the right.

Fig. 332.—Second maneuver. With the deformity increased the head is bent or flexed laterally sharply away from the dislocated side.

Fig. 333.—Third maneuver. The chin is returned to the midline and the neck is hyperextended.

Walton's Method.—In a complete unilateral cervical dislocation on the left side, the patient will present a torticollis with the chin rotated to the right shoulder and the head inclined to the left. In order to reduce this dislocation, the patient should be placed supine on a table with his head hanging over the end of the table and supported by the surgeon while an assistant grasps his shoulders to make countertraction and steady him on the table. Then the head should be lifted slightly (Fig. 331), thus flexing the cervical spine and the rotation of the chin to the right should be increased slightly. This slight flexion and increase of the deformity should be accompanied by moderate traction on the head (Fig. 332). This tends to unlock the articular facet. When this has been accomplished the head should be forcibly inclined to the right and the chin rotated to the left or to the midline and then hyperextended (Fig. 333). Inclining the head to the right lifts the displaced facet up to the level of the top of the one below, and the rotation to the left, performed while the head is inclined to the right and the facet lifted, carries the facet back into its normal position. If this movement can be performed freely, the reduction may be regarded as complete; but when possible, it should be controlled by lateral x-ray pictures taken before the cast is applied.

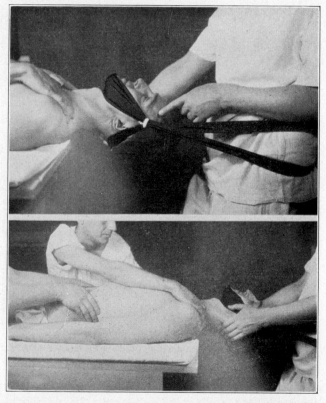

Fig. 334.—Taylor's method used in the reduction of dislocations and fracture dislocations of the cervical vertebra. Traction is made by the surgeon's body with a sling around the patient's head and chin while countertraction on the shoulders is made by an assistant.

Fig. 335.—The head is steadied by the surgeon's hand. When the neck is felt to elongate, the cervical spine is gently hyperextended.

Langworthy in performing the manipulation uses the edge of his hand as a fulcrum on the opposite side of the neck and bends the head laterally against this hand to disengage the facet. He states that in most of the older cases great force is required in this part of the manipulation and that the hand, acting as a fulcrum, prevents a lateral pushing of the head and neck

toward the shoulder which is not an effective maneuver in the reduction. In
some cases he has used practically his full strength in this maneuver without
harm. As soon as the dislocation is reduced, he throws the head back into
hyperextension and keeps it there in order to prevent redislocation. In old
dislocations on the left side he bends the head to the right as far as it will go;
then applies quick force to bend the head still farther to the right and at the
point of maximum application of force rotates the head sharply to the left.

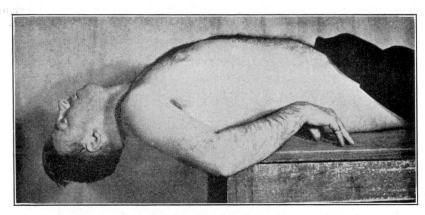

336.—Watson Jones' method for hyperextension of the cervical spine. A thin board
is nailed to and projects from the table. The patient's spine up to the site of the fracture
rests on this board and head and spine cephalad of the fracture are hyperextended over the
end of the board. (J. Bone and Joint Surg., 1934.)

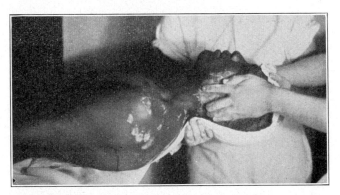

Fig. 337.—Application of a posterior plaster mold to back of neck, head and upper chest
for the immediate immobilization after reduction of dislocation of the cervical vertebra. The
circular cast around head, neck and body is applied as soon as this sets.

Taylor's Method.—In Taylor's method slow, steady traction combined
with hyperextension is used to effect the reduction. The principle consists of controlled traction exerted on the head with countertraction on the shoulders
or lower extremities until the contracted cervical muscles have relaxed sufficiently to permit a successful manipulative reduction on the part of the
operator.

Taylor recommends that traction be applied by a suspension sling for
the head which is fastened to a band of clothesline passed around the operator's pelvic girdle and of such a length that the patient's vertex is only a
short distance from the operator who faces the patient and grasps his neck

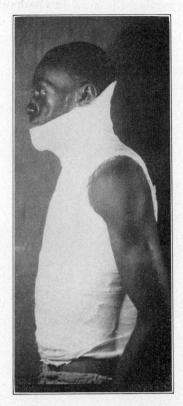

Fig. 338.—Plaster jacket for immobilization of fractures and fracture dislocations of the cervical spine. Note that the plaster extends well down below the iliac crests.

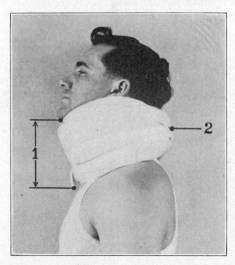

Fig. 339.—Thomas collar. *1*, Stockinette—8 inches wide, 6 feet long. *2*, Filler—twelve layers of 8 inch sheet wadding. *3*, Cotton tape to tie. *4*, Start under chin, wrapping snugly around neck. Conform to maintain necessary degree of hyperextension. (Courtesy Dr. Arthur G. Davis.)

in the damaged area, supporting the head in the hands. When everything is ready, the operator applies traction on the neck muscles gradually and increasingly by backing the body away while holding the neck with his two hands, thus maintaining control of the whole procedure (Fig. 334). The traction is first exerted in the axis of that portion of the cervical spine above the injury so as to unlock the articular processes of the damaged vertebra.

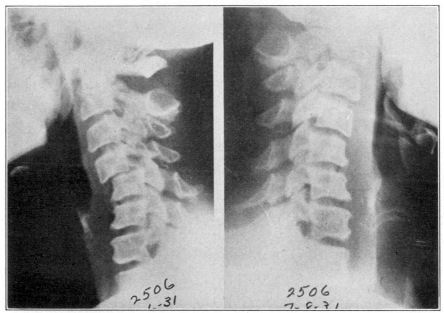

Fig. 340.   Fig. 341.

Fig. 340.—Dislocation fourth cervical vertebra. (Courtesy Dr. Theodore Brookes.)
Fig. 341.—Same case after reduction and immobilization in a plaster cast. (Not adequate hyperextension.)

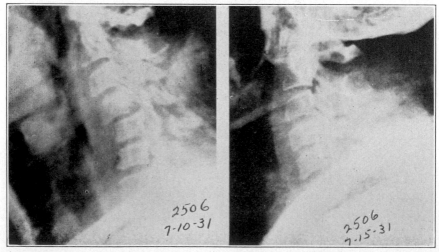

Fig. 342.   Fig. 343.

Fig. 342.—Same case two days later. Patient got chin inside cast, flexed head, and dislocation recurred.
Fig. 343.—Same case after second reduction. (With adequate hyperextension.)

After traction for a period varying with the degree of strength and muscle spasm (five to ten minutes) the neck is felt to elongate, the bones unlock; then the head and upper spine are allowed to sag downward while still under traction (Fig. 335). Reduction is indicated (a) sometimes by the patient who feels the bone slide into place with immediate relief of previous discomfort; (b) by finding the spinous processes in proper alignment; and (c) by a plate taken by a portable machine and developed while the patient remains on the table.

Immobilization.—After the reduction lateral x-rays should be taken to determine whether or not the reduction is satisfactory. Then the head and neck should be immobilized in hyperextension in a neutral position as regards rotation in a plaster-of-Paris jacket. In dislocations of the atlas on the axis this jacket should include the head, but in dislocations of the lower cervical vertebrae it need extend only to the occiput and be well molded under the chin to prevent flexion of the head, which may result in redislocation. It should include the shoulders and chest, but need not extend to the pelvis.

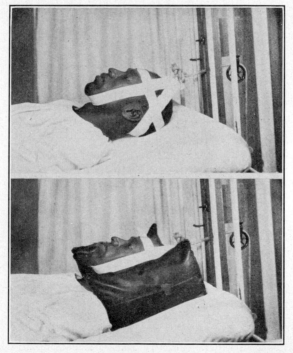

Fig. 344.—Simple type of head traction used in the treatment of fracture dislocations of the cervical spine. This traction is useful in cervical traumatic arthritis or muscle spasm or nontraumatic dislocation of the atlantoaxial joint. Sandbags stabilize the head.

It may be applied by the method of Watson Jones of having a thin board nailed to and projecting from the table to support the upper dorsal region or by having a long thin metal strip on the table under the patient. This is pulled out as far as necessary and after the cast is applied it is withdrawn. The patient's body weight keeps the strip from tilting downward. The plaster jacket may be begun by placing a wide vertical plaster slab or mold up the back, molding it to the neck and occipital region, as this affords sufficient immediate immobilization, and the jacket can be finished with relatively little discomfort to the patient (Figs. 337 and 338). The plaster cast should be left on four or five weeks in cases of simple dislocation without fracture. At the end of this time it should be removed and the patient should be fitted with a leather or padded pasteboard Thomas collar which should be worn for two weeks or longer as necessary.

In cases with small chip fractures or slight crushing fractures of the vertebra with no cord injury the plaster jacket must be worn longer, usually two months, and can then be followed by a brace or Thomas collar for several weeks, the immobilization depending upon the severity of the fracture. (Fig. 339.)

Treatment of Fracture Dislocations in the Cervical Spine

We believe that these cases are best treated by immediate reduction by traction as advocated by Taylor, followed by immobilization in a plaster-of-Paris cast as described above. This is true even in those cases with cord injury, since once the fracture dislocation is reduced and the cast applied, further damage to the cord is prevented and the patient can be handled with greater ease.

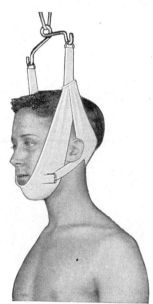

Fig. 345.—Head halter. (Courtesy Zimmer Manufacturing Company.)

This opinion, however, is not generally accepted. Many surgeons prefer to treat these cases by traction in bed. Traction can be applied by means of a head sling in which the head of the bed is elevated to permit the body to act as counterweight (Fig. 345), or by means of the special pillow head support of Hanflig, or by skeletal traction with special head calipers or wires through the outer table of the cranium. The difficulty with treating these patients by traction in bed is that they cannot be turned over and if paralysis is present, bed sores cannot be prevented, and if paralysis is not present the patient is much more uncomfortable

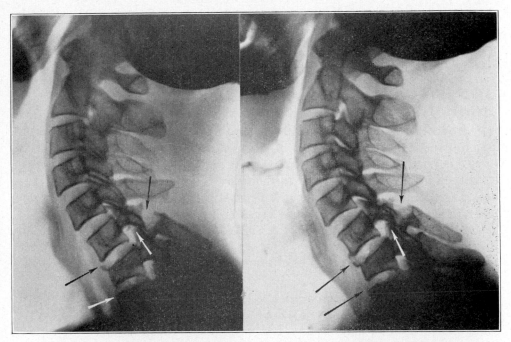

Fig. 346.—Fracture dislocation through the lamina of the sixth cervical vertebra with compression of the seventh followed by union and fusion. There were no neurological symptoms.

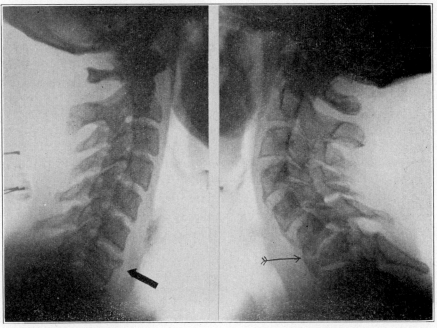

Fig. 347.   Fig. 348.

Fig. 347.—Mild crushed fracture of the seventh cervical vertebra. These fractures may accompany dislocations and demand prolonged immobilization and freedom from motion.

Fig. 348.—Old fracture dislocation of the seventh cervical vertebra seen by Conwell one year after the injury. Anterior union. No treatment following injury except few days' rest and local heat. Such treatment not recommended. Moderate pain at intervals in neck one year after injury. Treated by local heat and support with improvement.

than if the fracture dislocation is reduced immediately and immobilized in a plaster cast. Occasionally dislocations of the cervical vertebra can be reduced by placing the patient in bed with traction to the head in a position of hyperextension. We believe, however, that manual reduction is more likely to be successful and is much more comfortable for the patient. The only reason for treating such a patient by traction is that the surgeon is afraid to attempt reduction or is afraid of the effect of the anesthetic on the patient.

Prognosis.—In a case of simple dislocation, either unilateral or bilateral, which is successfully reduced soon after the accident, the patient may expect to have a normal neck. In cases in which reduction is delayed for several weeks, some pain in the neck from time to time may be expected, and cases of bilateral dislocation are said to develop union between the vertebral bodies at the site of the dislocation where the intervertebral disc has been torn (Figs. 348 and 349). This nearly always occurs in cases of fracture and may occur in dislocations without fracture, but as yet we have no statistics of a large number of cases and are not able to say how frequently it does occur in these uncomplicated cases.

In cases in which the dislocation is or is not reduced and in fracture dislocations even when cord symptoms are not present at the time of injury, a compression myelitis may occur a few days or some months after the injury and may result fatally.

FRACTURES AND DISLOCATIONS OF THE ATLAS AND AXIS

Fractures and dislocations of the atlas and axis deserve special attention, since, because of their location, they have a considerably higher mortality than do similar injuries of the lower cervical vertebra. However, they are by no means necessarily fatal. In addition to the cases which result from trauma, definite dislocations of the atlas or the axis may occur without a preceding injury (Fig. 350). Berkheiser* has reported five such cases, all occurring in children, and in each instance the dislocation occurred after an acute upper respiratory infection. Berkheiser believed these to be pathologic dislocations caused by inflammation in, and distention of, the joint capsule or of the bursa between the odontoid process and the atlas.

Simple Rotary Dislocation of the Atlas.—The most frequent lesion in this region is a simple rotary dislocation of the atlas on the axis. This injury is similar to that described above as a simple rotary dislocation of the cervical vertebra, in that the articular process of the atlas slides forward on that of the axis below and gets caught in the intervertebral notch (Fig. 350). The symptoms and treatment are identical with those of simple dislocations of the cervical spine, and the displacement can be reduced by manipulation by the method of Walton or of Taylor. The only difference between these lesions and those in the other cervical vertebra is that before the manipulation is undertaken, it should be determined whether or not the odontoid process is fractured; since, if it is fractured, manipulation may result in sudden death because of the displacement and compression of the medulla.

*Berkheiser: J. A. M. A. 96: 517, 1931.

In Berkheiser's series of nontraumatic dislocations, four of the five cases were successfully treated by traction. The patient was immobilized on a Bradford frame and light traction was applied to the head. In the beginning the traction was applied in the horizontal plane and then the head was hyperextended by placing a pad under the back of the neck. The period of traction varied from eight days to five months. After reduction the head was immobilized in a plaster cast.

Dislocation of the Axis With Fracture of the Odontoid Process is, as a rule, fatal, since it is only in cases with little or no displacement that the medulla escapes. Yet occasionally the patient survives and may even escape paralysis and live indefinitely.

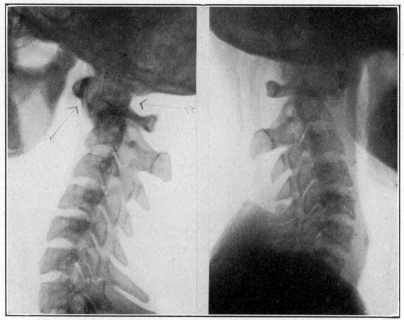

Fig. 349.   Fig. 350.

Fig. 349.—Old nontraumatic anterior dislocation at the atlantoaxial joint with ankylosis. It was an acute nontraumatic dislocation when first seen. Patient had paralysis of right upper and lower extremities when first seen. Recovered motor and sensory power in six weeks following application of traction to head. Treated by traction for three months, then a plaster cast followed by a metal brace. Good results in eleven months. The dislocation followed tonsillitis with infection about the atlantoaxial joint.

Fig. 350.—Anterior dislocation of the atlas. Treated by manipulative reduction and immobilization in plaster and later metal brace. Good results.

Diagnosis of Fractures and Dislocations of the Atlas and Axis.—The etiology and symptoms are those of other cervical dislocations and fractures, usually a fall upon the head followed by pain and stiffness in the neck and fixation of the head in an abnormal attitude. If the patient is not paralyzed, he will tend to support the head with the hands and is unwilling to relinquish this support to another person. Sudden death may occur at any time from a sudden displacement of the head with a pinching off of the medulla. It is, of course, impossible to determine by physical examination whether or not the odontoid process is fractured in these upper cervical lesions. However, such a fracture should be suspected if the patient has a marked sense of instability of the head on the neck. The displacement can be made out in some cases by palpation, since an unusual prominence of the spinous process of the axis indicates a slipping forward of the atlas and of the head. Likewise, the transverse process of the atlas can be palpated about halfway between the angle of the jaw and mastoid, and rotatory displacement of this bone will result in abnormality in the positions of these processes.

It is unwise, however, to attempt to make the diagnosis of such a dislocation by physical examination; for when a dislocation or fracture dislocation of the atlas and axis is suspected, great care should be taken not to subject the patient to injudicious manipulations. He should be placed on a bed or stretcher at the earliest possible moment with the head in a position of hyperextension supported by sandbags. Then x-ray pictures should be taken of the region, both anteroposteriorly and laterally.

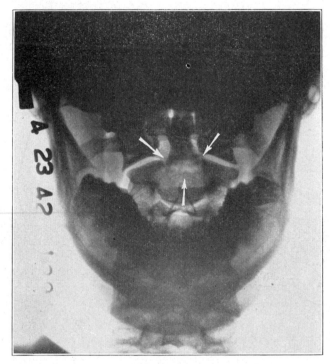

Fig. 351.—Transverse fracture of the base of the odontoid process.

In taking x-ray pictures of the atlas and axis, lateral pictures are taken in the usual manner while anteroposterior pictures are taken through the wide open mouth. It is important when taking them through the mouth to so direct the rays that the shadow of the occiput does not impinge upon that of the upper cervical vertebrae. The tendency is to slant the x-rays too far upward and backward, with the result that the occiput clouds the picture of the first and second cervical vertebrae. For this reason they should be carefully directed in such a manner that they run parallel with a line drawn from the edges of the upper incisor teeth to the base of the occiput.

Treatment

In case the x-ray pictures show a fracture of the odontoid process with displacement, the patient should be immobilized immediately in a plaster-of-Paris jacket which includes the head and gets its support on the pelvis, great care being taken not to let the head fall forward or slip forward during the application of the jacket. If there is displacement with fracture of the odontoid process, the patient will usually be killed immediately or at least paralyzed,

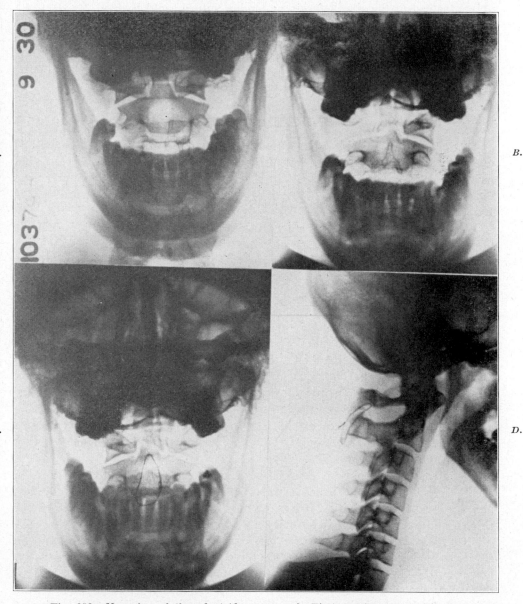

Fig. 352.—Nonunion of the odontoid process. *A*, First roentgenogram following accident showing questionable involvement in fracture. *B*. Two years later; definite nonunion with spasm and occipital radiation. *C* and *D*, Fusion of atlas and axis using wire and osteoperiosteal graft. Result: some limitation of motion in nodding but otherwise pain free. Patient returned to his occupation as truck driver. (Courtesy Dr. Arthur G. Davis.)

and nothing can be done except to fix the head in the position in which it is found. We know of no case with fracture displacement of the odontoid process that has been successfully reduced. The support should be worn for six months. At the end of this time it should be removed and x-ray pictures should be made to determine whether or not union has taken place.

Mixter and Osgood doubt whether fractures of the odontoid process ever unite by bone, and advise operative fixation. They suggest the method of passing a heavy silk ligature over the arch of the atlas, tying it to the spine of the axis. Instead of the silk, a fascia or tendon suture could be used for the same purpose. We have had no experience with this operation but would be inclined to attempt an arthrodesis of the first to the second cervical vertebra. The patient and family should be warned, however, that the operation may result in death from edema of the medulla or from some accidental movement during the operative procedure. (Fig. 352.)

SPONDYLOLISTHESIS

"Spondylolisthesis" is a term used to describe the forward displacement of one of the lumbar vertebrae on that of the one beneath. In most of the recorded cases the fifth lumbar is displaced upon the sacrum, but in occasional cases the fourth may be displaced upon the fifth or the third may slip forward on the fourth. (Fig. 353.)

The condition may or may not be traumatic and in some cases it is difficult to determine whether or not a given injury is really the cause of the condition or whether the injury has aggravated a preexisting condition. Recent studies by Hitchcock prove that spondylolisthesis is not a congenital anomaly, but is a fracture through the isthmus of the vertebral arch which is produced by hyperflexion of the fetus at birth. This does not heal by bone and results in a pseudarthrosis at the isthmus of the vertebral arch. If the vertebral body has not slipped forward, this is called a prespondylolisthesis or spondylolischesis. As a result of the pseudarthrosis the fifth lumbar is insecurely fixed upon the sacrum, and under the influence of body weight and normal activity may gradually slip forward to a variable degree. In Meyerding's* series of 121 cases, 38 per cent ascribed the condition to trauma. In the traumatic cases it is probable that the pseudarthrosis at the isthmus or even the slipping was present before the accident which caused the symptoms and that the accident merely strained an already weak spine.

Diagnosis.—The patient complains of sensation of pain and weakness in the back and inability to bend forward. The pain is usually relieved by rest and aggravated by activity. It may or may not be referred to the buttocks or thighs, and varies greatly in severity and duration.

On physical examination the most striking feature is lordosis, and in severe cases there is a shortening of the torso and a waddling gait. Occasionally, however, this lordosis is not obvious. The next most striking feature is a depression of the spine of the fourth lumbar vertebra; that is, when palpated, the spine of the fourth lumbar can be felt to be abnormally anterior to the spine of the sacrum. There is usually limitation of motion in the lumbosacral region,

---

*Meyerding: J. Bone and Joint Surg., p. 33, 1931.

especially on forward bending; this may or may not be accompanied by muscle spasm and pain. In severe cases the patient may walk with a guarded gait. The definite diagnosis depends upon the x-rays, especially those pictures made in the lateral plane which show the anterior displacement of the body of the vertebra on that of the sacrum, or, in rare instances, anterior displacement of the third or fourth lumbar on that of the one beneath. The x-ray picture may also show congenital anomalies, which were present in about 25 per cent of Meyerding's cases.

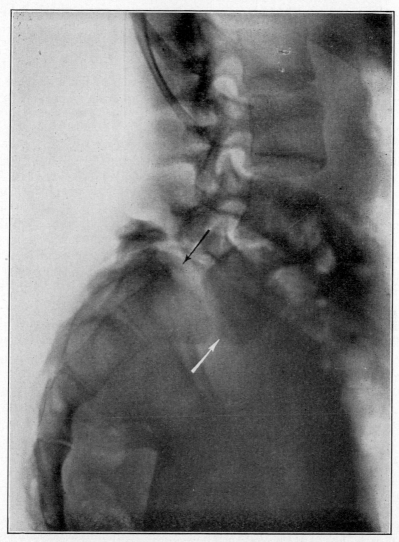

Fig. 353.—Spondylolisthesis of the fifth lumbar on the sacrum which became progressively worse during adolescence. No injury. Treated by lumbosacral fusion with satisfactory result.

Treatment of Spondylolisthesis

The treatment depends upon the condition of the patient and the severity of the symptoms. The symptoms can usually be relieved by rest in bed and in the average case they can be relieved by a well-fitting low back brace of the

Goldthwait type with an anterior pad or by a well-fitting corset or plaster-of-Paris jacket. In many cases a brace (Williams' back brace) or a wide lumbosacral belt will enable the patient to lead a normal life and no further treatment is necessary. In a man who must do heavy work and in patients who are not relieved by mechanical supports, operative intervention is indicated. It has been found that attempts to reduce the subluxation are useless; the operation of choice is a fusion of the third, fourth, and fifth lumbar vertebrae to the sacrum. It can be done successfully after the manner of Hibbs as described above or by any of the other fusion operations. Key explores for a protruding intervertebral disc and then fuses the area with notched slab grafts from the ilium supplemented by cancellous bone from the same area. After the fusion the patient should remain recumbent for six weeks. At the end of this time he may be permitted to be up, but the spine should be supported by a plaster-of-Paris jacket or a wide lumbosacral belt which should be worn for from four to six months.

LOW BACK STRAINS

One of the most perplexing problems in orthopedic and industrial surgery is pain in the low back. In this region of the spine we have the lower lumbar and lumbosacral articulations and the sacroiliac joints, any of which may be responsible for pain. In industrial and accidental cases we also have the difficulty of determining whether or not the patient's symptoms are faked or exaggerated, and if the patient has symptoms, whether or not they are due to postural defects, to trauma, or to arthritis. If arthritis is present, we are confronted by the question of whether or not the arthritis is caused by the strain or whether a preexisting painless arthritis has been aggravated by the trauma to such an extent that it now causes pain and disability.

Etiology of Low Back Strains.—In a series of 2,050 cases studied at Steindler's clinic, Miltner and Lowendorf[*] classified the cases as follows:

Etiology	No. of Cases
Osteoarthritis	1,050
Atrophic arthritis	300
Sacroiliac sprain	326
Sacrolumbar sprain	114
Combined sacroiliac and sacrolumbar sprain	85
Lumbar muscle strain	100
Lumbar myositis (myofasciitis)	25
Spondylolisthesis	22
Fracture of the transverse process	14
Fracture of articular facet	7
Fracture of lumbar vertebrae (undiagnosed)	5
Kümmell's kyphosis	2
Total No. of Cases	2,050

It is seen that of these there were 525 cases of lumbosacral and sacroiliac strains and that in 85 both sacroiliac and lumbosacral joints were involved. In addition to this it should be noted that 1,350 cases presented arthritis and 850 of this group had been originally diagnosed as low back strain. The question of arthritis will be taken up in another section. We are here concerned with those low back strains which are nonarthritic.

*Miltner and Lowendorf: J. Bone & Joint Surg., January, 1931, p. 16.

These 525 cases were classified as follows:

Etiology	No. of Cases	Per cent
Traumatic	240	45.7
Occupational	73	13.9
Postural	107	20.3
Others	105	20.0

It is interesting to note that Herndon (Industrial Surgical Clinics), in a series of 941 cases of back injuries in industrial employees, reports psychoneurosis in 17 per cent and malingering in 4 per cent, and in Miltner and Lowendorf's series of 525 cases there were 8 cases who had a definite psychoneurosis which was, according to all observers, entirely responsible for the pain.

It should be emphasized that the severity of the injury may bear little or no relation to the severity and duration of the symptoms. Some patients, after a relatively slight injury, may develop severe symptoms which are very resistant to treatment, while other patients with very severe injuries may clear up entirely after a relatively short period of treatment.

During the past four years one of us (J. A. K.) has radically changed his ideas on the etiology of low back strains or idiopathic low back pain and believes that in practically all of these cases which he formerly classified as lumbosacral or sacroiliac strain of the traumatic or postural type, the lesion is in the lumbosacral disc (Key, J. A.: Surgery 17: 291, 1945 and Annals of Surgery 121: 534, 1945).

This does not mean that all of these patients should be operated upon. As a matter of fact most of them recover under conservative treatment or even spontaneously without treatment and operative treatment is reserved for those who have not responded to conservative treatment and whose disabiltiy is so great that a major surgical procedure is justified in an effort to relieve the pain and disability. In practice this amounts to less than ten per cent of the patients with low back pain.

These patients correspond to the postural and traumatic types and are treated conservatively just as described here, only J. A. K. believes that he is treating lesions of the intervertebral disc rather than lumbosacral or sacroiliac strains. In the postural type of strain the protrusion is usually in the midline and in the traumatic type the protrusion is posterolateral.

Hypertrophic changes or arthritis of the spine is not accepted by him as a cause of low back pain, but may be present with a lesion of the intervertebral disc. If surgery becomes necessary the operation is on the offending disc or discs.

The old classification is continued in this edition because his (J. A. K.) views are not yet generally accepted.

Postural and Occupational Strains are more frequent in women than in men and are practically always chronic in nature. The symptoms vary from time to time, and either the sacroiliac or the lumbosacral joints may be involved. They are gradual in onset, usually mild in character, and tend to be worse when the patient is tired, frequently keeping him awake at night. The pain is often bilateral in the lumbosacral region, usually worse on one side. Occasionally it is sacroiliac, and may alternate from side to side.

On physical examination the patient is usually lordotic and stands with poor posture in a slumped position with round shoulders. The movements of the back are not, as a rule, restricted, and lumbosacral cases tend to have more pain on hyperextension than on flexion of the spine; with lateral motions the pain is more apt to be increased by bending away from the side of the lesion; that is, on bending to the left, the patient complains of pain in the right lumbosacral region. In the occupational type of low back strain the symptoms and physical findings are similar to the postural type except that it is usually possible in the history to connect the symptoms with some movement or position assumed while at work, and there is usually a history to the effect that this type of work results in exacerbation of the symptoms.

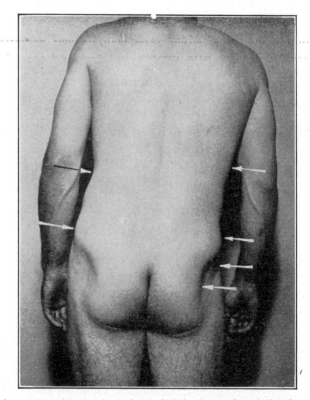

Fig. 354.—Typical posture with flat back bent slightly forward and listed to the right on account of acute low back strain, either lumbosacral or sacroiliac or an acute disc lesion.

Traumatic Low Back Strain.—In traumatic low back strain the patient can usually ascribe the onset to a definite injury or movement. It may be merely stooping over to tie the shoe, but at the time of the accident the patient feels a sharp pain or has a sensation of something giving way in the low back. In some cases there is immediate disability, the pain is very severe and persists; in others the patient is able to continue with his work and the pain comes on gradually, getting worse within a few hours or the next day. The patient may work for several days with the pain until he is eventually forced to give up on account of pain, weakness, and stiffness in the low back, the degree of pain and disability varying in individual cases. One patient may merely complain of slight pain in the low back from time to time with certain movements; another may be completely disabled with severe pain, and once he is able to assume a position of comfort, he objects very much to being moved at all. There are, of course, all gradations between the two extremes.

Differential Diagnosis Between Lumbosacral and Sacroiliac Lesions.—In the diagnosis of low back strains it is important to decide whether the symptoms are lumbosacral or sacroiliac in origin in order that treatment may be directed to the proper region. It should be pointed out that in certain cases both the lumbosacral and sacroiliac joints are involved and in these cases it is difficult or impossible to determine what proportion of the symptoms are the result of each lesion. In our experience it is not possible from the history to decide whether the pain is sacroiliac or lumbosacral, since either type may present pain in the low back, either type may present radiation of the pain along the distribution of the fifth lumbar and first and second sacral nerves; that is, the posterior and lateral aspects of the buttocks, thigh, and leg. Either type may be chronic in character and either type may be intermittent. Likewise in either type there may be great variation in the degree of disability.

On physical examination it should be remembered that the symptoms vary greatly in different cases, and on different days in the same case, and that the physical findings tend to vary directly with the acuteness of the pain. Either lumbosacral or sacroiliac strain may present a list, usually away from the side of the lesion, but in rare instances it may be toward the side of the lesion. On the other hand, in either type the patient may stand without a list.

In either type there may be muscle spasm and limitation of the motions in the low back when the patient is standing; it may be marked or the movements may be quite free. As a rule, bending the lumbar spine causes the pain. With the patient sitting, limitation of motion in the low back tends to be less in sacroiliac lesions than when standing, while in lumbosacral lesions limitation tends to be about the same with the patient sitting or standing.

The most important point in the differential diagnosis is, we believe, the localization of the acute tenderness. In lumbosacral strains the acute tenderness is most marked just above and mesial to the posterior superior spine of the ilium on the side of the lesion, while in sacroiliac cases the acute tenderness is most marked in the region of the posterior inferior spine and sacrosciatic notch. Either may present tenderness in the buttocks, thigh, or leg along the distribution of the superior gluteal and sciatic nerves.

With the patient supine, compression of the pelvis in either the anteroposterior or lateral plane may or may not elicit pain in sacroiliac lesions, but does not elicit pain in lumbosacral lesions if care is taken not to move the pelvis while applying the pressure.

Straight leg raising is apt to be more limited in an acute sacroiliac than in an acute lumbosacral lesion, but may be limited in either, or it may be free in either. Other movements of the hip, flexion with the knee flexed, internal and external rotation, abduction and adduction and hyperextension, may or may not cause pain, depending upon the severity of the symptoms, but give little evidence as to whether the lesion is lumbosacral or sacroiliac.

On rectal examination in sacroiliac lesions, it is almost always possible to demonstrate acute tenderness over the sacroiliac joint on the side of the lesion, while in lumbosacral lesions this tenderness is not present.

Distinguishing Assumed From Real Symptoms in Low Back Cases sometimes presents a very difficult question, since either the patients or their lawyers learn to imitate fairly well the low back syndromes, and in medicolegal cases may claim a great deal more disability than actually exists. As a rule, a fairly good estimate as to whether the patient is faking or whether he is psychoneurotic can be obtained while taking the history. In the malingerer the symptoms complained of do not fit those of any definite low back syndrome, but the patient frequently complains of symptoms in other parts of the body or of pain being brought on in ways which do not occur in the typical low back cases. Likewise the location of the pain varies from place to place and the pain is apt to be much more widely distributed than occurs in low back injuries.

On the other hand, the above is not always true and some malingerers have learned the clinical picture of low back strains and can give a typical history. The psychoneurotic patient is likely to be apprehensive during the examination and to complain of pain on almost any movement of the back or leg; the pain is not, as a rule, such as would be produced by a given movement in the true low back strain. Frequently the malingerer or psychoneurotic can be trapped by asking leading questions about symptoms and pains which could not be due to low back injuries.

On physical examination in a suspected case it is important for the surgeon to make a careful notation, first of the location of the site of the pain before the examination is started, then to examine the patient standing, noting the degree of movement in the back in flexion and hyperextension and bending to the right or left, carefully noting the location of the pain produced by the various movements. The entire back and buttocks should then be palpated and the tender areas marked with a skin pencil. Then, with the patient sitting, the same examination is repeated. After these findings have been jotted down, the patient is placed supine on the table and straight leg raising and the various hip movements with the knee flexed are carried out, and the locations of the pain and limitations of motion are noted on both sides. The abdomen is palpated and the compression of the pelvis in both the anteroposterior and lateral directions is carried out and the results noted.

The patient is then turned on the face, the knees are flexed, the hips are hyperextended and abducted, and the symptoms are noted. Then the back, buttocks, and legs are again palpated for areas of tenderness; it is to be noted whether or not the tender areas correspond with those found when the patient was standing.

Finally the patient is examined again standing and the findings of the second examination are checked against those of the first.

As a rule, the points of tenderness will be much more widely distributed in a malingerer or a psychoneurotic patient than in a true low back case. Likewise, the points of maximum tenderness will not coincide in the different examinations. A particularly suspicious point is that many of these patients complain of more pain when the hip is flexed with the knee flexed than they do on straight leg raising. Patients with back strains have more limitation and pain on straight leg raising than on flexion of the hip with the knee flexed.

The X-Ray in Low Back Strains.—The x-ray in low back strains is useful largely to rule out congenital anomalies, fractures, disease of the bone, and chronic arthritis and is not, as a rule, of great use in diagnosing the condition as the <u>changes are largely ligamentous and do not show in the picture</u>.

In old disc lesions the x-rays may show narrowing of the disc space, sclerosis of the adjacent bone and thickening of the posterior margins of the bodies of the vertebrae. Normal x-ray findings are the rule in acute disc lesions.

Low Back Strain and Chronic Arthritis

Many of these cases of low back strain present a variable degree of chronic arthritis which is almost always of the hypertrophic type. When confronted with a case of this type, a surgeon who has had much experience usually gives a guarded prognosis, especially in regard to time and completeness of relief of symptoms, because it is quite well known that these cases tend to hang on and become chronic even when properly treated for the acute strain, and that once they become chronic, they are frequently more difficult to relieve than are similar cases in which there is no evidence of arthritis. Consequently, in the very beginning <u>when the x-ray pictures show chronic hypertrophic arthritis, the patient should be treated more conservatively than should a similar case with a normal back.</u> The period of rest should be longer, the amount of support prescribed should be greater, and the resumption of work should be more gradual. In addition to the local treatment to the back, it is important that the surgeon do all that he can to relieve the arthritis. Unfortunately, we have no specific therapy for this type of arthritis, neither do we know its cause.

The matter of focal infection has been so stressed during recent years that it is important for the surgeon to seek and eliminate obvious foci such as abscessed teeth, chronically infected tonsils, constipation, gallbladder, large prostate, chronic sinuses, etc. On the other hand, in our experience it is rare indeed that the adequate treatment or removal of such foci will cure a chronic case of arthritis. Many surgeons report excellent results by putting these patients on a low protein diet. Our experience has not borne out this line of treatment, but we do believe that they should be put on an adequate diet which is high in vitamins. We give them a low fat diet containing relatively large amounts of sweets and starches, lots of green vegetables and fruits, from a pint to a quart of milk a day, two eggs a day, <u>six yeast tablets a day</u>, and, in many instances, we add <u>cod liver oil</u>.

high Protein

Free intestinal elimination is obtained by diet and mineral oil and saline cathartics or castor oil when necessary. We have these patients drink large quantities of water and prescribe hot baths or sweat baths to promote elimination through the skin. The general health must be built up in every way possible, and when they are having pain we give them enough salicylates to obtain relief with rest. We sometimes use aspirin, sometimes sodium salicylate. We sometimes shift to cincophen. The drug therapy is used, not because we believe that it cures, but because it makes the patient more comfortable until the symptoms quiet down. The back strain must be treated just as though no arthritis were present.

Medicolegal Status of Chronic Arthritis in the Low Back.—The question frequently arises as to whether or not the employer should pay compensation over an indefinite period to a workman who has a low back strain and in whom the x-rays show chronic arthritis of the spine. Not only does this question arise, but not infrequently the employer is actually sued and expected to compensate the workman, not only for his low back pain, but also for his arthritis, it being maintained by the workman and his counsel that the arthritis is the result of the injury. Excepting rare sharply localized lesions, the arthritis does not come from a low back strain, and in the great majority of cases the arthritis was present long before the back was injured. Not only is this true, but if x-ray pictures be taken of the entire spine it will be found that the arthritis is not confined to the injured area, but is usually present in other regions as well.

Consequently, the injury is not responsible for the arthritis. On the other hand, not infrequently we believe that we are right in saying that the arthritis is responsible for the injury, because a spine which is affected by hypertrophic arthritis is more liable to injury than is a similar spine which is not arthritic.

It would seem, therefore, that more leniency should be allowed in awarding compensation to low back cases with arthritis than in awarding compensation to similar cases without arthritis. Such is not the case, however, because the courts usually hold that if, through an injury, the patient's condition is rendered worse, the employer is still liable for compensation even though the disease may have been there over a period of years. This being true, it is conceivable that the time will come when applicants for work involving lifting or heavy labor of any kind will be subjected to a physical and x-ray examination, and will not be accepted if their spine shows chronic arthritis. This would not eliminate arthritis of the spine from the employees, because the arthritis may exist for some time before changes occur which can be seen in the x-ray, but it would undoubtedly cut down the number of industrial low back cases, and would also, in all probability, result in a certain amount of saving to the employer. It is questionable whether or not the amount saved would make up for the cost of the routine examination.

On the other hand, it would also lead to the rejection of a large number of workmen who are perfectly able and willing to work and may be expected to render a full day's work over a period of many years to come. This is true because the average man of the heavy type who has done hard manual labor will show some chronic arthritis in the spine by the time he has reached forty-five years of age. We do not believe these men should be rejected even should such examinations be put into force, but they should be given work with the provision that the employer will not be liable beyond a reasonable period of time, say three months, for any disability which may occur incident to any low back strain.

Treatment of Low Back Strains

It must first be decided whether the strain is postural or traumatic, and second, whether it is lumbosacral or sacroiliac in origin. From what has been said it may be seen that a careful history and physical examination will enable the surgeon to make a fairly accurate diagnosis.

Treatment of Postural Low Back Strains.—If the symptoms are purely postural in nature the treatment should consist of postural exercises and support to the low back. Support to relieve pain may be furnished by strapping with adhesive, by corset, or by a low back brace of the Goldthwait type. This brace consists of two steel uprights extending from the level of the trochanter to just below the angles of the scapula, united by three steel crossbars, one at the top, one at the bottom and one just below the iliac crest. This brace has an anterior pad and three straps and is a very good routine brace for all low back cases. In case of a sacroiliac, all that is needed is a belt around the pelvis, since a support higher up cannot affect the sacroiliac joint. One of us (J. A. K.) straps all acute low back lesions, if strapping is indicated, with a cross strapping extending from the lower ribs to the trochanters and for more prolonged support fits them with a corset or wide lumbosacral belt of about the same dimensions and fitted with stays similar to Fig. 362, but narrower in front.

In regard to exercises, those given vary with different surgeons. We use the following, none of which are original with us:

1. Rib Stretching: Lie on the back. Flatten the back. Retract the abdomen, hold, and inhale slowly, pulling the ribs apart. Exhale slowly and relax. Ten times, twice daily.
2. Straight Leg Raising: Lie on the back. Flatten the back. Retract the abdomen. Pull both feet up, turn them in and curl the toes and raise one leg slowly as high as possible, keeping the knees straight. Lower slowly and relax. Ten times each leg alternately, twice daily.
3. Back Stretching: Lie on the back. Flex one or both knees onto the chest pulling it up with the hands. Then straighten the knee and lower the leg slowly and relax. Ten times, each leg alternately, twice daily.
4. Side Stretching: Lie on the back. Place hands on hips. Flatten the back. Retract the abdomen. Inhale slowly raising the right side of the chest as high as possible and pressing down on the right hip. Do not elevate the shoulder. Exhale slowly and relax. Repeat on the left side. Do ten times alternately, twice daily.
5. Knee Flexion: Lie on the back. Flatten the back. Raise both knees to the chest. Then straighten the knees and lower the legs slowly keeping the knees straight. Ten times twice daily.
6. Trunk Exercise: Assume correct standing position with feet parallel and six inches apart. Pull up arches and curl toes, supporting the weight on the outer border of the feet. Place hands directly over head with thumbs clasped and palms forward. Bend slightly forward, then circle to left, slowly bending so that the hands, while extended above the head, describe a circle about eighteen inches in diameter. Ten times. Repeat circle to the right.

Rest in Hyperextension: Lie on the back with pillow crosswise beneath back at the level of the shoulder blades and no pillow beneath the head. Remain in this position for one-half hour after noon and evening meal.

Correct Standing: Back to wall. Head, shoulders, hips, and heels touching. Chin in and chest up with the weight resting on the balls of the feet and feet parallel. Flatten the back, retract the abdomen and stretch tall. Hold this position and walk away. Do at least ten times off and on during the day.

Correct Walking: Walk in the correct standing position with the toes turned slightly inward and the weight resting upon the outer borders of the feet. Cultivate the habit of curling the toes and pull-

ing up the inner side of foot off and on during the day while either
sitting or standing. Also get the habit of pressing downward with
the toes while walking, thus using the forefoot to propel the body
forward.

Correct Sitting: Sit well back in the chair with the head up, chin
in, chest up, and the abdomen retracted. In bending forward, bend
from the hips and avoid slumping at the waist.

In addition to the exercises the patient is directed to sleep on a fracture
bed which has boards between the mattress and the spring to prevent sagging
and if the patient has much pain at night he is directed to use a small pillow
beneath the spine. Local heat in the form of infrared, hot water bag, or an
electric pad may be used to relieve the pain.

Treatment of Traumatic Low Back Strain.—In traumatic cases treatment
is practically the same in the beginning whether one is dealing with a sacroiliac
or a lumbosacral. The primary requisites are rest to the low back with or
without traction and with or without immobilization and with or without
local heat and massage. If one is going to use physiotherapy, one cannot, of
course, strap the back with adhesive. On the other hand, one may use traction
and at the same time immobilize the low back with firm adhesive strapping
or use physiotherapy.

Most of these cases are not treated vigorously in the beginning and we
believe that this is one of the reasons so many of them develop a chronic condition which may persist in spite of treatment over a period of many months
and eventually demand operative fixation of the involved joints in order to
effect a cure. As a matter of fact, many low back strains recover without treatment. For this reason the average surgeon is inclined to take these patients
rather lightly in the beginning and to treat them in some ambulatory manner.
This type of treatment will work in the majority of cases, but it is impossible
in acute cases to decide which ones will get well and which ones will become
chronic. Especially is this true in industrial cases where the patient can claim
compensation, therefore we believe that the patients should have a thorough
physical and x-ray examination and that wherever possible they should be
put to bed with or without traction and kept in bed over a period of at least one
week; thus the injured ligaments are given an opportunity to heal. A quite
successful routine method of handling these patients is to put them to bed immediately in a bed with fracture boards between the mattress and spring, or
they may be put in Fowler's position with the back and knees flexed, and if
the pain is relieved, that is practically all that is necessary. If, however, the
patient is restless and complains of pain, the back should either be strapped
with adhesive (Figs. 355, 356 and 357) or the patient may be given physiotherapy in the form of infra-red or any other form of local heat and massage.

If the pain is still more severe, traction should be applied by Buck's extension to both legs, the foot of the bed being elevated and the body acting as
countertraction. The traction should in the beginning be about eight pounds and
this may gradually be increased to fifteen pounds to each leg. If this does not
give relief, the patient may be immobilized in a plaster-of-Paris jacket with
the lumbar spine flexed.

Certain cases of low back strain, especially those involving the sacroiliac joints, can be relieved by manipulation either without anesthesia or with an anesthetic. The type of manipulation advised varies in different clinics. The usual manipulation is to place the patient under an anesthetic until muscle spasm is relaxed and then perform the movement of straight leg raising; that is, flex the hip while the knee is held straight to at least 90 degrees. In slender patients the flexion can be carried farther. This manipulation stretches the hamstrings and is frequently accompanied by a snap as though some dislocation were being reduced. This snap is, we believe, not produced in the sacroiliac joint, but is due to the head of the femur slipping in the acetabulum. The patient is then turned on the back and the hip is manipulated into hyperextension.

Magnuson (Industrial Surgical Clinics) instead of turning the patient on the back, slides the patient over the edge of the table and sharply hyperextends the hip, thus obtaining the same effect.

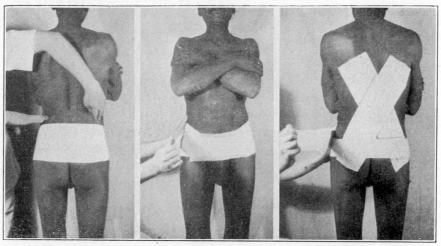

Fig. 355.   Fig. 356.   Fig. 357.

Fig. 355.—Method of strapping the back with adhesive, used in the treatment of acute sacroiliac strains. Note that the strapping is below the brim of the pelvis.

Fig. 356.—Same as preceding seen from front, one of the anterior pieces being applied.

Fig. 357.—One type of adhesive strapping used in the treatment of acute lumbosacral strains. The cross strapping should extend almost up to the axilla.

Conwell's manipulation is shown in the illustrations and consists of traction and countertraction assisted by a direct pressure on the pelvis by the surgeon (Figs. 358, 359 and 360).

II. II. Cox* manipulates the patient without an anesthetic by having him lie prone on a table and grasp the end of the table with his hands while an assistant stands on the table, picks up both feet, and lifts them to such a height that the hips are hyperextended and the pelvis is lifted from the table, the patient's weight being supported by the elbows and abdomen (Fig. 335). The body is held in this manner for several minutes with the legs in abduction and strong traction is made on the legs. The surgeon then makes firm pressure over the sacrum and the body is lifted up and down while the traction is made. He

*Cox, H. H.: Surg. Gynec. and Obst. 45: 637, 1927.

states that there is usually a sudden marked relief as the bones slip into place and that the normal lumbar curvature is in most cases restored at once.

Another type of manipulation is one in which the patient lies upon the side near and facing the edge of the table. With the patient lying upon the right side the right lower extremity is slightly hyperextended on the table and the left lower extremity is moderately flexed and permitted to hang over the edge of the table, thus rotating the pelvis to the right. The left shoulder is then pushed backward with the surgeon's left hand and with his right forearm on the patient's left iliac crest he suddenly pushes the pelvis forcibly downward, tending to rotate the pelvis to the right. This maneuver is re-

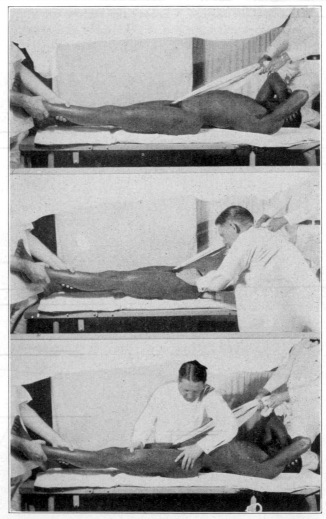

Fig. 358.—Conwell's maneuver for the manipulative reduction of acute sacroiliac strains. General or spinal anesthesia should be administered. Traction on the affected leg and countertraction with a folded sheet on the unaffected groin are carried out. (Noland and Conwell: J. A. M. A., Jan. 18, 1930.)

Fig. 359.—With the traction and countertraction continued the surgeon grasps the crest of the ilium on the affected side between his two hands and pushes it directly downward.

Fig. 360.—If there is inward rotation of the ilium the anterior superior spine is pushed directly outward.

peated on the opposite side. It is not very painful and can be done without an anesthetic. It is frequently accompanied by a crunching sound and may relieve the pain. It may be performed on the floor (Fig. 361). This maneuver was demonstrated to one of us (J. A. K.) about 20 years ago by Dr. Ned Bull of San Francisco and it, plus forcible hyperflexion of the knees on the chest and gradual hyperextension, are the only manipulations which he uses. All are done without anesthesia.

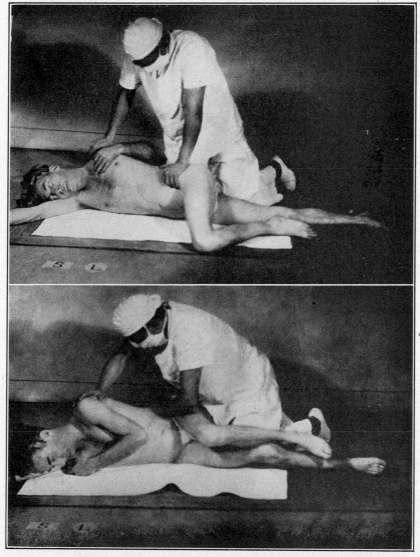

Fig. 361.—The rotary manipulation of the low back affecting both the sacroiliac and the lumbosacral joints used in the treatment of acute low back strain, presumably sacroiliac. In the top figure the wing of the ilium is pushed forward and downward and in the bottom figure it is pushed backward and downward. (Courtesy Dr. Frederick Jostes.)

After manipulation the low back is strapped firmly with adhesive. In patients in whom the manipulation is performed under general anesthesia the patient is then placed in bed for one week with a small pillow under the lumbar spine. He is then permitted up with a supporting belt with a sacral pad which is worn down low on the pelvis. The belt is worn for six months and can be removed at night, provided a small pillow is kept beneath the lumbar spine.

After any patient with acute low back strain is got up from the preliminary one or two weeks' rest in bed with immobilization, he should be given support. In the case of lumbosacral strain the support may be a wide canvas belt with steel stays or a low back brace of the Goldthwait type, or a heavy corset in cases in women (Figs. 362 and 363). In a sacroiliac strain all that is necessary is a narrow belt around the pelvis as illustrated in Fig. 343. If desired this may be fitted with a sacral pad. In most cases the support should be worn from three to six months.

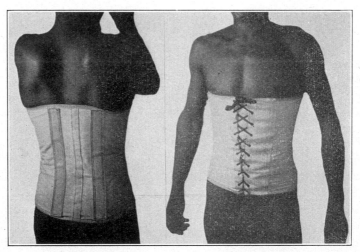

Fig. 362.   Fig. 363.

Fig. 362.—Canvas belt with steel staves used in treatment of lumbosacral strains.
Fig. 363.—Same as preceding seen from the front.

Treatment of Chronic and Recurrent Low Back Strains.—These cases are the bane of the industrial and orthopedic surgeon. The majority of them, however, can be relieved by exercises and support or by manipulation. We have not found that manipulation does any appreciable good in lumbosacral cases, neither have we found that it is of much value in the treatment of cases complicated by chronic arthritis.

As a rule, the treatment must be determined by the degree of disability and by the patient's status. Most of the cases must be treated in the ambulatory manner, because, first, rest in bed does not relieve the condition although it may relieve the symptoms while the patient is in bed, and second, most of the patients cannot or will not submit to hospital treatment.

If the pain is lumbosacral we prescribe either a wide heavy canvas belt, corset, or low back brace and give the patient postural exercises. If the pain is sacroiliac we do the same thing or use a narrow belt with the provision that **we may manipulate the joint either with or without an anesthetic if the pain is not relieved by the support.**

Under a course of postural exercises and moderate support, most cases gradually get well. Occasionally, however, symptoms may persist over a period of many months, and many patients may be completely and permanently disabled from resuming laborious occupations. Consequently in a small percentage of select cases, we believe that operative intervention is justified. The great difficulty is to decide absolutely whether the symptoms are sacroiliac or lumbosacral, since it does little good to arthrodese the sacroiliac joint for lumbosacral pain and vice versa. Consequently after a series of careful examinations a definite decision must be made by the surgeon before operation can be advised.

If repeated examination leads to a definite diagnosis of sacroiliac symptoms and the lumbosacral region can be eliminated with a fair degree of certainty, we believe that in these chronic cases the surgeon is justified in recommending arthrodesis of one or both sacroiliac joints, depending upon whether one or both of these joints is the cause of the symptoms. If the diagnosis is correct and if the operation is properly performed, the patient should obtain complete relief and be able to return to his original occupation in about four months. The sacroiliac joint may be arthrodesed by the method of Smith-Petersen.

In this operation the posterolateral surface of the ilium is exposed through a curved or straight incision and the sacroiliac joint is opened by cutting a window through the ilium opposite the joint. This plug of bone is then removed and the cartilage is cut from its deep (articular) surface. The window is then extended into the opposite side of the joint, that is, the sacrum, by removing the exposed portion of the sacrum, and the plug of bone from the ilium is driven in across the joint so that it firmly locks the two articular surfaces together.

After the operation, the patient's back and sacroiliac region are strapped with adhesive and the patient should remain in bed for about eight weeks. At the end of this time he may be permitted up with a sacroiliac belt and may gradually increase his activities until he is strong enough to go back to work.

If the symptoms are lumbosacral, and the sacroiliac joints can be excluded with a fair degree of certainty, the surgeon should recommend lumbosacral fusion. This can be done by the method of Hibbs as described above under Old Fractures of the Spine. After the operation the patient should remain in bed over a period of approximately eight weeks, when he may be got up with a high back brace which he should wear from three to four months.

In a certain percentage of cases both the sacroiliac and the lumbosacral regions are involved and in these cases it may be necessary to arthrodese both joints, but the most painful joint should be treated first with the hope that the rest in bed during the convalescence will result in a cure of the less troublesome joint.

Recently acquired knowledge of the symptoms caused by rupture and retropulsion of the nucleus pulposus makes it necessary that this condition be ruled out by physical and neurologic examinations and usually by spinograms before fusion of either the sacroiliac or the lumbosacral joint is recommended. Many surgeons now feel that the terms *sacroiliac* and *lumbosacral* strain should be discontinued, because it is their belief that the symptoms usually attributed to these conditions are caused by lesions of the intervertebral disc. One of us (J. A. K.) believes that all of these cases are due to intervertebral disc lesions and has discontinued sacroiliac or lumbosacral fusions except for definite disease (tuberculosis) or spondylolisthesis and operated upon the intervertebral disc instead.

LESIONS OF THE INTERVERTEBRAL DISCS

While it has been known for some years that an intervertebral disc might be ruptured and occasional cases have been reported in which cartilaginous material, presumably a new growth from the disc, protruded into the spinal canal and caused nerve root pain, it was not until recently that the work of Mixter and Barr demonstrated that the rupture of the posterior portion of the annulus fibrosus with retropulsion of some of the semiliquid nucleus pulposus was a fairly common cause of low back pain and sciatica and that these symptoms could be relieved by surgical removal of the displaced portion of the disc. They further demonstrated that the outline of the displaced material from the disc could be shown in the roentgenogram of the spinal canal after the injection of radiopaque oil. Since their original report the subject has been studied in many clinics, and it has been demonstrated repeatedly that this is a clinical entity which must be taken into consideration in the diagnosis of any case of chronic low back pain with or without sciatica.

Pathology.—The intervertebral disc which is placed between the body of each vertebra consists of a central semiliquid portion, the nucleus pulposus. This is separated from the cancellous bone of the vertebrae by thin plates of cartilage and bone and is surrounded by a fibrous ring, the annulus fibrosus. This fuses with the anterior and posterior common ligaments of the spine and is attached to the margins of the bodies of the vertebrae above and below. Due to degenerative changes or to injury, which may be a severe compression or a flexion strain, the posterior portion of this annulus fibrosus may be weakened or ruptured. When this occurs, the semiliquid nucleus pulposus material may be forced out from between the bodies of the vertebra and protrude into the spinal canal and may press upon and cause either friction or pressure neuritis in the root of the nerve which makes its exit from the spinal canal at the level of the protrusion. The protrusions which cause symptoms are usually those which are in the posterolateral portion of the disc and press upon the nerve root where it makes its exit from the spinal canal, and in this area the nerve is compressed between the displaced nucleus pulposus substance and the ligamentum flavum or the wall of the intervertebral canal.

Diagnosis.—A tentative diagnosis of a rupture of the annulus fibrosus with retropulsion of the nucleus pulposus is made from the history and the physical examination and is confirmed and localized by the spinogram or by operation. In a typical case the history and physical findings are so typical that many patients are operated upon successfully without resorting to a spinogram.

The condition is most common in active young adults and is about three times as frequent in men as it is in women, as would be expected if it is traumatic in origin. A history of an injury can be obtained in over half of the cases; in others the rupture occurs from the stress and strain of ordinary life and degenerative changes are a factor. This injury may be a fall on the feet or buttocks or the pain may arise during lifting or it may be caused by a sudden twist or awkward movement of the low back. In over half of the cases which are traumatic in origin, the pain follows the injury immediately. In others the onset of symptoms is delayed for a variable period of time. A not infrequent history is that the patient, while lifting, feels a sudden pain and sometimes a snap in the low back. This is followed by moderate pain in the lumbosacral region which is not sharply localized, but spreads outward on either side and down over the buttocks. The pain persists and increases in degree and in the extent of its radiation. Sciatic pain may come on immediately, but more often it makes its appearance one or two days, or even some weeks, later. In other patients, and these are usually the ones in the older age bracket, the pain begins gradually and with no known cause, and the patient can recall no known injury which may have accounted for the symptoms.

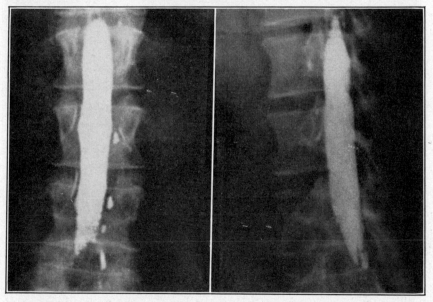

Fig. 364.—Anteroposterior and oblique views of a normal subarachnoid space in the lumbar region filled with lipiodol. Note uniform space opposite levels of the intervertebral discs. (Courtesy Dr. W. G. Scott.)

A characteristic feature in the histories of these patients is that the patient may have had several similar attacks—that is, the symptoms tend to be intermittent and may disappear entirely for a period of months or years, only to reappear again either with or without a subsequent injury. The pain resembles that of other low back strains of the traumatic type in that it is aggravated by movement, it is usually, but not always, relieved by rest, it tends to be unilateral, and the distribution varies considerably.

In approximately 90 per cent of patients with intervertebral disc lesions the rupture and displacement occur at the levels of the fourth and fifth lumbar vertebrae. The pain is nearly always present in the lumbosacral region of the low back and in the distribution of the sciatic nerve. The back pain is usually unilateral, but may be bilateral, and in these cases it tends to be more severe on the side of the lesion. It may be referred to the buttock, but is usually referred down the back of the thigh and to the lateral and posterior surface of the leg. In some patients the back pain subsides and only the sciatic pain persists.

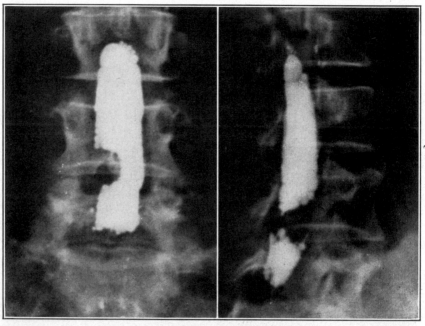

Fig. 365.—Unusually large protuberance of the nucleus pulposus between L4 and L5, antero-posterior and oblique views. (Courtesy Dr. W. G. Scott.)

The quality of the pain is not characteristic. It is variously described as a dull ache, a sharp shooting pain, or a burning pain. There is considerable variation in the degree and extent of the pain, and this also varies from week to week and may disappear entirely without known cause, or it may persist for weeks or months and confine the patient to bed in spite of various methods of conservative treatment. The pain is aggravated by bending, sneezing, straining or coughing, and sometimes by flexing the head on the neck. In cases of long standing there is apt to be some paresthesia and numbness in the distribution of the fourth and fifth lumbar and first sacral nerves. There also may be noted weakness of the leg and atrophy of the muscles of the thigh, and sphincter disturbances may be present. Rarely the symptoms are bilateral.

Physical Examination.—The condition found on physical examination will vary with the symptoms. The patient may walk in with no limp and give a history of pain in the low back and down one or the other leg in the sciatic distribution, but at the time of the examination he may have relatively few symptoms. On the other hand, a patient when first seen may have the lumbar spine rigidly fixed by muscle spasm and stand with a flat back and with a sciatic scoliosis or list to one side, have great difficulty in walking or bending in any direction, and suffer severe pain both in the back and down the posterior thigh and leg on the slightest movement, or bending may be normal for the individual and cause very little pain.

On palpation there may be marked spasm of all of the lumbar muscles and acute tenderness on pressure over the lumbosacral region and over the sacroiliac region—that is, between the spinous processes in this area of the spine and over the buttocks, posterior thigh and calf. With the patient sitting, forward bending may or may not be more free, depending upon the acuteness of the symptoms. With the patient lying on the back, tension on the sciatic nerve produced either by straight leg raising or by extending the knee after the hip has been flexed will nearly always cause pain and the movement of the leg will be limited. The degree of pain and the extent of the limitation of motion vary with the acuteness of the symptoms. Compression of the pelvis and flexion of the hip with the knee flexed, and also rotation and abduction of the hip, usually do not cause pain unless the patient is in a very acute stage.

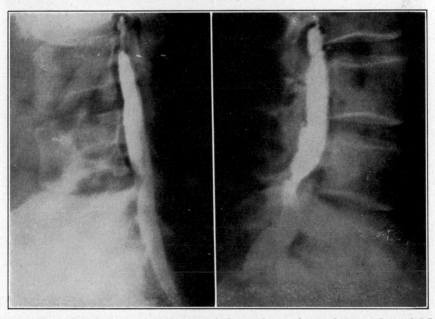

Fig. 366.—Lateral views of protrusion of the nucleus pulposus between L4 and L5. On the left in flexion which almost reduces the protrusion and on the right the spine is in hyperextension and the protrusion is increased. (Courtesy Dr. W. G. Scott.)

With the patient prone hyperextension of the hip may cause pain both in the sciatic region and in the low back. Likewise, palpation of the sciatic nerve may reveal acute tenderness. Nearly always there is tenderness on deep pressure over the lumbosacral joint on the affected side and usually over the interspinous ligament at the level of the lesion. There may be tenderness on deep pressure over the buttocks below and lateral to the posteroinferior spine of the ilium. Likewise, the lower end of the sacroiliac joint may be tender in this area. Ober's test for a tight iliotibial band may be positive.

On neurologic examination the knee jerks are usually normal. The ankle jerk on the affected side is diminished or absent in over half of the cases. The hamstring reflex may be diminished. Sensory examination will reveal hypesthesia in the distribution of the fourth and fifth lumbar and first sacral nerves in a considerable number of cases, especially where the condition is of long standing. Likewise, in long-standing cases there may be definite muscle atrophy and muscle weakness both in the thigh and in the calf muscles. The pain may be aggravated or produced by jugular compression (Naffziger's sign), and this is evidence of an intraspinal lesion.

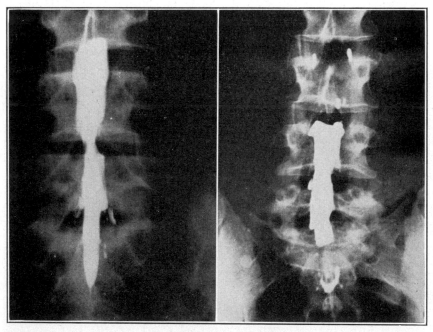

Fig. 367.—On left, bilateral protrusion of the nucleus pulposus between L4 and L5. On right, double unilateral protrusion on the right side between L4 and L5 and between L5 and S1. (Courtesy Dr. W. G. Scott.)

From what has been said above, it is obvious that the clinical picture and history presented by the patient with lesions of the intervertebral disc are similar to those presented by patients with traumatic low back strains of the lumbosacral or sacroiliac type, as discussed in previous sections. So similar is the picture that often it is not possible to make the differential diagnosis without a spinogram, and the frequency with which lesions of the intervertebral disc are suspected and found will vary directly with the interest of the examining physician. That is to say, if a physician is a neurologist or neurologic surgeon, he will find a good many more patients suffering from intervertebral disc lesions than will an orthopedic surgeon, and so true is this that many neurologic surgeons now believe that the conditions known as sacroiliac and lumbosacral strains no longer exist and that practically all of these patients with low back pain and sciatica are suffering from lesions of the intervertebral discs, and one of us (J. A. K.) concurs in this opinion.

On the other hand, many orthopedic surgeons believe that most of these patients with low back pain with or without sciatica can be relieved by conservative treatment and that it is probable that most of them are suffering from ligamentous strain, either of the sacroiliac or of the lumbosacral joint or fascial lesions, and they reserve the diagnosis of a rupture and retropulsion of the intervertebral disc to those patients who prove refractile to conservative treatment. Orthopedic surgeons, however, have reached the point where they do have lumbar punctures done on patients who do not respond promptly to conservative treatment and whose symptoms and physical signs suggest an intervertebral disc lesion. This is especially true in those cases which present definite neurologic signs—that is, absence or diminution of the ankle jerk and paresthesia and hypesthesia in the distribution of the sciatic nerve.

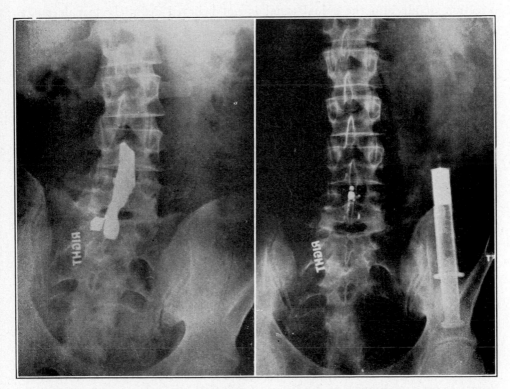

Fig. 368.—Anteroposterior view showing large unilateral intraspinal protrusion of intervertebral disc between L5 and S1 with the needle in place. On the right is shown the lipiodol which has been removed in the syringe and a very small amount of lipiodol remaining in the spinal canal. (Courtesy Dr. W. G. Scott.)

Examination of the Spinal Fluid.—From the lumbar puncture the only abnormal finding to be expected is an increase in the total protein of the spinal fluid. If the total protein is found to be over 40 mgm. per 100 c.c. of spinal fluid, it is further evidence that an intervertebral disc lesion is present. On the other hand, if the total protein is under 40 mgm. per 100 per cent, an intervertebral disc lesion may or may not be present. The increase in spinal fluid protein is found in about 60 per cent of the cases.

X-ray Examination.—Routine x-ray examination of the spine in the anteroposterior and lateral views as a rule shows nothing to account for the symptoms. Occasionally, in cases of long standing there is a narrowing of the intervertebral disc in the area responsible for the pain. However, this is so inconstant and appears so often without being accompanied by the symptoms of a ruptured intervertebral disc that it is not considered to be of diagnostic value. The only x-ray examination that is of importance in the diagnosis of an intervertebral disc lesion is intraspinal myelography with a contrast medium (air or iodized oil may be used).

Air is of practical value only in thin patients and even then the image is less sharp than with the intraspinal iodized oil, or lipiodol, and requires interpretation by an expert in the air technic. A negative finding after the injection of air into the spinal canal is not believed definitely to rule out a disc lesion.

The injection of iodized oil in the spinal canal carries with it the danger that a mild leptomeningitis may result, because the oil if present for a long time is a mild irritant, and it becomes widely diffused through the spinal canal and may extend down the sheaths of the nerve roots for a considerable distance. This is of importance in medicolegal cases in which the patient may believe that the oil caused an aggravation of the symptoms or produced new symptoms. As a matter of fact, there is very little evidence to the effect that the oil, when left in the canal for a long time, causes any symptoms whatever, and it is believed that examination with lipiodol is the method of choice until something better has been found to take its place. Certainly it is the most accurate method which we now have for the diagnosis and localization of these lesions.

During the past few years a technic for the injection and the subsequent removal of the oil immediately after the x-ray examination has been devised by Kubie and Hampton; it is believed that this should be done when possible. This method is illustrated in Fig. 368 and will be mentioned below. The lumbar puncture is done with the patient in the prone position and the needle is inserted between the third and fourth lumbar vertebrae—that is, in the deepest part of the dorsal concavity of the lumbar spine. This needle is equipped with a special stylet with a blunt point and about $\frac{1}{16}$ of an inch longer than the needle. When the needle enters the dura 10 c.c. of spinal fluid is removed for examination and from 3 to 5 c.c. of lipiodol is slowly injected into the spinal canal, and the stylet is replaced in the needle and it is left in situ. The patient is then placed on a tilting table in the prone position and is examined under the fluoroscope while the oil is permitted to flow up and down in the spinal canal. Likewise, the patient may be tilted to the right or left in order that oblique views of the spinal canal may be obtained. When the opaque material flowing over the projecting nucleus pulposus shows a defect in the outline of the spinal canal a spot film is made in this position. The patient is examined in the anteroposterior and oblique and lateral positions.

After the examination is completed, the patient is again placed in the prone position to permit the lipiodol to puddle around the needle. The special stylet with a blunt point and 1/16 of an inch longer than the needle is then pushed inward until the stylet touches the anterior wall of the dural sheath. This will cause the stylet to project slightly from the base of the needle. The stylet is then withdrawn and the syringe is attached to the needle, and the lipiodol is slowly withdrawn into the syringe. As a rule, it is possible to recover almost the entire amount. When this is done, it eliminates the objection of leaving the oil in the canal, and we believe that this is a great improvement over the original technic.

The outline of the defects varies considerably in size and in shape, as can be seen from the accompanying illustrations. Likewise, more than one intervertebral protrusion may be present. These may be two on one side, or they may be bilateral. Multiple disc lesions have been found in about 15 per cent of the patients operated upon.

As stated above, one of us (J. A. K.) believes that in practically all of these patients with idiopathic low back pain or low back strain the lesion is in the disc. He accepts and has repeatedly confirmed the facts reported by Dandy, that many of these discs are concealed (soft and perhaps protruding but not ruptured) and are not shown by intraspinal myelography. Consequently, in his practice this is used only in an exceptional case. As a rule a diagnosis can be made by the history and physical examination and a spinogram is not necessary.

Treatment.—The treatment of lesions of the intervertebral discs in the low back is first the conservative treatment of low back strain by rest, support, manipulation and postural exercises as described above. One of us (J. A. K.) now believes that the conditions which he formerly diagnosed lumbosacral strain or sacroiliac or subluxation are really lesions of the intervertebral discs and these lesions may cause low back pain with or without sciatic pain. The conservative treatment of these conditions is about the same as in the past.

When conservative treatment fails and the symptoms are so troublesome that the patient is disabled or demands relief from pain, operative treatment should be considered. The difference is that now the operation is directed at the removal of the protruding disc or discs and lumbosacral or sacroiliac fusions are no longer performed for the relief of low back pain unless spondylolisthesis is present, and in many cases of spondylolisthesis it is believed that the symptoms are due to a disc lesion and not to the spondylolisthesis.

In operating for the relief of low back pain the surgeon should localize the protruding disc or discs as accurately as possible by the history and physical examination and should then explore the spinal canal with the expectation of finding and removing the cause of the pain. In order to accomplish this both skill and experience are necessary. Consequently the operation is not to be undertaken lightly. It is to be emphasized that Dandy's concealed discs are relatively frequent causes of persistent low back and sciatic pain and that multiple disc protrusions are more frequent than is commonly known. For this reason it is often necessary to remove two and sometimes necessary to remove three protruding intervertebral discs before relief is obtained. The operation is really an exploration of the spinal canal in the lumbosacral region.

In some clinics the operation for removal of a ruptured or bulging intervertebral disc is combined with lumbosacral fusion in certain instances. This has not been satisfactory in the hands of one of us (J. A. K.). If the intraspinal cause of the trouble is removed fusion is not necessary and if it is not removed fusion is futile. This opinion may be modified by further experience.

Prognosis.—About 90 per cent of the patients are relieved by conservative treatment. In about 10 per cent operation is indicated. Of those operated upon about 70 per cent are completely relieved or markedly improved and about 25 per cent moderately improved. In a few patients little or no relief is obtained. Many of these should be reoperated upon and a further attempt should be made to find and remove the cause of the pain and disability.

CHAPTER XIV

FRACTURES AND DISLOCATIONS OF THE HYOID, LARYNX, AND TRACHEAL CARTILAGES

FRACTURES OF THE HYOID BONE

Surgical Anatomy

The hyoid is a small U-shaped bone which lies between the base of the tongue and the larynx and is not in contact with any other bone. It consists of a central body which is elongated transversely and has greater and lesser horns on each side. It gives origin to much of the musculature of the tongue, and by virtue of its suspension from the skull, supports this organ and the larynx.

Mechanism and Pathology

Fractures of the hyoid bone are very rare, but occasionally occur as a result of direct violence—direct blows, throttling, or attempts at suicide by hanging. They are frequently associated with fractures or injuries of the larynx. The fracture of the hyoid usually occurs at the junction of one of the greater horns with the body, but may involve the body itself.

Diagnosis

With the history of an injury in this region followed by acute pain and swelling and accompanied by difficulty in swallowing and talking and inability to protrude the tongue, a fracture of the hyoid should be suspected. There may be attacks of suffocation or dyspnea and the fracture may be complicated by a rupture of the larynx or trachea with resulting subcutaneous emphysema. The fracture may be visible in the x-ray (Fig. 369).

DISLOCATION OF THE HYOID BONE

Instead of being broken, the bone may be dislocated from the same type of violence as results in fractures or the dislocation may result from attempts to swallow large bodies, such as a large piece of meat. If the dislocating force is from the outside, the major horn is displaced inward; and if from the inside, as in swallowing, it is displaced downward against the superior horn of the thyroid cartilage. In cases with dislocation there is marked difficulty in swallowing but the voice and respiration need not be affected. It should be possible to detect the displacement by palpation.

Treatment

With fracture the treatment is symptomatic, since displacement is, as a rule, not important, and if reduction be accomplished, there is no means of maintaining it. Dislocation should be reduced either by hyperextending the head and depressing the jaw or by direct pressure over the displaced greater

459

horn. In obstinate cases it may be necessary for the surgeon to insert his fingers into the mouth and make pressure downward and forward against the displaced fragment. In instances complicated by severe injuries to the larynx or trachea there may be edema of the glottis, and immediate tracheotomy may be necessary.

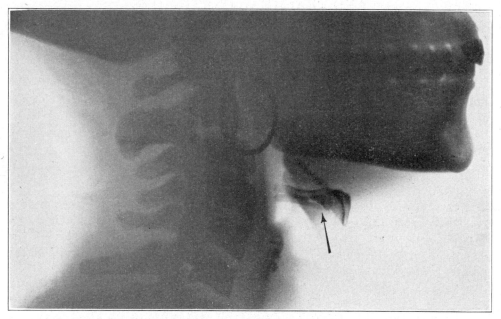

Fig. 369.—Fracture of the hyoid bone which healed without undue complications.

FRACTURE OF THE LARYNX AND TRACHEAL CARTILAGES

The mechanism of these rare fractures is similar to that of fractures of the hyoid. They are important because of the respiratory complications which may ensue and should be regarded as grave injuries which carry a guarded prognosis.

Diagnosis

There is a history of direct injury to the neck, followed by acute pain and spasmodic coughing with cyanosis and the expectoration of frothy blood. Swallowing is painful, and the voice may be hoarse or it may be impossible for the patient to speak. In cases in which there is a rupture extending from within the larynx or trachea into the adjacent tissues, subcutaneous emphysema may be a prominent feature and may demand tracheotomy. On palpation there is extreme tenderness over the injured area and a soft cartilaginous crepitus may be obtained. With acute edema there may be marked respiratory difficulty, and immediate tracheotomy may be necessary. The fracture may be visible in the x-ray (Fig. 370).

Treatment

Treatment is in most cases symptomatic. The most important point is that in severe cases tracheotomy may be necessary at any time and preparations should be made to perform this operation on short notice. In uncomplicated cases, the application of cold may serve to keep down swelling, or a soft bandage or cotton pad reinforced by a bandage and of such volume that it makes a dressing about an inch thick, extending from the base of the neck to the angles of the jaws, may serve as a very comfortable splint (a mild Thomas collar). It not only tends to immobilize the neck, but also tends to decrease the swelling and emphysema.

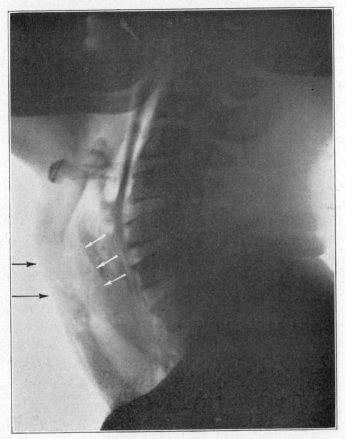

Fig. 370.—Subcutaneous emphysema following rupture of trachea from fall against edge of step. Tracheotomy necessary.

Attempts at reduction of the displacement are as a rule not advisable, since they may result in increasing edema or hemorrhage into the trachea and lungs. Such attempts may be made, however, at the time a tracheotomy is performed if this should become necessary. In some instances infection begins around the fracture and spreads into the soft tissues of the neck and demands incision and drainage. In some patients who recover, there may be a variable degree of disturbance in the voice due either to scar tissue formation around the vocal cords or to stenosis of the larynx.

CHAPTER XV

INJURIES OF THE THORAX

SURGICAL ANATOMY

The thorax is an expansile truncated cone which constitutes the upper part of the trunk and serves to contain and protect the lungs, heart, and great vessels as well as the structures passing between the neck and the abdomen. It is bound posteriorly by the twelve thoracic vertebra and the posterior portions of the ribs, laterally by the middle portions of the ribs and anteriorly by the sternum, costal cartilages and anterior portions of the ribs (Figs. 371 and 372).

The Ribs

A typical rib is a long, slender, curved, elastic bone which presents a head, neck, tubercle, and shaft. There are twelve ribs on each side. All are attached to the spine posteriorly and the upper seven are attached to the sternum anteriorly by means of costal cartilages, while the anterior ends of the eighth, ninth, and tenth are attached to the cartilage of the seventh rib. The anterior ends of the last two ribs are not fixed; hence, they are called "floating ribs."

The head presents two articular facets for the bodies of the corresponding dorsal vertebrae and the tubercle presents an articular facet for the transverse process of the corresponding vertebra. The neck is the compressed portion of the rib between the head and the tubercle, and the shaft is the continuation of the rib around the body to its anterior extremity where it unites with the costal cartilage. The shaft is flattened and smooth on its inner surface and roughened on its outer surface. In direction it first runs backward and outward and then twists downward and forward at the angle and after it crosses the midaxillary line it curves inward toward the midline of the chest.

The Sternum

The sternum, or breastbone, is a broad flat plate of bone which lies in the midline of the chest. It is divided into an upper portion, the manubrium sterni, a middle portion or body, the gladiolus, and an inferior portion or tip, the ensiform cartilage. The manubrium is thickened and presents facets for articulation with the clavicles. On its upper border there is a notch, the interclavicular notch. The body presents articulations on either side for the costal cartilages of the second to the eighth ribs. The ensiform cartilage is a small wedge-shaped cartilaginous plate which projects downward from the lower end of the body of the sternum. The manubrium is usually united to the body by a synchondrosis, but in adult life this joint may ossify. The upper portion of the body is marked by a prominent transverse ridge, the sternal angle which is an important landmark as it is at the same level the second costal chondral junction.

The Costal Cartilages

The costal cartilages are flat plates of hyaline cartilage which serve as prolongations of the anterior ends of the ribs and unite these bones to the sternum. The first costal cartilage is continuous with the manubrium sterni, while the second to the eighth costal cartilages are united to the sternum by true joints. The eighth, ninth and tenth costal cartilages are united to the costal cartilages of the seventh rib by fibrous tissue.

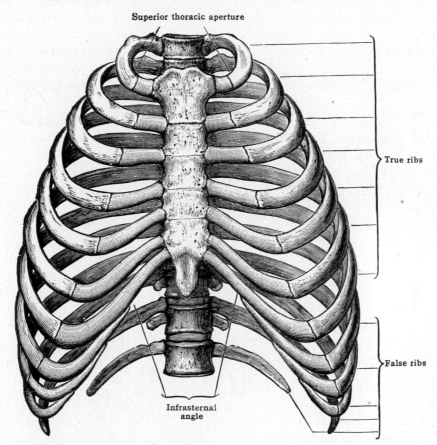

Superior thoracic aperture

True ribs

False ribs

Infrasternal angle

Fig. 371.—The thorax, front view. (From Morris: *Human Anatomy*, P. Blakiston's Son & Co., Inc., Publishers.)

FRACTURES OF THE RIBS

Fractures of the ribs are relatively frequent injuries and tend to be multiple, while double fractures may occur; that is, several ribs may be broken at one time or one or more ribs may be broken in two or more places. Not only are these fractures frequent as isolated injuries, but they are also relatively frequent complications of other severe fractures, particularly those due to falls or crushing injuries or to automobile accidents. Because of the great elasticity of the ribs in children, fractures of these bones are relatively rare below the age of puberty, but they may occur in severe crushing accidents.

Mechanism and Causes of Fractures of the Ribs.—Ribs may be fractured either by direct or indirect violence, and occasionally by muscular action, as from a cough or sneeze or from laughing. In fractures which are the result of direct violence, the fragments tend to be driven inward into the pleural cavity and may not only rupture the parietal pleura, but also penetrate the visceral pleura and damage the lung. These fractures tend to occur at the point of impact of the fracturing force and in such instances the extent of the displacement and the number of ribs broken vary directly with the degree of the force and with the size of the area subjected to direct trauma. (Figs. 373 and 374.)

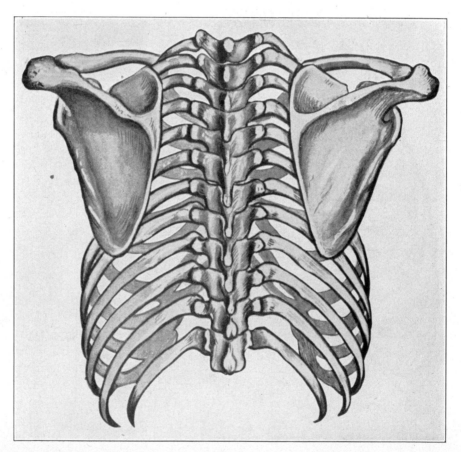

Fig. 372.—The thorax, back view. (Morris, *Human Anatomy*, P. Blakiston's Son & Co., Publishers.)

Fractures due to indirect violence are usually the result of crushing injuries to the chest or of severe blows in which the fracturing force is distributed over a considerable area, so that the ribs are bent inward at the point of impact and tend to break from being bent, the break usually occurring just in front of the angle of the rib (Figs. 375 and 376). In these indirect fractures the ends of the fragments tend to be forced outward and the pleura is not ruptured unless there is considerable displacement. The mechanism of a double fracture is usually a fracture from direct violence at the point of impact and fracture from indirect violence near the angle of the same rib.

Pathology of Fractures of the Ribs.—Greenstick fractures may occur in children and subperiosteal or incomplete fractures may occur in adults where the fracturing force is not sufficient to cause displacement. As a rule, however, most rib fractures occur in adults and the fractures are complete and may be comminuted. The plane of the fracture may be transverse, oblique, or irregular; and if complete displacement occurs, a small amount of overriding is the rule. In fractures in which several ribs are involved, and especially if these are double fractures, the side of the chest may be flattened or even caved in (Fig. 377).

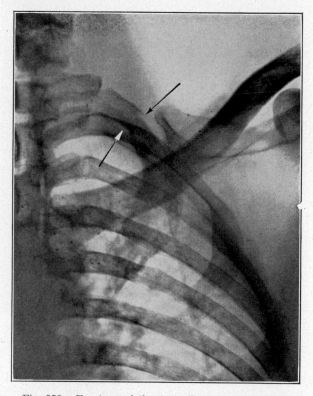

Fig. 373.—Fracture of the first rib; a rare fracture.

Compound fractures, with the exception of those due to gunshot wounds, are quite rare, but may occur, and in such instances the corresponding side of the chest is usually opened by the wound (Fig. 378). The first two ribs are rarely broken because they are protected by the shoulder and clavicle, and the last two are rarely broken because their distal extremity is free and may be moved widely in any direction before a fracture can occur. The majority of fractures involve the fifth to the ninth rib.

Diagnosis of Fractures of the Ribs.—There is usually a history of an injury either of a fall against the corner of a table or some other object or of a blow or crushing injury to the chest, followed by a sharp pain in the side. The pain persists and the patient is able to localize the pain very exactly; if the fracture is at all severe, the patient tends to lean to the affected side and support and immobilize the area of the fracture with the hands (Fig. 379). The breathing is shallow; deep breathing causes sharp pain in the chest, which is particularly aggravated by coughing, sneezing or laughing.

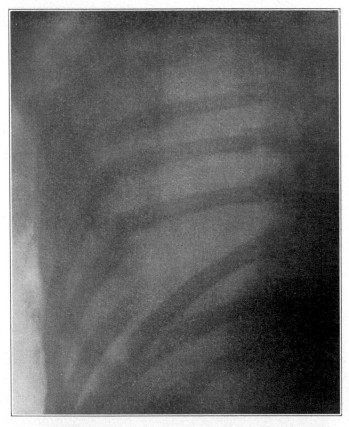

Fig. 374.—Multiple and double fractures of the ribs with wide separation. Treated by rest in bed; semireclining, no strapping, morphine gr. ⅙ when necessary, and local dry heat, with no attempt to reduce the fractures. Good results.

On physical examination there may or may not be localized swelling and evidences of contusions and lacerations of the skin. The patient should first be asked to localize with the fingers the points of greatest pain. Then the surgeon should place one hand on the back of the chest well away from the painful area and the other hand on the front of the chest and gently compress the chest by springing the anterior extremity of the ribs inward (Fig. 380). If there is a fracture, this maneuver will elicit sharp pain at the site. The surgeon should then palpate the ribs in the painful area, beginning in the front and working backward on the chest until the point of fracture tenderness is reached (Fig. 381). If displacement is present and the patient is not too fat, it may be possible to palpate the ends of one or more fragments.

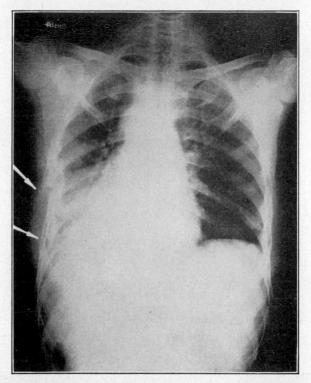

Fig. 375.— Chest film taken at six-foot distance to bring out fractures of the ribs in the axillary line.

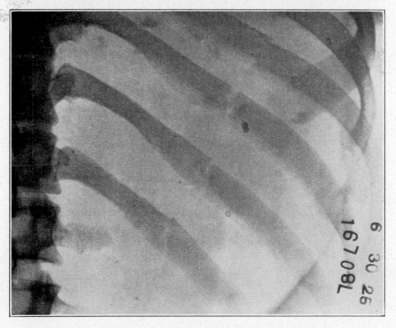

Fig. 376.—Fractures of the four lower ribs. Treated by strapping with adhesive. Good resluts in seven weeks.

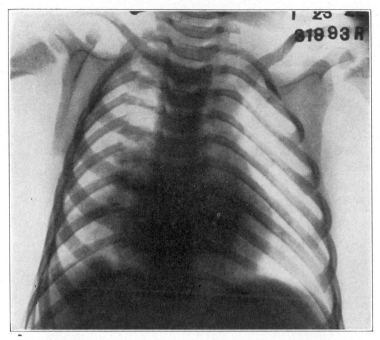

Fig. 377.—Multiple fractures of the ribs in a child run over by an automobile. Chest was double strapped forty-eight hours after the injury, when the patient had recovered from the shock. Good results in three months.

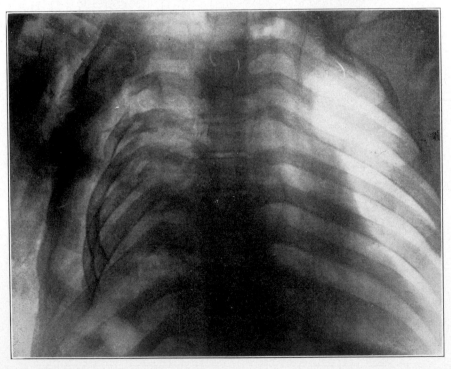

Fig. 378.—Compound multiple fractures of the ribs with the side of the chest open by a large wound. Treated by débridement under local anesthesia and partial suture of chest wound followed by irrigation of soft structures with Dakin's solution. Good result fourteen weeks following injury, although no attempt was made to reduce the displacement in the rib fractures. No strapping.

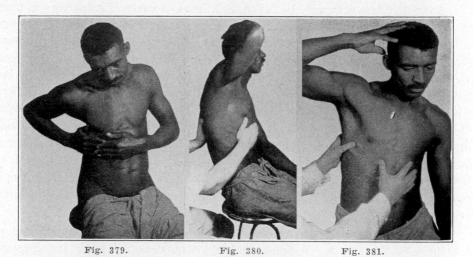

Fig. 379.   Fig. 380.   Fig. 381.

Fig. 379.—A patient with multiple fractures of the ribs showing posture assumed by the patient in an effort to relax and splint the side of the chest.

Fig. 380.—Examination of patient with suspected fracture of the rib. By pressing the two hands together the side of the chest is sprung and pain is elicited at the point of the fracture.

Fig. 381.—Palpation in order to determine points of maximum tenderness in a patient with a fracture of the rib.

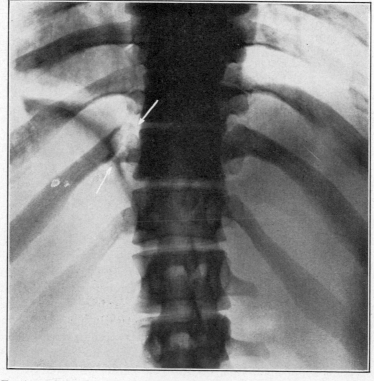

Fig. 382.—Fracture of the eleventh rib near its attachment to the spine. Treated by strapping with adhesive.

An x-ray should usually be taken, and in most cases if a fracture is present it can be seen in good anteroposterior x-ray pictures of the chest. However, if the fracture is in the region of the axillary line, the anteroposterior picture may not show it. If the anteroposterior picture is negative a lateral or oblique view should be made. This will not only show the lateral aspects of the ribs, but will also show the dorsal vertebrae, and it should be remembered that a patient with pain along a costal margin may be suffering from a compression fracture of the body of one of the dorsal vertebra. Even if the x-ray is negative, a fracture of the rib should be diagnosed with persistent pain and point tenderness and localized pain on compression of the chest, and the patient should be treated for the fractured rib regardless of the x-ray findings. A stethoscopic examination of the chest should be done to determine the possibility of pleural or lung injury.

Complications of Chest Injuries.—In many instances the complications of fractures of the ribs are a great deal more important than is the fracture itself, since they concern injuries to the lung, pleura, and intercostal arteries. In addition to the surgical shock which is present in all severe injuries (Fig. 383), and fractures of other bones which may be present (Fig. 384), chest injuries are subject to the following complications:

1. Massive collapse of the lung.
2. Pneumothorax.
3. Interstitial or surgical emphysema.
4. Hemothorax.
5. Hemorrhage into the lung.
6. Empyema.
7. Traumatic asphyxia or cyanosis.
8. Paralytic ileus.
9. Contusion of the heart.

In severe injuries to the chest, where several ribs are broken, the patient is usually in a state of considerable shock, which may be the dominant feature of the picture, while the injuries of the bone are of relatively little importance and may be ignored until the shock is combated.

1. Massive Collapse of the Lung.—(Figs. 385, 386, 387, 388, and 389.) Massive collapse of the lung is a condition which occasionally follows surgical operations or injuries to other parts of the body or may follow an injury to the chest. Two types are described by Sante.* The first type is one with sudden onset, dyspnea, rapid pulse, fever and a moderate leucocytosis. Cyanosis may or may not be present or there may or may not be profuse mucopurulent sputum. In the second type collapse occurs with practically no chest symptoms or cardiac or respiratory embarrassment, and the pulmonary condition is discovered accidentally. The mechanism is unknown and does not seem to be dependent upon a pneumothorax, because the chest wall is drawn in and the diaphragm elevated and the mediastinum drawn over to compensate for the space occupied by the collapsed lung (negative pressure in the pleural cavity).

---

*Sante: J. A. M. A. 88: 1539, 1927.

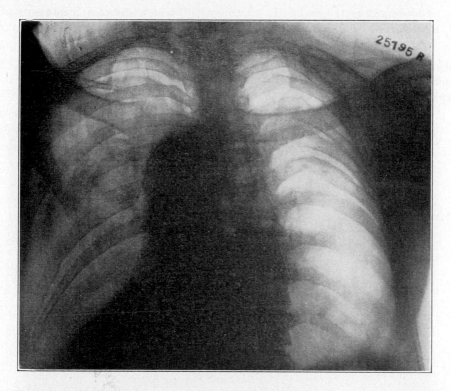

Fig. 383.—Multiple fractures of the ribs on both sides of the chest. Initial treatment for shock and adhesive strapping four days later, on the right side. No strapping on left chest with good result thirteen weeks following injury.

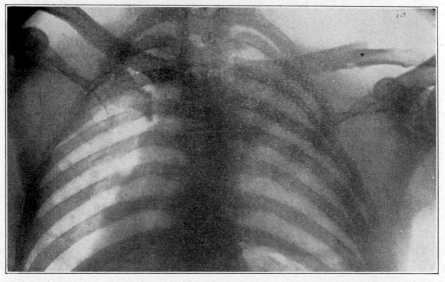

Fig. 384.—Fractures of the five upper ribs with fracture of the clavicle. Treated by double strapping with adhesive over the shoulders. Good results in eight weeks.

The diagnosis is best made by the x-ray, which shows the dense shadow of the collapsed lung and the rest of the pleural cavity empty.

Sante states that the most efficient treatment is to roll the patient back and forth on the involved side; this usually reestablishes aeration of the lung. The condition, if unilateral, is rarely fatal and usually lasts from ten days to three weeks.

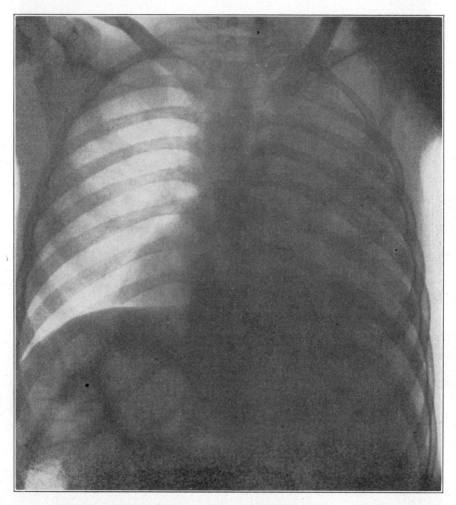

Fig. 385.—This photograph shows a massive collapse of the lung following a contusion of the chest as result of an automobile accident. Patient admitted to the hospital immediately after injury, developed the collapse about thirty-six hours following injury. Patient recovered without any complication within ten days. Lung cleared up entirely.

2. **Pneumothorax.**—In pneumothorax the pleural cavity is filled with air, which may have been drawn in through an opening in the chest wall or may have entered the pleural cavity through some injury of the lung. As the air enters the pleural cavity, the lung on that side collapses unless it is fixed to the chest wall by adhesions. The presence of a pneumothorax is suggested by respiratory embarrassment and displacement of the mediastinum to the opposite side. It is diagnosed by the presence of a tympanitic percussion note

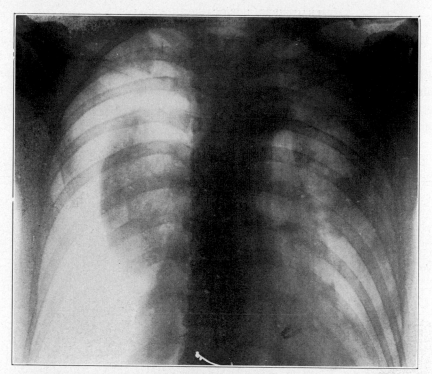

Fig. 386.—Collapse (pneumothorax from within) of the left lung following a contusion of the chest in which no fracture was demonstrated. There was very slight immediate disability and the patient was sent home, but a physician was called twenty-four hours later, when the patient was in a severe state of shock with air hunger, rapid pulse, and respiration.

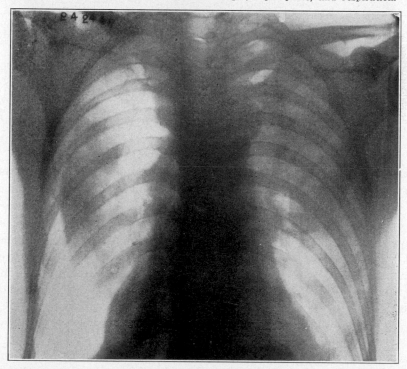

Fig. 387.—Same case as preceding. Partial expansion of the lung following aspiration of the chest with a suction machine. Air escaped through the needle when it entered the pleural cavity, and the patient's condition was much improved. Later aspiration by 50 c.c. syringe was followed by complete expansion of the lung.

over the area occupied by the air. If the air is under positive pressure, as may occur in either a wound of the lung in which there may be a valve effect so that the air is forced out into the pleural cavity on inspiration and cannot enter the lung on expiration, or a similar wound in the chest wall; the pressure may be so great as to seriously impair respiration and cause respiratory embarrassment and cyanosis.

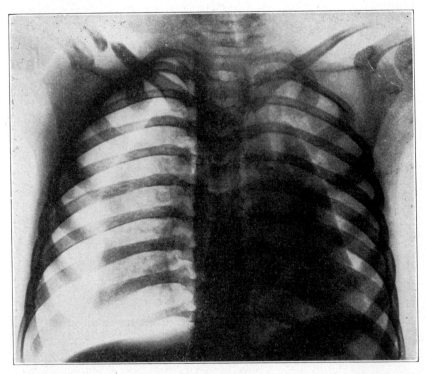

Fig. 388.—Bilateral collapse of the lungs in a child following a severe injury with contusions of the chest and fracture of the clavicle. The patient died from shock four hours after the injury.

In instances in which the positive pressure in the pleural cavity is the cause of respiratory embarrassment, the symptoms may be relieved by aspirating the chest and it may be advisable to suck out as much of the remaining air as possible. In two cases we have inserted a needle in the chest and the positive pressure in the thorax was so great that the plunger of the Luer syringe was shot out of the barrel and landed on the floor some distance away. The aspiration was followed by immediate relief of the respiratory embarrassment. One of us (H. E. C.) has used a sucking machine in these cases. Elkins* inserts a catheter into the pleural cavity and submerges the other end of the tube in a jar of water. The positive pressure in the chest forces the air out through the tube and the water prevents air being drawn into the tube during inspiration.

3. **Interstitial or Surgical Emphysema.**—Not infrequently in fractures of the ribs with pneumothorax, the air is forced out into the tissues of the chest

*Elkins: Southern Med. J. 28: 4, 1935.

wall through the rent in the parietal pleura and interstitial emphysema may occur. As a rule this interstitial emphysema is not marked in degree or of much importance. It can be recognized by soft crepitus when the involved area is palpated. In occasional cases the degree of emphysema may be very marked and the air may spread up and down the chest wall, into the neck, involve the face and even involve the extremities and cause considerable pain and discomfort. In instances where it is very marked, small incisions through the skin may be made under antiseptic precautions in order to relieve the tension. As a rule the opening in the chest or in the lung heals and the air in the tissues is gradually absorbed.

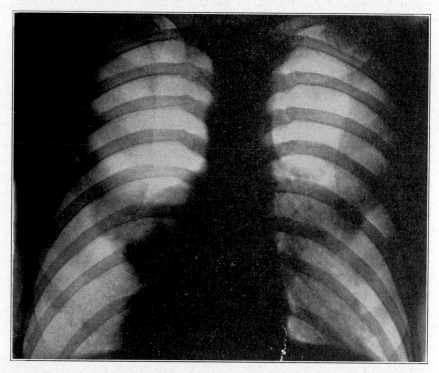

Fig. 389.—Bilateral collapse of the lungs (pneumothorax from within) following a contusion of the chest in an automobile accident. Recovery under conservative treatment, no aspiration; rest in bed with sedatives. Returned to work two months after the injury.

A very dangerous type of interstitial emphysema and one that is difficult to combat is one in which a bronchus is torn or ruptured and in which the air escapes into the tissue of the lung itself rather than into the chest wall and then travels up the mediastinum and into the neck; in this type expectant and supportive treatment are all that one can administer.

4. **Hemothorax.**—Hemothorax is blood in the pleural cavity. It may be due either to a tear or rupture of the lung or to an injury of an intercostal artery or vein. In simple fractures of the ribs hemothorax is rarely a troublesome feature, but it may occur; in compound fractures due to gunshot wounds it is practically always present. The amount of blood, however, is usually small and need cause no concern, but in some instances the amount of blood

may be considerable or even fatal hemorrhage may occur when a large vessel is injured.

Blood in the pleural cavity does not clot as it does in other localities, but tends to be absorbed. Consequently, it should not be aspirated unless the amount is sufficient to cause respiratory embarrassment. If after two or three weeks, however, physical examination should reveal the fact that a considerable amount of blood is present in the pleural cavity, it should be aspirated.

If the patient is exsanguinated, transfusion is, of course, in order. It is usually wise, however, to defer the transfusion until one believes that the bleeding has stopped; otherwise the transfusion may cause the bleeding to continue and necessitate aspiration to relieve respiratory embarrassment. In cases with evidence of severe hemorrhage, operative intervention should be undertaken to stop the hemorrhage. Before exploring the pleural cavity, the chest wall should be investigated, since the hemorrhage may be from an intercostal or internal mammary artery.

It should be remembered that when air is present in the pleural cavity some blood is also present and that hemopneumothorax is more frequent than either pneumothorax or hemothorax.

5. Hemorrhage into the Lung may occur as a result of a blow or compression of the chest even without a fracture of the ribs. The symptoms arise immediately after the injury and consist of severe pain deep in the chest, dyspnea, and a rapid, weak pulse. According to Sante the x-ray picture reveals a definite haziness of the involved area with large irregular blotchy areas of increased density.

6. Empyema.—Empyema or pus in the pleural cavity may result from any compound fracture of the ribs, one due to a bullet wound or one due to direct violence, or the infection may occur in a simple fracture of the ribs, the bacteria being transmitted through a tear in the lungs. Fortunately the pleura has a high resistance to infection, and infection in traumatic hemothorax is rare. The clinical findings are fever, leucocytosis, general toxemia and the physical signs of fluid in the chest.

The treatment is rib resection and drainage at the most dependent point.

7. Traumatic Asphyxia or Cyanosis (Fig. 390) occasionally follows severe compression of the abdomen or thorax or of both with complete or partial cessation of respiration for a variable period of time. It is characterized by a vivid blood red coloration of the conjunctivae and a purple coloration of the face, upper chest and upper arms. The color of the skin varies from violet or purple to black and is due to minute petechiae. The coloration of the conjunctivae is the result of subconjunctival hemorrhages. Apparently the condition is due to sudden backward pressure of the blood in the veins of the affected areas.

Unless the patient dies as a result of the injuries sustained at the time of the accident, the discoloration gradually disappears in from ten to twenty days, the conjunctivae being the last tissues to clear up. Permanent damage to the eyes and even blindness from optic atrophy have been recorded as sequelae in certain severe cases.

8. Paralytic Ileus.—Paralytic ileus is a rare, but occasionally a very severe, complication of rib fractures. For this reason the gastrointestinal tract should receive particular attention in these cases and free movements of the bowels should be maintained during the first few days after the injury.

9. Contusion of the Heart.—The heart, being placed between the spine and sternum, is apt to be compressed in chest injuries in which the force is applied to the front of the chest, as in steering wheel accidents, and may be contused or even ruptured. Beck* has reported three cases. With severe rupture of the heart sudden death would occur. With contusion precordial pain and surgical shock are the prominent symptoms. The treatment is symptomatic with rest in bed until the circulation is normal.

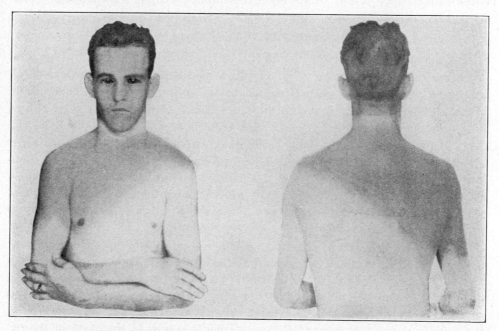

Fig. 390.—Case of traumatic asphyxia. Patient recovered.

Prognosis of Fractures of the Ribs.—The prognosis in fractures of the ribs must include a consideration of the fracture itself and the injury to the patient as a whole. The fractures practically always heal despite the fact that it is not possible to immobilize the fragments. If the fragments are displaced, healing takes place with deformity and not infrequently synostosis may occur between two or more ribs. In spite of the deformity, the functional result is practically always good. (Fig. 398.)

The general prognosis depends upon the severity of the injury including any complications which may arise, and the general condition of the patient. In old persons the prognosis is less favorable than in young, because they are more apt to succumb to respiratory infections. In extensive multiple fractures of the ribs there is always some damage to the intrathoracic viscera and these

*Beck: J. A. M. A., January, 1935, p. 109.

injuries are accompanied by considerable shock. Consequently the complications mentioned above are apt to ensue and may cause death.

The prognosis in these severely crushed chests is always grave during the first few days after the injury; if the patient survives the initial shock and hemorrhage, there is still the danger of empyema.

Treatment of Fractures of the Ribs

Just as in the prognosis, treatment of fractures of the ribs must be divided into the treatment of the fracture and the treatment of the patient. Consideration of the patient should come first, because the treatment of the fracture is of secondary importance and its only objective is to make the patient more comfortable, since it has relatively little influence upon the healing of the fracture.

Treatment of the Patient

In severe chest injuries with multiple fractures of the ribs, the general condition of the patient should be the first consideration and surgical shock should be combated. These patients do better and are more comfortable and breathe easier if kept in a sitting or semi-sitting position. Enough morphine should be given to keep them quiet. External heat should be applied in sufficient amounts to bring the body temperature to normal. If there are signs of exsanguination, transfusion may be considered; but with extensive bleeding into the pleural cavity, transfusion should be delayed as long as possible. Otherwise it will simply serve to increase the intrathoracic hemorrhage and result in respiratory embarrassment. In this type of case the decision as to whether or not to use transfusion is a very delicate one.

In gunshot wounds of the chest nothing should be done except to treat the patient along the lines mentioned above and apply an antiseptic dressing to the external wound or excise the wound and suture it under local anesthesia. A sucking wound should always be excised and sutured with drainage. It is very bad practice to attempt to remove a bullet from the lung or anywhere in the chest in these cases, since the attempt usually results in the death of the patient, whereas conservative treatment will result in the saving of many of these patients. Severe or persistent hemorrhage should be sought and stopped by operation, the chest wall being examined first and the chest being opened widely only when the bleeding has been found not to be from the chest wall.

If there is a compound fracture with a gaping wound in the chest, it is advisable to excise and suture the wound under local anesthesia.

If extensive multiple fractures of the ribs are present and the side of the chest is caved in, strapping with adhesive is usually to be avoided, since it serves to increase the pain and respiratory distress. It is always a good rule to remove strapping immediately if the patient is not more comfortable and if the general condition is not better after the adhesive has been applied. In such cases no dressing at all or the heavy muslin swathe or elastic stockinet bandage as described below under Management of the Breast in Women, should be used.

Treatment of Simple Fractures of the Ribs

Most patients with simple or minor multiple fractures of the ribs are more comfortable and do better if the chest is strapped (Fig. 391). This is particularly true of fractures below the fourth rib. In fractures of the upper four ribs, patients get along almost as well without strapping and sometimes are more comfortable. Horizontal strapping, especially, proves ineffective; however, in certain fractures of the upper ribs, vertical strapping over the shoulder and down the back may be of distinct advantage and may make the patient much more comfortable.

Method of Strapping the Chest.—Two distinct sets of adhesive are used; one vertical, the object of which is to hold the ribs up; the other, horizontal, the object of which is to hold the ribs down. The two opposing forces tend to limit respiratory excursion and to immobilize the fragments. (Fig. 392.)

If x-ray and physical examination discloses relatively transverse fractures with overriding of the fragments, an attempt may be made to reduce them by direct pressure while the patient inspires as fully as possible. But such attempts are, as a rule, not successful and should not be persisted in unless the reduction is effected with relative ease, because the displacement does not interfere with the prognosis, and attempts at reduction may injure the pleura.

The chest wall is cleaned with soap and water if it is dirty. Then it is shaved and washed with alcohol and ether. Two strips of adhesive three inches wide and long enough to extend from the lower back across the shoulder and down on the abdomen, and shorter strips of a length to extend about two-thirds of the distance around the chest and sufficient in number to cover the lateral chest wall are then prepared. Some surgeons carry the adhesive entirely around the chest.

The patient assumes the sitting posture with his arms at his side. He is instructed to take as full an inspiration as possible and to hold his breath with the chest elevated. The operator then applies the vertical strips, beginning low lown on the back, pulling the adhesive upward across the shoulder and then down to the front of the injured side of the chest as far as the upper abdomen, the skin being pulled upward. The second strip is applied at a slightly different angle from the first, but in the same manner. The arms are now elevated and the patient is told to expire as fully as possible and to hold his breath with the chest in expiration. Then, beginning at the lower ribs and slightly beyond the midline in the back, the operator applies the first strip of adhesive from behind forward; it should extend slightly across the midline in front. It is pulled tightly; then the second and third, and if necessary, fourth or fifth strips are applied in the same manner from below upward and from behind forward, each overlapping the one below by about an inch. Immobilization is more complete if the adhesive encircles the chest; this is advisable in some cases. If the nipple is covered by the adhesive, it should be protected by gauze or cotton.

At the end of four or five days the adhesive will have become loose and rather inefficient. It should be reinforced by fresh adhesive over the old, applied in the same manner. The old adhesive should, if possible, be left on

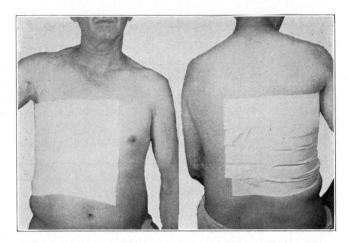

Fig. 391.—Usual method of strapping the chest with the chest contracted in fractures of the lower eight ribs. Note that adhesive extends slightly beyond the midline of the chest in front and back and is applied from below upward.

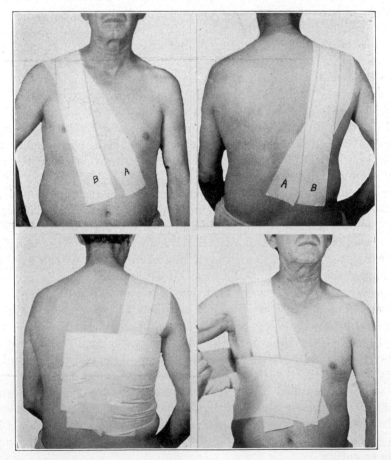

Fig. 392.—Double strapping of the chest in more severe fractures of the ribs and in fractures of the upper ribs. The vertical straps over the shoulder are applied with the chest in a position of full expansion, while the horizontal straps are applied to the chest in a position of full contraction.

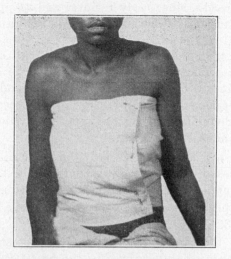

Fig. 393.—Binder used in treatment of fractures of the ribs in obese individuals and in persons with skin sensitive to adhesive, and in severe fractures of the ribs in which strapping with adhesive is not advisable.

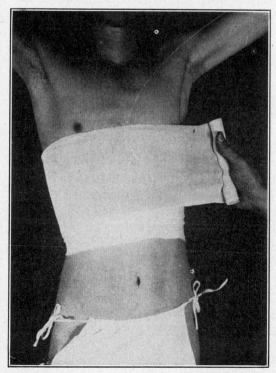

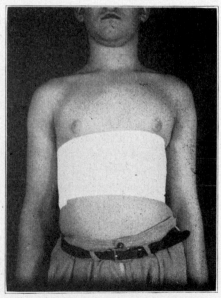

Fig. 394.   Fig. 395.

Fig. 394.—Application of a six- or eight-inch woven elastic bandage around the lower chest for comfort in fractures of the ribs. Adhesive may be used in the same manner for fractures at any level.

Fig. 395.—Circular strapping of the lower chest for fractures of the ribs at any level.

for ten days or two weeks, since early removal and reapplication of adhesive not only causes pain and discomfort to the patient, but also results in increased irritation of the skin. At the end of ten days or two weeks it will probably be necessary to remove the adhesive and reapply it. This should not, however, be done until it is necessary. New adhesive should be applied in the same manner after the skin has been washed with alcohol and ether. At the end of four weeks, strapping will in most cases not be necessary, since the ribs will be fairly well immobilized by callus and the patient will be more comfortable without the adhesive.

One of us (J. A. K.) usually straps only the lower ribs—that is, below the breast—and the adhesive goes entirely around the chest. This is done even for fractures of the upper ribs. In severe injuries with multiple fractures infiltration of the fractured areas with novocain will relieve the pain and respiratory distress. (Fig. 394.)

Management of the Breast in Women.—In women, and especially in obese women with large pendulous breasts, the breast is a nuisance and prevents efficient strapping of the chest, and only the lower part of the chest can be strapped. The natural thing to do is to elevate the breast and extend the adhesive up over its lower portion. But when this is done, the breast drops down over the edge of the adhesive and within a few hours the patient is very uncomfortable and demands that the adhesive be removed. In such cases if the breasts are held up with a tight brassiere the adhesive can be extended slightly higher, but here the lower margin of the breast should be protected by cotton or gauze pads.

A large, heavy muslin binder which can be pinned tightly around the chest (Fig. 393) proves much more comfortable and effective. Even better than the binder is a stockinet bandage applied to the chest quite firmly. This bandage, which is very elastic, is made by splitting stockinet used next to the skin under plaster-of-Paris casts. A four-inch strip makes an eight-inch bandage—a good width. It should be wound round and round from the lower chest upward and over one or both shoulders, until enough is applied to give the patient some comfort and a feeling of security.

Patients with simple fractures involving only one rib and whose general condition is good need not be confined to bed at all. On the other hand, patients with severe fractures must, of course, be kept in bed in a semireclining position until their general condition warrants allowing them up, first in a chair and then on their feet. In a simple fracture of one or two ribs the side may be expected to be painful and tender from four to eight weeks after the injury, and the patient may be expected to experience pain when lifting or applying force in any other manner with the arm on that side over about the same period. If the patient is troubled with a cough, a sedative cough mixture strong enough and given often enough to afford quick relief should be prescribed.

DISLOCATION OF THE RIBS AT THE VERTEBRA

Dislocation of the ribs at the vertebra is a very rare injury, but may occur as a result of severe direct violence, one or more ribs being torn off from their intervertebral attachment. The symptoms are similar to those of a fracture of the rib in its posterior portion, and the differential diagnosis can be made by means of the x-ray.

The treatment is the same as that for a simple fracture of the rib, and open reduction should not be considered, while attempts at manipulative reduction are usually futile. The prognosis is good after conservative treatment even though the dislocation is not reduced.

FRACTURES AND DISLOCATIONS OF THE COSTAL CARTILAGES

The mechanism of the injuries of the costal cartilages is the same as that of fractures of the ribs, the costal cartilage fractures tending to occur more frequently in young adults, while the rib fractures occur more frequently in patients over thirty years of age. One or more ribs may be separated from its cartilage at its costochondral junction; the cartilage may be dislocated from its attachment to the sternum; the cartilage may be broken across at any point; or two cartilages may be separated from one another.

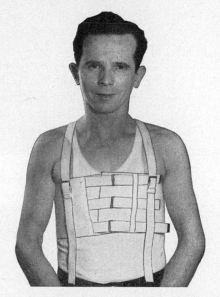

Fig. 396.—Zimmer rib splint. (Courtesy of Zimmer Manufacturing Co.)

The symptoms are similar to those of a fracture of the rib, except that the localizing symptoms point to a lesion in the area occupied by the costal cartilage. It is important to remember that unless they have become calcified, the costal cartilages are not visible in the x-ray picture; consequently, in most instances, the diagnosis of a fracture of a costal cartilage must be made from the history and physical findings, and the x-ray should not be expected to show the lesion. If there is obvious dislocation with deformity, attempts may be made to reduce the dislocation or displacement by having the patient inspire fully while the shoulders are drawn backward by assistants and the surgeon manipulates the displaced cartilage, and by direct pressure attempts to restore the normal contour of the chest. Whether or not the displacement is re-

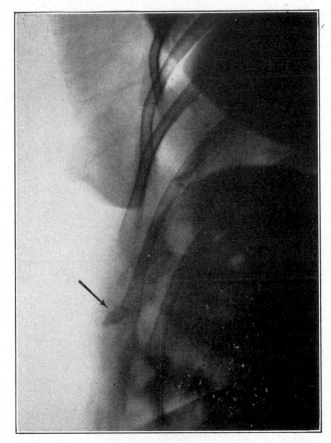

Fig. 397.—Fracture of a calcified costal cartilage following severe coughing seizure. Treated by strapping with adhesive and physiotherapy, with good result.

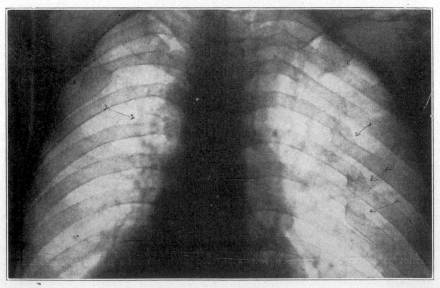

Fig. 398.—Old multiple fractures of the ribs in a man eighty-one years of age treated by double adhesive strapping. Healed with deformity, but with no impairment of function.

duced the prognosis is good, since, even in cases which have healed with considerable deformity, there is rarely any functional disability.

After the reduction or attempted reduction, the chest should be strapped by cross-strapping of adhesive as described under "Strapping of Fractures of the Ribs."

Slipping Rib.—Occasionally after a fracture or dislocation of a costal cartilage, firm union may not occur and the cartilage may slip with certain movements and be the cause of considerable pain. The symptoms can be relieved by resecting the end of the offending cartilage under local or general anesthesia.

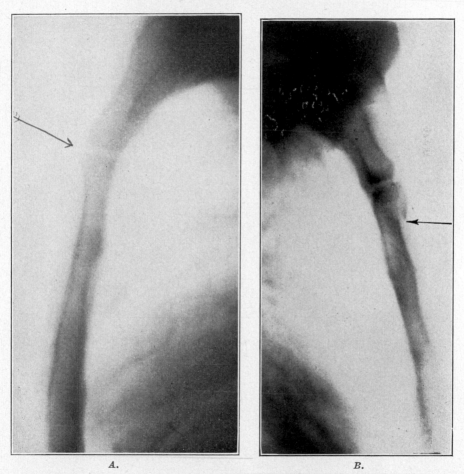

A.   *B.*

Fig. 399.—*A.* Separation at junction of manubrium with gladiolus of the sternum. Treated by ambulatory dressing with adhesive strapping pad with good result.
B. Fracture of the sternum. Treated as described in the text.

FRACTURES OF THE STERNUM

Fracture of the sternum is a rare injury, but it may occur either as a result of direct violence, as in blows upon the front of the chest, from crushing injuries, or from hyperflexion injuries, such as result in compression fractures of the spine.

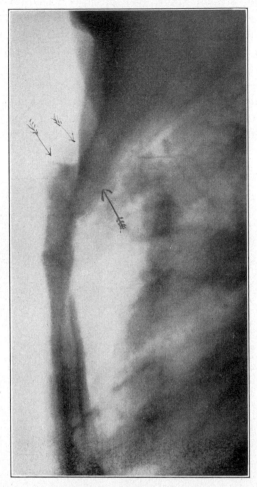

Fig. 400.—Fracture of the sternum with anterior displacement of the lower fragment. Treated by manipulative reduction followed by immobilization in recumbency, with sandbag on chest. Good result.

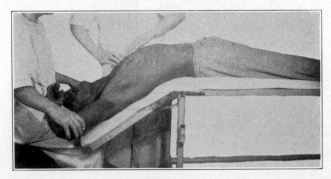

Fig. 401.—Position of patient and method of manipulating fragments in reducing a fracture dislocation of the sternum.

Pathology.—The majority of the fractures occur in the body of the bone near its junction with the manubrium or there may be a separation of the synchondrosis between the manubrium and the body (Fig. 399A). The line of fracture is usually transverse, but it may be oblique, while vertical fractures are almost unknown.

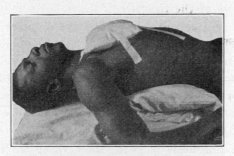

Fig. 402.—Position of patient with pillow under shoulders and sandbag strapped over sternum.

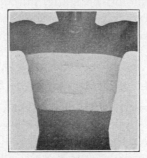

Fig. 403.—Adhesive strapping across chest with thick felt par over the injury as applied in ambulatory dressings in fractures of the sternum.

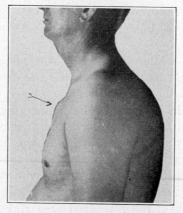

Fig. 404.—Old fracture dislocation of the sternum which united without reduction of the displacement. Recovery with slight deformity and no disability.

When displacement occurs, the lower fragment is usually displaced forward, and its upper end overrides the lower end of the upper fragment (Fig. 400). The periosteum on the posterior surface is reinforced by the intrathoracic ligaments and is rarely torn.

Diagnosis.—There is a history of injury to the chest with pain localized over the sternum. A moderate amount of swelling is present, and if displacement has occurred, the swelling may be considerable. The patient tends to assume an attitude with the head and shoulders drooped forward, respiration is shallow, and deep respiration and coughing or sneezing are accompanied by intense pain at the site of the fracture.

On palpation it may be possible to feel the displaced fragments and determine the displacement, and mobility of the fragments may be observed during breathing. In case a fracture of the sternum without displacement is suspected, the diagnosis can be confirmed by an x-ray picture, which should be taken in the lateral plane. It will show any displacement as well as the line of fracture. Anteroposterior x-rays of the chest are useless in the diagnosis of fractures of the sternum.

Prognosis.—The prognosis is good, since these fractures, being through cancellous bone, tend to heal rapidly. If deformity is present, an attempt to reduce it by manipulation should be made, but open reduction need not be resorted to, since even if the fracture heals with overlapping, the functional prognosis is good, although there may be some visible deformity on the front of the chest. (Fig. 404.)

Treatment of Fractures of the Sternum

If there is no displacement of the fragments, the patient should simply be placed in bed with a small pillow under the shoulders and a small sandbag on the front of the chest over the sternum (Fig. 402). The sandbag serves to immobilize the fragments more securely than does any form of adhesive dressing yet devised. It may be strapped on the chest with adhesive. This position should be maintained for from two to three weeks, at the end of which time the patient may be got up with a cross-strapping over a felt pad over the site of the fracture (Fig. 403) and a posterior figure-of-eight bandage on the shoulders.

Reduction.—Where displacement and overriding of the fragments are present, an attempt should be made to reduce the displacement. This is most satisfactorily accomplished if the patient is placed in a position of hyperextension as illustrated in Fig. 401. The hyperextension should involve particularly the cervical and upper thoracic spine. Likewise, the arms should be placed above the head and the shoulders drawn backward. If necessary, traction should be used with countertraction on the feet. With the patient in this position, the surgeon should attempt by downward pressure on the upper end of the lower fragment to push it backward into its normal position. If this is very painful the fractured area may be anesthetized by infiltration with novocaine, but a general anesthetic should not be given. If it is found to be impossible to reduce the displacement by the closed method the fracture may be exposed (preferably under local anesthesia), and the depressed fragment can be levered up into place, but this is not necessary for a good functional result.

The aftertreatment is the same as that described above.

CHAPTER XVI

INJURIES IN THE REGION OF THE SHOULDER GIRDLE AND SHOULDER

SURGICAL ANATOMY

The Shoulder Girdle.—The shoulder girdle, which serves to attach the upper limbs to the trunk, is formed by the scapulae and clavicles. It is open behind, but it is closed in front by the upper end of the sternum with which the inner ends of the clavicles articulate.

The Clavicle is a long doubly curved bone which is placed almost horizontally at the upper and anterior part of the thorax immediately above the first rib and serves as a prop to support the shoulder and hold it away from the chest wall (Fig. 405). The inner two-thirds are roughly cylindrical in shape and the outer third is flattened from above downward. The mesial half of the bone is convex forward, and the lateral third is concave forward. The enlarged mesial or sternal extremity articulates with the manubrium sterni while the outer or acromial end articulates with the mesial border of the acromion. The bone is subcutaneous throughout its length, and lies in the plane between the sternomastoid and anterior part of the trapezius muscles above and the pectoralis major and anterior part of the deltoid below.

Scapula.—The scapula is a large irregular bone the chief function of which is to serve as a socket for the humerus and to furnish leverage for the attachment of muscles which move the arm and the shoulder. It is attached to the trunk entirely by muscles except for its articulation with the clavicle. It consists of a body, head, neck, spine, acromion, and coracoid process.

The body is a large thin triangular plate of bone which is strengthened by a thickening of its borders and is slightly convex backward to conform roughly to the contour of the thorax. Its posterior surface is divided into infraspinous and supraspinous fossae by the spine, which is a triangular plate of bone projecting backward and upward from the posterior surface of the body and lying in the plane between the posterior portions of the trapezius and deltoid muscles. It extends transversely across the upper third of the bone, and its outer extremity is thickened, flattened, and curved forward to form the acromion which is the summit of the shoulder. The mesial border of the acromion presents an elongated facet which articulates with the clavicle.

The head of the scapula presents a concave articular surface, the glenoid, which is directed outward and forms a shallow socket for the head of the humerus. It is situated directly beneath the acromion and attached to the upper portion of the thickened inner border of the body by a short constricted neck. The coracoid is a thick beak-like process which arises from the anterior part of the neck and curves upward, forward, and outward in front of the glenoid.

The Sternoclavicular Joint.—This joint is the only articulation between the shoulder girdle and the trunk. It is formed by the enlarged inner extremity of the clavicle and a smaller facet at the posterolateral angle of the manubrium. A fibrocartilage is interposed between the two bones and the integrity of the joint is maintained entirely by ligaments which are thickenings of the joint capsule and entirely surround it. It is further strengthened by the interclavicular ligament which stretches across the top of the sternum between the two clavicles and by the very strong costoclavicular and rhomboid ligaments which bind the inner fourth of the clavicle to the first rib. This articulation permits a limited amount of motion in practically every direction including circumduction, and forms the center from which all movements of the shoulder on the trunk originate.

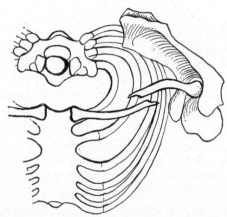

Fig. 405.—A diagrammatic drawing to illustrate that when the clavicular prop is broken and the support of the clavicle is removed the whole shoulder falls inward and forward and the scapula tilts outward. (From Scudder after Davis-Peotti. Scudder: Treatment of Fractures, W. B. Saunders Co.)

The Acromioclavicular Joint.—(Figs 406 and 407.) This is a simple gliding joint between the outer end of the clavicle and a flattened articular facet on the inner border of the acromion. It lies almost in a sagittal plane and is surrounded by a thin capsular ligament which is strengthened above and below by the acromioclavicular ligaments. The integrity of the joint is further strengthened by the strong coracoclavicular ligaments, the conoid and the trapezoid, which bind the clavicle to the coracoid process; and in addition, there is a strong coracoacromial ligament which stretches from the tip of the acromion to the coracoid process. The joint permits backward and forward rotation of the scapula on the clavicle.

Upper End of the Humerus.—The upper end of the humerus consists of a large round head which is joined to the shaft by a slightly constricted anatomic neck, and two processes—the greater and lesser tuberosities which are situated on the proximal portion of the shaft. The convex head is directed upward, inward, and backward to articulate with the shallow glenoid cavity of the scapula. Around its circumference is a shallow groove, the anatomic neck to which the articular capsule is attached. Lateral to this groove the upper end of the shaft is thickened to form the greater tuberosity which faces directly outward and upward, while below and in front is the smaller, more prominent lesser tuberosity. The bicepital groove which lies between the two tuberosities lodges the long tendon of the biceps muscle. Below the tuberosities the shaft of the bone is slightly constricted to form the surgical neck.

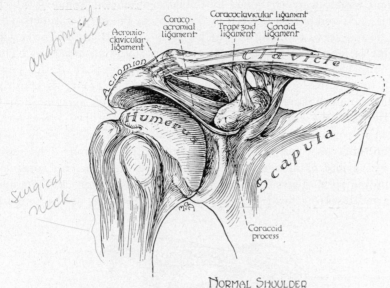

Fig. 406.—Normal shoulder showing the ligamentous attachments between the acromion and the coracoid processes of the scapula and the clavicle. (From Henry, M. O.: Minn. Med., July, 1929.)

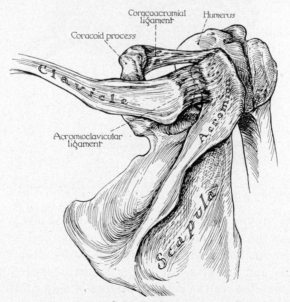

Fig. 407.—Normal shoulder viewed from above showing the acromioclavicular joint and the coracoacromial ligament. (From Henry, M. O.: Minn. Med., July, 1929.)

The upper end of the humerus is developed from three centers, one for the head, and one for each tuberosity which unite about the fifth year to form the caplike upper epiphysis which in turn unites to the shaft at about the twentieth year.

The Shoulder Joint (Figs. 406, 407, and 408) is a ball and socket joint formed by the large hemispherical head of the humerus and the relatively small and shallow glenoid cavity. It is entirely surrounded by a rather loose capsular ligament which is strengthened by the coracohumeral ligament which extends from the coracoid across the top of the joint to the greater tuberosity. The ligaments do not serve to maintain the bones in apposition and the integrity of the joint is largely dependent upon the surrounding muscles. The tendon of the long head of the biceps traverses the upper part of the joint cavity and is attached to the margin of the glenoid. The cavity is slightly deepened by the glenoid ligament which is attached around its margin outside the capsule. Between the capsule and the overlying structures are several bursae, the most important of which is the large subdeltoid bursa which lies over the greater tuberosity and is prolonged under the acromion. The joint permits of every variety of movement including circumduction and rotation. Abduction is limited to 90 degrees by the overhanging acromion, and the elevation of the arm above the head is accomplished by rotation of the scapula on the clavicle.

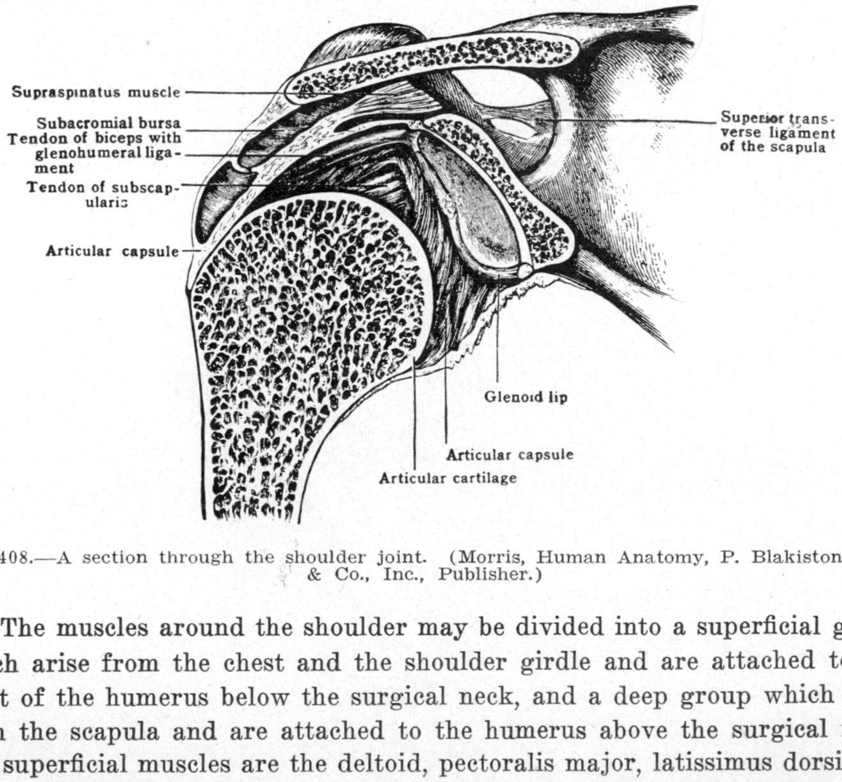

Fig. 408.—A section through the shoulder joint. (Morris, Human Anatomy, P. Blakiston's Son & Co., Inc., Publisher.)

The muscles around the shoulder may be divided into a superficial group which arise from the chest and the shoulder girdle and are attached to the shaft of the humerus below the surgical neck, and a deep group which arise from the scapula and are attached to the humerus above the surgical neck. The superficial muscles are the deltoid, pectoralis major, latissimus dorsi, and the teres major. The deep muscles are the supraspinatus, infraspinatus, subscapularis, and teres minor.

EXAMINATION OF THE SHOULDER GIRDLE AND SHOULDER

As accurate a history as possible should be obtained, emphasis being laid upon the mechanism of the accident, the manner in which it occurred, what injury the patient believes he suffered, the exact location of pain, and the extent of disability resulting from the accident.

The patient should then be stripped to the waist, and if his general condition permits, should be seated upright upon a stool. The surgeon should inspect both shoulders carefully, noting their relative positions and whether or not one shoulder is displaced downward, forward, or inward. Any abnormality in the contour of the shoulder or shoulder girdle and any swelling in the region of the shoulder should be noted. He should then ask the patient what movements he can perform without pain and have the patient try to abduct, adduct, rotate and move the shoulder backward and forward, in order to ascertain the amount of function and disability.

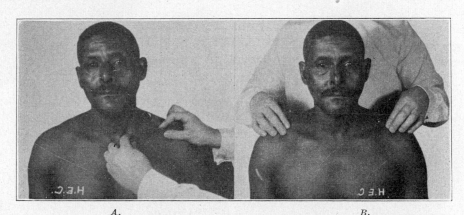

A. B.

Fig. 409.—*A*, Direct palpation and manipulation of the clavicle. *B*, Comparison of the contour of the clavicle on the injured side with that on the uninvolved side.

Having learned what he can from the history, inspection and amount of disability, the surgeon should palpate the entire shoulder in a systematic manner. It is well to begin with the clavicle. This bone is subcutaneous and should be palpated carefully with the fingers throughout its entire length, the positions of its two extremities and regularity of its contour being noted and compared with that of the other side (Figs. 409, *A* and *B*). In palpation point tenderness should be carefully noted wherever it occurs. Having ascertained the condition of the clavicle the surgeon should palpate the acromial ends of the clavicles and acromial processes in the manner shown in Fig. 410. The palpation should be continued over the scapula, the operator making bimanual examination of the body and spine of this bone as in Fig. 411. The head and upper end of the shaft of the humerus are then examined by grasping the outer portion of the two shoulders as in Fig. 412. The humerus is then palpated bimanually as shown in Fig. 413.

Manipulation.—As in the examination of any other region of the body, all manipulations should be begun gently and carried out slowly, and the force gradually increased as indicated. When false motion or crepitus occurs, it should be carefully noted, but undue force should not be used in trying to elicit these signs. In this manner severe pain is not inflicted on the patient.

If a fracture of the clavicle is suspected, the surgeon should stand behind the patient and pull the two shoulders upward and backward in order to determine whether or not the deformity can be corrected. If a fracture of the body of the scapula is suspected, he should grasp the lower angle of this bone with one hand and immobilize its upper portion with the other, and slowly but strongly manipulate the body of the bone between his two hands, noting whether or not pain or abnormal mobility occurs. He should then grasp the

Fig. 410.   Fig. 411.

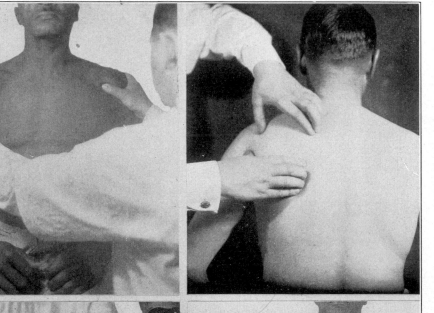

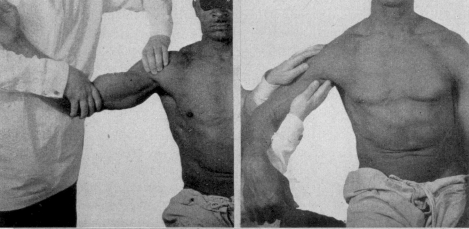

Fig. 412.   Fig. 413.

Fig. 410.—Palpation of the upper end of the humerus, the coracoid process, and the acromioclavicular articulation.

Fig. 411.—Method for bimanual palpation of the scapula.

Fig. 412.—Method for examination of the upper end of the humerus. Note that the patient's forearm is supported by the forearm of the surgeon.

Fig. 413.—Bimanual palpation of the upper end of the humerus. The patient's arm is supported by the surgeon's arm.

lower end of the humerus in the manner shown in Fig. 412 so that the patient's forearm is supported on the surgeon's forearm. With his other hand palpating the upper end of the humerus, he should execute gently motions of abduction, adduction, and rotation, taking particular note as to whether or not the upper end of the bone moves with the shaft. The range of passive rotation, abduction and adduction (Fig. 414*A*), flexion, and extension should be determined. Then by seizing the elbow with one hand and supporting the shoulder with the other, the effect of axial pressure on the humerus should be noted and it should be determined whether or not there is any telescoping of the bone. Finally the length of the arm as measured from the tip of the acromion to the external condyle of the humerus is determined and compared with that on the other side. (Fig. 414*B*.)

Anesthesia.—We do not believe that an anesthetic should be administered in order to examine the shoulder. If the surgeon cannot make a diagnosis without an anesthetic he may resort to x-ray examination.

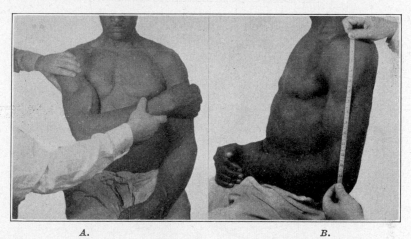

A.   B.

Fig. 414.—*A*, Method of determining the range of adduction at the shoulder. This is especially important in dislocations. *B*, Method of measuring the length of the arm from the tip of the acromion to the external condyle of the humerus.

X-Ray Examination.—Even after the surgeon has made his diagnosis, it is wise to procure an x-ray picture of the shoulder, especially if the lesion is anything except a simple fracture of the clavicle, because it is impossible to determine the details of most of the injuries in this region by physical examination alone, and it is important that the details be known in order that correct treatment may be instituted. Usually one flat plate in the anteroposterior plane is all that is necessary. However, in certain fracture-dislocations and fractures of the upper end of the humerus stereoscopic x-ray pictures are necessary for an accurate diagnosis, and in lesions of the upper end of the humerus, plates taken in the lateral plane should be made in order to determine the type of lesion.

FRACTURES OF THE CLAVICLE

Causation.—The clavicle is one of the most frequently broken bones in the body, and statistics show that it is involved in from 5 to 10 per cent of all fractures. This is especially true in childhood when many of the fractures are incomplete and are often not recognized. The reason this bone is so frequently broken is that it serves as the only connection between the shoulder girdle and trunk, and so must withstand any force tending to push the shoulder inward against the chest. Usually the injury is a fall, either from a height

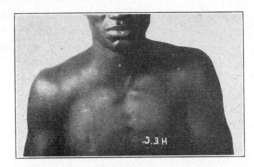

Fig. 415.—Fracture of the right clavicle with typical displacement. Note the downward, forward, and inward droop of the shoulder and the swelling over the clavicle.

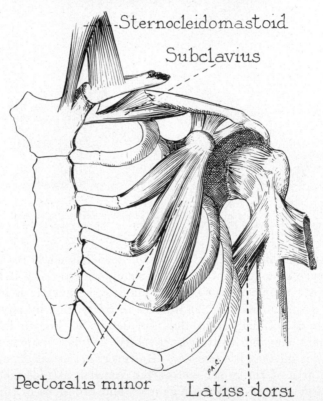

Fig. 416.—Drawing showing effect of muscle pull on displacement in fracture of the middle third of the clavicle.

or on the outstretched hand, elbow, or shoulder, the shoulder being pushed violently inward against the chest. The clavicle may also be broken by crushing injuries or by direct violence from in front and above. Very rarely the bone may be broken by muscular action.

Pathology and Displacement.—The clavicle may be broken in any part, but in the great majority of cases the break occurs in the middle third just internal to the attachment of the coracoid ligament. This is the vulnerable region of the bone because it contains the junction of the two curves and because it is unsupported by ligaments, and also because an elastic rod, broken

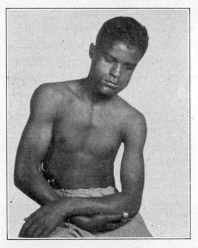

Fig. 417.—Fracture of the left clavicle. Typical posture assumed by a patient with this lesion. Note the downward, forward and inward droop of the shoulder. There is also a fracture of the left mandible.

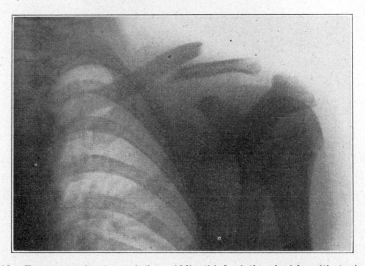

Fig. 418.—Transverse fracture of the middle third of the clavicle with typical displacement of the fragments. There is also a slight separation at the acromioclavicular joint. Treated by recumbency with traction, arm at right angle to shoulder, for eighteen days, and later Conwell's ambulatory adhesive dressing, with good results.

by compression from its ends, tends to break near its middle. In adults the fracture line is usually oblique, but it may vary from transverse to almost longitudinal and may take almost any direction. In older subjects the bone is often comminuted.

As the function of the clavicle is to hold the shoulder up and away from the chest, complete fracture of the bone results in shortening with overriding of the fragments and the shoulder drops downward, forward, and inward, and the outer fragment goes with the shoulder (Figs. 415, 416, and 417). This displacement is partly due to gravity when the patient is in the upright position and partly due to the pull of the muscles which pass from the trunk to the shoulder, especially the pectoral and the serratus magnus which pull the outer fragment inward and tend to rotate it in such a manner that its inner end is directed backward (Fig. 418).

The sternomastoid muscle tends to pull the inner fragment upward and backward, but its displacement is limited by the costoclavicular ligament. However, even without much displacement, the end of the inner fragment may be quite prominent because the displacement of the shoulder stretches the skin over it.

In children the fracture line tends to be roughly transverse and is often incomplete, when it may be of either the greenstick or infraction type. In either case, the bone tends to be bowed forward at its middle third, thus exaggerating the normal anterior convexity and shortening the bone to a variable degree.

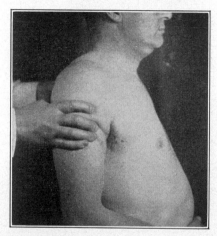

Fig. 419.—Method of reducing displacement in fracture of the clavicle by pulling the shoulders upward and backward.

Fractures of the inner third are quite rare, and if the costoclavicular ligament remains intact and attached to the outer fragment there is little or no displacement, but if this ligament is torn, the outer fragment may be pushed inward and pass in front of, behind, or above the inner fragment, and this fragment may be comminuted.

When the outer third of the clavicle is fractured the lesion is usually a transverse break and as the outer fragment is fixed to the acromion and the inner fragment is bound to the coracoid, there is little displacement unless this ligament is ruptured, but the scapula may swing forward and cause an angular deformity at the site of the fracture. If the coracoclavicular ligament is ruptured, the outer fragment is displaced downward and inward, the scapula being carried with it, and the displacement is similar to that which occurs in an acromioclavicular dislocation with a tearing of the coracoclavicu-

lar ligament. These fractures of the outer third are often due to direct violence and the bone may be comminuted.

Diagnosis.—In cases of complete fracture with overriding of the fragments, the diagnosis is relatively easy. The patient assumes a characteristic
attitude with the limb on the affected side supported by the other hand, and
the head is inclined to the affected side with the chin rotated to the opposite
side to release the tension of the sternomastoid on the inner fragment. On inspection the contour of the shoulder is normal, but it is found to be lower
than the one on the other side, slightly closer to the midline of the body, and
displaced slightly forward (Figs. 415 and 416). The displacement is especially well seen from behind. In a thin subject the break in the contour of
the bone may be visible, or it may be obscured by the swelling which occurs
after the accident.

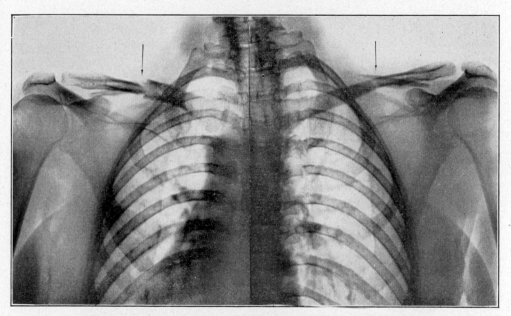

Fig. 420.—Fracture of both clavicles. Treated by adhesive dressing with good results.

On palpation there is tenderness over the site of the fracture, and it is
possible to feel the prominent outer end of the inner fragment beneath the skin.
The displacement of the shoulder can be reduced by pushing upward, outward,
and backward on the elbow, or by pulling the shoulder in this direction, but
it tends to recur as soon as the pressure is released (Fig. 419). With the
patient lying on the back, the forward and downward displacement tends to
be corrected by gravity, but the overriding of the fragments (inward displacement) persists.

In fractures without overriding or displacement the history of injury
followed by disability in the arm and the location of the pain and point tenderness are usually sufficient for a diagnosis.

In children with incomplete fractures (Figs. 421 and 422) there may be no
displacement and the history may be indefinite, it simply having been noted
by the parents that the child complained of pain or cried when lifted by the

arm and did not use the arm normally. On physical examination the shoulder may be normal to inspection, but usually the child will be unable to raise the affected arm above the level of the shoulder, and point tenderness may be elicited at the site of the fracture. There may be slight swelling over the fracture and the diagnosis can be confirmed by the x-ray, or some days later, by a small amount of callus at the site of the fracture. If there is increased anterior convexity of the middle third as compared with that of the outer side, the diagnosis is less difficult.

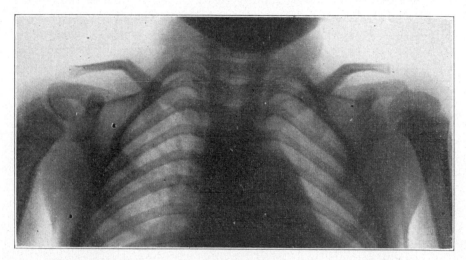

Fig. 421.—Typical greenstick fracture of the left clavicle in a child. Treated by reduction, under anesthesia, and adhesive dressing for eighteen days. Then sling to forearm for ten days. Good results in five weeks.

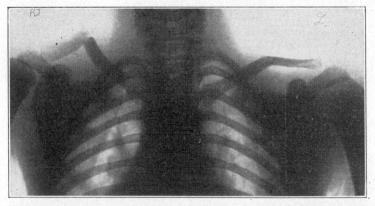

Fig. 422.—Fracture of both clavicles in a child. Reduction under ether anesthesia and application of adhesive dressing. Good results in six weeks.

In fractures of the inner third there may be relatively little displacement of the shoulder, and the diagnosis is made by the point tenderness, loss of function of the shoulder, and in some instances it is possible to palpate the displaced fragments.

In fractures of the outer third there may be no deformity and the diagnosis is made by the history of the injury, loss of function, and point tenderness, but if the coracoclavicular ligament is torn and the outer fragment is displaced, there is a definite dropping down of the point of the shoulder with prominence of the distal end of the proximal fragment, and the deformity may be visible and palpable, resembling that of an acromioclavicular dislocation, but slightly closer to the midline of the body.

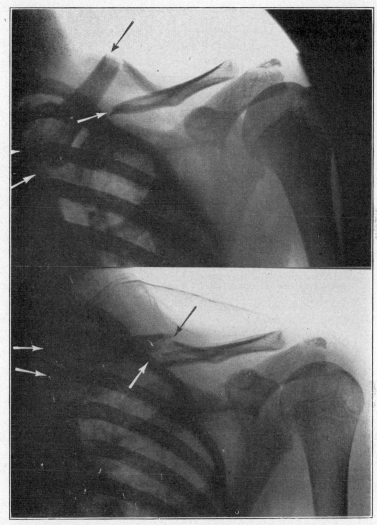

Fig. 423.—Comminuted fracture of clavicle and sternoclavicular dislocation. Reduced under general anesthesia and immobilized in an adhesive dressing.

X-Ray Examination.—In the great majority of instances an x-ray picture is not necessary for a diagnosis of fracture of the clavicle, but it is very useful in determining the exact line of the fracture and the amount of displacement. In fractures without displacement the x-ray is useful in confirming a clinical impression or in ruling out a fracture. This is especially true of injuries near either extremity of the bone. In fractures of the outer third an x-ray picture is often necessary to differentiate the lesion from an acromioclavicular dislocation. In lesions of the middle and outer third an anteroposterior view is all that is necessary, but in lesions of the inner third it is better to have the patient prone and make the exposure posteroanterior in such a manner that the shadow of the spine clears that of the sternoclavicular joint on the affected side.

If in doubt as to the diagnosis, the surgeon should insist upon an x-ray picture. After treatment has been instituted, the x-ray should be used to check its efficiency.

Complications.—Fortunately complications are rare in fractures of the clavicle. In spite of the subcutaneous location of the bone these fractures are rarely compound (1 per cent in Conwell's series), and when so the trauma is of the direct type as from gunshot wounds or direct severe crushing injuries. Very rarely in severe injuries with fracture of the clavicle there may be injury to the great vessels, brachial plexus, or pleura or lung.

Not infrequently, however, the clavicle is comminuted (Fig. 423) or the fracture is accompanied by a dislocation of one extremity or by some other lesion of the shoulder. In a series of five hundred cases reported by Eliason* there were thirteen associated fractures of the scapula, six acromioclavicular dislocations, six fractures of the humerus, nine fractures of one or more ribs. three dislocations at the shoulder, and three fractures of the olecranon.

Treatment

According to Lester† more than two hundred different methods have been described and recommended for the treatment of fractures of the clavicle. This is, of course, evidence that we have no method which is satisfactory to the majority of surgeons. As was stated above, the displacement can be reduced by simply pulling the shoulder backward, outward, and upward; but this reduction is almost impossible to maintain in an ambulant patient because any form of dressing or apparatus which maintains anatomic reduction will be intolerable to the patient. We shall describe the methods which we use and discuss their indications.

1. **Posterior Figure-of-Eight Bandage.**—(Figs. 424 and 425.) Thin felt or cotton pads of suitable size are placed over the front of each shoulder and axilla. One or more gauze or muslin bandages, three or four inches wide, are then applied as a posterior figure-of-eight to the two shoulders. The bandage must be applied tightly enough to hold the shoulder back and yet not so tightly that it constricts the axillary vessels. Sufficient bandage must be used to make a firm dressing and this should be reinforced by long strips of adhesive and the forearm supported by a sling. Billington uses a posterior figure-of-eight plaster-of-Paris bandage and makes a plaster yoke, providing a very efficient dressing.

2. **Axillary Pad, Swathe and Sling.**—A piece of absorbent cotton is folded to make a pad about 16 by 8 inches and about 2 inches thick. A strip of adhesive tape ½ inch wide and 18 inches long is placed across one side of the pad and the opposite side is well powdered with talcum. A pad of felt about 2 inches

---

*Eliason: J. A. M. A. **19**: 1974, 1928.
†Lester: Am. Surg. **89**: 600, 1929.

in diameter and ½ inch thick is placed over the site of the fracture. The deformity is then reduced by pushing the shoulder upward, outward, and backward, using the slightly abducted arm as a handle to control the shoulder. A long strip of adhesive 2 inches wide, is then placed vertically over the pad over the fracture. The adhesive begins well down on the chest and is pulled tightly over the shoulder and down the back to the level of the angle of the scapula. The cotton pad is then doubled with the powdered surface outside and pushed well up in the axilla and the ends of the strip of adhesive are crossed over the shoulder to hold the pad snug. The arm is then brought to the

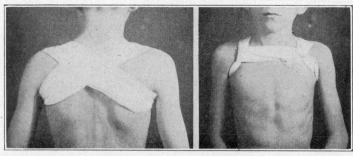

Fig. 424.   Fig. 425.

Fig. 424.—Posterior figure-of-eight bandage; useful in children and in adults where there is no displacement or as a convalescent dressing.

Fig. 425.—Posterior figure-of-eight bandage seen from the front. Note the anterior cross strap to prevent slipping.

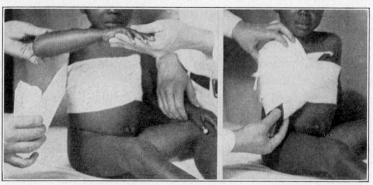

Fig. 426.   Fig. 427.

Fig. 426.—First roll of a modified Velpeau bandage useful in children when adhesive is liable to irritate the skin and in obese adults.

Fig. 427.—Completion of the modified Velpeau bandage. This dressing does not maintain reduction if there is a tendency to displacement.

side with the elbow slightly forward and a strip of adhesive 3 inches wide is passed around the arm and chest. The elbow and forearm are then supported in a modified Velpeau bandage (Fig. 427) or in a triangular sling. The sling must be large enough to project beyond the elbow in order that its ends can be folded and pinned snugly about the elbow. The sling may be tied or pinned at the back of the neck, or tapes may be attached to its ends and crossed behind and brought around under the arms and tied over the chest, thus taking the weight on the shoulders rather than on the neck.

3. **Conwell's* Adhesive Dressing.**—''The material consists of four pieces of adhesive (4 inches wide by 48 inches long), one pad of cotton, and a small circular pad of felt (3 inches in diameter). For children, these dimensions vary according to the size of the child.

''Application of the dressing is made as follows: After the chest has been shaved and cleansed with ether, the patient is placed in a sitting position with the hand of the uninvolved side on top of the head. The arm of the injured side is against the side of the chest with the forearm resting in the patient's lap. Adhesive strip 1 is then applied. This strip (Fig. 428) commences in front, just at the point of fracture of the distal fragment. With the aid of an assistant and with the patient's cooperation, the shoulders are pulled backward, tension being made on adhesive strip 1, which is carried out and around the upper part of the arm on the injured side, then in and diagonally across the back to the opposite axilla, extending underneath the latter, then around in front, crossing both sides of the chest and terminating about 2 inches below the nipple line on the injured side. This strip pulls the injured shoulder backward, thereby tending to approximate the fragments by correcting any overlapping.

''The felt pad is applied directly over the fracture, the pad being held in place with a small piece of adhesive tape. (Fig. 429.)

''Adhesive strip 2 (Fig. 429) commences in the medial line of the abdomen, a few inches above the umbilicus, and extends diagonally up the chest on the injured side, and over the felt pad. With the application of considerable tension the adhesive is then extended diagonally down the back to the median line, terminating usually at the lumbosacral region. This strip should be applied only after the patient has taken a deep expiration. Adhesive strip 2 aids in preventing any tendency of an upward displacement of the fragments, this displacement usually being more marked in the proximal fragment as a result of the action of the sternocleidomastoid muscle.

''A large cotton pad is now applied in the axilla (Fig. 430) which aids in pulling the distal fragment outward and at the same time separating the skin surfaces of the arm and chest. The forearm is flexed nearly to an acute angle at the elbow and placed against the chest. While the opposite ends of strip 3 are held widely apart, it is first applied (Fig. 431) to the inferior surface of the elbow, after a small piece of cotton has been applied to the latter. With considerable tension, the front and back halves of the adhesive strip are brought up the corresponding surfaces of the arm, meeting and overlapping over the shoulder near the middle third of the clavicle (Fig. 432). This strip pulls the shoulder upward, thereby aiding further approximation of the distal fragment which is usually displaced downward.

''Strip 4 commences on the back, at the midaxillary line of the opposite side in the region of the ninth and tenth ribs (Fig. 433). It extends horizontally across the back to the involved side around the arm about 4 inches above the olecranon process, then across the forearm and base of the wrist, ending where it commenced; that is in the midaxillary line of the opposite side. Cotton should be placed between the skin surfaces of the forearm and chest, and

---

*Conwell: J. A. M. A. **90**: 838, 1928.

also between the adhesive strip and the forearm (Fig. 434). When moderate tension is applied to strip 4, the distal fragment is pulled outward, the cotton pad in the axilla acting as a fulcrum. This piece also aids in stabilizing the arm and forearm, making a support for the latter.'' The dressing should be

Fig. 428.   Fig. 429.·

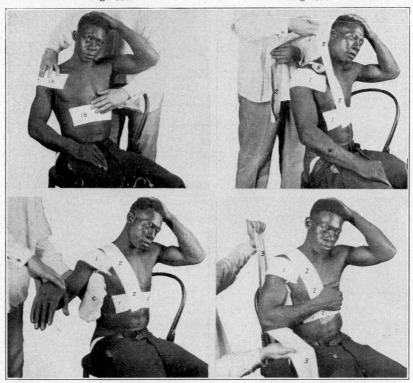

Fig. 430.   Fig. 431.

Figs. 428-431.—Conwell's adhesive dressing.

Fig. 428.—Application of first strip of adhesive.   Fig. 429.—Application of second strip.
Fig. 430.—Insertion of axillary pad.   Fig. 431.—Application of third strip.

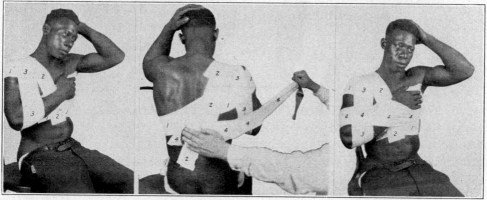

Fig. 432.   Fig. 433.   Fig. 434.

Fig. 432.—Completion of third strip. Fig. 433.—Application of fourth strip. Fig. 434.—Completion of dressing.

worn for about from four to six weeks, depending upon the severity of the injury, and should be reinforced about every five to seven days or as often as it becomes loosened and inefficient. None of the dressing has to be removed for reinforcement except strip 4. All the reinforcements are done by applying similar pieces of adhesive over the original ones. The dressing is very comfortable, cool, and efficient.

4. **Clavicular Cross.**—Several types of this splint are on the market and can be purchased from surgical supply houses (Fig. 435 and 436). A very serviceable one can be made from ordinary splint wood. The cross-piece should extend the width between the shoulders, and should be at least as wide or slightly wider than the distance between the top of the acromion and the axilla. The upright piece should be about 3 inches wide and reach from the level of the shoulder to about the first lumbar vertebra. A piece of felt is placed over the front of each shoulder, and the cross which has been nailed together and padded is placed behind the shoulder, and strapped first on the uninjured side. The affected shoulder is then lifted upward and backward and strapped. The vertical piece of the cross is then pushed against the back and fastened close to the body by an adhesive swathe or wide webbing strap. As the shoulder straps tend to slip outward and downward, a cross strap is placed in front to hold them in position.

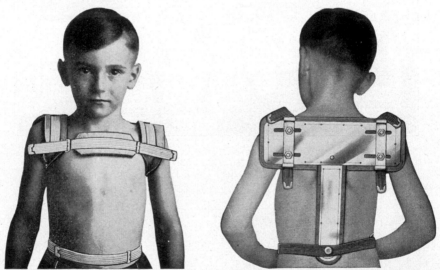

Fig. 435.—Front and back views of a commercial clavicular cross. (Courtesy Zimmer Manufacturing Co.)

5. **The Billington Plaster Yoke.**—This is a simple and effective method and is the one used routinely by one of us (J. A. K.). The area of the fracture is anesthetized with novocain and with the shoulder held up back and out to reduce the fracture the cast is applied over a foundation of felt or cotton padding, as illustrated. It is then trimmed to permit lowering of the arms to the sides and need not be changed until the fracture is healed. (Fig. 437.)

6. **Recumbency With Traction.**—Where treatment in recumbency is indicated traction should be applied to the arm in order to correct the overriding

and to make the patient more comfortable. The patient is placed flat on his back on a bed with a hard mattress and firm springs or fracture boards under the mattress. The arm and forearm are then shaved, and four strips of adhesive 3 inches wide and from 18 to 20 inches long are prepared for traction strips by tearing a half-inch strip along each edge for a distance of 8 or 10

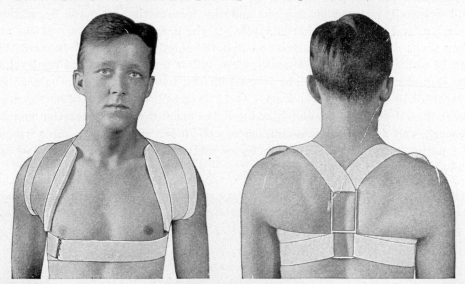

Fig. 436.—Clavicular support for convalescence and fractures in which the position is not difficult to maintain. (Courtesy Zimmer Manufacturing Company.)

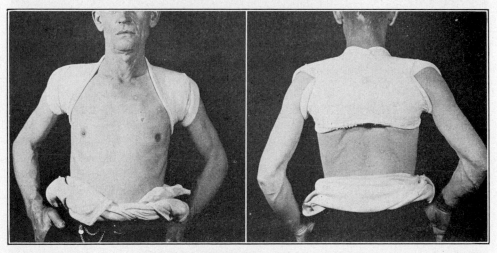

Fig. 437.—Billington plaster yoke applied for fracture of the right clavicle. (Courtesy Dr. Wallace Billington.)

inches, making three-tailed strips. The center of the strip 2 inches wide is laid along either side of the arm and the half-inch border strips are then wound spirally around the arm and the whole is bound on firmly with a gauze bandage. This bandage should be applied carefully and reinforced freely with adhesive; since it is expected to remain in place about three weeks. The other two three-tailed strips are placed on the dorsal and volar surfaces of the forearm and carefully bandaged. The free ends of the adhesive strips are prepared for the attachment of the traction ropes or spreader by folding in either edge to make a strip 1 inch wide.

The Conwell lateral traction frame or some other similar apparatus is attached to the bed and the arm on the affected side is abducted 90 degrees and externally rotated 90 degrees, and the forearm is suspended by vertical traction, and lateral traction is applied to the arm as in Fig. 439. If the patient sinks down in the mattress so that the shoulder is pressed forward this can be corrected by placing a small pad or pillow under the back at the level of the shoulders. Enough weight is used on the forearm to counterbalance its weight (3 to 6 pounds) and from 4 to 12 pounds traction is used on the arm. After the deformity is completely reduced, the amount of lateral traction may be lessened, and as soon as consolidation is well under way (two to three weeks) the patient may be permitted up in an ambulatory dressing, preferably an abduction plaster jacket.

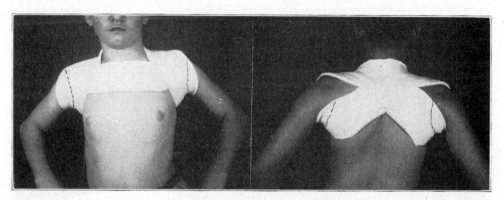

Fig. 438.—Plaster yoke with anterior crosspiece. This increases the stability of the dressing. This yoke needs to be cut out under each arm.

Plaster-of-Paris Spica Jacket.—The patient should be recumbent either on a fracture table permitting the application of a jacket or on the Goldthwaite irons. Both shoulders should be abducted and drawn backward, and traction should be maintained on the arm on the fractured side sufficient for complete reduction of the displacement. The jacket is then applied in the usual way, over stockinet or sheet cotton and felt, to include both shoulders and the pelvis down to the level of the trochanters. Very thin padding is placed around the affected shoulder and upper arm, and the plaster is carefully molded in this region. After the plaster is finished down to the lower arm, the traction is released and the cast is completed down to the wrist, the elbow and forearm being well padded.

Open Reduction.—We believe that it is rarely necessary to perform an open operation for the reduction of a fresh fracture of the clavicle. The bone is subcutaneous and easily reached, but this subcutaneous location makes it especially liable to suppuration after any suture or plating of the bone. Reduction of these severe fractures by recumbency with lateral traction is less spectacular, but it is more efficient and less dangerous.

Very rarely in fractures of the inner third with a short mesial fragment and marked displacement it may be necessary to perform an open reduction (Fig. 440). The site of the fracture is easily exposed by a curved incision which is convex downward and is placed below the bone. When the flap is lifted, the fragments can be manipulated into their normal positions, and after a small hole has been drilled in each, they should be tied together with chromic catgut. No plates or wire are necessary and it is dangerous to place metal in bones which lie just beneath the skin. The flap is then pulled down and sutured, thus leaving the site of the fracture covered by intact skin. Then treatment with recumbency and lateral traction is resumed and some form of ambulatory dressing is applied after from seven to fourteen days.

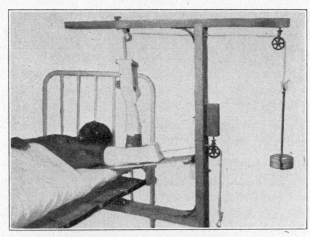

Fig. 439.—Conwell's lateral traction frame for the treatment of fractures of the clavicle with displacement in which a good cosmetic result is important.

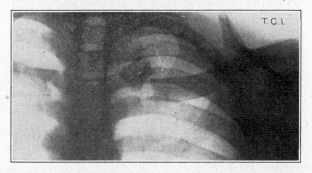

Fig. 440.—Fracture of the inner third of the clavicle with typical displacement. Open reduction was performed in this case with satisfactory result. Sutured with chromic catgut. Plaster spica to the shoulder with Hoke's upper extremity traction apparatus and adhesive to arm for three weeks; then adhesive dressing for two weeks. Forearm in sling for ten days. Good results in eleven weeks.

The above operation should be performed only after treatment with lateral traction has failed, and then only under conditions of rigid asepsis.

Choice of Method of Treatment.—The object of treatment is to obtain a satisfactory functional and cosmetic result, make the patient comfortable, and restrict the patient's activity as little as necessary. In deciding upon a method of treatment both the character of the fracture and of the patient must be considered.

Greenstick Fractures in Children.—The clavicle is bowed forward, and as the deformity tends to persist, it should be corrected. This can be done by placing the patient recumbent and pressing backward at the apex of the deformity. One of us (H. E. C.) administers a general anesthetic and overcorrects the deformity, thus completing the fracture, and applies his adhesive dressing; the other (J. A. K.) by pressure and outward traction on the shoulder without an anesthetic endeavors to just barely correct the deformity without completing the fracture and then applies a pad over the fracture with axillary pad, swathe, and sling. Time three weeks.

Fractures Without Displacement in Children.—The second, third and fourth adhesive strips of Conwell's dressing or the modified Velpeau dressing (Figs. 426 and 427) or the posterior figure-of-eight bandage are simple, comfortable, and adequate. Time three weeks.

In Fractures With Slight Displacement in patients of any age, except those who are quite fat or very old and feeble, the adhesive dressing of Conwell or the Boehler splint may be used. The clavicular cross is favored by many competent surgeons in this type of case, but in our experience it is difficult to make comfortable if it is applied tightly enough to be efficient. Time, three to five weeks, followed by a sling for two weeks.

Fractures in Fat or Senile Patients.—Axillary pad, swathe, and sling. This dressing is not very efficient, but it can be made fairly comfortable and gives a good functional and usually a good cosmetic result. The Boehler splint is more efficient and may be used. Time, from three to five weeks, followed by a sling for two weeks.

In these patients there is often more or less damage to the soft parts of the shoulder, even in the absence of bone injury and gentle passive motion, massage, and moist or dry heat over the deltoid region should be begun early, else considerable difficulty may be encountered in restoring abduction and rotation.

In Fractures With Marked Displacement in any type of patient or fractures with mild or moderate displacement in young girls or women in whom a good cosmetic result is of importance, recumbency with lateral traction is the method of choice. This will reduce practically any displacement and assure an almost perfect result in almost every case. Time, from two to five weeks, followed by ambulant adhesive dressing or swathe and sling for from three to five weeks, and a sling for a week or so longer.

We are of the opinion that a greater percentage of the clavicular fractures with marked displacement should be treated by recumbency with lateral traction. The reasons are: (1) During the first week or two after a severe fracture of the clavicle with displacement the patient is not of much use, even when ambulant, and might just as well be in bed as wandering around complaining. (2) If the patient is in bed, lateral traction will reduce the deformity and assure an almost perfect result, and avoids an operative scar. (3) Due to the local trauma over the site of the fracture, it is frequently impossible to apply pressure over the fracture site because of pain and danger of local slough from pressure.

In certain cases with marked displacement where for economic reasons it is necessary to treat the patient in an ambulant dressing, and a good result is of importance, the plaster-of-Paris jacket with shoulder spica either with or without Hoke's traction apparatus is useful.

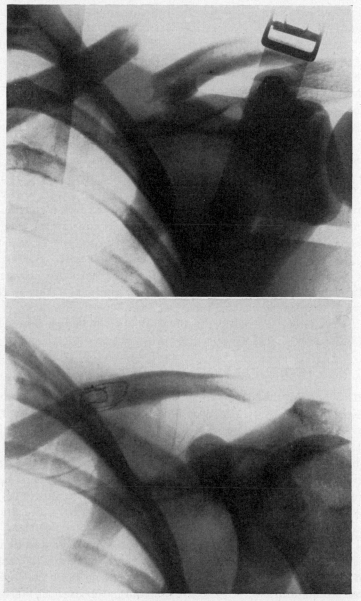

Fig. 441.—Fracture of the clavicle with marked displacement. Open reduction and wiring with excellent result. (Courtesy Dr. Joseph Lembeck.)

Compound Fractures.—The wound should be carefully débrided and closed or left open, depending upon its condition as noted in the chapter on compound injuries, and the fracture should then be treated in recumbency with lateral traction for the first two or three weeks, as immobilization is very important in preventing infection. When this danger has passed an ambulatory dressing may be used.

Complications should be looked for and treated as indicated. Recumbency with traction in abduction is efficient for any fracture of the scapula or upper end of the humerus except that of the coracoid process, and this can be treated by the ambulant adhesive dressing. In dislocations of the shoulder, abduction of the arm tends to cause recurrence of the dislocation; consequently, with this complication, the dislocation must be reduced and the fracture of the clavicle treated with the arm at the side in the adhesive dressing or swathe and sling for five or six days and at the end of this time the lateral traction can be applied if necessary to reduce the deformity in the clavicle.

Rupture of large vessels, fortunately, is a very rare complication of clavicular fractures. When it occurs, the diagnosis is evident from the large, rapidly increasing hematoma and immediate surgical intervention is necessary. With the arm abducted an incision of adequate length is made below and parallel to the clavicle, and the bleeding vessel is located and ligated. If it is the subclavian artery the vein should also be ligated. The wound is then closed with a rubber tissue drain which is removed at the end of forty-eight hours and the fracture of the clavicle is treated with recumbency and lateral traction.

Prognosis.—Fractures of the clavicle tend to unite quickly and firmly and nonunion is rare unless there is marked loss of substance or interposition of soft parts or marked displacement and inefficient treatment. However, many of these fractures unite with more or less deformity and this is the rule in fractures with displacement which are not treated in recumbency with lateral traction. Fortunately a fracture of the clavicle which has united with considerable deformity almost always gives a good functional result.

STERNOCLAVICULAR DISLOCATION

Varieties and Mechanism.—Sternoclavicular dislocation is an uncommon injury which may result from falls or blows upon the shoulder or direct force applied over the inner end of the clavicle. The inner end of the clavicle usually passes anteriorly beneath the skin, but it may be displaced backward into the chest, upward or downward. The final displacement is largely due to the direction of the force causing the dislocation rather than to muscle pull. Violent depression of the shoulder either from a blow or a fall upon it tends to lever the sternal end of the clavicle upward and anteriorly, the first rib serving as the fulcrum.

In all acute dislocations at this joint the sternoclavicular ligaments are ruptured and the intraarticular fibrocartilage tends to retain its attachment to the end of the clavicle and be displaced with it, while the costoclavicular ligaments usually remain intact. In chronic nontraumatic cases the sternoclavicular ligaments are stretched rather than torn.

Diagnosis.—As the joint is subcutaneous and the sternal end of the clavicle is quite large the diagnosis is not difficult (Fig. 442). Unless the sternal end of the clavicle has been forced backward it can be felt beneath the skin in its abnormal location. If it has been forced backward, palpation will reveal the fact that it is absent from its normal location. When it is forced backward

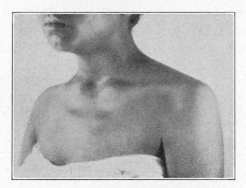

Fig. 442.—Bilateral sternoclavicular dislocation (chronic), viewed from the side. Note the upward and anterior dislocation of the clavicles.

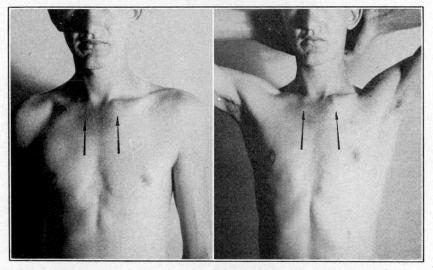

Fig. 443.—Left sternoclavicular subluxation, chronic. Operative fixation was necessary for relief.

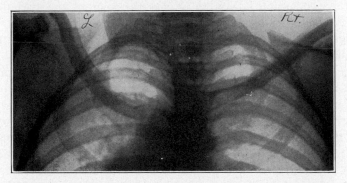

Fig. 444.—Sternoclavicular dislocation (upward) on the right and fracture of the sternal end of the clavicle on the left. Reduction under anesthetic by bilateral traction for eighteen days. Then adhesive strapping was applied to both clavicles and arms for two weeks. Good results.

behind the sternum it may cause pressure on the trachea. In cases with considerable swelling, an x-ray picture should be taken with the patient lying upon his face, the rays coming from behind and at an angle to avoid the vertebrae (Fig. 444).

Treatment

In most cases the dislocation can be reduced by making traction on the clavicle and manipulating the sternal end of the bone into its normal position. The necessary traction can be accomplished either by pulling on the abducted arm or by pushing the shoulder upward, outward, and backward, and is most efficient when the patient is lying upon his back:

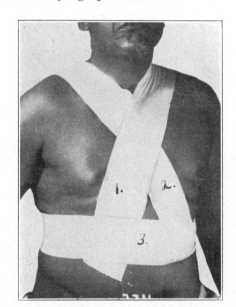

Fig. 445.—Ambulant sternoclavicular dressing on the right side. The right arm should be carried in a triangular sling.

While the dislocation is easy to reduce, the form of the articular surfaces is such that the stability of the joint depends upon the integrity of the sternoclavicular ligaments, and since these are torn, the dislocation tends to recur as soon as the pressure is relaxed. Consequently it is necessary to apply some form of retaining dressing. A simple and effective one is illustrated in Fig. 445. It is applied as follows: The dislocation is reduced by manipulation as was described above and a pad of felt 1 inch thick and 2 inches in diameter is placed over the sternal end of the clavicle. A strip of adhesive 3 inches wide is then placed over this pad and pulled over the shoulder and down the back. A similar strip is crossed over this as high as possible and pulled over the opposite shoulder. A third strip is then passed around the lower part of the chest and over the ends of the crossed strips to keep them from slipping. It is important to apply all three strips after the patient has exhaled deeply and while the chest is contracted. A triangular sling should then be applied tightly enough to support the arm on the affected side. This ambulant adhesive dressing should be worn for six weeks with frequent reinforcements, adhesive strips applied over the corresponding strips, and the sling for two weeks longer. At the end of this period, the patient may begin to use the hand on the affected side, but should avoid heavy lifting for some weeks longer.

If the above ambulant dressing will not maintain reduction, it will be necessary to treat the patient in recumbency with traction on the abducted arm and a sandbag over the joint as in Fig. 446. This should be continued for two or three weeks and at the end of this time the ambulant adhesive dressing can be applied and the patient may be allowed to be up.

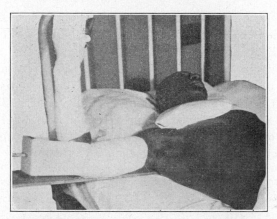

Fig. 446.—Lateral traction for right sternoclavicular dislocation with sandbag over the lesion. Recumbency over a period of two or three weeks; ambulatory adhesive dressing for two weeks.

Open reduction and suture of the capsule is rarely necessary in acute cases, but may be necessary in chronic cases or in the chronic nontraumatic subluxations which are sometimes seen in debilitated individuals. However, in many of these, rest and support to the shoulder with improvement in general health will often result in a cure. Nevertheless, if the condition persists, it can be cured by making a small incision over the joint, reefing or repairing the relaxed capsule and tying the clavicle down to the first rib, or sternum, with a strip of living fascia or chromic catgut.

ACROMIOCLAVICULAR DISLOCATION

Varieties and Mechanism.—As the joint is situated near the point of the shoulder, it is exposed to frequent trauma; injuries here are more frequent than at the sternal end of the clavicle. The acromion may be dislocated either downward or upward on the clavicle. A fall or blow on the point of the shoulder with the force directed downward and inward tends to tear the acromion loose from the clavicle and displace it downward and inward. The weight of the upper extremity and the pull of the pectoralis major and latissimus dorsi tend to maintain the displacement.

If the force is not great, the injury is limited to a tearing of the articular capsule and the coracoclavicular ligaments remain intact and prevent the dropping down of the acromion, but a slight displacement results from the rotation of the scapula around the coracoid process. With severe trauma the coracoclavicular ligaments are torn and the acromion is completely separated from the clavicle and is displaced downward and inward. Not infrequently a small portion of the outer end of the clavicle is torn off and displaced with the acromion.

Upward dislocation at this joint is a very rare injury, but occasionally occurs from force transmitted upward through the humerus from falls or blows on the elbow or hand. The acromion is pushed up over the end of the clavicle and caught in this position. As soon as it is loosened it tends to drop downward.

Diagnosis.—Since the joint is subcutaneous, the diagnosis can usually be made by palpation and inspection (Figs. 447 and 448). The history of an injury followed by pain, tenderness, and swelling over the acromioclavicular joint with inability to actively abduct the arm, leads the surgeon to suspect either an injury to the outer third of the clavicle or an acromioclavicular dislocation. Careful palpation of the line of the point tenderness and the distance of this line from the outer border of the acromion will determine whether or not the location of the injury corresponds to that of the joint as determined by examination of the opposite shoulder.

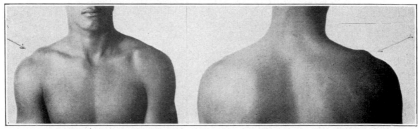

Fig. 447.   Fig. 448.

Fig. 447.—Right acromioclavicular dislocation with downward displacement of the acromion. Note the typical deformity.
Fig. 448.—Same case as the preceding, back view. Generally the posterior view of this type of case is of greater diagnostic importance than the anterior view.

In cases with slight displacement palpation will reveal a slight sulcus at the site of the joint. With complete dislocation, the outer end of the clavicle is unusually prominent, while the point of the shoulder is displaced downward and a definite sulcus is palpable and even visible between the two. The deformity can be reduced by pushing upward on the elbow while the outer end of the clavicle is pressed downward, but it tends to recur as soon as the pressure is released. Whether or not a small bit of the clavicle has been torn off with the acromion cannot as a rule be determined in the absence of an x-ray picture.

The rare upward dislocation can be diagnosed by the presence of the unusually prominent inner border of the acromion riding up on the outer end of the clavicle.

As the contours of the acromioclavicular joint are such that its integrity depends entirely upon the ligaments, it is necessary not only to reduce the dislocation, but to hold it reduced until the ligaments have healed. This is accomplished by any dressing which supports the shoulder up against the outer end of the clavicle.

Several types of acromioclavicular slings have been devised. A very satisfactory method of treatment is a slight modification of the figure-of-eight adhesive dressing of Stimson. It is applied as follows: The elbow is flexed to
about 80 degrees and the wrist is suspended by a clove hitch and sling around
the neck. A small pad of absorbent cotton is placed in the axilla, and with the
displacement reduced by upward pressure upon the elbow, a strip of adhesive
is then passed around the arm and chest, binding the arm firmly to the chest.

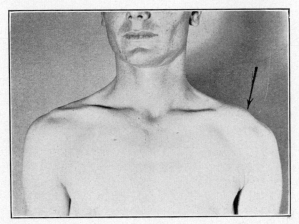

A.

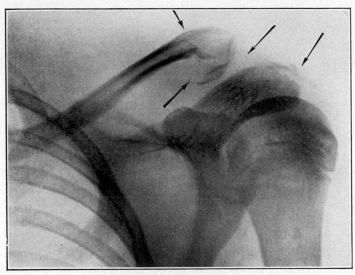

B.

Fig. 449 *A* and *B*.—Acromioclavicular dislocation with fractures of the clavicle and
acromion. Treated with lateral traction for two weeks; then plaster spica with arm abducted
three weeks; and strapping and sling for four weeks. Good result.

This strip should be tightened with the chest in full expiration. A small felt
pad is placed over the outer third of the clavicle and a pad of absorbent
cotton over the upper third of the ulna; a second strip of adhesive 3 inches
wide is placed under the forearm and elbow and crossed over the shoulder in
such a manner that the elbow is supported against the shoulder as in Fig. 451.

The dislocation is reduced and held by an assistant, while the adhesive dressing is applied. The dressing should be worn for about eight weeks, and it is necessary to reinforce it as often as it becomes loosened and inefficient. This can be done by simply strapping fresh adhesive over the old every four or

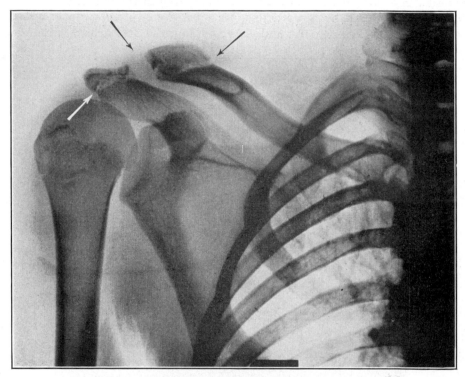

Fig. 450.—Acromioclavicular separation with fractures. Treated by plaster spica with arm abducted 90 degrees for three weeks; then adhesive strapping for three weeks; and sling for three weeks.

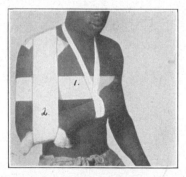

Fig. 451.—Modified Stimson figure-of-eight adhesive dressing for acromioclavicular dislocation.

five days. At the end of two or three weeks it is usually necessary to replace the entire dressing, and the shoulder should be carefully supported while this is done. A posterior figure-of-eight bandage and sling can be used as a convalescent dressing.

The Abduction Plaster Jacket.—It has been our experience that in acromioclavicular dislocations the extremity must be held up for from six to eight

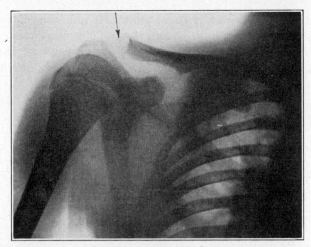

Fig. 452.—Moderately severe acromioclavicular dislocation (left). Traction two weeks, then plaster spica abduction cast to shoulder for two weeks; adhesive dressing for fifteen days. Forearm in sling for two weeks. Good result.

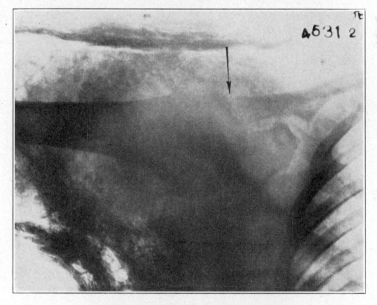

Fig. 453.—Position in cast.

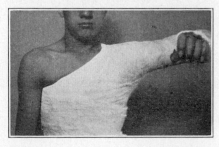

Fig. 454.—Type of cast used in preceding case.

weeks if a satisfactory result is to be obtained and that not only does the adhesive dressing described above tend to slip, but it is very uncomfortable and few patients can stand it. For these reasons we usually apply a plaster spica jacket similar to that illustrated in Fig. 454. This gets a firm grip on

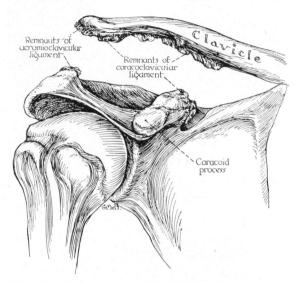

COMPLETE ACROMIOCLAVICULAR DISLOCATION

Fig. 455.—Complete acromioclavicular dislocation with tearing of the ligaments. (From Henry, M. O.: Minn. Med., July, 1929.)

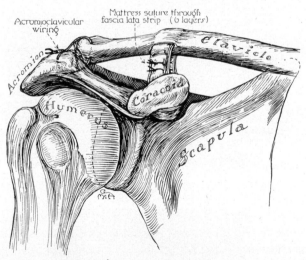

LIGAMENTO-PLASTY

Fig. 456.—Henry's operation for chronic acromioclavicular dislocation. (From Henry, M. O.: Minn. Med., July, 1929.)

the pelvis and supports the arm in abduction and is well molded over the sternal half of the clavicle. It is worn for from four to eight weeks, depending upon the severity of the injury, and is followed by a posterior figure-of-eight bandage which is worn until the shoulder is quite firm.

Chronic Acromioclavicular Dislocation.—A complete dislocation in which the displacement has been present for two weeks or more may be considered chronic as the power of the ligaments to heal by simple reduction and immobilization has ceased. In these cases it is useless to attempt cure by conservative methods, and if the disability is very great an open operation is indicated. Several such operations are described in the literature. A very satisfying one is that devised by M. O. Henry.* (Figs. 455 and 458.) It endeavors to reconstruct the coracoclavicular ligament by means of living fascia.

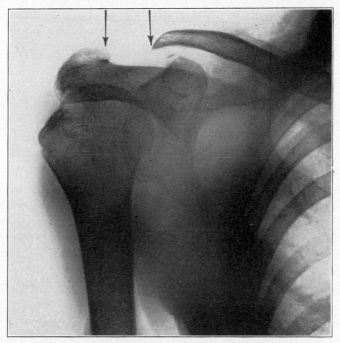

Fig. 457.—Mumford's method of resection of the outer portion of the clavicle for chronic acromioclavicular dislocation. Satisfactory result.

The operation is performed as follows: A curved incision is made just below the middle of the clavicle sweeping laterally over the acromioclavicular joint. The periosteum is carefully raised from the clavicle about the coracoid tuberosity. The base and neck of the coracoid process are exposed subperiosteally as far as possible, cleaning it of remnants of the ligaments. Next a strip of fascia lata 2 cm. in width and 14 cm. in length is removed from the thigh. This is folded upon itself lengthwise and passed beneath the base of the coracoid process one end being brought over the clavicle subperiosteally at the site of the coracoid tuberosity. While an assistant holds the dislocation reduced the ends of the fascial band are held taut and two mattress sutures of heavy silk are inserted through it. A suture is then passed around the acromioclavicular joint, after small drill holes have been made in the adjacent portions of the clavicle and acromion. For this suture, Henry uses Krupp steel wire, while the authors prefer chromic catgut or kangaroo tendon. After the wound

*Henry, M. O.: Minn. Med. 12: 431, 1929.

is closed, the arm is placed in a plaster spica jacket which has been previously prepared. This holds the arm abducted about 90 degrees. It is worn for a period of about eight weeks. Heavy lifting is avoided for eight weeks longer. Normal function may be expected.

Resection of the Outer End of the Clavicle.—Mumford has shown that resection of the outer end of the clavicle will relieve the symptoms caused by an acromioclavicular dislocation and result in a useful and painless shoulder. The operation is relatively simple and the convalescence relatively short. One of us (H. E. C.) has used this procedure in many instances with excellent result. The other author (J. A. K.) still prefers to restore the joint and now uses the Bunnell operation in which a single long strip of fascia lata is used to pull the clavicle and the coracoid together and to reinforce the acromioclavicular joint.

FRACTURES OF THE SCAPULA

Occurrence.—In the older statistics fracture of the scapula is regarded as a rare injury, and it is said to constitute less than 1 per cent of all fractures. With the increasing use of the x-ray, however, more of these lesions are being diagnosed, and it is evident that scapular fractures are not so rare as was formerly believed.

One would expect this broad, thin plate of bone which occupies such an exposed position on the shoulder and back to be one of the most frequent sites of fracture. But compared to the clavicle, it is relatively free from injury, partly because its edges are thickened, thus reinforcing the plate of bone, and partly because it is freely movable on the chest wall and lies between thick pads of muscle.

Mechanism.—In some instances the body of the scapula is broken as a result of direct violence and there is more or less damage to the overlying soft parts, though the break is rarely compound. However, most of the fractures of the scapula are the result of indirect violence, such as falls upon the hand, elbow, or shoulder with force transmitted through the humerus, while the scapula is pulled forward by the serratus magnus. This results in a fracture of the surgical neck or glenoid cavity or a buckling and fracture of the body of the bone. The bone may be broken in any of its parts, but the most frequent fractures are those of the body, neck, and glenoid.

1. Fractures of the Body

There may be a single transverse or oblique break in the bone, but more frequently it is comminuted by fracture lines running in various directions. The break is more often in the region of the lower angle and very rarely near the upper angle of the body. In extensive fractures there may be more or less overlapping or separation of the fragments, but as a rule the muscles on either side hold the pieces in position and there is little or no displacement. (Fig. 458.)

Diagnosis.—Diagnosis is made from the history of an injury either directly over the bone or indirectly from force transmitted through the humerus, followed by local pain, swelling, tenderness and usually an inability to raise the arm fully on the affected side. Disability is due to the fact that pain occurs when the scapula is automatically fixed in the attempt to raise the arm. On physical examination there is tenderness over the scapula, but this may be diffuse, and as the bone is quite deep-seated, it is usually impossible to elicit point tenderness. If either the vertebral or axillary borders are broken, and the fragments are displaced, it may be possible to detect the irregularity by palpation along the border of the bone. A fracture of the scapula may best be detected by fixing the bone by grasping the spine and upper border with one hand and then gently manipulating the lower angle with the other hand (Fig. 411). In this manner, if the bone is broken, definite pain can be elicited and it may be possible to detect false motion and crepitus. An x-ray picture is necessary to learn the details of the fracture.

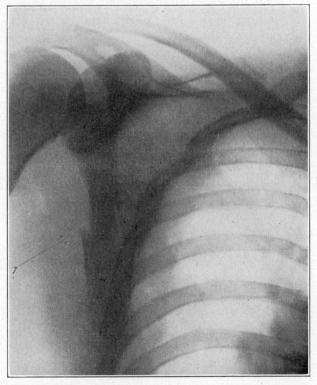

Fig. 458.—Fracture of the body of the scapula with involvement of the axillary border. Treated by cross strapping and a sling for the arm for three weeks with good result.

Complications.—Not infrequently fractures of the body of the scapula are part of extensive crushing injuries of the chest with multiple fractures of the ribs or spine or both, and the fracture of the scapula may be overlooked or ignored because of the gravity of the other injuries and their accompanying shock, surgical emphysema, or pneumothorax.

In other instances the direct trauma which causes the fracture may produce severe injuries to the soft parts, and the lacerations may communicate with the fracture and render it compound, although usually they do not do so.

Treatment

As there is little tendency for the fragments to be displaced, all that is necessary is to make the patient as comfortable as possible until the bone has healed. This is accomplished by immobilizing the shoulder and the soft parts over the scapula. A very efficient and comfortable dressing is illustrated in Fig. 463. A criss-cross strapping with adhesive is applied over the scapula as in the illustration, care being taken to have the strips of adhesive long enough to reach from the front of the affected shoulder well down around the opposite side of the chest, and to apply them tightly after the patient has exhaled completely.

After the criss-cross strapping has been applied over the scapula, a pad of absorbent cotton is placed in the axilla and the arm on the affected side is fastened to the chest by a single strip of adhesive three inches wide and long enough to reach around the arm and chest. The wrist is then supported by a clove hitch or a loop of bandage which passes around the neck.

This dressing is worn for a week or ten days and then reapplied, or if the fracture is not very painful at this time, the criss-cross strapping is applied and the arm is supported in a triangular sling. The strapping is continued for two weeks, or until the patient is comfortable without it. Function is gradually resumed about four weeks after the injury, and complete recovery is to be expected.

In cases with lacerations over the scapula, the criss-cross strapping cannot be applied until the wounds have healed, and the surgeon will treat the wounds of the soft parts and then place a cotton pad in the axilla, immobilize the shoulder by a circular bandage around the upper arm and chest, and support the wrist with a clove hitch or loop of bandage around the neck. Usually these lacerations do not communicate with the fracture and they can be treated as simple wounds of the soft parts.

If there is considerable displacement of the fragments, the surgeon should attempt to reduce this by manipulation of the arm or shoulder and of the inferior angle of the scapula. Usually adduction or abduction and traction of the arm will reduce the displacement. If the displacement recurs when the arm is lowered to the side, it will be necessary to treat the fracture with the arm in abduction, either with an abduction splint, or plaster jacket and shoulder spica, or by recumbency with lateral traction as will be mentioned below in the treatment of fractures of the surgical neck of the scapula.

2. Fracture of the Spine of the Scapula

Fracture of the spine of the scapula is practically always the result of direct violence and is usually accompanied by a comminuted fracture of the body of the scapula; an isolated fracture of the spine does occasionally occur. Diagnosis is made by the local tenderness and swelling with a palpable change in contour and the ability to detect loose fragments or false motion. There is little tendency to displacement, but false motion and crepitus may be elicited.

Treatment.—In these injuries also there is little or no tendency to displacement of the fragments, and they are treated exactly as are fractures of the body of the bone.

3. Fracture of the Acromion

Since the acromion forms the top of the shoulder, it is exposed to direct violence and also to indirect force transmitted upward through the head of the humerus or by leverage action through the tuberosity in abduction injuries. It is so strong, however, that it is rarely broken, and injuries tending to fracture the acromion usually result in fractures of the clavicle or dislocation at the shoulder or acromioclavicular joints. The process may be broken at its base, or in the region lateral to the acromioclavicular joint.

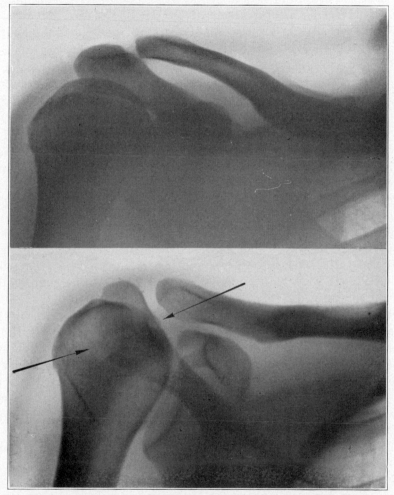

Fig. 459.—Fracture of acromion well shown only in the oblique view as seen in the lower x-ray.

When the break is through the base, the separated process is pulled downward and inward by the deltoid and the weight of the shoulder (Fig. 466). On inspection the shoulder is flattened and the patient is unable to raise or abduct the arm. By careful palpation along the outer portion of the spine, the fracture line can be felt as an irregularity in the bone or located by the presence of point tenderness, and false motion may be obtained by manipulating the acromion, or by pushing upward on the humerus while the scapula is fixed.

When the fracture is lateral to the acromioclavicular joint, there is little tendency for displacement of the small free fragment, and a diagnosis must be made by point tenderness and ability to produce false motion of the tip of the acromion. Usually the small detached fragment cannot be palpated and an x-ray examination is necessary for the diagnosis.

Treatment.—In fractures through the base without displacement and in those instances in which the fracture line lies lateral to the acromioclavicular joint, the tip of the process being detached, a criss-cross strapping should be applied over the deltoid in such a manner that the adhesive, being pulled from below upward, tends to force the fragment back in place. The arm is then immobilized by a circular swathe and sling as in fractures of the body.

In fractures through the base of the acromion or through the acromioclavicular joint with flattening of the shoulder and dropping down of the detached fragment, the condition is similar to an acromioclavicular lesion, and the acromioclavicular adhesive dressing should be applied as illustrated in Fig. 451.

4. Fractures of the Coracoid Process

Fracture of the coracoid process rarely occurs as an isolated lesion, but is not infrequently present in severe injuries to the shoulder with multiple fractures. When it occurs alone it may be caused by direct violence, but the fracture is usually the result of muscular action, the coracoid being broken across near its base and the distal fragment displaced downward for a short distance. The mechanism is an abduction of the arm which puts tension on the short head of the biceps and the coracobrachialis. The symptoms are swelling and tenderness over the process and localized pain when the arm is abducted or actively adducted against resistance. False motion and crepitus cannot always be obtained because the process is so deep-seated.

Treatment.—As the pectoralis minor, coracobrachialis and short head of the biceps tend to draw the loose fragment away from its base, the indications in treatment are to relax these muscles and make pressure over the process.

A convenient and efficient method of treatment is to place a pad of saddlers felt 3 inches in diameter and $1\frac{1}{2}$ inches thick over the fractured process. This is held in place by a strip of adhesive 3 inches wide which is started on the posterolateral aspect of the shoulder and pulled forward and downward across the pad and fastened around the opposite side of the chest. After padding the axilla and protecting the chest by a circular bandage, the hand on the affected side is then placed on the opposite shoulder and immobilized in the third and fourth strips of Conwell's adhesive dressing or in a Velpeau bandage. This dressing is worn for about three weeks and then the arm is carried in a sling for two weeks longer.

Prognosis.—If the above method of treatment is used, a normal shoulder is to be expected. Even in instances where the process fails to unite there is usually a good functional result.

5. Fractures of the Surgical Neck and Glenoid Cavity of the Scapula

These fractures may result indirectly from force transmitted to the glenoid through the humerus, or from falls or blows on the shoulder. The most com-

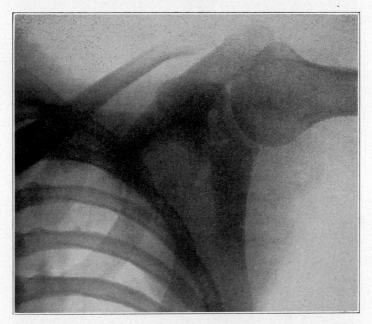

Fig. 461.—Comminuted fracture of the body of the scapula and glenoid with slight displacement. Treated the same as case shown in Fig. 460, with good result.

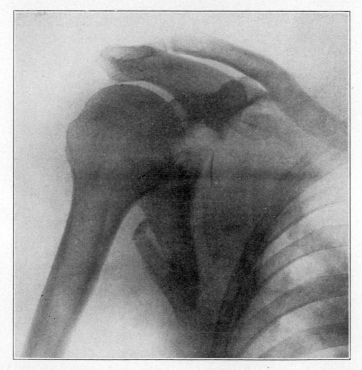

Fig. 462.—Severely comminuted fracture of the body of the scapula and glenoid. Treated the same as case shown in Fig. 460, except recumbency was twenty-five days and plaster spica cast for eighteen days. Only fair result.

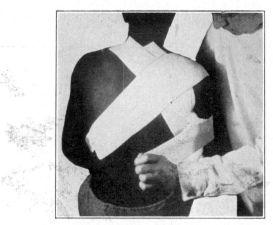

Fig. 463.—Ambulatory adhesive dressing for fracture of the body of the scapula. Simple cross strapping of the scapula. Axillary pad and adhesive swathe around arm. The forearm should be supported by a sling.

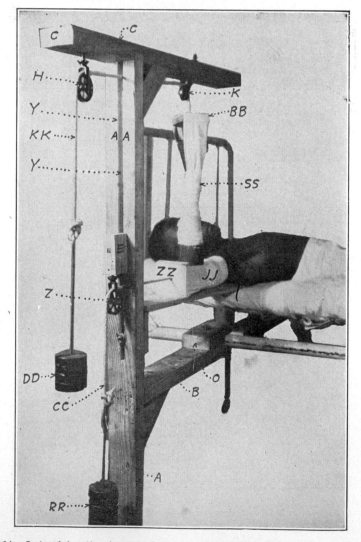

Fig. 464.—Lateral traction in recumbency for fractures of the surgical neck of the scapula or glenoid fossa (also for fractures of clavicle or upper third of humerus or acromioclavicular dislocations).

In fractures of the neck with considerable damage to the ligaments and downward displacement of the shoulder but no damage to the glenoid, the above adhesive dressing should be tried, but the results should be carefully checked by the x-ray, and if the position of the fragments is not satisfactory, the patient should be treated in an abduction plaster jacket or in recumbency with lateral traction as will be described below.

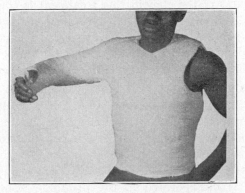

Fig. 465.—Ambulatory plaster-of-Paris spica jacket for fractures of the surgical neck of the scapula or glenoid. This dressing is excellent for moderate glenoid fractures or fractures of the neck of the scapula. It is excellent for follow-up dressing in cases requiring recumbency.

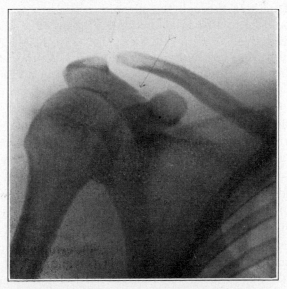

Fig. 466.—Fracture of the acromion with very little displacement. There is also a slight acromioclavicular luxation. Treated by acromioclavicular dressing for three weeks and cross strapping to scapula for two weeks with forearm in sling for one week. Good result.

If the fracture line involves the glenoid cavity and there is comminution and separation of the fragments, the fracture must be treated with traction and with the arm in abduction, and preferably, with the patient recumbent, if a stiff and painful shoulder is to be avoided. The traction tends to pull the fragments of the glenoid back into position and hold them there.

The patient is placed on a firm mattress and a lateral traction apparatus is set up (Fig. 464). Then the traction strips are applied to the forearm and it is suspended with the arm abducted 90 degrees and externally rotated 90 degrees. Traction strips are then placed on the arm and from 6 to 12 pounds traction is instituted. A Thomas ring splint or thick support beneath the shoulder should be avoided as they are not only uncomfortable, but tend to displace the fragments. The arm really needs no support, but if immobilization is desired, a small thin board may be placed under it.

In severe fractures of the glenoid this treatment is continued for from six to eight weeks, and the patient is permitted to use the arm when such movements do not cause pain. At the end of this time the arm can be brought down gradually to the side and carried in a sling, but physiotherapy and abduction and rotation exercises should be continued for some weeks longer.

In certain instances in which it is highly desirable to treat the patient in an ambulant apparatus, the abduction splint with traction or the plaster jacket and shoulder spica with the traction apparatus of Hoke may be used. In either case the adhesive traction strips are fastened to the arm and traction is made on the abducted arm with the elbow flexed. In the case of the Hoke apparatus the plaster spica jacket is applied over the traction strips and the traction apparatus is incorporated in the plaster. Then the plaster is cut away over the elbow and upper half of the ulna and the strips are fastened in the apparatus and traction is applied.

In simple fractures through the glenoid with little or no displacement, the fracture should be treated in abduction for about four weeks, with a traction splint or plaster jacket with shoulder spica (Fig. 465). The jacket can be applied with the patient either sitting or standing. At the end of four weeks the splint or plaster is removed, the arm is carried in a sling, and massage, local heat and graded exercises are begun and continued until function is restored (two to six weeks).

In small chip fractures of the glenoid, simple immobilization of the shoulder and arm in about 30 degrees abduction by means of an axillary pad swathe and sling for from three to four weeks are all that is necessary.

Prognosis.—In fractures of the neck which do not involve the glenoid, a normal shoulder may be expected in three months unless there is severe damage to the soft parts and traumatic arthritis or periarthritis develops. These may prolong the disability indefinitely.

In fractures of the glenoid without displacement one usually obtains a practically normal shoulder. If the bone is comminuted, there is apt to be more or less limitation of motion and occasional twinges of pain from time to time, especially with changes of weather.

DISLOCATION OF THE SCAPULA

Etiology.—Dislocation of the scapula is a very rare injury, but by outward traction on the arm or by direct violence from behind the entire scapula may be dislocated outward and rotated outward so that its lower angle or vertebral border becomes caught between the ribs and fixed in an abnormal position. The rhomboid muscles attached to the vertebral border are either stretched or torn.

Diagnosis.—The diagnosis is relatively easy as the axillary border of the scapula, especially in its lower portion, is unusually prominent and the vertebral border is displaced outward or cannot be palpated especially in its lower portion. The bone is fixed in its abnormal position and severe pain is produced by attempts to manipulate it or the shoulder (Fig. 467).

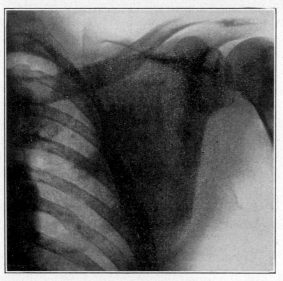

Fig. 467.—Dislocation of the scapula. Reduced by manipulation and immobilized by adhesive strapping for three weeks with forearm in sling for ten days, with guarded motions for three weeks longer, with good result.

Treatment

In order to reduce the dislocation, the lower portion of the vertebral border must be freed from between the ribs. This can usually be done by having an assistant make traction on the hyperabducted arm while the surgeon grasps the axillary border of the scapula and rotates the bone forward at the same time that he pushes it directly backward. As soon as it is released, the scapula tends to slip back to its normal position.

After reduction is accomplished the scapula is pushed as far as possible toward the midline and strapped firmly in place by wide strips of adhesive which begin in front, pass under the arm on the affected side, and are carried over the scapula and around the chest or over the opposite shoulder. A pad is placed in the axilla and the arm strapped to the side by a single wide band of adhesive which passes entirely around the chest. The forearm and wrist should be supported by a clove hitch or sling. This dressing is worn for four weeks and the arm is carried in a sling for a week or two longer.

In very rare instances it may be necessary to perform an open reduction and suture the bone in place.

DISLOCATION AT THE SHOULDER

Frequency.—Dislocation occurs more frequently at the shoulder than at any other joint in the body, and statistics show that this lesion comprises approximately 50 per cent of all dislocations. The great majority of the cases occur in robust adult males, but the accident may occur in patients of any age or sex, though it is extremely rare in children.

Predisposing Causes.—The relative frequency with which dislocation occurs at the shoulder may be explained by the following anatomic characteristics of the joint: (1) The head of the humerus is relatively much larger than the shallow glenoid cavity in which it rests; (2) the capsule and ligaments are relatively loose and weak and the integrity of the joint is largely dependent upon the muscles, which may be easily stretched; (3) the joint has a very wide range of movement and leverage can be exerted upon it through the upper extremity; and (4) the joint occupies an exposed position upon the body.

Types of Dislocation.—Depending upon the final position of the head of the humerus as related to the glenoid cavity, dislocations at the shoulder may be classified as anterior, downward, posterior, and upward dislocations.

Depending upon the anatomic position of the humeral head, the various dislocations are also given special names, such as subcoracoid, subclavicular, etc. These are all varieties of the four primary types mentioned above and will be described in their proper places.

Anterior Dislocations at the Shoulder

Subcoracoid.—In the great majority of anterior dislocations the head of the humerus rests beneath the coracoid process and this is the most frequent type of dislocation at the shoulder.

Mechanism of Production.—In the majority of instances subcoracoid dislocations are caused by a fall or blow upon the abducted arm, the force acting in a direction tending to increase the abduction. In a position of full abduction, the head of the humerus tends to leave the glenoid and rest upon the inferior portion of the capsule of the joint. Consequently when force is applied through the humerus, the inferior portion of the capsule is torn from the margin of the glenoid or ruptured and the head is forced directly through the rent by axial pressure, or levered through on the acromion as a fulcrum, or levered through by rotation of the shaft of the humerus around the attachments of the strong adductor muscles. In any event the head tends to be displaced downward and inward, and after it leaves the capsule, the pull of the pectoralis major and subscapularis muscles tend to move it forward beneath the coracoid.

In addition to the mechanisms of hyperabduction and axial pressure on the abducted arm described above, a subcoracoid dislocation may be caused by a fall or blow on the point of the shoulder while the arm is at the side. In this type of injury the humeral head is driven downward, forward, and inward by direct trauma. Very rarely a dislocation at the shoulder may result from muscular action, as in throwing.

Pathology of Subcoracoid Dislocation.—The joint capsule is torn in its anterior and inferior portions, the tear extending for a variable distance along the rim of the glenoid, and the head of the humerus having passed through, the margins of the tear surround the upper portion of the shaft. The strong coracohumeral ligaments usually remain intact and tend to limit the displacement of the humerus.

The arm is maintained in a position of slight abduction and its axis is displaced inward and downward. The head of the humerus usually lies on the anterior surface of the neck of the scapula just beneath the coracoid, but with extensive tearing of ligaments and capsule it may be displaced farther inward and lie mesial to the coracoid.

The deltoid and posterior scapular muscles are stretched over the glenoid and the subscapularis is stretched over the head of the humerus and any of the deeper muscles may be torn or avulsed from their insertion.

Not infrequently the anteroinferior lip of the glenoid is injured and small fragments of cartilage or bone may be broken off. In a considerable percentage of cases with severe injury and marked displacement the greater tuberosity is broken off and the separated fragment may remain close to its original position because of intact periosteum, or it may be widely separated and drawn up beneath the acromion by the posterior scapular muscles.

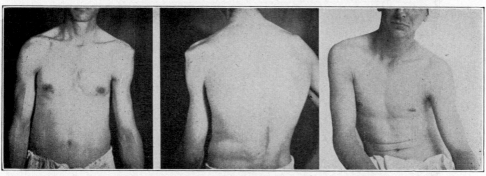

Fig. 468.   Fig. 469.   Fig. 470.

Fig. 468.—Subcoracoid dislocation at the left shoulder. Note the flattening of the shoulder, prominence of the acromion, and swelling in the subcoracoid region.

Fig. 469.—Same patient seen from behind. The flattening of the shoulder is even more evident.

Fig. 470.—Typical position of patient with subcoracoid dislocation at the left shoulder. Note the moderate abduction of the arm with flattening of the shoulder as in the previous photograph.

As the greater tuberosity forms the posterior lip of the bicipital groove, when it is broken and displaced the biceps tendon may slip out of its groove and get caught on the area of raw bone and offer a serious obstacle to reduction.

Diagnosis of Subcoracoid Dislocations.—There is the history of an injury followed by pain and disability in the shoulder, and the arm is fixed in a position of slight abduction (about 30 degrees). Attempts to bring it to the side or to move it more than a few degrees in any direction cause pain and are resisted by an elastic-like force.

On inspection the arm appears to be lengthened and its axis is displaced inward and downward and passes below and anterior to the glenoid. The axilla is broadened and the anterior axillary fold is displaced downward.

The normal contour of the shoulder is disturbed in that the acromion is unusually prominent and the deltoid is flattened. In any except very fleshy individuals an unusual fullness is visible in the region below the coracoid. (Figs. 468, 469, and 470.)

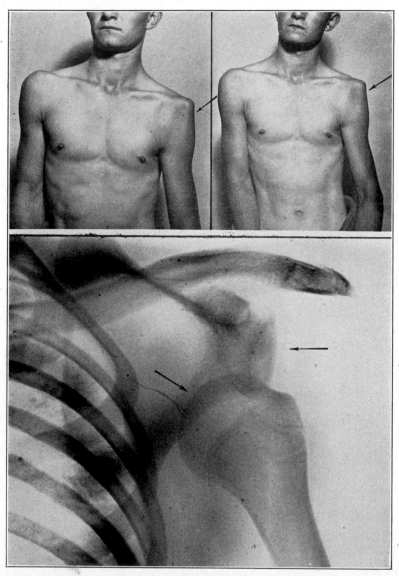

Fig. 471.—Subcoracoid dislocation with only slight displacement inward. Reduction under an anesthetic. Immobilization with adhesive dressing for twelve days after which the forearm was carried in a sling for ten days. Good result.

On palpation the fingers sink into the space beneath the acromion and the head of the humerus is felt to be absent from its normal position and can be palpated on the front of the shoulder near the coracoid as a rounded mass which rotates with the shaft of the humerus. The length of the arm as measured from the tip of the acromion to the external condyle of the humerus is slightly increased or decreased.

There is practically no active motion, but passive rotation is fairly free although it may be painful. Other motions are markedly limited and this is especially true of adduction unless there has been extensive tearing of ligaments. Duga's sign, inability to place the hand on the opposite shoulder while the elbow is held against the chest, may fail in the presence of extensive tearing of ligaments and muscles.

The X-Ray.—While not necessary for the diagnosis, an x-ray picture is desirable before instituting treatment in order to rule out fractures which may be present and which may modify the treatment. (Figs. 471 and 472.)

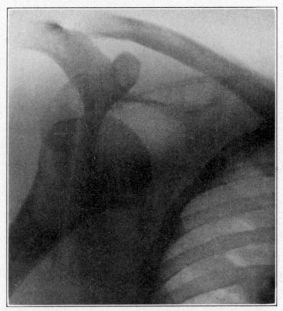

Fig. 472.—Subcoracoid dislocation in which the inward displacement is more marked than in the preceding case. Reduction under an anesthetic, adhesive dressing two weeks, forearm in sling ten days. Good result.

Complications of Dislocations at the Shoulder

Complications are rather frequent in dislocations at the shoulder and may be very severe. The most frequent types are those in which fractures of either the humerus or the scapula are produced at the time of the original injury or by strenuous attempts at reduction. These fractures during reduction are particularly apt to occur when the dislocation has been present for some time and scar tissue formation and bone atrophy have developed. The fractures which have occurred with dislocations of the shoulder are glenoid, coracoid, and acromion of the scapula, anatomic or surgical neck, or either tuberosity of the humerus. The most frequent is fracture of the greater tuberosity.

1. Bone Lesions

1. **Fractures of the Glenoid.**—One of the most frequent complications is fracture of the glenoid which consists of a chip off the lower part of the anterior lip of the glenoid cavity. This injury can be positively diagnosed only

by the x-ray. It is to be suspected if during reduction bony crepitus is felt at the point when the head slips into the cavity or if the dislocation recurs very readily after reduction.

2. **Fractures of the Coracoid and Acromion** are both rare injuries and give rise to local tenderness and swelling over the site of the fracture. In the case of the acromion, false mobility and crepitus may be obtained by manipulating the detached fragment. In the case of the coracoid process, the fracture is usually diagnosed only by means of the x-ray.

3. **Fractures of a Tuberosity of the Humerus.**—Fracture of the greater tuberosity is a frequent complication and it may be possible to palpate the detached fragment in the tissues beneath the acromion where it has been drawn by the posterior scapular muscles. As a rule, however, the fragment remains attached to the humerus by periosteum and there is little tendency for it to be widely separated.

The lesser tuberosity is rarely fractured, but when it is torn off, the biceps tendon may slip out of its groove and interfere with reduction. Here, too, there is little tendency to displacement of the detached fragment and it does not interfere with reduction. The diagnosis of a fracture of the tuberosity is difficult to make in the absence of a positive roentgenogram.

4. **Fracture of the Anatomic Neck of the Humerus** is a very rare lesion in connection with dislocation of the shoulder, and can only be differentiated from fractures of the surgical neck with dislocation by the x-ray.

5. **Fracture of the Surgical Neck (Fracture Dislocation at the Shoulder)** is a severe and rather rare complication of dislocation of the shoulder. The head of the humerus is absent from its normal position and can usually be palpated in the tissues beneath the coracoid. The clinical picture resembles that of a fracture of the surgical neck of the humerus in that the arm is not fixed in abduction, and false motion can be demonstrated, but the glenoid is felt to be empty and the head of the humerus can be palpated in its abnormal position. It is very important to recognize this complication before attempting reduction as energetic manipulation may cause considerable permanent damage to the soft tissues in the vicinity.

2. Nerve Injuries

The brachial plexus or some of its branches, especially the circumflex, may be stretched or torn by the depression of the shoulder caused by the dislocating force, or may be stretched over the dislocated head of the humerus, or may be directly injured by the head of the humerus. In cases in which the humeral head is widely displaced the circumflex nerve is apt to be torn or stretched because it is in such intimate relation with the upper end of the bone. (Fig. 473.)

These nerve injuries are more common than is generally known, but they may be produced by attempts at reduction of the dislocation. Consequently, it is advisable for the surgeon to make a rough motor and sensory examination of the extremity before he attempts to reduce the dislocation, because if the nerve lesion is not discovered until after the reduction, the patient and perhaps his lawyer too, may conclude that the nerve injury was produced by the surgeon when he effected the reduction. In the case of the circumflex it may be impossible to decide whether or not that nerve is injured, because the trauma to the deltoid may cause a temporary paralysis of the muscle.

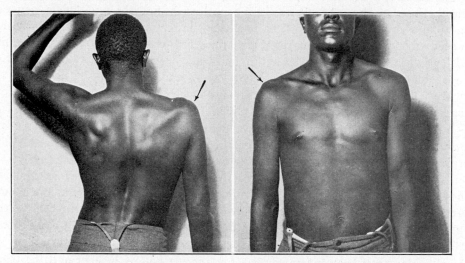

Fig. 473.—Paralysis of the right deltoid following a traumatic dislocation of the shoulder, showing atrophy and inability to abduct the arm.

3. Vascular Injuries

Fortunately vascular injuries are very rare. Occasionally, however, the axillary artery or vein may be torn at the time of the injury or by violent attempts at reduction. When the artery is torn the radial pulse is absent and a large hematoma, which may pulsate, appears rapidly in the front of the shoulder and axilla. When the vein is torn, the hematoma appears more slowly and the extremity is swollen and cyanotic.

4. Compound Dislocations at the Shoulder

Compound dislocations at the shoulder are very rare but may result from great violence. The head of the humerus may be driven through the skin of the axilla, in the pectoral region, or even behind the shoulder. Because of the marked displacement these injuries are usually accompanied by injury to the circumflex nerve.

Treatment of Subcoracoid Dislocations

In an uncomplicated dislocation at the shoulder the indications are to reduce the dislocation as soon as possible. Immediate reduction is advisable, not only to relieve the pain, but also to facilitate reduction, since the longer the dislocation is present, the more difficult it is to reduce.

Question of an Anesthetic.—The surgeon must decide the question of an anesthetic as soon as he has made his diagnosis. We give ⅙ to ¼ grain of morphine hypodermically and then base our decision upon the cooperation of the patient, musculature of the patient, and the duration of the dislocation.

Some patients are cooperative and are willing to stand a few seconds of sharp pain in order to avoid an anesthetic. Others are uncooperative and demand an anesthetic before any reduction is attempted. In the latter an anesthetic is necessary; usually nitrous oxide is sufficient. If the musculature is weak, reduction is less difficult and can usually be accomplished without a general anesthetic. On the other hand, if the patient is heavily muscled, a general anesthetic is advisable. The time is a very important factor. If the patient is seen within an hour after the dislocation, reduction can usually be accomplished without an anesthetic, but if he is not seen until several hours after the accident a general anesthetic is advisable, and ether may be necessary to secure muscular relaxation. If a previous unsuccessful attempt at reduction has been made, an anesthetic is advisable.

The argument for always using a general anesthetic is that the surgeon may fracture the humerus or damage the soft parts in attempting reduction in the presence of muscle spasm. The argument against it is that there is a certain amount of danger, discomfort, and inconvenience in every general anesthetic, and that experience has shown that fresh dislocations at the shoulder in patients who are cooperative and not too heavily muscled can be reduced without an anesthetic and with the application of relatively little force.

Choice of Method.—Many methods for reducing anterior dislocations at the shoulder have been recommended, but the method of Kocher and the traction and leverage method are the only ones which we shall describe.

Kocher's Method.—This is the most efficient and least traumatizing method yet devised for the reduction of subcoracoid dislocations. As subcoracoid dislocation occurs far more frequently than any other type at the shoulder, and as dislocations at the shoulder comprise about 50 per cent of all dislocations, every surgeon should learn and understand this method, because he may be called upon to reduce a subcoracoid dislocation and not have an opportunity to look it up.

Preliminary Maneuver.—Kocher's method causes the head of the humerus to retrace its path into the glenoid and is most easily performed when the head of the humerus lies close to the anterior and lower border of the glenoid; that is, near the rent in the capsule. Consequently, before beginning the classical maneuver, it is advisable to get the head in the most favorable position possible. With this end in view the patient is placed on his back and with the elbow flexed to a right angle an assistant makes firm but slow and steady traction in the direction of the long axis of the humerus while the surgeon grasps the humerus as high up in the axilla as possible and pulls its upper end directly outward with the same slow, steady traction. The amount of traction exerted should be just enough to overcome the muscle spasm and there is no necessity for great force. This maneuver causes the head of the humerus to approach the glenoid and may even effect reduction, though it should not be carried out with great force in the hope that it may do so. It is far better surgery to proceed gently with the three stages of Kocher's method as described below.

1. **External Rotation** (Fig. 474).—The surgeon now grasps the patient's elbow with one hand and his wrist with the other, and while pressing the

patient's arm against the chest wall very slowly, but firmly, rotates the arm and forearm outward until the forearm points almost directly away from the side of the body (about 75 degrees). Cotton recommends that this external rotation be performed so slowly that from two to five minutes be consumed in its accomplishment.

This outward rotation slowly overcomes the spasm of the subscapularis muscle and causes the head to move outward against the lip of the glenoid.

2. **Adduction Forward** (Fig. 475).—With the external rotation and slight traction maintained the patient's arm is now carried forward across the chest in such a manner that the point of the elbow tends to approach the ensiform cartilage or midline of the abdomen. The movement should be slow, firm, and steadily progressive, and the elbow should be kept as close to the chest as possible and the arm sort of levered over the ribs in order to lift the head of the humerus and cause it to slip over the edge of the glenoid. In the majority of instances the head slips into the glenoid during this second maneuver of forward adduction, and the reduction may be so gently accomplished that the surgeon does not know when it happens.

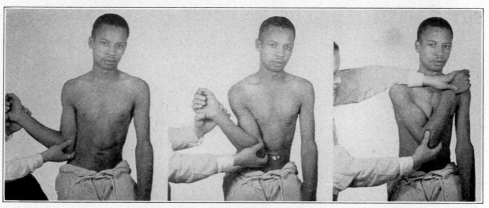

Fig. 474.   Fig. 475.   Fig. 476.

Fig. 474.—Kocher's first maneuver for the reduction of anterior dislocation at the shoulder. The arm is carried into full external rotation while the elbow is held against the chest and moderate traction is made on the humerus.

Fig. 475.—Kocher's second maneuver. While rotation and traction are maintained, the humerus is adducted across the chest.

Fig. 476.—Kocher's third maneuver. Still maintaining the traction, the arm is rotated inward until the hand is placed on the opposite shoulder.

3. **Internal Rotation** (Fig. 476).—With the point of the elbow held as close to the midline of the body as possible, the arm is rotated internally, using the forearm as a lever, and the hand is placed upon the opposite shoulder. This maneuver completes the reduction and restores the head to its normal position.

If much resistance is encountered in performing the third maneuver, the attempt has probably failed and the surgeon should start again at the beginning.

In the second attempt it is advisable to place some sort of fulcrum in the patient's axilla before starting the second maneuver. A fist or forearm of an assistant or a folded sheet or large towel is enough and gives the surgeon a fulcrum over which he can lever the shaft of the humerus and lift the head outward and into the glenoid.

If this second attempt with an axillary pad or fulcrum fails, then the surgeon should examine the shoulder carefully, make sure that his diagnosis is correct and that he is not dealing with a fracture-dislocation of the shoulder. If no obstacle other than muscle spasm or adhesions in the case of an old dislocation can be found, the surgeon should start again, first pulling the head of the humerus down and out as close to the glenoid as possible. Then he should relegate the manipulation of the arm to an assistant who can be trusted to proceed slowly and follow directions and not violently manipulate it and either break the humerus or damage nerves or vessels.

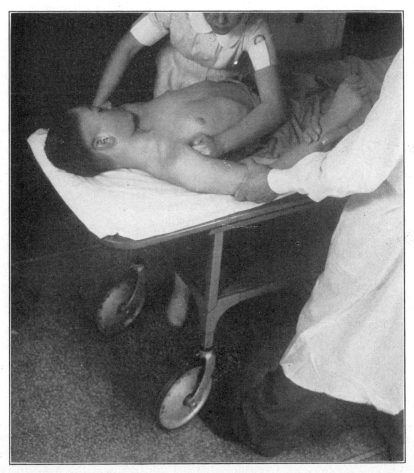

Fig. 477.—Using the fist of an assistant in the axilla as an aid in reducing dislocations of the shoulder. The stockinged foot of the surgeon is even more efficient. (Courtesy Dr. Benjamin Meyer.)

The arm is now externally rotated and the fulcrum is placed in the axilla. As the assistant slowly adducts the humerus forward over the fulcrum, maintaining the full external rotation, the surgeon grasps the acromion and spine of the scapula with one hand and presses the scapula inward and backward while with the other hand he endeavors to push the head of the humerus into the glenoid.

If this third effort fails in a fresh subcoracoid dislocation, we believe it is time to quit and either do an open reduction or let some other surgeon try his hand at it, as violent manipulations may do more harm than good.

The Traction and Leverage Method.—This is one of the oldest and still one of the most efficient methods. The surgeon's heel in the axilla is a satisfactory fulcrum for the lever. In using this method the patient lies on his back and the surgeon places his unbooted heel in the axilla and, grasping the patient's wrist, makes traction on the arm in line with the humerus, at the same time adducting the arm slightly, thus levering the head of the humerus outward over the margin of the glenoid. If reduction does not occur immediately, the arm is rotated outward to lift the head of the humerus over the margin of the glenoid. The surgeon's right heel is used for a dislocation of the right shoulder and the left heel is used for a dislocation of the left shoulder. The traction should be slow and steady as violent manipulation may damage the soft tissues.

This method has the advantage that it is equally efficient for subglenoid dislocations while Kocher's method is primarily for anterior dislocations.

Operative Reduction of a Recent Anterior Dislocation.—If the application of the methods described above fails to effect reduction, and if there is no fracture of the humerus, then there must be some obstacle to reduction which does not show in the roentgenogram and an open operation is justified.

The anterior region of the shoulder is exposed by an incision about 5 inches long over the groove between the deltoid and pectoralis major muscles. When these muscles are retracted the glenoid, torn capsule, and upper end of the humerus can be exposed and whatever is interfering with reduction (usually the biceps tendon or fragments of bone in the glenoid) can be removed or pulled aside and the shoulder reduced by the Kocher method. Then the wound is closed in layers and the case is treated as though the dislocation had been reduced by the closed method.

Treatment After Reduction.—After the shoulder dislocation has been reduced the arm must be bound to the side with the humerus rotated inward to guard against a recurrence of the dislocation and to permit the torn ligaments and capsule to heal.

For this purpose a Velpeau bandage or an adhesive dressing with a clove hitch for the forearm as illustrated in Fig. 478 is fairly comfortable and quite simple to apply. A pad of absorbent cotton is placed in the axilla and a three-inch strip of adhesive long enough to encircle the upper arm and chest is strapped tightly around the upper arm to encircle the chest just beneath the opposite axilla. A similar strip is passed around the lower arm and chest and a third strip around the lower arm, flexed forearm, and chest, and the wrist is suspended by a clove hitch or cravat sling. The dressing should not be tight enough to obstruct the circulation in the arm.

Another efficient and comfortable method is the application of the acromioclavicular adhesive dressing as illustrated in Fig. 479.

The dressing should be worn for from one to two weeks. At the end of this time it may be removed, the arm carried in a sling, and exercises begun in an effort to hasten the restoration of function. The sling should be continued for from one to three weeks or until the shoulder is stable, fairly strong, and not painful when the sling is omitted.

During this period the patient should be cautioned to keep the arm at the side except while taking prescribed exercises and especially to avoid reaching out and up for objects, particularly the guards on a streetcar or bus which may jerk the arm and cause recurrence of the dislocation.

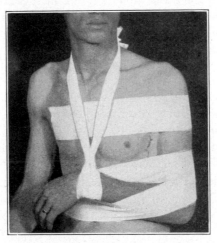

Fig. 478.—Simple fixation dressing to be used after reduction of a dislocated shoulder.

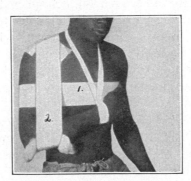

Fig. 479.—Acromioclavicular adhesive dressing for use after reduction of a dislocation at the shoulder. (See also Fig. 451.)

Restoration of function usually occurs spontaneously and a normal shoulder results after two months or so with no particular effort on the part of the surgeon. On the other hand, especially in older patients, a stiff and painful shoulder with limited abduction and rotation may persist for several months despite strenuous efforts on the part of the surgeon. The latter course is apt to be followed in older patients, particularly those with arthritis. Consequently, as soon as the retention dressing is removed, exercises are begun and continued until a satisfactory result is secured.

In the beginning, heat (dry, moist, or diathermy) should be applied to the shoulder and followed by gentle massage and passive motion. As the tenderness disappears, active exercise should be instituted, the abduction being limited at first and gradually increased. In the early stages abduction is best accomplished by having the patient lie upon the back and abduct the arm as far as possible with the deltoid and then continue the motion by working the hand out with the fingers. As the movement improves, the patient is taught to stand with the shoulder facing the wall and the hand against the wall. Then by means of the fingers "crawling up the wall" the abduction is gradually increased (Fig. 480). In order to stimulate the patient and to check the results, daily records of the height reached should be kept.

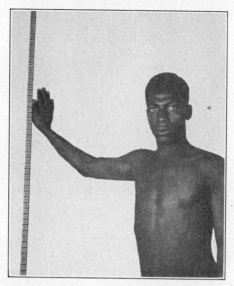

Fig. 480.—Exercise to aid in restoring abduction of the arm at the shoulder after a dislocation.

Other Anterior Dislocations

Depending upon the final resting place of the head of the humerus, intracoracoid, supracoracoid and subclavicular dislocations have been described. These are all identical with the subcoracoid except that there is more extensive ligamentous injury and the head of the humerus has been displaced farther inward. They should be reduced by the Kocher method as described above, but in these the preliminary downward and outward traction are especially important because the head must first be brought to the subcoracoid position.

The same is true of the very rare intrathoracic dislocation. In this lesion the head of the humerus must be pulled out of the chest and then reduced by the usual method.

Downward Dislocation at the Shoulder

Subglenoid Dislocation.—Next to the subcoracoid, the subglenoid is the most frequent form of dislocation at the shoulder and it is probable that many subcoracoid dislocations are first subglenoid and then become subcoracoid by slight inward and anterior movement of the head. All transitions between the two types may be met.

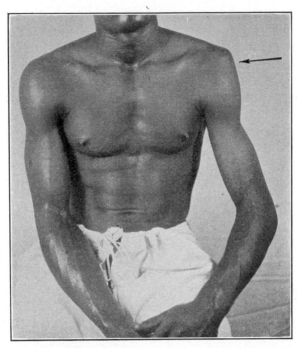

Fig. 481.—Subglenoid dislocation at the left shoulder. Note the abduction, flattening of the shoulder, displacement of anterior axillary line, and absence of swelling near the coracoid.

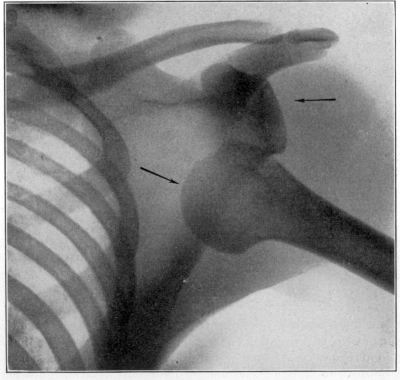

Fig. 482.—Roentgenogram of preceding case.

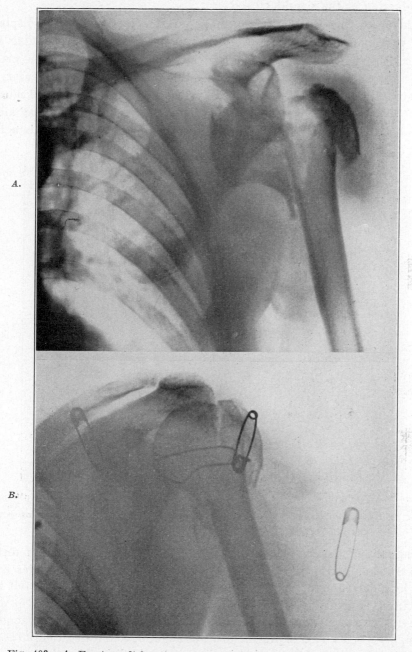

Fig. 483.—*A*, Fracture dislocation of left shoulder. Closed reduction unsuccessful.
B, Same as preceding after open reduction and wiring fragments to maintain position with arm dressed at side to maintain reduction of dislocation. Wire is not through articular surface. Safety pins, in dressing. Recent case.

Cause.—As in the subcoracoid type this dislocation is usually caused by hyperabduction at the shoulder.

Pathology.—The capsule is torn in its inferior portion and the displaced head of the humerus rests upon the triceps tendon and the triangular area of the axillary border of the scapula just beneath the glenoid with the greater tuberosity opposed to the lower border of the glenoid. The teres major and minor muscles tend to be relaxed, but all of the other scapulohumeral muscles are stretched or torn. The coracohumeral ligaments are intact and aid in maintaining the arm in its abnormal position of about 45 degrees abduction.

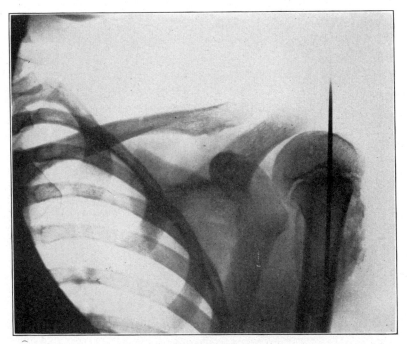

Fig. 484.—Fracture dislocation of shoulder in a child after an unsuccessful attempt at open reduction and after open reduction and fixation with a single Kirschner wire. The wire was bent at a right angle close to the skin and was removed four weeks postoperatively. Normal shoulder obtained. (J. A. K.)

Diagnosis of the Subglenoid Dislocation.—The cardinal signs of dislocation at the shoulder are present. The normal contour of the shoulder is disturbed by a flattening of the deltoid and the head of the humerus is felt to be absent from its normal position (Figs. 481, 482, 483, 485, and 486). The depth and circumference of the axilla are increased, the arm is fixed in an abnormal position, and Dugas' sign is present just as in subcoracoid dislocation. The only differences between the two are that in the subglenoid dislocation the head of the humerus can be palpated in the axilla and the axis of the humerus is displaced directly downward and the arm tends to be maintained in a position of about 45 degrees abduction.

Treatment of Subglenoid Dislocation.—This dislocation can be reduced by the traction and leverage method with the heel in the axilla as described above.

However, it is usually simpler merely to lift the head back into the glenoid. Ordinarily this can be done by having an assistant make moderate slow continuous traction on the arm in the direction of the long axis of the humerus, while the surgeon grasps the upper arm with his fingers in the axilla and gently lifts the head of the humerus directly outward and lets it slide up over the rim of the glenoid and into the socket.

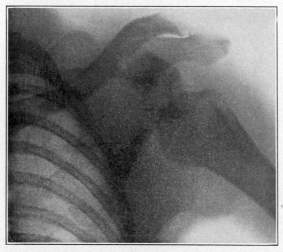

Fig. 485.—Subglenoid dislocation at the shoulder. Reduced under an anesthetic, immobilized with adhesive dressing for twelve days; then arm carried in a sling for one week. Good result.

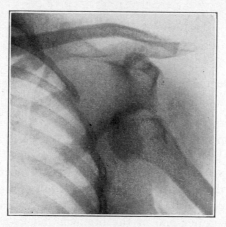

Fig. 486.—Subglenoid dislocation with fracture of the greater tuberosity. Reduced under an anesthetic, treated by adhesive dressing for ten days, then lateral traction with 90 degrees abduction and 180 degrees external rotation for three weeks, after which the arm was put in a sling and exercises were begun. Good result in twelve weeks.

After reduction the treatment is the same as for subcoracoid dislocation.

Luxatio Erecta is a rare type of downward dislocation in which the arm is directed directly upward and is fixed in this abnormal position and cannot be lowered. Usually the humerus is rotated in such a manner that the forearm rests on the top of the head. It is an exaggerated subglenoid dislocation produced by hyperabduction with downward pressure on the humerus. There

is extensive tearing of the capsule, ligaments, muscles, and the nerves, especially the circumflex, may be injured. Likewise one or both tuberosities may
be torn off. The diagnosis is obvious. In addition to the erect deformity the
head of the humerus can be felt in the axilla at some point on the axillary
border of the scapula.

Treatment is reduction by traction upward and slightly outward. After
the head of the humerus slips into the glenoid the arm is gently lowered to
the side and treated as is a subcoracoid dislocation.

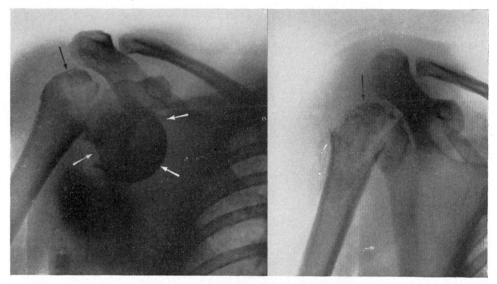

Fig. 487.—Fracture dislocation of the shoulder. Fair result after removal of the head of the
humerus.

Posterior Dislocations at the Shoulder

These are rare injuries in which the head of the humerus is forced directly
backward through the posterior capsule and comes to rest upon the posterior
surface of the neck of the scapula either beneath the acromion or the spine.
Depending upon the position of the head, these dislocations are classified as
subacromial and subspinous, the latter being the more extensive displacement. The posterior dislocations are caused by force applied to the adducted
arm as in falls forward on the hands, or by direct trauma to the front of the
shoulder, forcing the upper end of the humerus backward.

The capsule is extensively torn in its posterior portion and the subscapularis is torn or stretched across the glenoid. The posterior scapular
muscles are torn off or stretched over the upper end of the humerus.

The diagnosis is not difficult but the subacromial dislocation may be
overlooked because the displaced head is shielded by the acromion and masked
by the swelling. The shoulder is markedly swollen behind and flattened in
front and the acromion is prominent. The arm is usually fixed in a position
of adduction with the elbow against the chest and attempts at abduction cause
pain. The position of the arm varies considerably in different cases and in

the subspinous type it may be abducted and forward. The glenoid may be partly filled by the shaft, and the head is largely responsible for the swelling behind the shoulder and may be palpable here. However, the extensive swelling may mask the displaced head of the humerus and it may be necessary to slightly rotate the shaft in order to identify the head in its abnormal position.

Treatment.—Reduction is by traction in the long axis of the humerus assisted by pressure on the displaced head with the thumbs. When the head has reached the rim of the glenoid it may be assisted over this by gently adducting the arm, thus levering the head outward, and gently rotating it inward.

After reduction, treatment is the same as for subcoracoid dislocation except that the arm should be immobilized directly downward against the chest and not brought forward.

Dislocation Upward

These are extremely rare injuries in which the head of the humerus rides upward in front of the acromion which may or may not be fractured. All of the recorded cases are in the older literature and most of these were old unreduced dislocations. In a recent case the diagnosis would be obvious and reduction would be accomplished by downward and outward traction assisted by pressure on the head with the thumbs.

Treatment of Complications of Dislocation at the Shoulder

1. **Fracture of the Greater Tuberosity of the Humerus.**—When the greater tuberosity of the humerus is broken off the indications are to treat the fracture by placing the arm in a position of full abduction and external rotation, but if the arm is placed in this position immediately after the reduction of a dislocation at the shoulder the dislocation will probably recur. Consequently, when a dislocation at the shoulder is complicated by a fracture of the greater tuberosity, the fracture of the tuberosity must be ignored at first and the arm immobilized at the side until the acute danger of recurrence is over. As a matter of fact, if a large cotton pad is placed in the axilla and the arm is immobilized in a large Velpeau bandage with the hand near the opposite shoulder, it will usually be found in the postreduction x-rays that the fragment of the tuberosity has settled or been pushed back into place and that the fracture needs no special treatment.

If the fragment remains displaced the arm may be slowly abducted and externally rotated about a week after the reduction, and the shoulder immobilized in this position in a plaster spica jacket.

Fractures of the edge of the glenoid and fractures of the lesser tuberosity do not demand any special treatment and can be ignored unless they cause symptoms later, when the loose fragments should be removed if necessary.

Fracture of the Neck of the Humerus (Fracture Dislocation at the Shoulder) is a very serious complication of dislocation of the shoulder which, fortunately, does not occur frequently; however, since its presence changes both the clinical picture and the treatment, it is important that those who treat fractures be familiar with its diagnosis, which has been given above under complications, and with its treatment which is given below.

Treatment.—The indications are to reduce the dislocation and fracture as soon after the injury as possible. It is very bad practice to permit the fragments to unite with the head out of its socket and expect to reduce the dislocation after union has been obtained, because reduction will then probably be impossible without an extensive and difficult operation, and because the callus incident to union may seriously damage the brachial plexus.

Reduction may be accomplished by manipulation or by open operation.

Reduction by Manipulation.—In a recent case, reduction by manipulation offers a fair chance of success, but requires considerable skill.

The fracture of the humerus eliminates the possibility of using that bone as a lever and consequently it is useless or even dangerous to attempt reduction by Kocher's method or by any other method which uses the humerus as a lever.

Closed Reduction by Traction and Manipulation.—As this is a difficult procedure anesthesia is necessary and we prefer ether. Boehler uses novocaine. Reduction can only be accomplished by a combination of traction and direct manipulation of the separated head of the humerus. The object of traction is to pull the upper end of the shaft of the humerus so far away from the glenoid that it does not interfere with the passage of the head into the socket, and this amount of traction must be maintained until the reduction is accomplished.

Because the traction must be slow, steady, powerful, constant, and under the control of the surgeon, it should, if possible, be obtained by mechanical means. Efficient methods of obtaining this traction are the screw traction apparatus of Boehler or the Soutter traction apparatus. With the Boehler apparatus the traction is obtained by means of a pin passed through the olecranon and regulated by a long traction screw, while the frame makes counterpressure against the chest wall. So efficient is this method that Boehler has reported eight consecutive cases of fracture dislocations at the shoulder in seven of which he was able to effect reduction. Lacking such an apparatus the surgeon may apply countertraction with a sheet around the chest and obtain traction on the arm by means of the screw footpiece on the Hawley table or by a block and tackle or by a husky assistant. In the case of mechanical traction, the traction may be applied to the arm by means of a pin through the olecranon or by a double clove hitch around the arm, the elbow being protected with saddler's felt. The direction of the traction should be directly outward (90 degrees abduction).

When the upper end of the shaft has been drawn well away from the glenoid by a slow, steady pull, the head should be pushed outward and upward by direct pressure and forced over the rim of the glenoid and into the cavity. Intact shreds of periosteum may cause the head to be drawn out with the shaft and then reduction by upward pressure in the axilla is relatively easy. If the head does not follow the shaft reduction is more difficult and may fail entirely. It is impossible to describe the method of getting the head into the glenoid. The surgeon must use his fingers and thumbs and gradually push it outward and upward and over the glenoid rim.

After reduction has been accomplished immobilization of the **fracture** and of the dislocation must be maintained. For this purpose Boehler uses an abduction arm splint with traction. We prefer to treat these patients in a plaster spica jacket or in recumbency with the lateral traction frame (**Fig.** 464) abducting the arm about 60 degrees and using just enough weight to maintain position of the fracture (five to eight pounds). The shoulder is further immobilized by a large cotton pad in the axilla and a figure-of-eight elastic bandage over the shoulder. At the end of four or five weeks union will be sufficiently firm to begin gentle active and passive motion and the **arm** can be lowered to the side and carried in a sling.

In cases several days old, we believe that it is useless to attempt closed reduction.

Open Reduction.—If closed reduction fails or is not deemed advisable, an open reduction is indicated. An incision about five inches long is made over the sulcus between the pectoralis major and the deltoid muscles. The muscles are retracted and the dislocated head and upper end of the shaft are exposed. The shaft is pulled outward and downward to expose the rent in the capsule and the glenoid which is then cleared of débris. In order to do this it may be necessary to divide the insertion of the pectoralis major muscle. After the glenoid is cleared, the head is lifted into place, care being taken to preserve its muscular attachments if possible. It may be necessary to divide the insertion of the subscapularis muscle. In handling the head, care should be taken not to injure its articular surface. It can usually be lifted into place with a pair of lion-jawed bone forceps applied to its nonarticular portion, or a strong hook can be placed in the medullary cavity or cancellous tissue of its broken surface. If this fails a small drill hole may be made in the cortex and a hook passed through this. (Fig. 483, *A* and *B*).

After the head is back in the glenoid in its normal position, the fracture is reduced, and the capsule and severed or torn muscles are sutured. Small holes are then drilled through adjacent portions of the two fragments and they are tied together with wire.

The wound is now closed in layers and dressed with the arm at the side and the hand on the opposite shoulder (Velpeau bandage). The wiring of the fragments will maintain reduction of the fracture. At the end of four weeks active and passive motions should be begun cautiously and increased gradually. These should be supplanted by local heat and massage to hasten the restoration of function.

One of us (J. A. K.) now uses Kirschner wires to fix the head to the shaft and even to the glenoid if necessary.

Removal of the Head of the Humerus.—In instances where the head of the humerus is found to be completely or almost completely free in the wound, it should be removed because aseptic necrosis and possible nonunion would follow its reduction. In other instances where the head of the humerus is severely comminuted it may be removed.

When the head of the humerus is removed, an effort should be made to attach the deep shoulder muscles to the proximal portion of the shaft which is smoothed off and placed in the glenoid. This will give a fairly useful, but by no means a normal, shoulder.

Injuries to Blood Vessels.—If a large blood vessel is ruptured and a large and growing hematoma is present, the region must be explored immediately and the bleeding vessel ligated.

Nerve Injuries should be watched carefully and if the injury involves the brachial plexus and there is no evidence of recovery at the end of a few weeks, the plexus should be exposed and an attempt made to repair the damage. If the paralysis involves only the circumflex nerve, an abduction splint should be worn as soon as it can be applied without danger of causing a recurrence of the dislocation. In either case the paralyzed muscles must be supported and protected from stretching and as power begins to return, they should be helped by graded exercises. If a cord of the plexus is severed, it should be sutured, but the prognosis is poor. Most of these nerve injuries are due to contusion or stretching and recovery is spontaneous.

Old Dislocations at the Shoulder

Occasionally one sees a dislocation at the shoulder which has been present for a considerable time and such a case offers a serious problem to the surgeon.

The patients usually have marked deformity and disability in the shoulder and more or less pain, and there may be definite evidence of pressure on the brachial plexus. Consequently, the surgeon should attempt relief of the symptoms and restoration of function and contour if the general condition of the patient is satisfactory. However, if the condition has existed for six months or longer, and there is little or no pain and a fair function of the extremity it is usually wise to let well enough alone.

Obstacles to Reduction in Old Dislocations at the Shoulder.—The obstacles to reduction consist of shortening and fibrosis of the muscles, especially the pectoralis major and subscapularis, the formation of scar tissue around the head of the humerus which binds it firmly in its abnormal location and to the surrounding structures, healing and contraction of the capsule, filling of the glenoid with scar tissue or bone fragments, atrophy of the humerus, and overgrowth of the glenoid margin. All of these obstacles tend to increase progressively with the duration of the dislocation.

Choice of Method.—If the dislocation has existed for eight weeks or less it can usually be reduced by the closed method. If it has existed longer than twelve weeks an open reduction is nearly always necessary. Those of eight to twelve weeks' duration are borderline cases, and the surgeon will base his decision upon the amount of movement of the humerus and his own skill in manipulation or open operative surgery. Those cases in which the humerus has a considerable range of movement are more favorable for manipulative reduction.

Manipulative Reduction of Old Dislocation at the Shoulder.—This method is dangerous in the hands of an unskilled surgeon because the procedure cannot be a gentle one, and the margin between successful reduction and considerable damage may be a very narrow one. The dangers to be avoided are rupture of the axillary artery or vein, rupture of the brachial plexus, and fracture of the humerus.

The patient is anesthetized with ether and placed upon the floor. The humerus is first loosened from its adhesions by being slowly rotated outward and inward. This should be done very carefully using the flexed elbow as a lever. Then the arm is slowly abducted and rotated outward to stretch the pectoralis major and subscapularis muscles.

Having loosened the humerus as much as seems necessary by the rotation and abduction movements, the surgeon removes his shoes and sits on the floor facing the dislocated shoulder. He then places one foot in the patient's axilla against the border of the scapula and the other against the acromion and grasps the patient's arm just above the elbow and makes traction on the arm. The traction should be slow, steady, and powerful. An assistant may assist the operation by pushing outward on the head of the humerus.

If the head of the humerus can be drawn outward to the margin of the glenoid, the assistant should then push it upward and over the rim. This powerful lateral traction is dangerous to vessels and nerves, but cannot be avoided.

If the head seems to have been pulled outward a sufficient distance and reduction has not been accomplished by pushing it upward and backward, then the surgeon should use Kocher's maneuvers: external rotation, adduction, and internal rotation. It is here that one is especially apt to fracture the humerus and the surgeon should not attempt to execute the maneuvers against too great resistance.

If reduction is secured, a retention dressing should be applied and the lesion treated as a fresh dislocation except that more physiotherapy and exercises are necessary to restore function.

It sometimes happens that the head can be brought to the anterior margin of the glenoid but cannot be gotten into the socket. In such a case the hand should be placed on the opposite shoulder and the arm and forearm bound across the chest and the anesthetic discontinued. In one of our cases (J. A. K.) this procedure was followed, and an x-ray picture taken two weeks later when the patient returned for an open reduction showed the reduction complete and a good result was obtained despite the fact that the dislocation had existed for three months.

Operative Reduction of Old Dislocation at the Shoulder.—If the dislocation has persisted for more than three months, the open operation is the method of choice. If the attempt at manipulative reduction has been unsuccessful, an open reduction is indicated. But the patient should be given a rest period of a week or two before the operation. The method of attempting a closed reduction and then proceeding immediately to the open operation is, we believe, poor surgery because, if the attempt has been serious, not only has the patient had enough for one session, but asepsis is poor and the surgeon is apt to be tired and in no condition to proceed immediately with a difficult operation.

Operative Technic.—An anterior incision about five inches long is made over the sulcus between the deltoid and the pectoralis major. These muscles are separated and retracted to expose the upper end of the humerus and the region over the glenoid. If necessary the anterior margin of the deltoid can be cut for a variable distance close to its origin from the clavicle. The scar tissue and remains of the capsule are cleared from the anterior inferior margin of the glenoid, and an opening large enough to admit the head is made. The glenoid is then cleared of scar tissue. The insertion of the pectoralis major is now exposed and this muscle is divided by the Z method close to its insertion.

Attention is now directed to the head of the humerus. It is freed of the overlying scar tissue and loosened from its bed by rotation of the arm and by sharp dissection. If the subscapularis muscle cannot be stretched sufficiently to permit reposition of the head, and this is usually the case, the humerus is rotated outward to bring the insertion of this muscle into view, and it is divided by the Z method. After the muscle has been cut, reduction is comparatively easy and the head of the humerus is either levered into the glenoid with a bone skid or manipulated into position.

After reduction has been accomplished the capsule is repaired with whatever tissue is left around the margin of the opening, the divided subscapularis and pectoralis major are sutured, the anterior margin of the deltoid is replaced and sutured to the clavicle, and the wound is closed in layers.

The arm is then immobilized at the side with an adhesive dressing and the after-treatment is the same as in a fresh dislocation except that the physiotherapy must be continued longer.

Prognosis.—Reports in the literature indicate that better results are obtained by the closed method, but this is probably due to the fact that the closed method is usually applied to fairly early cases. Other things being equal, the longer the dislocation has existed before reduction, the poorer the result will be. In most cases the shoulder will be stable, strong, and free from pain, but limited in abduction and rotation.

Recurrent Dislocation at the Shoulder

Compared to the number of traumatic dislocations at the shoulder, recurrent dislocation is rare. One occasionally encounters a patient, however, in whom dislocation at the shoulder occurs so frequently as to be classed habitual, and such a patient is conscious of the instability of the joint and avoids any movement in abduction. A very large percentage of these patients are epileptics and the dislocations occur during seizures.

Cause.—Much stress has been laid upon defects in the glenoid or the head of the humerus either congenital or acquired at the time of a traumatic dislocation as being responsible for the recurrence. However, roentgenograms of the shoulder of these patients are usually negative and the glenoid is normally so shallow that it has relatively little to do with the stability of the joint. The recurrences are probably due to incomplete healing and tightening up of the capsule and muscles after a traumatic dislocation. This is particularly to be expected in an epileptic where a fresh severe strain is apt to be inflicted during convalescence from a traumatic dislocation, and with repetition the tissues become more lax and the shoulder more unstable.

Treatment.—The dislocation is practically always anterior and reduction is usually easy. In an otherwise normal individual in whom the shoulder has been out only three or four times over a period of years, exercises to strengthen all of the muscles of the shoulder girdle should be prescribed and the patient cautioned against strains on the abducted arm. If the patient is an epileptic or if the dislocations occur so frequently as to greatly inconvenience the patient, operative treatment should be resorted to.

Types of Operation.—The considerable number of operations which have been devised for the cure of this relatively rare condition is evidence that we have no procedure which can be depended upon to yield uniformly satisfactory results in the hands of the average surgeon.

The object of all of the operations is to prevent the head of the humerus from moving downward and forward when the arm is abducted.

The operations fall into three groups: (1) Plication or reefing of the capsule, (2) bone block; (3) muscle or fascial slings; and (4) the Nicola operation. Since its introduction one of the authors (J. A. K.) has used and prefers the Nicola operation.

The capsule operations have given good results in the hands of Thomas, Cotton, and others, but not in the hands of the average surgeon. The capsule should be exposed by a posterior axillary incision and a crucial plication should be performed on the anteroinferior portion. It is also advisable to lengthen the pectoralis major muscle.

Bone Block.—The simplest method of bone block is that of Kellog Speed. The technic follows: A vertical incision four inches long is made below the coracoid. The pectoralis major is isolated and cut across and the axillary vessels and nerves are retracted inward to expose the margin of the glenoid. With a broad drill or chisel a hole is made in the scapula just anterior to the glenoid near its lower margin. Into this hole or slot a transplant removed from the tibia is driven home ''and about three-fourths inch is left projecting anteriorly and obliquely across the lower anterior margin of the shoulder joint.'' This method is simple and efficient. We would expect a painful shoulder to result, but such apparently is not the case.

Slings.—The first of these was the strip from the posterior border of the deltoid which was detached with its nerve supply intact and passed under the shoulder to be sutured in front (Clairemont). With the vogue for sutures of living fascia and tendons several operations have been devised. Plummer and Potts and Henderson pass a suture of living fascia or peroneal tendon through the acromion and through the greater tuberosity.

The Nicola[*] Operation.—In this operation the long head of the biceps is converted into a ligamentum teres to hold the head of the humerus in the glenoid. It is performed as follows: The incision begins at the acromion just lateral to the coracoid and passes downward for three inches. The deltoid fibers are separated, care being taken not to injure the circumflex artery and nerve which may appear beneath the muscle in the lower part of the incision. The bicipital groove is located by palpation and the transverse humeral ligament is divided. This incision is extended upward into the shoulder to

---

[*]Nicola: J. Bone & Joint. Surg., 1929, p. 128.

expose the biceps tendon. The elbow is now flexed and the tendon of the long
head of the biceps is divided one-half inch above the tendon of the pectoralis
major.

By means of a quarter-inch drill or gouge a tunnel is made from a point
in the bicipital groove one inch distal from the lesser tuberosity to emerge
on the articular surface of the head of the humerus in line with the groove
and from one-half to three-fourths of an inch from the articular margin.

A flexible probe is then passed through the tunnel and the proximal part
of the cut biceps tendon, which has been denuded of its synovial covering, is
drawn through the tunnel and sutured to its distal part. The arm is then
abducted to 90 degrees and the transverse humeral ligament is sutured to the
tendon and the wound is closed and the arm immobilized in a Velpeau bandage for two weeks. Then it is placed in a sling and exercises are started to
restore function. (Fig. 488.)

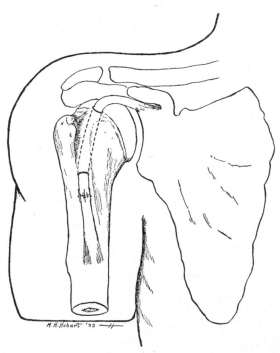

Fig. 488.—Modified Nicola operation for recurrent dislocation of shoulder, showing the
tunnel for the long tendon of the biceps muscle through the humerus under the bicipital groove.
(From Marcus H. Hobart, J. Bone & Joint Surg. 15: 733, 1933.)

FRACTURES OF THE UPPER END OF THE HUMERUS

Classification.—In surgical literature the upper end of the humerus is
that part of the bone which is proximal to the insertions of the teres major
and latissimus dorsi muscles. It includes a constricted portion of the shaft
(the surgical neck), the tuberosities, the anatomical neck, and the head. It
is usual to classify the fractures which occur in this region as follows: 1.
Fracture of the Surgical Neck. 2. Fracture of the Anatomical Neck. 3. Separation of the Upper Humeral Epiphysis. 4. Fracture of the Greater Tuberosity. 5. Fracture of the Lesser Tuberosity. 6. Fractures of the Head.

In practice we are not able to make a sharp distinction between fractures of the anatomical and surgical necks but find that fractures through the cancellous region of the bone may involve the anatomical neck, surgical neck, and the tuberosities. Furthermore, the treatment of fractures of the surgical neck and fractures of the anatomical neck is identical. Whether or not the fracture is impacted does, however, make considerable difference in the treatment; consequently we shall use the following classification:

1. Complete Fractures Through the Upper End of the Humerus.
2. Impacted Fractures Through the Upper End of the Humerus.
3. Fractures of the Head of the Humerus.
4. Fractures of the Greater Tuberosity.
5. Fractures of the Lesser Tuberosity.

Complete Fractures Through the Upper End of the Humerus

Occurrence and Causation.—Complete fractures through the upper end of the humerus include fractures of the surgical neck of the humerus and are rather unusual in children in whom the usual lesion in this area is an epiphyseal separation, but are frequent in adults of all ages and of both sexes. They may be produced by direct violence, such as a blow or fall on the shoulder or upper arm; but they are more often caused by indirect violence, such as a fall upon the outstretched hand.

Pathology.—The fracture line tends to be roughly transverse and rather irregular in character. It may lie completely in the compact bone of the surgical neck or in the cancellous bone of the anatomical neck and tuberosities, or it may occupy the transition zone between the compact and cancellous bone. Not infrequently the fracture line is deeply serrated or oblique and involves both regions and in many cases the bone is comminuted with the separation of one or more relatively large fragments. In children the fracture may be subperiosteal or incomplete.

Displacement.—Occasionally, even without definite impaction the bone ends remain in contact and there is relatively little displacement, but in the majority of instances there is a characteristic displacement. The proximal fragment is abducted and the distal fragment is drawn upward, inward, and usually forward. (Fig. 489.)

The abduction of the proximal fragment is due to the posterior scapular muscles, especially the supra spinatus. Those muscles which are attached to the greater tuberosity also tend to rotate the upper fragment outward, but this force is partly neutralized by the subscapularis which is a strong internal rotator so that only moderate outward rotation of the upper fragment occurs.

The upward displacement of the distal fragment is due to the fracturing force and to the pull of the muscles which cross the fracture line (deltoid, biceps, triceps, and coracobrachialis). The inward displacement is due to the pectoralis major, latissimus dorsi and teres major. The anterior displacement of the lower fragment is largely due to the pectoralis major, short head of the biceps, and coracobrachialis muscles.

The position of the lower fragment as regards rotation is independent of muscle pull and depends upon gravity. Consequently it is inconstant. In rare instances a continuation of the fracturing force may displace the distal fragment backward or even outward and it may remain in the unusual location.

Diagnosis.—Following the injury there is complete disability of the extremity, and the arm, unless supported, hangs useless at the side or may be twisted in an abnormal manner. There is a variable amount of local pain and swelling. The swelling tends to increase rather rapidly and may involve the entire arm and shoulder region. Ecchymosis usually appears on the front and inner side of the arm within twenty-four hours and may be very extensive, even involving the forearm.

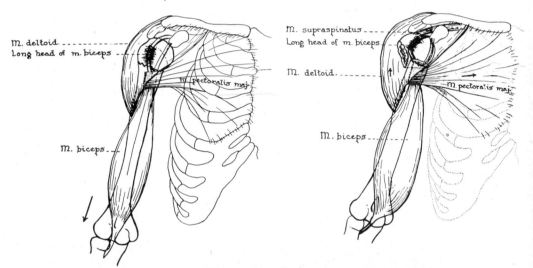

Fig. 489.—The forces causing displacement in fractures of the humerus above the insertion of the pectoralis major. (Courtesy of Dr. Arnold Griswold, Am. J. Surg., January, 1939.)

On inspection the contour of the shoulder is normal but the swollen upper arm appears to be shortened and displaced inward, and the outer surface of the deltoid may be flattened or even concave in its middle and lower portion. The anterior axillary fold is deepened and distorted and there is a slight prominence on the front of the shoulder which is most evident when viewed from the side. The above signs are absent in the cases without displacement.

On palpation there is acute point tenderness over the ends of both fragments and the rough proximal end of the distal fragment may be felt in the anterior axillary region lateral to the coracoid process. Deep palpation of the outer border of the deltoid may reveal the end of the abducted proximal fragment. Measurement of the distance from the tip of the acromion to the external epicondyle of the humerus when compared with that on the other side will reveal the amount of shortening or upward displacement of the lower fragment.

On manipulation it will be found that the head of the humerus does not move when the shaft is rotated, and there may or may not be crepitus. Abnormal mobility can be demonstrated by grasping the upper end of the humerus

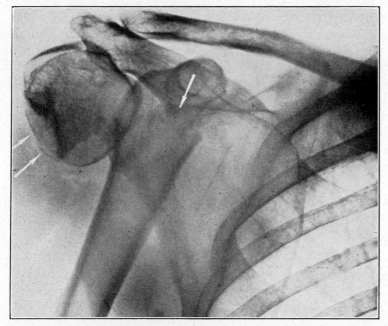

A.

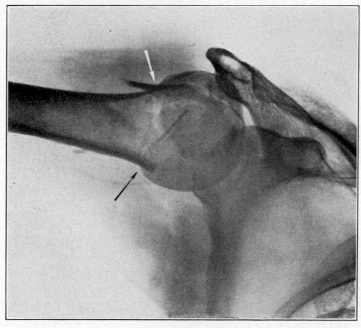

B.

Fig. 490 *A* and *B*.—Fracture of the upper end of the humerus reduced by closed manipulation, traction in abduction for three weeks, then cast at 45 degrees for three weeks and sling for five weeks. Good result. (H. E. C.)

with one hand and gently moving the lower end from side to side or telescoping it (alternately pushing it up and pulling it down).

The diagnosis should be confirmed by the x-ray, and in most instances lateral as well as anteroposterior views should be made. The lateral view of the upper end of the humerus can be obtained by abducting the arm, placing the casette on top of the shoulder, and directing the rays upward through the axilla or through the chest with the arm at the side.

Complications.—As was noted above, this fracture may occur in conjunction with a dislocation at the shoulder. Consequently the surgeon should identify the head of the humerus in its socket.

Occasionally the sharp distal fragment may injure the brachial plexus or its branches, especially the musculospiral nerve. This is more apt to occur when the fracture line lies in the compact bone of the surgical neck. Consequently a rough neurological examination should be made before treatment is begun.

Compound fractures in this region are rare.

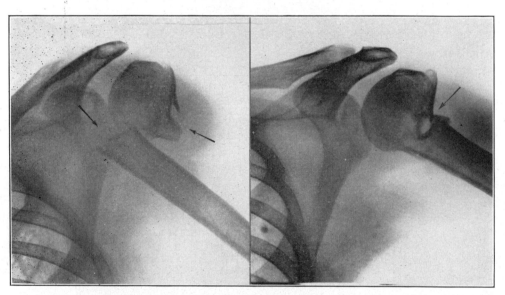

Fig. 491.—Fracture of the surgical neck of the humerus reduced by closed manipulation and a hanging cast applied. Good functional result obtained. (Conwell.)

Treatment.—Experience with the hanging cast as introduced by J. A. Caldwell (*Ann. Surg.* 97: 161, 1933) has convinced us that Howard and Eloesser (*J. Bone & Joint Surg.* 16: 1, 1934) are correct in their statement that the fracture should be reduced and immobilized with the arm at the side and, contrary to the opinions expressed in former editions, we now rarely use the abduction plaster cast or treat these fractures by lateral traction. If displacement is present, an attempt is made to correct it by manipulation and then the hanging cast is applied. If we are not satisfied with the position in a week or ten days, the fracture is reduced by open operation, and the hanging cast is used in the postoperative treatment. We find that the free exercise of the shoulder which this method permits more than compensates for the possible loss in abduction which we feared when we abandoned the abduction treatment of these fractures, and

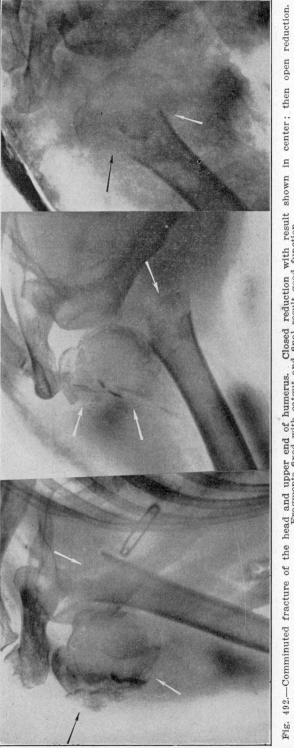

Fig. 492.—Comminuted fracture of the head and upper end of humerus. Closed reduction with result shown in center; then open reduction. Fragments fixed with catgut and final result good function.

the patients are much happier and regain the use of their arms sooner than with the older methods.

The Hanging Cast Method.—With the elbow flexed to 90 degrees and the forearm in the mid-position between pronation and supination a plaster-of-Paris cast is applied from the upper arm to the wrist or base of the fingers. It is applied over a moderate amount of padding and the weight of the cast varies with the musculature of the patient; that is, light casts with weak muscles and heavy casts for patients with strong muscles.

After the plaster has set, the forearm is supported across the lower chest by a cravat sling which is looped around the cast at the wrist, thus permitting the weight of the cast and the extremity to reduce or maintain reduction of the fracture. In fractures with little or no displacement the hanging cast is applied without anesthesia.

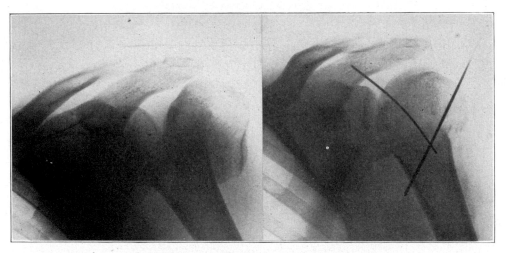

Fig. 493.—Fracture of the proximal portion of the humerus in which closed reduction was unsuccessful. Treated by open reduction and fixation with two Kirschner wires. The wires should be bent close to the skin to prevent drifting inward. Excellent result. (J. A. K.)

Reduction.—If complete displacement is present and the fragments are not badly comminuted, reduction under local or general anesthesia is advisable. If comminution is present the traction of the cast may be depended upon to effect reduction.

When satisfactory anesthesia has been obtained, the elbow is flexed to 90 degrees and with the forearm supinated slow steady traction is made in line with the shaft of the humerus until the fragments have slipped by one another. During this maneuver the long head of the biceps tends to pull the distal end of the proximal fragment down to the side. It may be necessary to make counter traction by means of a band in the axilla.

When the distal fragment has been pulled down beyond the proximal one, its proximal end can be pulled or levered outward and backward until it is in line with the proximal fragment, and when the traction is released, the two will engage.

This manipulation may be performed by the method of Cotton and Morrison who use the surgeon's forearm as a fulcrum as follows: With the patient recumbent the surgeon places his forearm in the patient's axilla with his hand resting on the table. The assistant maintains the traction and swings the arm inward across the chest while the surgeon presses the proximal end of the upper fragment outward and backward with his forearm.

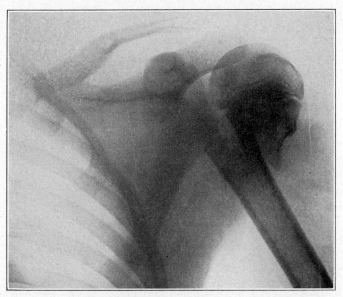

Fig. 494.—Irregular fracture through the upper end of the humerus with inward and interior displacement of the distal fragment.

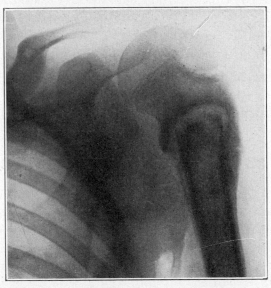

Fig. 495.—Result in previous case after open reduction and immobilization in plaster cast in 55 degrees abduction and 15 degrees anterior flexion of arm at the shoulder for eight weeks. Arm and forearm strapped to chest for ten days then sling to forearm for one week. Good results in three months. (H. E. C.)

Another method is for the surgeon to grasp the patient's upper extremity with both hands so that his thumbs rest on the outer surface over the tuberosity and his fingers on the axillary surface. Then as the traction pulls the distal fragment down the surgeon pulls or squeezes the proximal end outward or backward until it is in line with the proximal fragment. As the traction is decreased, the fragments are engaged and their stability is tested by pushing upward on the elbow. The hanging cast is then applied and suspended across the body by a sling which supports it at the wrist.

Aftertreatment.—The patient is instructed to remain upright as much as possible and to let the arm hang from the shoulder. While sitting he is cautioned not to rest the elbow on the arm of the chair. During the first few days he sleeps propped up in bed in a semireclining position or if he remains in bed about five pounds weight is fastened to the cast at the elbow and hung over the foot of the bed for traction. After the first week or so this is not necessary, if he is upright most of the day. The sling is so adjusted that the forearm is horizontal.

Exercise.—After the first day or so the patient is instructed to lean forward so that the arm swings free from the body and with the muscles relaxed to swing it gently to and fro across the body. As the tenderness subsides the rotary movement of the elbow is added and the range of movement and frequency of the exercise are increased.

The cast is left on for from four to six weeks until union is fairly solid. It is then removed and the wrist sling is continued until the patient is comfortable without it.

X-rays are not taken until a week or more after the cast has been applied.

If the proximal end of the distal fragment is displaced forward or inward, the sling is shortened; if backward or outward it is lengthened.

Sometimes the head of the humerus tends to subluxate downward. It will return to its normal level after the cast is removed and the muscles regain their tone.

The Abduction Treatment of Complete Fractures of the Upper End of the Humerus

Simple Immobilization.—The arm should be abducted from 60 to 90 degrees and so rotated that the flexed elbow is horizontal. It should not extend directly outward from the shoulder, but should be flexed forward about 35 degrees so that with the elbow flexed to a right angle the hand is in front of the shoulder or chest.

Immobilization may be obtained by a plaster-of-Paris spica jacket or by an abduction splint. The plaster-of-Paris jacket is more troublesome to apply, but once on properly, it is more comfortable than an abduction splint, more efficient, and needs no adjustment (Fig. 496).

The Plaster-of-Paris Spica Jacket can be applied in recumbency (Figs. 497 and 498), but is most conveniently applied with the patient sitting upright on a stool with the opposite arm elevated and resting on his head. The injured arm is supported by an assistant. The body and affected arm are covered with stockinet or sheet wadding. Felt pads are placed over each iliac crest and over each clavicle, and a strip of felt is placed along the entire ulnar surface of the forearm, from the internal epicondyle of the humerus to the base of the little finger, as the plaster is applied with the forearm supinated.

The patient having been prepared as above, and the arm placed in the correct position, the plaster jacket is applied and with a spica over the affected shoulder it is extended down the arm and forearm to the bases of the fingers. It is of some advantage to extend the plaster over the opposite shoulder in the form of a wide strap as this aids in the balance of the cast and renders it more efficient and comfortable. If the spica around the shoulder is properly constructed struts or braces extending from the side of the cast to the arm or elbow are not necessary.

Reduction by Manipulation should not be attempted without anesthesia, either general or local. The patient may be in the recumbent or upright position, depending upon whether general or local anesthesia is used. With the arm in a position of from 45 to 60 degrees abduction and the forearm flexed to a right angle and in the horizontal plane if the patient is sitting upright, lateral traction is applied. The traction should be slow and steady, but strong enough to pull the distal fragment out beyond the proximal one. The traction should be made by an assistant or mechanical device, and is most effective when the elbow is flexed to 90 degrees, since this relaxes the biceps muscle. Countertraction is made by a band around the chest or by another assistant.

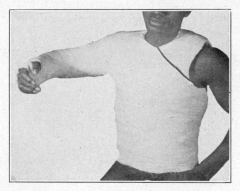

Fig. 496.—Plaster spica jacket with shoulder in 90 degrees abduction and 90 degrees external rotation used in treatment of complete fractures through the upper end of the humerus. The portion extending over the left shoulder may be removed if desired.

When the shortening is overcorrected; that is, when the ends of the fragments have slipped by one another, the surgeon should attempt to so manipulate the two fragments that when the traction is released, the ends will engage with as little lateral displacement as possible. This is most easily done by grasping the upper arm with both hands in such a manner that the thumbs rest on the lateral surface of the deltoid over the end of the upper fragment, while the fingers rest on the axillary surface over the end of the lower fragment. Squeezing the fingers and thumbs together tends to correct the lateral deformity. When the two fragments are felt to be in line, the traction is gradually lessened and the ends are permitted to engage.

If the reduction is adequate and the fracture is of a type that can be treated without traction, the shortening does not recur and the fracture is fairly stable.

The question of adequate reduction and stability of the fragments must be decided by the surgeon as the traction is relaxed. If the ends tend to slip by one another, the fracture should be treated by traction. If the position and stability seem satisfactory, the fracture is immobilized in a plaster jacket or splint in from 50 degrees to 90 degrees abduction and forward flexion of about 35 degrees and the elbow flexed to 90 degrees and the forearm horizontal as described above. The degree of abduction necessary is determined by the position in which the fragments are most stable.

In applying the plaster or splint, care must be taken not to disengage the fragments, and it is advised that the surgeon hold the arm while his assistant applies the plaster or splint. If a general anesthetic has been used, the plaster must be applied with the patient recumbent; for this a fracture table is necessary, or the sheet metal support may be used as illustrated in Fig. 497.

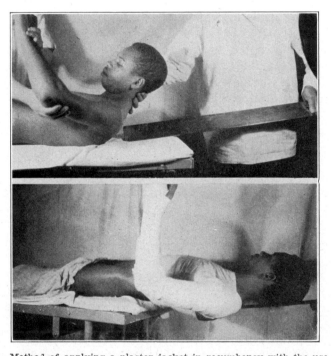

Fig. 497.—Method of applying a plaster jacket in recumbency with the use of an ordinary operating table. The sheet of metal, 3 feet long and 4½ inches wide and ¼ inch thick is permitted to project beyond the end of the table and is supported by an orderly or another table.

Fig. 498.—The patient pulled up and supported on the metal strip which is pulled out after the cast has been applied. If a Hawley table (Fig. 36) is available the patient can be reversed on the table and the metal strip supported by the pelvic rest. This eliminates moving the patient after the anesthetic is started.

Treatment of Complete Fractures of the Upper End of the Humerus by Lateral Traction is used for those fractures which cannot be satisfactorily reduced or in which the fragments tend to slip after adequate reduction.

The most efficient and satisfactory method is recumbency with lateral traction. The disadvantage is that the patient must remain in bed.

In a fresh case the patient is placed in a bed equipped with a lateral traction frame. The arm and forearm having been shaved, traction strips of adhesive are placed on the forearm and extended beyond the finger tips and fastened to a block or spreader. A bandage is placed over these strips, and the elbow is flexed to 90 degrees and suspended, just enough weight being used to counterbalance the extremity. (Fig. 499.)

Traction strips of adhesive are now applied to the inner and outer surfaces of the arm and passed over a block or spreader beyond the flexed elbow. These are bandaged on, a rope is passed from the spreader through the pulley on the traction frame, and a weight of from five to ten pounds is fastened to the rope. The amount of weight varies directly with the musculature of the patient. An anesthetic is usually necessary. The arm is placed in about 45 degrees of abduction, the angle being determined by the position of the upper fragment.

The position of the fragments should be checked at the end of forty-eight hours by means of a portable x-ray machine. If the position is not satisfactory, then a general anesthetic may be administered to the patient in bed without disturbing the traction, manual traction can be applied, and the surgeon can mold the fragments into better position. This molding may be repeated if necessary. The traction remains and tends to maintain the position obtained.

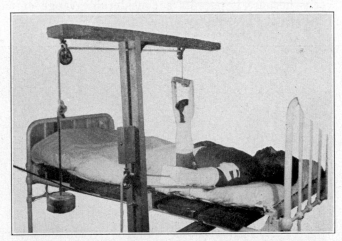

Fig. 499.—Treatment of fractures at the upper end of the humerus in recumbency with lateral traction. Note the accessibility of the shoulder region for dressing. This is also of great advantage when compound fractures are present.

The Thomas Arm Splint is a very popular splint and is much used for the application of lateral traction in recumbency because it can be rested upon the back of a chair or slung from an ordinary Balkan or fracture frame, and most hospitals are not equipped with lateral traction frames of any sort.

We do not recommend the Thomas arm splint for two reasons: 1. The arm is treated with the elbow extended, and this not only tends to prolong disability from the resultant stiffness in the elbow, but it renders the traction less efficient because the biceps is not relaxed. 2. The ring is a very uncomfortable thing to lie upon for twenty-four hours a day; this is particularly true in fractures of the upper end of the humerus, and no amount or arrangement of padding will make it comfortable.

Duration of Treatment in Complete Fractures of the Upper End of the Humerus.—In fractures which are not displaced and require simple immobilization in abduction and external rotation, a plaster cast or splint should be continued for about two weeks. In fractures in which satisfactory reduction has been accomplished the immobilization in abducton and external rotation should be continued for from three to five weeks, depending upon the character of the fracture.

Fractures through the cancellous portion of the bone heal more rapidly than do those through cortical bone, and consequently these may be taken down sooner. In fractures where it is necessary to use traction the traction should be applied over a period of approximately three weeks. At the end of this time a plaster spica jacket or abduction splint can be applied and continued from two to three weeks longer. In many instances, however, when it is necessary that the patient remain in a hospital and when there is considerable danger of stiffness at the shoulder, it is favorable to continue the traction during the full period of immobilization. And in many cases where bed traction has been used and there is no important reason why the patient should not remain in a hospital, it is favorable to continue this treatment for some five to six weeks because it permits a considerable range of motion at the shoulder and lessens the probability of stiffness.

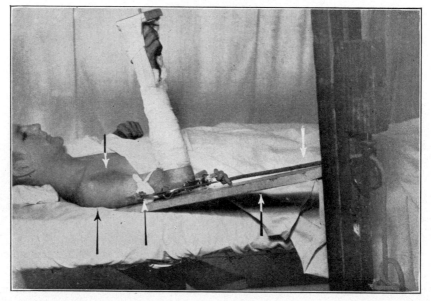

Fig. 500.—Lateral traction for fracture of the humerus with wire through the lower third of the shaft and arm abducted 45 degrees.

Aftertreatment.—In all injuries around the shoulder one must be constantly on guard against long-continued or even permanent limitation of motion, especially abduction and internal rotation. This is not due so much to the fracture as to the injury of the soft parts, especially the tissues beneath the deltoid muscle in the region of the subdeltoid bursa. Consequently these fractures should be treated by the application of local heat, massage and active and passive movement. Where a plaster cast has been used the arm part of the cast can be bivalved at the end of the second week and the top removed daily for exercise of the arm. With the abduction splint or with lateral traction in recumbency, the heat can be begun immediately, massage as soon as the tenderness has disappeared, and active movement within a few days.

After the plaster or splint or lateral traction has been removed, the arm may be carried at the side with the wrist supported by a sling, but the surgeon must insist that the patient exercise it daily, and that the full range of abduction be obtained as soon as possible. In the beginning this is best done by having the patient swing the arm backward and forward and across the body as used with the hanging cast. Within two or three weeks, as union becomes more solid and muscle tone increases, the patient should practice abduction exercises and should increase abduction by standing opposite a wall, placing the hand on the wall and slowly crawling up the wall with the fingers. The amount gained should be measured daily; thus the patient is stimulated to excel his previous record and gradually obtain full abduction.

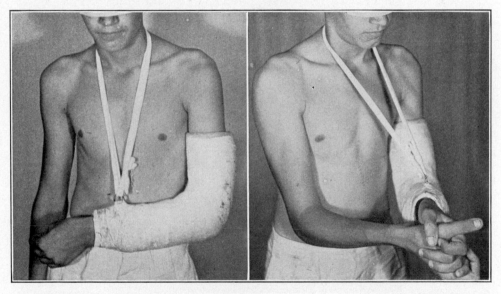

Fig. 501.—The hanging cast as applied for fractures of the shaft of the humerus. It is also useful for fractures of the proximal third. (Courtesy Dr. John A. Caldwell, Cincinnati.)

Rotation must not be ignored. It is best accomplished by having the patient lie upon his back on the bed, abduct the arm to 90 degrees, flex the forearm, and practice internal and external rotation in this position. In a child or young adult full range of motion may be expected in from eight to ten weeks after the injury and a practically normal shoulder in approximately three months. This time increases, of course, when the degree of soft structure involvement is increased. In an older adult there may be some permanent restriction of abduction and rotation at the shoulder and the period of partial disability will probably be doubled, but if the exercises and local heat are persisted in, surprisingly good results may be obtained.

Impacted Fractures Through the Upper End of the Humerus

Impacted fractures through the upper end of the humerus tend to occur in patients beyond middle life, but may occur in adults of any age, and are very rare in children. They are largely the fractures which are usually classified as those of the anatomic neck. Most of them are the result of indirect violence, being caused by a fall on the elbow or outstretched hand, the force being transmitted upward through the shaft of the humerus. The fracture usually occurs in the transition zone between the compact and cancellous bone and a continuation of the force drives the end of the compact bone up into the cancellous portion. The fracture line tends to be roughly transverse or slightly oblique beginning on the inner side near or in the anatomic neck and passing outward through the tuberosity (Fig. 502). In rare instances the fracture may follow the line of the anatomic neck. Ordinarily with the impaction there is a slight adduction deformity.

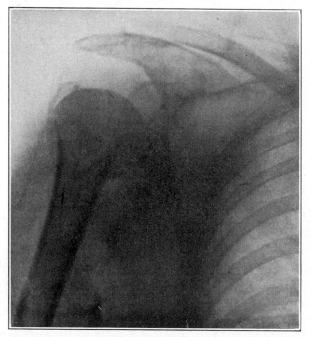

Fig. 502.—Impacted fracture of the upper end of the humerus in a woman of sixty yeras. Fracture not recognized for three weeks. Treated by adhesive dressing for three weeks; then arm and forearm in sling for one month. Only fair function. Very little pain. When a feeble individual of sixty years or thereabouts receives such a fracture, no breaking up of the impaction should be done, but the arm should be fixed in some ambulatory dressing.

Diagnosis.—The diagnosis of these fractures is not so easily made as in those without impaction and may be impossible in the absence of a roentgenogram. There is a history of an injury, followed by severe pain and disability in the shoulder with local tenderness which is rather general over the upper end of the humerus. The swelling is relatively slight and there may be a slight flattening of the deltoid. Ecchymosis appears within a few days usually down the side of the arm over the biceps, all motions of the shoulder are limited and painful, especially abduction and rotation, but there is little demonstrable shortening, no perceptible deformity, and no false motion. When the shaft of the humerus is moved, the head tends to move with it. Pressure transmitted through the long axis of the humerus by pushing upward on the elbow tends to cause pain in the region of the shoulder.

The diagnosis is made by the presence of a rather severe injury to the shoulder with the signs of a fracture and by excluding the clavicle, scapula, and the complete fractures through the upper end of the humerus without impaction.

X-Ray.—Diagnosis should always be confirmed by an x-ray examination and it is to be pointed out that even in a good roentgenogram the fracture line may not be obvious; in fact it may not be visible and it may be necessary to take a roentgenogram of the opposite shoulder and make the diagnosis on the basis of a slight distortion of the upper end of the humerus. In addition to the routine view in the anteroposterior plane a lateral view of the humerus should be made as the lower fragment is often displaced interiorly. This view is easily obtained by abducting the arm, placing the casette on top of the shoulder and directing the rays upward through the axilla.

Treatment.—The treatment to be instituted depends to a considerable extent upon the age, physique, and temperament of the patient, and the amount of deformity. If the patient is a comparatively young adult or middle-aged adult with the expectation of many years of active life ahead of him, and if there is considerable deformity, the surgeon should break up the impaction and treat the fracture as described in the preceding section on complete fractures through the upper end of the humerus. If the patient is an aged and debilitated individual, even in the presence of considerable deformity, no attempt should be made to break up the impaction, but the fracture should be treated by simple immobilization. This may be accomplished by placing a large triangular pad in the axilla, binding the arm to the side and supporting the forearm by a sling. If the patient is a young or middle-aged adult in apparently good health, and there is little or no demonstrable deformity, the fracture should be treated by immobilization, preferably in a position of abduction and external rotation, either in a plaster spica jacket or in an abduction splint just as has been described in the previous section on the treatment of fractures through the neck of the humerus.

In any case, the period of immobilization can be comparatively short, and every attempt at the restoration of function should be made. This means that immobilization may be discontinued at the end of two or three weeks and the arm carried in a triangular sling.

Active and passive motion should be begun at the end of two weeks and the patient should be given abduction and rotation exercises as described in the after-treatment on complete fractures through the neck of the humerus.

We now treat most of these fractures in the hanging cast as described in the preceding section, and the period of disability is less and the functional result is better.

Fractures of the Head of the Humerus

These are very rare injuries because the head of the humerus is much denser than the surrounding bone. Fractures may be caused by indirect violence, such as a fall on the hand or elbow, or the force **may be transmitted** through the tuberosity from a blow or fall on the shoulder. Occasionally they occur in the presence of a dislocation. In the main, the fractures of the head are of two types. A small piece of the head may be chipped off and remain loose in the joint, or in extensive comminuted fractures of the upper end of the humerus the head may be split into two or more fragments.

If a small piece is broken off, the arm should simply be immobilized in a sling and active and passive motion should be begun early. If the fragment gives trouble such as locking or pain in the joint, it should be removed by simple arthrotomy which can be performed through the anterior or axillary route, depending upon the choice of the surgeon.

Extensive comminuted fractures with fragmentation of the head are serious injuries and offer a poor prognosis as regards function. They are treated with lateral traction, abduction, and external rotation, and the surgeon should make an effort to secure anatomic reduction by manipulation under an anesthetic. If approximate anatomic reduction cannot be obtained, an open reduction is indicated. This is particularly true in those instances where the head is split and impacted in such a manner that one portion of it projects definitely beyond the other so that there is an inequality in its articular surface. At the open reduction, which is best done from seven to ten **days** after the injury, the fragments should be loosened, anatomic reduction obtained, and if necessary, small drill holes made in their extraarticular portions, and they should be sutured or pegged together. Separated fragments which cannot be immobilized in approximately their normal position should be excised. After the operation a plaster spica jacket should be applied with the arm in abduction, and external rotation or lateral traction in recumbency may be instituted. Active and passive motion and intensive local heat and massage should be begun early and continued until motion is either restored or despaired of. We now treat most of these injuries in the hanging cast.

Prognosis.—With the slight chip fractures a practically normal shoulder should result after the fragment is removed. With the extensive comminuted fractures one may by efficient and skillful treatment obtain a practically normal shoulder. On the other hand, if anatomic reduction is not secured, a traumatic arthritis will probably result and it may occur with the fragments in good position; either complete ankylosis will occur or a stiff and painful shoulder with slight motion will result.

In these instances the shoulder should be supported in a position of 90 degrees abduction and 90 degrees external rotation over a period of several weeks in order to prevent ankylosis with the arm at the side. If the pain persists it is wise to perform an arthrodesis of the shoulder.*

Fractures of the Greater Tuberosity

Fractures of the greater tuberosity may accompany dislocation of the shoulder or may occur as isolated injuries from direct violence, such as a blow upon the shoulder or from compression by the acromion in hyperabduction injuries, or rarely by muscular action. The tuberosity may be torn off, broken across,

*Key, J. A.: Surg., Gynec. and Obst. 1930, p. 468.

mashed in, or a small chip may be pulled off. As a rule there is little tendency to displacement of the fragments. Very rarely a large fragment may be torn off and pulled up under the acromion.

Diagnosis.—There is a history of an injury with acute tenderness and swelling over the lateral surface of the shoulder and especially around the greater tuberosity. Passive movements of the shoulder, especially internal rotation, aggravate the pain and there is total inability to abduct or externally rotate the arm. In some cases slight crepitus may be obtained on passive abduction or rotation of the arm and in rare instances where a large fragment is completely separated this may be palpable and movable. Upward pressure on the elbow demonstrates the fact that the shaft of the humerus is intact. The diagnosis should be confirmed by x-ray examination. (Fig. 503.)

Treatment.—We formerly treated these fractures in a plaster spica cast with the shoulder immobilized in a position of abduction and external rotation. We now treat them much more simply, placing the arm in a sling or in a hanging cast and insisting on daily pendulum or swinging exercises, as described below in the treatment of fractures of the shaft of the humerus.

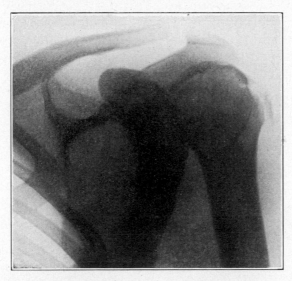

Fig. 503.—Isolated fracture of the greater tuberosity, treated in a plaster cast in 90 degrees abduction and 180 degrees external rotation two weeks; later a simple ambulatory plaster abduction splint for two weeks; then a sling for one week. Good results.

If the fragment is relatively large and so displaced that it interferes with movement of the shoulder, it is exposed through a short vertical anterolateral incision through the proximal portion of the deltoid, reduced, and fastened with a Kirschner wire which is driven through the intact skin. The wire is pulled out in four weeks and the exercises are then increased.

Fracture of the Greater Tuberosity with Dislocation of the Shoulder.— When the shoulder is dislocated anteriorly or downward, it is imperative that the arm be immobilized in a position of adduction because recurrence of the dislocation tends to occur in a position of abduction. For this reason the fracture of the tuberosity must be ignored in the early part of the treatment and the shoulder must be immobilized at the side in the usual manner. It usually will be found that the fragment of the tuberosity will settle back into place and offer little obstruction to the restoration of function. If it remains widely separated, it should be exposed and replaced by open operation and fixed with a Kirschner wire, as described in the preceding section.

Fractures of the Lesser Tuberosity

Fracture of the lesser tuberosity is a rare injury as an isolated lesion, but may result from forcible external rotation of the arm or violent contraction of the subscapularis muscle. The symptoms are inability to internally rotate the arm and localized pain which is aggravated when active adduction or internal rotation are attempted. The patient tends to support the arm in a position of internal rotation and adduction, there is moderate swelling and tenderness over the anterior and inner portion of the upper end of the humerus, and it may be possible to palpate the detached fragment in the subcoracoid region. More frequently the injury occurs in connection with dislocation of the shoulder or extensive comminuted fractures of the upper end of the humerus.

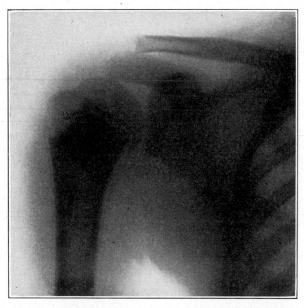

Fig. 504.—Epiphyseal separation with slight displacement. With only this amount of displacement no attempt should be made to improve the position. Treated by simple adhesive fixation of arm and forearm to chest and abdomen (with pad in axilla) for three weeks, being renewed when necessary. Sling to forearm for two weeks. Good results.

Treatment.—As the subscapularis muscle is inserted into the lesser tuberosity and as the action of this muscle is to internally rotate and adduct the arm, treatment should be immobilization of the arm in a position of adduction and internal rotation. This is best accomplished by placing the hand on the affected side on the opposite shoulder and immobilizing the arm in this position with adhesive and bandages for a period of about there weeks. At the end of this time the arm can be carried in a sling for two weeks longer and then use gradually resumed. No special exercises are necessary and a normal shoulder is to be expected. When the injury occurs in connection with dislocation of the shoulder or comminuted fracture of the upper end of the humerus the fracture of the lesser tuberosity may be ignored and the shoulder dislocation or humerus fracture treated as described in the preceding sections. It will be found that the fracture of the lesser tuberosity will not increase the disability incident to the accompanying grave injury.

Separation of the Upper Epiphysis of the Humerus

The upper end of the humerus develops from three centers of ossification—one for each tuberosity and one for the head. These unite at about the seventh year to form a cap-like mass of bone which surmounts the conical end of the diaphysis. In its inner half the epiphyseal line follows the line of the anatomic neck to about the middle of the bone and then passes outward and downward to the lower border of the greater tuberosity. Ossification is completed at about the twenty-fifth year, but epiphyseal separations of the upper end of the humerus have not been recorded after the twentieth year.

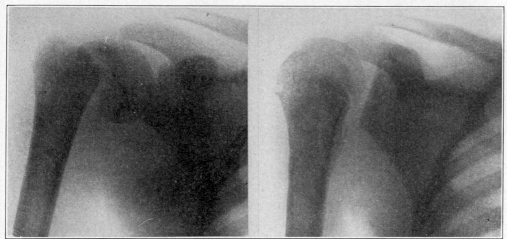

Fig. 505.   Fig. 506.

Fig. 505.—Epiphyseal separation at the upper end of the humerus with rather marked displacement. Treated by closed manipulative reduction under an anesthetic and immobilized in a plaster spica jacket in 45 degrees abduction and 90 degrees external rotation for twenty-four days then forearm in a sling for two weeks, with good result.

Fig. 506.—Preceding case after reduction. Note the new bone formation the result of stripping up of periosteum from the shaft.

Occurrences and Cause.—Separation of the upper epiphysis is probably the most frequent injury to the upper end of the humerus in children, especially in those between the ages of four and fourteen. It may result from indirect violence such as a fall upon the elbow or outstretched hand, the force being transmitted upward through the shaft of the humerus or it may result from direct violence such as a fall or blow on the outer surface of the shoulder. Occasionally the injury results from forcible abduction or outward rotation of the arm with traction.

Displacement.—The epiphysis may be simply loosened and practically no displacement occur (Fig. 504), or the shaft may be completely separated and displaced upward as in the complete fractures through the upper end of the humerus described above (Fig. 505). When this occurs there tends to be abduction and external rotation of the upper fragment and the diaphysis tends to be drawn upward, forward, and inward, just as occurs in fractures through the upper end of the humerus. In other instances the displacement is incomplete; that is, the diaphysis is only partly displaced. Usually in cases with separation there is more or less stripping up of the periosteum of the shaft, but this being unusually tough in children, tends not to be completely ruptured and binds the fragments together and renders the reduction by traction relatively difficult. In older children a portion of the upper end of the shaft is often split off with the epiphysis and occasionally the upper end of the shaft is driven into the epiphysis and impacted.

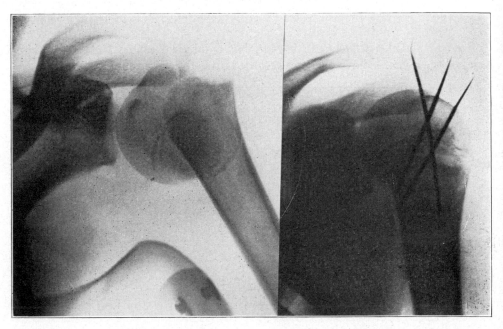

Fig. 507.—Epiphyseal separation of the humerus, two weeks' duration. Open reduction and fixation with three Kirschner wires. The projecting ends of the wires were bent to 90 degrees close to the skin and the wires were removed in four weeks. Normal shoulder obtained. (J. A. K.)

Diagnosis.—In cases without displacement the diagnosis rests upon the history of the injury, the age of the patient, and the swelling, tenderness, disability, and local pain. In such instances the x-ray picture may show a slight displacement or may be completely negative. In displacement the upper end of the shaft tends to project anteriorly and cause a prominence under the anterior portion of the deltoid which is usually palpable and may even be visible. The head of the bone can be palpated in its normal position in the glenoid.

With complete displacement the diaphysis is pulled upward and forward and causes a prominence in the front of the axilla near the coracoid which can be palpated and even seen. The arm is shortened, the axis of the humerus is altered, the anterior axillary fold is distorted, false motion is demonstrable, and the head of the humerus can be palpated in its normal position. In doubtful cases with slight displacement, the diagnosis can be confirmed by the x-ray taken in both the anteroposterior and lateral directions.

Treatment.—We now routinely treat these cases in the hanging cast as described in the preceding section (p. 564).

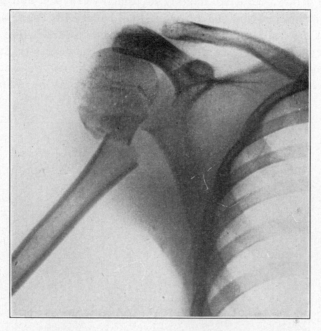

Fig. 508.—Fracture through upper portion of humerus in a child. Treated by closed reduction and lateral traction four weeks, plaster spica two weeks, and sling two weeks. Good result in ten weeks.

Alternate methods of treatment are as follows: In cases with only slight displacement (Fig. 504) all that is necessary is to immobilize the arm at the side as there is no tendency to spontaneous displacement or later limitation at the shoulder. This can be accomplished by placing a pad of absorbent cotton in the axilla and a wide band of adhesive around the chest and arm and supporting the forearm and elbow in a sling for about ten days. With moderate or considerable lateral displacement (Figs. 505, 506, 508, and 509) it is necessary to reduce the displacement, and this should be done under an anesthetic. After the patient has been anesthetized, the arm is abducted, and moderate traction in abduction is made by the assistant, while the surgeon, with his thumbs on the greater tuberosity and his fingers on the upper end of the shaft, endeavors to push the shaft outward and backward into its normal position.

Reduction having been completed, the arm should be immobilized for three weeks in a position of from 60 to 90 degrees abduction and flexed forward about 35 degrees with the forearm horizontal. At the end of this time it can be lowered to the side and carried in an ordinary triangular sling for two weeks longer. Then the sling can be removed and the patient begin to use the arm, gradually increasing the use as the muscle tone increases. Exercises and physiotherapy are not necessary in children, but the child should be cautioned against falling upon or straining the arm.

In cases with displacement reduction under an anesthetic should be attempted as described above, but more traction is necessary, and if the fragments are impacted, it is necessary to break up the impaction within a few days after the injury. This can usually be done by traction and manipulation.

If this does not succeed the surgeon should place his thumbs on the head of the bone in the axilla and press it upward and inward while his assistant abducts the arm directly above the head, and with moderate traction attempts to pry the fragments loose by levering the shaft against the acromion. Too much force should not be exerted, since the shoulder may be dislocated in this manner.

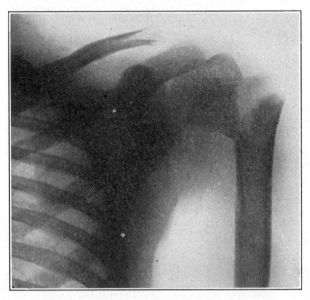

Fig. 509.—Fracture through the upper portion of the humerus extending into the epiphyseal line.

Reduction having been accomplished, the arm should be immobilized in from 60 to 90 degrees abduction and 90 degrees external rotation for a period of three weeks. It can then be lowered to the side and carried in a sling for two weeks, when all support may be removed and the patient encouraged to use the arm.

If satisfactory reduction cannot be accomplished and if the fragments are not impacted, the lesion is best treated with recumbency and lateral traction as described under complete fractures through the upper end of the humerus. But this treatment must be begun early, since union tends to occur very rapidly and it will be impossible to correct deformity by traction if the fragments are permitted to unite in their abnormal positions.

Open Reduction.—If the impaction cannot be broken up, if it is impossible to secure approximately anatomic reduction, or if the fragments have united with deformity, open reduction is indicated. We are inclined to perform open reduction for epiphyseal separation at the shoulder in children more frequently than we are for fractures in the same region in adults because we feel that it is important that approximately anatomic reduction be secured. (Figs. 510 and 511.)

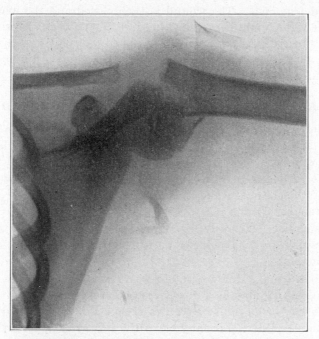

Fig. 510.—Same case as preceding after manipulation and lateral traction with failure to accomplish reduction. An open reduction was done seven days later.

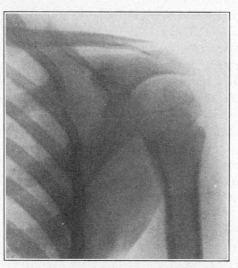

Fig. 511.—Same case as preceding after open reduction.

The site of the lesion is exposed through a vertical anterolateral incision which is carried down through the proximal portion of the deltoid muscle, care being taken not to injure the circumflex nerve at or near the distal end of the incision. The displacement is then reduced by a combination of manipulation and leverage, and if the fragments are quite stable, the wound is closed and the extremity immobilized in a Velpeau bandage with the hand on the opposite shoulder. If it is not stable, one or more Kirschner wires are passed through the intact skin and proximal fragment and across the fracture line into the distal fragment. The wound is then closed and the wires are cut off and bent to a right angle near the skin, and the Velpeau dressing is applied. In from four to eight weeks the wires are pulled out and the arm is placed in a sling and pendulum exercises are started. The sling is discarded when the patient is comfortable without it.

TRAUMATIC PERIARTHRITIS OF THE SHOULDER

In addition to the definite fractures and dislocations in the region of the shoulder, we are confronted with a large group of cases which we find it impossible to diagnose accurately or satisfactorily classify. All the industrial and insurance surgeons are familiar with these cases, and most of them are quite wary of them because they may be very discouraging from the standpoint of treatment.

These lesions are variously classed as periarthritis of the shoulder, subacromial bursitis, sprain fractures of the acromion, rupture of the supraspinatus tendon, etc.

The patient, usually forty or more years of age, suffers an injury to the shoulder. This injury may be a direct contusion as from a blow or fall on the shoulder, or it may be an indirect trauma from a fall on the hand or wrenching or strain of the shoulder. In many cases the injury is apparently trivial, but the shoulder remains sore, stiff, and painful, and the pain may be referred down the arm even to the fingers.

On physical examination there is little or no swelling and no disturbance of the bony landmarks. There is a variable amount of tenderness to deep pressure and this varies greatly in location. The most frequent site of tenderness is below the anterior margin of the acromion over the subacromial bursa and tuberosity of the humerus. In some cases the tenderness is posterior and below the margin of the acromion; in others it is around or even on top of the acromion; and again it may be over the coracoid.

Motion of the shoulder in the anteroposterior plane is generally free and painless, but abduction, internal rotation and external rotation are limited and painful. In chronic cases there is marked atrophy of the shoulder girdle muscles and the above motions are markedly limited. The roentgenogram is usually negative, but may show chronic arthritis or calcareous deposits in the subacromial bursa.

In a small percentage of these cases with the arm at the side, the patient finds it impossible to start the movement of abduction, but if he is assisted through the first 15 degrees of abduction he is able to continue the movement for some distance. Codman has shown that these patients are suffering from a rupture of the supraspinatus tendon, and it may be possible to palpate the thickened distal end of the tendon beneath the deltoid.

Treatment.—The most important factor in the treatment of these patients is for the surgeon to bear in mind the fact that a great many patients who have had no injury to the shoulder develop a practically identical train of symptoms. In these patients we are inclined to regard the condition as a manifestation of chronic arthritis. Consequently, in our treatment of a similar condition following an injury to the shoulder, we must not limit our efforts to the local condition, but must treat the patient as a whole.

Locally we put the shoulder at rest and apply local heat or cold. Rest may be obtained by strapping with adhesive or by an axillary pad, swathe, and sling. Heat may be applied by means of hot fomentations, a hot water bag, an electric pad, infra-red lamp, diathermy, or any other convenient method.

As measures of general treatment we advise a relatively low calorie diet, low in fats, and rich in green vegetables and fruits, and a teaspoonful of sodium phosphate in a glass of water on arising in the morning. For the relief of pain we give salicylates, aspirin, gr. 10, every four hours.

After the acute pain has subsided, the sling is continued as are the other measures, but the swathe is removed and abduction and rotation exercises are given to restore movement in the shoulder.

X-Ray Treatment.—Several authors have reported excellent results after deep x-ray therapy in these cases. The dosages vary from 100 to 350 R. and the intervals between doses vary from three days to two weeks. In our hands this method has failed more often than it has afforded relief.

Novocain Injection.—This is most successful in the patients with an acute bursitis with a calcium deposit in the bursa. This deposit is of the consistency of tooth paste, and when diluted with novocain or salt solution, it can be washed out or aspirated in the syringe. The skin and tissues over the point of acute tenderness are infiltrated with 1 per cent novocain. Then a Wassermann needle is inserted, and with a 10 c.c. syringe 1 per cent novocain is injected into the bursa and the tissues around it. Then salt solution or ½ per cent novocain is injected into the bursa and reaspirated in the syringe if calcified material is present. If not, multiple punctures are made in the bursa, and about 20 c.c. of the novocain is left in the tissues. We now rarely use the through-and-through washing with two needles as recommended by Smith-Petersen.

This method is excellent for the moderately acute cases and cures some of the chronic cases. When it fails, operation is indicated.

In our hands the injection of novocain is often followed by a day or two of severe pain, and we prefer that the patient remain in the hospital at least overnight after the injection.

In chronic cases there is a variable degree of atrophy of the muscles of the shoulder girdle and abduction and rotation are limited by adhesions. In rare severe cases a general anesthetic should be administered and the shoulder manipulated into full abduction, full internal rotation, and full external rotation. The movements should be carried out only once in each direction in order to avoid useless trauma, and then lateral traction or an aeroplane splint or plaster-of-Paris spica jacket should be applied with the shoulder in 90 degrees abduction and 180 degrees external rotation. The patient is then started on the regime recommended for the acute cases. At the end of two weeks exercises are begun to restore function in the shoulder.

Operative Treatment.—This has a definite place in the treatment of sub-acromial bursitis. It will relieve the pain in an acute case in a day or so and will frequently relieve pain and restore movement in a chronic case in a relatively short time. We prefer to perform the operation under general anesthesia, as this permits free movement of the arm and wide excision of the bursal wall.

An incision two or three inches long is made downward from the antero-lateral border of the acromion and the fibers of the deltoid are separated to expose the anterior wall of the bursa. This may or may not be thickened. The muscle fibers are separated from it, and as much of the anterior wall as can be exposed is excised. Care is taken not to extend the incision far enough downward to cut the circumflex nerve. After the anterior wall is removed, any calcified material in the bursa or blisters in the floor of the bursa is evacuated. Granulation tissue or necrotic tissue in the fibrous floor of the bursa is excised. The humerus is rotated inward and outward, and any adhesions found are cut. The wound is sprinkled with sulfonamide powder, and the skin and subcutaneous tissue are closed with silk. Swinging exercises are started within a few days.

Prognosis.—In practically all of these cases the pain subsides eventually, and the motion can be restored by exercises or by manipulation. However, many cases persist for weeks or months and we find it impossible in any given case to say whether or not the man will be back at work in a week or in six months. In general, the older and more rheumatic the patient, and the longer the symptoms have been present, the poorer the prognosis for prompt recovery, and the greater the probability that the symptoms will recur.

Many of the acute cases recover and are back at work within two weeks.

Rupture of the Supraspinatus Tendon

If a definite rupture of the supraspinatus tendon can be diagnosed, Codman advises immediate suture of the torn tendon. The cardinal signs of a rupture of this tendon are inability to perform the first fifteen degrees of abduction and in a chronic case the ability to palpate the thickened distal end of the tendon below and lateral to the tip of the acromion. Tenderness in this region is suggestive of a tearing of the tendon, but this alone is not sufficient evidence to warrant operative interference, since the operation is a difficult one.

Philip Wilson* has recently modified Codman's operation by repairing the tendon with strips of living fascia which are woven into the tendon. If necessary a transverse groove is cut in the greater tuberosity of the humerus and the fascial strips are passed through drill holes emerging at the bottom of this groove, thus reattaching the tendon to its insertion. After the operation the arm is immobilized in 90 degrees abduction and 90 degrees external rotation for two weeks, and active exercises in abduction and external rotation are begun at the end of the second week. L. C. Abbott has greatly simplified the operation by doing it under local anesthesia and using a small anterolateral incision through the deltoid with the patient sitting upright. This position permits free movement of the humerus and consequent thorough examination

---

*Wilson, P. D.: J. A. M. A. 96: 433, 1931.

of the bursa. We diagnose and operate upon this condition so rarely that we believe that most of the cases get well without operation and that function of the shoulder is restored without the supraspinatus.

DIFFERENTIAL DIAGNOSIS OF INJURIES TO THE SHOULDER AND SHOULDER GIRDLE

The history, symptoms, and location of the pain as stated by the patient may lead the surgeon to suspect some definite injury but the differential diagnosis should be made by the physical examination and x-ray.

A rough estimate of the injury may be determined from the amount of disability present. If the patient with the elbow extended can raise the arm vertically over the head and lower it slowly, it is probable that there is no serious injury to the shoulder or shoulder girdle. However, full movement may be present in subperiosteal or incomplete fractures of the clavicle in children.

If the arm can be raised to the horizontal position only with difficulty and if the patient then lets it drop suddenly and experiences a sharp pain over the clavicle, there is probably a fracture of the clavicle without displacement. The diagnosis is confirmed by point tenderness and a positive roentgenogram.

On inspection the surgeon first notes the position of the shoulder. If the shoulder is displaced downward, inward, and forward there has been some disturbance in the supporting function of the clavicle. This may be either a complete fracture with displacement or a dislocation of its inner end. As the bone is subcutaneous throughout its length, the type and location of the lesion can be determined by palpation, but in lesions around the sternoclavicular joint a roentgenogram may be necessary to determine the exact nature of the injury.

In examining a patient for displacement of an intact shoulder it must be remembered that in many normal individuals one shoulder, usually the right, is slightly lower than the other and that the shoulders are always asymmetric in patients with curvature of the spine.

The contour of the shoulder as determined by inspection and palpation is compared with that of the other side. A slight depression of the acromion with an abnormal prominence of the acromial end of the clavicle indicates either an acromioclavicular dislocation or a fracture very close to the joint. Local tenderness and ability to reduce the deformity temporarily by pressing upward on the elbow while the clavicle is immobilized with the surgeon's other hand confirms the diagnosis.

A flattening of the lateral surface of the deltoid below the acromion suggests a dislocation at the shoulder or a fracture of the surgical neck of the scapula with displacement or an epiphyseal separation or fracture of the upper end of the humerus with displacement.

If there is a dislocation, the fingers can be made to sink into the space beneath the acromion which is usually occupied by the upper end of the humerus. It should be noted, however, that the presence of great swelling may obliterate the flattening and even make it difficult to determine whether or not the upper end of the humerus is in its normal position. Consequently, the axis of the shaft of the humerus should be projected upward, and it should be noted whether or not this axis tends to intersect the glenoid cavity. If the axis of the humerus does not intersect the glenoid and the arm is maintained in an abnormal position by muscle spasm, there is a dislocation at the shoulder and the type can be determined by palpating the head of the humerus in its abnormal location.

If the humerus is intact and its head can be felt deep in the tissues beneath the acromion and if the deformity can be reduced by upward pressure on the elbow and recurs when the pressure is released, there is a fracture of the surgical neck of the scapula with displacement.

If the head of the humerus is in its normal position and if there is point tenderness of the upper end of the humerus and the head of the bone does not move with the shaft, there is an epiphyseal separation or a fracture through the upper end of the humerus with displacement. It is usually possible to palpate the upper end of the distal fragment in the anterior axillary region.

If the signs of a fracture through the upper end of the humerus with displacement are present and the glenoid is felt to be empty, there is a fracture dislocation at the shoulder, and the head can usually be palpated in its abnormal position.

Marked swelling behind the shoulder suggests either a posterior dislocation, a fracture of the scapula, or a fracture of the upper end of the humerus with posterior displacement.

In fractures of the spine or body of the scapula with displacement, it is usually possible to detect irregularities in the contour of the spine or vertebral border of the bone. In obese subjects or in patients in whom the accident has occurred some hours or days previously the disturbances in contour mentioned above may be obscured. The two shoulders should then be palpated systematically as described in the section on examination of the shoulder. In fractures without demonstrable displacement, the surgeon has to depend upon point tenderness and local pain elicited by axial pressure, torsion, cross strain, or muscle pull on the suspected bone which can be produced by manipulating the extremity. These lesions are fractures of the clavicle, fractures of the coracoid, acromion, glenoid, or neck of the scapula and fractures of the upper end of the humerus, especially of the tuberosities. In most instances an x-ray is necessary to determine the details of the lesion.

The diagnosis of sprain, contusion, or periarthritis should be made only after careful physical and x-ray examinations have ruled out definite anatomic lesions. Even in the presence of negative roentgenograms and a history of recent injury, if pain and tenderness and limited motion are present, the shoulder should be treated by rest and heat and protection until improved.

CHAPTER XVII

FRACTURES OF THE SHAFT OF THE HUMERUS

SURGICAL ANATOMY

Surgically the shaft of the humerus may be considered as extending from the upper border of the insertion of the pectoralis major muscle above to the supracondylar ridges below (Figs. 512 and 513). It is roughly cylindrical on cross-section and practically straight in its long axis. The anterior surface is covered by the deltoid, biceps, and brachialis anticus muscles and the posterior surface is covered by the deltoid and triceps. Consequently, the bone is most successfully palpated on its lateral and mesial aspects where the intermuscular septa dip down between the muscles to be attached to the bone.

The intermuscular septa divide the arm into anterior and posterior compartments. The anterior compartment contains the biceps, coracobrachialis, and brachialis anticus muscles, and the neurovascular bundle which has its course along the mesial border of the biceps and is separated from the bone by the other muscles. The posterior compartment contains the triceps muscle and the radial nerve. This nerve lies in a shallow groove in the posterior and lateral surfaces of the middle and upper thirds of the shaft. The direction of the groove and of the nerve is from within, outward, downward and forward, and they lie between the origins of the inner and outer heads of the triceps muscle.

FRACTURES OF THE SHAFT OF THE HUMERUS

Occurrence and Cause.—Fractures of the shaft of the humerus are not as common as are those of the upper end of the bone, but are by no means rare. In the majority of cases they are the result of direct violence such as falls on the arm at the side, blows, and crushing injuries and for this reason are frequently compound. Occasionally the shaft of the humerus is broken by indirect violence such as a fall on the elbow or hand. It may also be broken by muscular action and the shaft of the humerus is said to be the most frequent site of fracture from this cause.

Pathology and Displacement.—The fractures from direct violence tend to be roughly transverse or comminuted, while those from indirect violence or muscle action tend to be oblique or spiral.

In rare instances the ends of the fragments may remain in contact and some angulation, but little or no displacement occurs. Usually, however, the ends are displaced and slip by one another and the lower fragment is drawn upward by the contraction of the muscles of the arm. The shortening is usually less than 1 inch, but may be more than an inch.

The outward or inward displacement of the lower fragment depends largely upon whether the fracture line lies above or below the insertion of the deltoid. If the shaft is broken above the deltoid insertion, this muscle, being attached to the lower fragment, tends to draw it outward; while the pectoralis major, latissimus dorsi and teres major pull the upper fragment inward. If the fracture line lies below the deltoid insertion, this muscle and the coracobrachialis tend to draw the upper fragment outward and forward, while the lower fragment is simply drawn upward by the arm muscles. Gravity and position also influence the displacement, particularly in rotation, as the forearm is usually carried across the chest and the lower fragment is thus rotated inward while the upper fragment remains in the midposition.

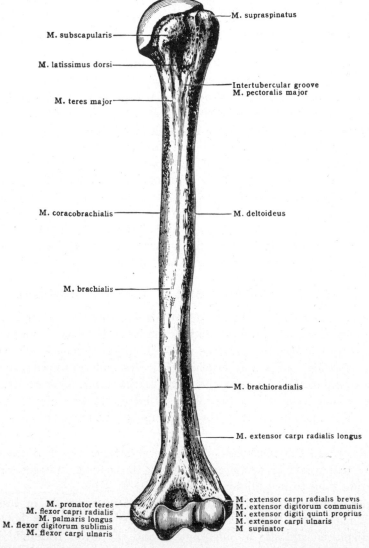

M. supraspinatus

M. subscapularis

M. latissimus dorsi

Intertubercular groove
M. pectoralis major

M. teres major

M. coracobrachialis

M. deltoideus

M. brachialis

M. brachioradialis

M. extensor carpi radialis longus

M. pronator teres
M. flexor capri radialis
M. palmaris longus
M. flexor digitorum sublimis
M. flexor carpi ulnaris

M. extensor carpi radialis brevis
M. extensor digitorum communis
M. extensor digiti quinti proprius
M. extensor carpi ulnaris
M supinator

Fig. 512.—Drawing of humerus, anterior view, showing muscle attachments. (From Morris: Human Anatomy, P. Blakiston's Son & Co., Inc., Publisher.)

The above displacements from muscle action are by no means constant because a continuation of the fracturing force may cause the displacement and the distal fragment may move upward and in any direction around the proximal one.

Diagnosis.—In a complete fracture of the shaft of the humerus with displacement the diagnosis is usually obvious at a glance. If there is any doubt, the arm may be measured from the tip of the acromion to the external condyle to determine shortening and gently manipulated to demonstrate abnormal mobility or crepitus. The extensive swelling may render it difficult to determine the displacement.

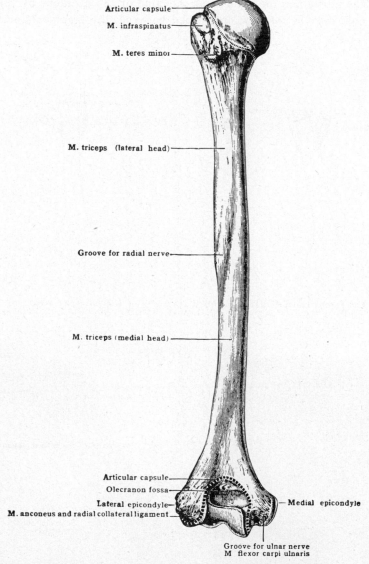

Fig. 513.—Drawing of humerus, posterior view, showing muscle attachments. (From Morris: Human Anatomy, P. Blakiston's Son & Co., Inc., Publisher.)

In incomplete fractures in children or fractures without displacement, the diagnosis is more difficult and is made from the disability, point tenderness, and angulation or abnormal mobility, if present. In some instances a roentgenogram may be necessary.

Complications

As was stated above, since a large percentage of these fractures are the result of direct violence, many of them are compound.

Other than compound fractures radial nerve paralysis is the most frequent and serious complication of fractures of the shaft of the humerus because of the intimate relation of the nerve to the bone where it lies in the musculospiral groove. The nerve may be injured at the time of the accident by the fracturing force or it may be torn by, or crushed between, the fragments or it may be

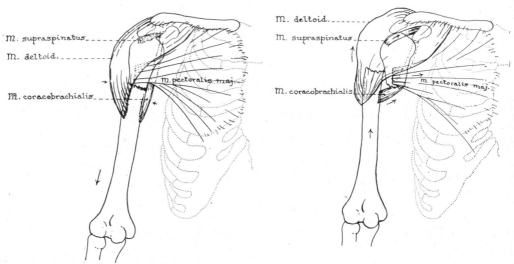

Fig. 514.—The forces causing displacement in fractures of the humerus below the insertion of the pectoralis major. (Courtesy of Dr. Arnold Griswold, Am. J. Surg., January, 1939.)

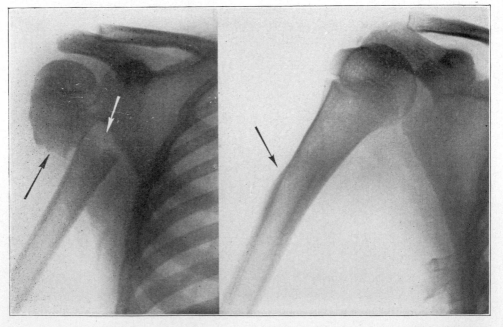

Fig. 515.—Fracture of proximal third of humerus. Closed reduction failed. Open reduction fixed with catgut and hanging cast. Normal shoulder obtained. X-ray four years later shows normal growth of shaft.

injured secondarily by movements of the fragments or by being stretched over the displaced fragments. In other instances the radial (musculospiral) paralysis appears some weeks after the accident and is the result of pressure on the nerve by scar tissue or callus.

The symptoms of radial nerve injury are wrist drop and loss of supination of the forearm and extension of the fingers and thumb. There is also some sensory disturbance of the dorsum of the forearm, hand, and thumb. The triceps is not affected because the nerves to this muscle leave the radial before it enters the musculospiral groove.

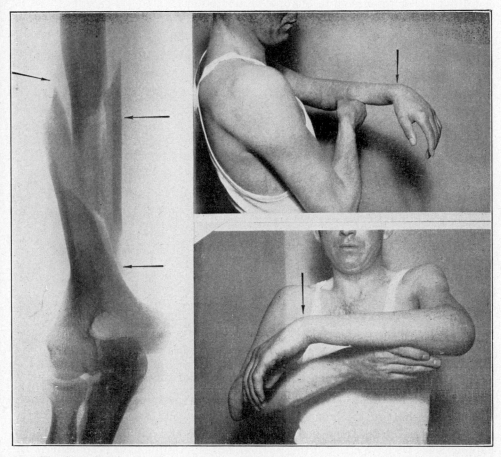

Fig. 516.—Fracture of humerus with radial nerve paralysis. At operation nerve found partially severed. It was repaired and bones fixed with kangaroo tendon and cast. Functional recovery followed after some months.

More rarely the median or ulnar nerves may be injured. With the median nerve paralysis, there is loss of pronation of the forearm, flexion of the wrist, fingers, and thumb is impaired, and there is inability to oppose the thumb and little finger. There is also sensory disturbance on the volar surface of the hand, thumb, and index and middle fingers. With ulnar paralysis there is impairment of flexion of the ring and little fingers and inability to spread the fingers or adduct the thumb and loss of sensation on the ulnar side of the dorsum of the hand and of the ring and little fingers.

In rare instances the brachial artery or vein may be torn or so injured that thrombosis occurs with resulting swelling, loss of the radial pulse or even gangrene.

Nonunion is said to occur more frequently in fractures of the shaft of the humerus than in any other location. The cause is not known. The causes usually given are: 1. Extensive damage to the surrounding soft parts. 2. Injury to the nutrient artery. 3. Interposition of muscle between the fragments (Fig. 517). 4. Inefficient immobilization due to the practice of fixing the elbow in 90 degrees flexion while the shoulder and upper fragment are not immobilized. (See discussion in chapter on nonunion.)

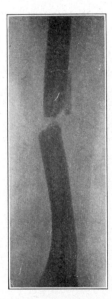

Fig. 517.—Fracture of the humerus with nonunion due to interposition of muscle between the fragments. Successfully treated by open operation. The muscle was removed from between the bones, the medullary canal was drilled open, the ends of the bones were freshened and sutured together with chromic catgut. Fixation in plaster for nine weeks; molded plaster splint for two more weeks; sling to forearm thereafter for three weeks. Good results.

Treatment of Fractures of the Shaft of the Humerus

The Hanging Cast.—We now routinely treat practically all of our fractures of the shaft of the humerus in the hanging cast, as described in the preceding chapter (p. 564) and not only have both we and our patients been much happier since we have adopted this method, but our results have been better. In fractures of the distal portion of the shaft the forearm is immobilized in full pronation in order to compensate for the tendency of the supinators to tilt the distal fragment outward. Forward or backward bowing at the site of the fracture is controlled by shortening or lengthening the sling which supports the wrist. When this fails, we resort to open reduction.

Dr. Richard T. Hudson suggests the following "Dont's" when using a hanging cast in treating fractures of the humerus:

> Don't worry about some pain and crepitation the first week.
> Don't worry that the fragments move.
> Don't let the patient disturb the length of the support.

Don't apply too heavy a cast.

Don't neglect to see that the humerus hangs vertically.

Don't fail to make the patient ambulatory.

Don't allow the patient to attach the cast to the body or wear a sling.

Don't fail to start circumduction exercises of the shoulder as soon as possible.

Don't fail to check with x-ray picture after one week with patient sitting or standing.

Don't expect the cast to reduce fractures of the surgical neck.

Alternate methods of treatment are the following:

1. Fractures of the Shaft of the Humerus in Which the Fragments Are in Good Position and Exhibit Little Tendency to Displacement.—(a) In this type of fracture, which is usually transverse, and in children may be subperiosteal in character, all that is necessary is to splint the arm with coaptation splints and immobilize it at the side with a cotton pad in the axilla while the forearm is supported by a clove hitch around the neck with the elbow flexed to 90 degrees. The coaptation splints may be purchased readymade or can be made in a few minutes by laying a piece of splint board of the proper length on a wide strip of adhesive and splitting the splint board longitudinally into strips about ⅓ of an inch wide, leaving the strips attached to the adhesive. One of these should be long enough to reach from the external condyle to the upper end of the humerus and the other long enough to reach from the internal condyle to the axilla. One is placed on the inner side, one on the outer side of the arm, and they are fastened with adhesive (Fig. 519*A*). A triangular pad at least 3 inches thick at its base and long enough to reach from the axilla to the tip of the elbow is made of absorbent cotton and slung in the axilla by a band of adhesive which passes over the shoulder. The arm is then bound to the side by two or more wide strips of adhesive which pass completely around the chest, the elbow is brought across the chest, the wrist is supported by a clove hitch fastened around the neck.

(b) A more efficient method of supporting this same type of fracture, affording greater comfort, is to place the arm in the desired position close to the side and so rotate it inward that the forearm extends across the lower chest. A posterior plaster mold, long enough to extend from the base of the neck over the shoulder, down the arm, around the elbow, and along the forearm to the base of the fingers, is now made and applied. The plaster splint is molded to the shoulder and extremity and fastened with gauze bandage until it is quite dry, when it can be strapped on with adhesive and the forearm supported in a cravat sling or clove hitch. This posterior plaster mold has the advantage of tending to immobilize the shoulder and elbow (Fig. 519*B*).

2. Fractures Without Marked Displacement But in Which There Is a Tendency for Angulation of the Lower Fragment to Occur.

(a) These fractures should be immobilized in the neutral position as regards rotation and the shaft of the humerus must be supported to prevent angulation. By neutral position for the humerus we mean that with the elbow flexed to 90 degrees the forearm points forward and inward across the lower chest. We formerly had the forearm pointing directly forward, but find that a position of apparent moderate internal rotation is a more natural one. The best method of obtaining this type of immobilization is to have the arm supported in a position of slight abduction and anterior flexion with the forearm flexed to 90 degrees and pointing forward and inward, and then apply a plaster spica cast which includes the shoulder and trunk and extends downward on the extremity to the finger tips. Since the humerus usually tends to angulate

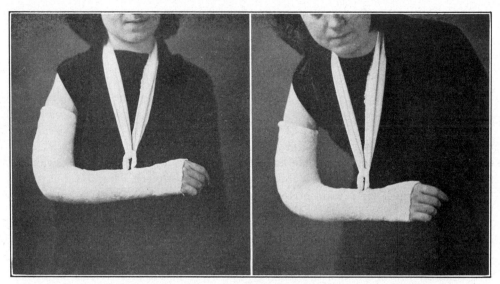

Fig. 518.—The hanging cast as used in fractures of the shaft of the humerus. On the right the patient is shown exercising the arm. (Courtesy of Dr. Arnold Griswold.)

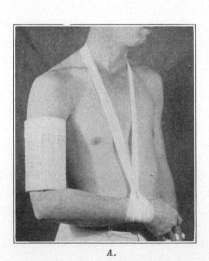
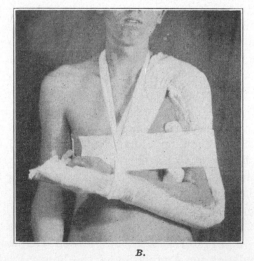

A.   B.

Fig. 519.—A, Application of coaptation splints to the arm and forearm, supported by a sling. Used as a convalescent dressing in certain fractures of the humerus. Does not give support and fixation as does splint shown in Fig. 519 B.

B, Long plaster mold extending from base of neck over shoulder, down arm, around elbow, down the forearm to the base of the fingers for postoperative immobilization of fractures of the humerus. Suspended by clove hitch around wrist.

outward we pronate the forearm to correct this angulation and shaft of the humerus fractures are habitually immobilized with the forearm fully pronated. For the purpose of immobilization, it is of advantage to first apply a posterior mold extending from the shoulder and downward around the elbow to include the forearm before the circular plaster is put on, since it is always difficult to avoid angulation during the application of a circular plaster bandage. (Fig. 520.)

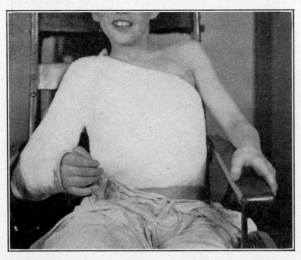

Fig. 520.—Spica plaster cast as used in the treatment of fractures of the shaft of the humerus.

A lighter and more comfortable method is simply to apply the cast from the axilla to the knuckles with the elbow flexed and the forearm pronated and support the wrist in a sling.

(b) Instead of the plaster-of-Paris dressing as described above the Magnuson humerus splint can be used or a triangular splint can be constructed of splint board. The triangle, sufficiently long to extend from the axilla to the elbow, is made and the ends bound together with adhesive; then a crosspiece to support the forearm is attached to one side at the base of this either with adhesive or nails and the splint is padded and strapped to the chest. The arm is then placed upon it and fastened with bandage and adhesive.

(c) As a substitute for the axillary splint of wood a triangular splint may be made of cardboard. The disadvantages of this splint are that it is weak and that the lower fragment is supported in the position of moderate internal rotation; consequently it is not so efficient as either the wood or plaster dressing.

(d) An adjustable abduction splint which can be adjusted to support the arm in not more than 30 degrees abduction from the side may be applied as a substitute for any of the above.

3. **Fractures With Displacement.**—In fractures with displacement either with or without shortening and in which the fracture line is roughly transverse or of such a nature that it seems probable that if reduction can be accomplished, the ends of the bone can be made to engage and not slip by one another, it is better to reduce the displacement and apply one of the forms of dressing enumerated above under section 2.

The reduction is best accomplished under an anesthetic (local or general) with the patient recumbent. When muscular relaxation has been obtained, with the arm close to the side, the elbow is flexed to approximately 90 degrees and one assistant immobilizes the shoulder while another assistant makes traction on the arm in the line of the shaft of the humerus. When this traction, which should be slow, steady, and strong, has completely corrected the shortening so that the ends of the bone have slipped by one another, the surgeon can mold the fragments with his fingers until they seem to be in line or until the shortening does not reappear, when the traction is released (Fig. 522). Then, care being taken not to reproduce the displacement, the plaster dressing or triangular board splint or abduction splint can be applied.

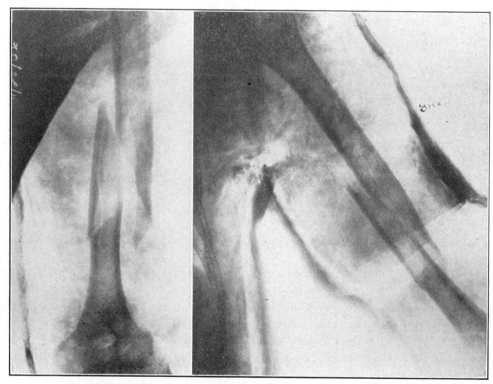

Fig. 521.—Left, fracture of humerus after reduction and immobilization in a plaster-of-Paris spica. Right, same after cutting cast and shifting distal portion outward and fixing it with a plaster bandage around the cast at the cut. Union occurred promptly.

4. Oblique Spiral or Comminuted Fractures With Displacement. (Figs. 523, 524, and 525.) In these fractures, even though the displacement is completely reduced under an anesthetic, it tends to recur unless traction is maintained; consequently the fracture should be treated in traction until the bones have united. This may be obtained either in an ambulant splint or in recumbency or in a hanging cast.

(a) *Plaster Cast Without Traction.*—We formerly treated these fractures in a plaster-of-Paris spica jacket which extends to the bases of the fingers and gets a good grip on the pelvis. In applying this cast the elbow is flexed and the forearm pronated and the displacement is reduced by traction in line with the proximal fragment, and the traction is maintained while the plaster is being applied and until it has set. Radiographs in two planes to determine the position of the fragment are then made and if they are not satisfactory, the cast is cut through at the level of the fracture and the lower fragment is manipulated or angulated until the position is satisfactory and the two sections of the cast are then united with a plaster bandage. (Fig. 521.)

(b) *The Jones Humerus Splint and the Thomas Arm Splint* are very popular types of splints which one often sees used and which we mention, but rarely use. The Jones humerus splint is uncomfortable and difficult to keep adjusted. We object to the Thomas arm splint because most fractures of the shaft of the humerus should be treated with the elbow flexed. If traction is made on the arm with the elbow extended, the brachialis anticus and the

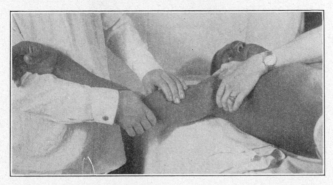

Fig. 522.—Method of manipulation in reduction of fracture of the shaft of the humerus.

flexor muscles of the forearm tend to pull the distal fragment forward so that complete displacement or marked anterior bowing at the site of the fracture occurs. This difficulty may be modified by keeping the patient in bed and making traction on the arm from the end of the splint, while the forearm is suspended in a position of 90 degrees flexion at the elbow, but in this position the arm must be abducted in order to use the splint at all, and abduction tends to result in internal bowing because of the pull of the pectoralis major, teres major, and latissimus dorsi on the upper fragment. This difficulty can be met by the hinged modification of the Thomas arm splint, but if this is used the patient's arm must rest upon the posterior bar of the splint, which is, of course, uncomfortable. Consequently the only use that we see for the Thomas arm splint is as an emergency transportation splint for the immobilization of a fresh fracture until it can be properly treated.

(c) *Abduction Traction Splint.*—An adjustable abduction traction splint which can be set with the arm at not more than 30 degrees abduction is a good method for the treatment of fractures of the shaft of the humerus and has the advantage over the Jones splint of controlling rotation at the shoulder. Satisfactory traction and immobilization can also be obtained with the Magnuson splint.

(d) *The Hoke Traction Apparatus* probably affords the most efficient ambulant method of obtaining traction for immobilization in fractures of the shaft of the humerus. Adhesive traction strips are applied to the

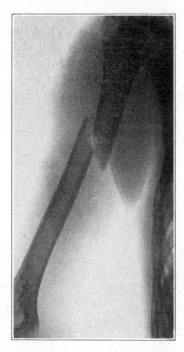

Fig. 523.—Oblique fracture of the shaft of the humerus treated by reduction under an anesthetic and immobilization in a plaster spica cast for eight weeks; molded plaster splint for three weeks; sling for two weeks. Good results.

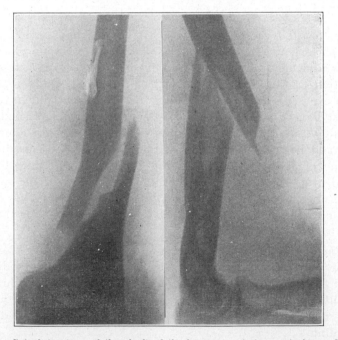

Fig. 524.—Spiral fracture of the shaft of the humerus. Anteroposterior and lateral views. Lateral traction (skeletal) for three weeks with arm in 30 degrees abduction; then plaster spica cast for six weeks; molded splint for two weeks; sling for three weeks. Good result.

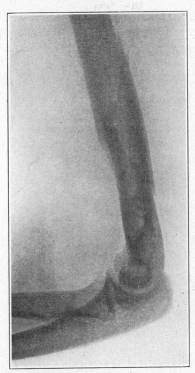

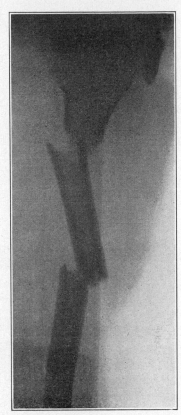

Fig. 525.   Fig. 526.

Fig. 525.—Preceding case after treatment by skeletal traction followed by immobilization in a plaster spica.

Fig. 526.—Double fracture of the shaft of the humerus treated by skeletal traction through upper end of ulnar shaft with arm in 45 degrees abduction for twenty-five days; plaster spica cast for eight weeks and posterior plaster splint for three weeks. Sling to forearm two weeks. Good result. Treatment by traction is usually necessary in this type of fracture.

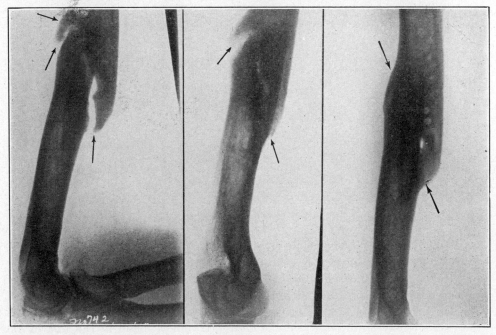

Fig. 527.—Fracture of the shaft of the humerus with nonunion before and after bone drilling.
Union occurred.

upper arm and bound in position with adhesive and bandage. A plaster spica jacket which includes the upper extremity down to the base of the fingers is applied with the arm in slight abduction and anterior flexion and the forearm pointing straight forward and the elbow flexed to 90 degrees. The Hoke traction apparatus is incorporated in the plaster cast and a large window is cut over the elbow and ulnar surface of the forearm and the traction strips

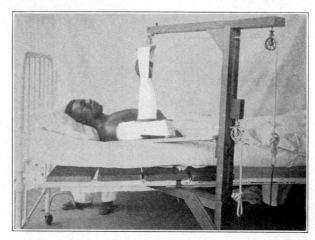

Fig. 528.—Adhesive traction (with lateral traction frame) in recumbency with arm slightly abducted and supported on board; forearm suspended.

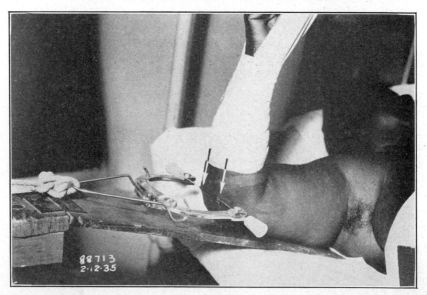

Fig. 529.—Lateral traction with wire through ulna for fracture of the shaft of the humerus.

are brought out and fastened to the apparatus. With this method any degree of traction desired can be obtained and maintained until union is firm.

(e) *Traction With Recumbency.*—(Fig. 528.) With the patient in bed on a firm mattress adhesive traction strips are applied to the arm and forearm. The forearm is then suspended with the elbow flexed 90 degrees and with the arm slightly abducted from the side, traction is made in the line of the

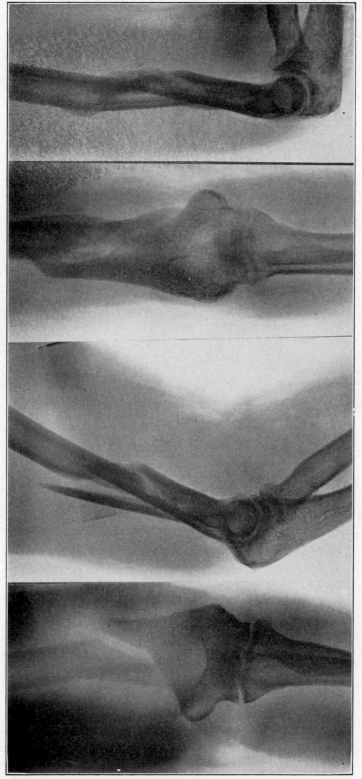

Fig. 530.—Fracture of lower third of the humerus. Treated by lateral traction with wire through the ulna.

humerus. In this treatment it is necessary that the arm be supported. This is best accomplished by a thin splint board which is placed under it and on which the arm rests and is fastened by bandages.

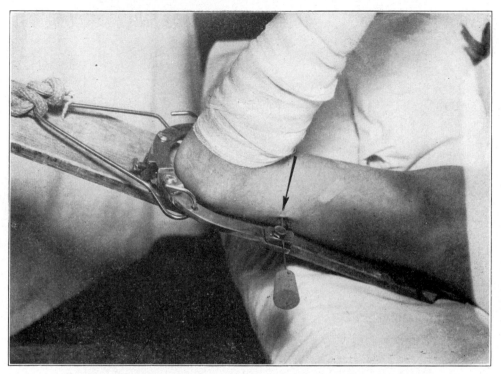

Fig. 531A.—Improper application of Kirschner wire showing the pull on the skin. In every case when the Kirschner wire is applied the skin should be incised distally to the pin or wire to prevent painful pull on the skin, where most of the discomfort in skeletal traction is experienced.

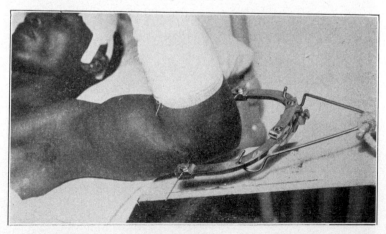

Fig. 531B.—Application of skeletal traction to humerus by wire through the lower fourth of the bone. Used in fractures involving the upper half of the humerus when traction is indicated. (DePuy Clamp.)

5. Compound Fractures With Displacement.—If there is considerable damage to the soft parts so that it is not possible to apply adhesive traction strips to the skin, traction may be obtained by two methods: (1) A broad band around the upper forearm. (2) Skeletal traction to the arm, best obtained by means of a Kirschner steel wire or a small Steinmann nail or drill passed through the bone, since ice tongs are apt to slip and cause damage to the soft parts. One of us (H. E. C.) passes the wire through the lower end of the shaft of the humerus just above the elbow (Fig. 531 B). The other puts the wire through the thick part of the upper end of the shaft of the ulna just posterior to the coronoid process.

6. **Time of Immobilization and After-Treatment.**—Fractures with little displacement should be immobilized from three to five weeks, when a coaptation splint can be applied and the forearm supported by a clove hitch around the neck. If the triangular sling is used in the treatment of fractures of the shaft of the humerus care should be taken that the upward pressure on the elbow does not cause angulation, displacement, and overriding of the fragments. This should be continued from two to four weeks and then the patient may be allowed to resume use of the arm. As a rule no physiotherapy is necessary or even indicated. In fractures with displacement or which have been comminuted, the period of traction or immobilization should be continued for from six to eight weeks and then followed by a cylinder cast or coaptation splints and a support for the wrist for from two to four weeks longer, depending upon the amount of damage to the bone and soft parts and the rapidity of union. At the end of this time the patient can be permitted to begin to use the arm and a practically normal arm may be expected in from ten to twelve weeks.

CHAPTER XVIII

FRACTURES IN THE REGION OF THE ELBOW

SURGICAL ANATOMY

The Lower End of the Humerus.—In its lower fourth the shaft of the humerus is broadened and flattened from before backward and terminates in the internal and external condyles which are separated by the coronoid and olecranon fossae. The articular surface lies below and between the condyles and is directed downward and forward at an angle of about 45 degrees. It is unequally divided by a median ridge into a larger internal surface, the trochlea, and a smaller lateral surface, the capitellum. The trochlea which articulates with the greater sigmoid fossa of the ulna is concave from side to side and convex from before backward and is continued around the end of the bone on to the posterior surface where it terminates in the broad, rather deep olecranon fossa. The capitellum is rounded to articulate with the head of the radius and faces forward to such a degree that it is not visible from behind.

On the anterior surface of the shaft just above the trochlea and capitellum there are shallow depressions for the coronoid and the head of the radius. These are superimposed on the olecranon fossa behind and cause the bone to be very thin in this area.

Surgically the lower end of the humerus may be divided into an external and internal condyle, each of which is surmounted by an eminence, the epicondyle. The external condyle includes the rounded capitellum and the bone above it. Its most prominent portion is called the "external epicondyle." The internal condyle includes the trochlea and the bone above it. Its most prominent portion is called the "internal epicondyle." This is much more prominent than the external epicondyle and its posterior and inferior surfaces present a groove for the passage of the ulnar nerve.

In anatomical literature the epicondyles are called "condyles."

The Upper End of the Ulna.—The shaft of the ulna is thickened in its upper half and terminates above in the coronoid and olecranon processes which are separated by the sigmoid fossa. This is hollowed out of the adjacent anterior surface of the olecranon and superior surface of the coronoid. It is convex laterally and deeply concave in its longitudinal direction to articulate with the trochlea surface of the humerus.

The olecranon is a heavy process of bone which projects upward in the line of the shaft and presents a broad proximal end for the insertion of the triceps muscle. Its posterior surface is subcutaneous and its anterior surface forms part of the floor of the greater sigmoid cavity. The coronoid is a thick pyramidal process which projects from the anterior surface of the shaft of the ulna and is roughened for the insertion of the brachialis anticus muscle. Its superior surface is articular and forms part of the floor of the greater sigmoid cavity. On its lateral side there is a small articular surface, the lesser sigmoid fossa, for the border of the head of the radius.

The Upper End of the Radius.—The upper end of the radius consists of a disc-shaped head and a short cylindrical neck which unites the head to the shaft of the bone. The upper surface of the head is slightly concave and articulates with the capitellum and the rounded border articulates with the lesser sigmoid cavity on the side of the coronoid process of the ulna. The bicipital tuberosity is a prominent process on the mesial side of the shaft of the radius just below the neck of the bone for the insertion of the tendon of the biceps muscles.

Ossification of the Bones at the Elbow.—At birth the lower end of the humerus is entirely cartilaginous and later this becomes ossified from four centers. The largest of these is for the capitellum and the outer part of the trochlea. It appears at about two years and the ossification extends inward across the strip of cartilage to unite with the small center for the inner portion of the trochlea which appears about the eleventh year. This entire strip which forms the articular end of the bone fuses with the shaft about the sixteenth year. The centers for the mesial and lateral condyles (epicondyles) appear at about the fifth and twelfth years respectively. That for the lateral condyle (epicondyle) rapidly coalesces with those for the capitellum and trochlea to form the lower epiphysis while the center for the mesial condyle (epicondyle) forms a separate epiphysis which unites to the shaft about the eighteenth year.

The Ulna and Radius.—The upper end of the ulna is practically all developed from the shaft of the bone except a small epiphysis for the tip of the olecranon which appears about the tenth year and fuses with the shaft about the sixteenth year. The head of the radius is developed from a single center which appears at from five to seven years and fuses to the shaft at from eighteen to twenty years.

The Elbow Joint is really composed of two separate joints, a main hinge-like joint between the humerus above and the head of the radius and the greater sigmoid of the ulna below, and a smaller joint between the border of the head of the radius and the lesser sigmoid of the ulna which permits rotation of the head of the radius in the orbicular ligament.

The stability of the elbow joint is largely dependent upon the contour of the articulation between the trochlea of the humerus and the greater sigmoid of the ulna. This is, however, reinforced by strong lateral ligaments which bind the ulna to the condyles of the humerus (Figs. 532 and 533). The internal of these is considerably stronger than the external, which is not inserted into the radius, but splits to blend with the orbicular ligament and ultimately to be attached to the upper end of the ulna. The synovial cavities of the two joints communicate and the capsule is relatively thin except where it is reinforced by the lateral ligaments. The stability of the joint between the head of the radius and the ulna is almost entirely dependent upon the orbicular ligament which encircles about three-fourths of the radial head and is attached at either end of the lesser sigmoid cavity, thus binding the radius firmly to the ulna.

Movements of the Elbow Joint.—The axis of the elbow joint is obliquely transverse so that in the extended position the humerus and ulna form an angle of from five to twenty degrees which is open outward and is known as the carrying angle, while in the flexed position the ulna swings inward toward the mouth (Figs. 534, 535, and 536). The carrying angle is most evident when the forearm is supinated because with pronation the radius swings inward around the ulna and apparently obliterates the angulation, but the line of the ulna and the humerus remains unchanged. The joint between the head of the radius and the ulna permits free rotation of the head of the radius in supination and pronation.

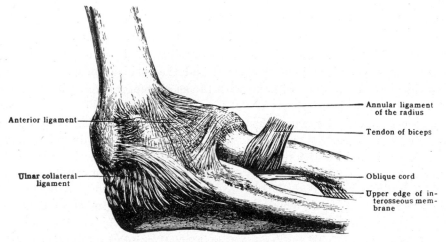

Fig. 532.—Left elbow joint showing anterior and internal ligaments. (From Morris, Human Anatomy, P. Blakiston's Son & Co., Inc., Publisher.)

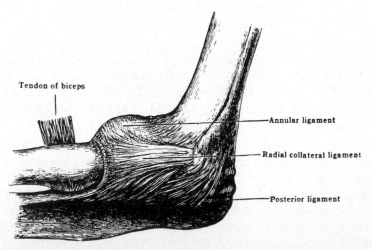

Fig. 533.—Left elbow joint showing posterior and external ligaments. (From Morris, Human Anatomy, P. Blakiston's Son & Co., Inc., Publisher.)

Structures in the Region of the Elbow.—Just beneath the skin in the superficial fascia over the front of the elbow are the median cephalic and basilic veins which return a considerable portion of the blood from the forearm and consequently should not be compressed by dressings. At the bottom of the depression or cubital fossa in front of the joint is the biceps tendon which is inserted into the bicipital tuberosity of the radius. The brachial artery lies mesial to the tendon and divides into the radial and ulnar artery in the lower portion of the cubital fossa. The median nerve lies just mesial to the artery. The radial nerve courses downward between the brachioradialis and brachialis anticus and terminates in the posterior interosseous nerve which

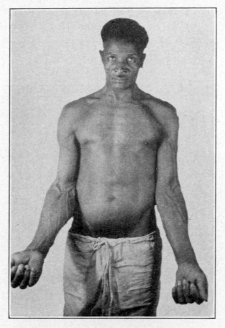

Fig. 534.—Normal carrying angle in a laborer.

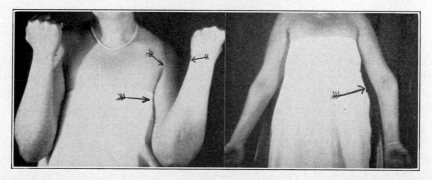

Fig. 535.—Reversal of carrying angle (gun stock deformity on the left) due to a fracture improperly reduced of the lower end of the humerus in childhood.

passes outward and backward around the neck of the radius. The ulnar nerve passes backward through the internal intermuscular septum a short distance above the elbow and lies in the groove on the posterior surface of the internal condyle when it is encased in a sheath of dense fibrous tissue. After its emergence from this tunnel-like sheath it enters the forearm between the heads of the flexor carpi ulnaris.

The muscles of the elbow are usually divided into flexor and extensor groups. The flexors are the biceps, brachialis anticus, brachioradialis, and the flexor carpi radialis. These muscles flex the forearm and the biceps, by virtue of its attachment to the tubercle on the inner side of the shaft of the radius, acts as a powerful supinator of the forearm. The extensor group consists of the triceps and anconeus and their action is to extend the forearm on the arm. The medial condyle and the ridge above it give origin to the flexors of the wrist and fingers and to the pronator radii teres, while the lateral condyle and ridge give origin to the extensors of the wrist and fingers, but the leverage of these muscles is so poor at their origin that they have little or no effect upon the movements of the elbow.

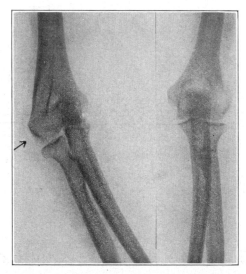

Fig. 536.—X-ray pictures of the preceding case taken twenty years after the injury.

EXAMINATION OF THE ELBOW

Both elbows are exposed and the injured elbow is inspected from the front, back, and sides and compared with that on the other side in order to determine the amount of the swelling and the character of the deformity if present. Then the patient is asked to attempt to flex and extend the elbow and pronate and supinate the forearm in order to determine the amount and character of the disability.

The surgeon should palpate the elbow and definitely locate the three cardinal bony landmarks (Figs. 537 and 538). These are the tip of the olecranon and the epicondyles of the humerus. With the elbow flexed to 90 degrees they should form an equilateral triangle and with the elbow extended the tip of the olecranon should lie about the midpoint of the line uniting the two epicondyles. If these are obscured by swelling, this can be pressed aside by slow firm pressure or deep massage and this, if done carefully, is not very painful to the patient.

The integrity of the lower end of the humerus should be tested by fixing the shaft and gently pulling the forearm forward and pushing it backward,

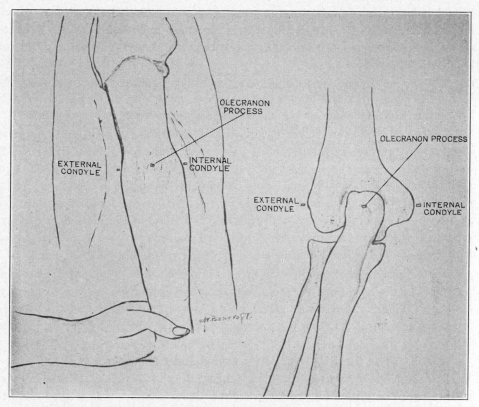

Fig. 537.—Drawing to show bony landmarks at the elbow with the forearm extended.

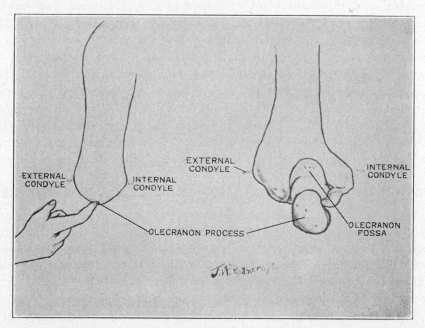

Fig. 538.—Drawing to show bony landmarks at the elbow with the forearm flexed.

thus demonstrating false motion if present. Having located the three cardinal bony landmarks and tested the humerus, the surgeon should carefully palpate the entire elbow and note any abnormalities in the bony contour or points of local tenderness.

Finally he should test the lateral stability of the joint by fixing the humerus and moving the extended forearm from side to side and should test the flexion and extension at the elbow and the supination of the forearm.

Unless the surgeon is perfectly sure of the diagnosis a roentgenogram should be made before treatment is instituted, and in children, unless he is quite familiar with the normal x-ray picture of the elbow at the given age, pictures of the opposite normal elbow should be taken for comparison. If no roentgenogram has been made before treatment it should be made afterward, as many of these injuries are multiple and the diagnosis of one does not exclude the others, as, for instance, a posterior dislocation is often accompanied by a fracture of the head of the radius or of the coronoid.

In the presence of much swelling the surgeon should palpate the radial pulse and carefully note the condition of the circulation in the extremity. He should also make a rough sensory and motor examination of the part in order to determine whether or not any of the important nerves have been injured.

The X-ray in the Diagnosis of Fractures and Dislocations at the Elbow.— While it is possible to make a fairly accurate diagnosis of most of the injuries in the region of the elbow by physical examination alone it is not possible to determine the exact lines of the fracture and the exact character of the displacement, and these are often of importance in prognosis and treatment. In severe injuries of the elbow there is a definite tendency for more than one lesion to be present, and in such instances it is frequently impossible to make an accurate diagnosis from physical examination alone. Consequently in all except the simplest injuries in which the diagnosis and character of the displacement are perfectly definite the surgeon should secure an x-ray picture before and after treatment. Both anteroposterior and lateral views should be taken and in children it is often advisable to take pictures of the opposite normal elbow for control because the epiphyseal lines may be very confusing and may lead to the erroneous diagnosis of fractures which do not exist.

POSITION OF OPTIMUM FUNCTION IN ANKYLOSIS OF THE ELBOW

While the surgeon should always endeavor to obtain the maximum amount of motion after injuries at the elbow, one occasionally encounters severe compound fractures in which more or less infection is present and in which it is practically hopeless to obtain motion. In such instances it is important that the elbow be immobilized in such a position that the patient will have as useful an arm as possible after the joint has become stiff.

There is considerable difference of opinion among various surgeons as to what this position should be. By many it is argued that the elbow should be immobilized with flexion slightly beyond a right angle and with the forearm supinated as with this position it is possible for the patient to get the hand to the face. However, we feel that it is even more important that he be able to use the hand in some gainful occupation. Consequently we advise immobilization with the elbow extended to about 120 degrees; that is, about 30 degrees extension beyond a right angle and with the forearm in the midposition between pronation and supination as illustrated in Fig. 540.

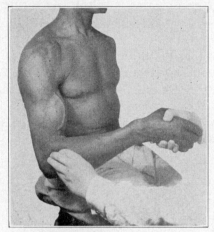
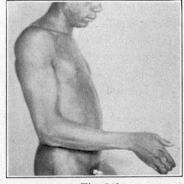

Fig. 539.   Fig. 540.

Fig. 539.—Method of palpating the head of the radius while the forearm is rotated with the other hand.
Fig. 540.—Position of optimum function for ankylosis at the elbow in a workingman.

COMPLETE FRACTURES OF THE LOWER END OF THE HUMERUS

Classification.—The complete fractures of the lower end of the humerus fall naturally into three groups: (1) Extension type; (2) intercondylar, T, or comminuted fractures; and (3) flexion type. The extension type of fractures are usually the result of backward thrust or hyperextension at the elbow and the distal fragment tends to be displaced backward. Depending upon the location of the line of fracture they are called supracondylar fractures, transverse dicondylar fractures, and epiphyseal separations. The intercondylar or T fractures may result from either hyperextension injuries, thrust injuries, or direct trauma and may be comminuted with no characteristic displacement of the fragments. The flexion type are caused by falls or blows on the flexed elbow and the distal fragment tends to be displaced forward.

1. Extension Type

Occurrence and Mechanism.—These extension fractures and epiphyseal separations are the most frequent traumatic lesions that occur in the region of the elbow and are especially common in children. The injury usually results from falls on the hand with the elbow flexed, and the lower end of the humerus being pushed backward by force transmitted upward through the bones of the forearm. Occasionally these fractures are due to forcible hyperextension at the elbow, the lower end of the humerus being pulled off by the lateral ligaments, while the olecranon, being locked in its fossa, acts as a fulcrum as in a fall on the extended hand with the forearm pronated.

Pathology

1. **Supracondylar Fractures of the Humerus: Extension Type.**—The fracture line usually begins close to the articular surface on the front of the shaft and tends to be roughly transverse in the frontal plane, but courses obliquely upward and backward in the sagittal plane (Fig. 541). The obliquity tends to be more marked in adults while in children the fracture line is often practically transverse. In rare instances the fracture line is spiral. As a rule the fracture is complete although occasional greenstick fractures occur in this region.

The displacement is characteristic in that the short distal fragment is displaced upward and backward. This is due partly to a continuation of the fracturing force, and partly to the pull of the triceps muscle which serves to maintain the displacement, while the end of the proximal fragment projects into the cubital space beneath the brachialis anticus and biceps tendons and may injure the brachial artery and vein or median nerve in this region.

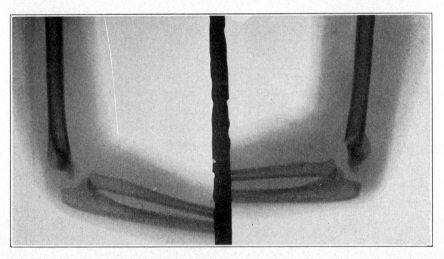

Fig. 541.—Supracondylar fracture of the humerus; extension type, with slight posterior displacement compared with the opposite normal elbow. Treated by manipulative reduction, under an anesthetic, and immobilization in moderately acute flexion in a posterior plaster mold for fourteen days. Then splint was removed daily for ten days following the injury and hot baths were used. Splinted for three weeks. Good result.

In addition to the typical upward and backward displacement the distal fragment is often forced laterally or mesially (Figs. 542 and 544) by the fracturing force and as it is controlled by the forearm it may be deviated outward (valgus) or inward (varus) by gravity or the pressure of splints. Furthermore it is often rotated inward by the custom of supporting the forearm across the chest. The forearm muscles which are attached to the condyles tend to pull the short lower fragment forward flexing it on the forearm.

In addition to the fracture of the bones there is usually considerable damage to the soft parts, and this may be so severe that it dominates the picture. The periosteum is stripped up from the posterior surface of the proximal fragment and from the anterior surface of the distal fragment; the joint capsule is usually torn; and there is a variable amount of hemorrhage into

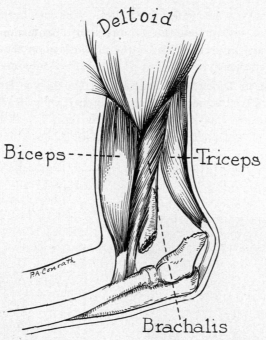

Fig. 542.—Supracondylar fracture of the humerus of the extension type showing the characteristic displacement and the pull of the muscles.

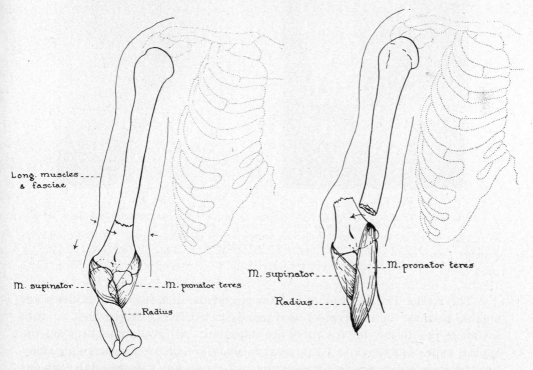

Fig. 543.—Fracture of the humerus in the lower third. On the right is shown the varus deformity which occurs unless the forearm is fixed in full pronation. (Courtesy of Dr. Arnold Griswold, Am. J. Surg., 1939.)

the joint and into the surrounding tissues. The hemorrhage and resultant swelling may be so severe that the venous return from the forearm and even the radial pulse are interfered with and immediate treatment may be necessary to save the extremity.

2. **Transverse or Dicondylar Fracture of the Lower End of the Humerus** has been described as a separate clinical entity by Kocher, Ashurst, and Chutro. The fracture line lies just above the epiphyseal line, courses transversely across the lower part of the bone, passes through one or both condyles, and is always partly intraarticular as it passes through the coronoid and olecranon fossae (Fig. 546). The lower fragment includes all of the articular surface and usually the internal condyle (epicondyle).

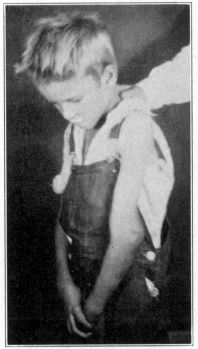
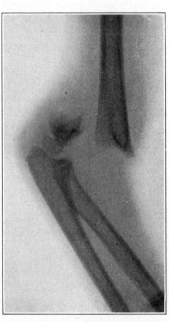

Fig. 544.   Fig. 545.

Fig. 544.—Typical posture and deformity in a severe supracondylar fracture of the humerus of the extension type with marked posterior displacement.

Fig. 545.—Lateral x-ray of the fracture shown in the preceding figure. Treated by manipulative closed reduction and immobilization in moderately acute flexion at the elbow in a posterior plaster mold and plaster swathe around the chest with the forearm pointing forward for eighteen days. Then a molded posterior plaster splint to arm and forearm for three weeks. Good result.

The mechanism of production, displacements, and soft part injuries are similar to those in the typical supracondylar fracture, except that in rare instances the dicondylar fractures are impacted. All gradations between the typical supracondylar and the typical dicondylar fractures occurs and many authors do not distinguish between the two types, but the dicondylar lesions deserve separate mention because the fracture line is intraarticular and the callus may interfere with the movements at the elbow joint.

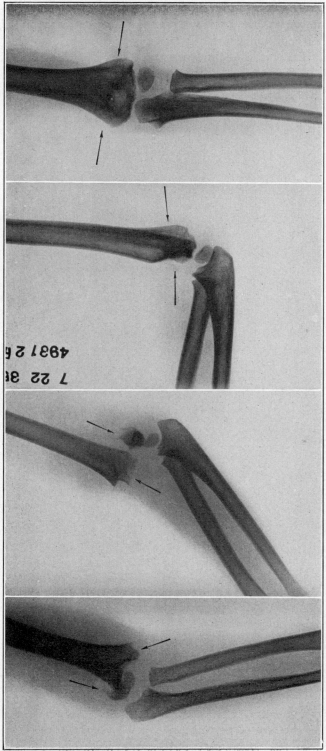

Fig. 546.—Typical low supracondylar (extension type) or transcondylar fracture of the humerus in a child before and after reduction with union.

3. Epiphyseal Separation of the Lower End of the Humerus.—Up to the age of four or five years the entire cartilage plate of the articular surface of the lower end of the humerus tends to be separated in one piece (Figs. 547 and 548), but after this time in lesions at the epiphyseal line the external condyle is broken off from the shaft and the epiphyseal cartilage is split, leaving the thin trochlear portion attached to the shaft. Not infrequently, espe-

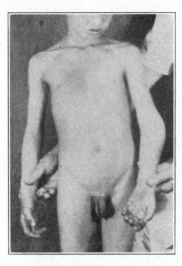

Fig. 547.—Separation of the lower epiphysis of the humerus of the extension type with posterior and mesial displacement. Note the reversal of the carrying angle.

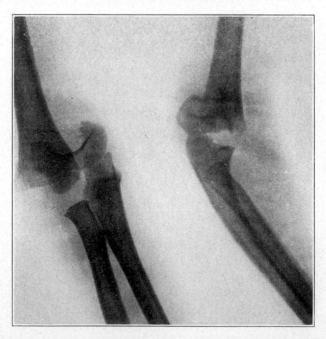

Fig. 548.—Roentgenogram of preceding case. Note that the epiphysis is fractured and dislocated backward and inward. In this case it was necessary to aspirate the elbow to relieve the intra-articular tension and restore the circulation. The displacement was then reduced under an anesthetic and the extremity immobilized in moderately acute flexion by means of a posterior plaster mold and a plaster swathe around the body; forearm and hand placed forward for three weeks. Molded posterior plaster shell to arm and forearm for fourteen days. Good result.

cially in older children, a portion of the shaft is broken off and displaced with the epiphysis. Consequently in older children these epiphyseal injuries are really separations of the external condyle and are considered under that heading.

From the surgical standpoint the small center of ossification in the trochlear portion of the epiphyseal cartilage is of no importance, since it is practically never injured alone and rarely separated with the center for the capitellum.

The mechanism of production, displacements, and soft part injuries in these epiphyseal injuries are similar to those of the supracondylar fractures described above, but the epiphyseal lesions differ slightly in that they exhibit a greater tendency to stripping up of the periosteum from the posterior surface of the shaft of the humerus.

Diagnosis of Hyperextension Fractures of the Lower End of the Humerus

1. **Supracondylar Fractures of the Humerus.**—The appearance of the arm depends upon the degree of swelling and displacement. With relatively little swelling and incomplete displacement the patient presents simply a swollen, tender, painful elbow which, with the history of the injury followed by complete disability, leads the surgeon to suspect a supracondylar fracture.

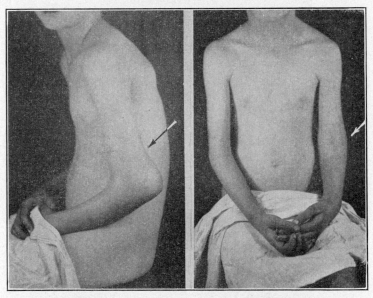

Fig. 549.   Fig. 550.

Fig. 549.—Supracondylar fracture of the humerus of the extension type with posterior displacement, viewed from the side to show the deformity.
Fig. 550.—Same patient as in preceding figure, viewed from the front.

This suspicion is strengthened if there is point tenderness above the condyles and if the three bony landmarks (olecranon, internal and external epicondyles) are in their normal relationship. However, a roentgenogram may be necessary to confirm the diagnosis.

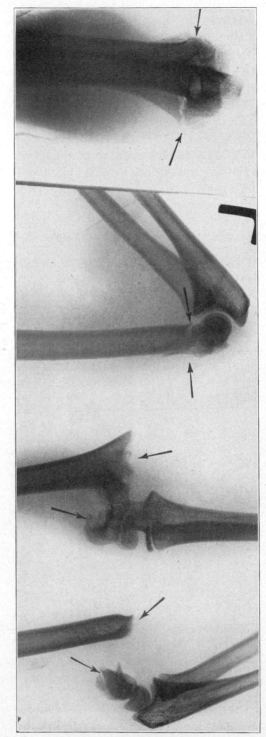

Fig. 551.—Supracondylar fracture with complete displacement. Before and after manipulative reduction.

With only moderate swelling and upward and backward displacement of the lower fragment the deformity is characteristic and resembles that of a posterior dislocation at the elbow (Fig. 549). The forearm appears to be shortened and the region over the triceps tendon on the posterior surface of the lower third of the arm is concave when viewed from the side. This concavity may be obliterated by the swelling and the patient's tendency to support the forearm in a position of slight flexion with the uninjured hand.

Palpation will reveal point tenderness above the condyles, and it may be possible to feel the sharp lower border of the proximal fragment beneath the biceps tendon and above the fold in the front of the elbow. The epicondyles and olecranon are in their normal relationship to one another, but posterior to the line of the shaft of the humerus, and measurement (acromion to external epicondyle) will reveal shortening of the humerus. Finally manipulation will show false motion in every direction except flexion which is usually limited to 90 degrees and this may be accompanied by crepitus which is most easily obtained by traction on the forearm, thus bringing the ends of the bones together. The deformity can be reduced by pulling the moderately flexed forearm downward and forward but it tends to recur when the elbow is extended.

With great swelling the diagnosis is more difficult as the entire elbow region may be converted into a tense, tender, spindle-like tumor and the swelling may involve the entire extremity. The bony landmarks are obliterated, but can be identified by continuous steady pressure which pushes the edema aside. False motion can, of course, be demonstrated, but it is difficult to determine its exact location. A roentgenogram is necessary to clear up the details of the fracture and should be taken before reduction is attempted.

2. **Transverse or Dicondylar Fracture of the Lower End of the Humerus.** —The clinical picture is similar to that of the supracondylar fracture except that the point tenderness is at a lower level and parts of one or both epicondyles may remain on the shaft and lead to an abnormal relationship between these bony landmarks and the olecranon. Furthermore the tendency to posterior displacement and shortening is less and to lateral displacement is greater in the dicondylar fractures.

3. **Epiphyseal Separation of the Lower End of the Humerus.**—The clinical picture resembles that of a dicondylar fracture except that the crepitus is soft and muffled (cartilaginous) in quality. In children over five years of age the epiphyseal separation usually involves only the external condyle and will be considered with the fractures of that portion of the bone.

Treatment of Extension Type of Fractures of the Lower End of the Humerus

The exact location of the fracture makes little or no difference in the treatment and what is written below applies equally to supracondylar or dicondylar fractures or epiphyseal separations. In each the treatment is reduction and immobilization in flexion.

1. **Fractures With Practically No Displacement.**—Occasionally one sees a supracondylar fracture in which the bones are in approximately their normal relations. In such instances all that is necessary is to flex the elbow and apply

some type of dressing which maintains the flexion. As there is relatively little swelling in this type of injury, acute flexion at the elbow may be instituted from the beginning.

Adhesive Dressing and Jones Sling (Fig. 552).—A simple convenient and safe method follows: The front of the elbow is dusted with talcum powder. The elbow is then placed in acute flexion and, with the forearm in the neutral position as regards rotation, a strip of adhesive tape 3 inches wide is placed across the angle between the arm and forearm and its free ends are applied to the lateral surfaces of the arm and forearm and partly around them. The ends of this strip lie obliquely on the arm and forearm and are permitted to fall where they will and are drawn taut without creases. A similar strip is placed across the inner side of the angle and applied to the mesial surfaces of the arm and forearm. The ends of the strips should be bound down with gauze bandage, which may be continued around the arm and forearm to reinforce and cover the adhesive if desired. A clove hitch is then placed around the wrist, and the forearm is placed across the chest and the wrist is suspended by a bandage tied around the neck. (This is the Jones sling.)

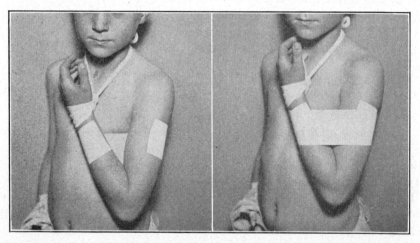

Fig. 552.—Adhesive dressing with Jones sling for mild fractures in the region of the elbow in which the fragments are not apt to become displaced.

This form of dressing is in disrepute because many surgeons attempt to apply it with one continuous band of adhesive and this is like winding adhesive horizontally around a cone; it cuts in on the edge next to the base and is loose on the edge next to the apex. Adhesive must be allowed to fall where it will and be applied where it falls.

This form of dressing does not prevent rotation of the lower fragment and should be used only in fractures where there is little tendency to displacement, because we have seen displacement occur in supracondylar fractures which were reduced and immobilized in an adhesive dressing and Jones' sling as described above.

Posterior Plaster Mold.—A plaster slab or mold long enough to reach from the upper arm around the elbow to the base of the fingers and wide enough to reach halfway around the arm is prepared and applied to the extensor surface of the arm and flexed and slightly supinated forearm. This is bound on with a gauze bandage and supported by a clove hitch around the wrist and a sling around the neck. After the plaster is dry, the bandage may be removed and the mold may be strapped on with adhesive or webbing straps.

The plaster mold is more efficient than the Jones sling with adhesive dressing because it prevents rotation of the forearm as well as motion at the elbow. It is more comfortable than the Jones sling with the adhesive dressing because it protects the sensitive elbow region from injury.

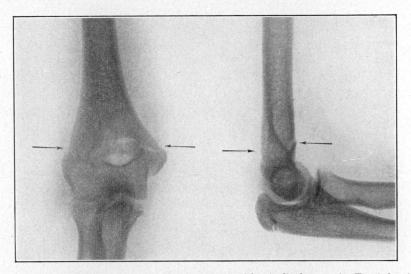

Fig. 553.—Supracondylar fracture of the humerus without displacement. Treated with adhesive strapping and Jones sling as shown in Fig. 552.

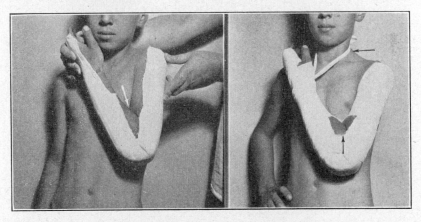

Fig. 554.—Posterior plaster mold with Jones sling as used for supracondylar fractures of the humerus which are not apt to get displaced.

A posterior angular splint of metal may be substituted for the plaster mold if desired, but it rarely fits as well.

Anterior angular splints are mentioned to be condemned. We do not believe that any splint should be placed over the front of the flexed elbow after a recent injury as it is liable to interfere with the return of blood from the forearm.

2. **Supracondylar Fractures of the Humerus With Displacement.**—If the swelling is not too great, these fractures should be reduced by manipulation under a general or local anesthetic as soon as possible after the injury and immobilized in a plaster cast or splint. Reduction is not only easier and more accurate when done early, but it also lessens the swelling as it decreases the constriction of the veins at the elbow and the bleeding ends of the fragments are sealed off when accurately fitted together.

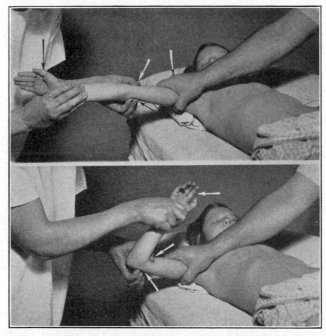

Fig. 555.—Manipulative reduction of supracondylar fracture of the humerus. First maneuver, slight hyperextension with traction on forearm and countertraction to the arm and backward pressure on the proximal fragment to engage the fragments. Second maneuver, maintaining traction and pressure; the forearm is slowly flexed while forward pressure is made on the distal fragment. Note that the forearm is pronated.

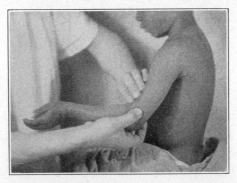

Fig. 556.—Reduction of supracondylar fracture by grasping the distal fragment and pulling it down and forward. Countertraction to the arm by an assistant is usually necessary.

Method of Reduction.—When muscular relaxation has been obtained by the anesthetic an assistant fixes the arm and the surgeon grasps the forearm with one hand and slowly hyperextends the elbow and applies moderate traction to pull the lower fragment down.   As the lower fragment is pulled down, the surgeon uses his other hand to manipulate the fragments into position, first correcting any lateral or rotary displacement and getting them in line, then he pushes the lower fragment forward and presses the lower end of the upper fragment backward and holds them in position while he gently flexes the forearm which is held in pronation or in the neutral position as regards rotation (midway between pronation and supination), because full supination tends to cause adduction of the lower fragment.   If the displacement has been reduced flexion will be free, except as limited by the swelling.   (Fig. 555.)

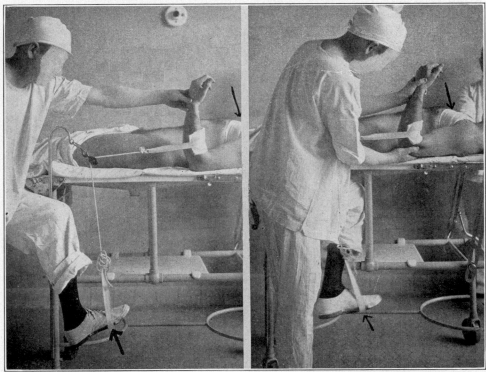

Fig. 557.   Fig. 558.

Fig. 557.—Method for obtaining powerful, slow, steady traction and countertraction (with sheet around body) in the reduction of supracondylar and shaft fractures of the humerus.   (Dr. E. L. Scott.)
Fig. 558.—Same showing manipulation of fracture.

Some surgeons use a slightly different and quite as efficient method of reduction; with the patient's elbow flexed to about 90 degrees the surgeon grasps the condyles of the humerus with one hand and pulls them downward while he presses the lower end of the upper fragment backward with the other hand (Fig. 556).   When reduction has been obtained the elbow is flexed to the position of maximum flexion with safety.

It is to be emphasized that these fractures are not reduced by the movement of flexion.   They are reduced by extension, traction in the long axis of the humerus and manipulation with the surgeon's thumb and fingers.   Where more traction is needed Scott's method is useful (Figs. 557 and 558).   After the fracture has been reduced the forearm is flexed to maintain the reduction,

This is accomplished by the tendon of the triceps which is applied firmly around the posterior surface of the lower end of the humerus when the elbow is flexed, and tends to hold the fragments in position.

Position of Maximum Flexion With Safety.—The degree of flexion in which to immobilize the forearm varies inversely with the swelling and must be determined by trial, as too much flexion not only interferes with the venous return from the forearm, but may even obliterate the radial pulse. A safe plan is to flex the elbow until the radial pulse is obliterated, then to extend it until a bounding radial pulse returns (approximately normal), and then to extend it about five degrees or more to allow for further swelling and immobilize it in this position. This will usually be a little less than a right angle. (Fig. 559.) After the immobilization the hand must be inspected every few hours, and if circulation is found to be dangerously impaired, the dressing must be loosened.

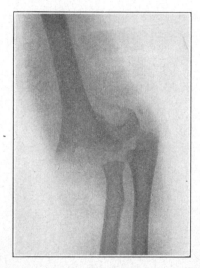

Fig. 559.—Supracondylar fracture of the humerus with marked swelling. Reduced by manipulation and immobilized at 15 degrees beyond a right angle (position of maximum flexion with safety) for eighteen days, then a posterior molded plaster splint for three weeks. Sling for two weeks. Good result in seventeen weeks.

A great deal of emphasis is put on the position of acute flexion in the treatment of these fractures of the lower end of the humerus. This is dangerous and may cause ischemic paralysis or even gangrene. The circulation must not be blocked by the position. The fracture is immobilized in as much flexion as can be maintained with safety and the acute flexion is obtained later after the swelling has decreased. Acute flexion will not accomplish reduction, and is not necessary to maintain reduction after it has been obtained. In certain cases the distal fragment may slip back a little or tilt back and these cases must have another anesthetic and the defect must be corrected, but it is much better to do this than to risk an ischemic paralysis or gangrene by jamming the acutely swollen elbow up into a position of acute flexion and holding it there while the patient's severe pain is ignored or relieved by morphine. (Figs. 564 and 565.)

Immobilization After Reduction.—For complete fractures through the lower end of the humerus which have been reduced nothing is as efficient as a plaster-of-Paris dressing properly applied. It is true that in the great majority of instances the position of hyperflexion (if it can be obtained with safety) and the adhesive dressing described above, or Lund swathe, posterior angular splint, or posterior plaster mold will maintain position after reduction, but occasionally they permit rotation, lateral deviation, or even total displacement of the lower fragment, and the careful surgeon should not take this chance in any except selected cases which are relatively stable when reduced.

The plaster-of-Paris dressing (Eliason*) is applied as follows: After the fracture has been reduced and the position of maximum flexion with safety determined, the forearm is supported in this position in pronation or in the midposition between pronation and supination and pointing directly forward with the arm slightly abducted. Sheet cotton is wound around the upper arm and chest and a plaster mold half again as long as the distance from the acromion to the wrist and wide enough to extend halfway around the arm and forearm is prepared and applied from the base of the fingers along the ulnar surface of the forearm around the elbow, up the posterolateral surface of the arm, over the shoulder, and obliquely down across the front of the chest.

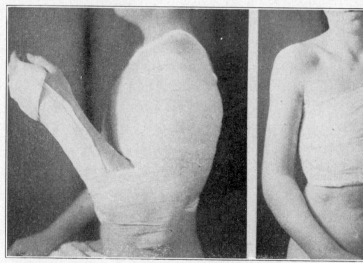 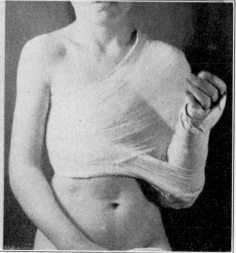

Fig. 560.   Fig. 561.

Fig. 560.—An excellent dressing for immobilization of severe supracondylar fractures which have been reduced. (Eliason.) The posterior plaster mold is incorporated in a light plaster cast which extends around the body and the involved arm, shoulder, and elbow, fixing the involved arm and elbow to the chest with the forearm placed forward and the forearm and hand near midpronation and supination. No bandage has been used in order to show detail on forearm.

Fig. 561.—Same dressing as preceding viewed from the front showing the plaster swathe around the chest.

In the Eliason* dressing a few turns of plaster bandage are wound around the chest and the arm is then adducted and with the forearm pointing directly forward the plaster is wound around the arm and chest thus forming a continuous plaster swathe which with the posterior mold and rope over the shoulder immobilizes the arm and prevents rotation of the lower fragment. (Figs. 560 and 561.) Gauze bandage is used to bind the mold to the elbow,

*Eliason: J. A. M. A. 82: 1934, 1924.

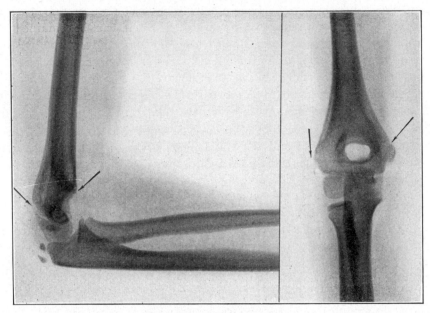

A.

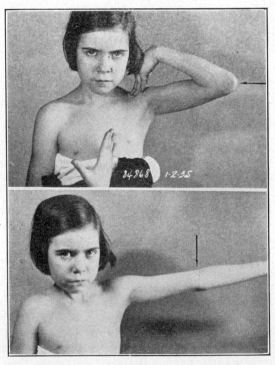

B.

Fig. 562 *A* and *B*.—Supracondylar fracture of the humerus with incomplete reduction. In spite of this, normal movement at the elbow was obtained.

forearm, and hand. The mold must be well padded over the wrist, forearm, and elbow because of the subcutaneous position of the ulna.

We prefer a light plaster spica cast over the plaster mold. One of us (H. E. C.) applies this with the arm abducted to 90 degrees at the shoulder in order to reduce the swelling. The other (J. A. K.) brings the arm forward and outward about 30 degrees and rotates it inward about 45 degrees to bring the fully pronated forearm across the right half of the chest.

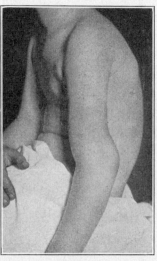

Fig. 563.—Severe supracondylar fracture of the humerus with marked swelling and damage to soft tissues.

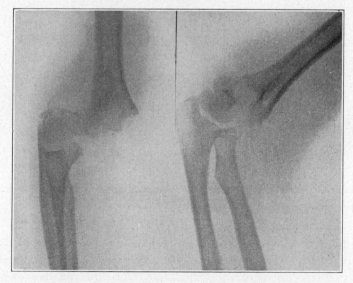

Fig. 564.—Roentgenograms of preceding case.

In an adult the plaster should extend down to the pelvis, but in a child the plaster is so light that pressure on the side of the chest is not troublesome and the plaster may stop at the lower ribs, and most of these fractures occur in children.

After the reduction a fluoroscopic examination and in many instances x-ray checks are made and if satisfactory the plaster dressing should be continued for from three to six weeks, depending upon the age of the patient and the severity of the fracture, after which time it can be discontinued and replaced by the adhesive dressing and sling or a simple posterior mold with the elbow in more acute flexion. This should be continued for from twelve to eighteen days longer according to the severity of the fracture. Then the arm can be supported in a triangular sling and graded active motion and exercises may be commenced. These should be continued until full motion is restored or despaired of and should be supplemented by local heat and graduated gentle massage, but passive motions are not to be used as they tend to prolong the disability and may be a contributory factor in the development of myositis ossificans which occurs more frequently around the elbow than anywhere else in the body and will be discussed below. In children confidence of the child is to be desired. Let the child do the work and not lose confidence in himself. If pain or tenderness develops let the child rest with his arm in a sling for a day or two; then recommence motion.

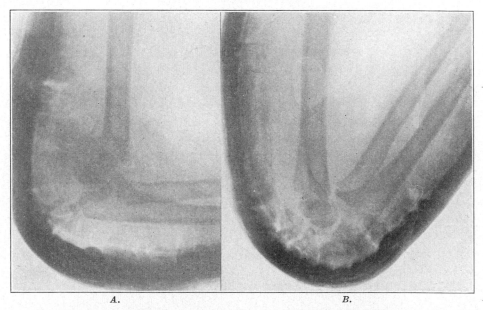

A. *B.*

Fig. 565.—*A.* Preceding case after closed manipulative reduction which was incomplete. Flexion of the forearm to acute angle is usually difficult or impossible when reduction is incomplete. Another attempt by closed method with good reduction. *B* shows good reduction after second manipulation.

If the position of the fragments is not satisfactory, the closed manipulation should be repeated. The plaster dressing may be left on in certain cases where the soft structures are severely traumatized for four or five days until the swelling has decreased and then the manipulation should be repeated and the elbow can be immobilized in more acute flexion. (Figs. 564 and 565.) However, it should be noted that in supracondylar fractures complete anatomical reduction is not necessary and a slight projection of the distal end of the lower fragment in the cubital space need cause no concern.

In an occasional case such as Fig. 567 it will be impossible to maintain satisfactory reduction in a splint or plaster. Such cases are often operated upon. We believe that some of these operations may be avoided if they are treated by lateral traction as described below under comminuted fractures of the lower end of the humerus.

Fractures of the Lower End of the Humerus With Great Swelling.—Occasionally one encounters a fracture of the lower end of the humerus in which the swelling is so great that the immediate concern of the surgeon is to save the arm rather than to reduce the fracture. These are severe fractures which have been present for several hours. The region of the elbow is enormously swollen and the swelling involves the arm and forearm and hand. The hand is cold and cyanotic and the radial pulse may not be felt.

It is necessary to relieve the tension in the elbow region. This can generally be done by aspiration. A spot is selected, usually over the lateral border of the tendon of the triceps, and painted with iodine. A rather large needle (20 gauge) is introduced into the hematoma or joint cavity and as much blood as possible is removed. If this is not successful, the skin and fascia should be incised under local anesthesia and the hematoma drained.

The tension having been lessened, reduction may be attempted or the arm can be suspended by traction with adhesive on the forearm or elevated on pillows for a few days (two to six) until the swelling has decreased and then reduction may be attempted in the manner described above. (Figs. 564 and 565.)

The Jones Sling and the Position of Acute Flexion

Since Sir Robert Jones has so strongly advocated the treatment of all injuries of the elbow, except fractures of the olecranon, in a position of acute flexion, this position has become generally known as the Jones position and is most conveniently maintained by a clove hitch around the wrist and a bandage around the neck. This dressing has become known as the Jones sling.

While it is true that the position of acute or hyperflexion is much better than the position of extension in the treatment of practically every fracture of the elbow except those of the olecranon, it must be emphasized that merely placing the elbow in a position of acute flexion and suspending the forearm from the neck in a clove hitch and sling is not an efficient method of immobilizing fractures at the elbow, and in many instances even after the fracture has been adequately reduced, if this is all that is done, the fragments are apt to become displaced. This is especially true of fractures of the internal condyle. Furthermore it must be emphasized that the fracture or dislocation must be reduced before the elbow is flexed as the movement of flexion does not effect the reduction, although a great many men seem to have this impression.

Lastly and of great importance is the fact that more important even than the maintenance of the reduction, once it has been accomplished, is the maintenance of the circulation of the forearm and hand, and the surgeon should ever be on his guard against Volkmann's contracture. For this reason the position of acute flexion should be used with great care in recent injuries where considerable swelling is present or may be expected to develop. In the section on supracondylar fractures of the elbow we have given our rule for the amount of flexion which may be maintained in these acute injuries. It is that the elbow should be flexed until the radial pulse is obliterated. It should then be extended until a full bounding pulse appears at the wrist and then extended about 5 degrees more to allow for swelling which may develop later and the elbow should be immobilized in this position.

Not only is displacement apt to occur when only the Jones sling is used, but due to the fact that immobilization is so inefficient most acute cases treated in this manner have considerable pain because of the inefficient immobilization. Consequently, we recommend it and use it as a convalescent dressing but not in acute injuries.

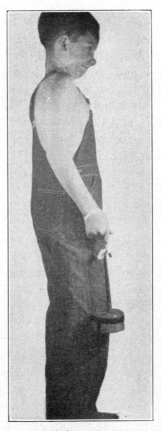

Fig. 566.—Suspended weight from arm to help restore extension of elbow after immobilization in flexion. This weight can also be replaced by different sizes of water pails.

Application of the Jones Sling.—It is applied as follows: The wrist is padded with a small amount of sheet cotton and this is covered with gauze bandage. A clove hitch is then made with a piece of muslin or cotton flannel or other bandage which will not stretch, and this is placed loosely around the wrist. The forearm is then placed in acute flexion and the ends of the bandage are tied or pinned around the neck.

Restoration of Motion After the Position of Acute Flexion at the Elbow.— When it is deemed advisable to have the patient begin motion at the elbow, the Jones sling can be gradually lengthened daily or several times a week and the wrist gradually lowered, thus decreasing the angle of flexion; but in order that full motion in flexion may be maintained, the patient should completely flex the forearm several times daily, and if it is noted that he is unable to obtain complete flexion at any time during convalescence, the sling should be tightened and the forearm maintained in acute flexion for a few days longer, when lowering of the wrist may be started again. When the angle has been increased to about 90 degrees, it is usually more comfortable to replace the Jones sling and clove hitch with a cravat sling which can be worn until the patient is comfortable without it. We then encourage the patient to exercise the arm in extension and to carry weights such as pails of water in an effort to straighten the elbow.

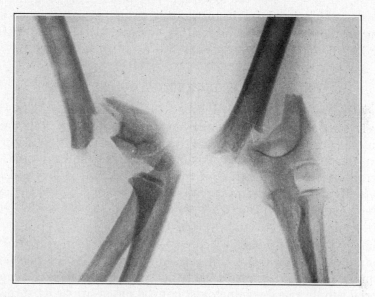

Fig. 567.—Supracondylar fracture of the humerus in which the fracture line is irregular and in which it is difficult to maintain reduction. Treated by open reduction after closed method had failed. Fixed with chromic sutures, a molded posterior plaster splint, and a plaster body swathe with forearm and hand forward for three weeks. Posterior plaster splint then applied for sixteen days.

In certain cases after a severe fracture it will be found that extension will be obtained with ease to a position of about 90 degrees and will then stop and little or no progress will be noted despite conscientious efforts on the part of the patient and of the surgeon. This is a grave situation which may arise after a supracondylar fracture in which practically perfect anatomical reduction has been obtained.

The limitation of motion is, we believe, due to the organization of the blood clot in the cubital fossa and to thickening and fibrosis of the anterior capsule of the joint.

It is very important to obtain further extension at the elbow, but the surgeon is in a quandary. He hopes that in time the elbow will gradually come down, but he is not sure. On the other hand, he knows that vigorous attempts to obtain extension by passive motion will do more harm than good. He would like to give the patient an anesthetic and manipulate the elbow into full extension, but he is afraid that if he does this he will refracture the humerus.

In a few selected cases one of us (J. A. K.) has manipulated these elbows under a general anesthetic with good results. The cases were those in which no progress in extension had occurred over a period of two weeks and in which there was no evidence of a bony block. The manipulations were performed ten to twelve weeks after the injury, and it was necessary to use great force. The thickened anterior capsule was ruptured or torn off from the humerus with a definite snap and then extension was easily obtained.

After the manipulation the arm was immobilized in full extension for two weeks in a posterior plaster mold and then flexion was gradually obtained by exercises, the patient continuing to use the plaster mold at night for several weeks. In other cases the extension was obtained by wedging plaster-of-Paris casts, and it is advisable to try this more conservative method before resorting to the dangerous manipulation. One of us (H. E. C.) tries lateral traction in bed, and if this fails, he divides the anterior capsule by open operation.

VOLKMANN'S ISCHEMIC CONTRACTURE

The progressive extremely resistant contracture of muscles which occasionally follows a fracture or dislocation was described by Volkmann in 1869 and is usually called Volkmann's ischemic contracture. It is also referred to as Volkmann-Leser paralysis, Volkmann's paralysis, and myositis. It is one of the most serious complications of fractures and dislocations and may result in a markedly deformed and practically useless extremity. That the condition is far too common is evidenced by the fact that 128 cases were seen at the Mayo Clinic during the period from 1910 to 1928.*

Etiology.—There are many theories as to the cause of this transformation of the muscles into dense fibrous tissue, but Brooks† has demonstrated that it can be produced by interference with the venous return from a muscle while the arterial supply remains intact, and clinical observations by surgeons everywhere bear out his experimental results.

S. J. Jones‡ notes that since 80 per cent of the cases follow a supracondylar fracture of the humerus, the anatomical structure of the forearm is necessary to produce a Volkmann's contracture and incriminates the deep fascia and especially the bicipital fascia which passes inward and downward from the biceps tendon, and he states that hemorrhage within this fascial envelope may result in tremendous pressure and that the time-honored belief that pressure from tight splints causes the contracture is a legend.

In corroboration of Jones' opinion, it is to be pointed out that the condition may occur without the assistance of tight dressings and many such cases are recorded in the literature. One of the most severe cases that one of us (J. A. K.) has seen was in a sailor who had suffered a severe fracture at the elbow while on a small sailing vessel at sea. No medical assistance was available and the man simply waited until the swelling went down and then carried the arm in a sling. In such a case the great swelling in the deep tissues

---

*Meyerding: J. A. M. A. 94: 394, 1930.
†Brooks: Arch. Surg. 5: 188, 1922.
‡Jones: J. Bone & Joint Surg., July, 1935.

causes the skin and fascia of the extremity to be stretched so tightly around it that the veins are compressed and the venous return is interfered with.

Since over 90 per cent of all cases of Volkmann's contracture occur in the forearm, surgeons should be on the alert for the early signs of the condition in all injuries of the elbow and forearm where swelling may be expected and should be prepared to relieve the internal pressure if it assumes dangerous proportions. This is true even in cases where no splint dressing or cast has been applied.

Pathology of Volkmann's Contracture.—According to Brooks, the primary change is an extravasation of blood into the muscles and an infiltration of these tissues with leucocytes. This is accompanied by degeneration and vacuolation of the muscle fibers and is followed by a marked proliferation of fibroblasts. This fibroblastic reaction results in the production of a large amount of collagenic fibers which infiltrate the involved muscle and largely replace the degenerated muscle fibers. This newly formed fibrous tissue then slowly contracts and in the flexor muscles of the forearm causes a flexion contracture of the fingers.

In old cases in which the process is completed the involved muscles are markedly shortened, very hard and tough in consistency, pale in color, and firmly adherent to the surrounding structures. Microscopically the muscle fibers are decreased in size and number and are surrounded by, and largely replaced by, dense fibrous tissue. The nerves in the vicinity may be involved in the fibrosis to such a degree that either because of constriction or of infiltration nerve impulses cannot pass through them and motor and sensory paralysis may result. This is especially apt to happen to the ulnar nerve.

Early Symptoms of Volkmann's Contracture.—Severe pain in the elbow with marked swelling with coldness and cyanosis of the hand and fingers are the earliest symptoms of Volkmann's contracture. In nearly every case the pain is intense, but in some instances, either because of nerve injury or because of large doses of sedatives, the pain is not a prominent symptom. The radial pulse is weak or absent. Subjectively there is first tingling and then numbness of the hand and fingers. After a few hours there is paralysis of the involved muscles and this paralysis is characteristic in that the muscles are not flaccid, but exhibit signs of contracture.

The contracture may begin within a few hours after the injury and in the early stages attempts to stretch the involved muscles as by forcibly extending the fingers cause intense pain. On palpation the involved muscles are very tender and unusually firm in consistency.

Diagnosis of Late Volkmann's Ischemic Contracture.—In a typical case there is a history of a fracture, usually at the elbow, which had been treated by tight splints, bandages or cast, and in which intense pain and swelling had followed the treatment. As a rule the contracture is not noted early, but becomes evident after the dressings have been removed and continues to progress over a period of months and may reach such a degree that the strongly flexed fingers press into the palm of the hand and cause pressure sores.

On inspection the forearm is markedly atrophied and may be shortened and the patient tends to carry it in a position of full pronation and slight flexion. The wrist is flexed, the hand is atrophic and the fingers are extended at the metacarpophalangeal joints and strongly flexed at the interphalangeal joints. Atrophy of the intrinsic muscles of the hand and trophic changes may be present. (Figs. 568, 569, and 570.)

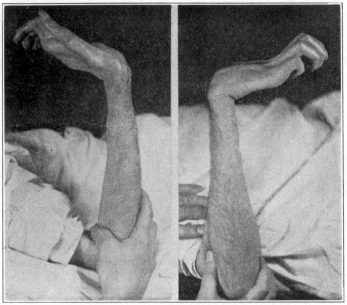

Fig. 568.   Fig. 569.

Fig. 568.—Volkmann's ischemic contracture first seen by Conwell fifteen years after a comminuted fracture of the lower end of the humerus.

Fig. 569.—Preceding case seen from ulnar aspect.

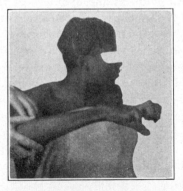

Fig. 570.—Typical case of Volkmann's paralysis following a fracture of the lower end of the humerus, the head of the radius, and the olecranon process.

Neurologic examination may disclose lesions of one or more of the nerves of the forearm. There may or may not be extensive impairment of circulation to the hand.

On manipulation it will be found that as the wrist is flexed, the contracture of the fingers is lessened, and as the wrist is extended, the contracture of the fingers is increased. As the flexed fingers or wrist are stretched in attempting to extend them, the flexor tendons stand out like hard cords under the skin of the forearm. Palpation of the muscles in the forearm discloses the fact that they are smaller in size than normal, but unusually hard and boardlike in consistency.

Treatment of Early Cases.—In cases of fracture with great swelling, cyanosis, pain, and numbness of the extremity, and absence of the radial pulse, it should be recognized that Volkmann's ischemic contracture is impending and immediate attention must be given the circulation in the extremity. If splints or dressings have been applied they should be removed regardless of the consequences. If the elbow has been placed in acute flexion, it should be extended to a point where the swelling decreases, pain is lessened, and sensation and circulation are improved regardless of the fracture. If there is no dressing on the arm and impairment of circulation is due to the pressure of hematoma from within, the surgeon should immediately take measures to relieve this internal pressure. In certain instances this can be accomplished by aspiration of the elbow joint or of the hematoma in its vicinity. If this is not successful an incision should be made into the tissue and the hematoma evacuated. The site of the incision will depend upon the fracture and upon the site of the swelling.

Jones advises a fasciotomy just mesial to the biceps tendon and cuts the biceps fascia also, and after the hematoma is evacuated, if the radial pulse does not return, he examines the brachial artery which in some instances he has found to be caught between the fragments or wrapped around the proximal fragment. The skin is then sutured loosely, but the fascial wound is not closed. The arm is immobilized in a long plaster mold and elevated on a pillow. The fracture is ignored and if position of the fragments is lost a reduction is attempted some days later.

In certain instances where no reduction has been performed it is advisable to administer a general anesthetic and attempt immediate reduction of the fracture as the continued displacement tends to cause increased hemorrhage and increased swelling around the elbow. Meyerding recommends that an open reduction be performed through a posterior incision splitting the triceps tendon and placing a lever between the fragments. This will not, as a rule, be necessary, as most of these cases can be reduced by the closed method.

After the pressure is relieved, a plaster mold should be applied and the extremity should be elevated and kept warm with dry heat and watched carefully to see that the symptoms do not recur.

Early Cases With Beginning Contracture.—In these cases the swelling should, of course, be relieved and the circulation be restored by measures as indicated above, but the damage to the muscles is done and the surgeon should endeavor to avoid the contracture. This can best be accomplished by placing the hand and wrist in an anterior plaster mold or splint with the wrist and fingers hyperextended. As the symptoms quiet down, massage, local heat, and exercises should be used to restore function.

Late Cases With Contracture.—In these late cases in which the contracture has persisted for months or years the problem is to correct the contracture and to restore as much motion as possible to the wrists and fingers. The tissues have undergone structural shortening and the muscle fibers have been more or less completely replaced by scar tissue.

The line of treatment attempted will depend upon the severity of the damage. The natural inclination is to administer a general anesthetic and manipulate the wrist and fingers into hyperextension, but experience has shown that not only is this not possible in the great majority of cases, but that it may actually do considerable harm. In the majority of instances in which there is no definite nerve involvement it will be possible to correct the deformities by gradual stretching. It is well to begin with the fingers and after they are corrected to stretch the wrist. The gradual stretching may be accomplished by traction on a banjo splint or by the Jones method with a molded splint fitted into the palm of the hand and below the surface of the forearm which can be extended from day to day, or by a wedging plaster. Personally, we use the wedging plaster, since it can be applied to exactly fit the crippled hand, can be changed frequently, and offers a maximum amount of pressure surface for the correction of the deformity.

Our method is to apply a plaster-of-Paris cast from the bend of the elbow to the tips of the fingers with the fingers in the greatest possible amount of extension and the wrist flexed. The plaster is then cut on the volar surface opposite the metacarpophalangeal joints leaving the dorsal surface intact to act as a hinge. The cut is then spread once or twice daily and small pieces of wood are put into the gap to maintain the correction. After hyperextension of the fingers has been obtained, the anterior cut is made opposite to the wrist joint and the wrist is gradually wedged into hyperextension. It will be found that by this method quite severe deformities can be corrected and useful hands obtained, although in severe cases there will be, of course, considerable permanent impairment.

If the condition is so severe that it is impossible to extend the fingers sufficiently to begin a wedging plaster, then surgical interference is indicated. Probably the best form of operation is one in which the forearm muscles and tendons are exposed and the muscles are stripped up from their beds, care being taken to preserve their nerve supply, and stretched as much as possible. If this does not give correction, the contracted tendons are lengthened sufficiently to permit extension.

In cases with nerve involvement the paralyzed nerves (ulnar and median) should be exposed and their condition determined. If they are encased in fibrous tissue they should be freed. If they are fibrosed their sheath should be split, and if they are severed their ends should be sutured. In severe cases it is advisable to shorten the radius and ulna.

After operation exercises should be begun relatively early in an attempt to restore motion. In these severe cases one cannot, of course, expect anything like a normal hand, but in nearly every instance it is possible to obtain a hand which will be much more satisfactory and useful than an artificial hand. Consequently, we have not advised amputation in any case which we have seen.

Prevention of Volkmann's Contracture.—The most successful treatment of Volkmann's contracture is prevention. If the following points are borne in mind, the cases will be very rare: (1) Reduce all fractures early as continued displacement of the fragments increases the tension and the extravasation of blood.   (2) If the radial pulse is not present before the reduction or after an attempted reduction, the forearm in front of the elbow should be incised and the tension relieved, and if necessary the brachial artery should be released from pressure.   (3) Avoid acute flexion of the elbow in the presence of swelling in this region.   (4) Inspect or get a definite reliable report on all cases of fracture in the elbow and forearm from four to eight hours after the dressing has been applied.   (5) In the presence of great swelling, relieve this by aspiration or incision before attempting reduction.

FLEXION TYPE OF SUPRACONDYLAR FRACTURES OF THE HUMERUS

Occurrence and Mechanism.—These fractures are as rare as the extension type are common.   They are due to direct trauma on the elbow in which the force is applied to the olecranon or posterior surface of the ulna, usually by falls upon the flexed elbow, the olecranon being thrust upward and forward and carrying the lower fragment of the humerus with it.

Pathology.—The lower end of the humerus is usually broken in an oblique manner, the fracture line running from below upward and forward and being situated a short distance above the epiphyseal line of the humerus.   True dicondylar fractures and epiphyseal separations of this type apparently do not occur.   The distal fragment is displaced upward and forward into the cubital fossa, while the lower end of the proximal fragment is displaced backward beneath the triceps tendon (Figs. 571 and 572).   There may be a variable degree of lateral displacement and rotation.   The periosteum tends to be stripped up from the front of the shaft and from the posterior surface of the distal fragment.   As a rule the damage to blood vessels is not so great as in the extension type of fracture, and the swelling is less.

Diagnosis.—The patient supports the arm in a position of moderate flexion and the deformity resembles that of an anterior dislocation at the elbow.   The forearm appears to be lengthened, the posterior surface of the lower third of the arm is convex, and the elbow is thickened in its anteroposterior diameter. On palpation the upper end of the distal fragment may be felt in front of the elbow beneath the biceps tendon.   The cardinal bony points of the elbow are not disturbed in their relationship to one another but are displaced anteriorly to the line of the shaft of the humerus and it may be possible to feel the lower end of the upper fragment beneath the triceps tendon which is stretched over it. There is false motion in every direction except extension which is apt to be limited by the soft tissues and crepitus may be obtained.

Treatment

The treatment of this type of fracture is reduction by manipulation and immobilization of the extremity in a position of approximately 90 degrees flexion at the elbow with no rotation of the arm or forearm, or in acute flexion if the fragments are stable in this position.   (Figs. 571 and 572.)

Method of Reduction.—When muscular relaxation has been obtained by either local or general anesthesia, the arm and upper fragment are fixed by

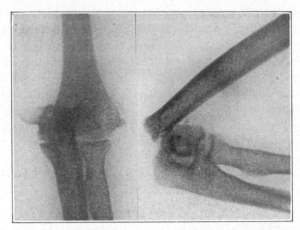

Fig. 571.—Flexion type of supracondylar fracture of humerus with complete anterior displacement of the lower fragment. (Courtesy Dr. John D. Sherrill.)

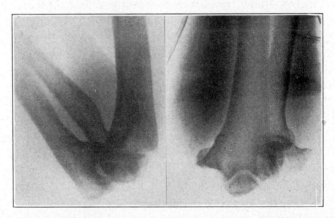

Fig. 572.—Same as preceding after manipulative reduction. Excellent functional result.

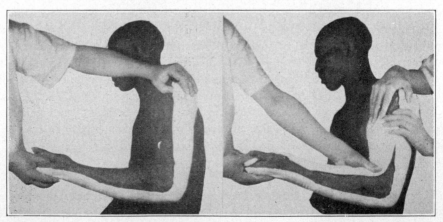

Fig. 573.   Fig. 574.

Fig. 573.—Application of posterior plaster mold used after the reduction of supracondylar fractures of the flexion type.

Fig. 574.—Application of the anterior plaster mold after reduction of a supracondylar fracture of the flexion type. This is well molded in the fold of the elbow and the two molds are then encased in a plaster swathe around the chest.

an assistant, preferably with the end resting upon and projecting over the edge of a sandbag placed on the table. The forearm is then flexed to approximately 90 degrees. The surgeon places his thumbs in the cubital fossae and grasps the forearm and condyles with his fingers. He makes traction in the long axis of the humerus to bring the lower fragment down beyond the end of the upper fragment at the same time correcting any deformity in rotation or lateral displacement. When this has been accomplished, the lower fragment is pushed directly backward and an attempt is made to engage it upon the upper one. The traction and then the backward pressure are gradually released. If the reduction is complete, it will be found that the fragments will be fairly stable with the elbow flexed 90 degrees. A long posterior plaster mold reaching from the base of the fingers up the forearm over the shoulder and down the front of the chest is applied as in the treatment of supracondylar fractures of the extension type (Fig. 573), care being taken not to displace the fragments. An anterior plaster mold extending from the upper arm to the base of the fingers is then applied and well molded into the fold of the elbow, obstruction of circulation being carefully avoided (Fig. 574). The forearm and arm are then encased in a plaster bandage to guard against the slipping forward of the lower fragment, and the plaster molds and upper arm are fixed to the chest by a circular swathe or plaster-of-Paris bandage just as was described above. This dressing is left on for three or four weeks, when it is removed and a posterior plaster mold applied for some two to three weeks longer, depending upon the age of the patient and the severity of the fracture; it is then replaced by an ordinary triangular sling, and the patient is encouraged to begin active exercises with the arm.

INTERCONDYLAR, OR T, OR COMMINUTED, FRACTURES OF THE LOWER END OF THE HUMERUS

Occurrence and Mechanism.—Intercondylar fractures are quite rare in children, but are not uncommon in adults. They are usually the result of severe injuries such as falls from a height on either the flexed or extended hand, the mechanism being similar to that in the production of the fractures of the extension type, or they may be produced by direct trauma to the elbow as in fractures of the flexion type. A severe type, the car window elbow, is illustrated in Figs. 584 and 585.

Pathology.—These fractures are really supracondylar or dicondylar fractures of the lower end of the humerus in which the distal fragment is split either by the ulna or by the distal end of the upper fragment. In the typical intercondylar fracture there is a transverse or oblique fracture through the lower end of the shaft of the humerus and a roughly vertical fracture between the condyles. In addition there may be more or less comminution, especially of the distal fragment (Figs. 575 and 576). In the simplest type there may be little or no separation of the condyles and the distal portion of the bone may be displaced backward; the picture is practically identical with that of the supracondylar fracture of the extension type. In the severe type the condyles may be widely separated and the upper fragment may be driven down between them or one of the condyles may be rotated or pushed far out to one

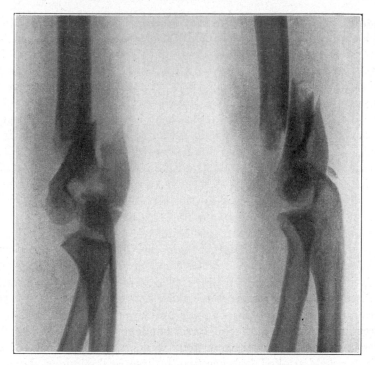

Fig. 575.—Severe comminuted intercondylar or T fracture of the humerus. The fragments will not remain in place after reduction and these fractures should be treated by lateral traction and extension or by operation. (Conwell: South. M. J. 20: 579, 1927.)

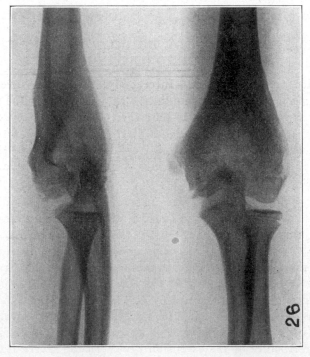

Fig. 576.—Same as above after treatment by lateral traction.

side. These fractures are often compound and are often complicated by other fractures of the upper ends of the radius and ulna; they are always accompanied by great swelling and damage to the soft tissues around the elbow.

Diagnosis.—In intercondylar fractures with little separation of the lower fragments, the clinical picture is identical with that of a supracondylar fracture of the extension or flexion type, depending upon the displacement, and the diagnosis can be made only by the x-ray. However, a split between the condyles may be suspected if with the arm and forearm carefully supported, slow, steady lateral pressure on the condyles causes pain, and especially if this pain occurs when the pressure is released without causing movement of the lower fragment. In cases with considerable separation of the condyles the broadening of the elbow is marked and palpation even in the presence of extensive swelling will reveal a definite broadening in the lower end of the bone; and unless the upper fragment is jammed down between the condyles, they can usually be squeezed together by lateral pressure of the fingers and thumb, and independent mobility of the condyles may be obtained by manipulation. The shortening of the arm and the deformity is similar to that in supracondylar fractures, and false motion is present in every direction.

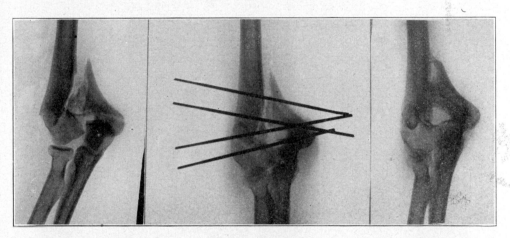

Fig. 577.—Comminuted fracture of the distal end of the humerus. Treated by manipulative reduction and transfixation and Kirschner wires. Good functional result eight months later.

Treatment

These fractures can be reduced with comparative ease by manipulation, but it is very difficult to maintain reduction because the position of acute flexion which is so efficient in fractures of the extensive type tends to force the ulna between the condyles and cause them to separate. Consequently, in all except those instances in which the fracture between the condyles is incomplete, they must be treated by either traction or open reduction.

Anyone who has operated upon these badly broken and comminuted fractures of the lower end of the humerus must have been impressed by the extreme difficulty of fixing the fragments in their proper positions, even where the free use of wire, nails, or plates is not frowned upon.

Consequently, the best treatment is by traction with support of the elbow and arm on a board and with lateral splints to make pressure upon the condyles. For this treatment recumbency is advisable. Lateral traction strips of adhesive plaster should be applied to the forearm. The patient should be placed on a firm bed, and a lateral traction frame of some sort (Figs. 578 and 579) should be set up and the forearm suspended in a position midway

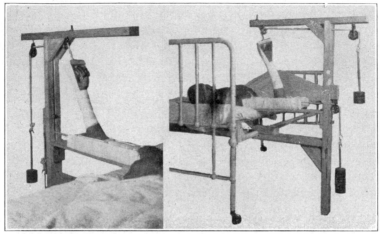

Fig. 578.   Fig. 579.

Fig. 578.—Conwell's lateral traction apparatus with arm board and lateral splints for the treatment of severe fractures at the elbow seen from foot of bed.
Fig. 579.—Same as above viewed from head of bed.

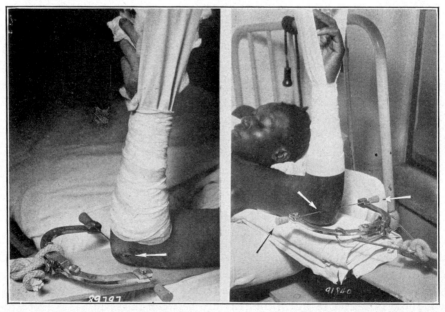

Fig. 580.—Traction through the olecranon, as used in the treatment of supracondylar fractures of the lower end of the humerus.

between supination and pronation. The forearm should be suspended at an angle of approximately 135 degrees of extension at the elbow; that is, midway between full extension and a right angle flexion, thus exerting a certain amount of traction on the lower fragments of the humerus.

Then traction should be applied to the traction strips on the **humerus** (five to eight pounds, depending upon the musculature of the patient). In applying traction to the lower end of the humerus a small pin or wire through the upper third of the ulna is the most efficient method. Lacking this, **a**

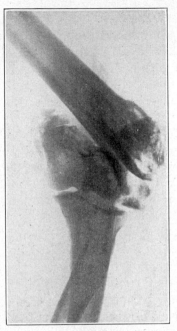

Fig. 581.—Severe compound comminuted fracture of the lower end of the humerus (flexion type) treated by lateral traction and suspension with lateral traction frame.

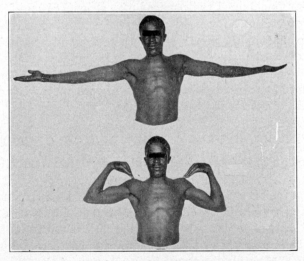

Fig. 582.—Functional result obtained in the preceding case.

broad band of heavy material may be placed across the upper half of the flexed forearm or lateral adhesive traction strips may be applied to either side of the lower arm. An anesthetic may be used from the beginning or after the traction has been applied and with the arm resting upon the board support preferably in a position of abduction of about 70 to 90 degrees at the shoulder. Either local or general anesthesia should be used and an attempt should be made to reduce the fragments by having an assistant fix the arm while the surgeon makes traction on the moderately flexed forearm, pushes the upper fragment backward, pulls the lower fragments forward, and squeezes them together. When satisfactory reduction has been accomplished, the well-padded lateral board splints, long enough to extend from the axilla well down below the elbow, should be placed on either side of the arm and bound quite firmly to it with adhesive tape.

This method of treatment will give better results than can be obtained by operative procedures on these severe fractures of the lower end of the humerus and in addition it does not complicate the recovery by exposing the patient to the possibility of infection. The traction should be maintained for from three to five weeks, depending upon the severity of the fracture, and it is necessary that the lateral splints be tightened as the swelling disappears. The position should be checked by portable x-rays, and if it is not found to be satisfactory a second or third reduction by manipulation should be attempted after the swelling has decreased. As the swelling subsides more flexion at the elbow can be accomplished every few days.

When the fragments are quite firmly united in good position, the patient should be encouraged to begin active motion at the elbow and local heat may be used. At the end of from three to five weeks, the patient may be got up and a posterior plaster mold may be applied to the arm and forearm and supported across the chest in a sling. This should be worn for from two to three weeks and can be followed by an ordinary triangular sling which should be worn until the patient can go without it without discomfort. The exercises should be continued until full motion is obtained or despaired of. (Figs. 581 and 582.)

The Hanging Cast.—Recently we have been using the hanging cast as described on p. 564 in the treatment of these fractures and believe that it is a simple and efficient method which has a wide application in practically all fractures of the shaft of the humerus. In comminuted supracondylar fractures, however, the position must be checked by x-ray within a week and if not satisfactory, traction or open reduction resorted to.

MULTIPLE FRACTURES IN THE REGION OF THE ELBOW

Occurrence and Mechanism.—Multiple fractures at the elbow are rare in children because here the ends of the bones are largely cartilaginous and the fractures in the region usually occur in the shaft of the bones near the joint; it is rare for more than one bone to be broken. But in adults it is not rare to find two or even all three of the bones broken at the elbow as a result of severe injuries, such as a fall from a height or an automobile accident.

Pathology of Multiple Fractures in the Region of the Elbow.—There is no rule as to the type of fractures or combination of fractures which one may expect to find in these severely injured elbows. Almost any combination of the lesions described in the preceding pages may be present and the bones may be extensively comminuted so that the elbow, as Cotton aptly remarked, "may be converted into a veritable bag of bones."

Diagnosis of Multiple Fractures in the Region of the Elbow.—While it may be possible to determine the presence of one or more major fractures, accurate diagnosis of the various lesions present can be made only by antero-posterior and lateral x-rays, and even then one is apt to overlook some of the fracture lines. At least that has been our experience.

Treatment of Multiple Fractures at the Elbow

In general these severe injuries should be treated as described above under the treatment of intercondylar or T fractures of the lower end of the humerus; that is, by recumbency with the forearm suspended and the elbow at from 90 to 135 degrees. Lateral traction is applied to the arm and lateral compression by board splints to the elbow and humerus.

The surgeon should attempt manipulative reduction under anesthesia with the patient in bed and the traction applied. By this means it is often possible to mold the fragments into place.

If the olecranon is fractured and the fragments are separated, the displacement should be reduced and the fragments sutured by open operation. This should be done immediately unless there is some definite contraindication. After the olecranon has been sutured, the elbow can be treated as described above.

When extensive comminution is present, we do not believe that it is advisable to try to reduce and suture or nail or screw in place the various fragments of the lower end of the humerus. Our experience has been that it is very difficult to fix these fragments by sutures or any other method and that conservative closed treatment gives better results. An exception is a fractured external or internal condyle which is rotated and which it is impossible to reduce by manipulation. These should be reduced by open operation.

Fractures of the head and neck of the radius in these complex injuries are best treated conservatively and may be more or less ignored for the time being.

In other words, the surgeon should treat the fracture of the humerus conservatively, suture the olecranon if necessary, and ignore the fractures of the upper end of the radius. All dislocations should, of course, be reduced.

After consolidation has taken place in the humerus and olecranon, if it is found that disability is due to some lesion in the upper end of the radius, the head of this bone should be removed.

COMPLICATIONS OF FRACTURES AND DISLOCATIONS AT THE ELBOW

The most serious complications after elbow injuries are the production of new bone often leading to myositis ossificans and Volkmann's ischemic contracture. Both of these conditions have been dealt with under separate headings.

The most frequent complication of fractures and dislocations of the elbow is the presence of other fractures and dislocations in addition to the dominant lesion and these multiple injuries have also been dealt with under a separate heading. Extensive hemorrhage into the soft tissues may be so severe as to demand immediate treatment. A discussion of this condition is given under the heading ''Fractures of the Lower End of the Humerus with Great Swelling.''

Injuries to the important blood vessels in fractures and dislocations of the elbow are rare, but in the absence of a radial pulse and brachial artery may be caught between the fragments, wrapped around the proximal fragment or thrombosed, and such cases should be explored immediately.

Nerve Injuries.—Injuries to the median nerve are rare. The deep muscular branch of the radial nerve is occasionally stretched and may even be torn in dislocations at the elbow and the upper end of the radius and in fractures of the radial head or neck. Most of these radial nerve injuries are temporary and clear up with rest. The most important nerve lesion in elbow injuries is a paralysis of the ulnar nerve which is especially prone to be stretched in dislocations (either posterior or posterolateral or directly lateral). It is also occasionally injured in fractures of the internal condyle or epicondyle.

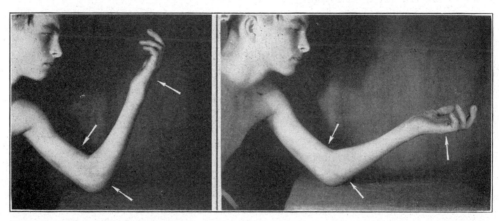

Fig. 583.—Limitation of movement at the elbow and paralysis of the median nerve following a supracondylar fracture of the humerus.

Late ulnar neuritis or paralysis may occur after fractures of the internal condyle or epicondyle or after supracondylar fractures in which union has occurred with a deformity of abduction at the elbow. In the fractures around the condyle, the ulnar nerve is injured by the production of callus or by true trauma from misplaced fragments, while in late injuries following supracondylar fractures with abduction deformity at the elbow; that is, exaggeration of the carrying angle, the ulna is injured by being pulled around the epicondyle.

The treatment of these late ulnar nerve paralyses is to expose the nerve, remove it from its canal behind the internal epicondyle and transplant it over the origins of the flexor muscles of the forearm in front of the internal condyle, thus shortening its course and freeing it from the irritation caused by the bone.

FRACTURES OF SINGLE CONDYLES AND EPICONDYLES OF THE LOWER END OF THE HUMERUS

Fractures of the Internal Epicondyle

This is also called epitrochlear fracture, sprain fracture of the internal condyle, or extraarticular fracture of the internal condyle, and before the age of eighteen years the lesion may be an epiphyseal separation rather than a fracture. The prominent tip of the internal condyle may be torn off by the internal lateral ligament in forcible abduction of the extended arm, or it may occur as a complication in dislocations of the elbow. Occasionally it may be knocked off by direct violence.

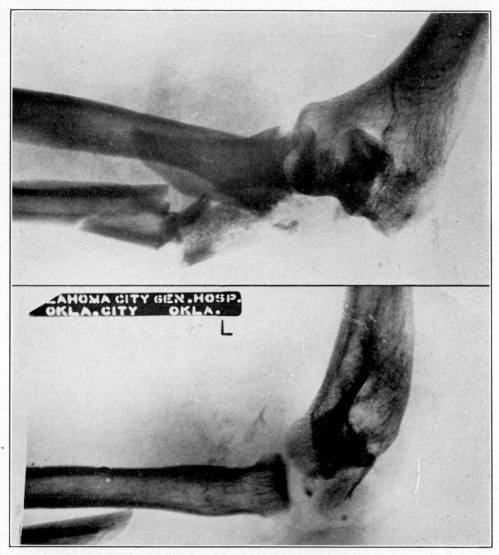

Fig. 584.—Severe compound comminuted fracture at the elbow due to collision with elbow extended out of automobile window, before and after débridement. Amputation was considered. Fairly good functional result. (Courtesy of Dr. H. B. Shorbe, Oklahoma City.)

Pathology.—The small piece of bone which is torn off or knocked off is usually displaced downward and forward and more or less rotated by the pull of the superficial flexor muscles of the forearm which take their origin from it. Not infrequently the avulsed fragment is displaced into the elbow joint and may be locked between the coronoid and the trochlear surface of the humerus. Occasionally there may be practically no displacement or it may be displaced directly outward or backward. The ulnar nerve which lies in the groove behind the internal condyle may be injured by the trauma or caught between the fragments or involved in the callus, but fortunately this complication is rare.

Diagnosis.—After the injury the patient has more or less pain, especially over the internal condyle, a variable amount of limitation of motion and disability at the elbow and weakness in pronation of the forearm and flexion of

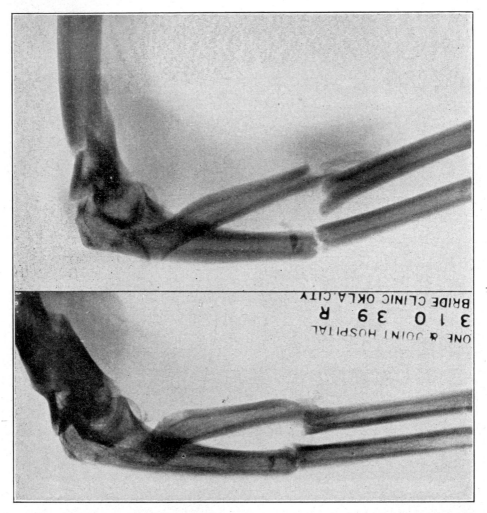

Fig. 585.—Automobile window elbow with fractures of forearm and elbow region before and after treatment. Fair result. (Courtesy of Dr. H. B. Shorbe.)

the wrist and fingers, and these movements are apt to cause pain at the site of the fracture. There is a moderate amount of swelling over the inner side of the elbow and there is local point tenderness over the internal condyle. It may be possible to palpate the displaced fragment, and if it is large enough comparison of the internal condyle with that on the uninjured side will reveal a definite difference in contour. The rest of the elbow is intact and usually crepitus is not obtained.

Treatment.—The treatment of this fracture varies with the amount of displacement. Because of its proximity to the ulnar nerve and because it is a point of origin for important muscles we believe that an effort should be made to obtain union in good position.

If the displacement is slight the elbow should be immobilized in a position of acute flexion with the forearm in full pronation over a period of from four to six weeks. This position relaxes the pull on the muscles of the forearm which arise from the internal condyle and permits the fragment of bone to settle into its place. At the end of this time the arm may be carried in a sling and active motion begun gradually.

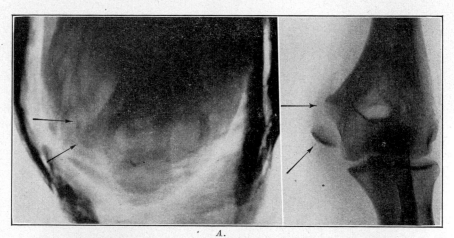

A.

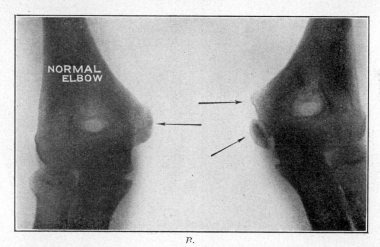

B.

Fig. 586 *A* and *B*.—Fracture of the internal epicondyle with apparent reduction in a plaster cast and showing failure of reduction after the cast was removed three weeks later.

If the fragment cannot be brought back to its normal position by flexion and pronation of the forearm or if the fragment is displaced into the elbow joint, it should be replaced and fixed by a suture or small wire nail or peg at open operation through a mesial incision just in front of the epicondyle.

After the operation the treatment is the same as without operation; namely, immobilization of the forearm in flexion and pronation. If, at the

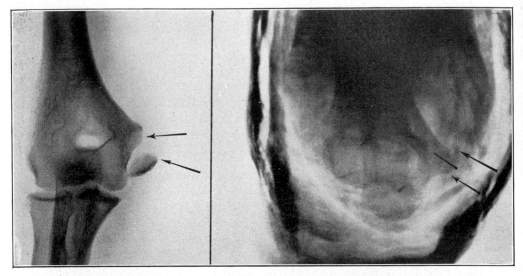

Fig. 587.—Fracture of the internal epicondyle before and after operation and fixation with a small wire nail.

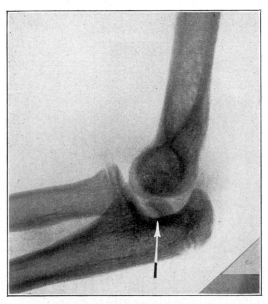

Fig. 588A.

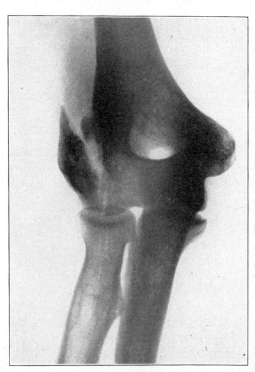

Fig. 588B.

Fig. 588A.—Fracture of the internal epicondyle of the humerus which is displaced into the elbow joint. Replaced at open operation and fixed with chromic catgut.

Fig. 588B.—Fracture of the external condyle from direct violence. The external condyle of the humerus is seldom fractured. It is usually produced by direct violence. In most instances such fracture, as shown, demands internal fixation which is not a difficult procedure to carry out by simple nailing or pegging. (Courtesy Dr. John D. Sherrill.)

operation, the ulnar nerve is found to be exposed or between the fragments, it should be removed from its canal on the posterior surface of the internal condyle and its course shifted so that it passes through the muscular tissue anterior to the condyle.

Fracture of the Internal Condyle of the Humerus

Fracture of the internal condyle of the humerus is a rare lesion which may result from a fall on the elbow and the dorsum of the forearm, the force being transmitted to the internal condyle through the ulna. This entire process is broken off, usually in an almost vertical plane, the fracture line beginning in the trochlea and passing upward to emerge at some point on the internal supracondylar ridge (Figs. 589 and 590). As the ulna remains attached to the separated portion, the displacement is not great unless the head of the radius is dislocated, but this often happens in these cases, and when it does, we have a fracture which is easily reduced, but in which displacement tends to recur as soon as the reducing force is removed, the entire forearm and fractured internal condyle tending to slip upward and backward.

Diagnosis.—There is complete disability at the elbow, and the arm is carried in a position of slight flexion. The swelling is at first limited to the region over the internal condyle, but soon becomes general around the region of the elbow. On palpation there is point tenderness over the internal condyle, and if there is displacement, the condyles may be broadened and the internal epicondyle occupies its normal position in relation to the olecranon, but is abnormal in its relation to the external epicondyle. Usually the displacement is so slight that it is not possible to detect it by physical examination.

If the head of the radius is dislocated it may be palpated in front of the external condyle. It may be possible to grasp the internal condyle with the fingers and demonstrate false motion and crepitus.

False motion in abduction, adduction, and extension can be obtained if the internal condyle is definitely loosened or displaced. The diagnosis should be checked by the x-ray.

Treatment.—If the fragment is not displaced, all that is necessary is to immobilize the forearm in a posterior plaster mold for about three or four weeks. This posterior plaster splint should reach from the upper arm to the fingers and should be applied with the forearm flexed from 90 to 110 degrees and in full pronation to relax the muscles attached to the internal condyle. The plaster should be well molded around the internal condyle. When the rigid support is removed, the arm can be carried in a triangular sling until the patient is comfortable without it. Active motion and local heat aid in the restoration of function.

With gross displacement of the internal condyle treatment is difficult because even after complete reduction the fragment is very unstable and a position of hyperflexion causes displacement to recur immediately (Figs. 589 and 590). Conservative treatment should be tried with traction in the line of the humerus and with the forearm flexed about 45 degrees. This means that the patient must be in bed and traction must be applied by means of a lateral

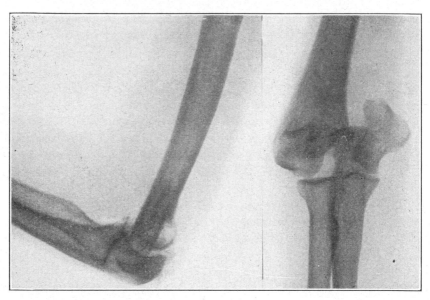

Fig. 589.—Fracture of the internal condyle of the humerus with upward displacement. Easy to reduce but difficult to hold. Manipulated twice, then treated by open operation, with nail fixation with fair functional results.

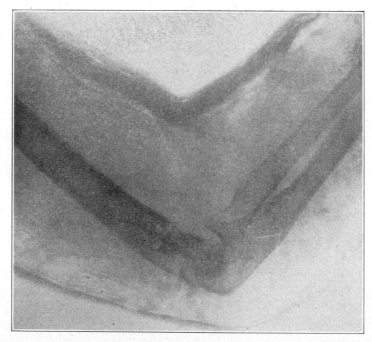

Fig. 590.—Same case; postoperative position good, but ultimate result was poor on account of traumatic arthritis.

traction frame with lateral pressure on the condyles. This fracture should be treated as described above in intercondylar, or T, fractures.

The result of the treatment must be controlled by x-ray examination by means of portable apparatus, and if it is not successful an open reduction should be performed, since in this type of fracture it is quite important to obtain approximately anatomical reduction. Otherwise the entire mechanics of the elbow joint are upset and a traumatic arthritis will result. If it is found necessary to operate, the fracture should be exposed through an incision along the inner side of the arm and especial care should be taken to identify the ulnar nerve before it is harmed accidentally. If the canal for the nerve is not involved in the fracture, it should not be interfered with, but if it is involved, the nerve should be removed and transplanted to the front of the elbow. The separated condyle must be reduced and firmly fixed in its original position on the main body of the humerus. In order to accomplish this it may be necessary to nail the fragment on with one or two small nails or Kirschner wires or to fasten it with screws. This is always rather difficult as the bone is hard and brittle and thin. In most cases it will be possible to suture it in place with chromic catgut, with or without drill holes.

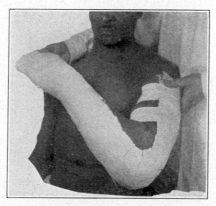

Fig. 591.—Posterior plaster mold applied with the forearm in complete pronation. Used in isolated fractures of the internal condyle or epicondyle.

After operation a posterior plaster mold or plaster cast is applied with the forearm pronated and flexed about 90 degrees (Fig. 591). This is molded firmly around the internal condyle. Immobilization is continued for about five weeks, at the end of which time the arm can be carried in a sling and active motion begun and gradual extension commenced at the elbow. After two or three weeks, the sling can be dispensed with and the patient encouraged to use the arm. It may be necessary to continue physiotherapy for months in an effort to restore motion at the elbow and this may fail almost completely. (Figs. 589 and 590.)

Fracture of the External Epicondyle

As the external epicondyle is much less prominent than the internal, it is rarely fractured. However, occasionally the tip of the condyle is knocked off by direct violence or torn off by forcible adduction of the extended forearm.

The displacements and symptoms are similar to those found in fractures of the internal epicondyle as described above except that they are present on the outer side of the elbow and the detached fragment is usually so small that it cannot be palpated. The diagnosis should be confirmed by the x-ray.

Treatment consists in immobilization of the forearm in a position of acute flexion and full supination for a period of three or four weeks in either adhesive dressing and sling or a posterior plaster mold as described in the treatment of supracondylar fractures of the humerus without displacement. At the end of this time the arm may be carried in a triangular or cravat sling and this can be dispensed with as soon as the patient is comfortable without it.

Fracture of the External Condyle

This lesion accounts for many of the cases of so-called epiphyseal separation of the lower end of the humerus because most of the lower epiphysis is included in the external condyle. The fracture may result from a fall on the outstretched hand with the elbow either in the flexed or extended position, the radius being driven upward and backward against the capitellum and breaking it off, or it may be caused by a fall on the hyperflexed elbow or from direct violence to the external condyle, or the external condyle may be pulled off by hyperadduction injuries to the extended elbow. Most cases result from a fall on the hand with the elbow in a position of moderate flexion.

Pathology.—The fracture line begins on the articular surface of the humerus just mesial to the capitellum or even mesial to the ridge on the trochlea and passes upward and outward to emerge at some point in the external supracondylar ridge. The fragment comprises the capitellum and external epicondyle and may include a portion of the trochlea. As the external lateral ligaments are rarely ruptured, there is little displacement when the forearm remains in its proper position, but with abduction of the forearm the fragment is displaced upward, outward, and backward, and with adduction of the forearm it is displaced downward, forward, and outward. There is a definite tendency for the separated fragment to be rotated in such a manner that its upper end tilts forward in a position of flexion and occasionally it is rotated transversely so that its articular surface faces inward and its fractured surface faces upward or even outward.

If this injury is complicated by a dislocation of the elbow, the broken-off external condyle remains attached to the upper end of the radius and is displaced with it. In rare instances the radial nerve which lies anterior to the external condyle may be injured.

Diagnosis.—Soon after the accident the swelling is localized in the region of the external condyle; but due to the severity of the injury and its intra-articular location, it soon becomes general and involves the entire elbow region. The tenderness is most marked over the line of fracture. If there is displacement, the lower end of the humerus is broadened; that is, the distance between the condyles is increased and the bony landmarks of the elbow may be disturbed in their relation to one another. The lower end of the humerus and the elbow joint are fairly stable, but there is usually some lateral mobility which is greater in adduction and it may be possible to grasp the detached fragment between the fingers and thumb and demonstrate false motion or crepitus. In cases with gross displacement or rotation the normal relations of the external condyle to the internal condyle and olecranon are disturbed, but it is not possible definitely to determine the type or extent of rotation by physical examination. In all cases with fracture of the external condyle an x-ray should be made before treatment is instituted as the rotation deformity cannot be corrected by manipulation or traction and demands an open reduction.

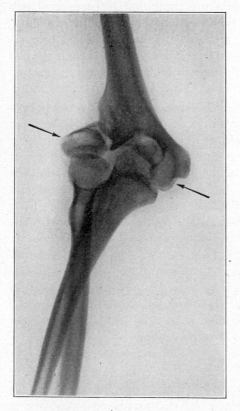

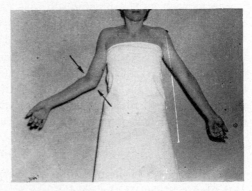

A.   *B.*

Fig. 592*A* and *B*.—Result of old unreduced, ununited fracture of capitellum. Ulnar nerve paralysis developed fifteen years later. Treated by anterior transposition of the ulnar nerve with improvement. (Courtesy Dr. John D. Sherrill.)

Treatment.—The method of treatment depends upon the displacement.

If the external condyle is simply cracked or broken off and not displaced to any appreciable degree all that is necessary in the way of treatment is to immobilize the forearm in moderately acute flexion and supination and suspend it by a Jones sling around the neck.

This is most efficiently done by a posterior plaster-of-Paris mold extending from the upper arm to the base of the fingers as described under supracondylar fractures without displacement. The plaster should be well molded around the external condyle in order to keep it in place. This should be worn for two or three weeks and then replaced by a triangular sling and the patient may begin active motion to restore the function at the elbow.

With displacement outward, downward, and backward, or forward an attempt should be made to reduce the fracture under either local or general anesthesia. This is best accomplished by direct manipulation of the fragment with the forearm in a position of almost complete supination and extension. If there is much swelling over the fracture, the edema should be pushed aside by slow, continuous pressure. Abduction or adduction of the extended forearm may aid in the reduction. The problem is to push the displaced fragment back where it belongs. When reduction appears to be satisfactory, the condyle is held in place with the thumb while the supinated forearm is slowly flexed to a moderately acute angle. In this position the capitellum tends to be held against the head of the radius by the tissues behind it and there is little tendency for it to be displaced. A posterior plaster mold is then applied to the arm and forearm to the base of the fingers and molded firmly around the condyle to exert lateral pressure and hold it in position.

The position of the fragment should be checked by post-reduction x-rays and if it is not satisfactory, the elbow should be operated upon and the fragment accurately replaced and fixed by sutures or a wire nail.

The plaster mold is worn for two or four weeks and then it can be removed and the forearm supported in acute flexion by a Jones sling around the neck. This can be gradually lengthened, and at the end of ten days or so, a triangular or cravat sling can be substituted. Active exercises should be begun as soon as the plaster splint is removed and gradually increased. The cravat sling is discontinued as soon as the patient is comfortable without it.

When the capitellum is rotated so that its fractured surface faces outward, attempts to reduce the displacement by manipulation are rarely successful. This fracture should be reduced by an open operation; otherwise severe deformity of the elbow will result. The displaced capitellum is exposed through a lateral incision, and after reduction, is sutured in place. After the open reduction the fracture is treated as described above.

Fractures of the Capitellum

Fracture of the capitellum is a very rare injury in which a piece of the articular surface of the capitellum is broken off and displaced anteriorly in front of the lower end of the proximal fragment or set free in the joint cavity where it may wander either backward or forward and block either flexion or extension. It was first described by Kocher as the fracture toruli humeri and is usually caused by indirect violence, the force being transmitted through the radius, but it may be caused by direct crushing injuries. In size the loose fragment varies from a thin sliver of bone and cartilage to a large piece comprising most of the capitellum. (Fig. 593.)

Diagnosis.—Unless the fragment is large or complicated by other injuries, the immediate symptoms are not severe and consist of pain and effusion into the joint with more or less limitation of motion which is characteristic in that it is free to a certain point and then suddenly blocked. The diagnosis is made by the absence of the signs of any other fracture and by the x-ray.

Treatment.—If the fragment is large it may be possible by direct pressure to push it back into place while the pronated forearm is adducted and slightly flexed. If this can be done, the elbow should then be immobilized in moderately acute flexion for three weeks with the hope that the large loose fragment will unite.

Small loose fragments free in the joint probably have no blood supply and are not likely to unite, even when accurately reduced and immobilized. The signs of a loose body in the joint with limitation or blocking of motion will persist as long as the fragment remains in the joint, and it should be removed by arthrotomy. The site of the arthrotomy depends on the location of the loose fragment as determined by a roentgenogram taken shortly before the operation.

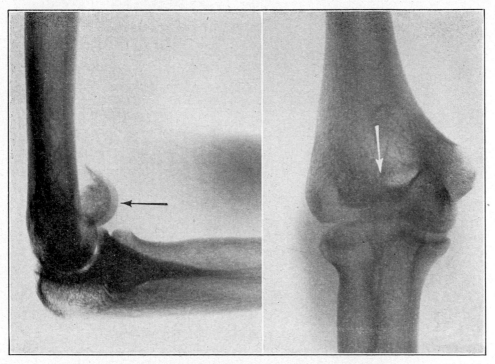

Fig. 593.—Fracture of the capitellum with displacement. Treated by excision of the loose fragment with satisfactory result.

FRACTURES OF THE UPPER END OF THE ULNA

Fractures of the Olecranon

Occurrence and Mechanism.—Despite the fact that it is a very heavy, strong process of bone, the olecranon is rather frequently fractured in adults. This is partly due to its exposed position on the point of the elbow where it receives most of the direct injuries to the elbow, and partly to the tremendous cross strain which is put upon it in falls upon the flexed and supinated forearm. The process is rarely broken in children because in early life it is short and thick and relatively much stronger than the lower end of the humerus.

The most common mechanism is a fall on the semiflexed and supinated forearm. As the hand strikes the ground, the muscles are tensed to break the fall and the powerful triceps snaps the olecranon over the lower end of

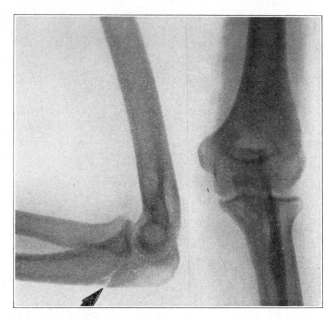

Fig. 594.—Oblique fracture of the base of the olecranon with very little separation. Treated by immobilization in a circular plaster for three weeks, then a posterior molded splint for two weeks with the elbow extended to 135 degrees. No manipulation necessary. Good result.

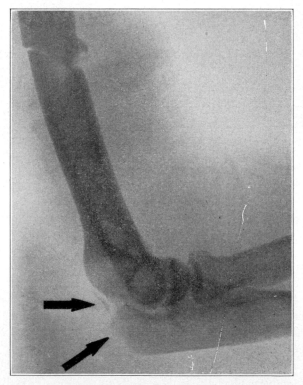

Fig. 595.—Chip fracture of the olecranon with avulsion of the triceps tendon. Treated by open operation, suture of the tendon to the olecranon, and immobilization with the elbow at an angle of 135 degrees in posterior plaster mold and spica jacket. There is also a fracture of the shaft of the humerus. Good result.

the humerus which acts as a fulcrum. The next most frequent cause is direct trauma as in falls or blows on the point of the elbow. More rarely the olecranon may be fractured by hyperextension injuries such as usually result in dislocation of the elbow in adults or supracondylar fractures in children. Very rarely it is broken by muscular violence as in throwing.

Pathology.—The usual fracture is a transverse or slightly oblique break near the base of the olecranon (Fig. 594). In the oblique fractures the fracture line tends to slope down and back and emerge on the posterior border of the ulna. In other instances a small piece of bone is pulled off the proximal end of the olecranon and the injury resembles a sprain fracture (Fig. 595). The fractures from direct violence are often compound and may be comminuted (Figs. 596 and 597).

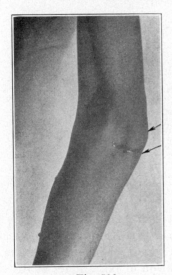
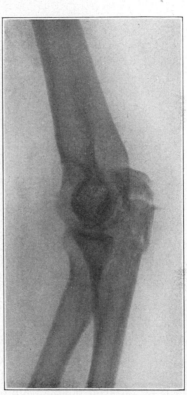

Fig. 596.   Fig. 597.

Fig. 596.—Photograph of a fresh compound comminuted fracture of the olecranon. Note the localized swelling over the olecranon process.

Fig. 597.—X-ray of preceding case. Treated by débridement and suture of aponeurosis with good result. Fixation in anteroposterior plaster shells for ten days, with forearm in full extension at elbow; then a circular plaster cast to arm and forearm for four weeks. Gradual active motion afterward with hot baths.

The displacement is largely due to the pull of the triceps muscle which tends to pull the separated fragment upward but it is resisted by the strong fibrous covering on the olecranon. This is formed by a blending of the fibers of the lateral ligaments and capsule of the elbow and of some of the fibers of the triceps tendon, all of which blend with the periosteum. If this fibrous sheath is not torn by the fracturing force there is little or no tendency to displacement even in the presence of considerable comminution, and as a matter of fact a considerable percentage of olecranon fractures show little or no displacement.

If the fibrous covering of the olecranon is torn the upper fragment is forced upward by the fracturing force and drawn upward by the triceps muscle which is inserted into it. However, in a fresh fracture, the displacement is rarely more than half an inch. The fractures of the olecranon in which there is wide separation of the fragments are usually old fractures with extensive tearing of the fibrous sheath in which the unopposed triceps has gradually contracted and drawn the separated fragment upward. The amount of separation of the fragments is increased by flexion and decreased by extension of the elbow.

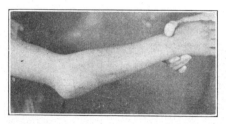

Fig. 598.—Simple fracture of the olecranon. The swelling is greater than in the compound fracture.

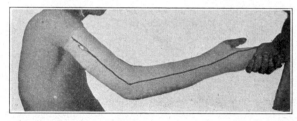

Fig. 599.—Circular plaster cast with the elbow extended 135 degrees, used in the treatment of simple fractures of the olecranon in which there is little tendency to displacement of the fragments. The cast is bivalved to permit swelling.

In addition to the displacement of the upper fragment there may be more or less anterior displacement of the bones of the forearm on the humerus. In such cases the upper end of the radius moves with the upper end of the ulna and there is an anterior subluxation or dislocation of both bones at the elbow which can be easily reduced, but tends to recur when pressure is released as in Fig. 605.

Since these fractures are practically all articular, there is more or less effusion into the elbow and there may also be effusion into the olecranon bursa. In severe injuries the fracture may be accompanied by dislocation or fracture of the head of the radius and fracture of the lower end of the humerus. In simple fractures of the olecranon there is as a rule relatively little damage to the soft parts.

Diagnosis.—The region of the elbow is moderately swollen (Figs. 596, 597, and 598), especially over its posterior surface and the patient usually supports the forearm in a position of slight flexion (about 135 degrees extension). In most cases of complete fracture there is a characteristic soft fluctuant tender swelling over the olecranon from effusion into the bursa and surrounding tissues.

Palpation reveals point tenderness over the line of fracture, and if there is separation of the fragments, it is usually possible to feel the sulcus between the fragments, and if the upper fragment is grasped with the thumb and fingers, false motion can be demonstrated and it can be noted that the fragment does not move with the forearm when the elbow is flexed and extended. If the elbow is extended, the separated fragment can be pushed down against its original attachment and crepitus can be demonstrated.

Active extension is, of course, abolished in fractures with separation of the fragments and is greatly weakened and accompanied by pain in fractures without displacement. This loss of active extension of the elbow with pain, tenderness, and swelling over the olecranon are sufficient for a diagnosis.

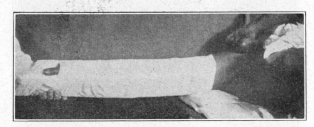

Fig. 600.—Emergency dressing for fracture of the olecranon.

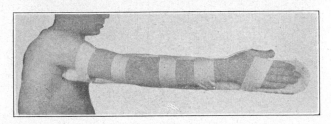

Fig. 601.—Anterior wooden splint used in treatment of fractures of the olecranon in which there is little or no displacement, but where marked swelling of the soft tissues is present. This should be replaced in a few days by the circular plaster cast or plaster molds which are more comfortable.

Treatment of Fractures of the Olecranon.—In fractures without separation of the fragments (Fig. 594) all that is necessary is to immobilize the elbow in a position of slight flexion over a period of four weeks (Fig. 596). This is most comfortably maintained by a light plaster-of-Paris cast reaching from the axilla to the wrist.

Comminuted Fractures Without Displacement or Transverse or Oblique Fractures With Little Displacement are best treated in slight flexion, but full extension may be necessary. This can be maintained by a long anterior splint reaching from the upper arm to the wrist (Figs. 600 and 601). It is made of splint board, well padded, and fastened to the arm with adhesive strips and a bandage. Oblique cross strapping may be used to immobilize the upper fragment and draw it downward (Fig. 602). It is not only useless, but detrimental to attempt to pull the lower fragment upward as the shaft of the ulna is fixed to the splint, and the adhesive simply forces the soft tissues upward and between the fragments.

A light plaster-of-Paris mold (Fig. 603) or splint applied to the arm and forearm in slight flexion or full extension is more comfortable and efficient than the long board splint described above.

The immobilization is continued for from three to six weeks depending upon the severity of the fracture. At the end of this time the elbow can be flexed to about a right angle and the arm carried in a triangular sling for two or three weeks or until the patient is comfortable without it. Restoration of function is hastened by graded exercises and hot baths.

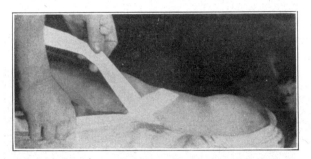

Fig. 602.—Oblique cross strapping with adhesive used in the conservative treatment in fractures of the olecranon with little or no separation. Not very good treatment.

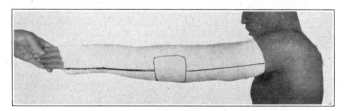

Fig. 603.—Circular plaster used in treatment of fractures of the olecranon in which full extension is necessary. A small window is outlined for the purpose of dressing an open wound which may be present. This cast should be bivalved or cut along the line as outlined after the plaster has set.

Fractures With Moderate or Considerable Displacement and Which Are Not Compound should be operated upon, since conservative treatment often results in fibrous union because the fragments cannot be brought together, and because shreds of the torn fibrous sheath tend to hang down between the fragments. However, a firm fibrous union with relatively slight separation of the fragments may give a fairly good functional result.

Operative treatment usually results in firm bony union and a good functional result if anatomical reposition is obtained and maintained, but it may be followed by a mild traumatic arthritis with resultant disturbance in function.

Operative Treatment of Fractures of the Olecranon.—When the space between the fragments is an eighth of an inch or more simple fractures of the olecranon should be subjected to operation. Occasionally it is necessary to operate in comminuted fractures with relatively little displacement, but in which it has not been possible to replace some of the fragments by manipulation. These fragments may become tilted into the joint and interfere with joint motion. The simplest possible type of operation should be performed.

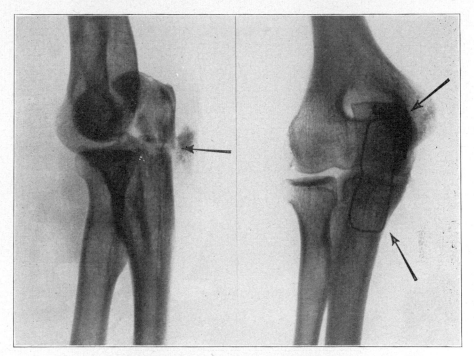

Fig. 604.—Comminuted fracture of the ulna with detached fragment. Open reduction and fixation with stainless steel wire.

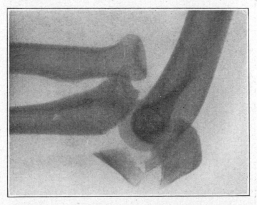

Fig. 605.—Severe fracture of the olecranon with anterior displacement of both bones at the elbow. Treated by open reduction, suture of the olecranon with wire fixation of the head of the radius with fascia lata, and immobilization with the elbow extended to 110 degrees. Fair result.

Technic.—The fracture is exposed through a posterior longitudinal or U incision and any completely loose fragments of bone are removed, and the upper fragment is reduced. A small hole should be drilled transversely through each fragment and the two fragments should then be tied tightly to-

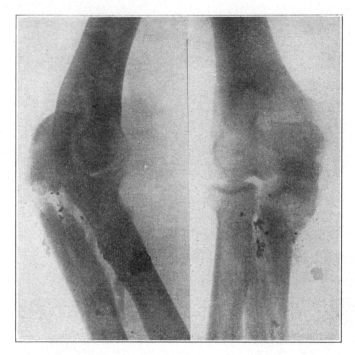

Fig. 606.—Gunshot fracture of the olecranon with severe damage to the soft parts. Treated by upper extremity traction frame with elbow extended to 120 degrees and four weeks later elbow at right angle in molded plaster cast. Good result considering the extensive soft tissue injury.

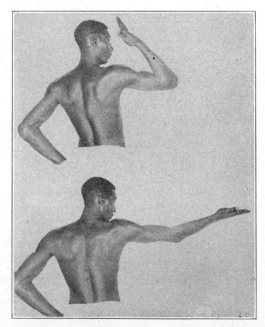

Fig. 607.—Result obtained in fracture shown in preceding figure.

gether with chromic catgut, kangaroo tendon, silver, or stainless steel wire (Figs. 608 and 609). In some cases it may be necessary to make two holes in each fragment and use two bone sutures in order to maintain accurate approximation of the fractured surfaces. The drill holes should be as far from the dorsal surface of the bone as possible in order that the sutures which are passed through them and tied or twisted will not be directly under the skin incision.

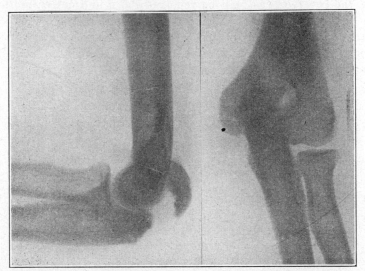

Fig. 608.—Fracture of the olecranon with wide separation of the fragments.

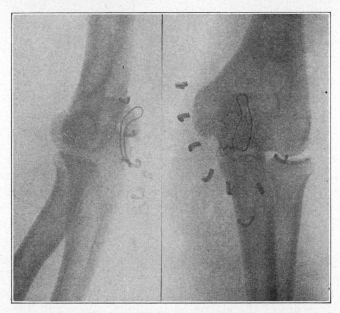

Fig. 609.—Same after open reduction and wiring of fragments.   Good result in ten weeks.

In cases with comminution in which some of the fragments retain sufficient attachment to assure them a blood supply, these fragments should not be removed but should be encircled by the suture which binds the main fragments together. In fractures near the apex of the process the proximal suture should be passed through the triceps tendon and around rather than through the loose upper fragment.

The wound is then closed in layers and a plaster cast is applied with the forearm in a position of moderate flexion (about 135 degrees). This is bivalved in ten days and the skin sutures are removed. Three weeks after the operation, the bivalved cast can be removed daily and active motion may be started. Five or six weeks after the operation the cast can be discarded and the arm carried in a sling with gradually increasing flexion at the elbow. This is worn for a week or two. Exercises and hot baths are continued until full motion and strength are restored.

Some surgeons prefer a screw or nail driven down through the process and into the shaft of the ulna. This is a more difficult operation than simply tying the fragments together with a suture. We prefer the easier and safer way and routinely use stainless steel wire.

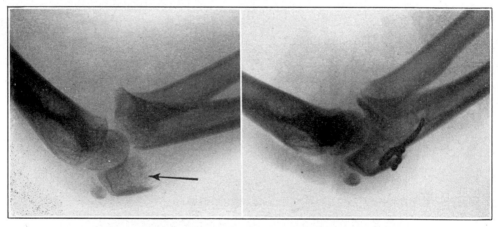

Fig. 610.—Fracture at the base of the olecranon in a child treated by open reduction and wiring. (Courtesy Dr. John D. Sherrill.)

Separation of the Epiphysis of the Olecranon

In early childhood the olecranon is entirely cartilaginous and the bony process is formed by growth upward from the shaft so that by the age of ten years the process is all bone with the exception of a small mass of cartilage at the tip. At about this time a small center of ossification appears in this cap of cartilage to form an epiphysis which unites to the shaft about the sixteenth year.

This epiphysis is small and covered by the insertion of the triceps tendon and is thus protected from injury. Occasionally, however, it is separated either by direct or indirect violence as the result of accidents similar to those which cause fracture of the olecranon in adults. As a rule the separation is slight because the main attachment of the triceps is into the bone of the olecranon.

Diagnosis and Treatment of Separation of the Epiphysis of the Olecranon. —Usually the symptoms are relatively mild. There are moderate swelling and tenderness around the tip of the olecranon with loss of power in extension and pain on flexion of the elbow.

Treatment is conservative. All that is necessary is to immobilize the elbow in full extension for two weeks and then place the arm in a triangular sling for a week or so and permit the patient to begin to use the extremity.

Fracture of the Coronoid Process

Fracture of the coronoid process is a relatively rare injury which usually occurs as a complication of posterior dislocation of the elbow, but it may occur as an isolated injury. The mechanism is hyperextension at the elbow, the coronoid being pulled off by the brachialis anticus or knocked off by the lower end of the humerus. In a personal case the injury resulted from a fall backward on the ice. The hand was thrown out and back and slapped the ground with the elbow extended and the forearm pronated. The elbow was definitely felt to hyperextend and then snap back into place. Both lateral ligaments were ruptured and the roentgenogram showed an oblique fracture including about a third of the process with slight separation of the avulsed fragment.

The fracture may also be caused by being forced up against the humerus as in falls upon the flexed forearm. The tip may be broken off or the fracture may be transverse or oblique in any part of the process and the separated fragment may be displaced into the joint and lead to bony block at the elbow.

Diagnosis of Fracture of the Coronoid.—The cardinal points in the diagnosis are pain on pressure over the front of the elbow directly over the coronoid and pain here on forcible flexion of the elbow or on attempts to flex the elbow against resistance. There is a moderate amount of effusion into the joint and if the lateral ligaments are torn, pain, swelling and tenderness are present over the torn ligaments. The diagnosis should be confirmed by the x-ray. (Figs. 611 and 612.)

Treatment of Fracture of the Coronoid.—In fractures with only slight separation no anesthetic is necessary. The elbow should be immobilized in a posterior plaster mold or cast in as much flexion as is permitted (usually an angle of 45 degrees). At the end of a week or so after the swelling and tenderness have disappeared, the elbow can be placed in acute flexion and immobilized for three or four weeks longer. After this time it can be carried in a triangular sling until the patient is comfortable without it and use may be resumed gradually.

In fractures with moderate or considerable separation, local or general anesthesia should be administered and the elbow forced into acute flexion while the surgeon's thumb makes pressure over the coronoid and endeavors to force the detached fragment back into position. The forearm should then be immobilized for four weeks in as acute flexion as can be maintained without endangering the circulation of the hand.

If bony block from a loose fragment or excess callus or myositis ossificans results, the fragment or excess bone should be removed after the process has ceased to progress. When the coronoid is fractured in connection with a dislocation at the elbow, the dislocation should be treated in acute flexion.

Traumatic Olecranon Bursitis is not very rare and may be confused with a fracture of the olecranon. It is usually due to a blow received on the elbow which is followed by immediate swelling over the posterior surface of the olecranon process with relatively little disability at the elbow. (Fig. 613.) On physical examination the patient presents a soft tissue swelling over the olecranon which is not especially tender and there is no tenderness on palpation along the lateral borders of the bone. Active extension of the elbow is, as a rule, very little disturbed, and this and the lack of tenderness along the lateral borders of the bone are the chief points of differentiation between the bursitis and a fracture of the olecranon without separation of the fragments.

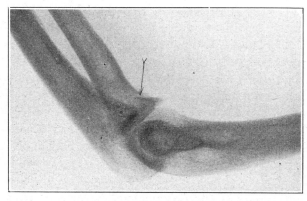

Fig. 611.—Simple fracture of the coronoid. Treated by plaster cast in acute flexion. No reduction was necessary. Good result.

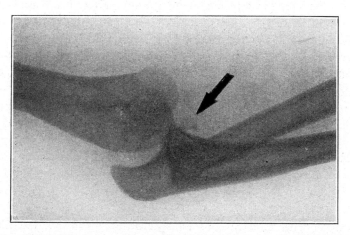

Fig. 612.—Fracture of the coronoid process complicating posterior dislocation at the elbow. Treated by reduction and immobilization in a posterior plaster mold to arm and forearm with as much flexion as could be maintained with safety (70 degrees) for a period of four weeks. Good result.

If the blood in the bursa has clotted since the injury, palpation elicits soft crepitus. The condition must, however, be differentiated from an infectious bursitis and this is usually possible from the history. In the traumatic cases aspiration yields bloody fluid and in infectious cases the fluid is usually purulent but may be bloody, and it may be necessary to culture the material in order to rule out infection.

Treatment of Traumatic Olecranon Bursitis.—The bursa is aspirated and a compression dressing is applied. If the effusion reappears the aspiration should be repeated. A chronic thickened bursa should be excised, and it is important that all of the sac be removed.

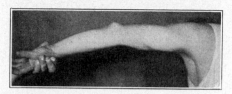

Fig. 613.—Traumatic olecranon bursitis. Treated by aspiration and compression dressing.

FRACTURES OF THE HEAD AND NECK OF THE RADIUS

Occurrence and Mechanism.—Fractures of the head and neck of the radius were formerly regarded as rare injuries, but with increasing use of the x-rays it is found that they occur rather frequently, not only as isolated injuries, but as complications of severe fractures and dislocations involving the elbow joint. (Figs. 622, 623, and 624.) The comminuted fractures of the head of the radius are usually the result of direct violence such as a fall or blow upon the lateral surface of the elbow, while the fractures of the neck and the fractures in which the head is split or a small piece is broken off are apt to be the result of an indirect violence, such as a fall upon the hand with the forearm pronated and partially flexed.

These lesions may be divided into fractures of the head of the radius, separation of the upper epiphysis of the radius, and fractures of the neck of the radius; but since they lie so close together and are occasionally combined we shall consider them under one heading.

Pathology.—The simplest type of fractures of the head of the radius is a vertical fissure which may extend into the neck of the bone. A variation of this is the breaking off from the margin of the head of a fragment varying in size from a small chip to practically half of the head of the bone. This is the so-called chisel fracture of the head of the radius (Fig. 614). Not infrequently the head of the bone is comminuted and it may be impacted upon the neck (Fig. 613). The separated fragments may be displaced into the elbow joint or driven outward or forward into the surrounding tissues.

The epiphysis of the head develops from a single center which appears at about the fifth year and unites to the shaft about the sixteenth year. Separation of the epiphysis is very rare but it may be split or comminuted or impacted upon the neck in the same manner as is the head of the bone in the adult.

In fractures of the neck the fracture line tends to be roughly transverse, and it usually involves the bone just behind the head, but it may be lower down close to the bicipital tuberosity. In other cases the fracture line may be oblique or comminuted and the head is frequently impacted upon the neck. The head of the radius may be displaced downward and impacted, or it may be tilted forward or to one side, and in unusual instances it may be completely displaced and remain imbedded in the flexor muscles of the forearm. In complete fractures through the neck of the radius the annular ligament tends to maintain the head in approximately its normal position while the biceps, by virtue of its insertion into the bicipital tuberosity, tends to pull the lower fragment forward and rotate it outward.

Diagnosis of Fractures of the Head and Neck of the Radius.—In an isolated fracture of the head or neck of the radius the pain is localized over the involved portion of the bone and there is moderate swelling on the outer side of the elbow and a variable amount of effusion into the joint (Fig. 616). Pronounced point tenderness is present over the head or neck of the radius and attempts to rotate the forearm either actively or passively cause local pain.

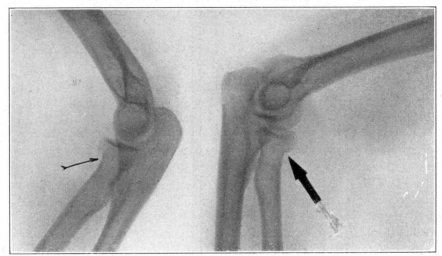

Fig. 614.   Fig. 615.

Fig. 614.—Chisel fracture of the head of the radius with very little displacement. Treated by posterior plaster mold for eighteen days and was removed daily for hot baths after ten days, with the elbow in acute flexion and the forearm in full supination. Sling to forearm and arm for two weeks. Good result.

Fig. 615.—Compression fracture of the neck of the radius with very little displacement. Treated by posterior plaster mold in moderate flexion of the elbow and full supination of the forearm. Good result.

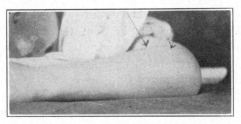

Fig. 616.—Recent fracture of the head of the radius in a child. Note the localized swelling.

This is especially pronounced with supination. If the fragments are not impacted, it may be possible to elicit crepitus by rotating the forearm, and by palpation over the head of the radius during rotation of the forearm, and it may be possible to demonstrate the fact that the head of the radius does not rotate with the shaft of the bone. Flexion and extension of the elbow may be fairly free, but are usually limited and painful.

In fractures of the neck below the annular ligament with forward displacement of the lower fragment, it may be possible to palpate the upper end of this fragment beneath the supinator longus. All elbows in which a fracture of the upper end of the radius is suspected should be subjected to careful study by the x-ray, since this is the only method of making an accurate diagnosis, and an accurate diagnosis of the exact type of lesion is necessary for treatment.

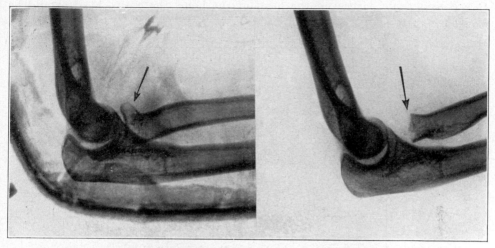

Fig. 617.—Comminuted fracture of the head of the radius. Developed pain and limitation of motion. Head of the radius removed with good result.

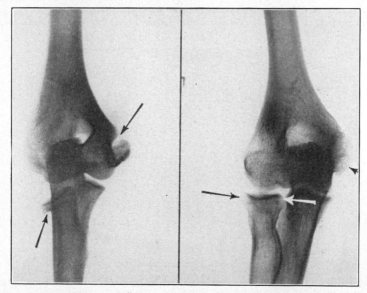

Fig. 618.—Fracture of the internal epicondyle of the humerus and of the neck of the radius. Treated by open reduction of both. On the right is shown an x-ray of the same elbow eight years later.

Treatment of Fractures of the Head and Neck of the Radius

In considering the treatment of fractures of the upper end of the radius the surgeon should be impressed by the fact that not only does the head move across the capitellum in flexion and extension of the elbow, but that it also

rotates approximately 160 degrees on the ulna and on the capitellum in pronation and supination of the forearm.　Consequently, in order that full motion
may be restored to the elbow joint, it is necessary that approximately exact
anatomical reposition be obtained.　If this cannot be obtained, the fragments
which cannot be exactly fitted into place should be removed; if this applies
to a considerable portion of the head of the bone, the entire head should be
excised.

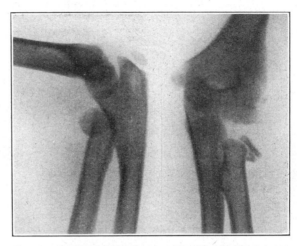

Fig. 619.—Fracture of the neck of the radius with displacement in a child.　Treated by operative replacement of the head.　Good result.　(Key, J. A.:　J. A. M. A. 94: 101, 1931.)

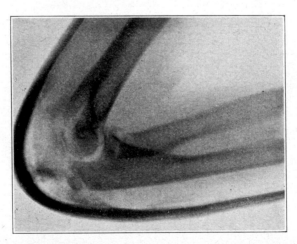

Fig. 620.—Same case after replacement of the head by open operation.　Then posterior plaster
mold for four weeks and sling for two weeks.　Good result.

It is further to be noted that the prognosis of these fractures in children
is much better than it is in adults and that considerably more leeway may be
allowed conservative treatment in children than in adults.

In discussing the treatment of fractures of the head and neck of the
radius we may divide these injuries into three groups:　(1) Those in which
conservative treatment is indicated; (2) those in which operative treatment is

indicated; and (3) those borderline cases which the surgeon is justified in treating conservatively with the expectation that it may be necessary to remove the head later on.

Conservative Treatment is indicated in all simple fissures of the head of the radius, in fractures of the head which involve less than one-third of the circumference, and in all fractures of the neck in which the fragments are not displaced; as a matter of fact this class will be found to include a considerable percentage of the fractures of the upper end of the radius. (Figs. 614 and 615.)

All that is necessary in these cases is to immobilize the elbow and forearm in a position of moderately acute flexion and full supination. This is most conveniently and most efficiently done by means of a posterior plaster mold applied upon the dorsal surface of the arm and forearm extending down to the base of the fingers.

The plaster mold should be left on for from two to four weeks, depending upon the severity of the fracture and the age of the patient. At the end of this time the mold can be removed and the wrist slung from the neck with a Jones sling, and active motion may be begun. The sling should be lengthened gradually and the flexion decreased as motion is restored.

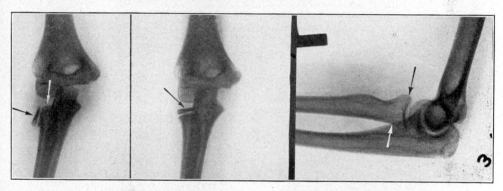

Fig. 621.—Fracture of the neck of the radius in a child. Reduced by open operation. Normal growth and function as shown by x-ray eight years later.

If the surgeon prefers, the arm can be placed in acute flexion with the adhesive and bandage dressing described under fractures of the upper end of the humerus, or it can be immobilized with a Lund swathe or posterior angular splint. However, these dressings do not control rotation of the forearm and for this reason are not so efficient as the posterior plaster mold.

Operative Treatment.—When the head of the radius is comminuted or when a piece including as much as a third of the head is broken off and displaced (Figs. 622 and 623), or when the neck is fractured and the head is displaced or tilted in such a manner that its surface no longer fits the capitellum and the lesser sigmoid of the ulna, the fracture should be operated upon unless it is possible to completely reduce the displacement by manipulation. Operative treatment is necessary because the continued displacement not only results in limitation of motion of the elbow and of the forearm, but is also apt to cause a definite traumatic arthritis, which may be the cause of considerable pain and permanent disability.

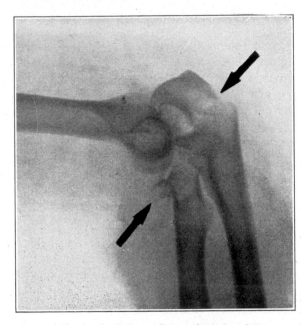

Fig. 622.—Fracture of the head of the radius and of the olecranon. The olecranon was sutured and the head and upper portion of the neck of the radius were removed. Fair result. (On compound fractures of the olecranon and simple fractures of the head of the radius we débride the wound, suture the olecranon, and remove the head of the radius some weeks later if necessary.)

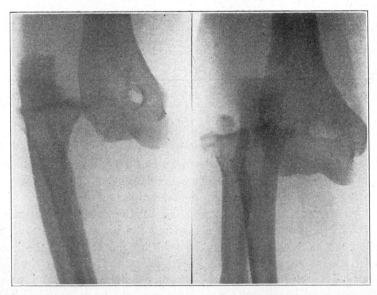

Fig. 623.—Posterior dislocation at the elbow with lateral displacement and chisel fracture of the head of the radius treated by closed reduction of the dislocation and removal of the loose fragment of the head of the radius. Fair flexion and extension at elbow. Poor rotation.

Unless there is some definite contraindication, such as shock from other injuries or local infected abrasions or lacerations, or other fractures in the vicinity, the operation should be performed as soon after the injury as possible. In other words, when the lesion is such that the surgeon knows immediately that conservative treatment will give a poor result he should advise immediate operation.

Technic of Operative Removal of the Head of the Radius.—The operative approach is by an oblique posterolateral incision which begins over the epicondyle of the humerus and extends downward and backward along the anterior border of the anconeus. This incision may be carried to the ulna and then extended downward along the subcutaneous border of this bone. The muscles are separated in line with the incision and the capsule of the joint is incised to expose the head of the radius. The posterior interosseous branch of the radial nerve is not exposed or injured. If the separated fragment is small, it may be removed and the remainder of the head may be left in place. If the head is comminuted or if it is impacted upon the neck in an adult with displacement, the entire head should be removed and with it should be included enough of the neck to insure free rotation and free flexion and extension at the elbow joint, the stump of the neck being rounded off by rongeur forceps and covered by a purse-string suture in the surrounding soft tissue. The periosteum is not stripped up and care is taken to leave no tags of periosteum attached to the stump of the neck. When enough of the stump of the neck has been removed to assure free motion the joint capsule is sutured and the wound is closed in layers without drainage. After the operation a posterior plaster mold or plaster cast is applied with the forearm flexed and supinated and the fracture is then treated as described above under conservative treatment.

In children with fractures of the neck in which the intact head is displaced, it is often possible to replace the head in its normal position by open operation and suture the tissues around it in such a manner that it will not be displaced during the closure of the wound and the molding of a posterior plaster splint to the arm and forearm, and, consequently, to obtain a normal elbow. The head of the radius should not be removed in growing children.

After removal of the radial head we expect a painless elbow with almost normal motion and strength. Sutro* has reported four cases with sufficient regeneration of bone after the excision to cause disability. This has not occurred in our experience, but his report stimulates us to make the excision clean cut and after smoothing the front of the neck to cover it with soft tissue.

Borderline Cases.—In those fractures in which a small portion of the bone is broken off or in which the displacement is slight, the surgeon is justified in using conservative treatment until it has been determined whether or not marked limitation of motion will result, but he should not wait until traumatic arthritis has developed in the elbow joint. Occasionally small detached fragments of the head of the radius become free in the elbow joint and act as loose bodies (joint mice) which block motion from time to time. These should

---

*Sutro: J. Bone & Joint Surg., October, 1935.

be removed not only because of the blocking of motion, but also because their continued presence in the joint causes irritation and may cause definite traumatic arthritis.

Another form of fracture in which he is justified in waiting is one in which the head of the radius has been widely displaced and lies under the flexor muscles of the forearm. The obvious thing to do is to remove this loose fragment immediately, but this type of case is usually a severely traumatized elbow which has been dislocated and reduced and in which operative interference is dangerous from the standpoint of infection. Consequently, the displaced head need not be excised unless it causes definite symptoms and usually the operation will not be necessary. (Fig. 624.)

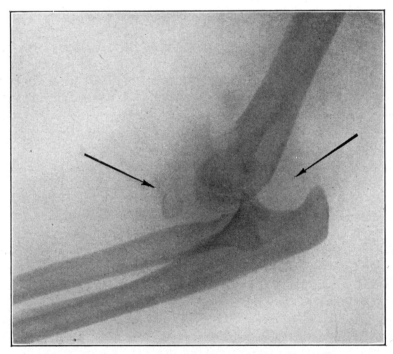

Fig. 624.—Posterior dislocation of the elbow with fracture of the neck of the radius and marked displacement of the head. Treated by closed reduction and later removal of the radial head. We do not remove the head in this type of injury unless it causes symptoms later.

TENNIS ELBOW

This condition is variously known as tennis elbow, radiohumeral bursitis, epicondylitis, and epicondylalgia. It is rather common and is often resistant to treatment. It is characterized by pain originating in and around the lateral epicondyle of the humerus. It is quite characteristic that the condition occurs after unusual use of the arm as in tennis players, painters, and occasionally in housewives.

Pathology of Tennis Elbow.—The pathology probably varies in different cases. In Osgood's* personal case there was a small bursa between the tendons of the extensor muscles and the tip of the condyle. It is probable that in other cases there may be localized periostitis or tears of the muscle origins.

———————————
*Osgood, R. B.: Arch. Surg. 4: 420, 1920.

Diagnosis of Tennis Elbow.—The symptoms usually begin after unusual exertion, gradually increasing in severity often to a point where the localized pain may be very acute, and then tend to assume a chronic state in which the pain and weakness is felt only with certain movements, especially in lifting objects with the pronated forearm extended or carrying a bag for a considerable time. The pain may radiate down the forearm or it may remain localized. On physical examination the elbow presents a variable amount of local tenderness over the tip of the external epicondyle or just below it, and in certain cases there may be a slight bulge or fullness in this region. Passive motions are free, but the pain can usually be elicited by having the patient make a fist and flex the wrist or attempt to lift an object with the elbow extended and the forearm pronated. The roentgenogram is usually negative but may show a slight periostitis in this region.

Treatment of Tennis Elbow

In mild cases relief and cure are obtained by cross strapping with adhesive applied over the bursa or by a posterior plaster mold or sling applied to the arm, elbow, and forearm, with daily heat—dry or moist—or diathermy. We have tried local injections of 1 per cent novocaine with indifferent success. In chronic cases in which there is a definite bulge or swelling, the region should be explored and the small inflamed bursa, if present, should be removed. If no bursa is found, and this is the rule in our experience, the incision is carried down to the tender point on the bone and a small area of periosteum is excised.

DISLOCATION AT THE ELBOW

Dislocations occur more frequently at the elbow than at any other joint in the body except the shoulder. This is probably due to the exposed position of the joint and to the fact that it is subjected to tremendous leverage in hyperextension injuries. It is further to be noted that in children and adolescents dislocations occur at the elbow much more frequently than they do at the shoulder. This is due to the fact that the coronoid and olecranon processes on which much of the stability of the joint depends are poorly developed in early life.

Types of Dislocations.—Backward dislocation of both bones of the forearm upon the humerus is by far the most frequent type of dislocation which occurs at the elbow. The next most frequent type is a forward dislocation of the head of the radius alone. All other forms of dislocation at this joint are rare injuries. They include backward or outward dislocations of the head of the radius alone, backward or inward dislocations of the upper end of the ulna alone, and forward, lateral, or divergent dislocations of both bones of the forearm upon the humerus.

Posterior Dislocation at the Elbow

Occurrence.—Posterior dislocation occurs more frequently than all other types at the elbow for six main reasons. (1) Both bones are usually dislocated because the radius is firmly bound to the ulna by the annular ligament and interosseous membrane, while it articulates rather loosely with the humerus.

(2) The lower end of the humerus is very wide in the lateral plane and rather narrow in the anteroposterior plane; consequently the bones of the forearm can be dislocated anteriorly or posteriorly much more easily than they can laterally. (3) The anterior and posterior portions of the capsule of the joint are relatively weak, while the lateral ligaments are relatively strong. (4) The normal motions of the joint occur in the anteroposterior plane and there is

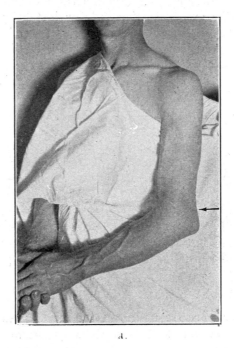

A.

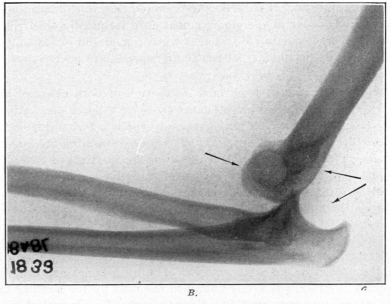

B.

Fig. 625 *A* and *B*.—Typical posterior dislocation of the left elbow.

practically no motion in the lateral plane. (5) The injuries which cause dislocation are usually forces which tend to force the forearm upward and backward. (6) Posterior dislocation is resisted by the coronoid process which is relatively small in children.

Mechanism of Posterior Dislocation at the Elbow.—This lesion is in most instances the result of a hyperextension injury at the elbow such as is incurred in a fall upon the outstretched hand with the elbow extended and the forearm supinated. The force is transmitted through the ulna, and as the olecranon is levered against the lower end of the humerus the upper end of the shaft of the ulna is forced backward and the lateral ligaments are stretched or ruptured. The upper end of the radius moves with the ulna and when it and the coronoid have been displaced backward to a point where they no longer rest upon the lower surface of the humerus the bones of the forearm slip upward behind the humerus and become locked in their new position by the coronoid which comes to rest in the olecranon fossa.

It is also to be noted that force in abduction as well as in hyperextension favors this type of dislocation, and that Malgaigne found that the internal lateral ligament could be torn and the ulna forced backward by forcible internal rotation of the semiflexed forearm.

Pathology of Posterior Dislocation at the Elbow.—The dislocation may be complete or incomplete. In the incomplete form the tip of the coronoid rests upon the trochlea and in the complete form it has traveled upward and rests in the olecranon fossa. Not infrequently there is a variable degree of displacement of the forearm in the lateral plane, either an abduction or adduction deformity being present, and the upper ends of the forearm bones are displaced in the opposite direction on the humerus. The most frequent type is a dislocation backward and outward in which the internal lateral ligament and anterior capsule are torn or detached from the humerus while the external lateral ligament may or may not be torn.

With complete tearing of all the ligaments the lateral displacement of the forearm is largely dependent upon gravity as there is considerable lateral instability at the elbow joint. The orbicular ligament remains intact and the upper end of the radius is firmly attached to the ulna and is displaced with it. The lower end of the humerus projects in the cubital fossa and the tendons of the biceps and brachialis anticus are stretched over it and may be lacerated. There may be considerable stripping up of the periosteum on the posterior surface and lateral borders of the lower end of the humerus.

In severe injuries due to great force there may be wide displacement with injury to the ulna, radial, and median nerves or brachial vessels and the flexor muscles of the forearm may be extensively lacerated and torn from their attachments. The dislocation may be complicated by fractures of the upper end of the radius or of the coronoid of the ulna or of the external condyle of the humerus or the internal epicondyle of the humerus. (Figs. 623 and 624.)

Diagnosis of Posterior Dislocation at the Elbow.—In a recent case the forearm is usually carried in a position of moderate flexion (about 135 degrees extension), but there is no characteristic position; it may be fully extended or even hyperextended, may be in any position as regards rotation, and a valgus or varus deformity may be present (Figs. 626 and 627). On inspection the anteroposterior diameter of the elbow is increased, while the lateral diameter is normal except for the swelling which varies in different cases. When viewed from the side, the forearm appears to be shortened, the olecranon is usually prominent and higher than normal, and the lower end of the arm appears to be bowed forward; that is, it tends to be concave behind and convex in front. There is a definite fullness in the cubital fossa over the front of the elbow, and if the extremity is viewed from the front, the shortening appears to be in the forearm; while if it is viewed from behind, the shortening appears to be in the arm.

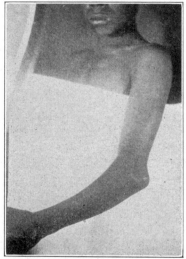

Fig. 626.—Posterior dislocation at the elbow with typical deformity.

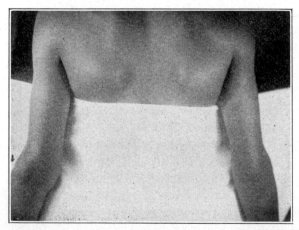

Fig. 627.—Same case seen from behind to show lateral displacement.

As a rule extensive swelling occurs rather rapidly after the injury and may involve the entire elbow region and obscure the characteristic picture described above. However, the diagnosis can be made by palpation, since it is always possible to identify the olecranon and epicondyles. When these are palpated, it will be noted that the olecranon is displaced upward and backward; that is, above and behind the line joining the epicondyles. It will usually be possible also to palpate the head of the radius in the tissues posterior to the external condyle and lateral to the displaced olecranon. This distortion of the bony landmarks of the elbow is characteristic and makes the diagnosis.

In thin subjects without much swelling it may be possible to palpate the inner border of the greater sigmoid fossa and the inner border of the trochlear surface of the humerus. False motion in extension and abduction or adduction may be demonstrated and voluntary motion and rotation of the forearm may be possible, but, as a rule, the spasm of the muscles of the arm holds the forearm bones firmly in their abnormal position, and only a few degrees of motion in any direction is possible, and this is accompanied by considerable pain. An x-ray picture should always be taken in elbow dislocations as in other dislocations when fractures are suspected.

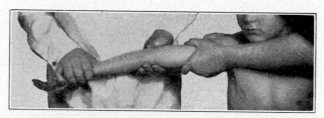

Fig. 628.—Manipulative reduction of posterior dislocation at the elbow. The surgeon slightly hyperextends the elbow and makes traction on the forearm while countertraction is made by an assistant.

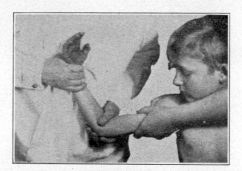

Fig. 629.—Second step in manipulative reduction of posterior dislocation at the elbow. With the traction maintained, the operator presses the lower end of the humerus backward and the upper end of the ulna forward, and slowly flexes the forearm over his thumb.

Complications in Posterior Dislocation at the Elbow.—Not infrequently in posterior dislocations the coronoid process is fractured (usually at its tip) and occasionally there is a fracture of the head of the radius or of the external condyle of the humerus. Vascular and nerve lesions are rare. A late complication is the development of myositis ossificans which will be discussed below.

Treatment of Posterior Dislocation at the Elbow.—The treatment of a recent posterior dislocation at the elbow is reduction by manipulation and traction and this should be done as soon after the injury as possible, both to relieve the pain which is severe, and to lessen the tension on the soft tissues with its resultant swelling.

Anesthesia.—In most patients either adequate local or general anesthesia is advisable and this is particularly true in strong muscular individuals. While it is possible to reduce the dislocation without an anesthetic, it is usually unwise to do so, as in addition to the pain inflicted the force necessary for the reduction may result in serious damage to the soft tissues or the fracturing of one of the bones.

Method of Reduction.—Muscular relaxation having been secured, an assistant grasps the patient's arm firmly with both hands and immobilizes it. The surgeon then grasps the wrist with one hand and places his other hand over the upper end of the forearm at the bend of the elbow. The patient's forearm is then supinated fully to relax the biceps and extended to the point where further motion is checked by the elastic resistance of the muscles (Fig. 628). At this time any lateral deviation of the forearm is corrected.

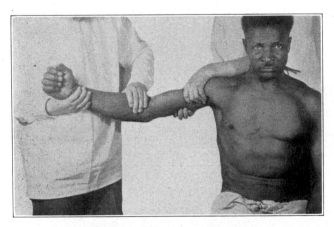

Fig. 630.—Another method for manipulative reduction of posterior dislocation at the elbow. When the forearm is maintained in a position of flexion, no attempt should be made to hyperextend the elbow, as this may cause damage to the soft parts, but traction can be made on the flexed forearm and the dislocation can be reduced in this manner and then flexed as shown in the preceding illustration.

Having placed the forearm in the above position, the surgeon is now ready to proceed with the actual reduction. This is accomplished by three maneuvers: (1) The upper end of the patient's forearm is pushed directly backward by the surgeon's hand which is placed at the bend of the patient's elbow. This will lift the coronoid out of the olecranon fossa and enable it and the head of the radius to slip over the expanded lower end of the humerus. (2) While the backward pressure is maintained, traction is made with the surgeon's hand which grasps the patient's wrist. This is slow, steady, and powerful enough to draw the forearm forward on the humerus. (3) Having unlocked the bones of the forearm and drawn them forward, the backward pressure and traction are continued, while the forearm is slowly flexed (Fig. 629).

Usually at the beginning of the flexion a slight click will be felt and after this practically no resistance will be encountered in flexion. When this occurs the reduction is complete. Sometimes reduction occurs without the click.

If undue resistance is encountered in flexing the elbow, reduction has not been accomplished, and the surgeon should start over again from the beginning because forcible flexion of an unreduced dislocation may cause considerable damage.

By the above method almost every recent posterior dislocation at the elbow can be reduced without further damage to the soft parts. But if the elbow is maintained in a position of flexion, reduction should be by traction on the flexed forearm, as in Fig. 630.

Aftertreatment of Posterior Dislocation at the Elbow.—Reduction having been accomplished, the elbow should be immobilized in as much flexion as it is safe to use in the presence of whatever swelling may have occurred. This will vary from slightly less than a right angle to acute flexion.

The position of flexion is safely, comfortably, and conveniently maintained by a posterior plaster mold extending from the upper arm to the base of the fingers (Fig. 631). This is supported by a clove hitch and sling around the neck. X-ray pictures should be taken after doubtful reductions in order to check the positions of the bones.

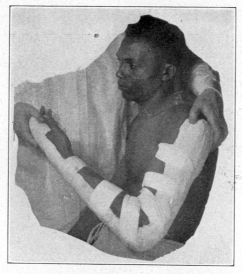

Fig. 631.—Posterior plaster mold strapped on with adhesive, used after the reduction of a posterior dislocation at the elbow.

If the surgeon prefers, the acute flexion may be maintained by an adhesive or bandage dressing and Jones' sling or posterior metal splint.

If acute flexion has not been obtained at the time of the reduction on account of the swelling, it can usually be obtained within a few days when the swelling has lessened. The immobilization in acute flexion is maintained for from ten days to three weeks depending upon the severity of the injury. It is a good policy to maintain immobilization as long as acute tenderness persists over the lateral ligaments and as long as these ligaments are relaxed.

When the immobilization is discontinued the elbow is gradually lowered to a right angle by applying a Jones sling and lengthening it a little each day, and active motion is permitted. After two weeks of this treatment, the patient may be permitted to begin to use the arm and discard all support if he is comfortable without it. During the process of lowering the arm, the patient must bring the forearm to a position of acute flexion at least twice daily in order to prevent permanent loss of flexion. In uncomplicated cases full extension will be obtained within a few weeks after support has been discontinued.

If there appears to be undue stiffness in the elbow, local heat and massage may be used to hasten the return of function, but the joint should not be manipulated as this encourages the development of adhesions and of myositis ossificans.

If tenderness and marked limitation of motion are present seven or eight weeks after the injury, roentgenograms should be taken to determine whether or not myositis ossificans is developing. If the x-rays show abnormal calcium shadows around the joint, the elbow should be immobilized and treated as described under myositis ossificans. If there is no calcium deposit around the joint and the flexion persists, the elbow should be extended by traction or a wedging plaster or by operation as described under the treatment of supracondylar fractures of the humerus.

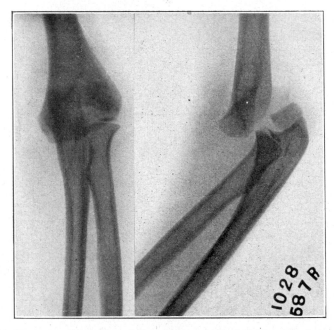

Fig. 632.—Posterior dislocation of the elbow complicated by a fracture of the external condyle. Treated by manipulative reduction and immobilization in a position of moderately acute flexion with a posterior plaster splint to arm and forearm for six weeks. Good result.

Treatment of Posterior Dislocation Complicated by Fracture.—A large percentage of the dislocations at the elbow are complicated by fractures. Those most frequently seen are: fractures of the head or neck of the radius (Figs. 623 and 624); fractures of one or both condyles of the humerus (Figs. 626, 627, and 632); fractures of the coronoid or olecranon of the ulna; fractures of both bones of the forearm; or a combination of two or more of the above. In most instances the presence of these fractures can be excluded only by the x-ray. Consequently every suspicious dislocation at the elbow should be examined by the x-ray.

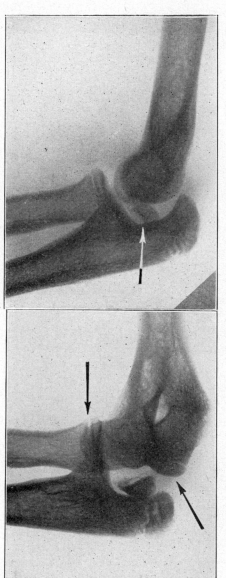

Fig. 633.—Lateral dislocation of the elbow with fracture of the epicondyle. After closed reduction the epicondyle, which remained in the joint, was excised.

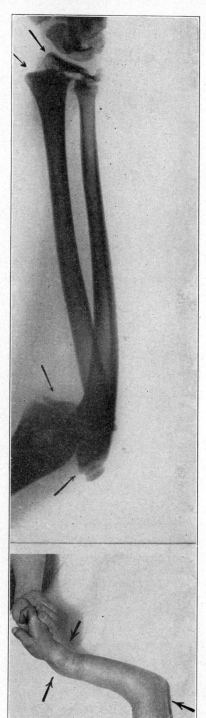

Fig. 634.—Posterior dislocation at the elbow and epiphyseal separation at the wrist. Treated by manipulative reduction of each and immobilization in a plaster cast. Good result.

In the presence of any of the above fractures the dislocation should be reduced by manipulation just as though the fracture did not exist. Then the surgeon should treat the fracture in most instances just as though the dislocation had not existed.

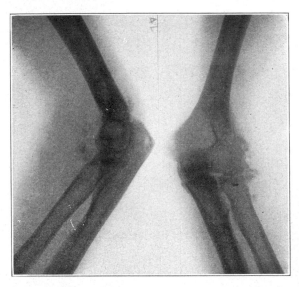

Fig. 635.—Myositis ossificans following dislocation of the elbow and fracture of the lower end of the humerus. Treated by fixation of arm and forearm in anterior plaster cast from upper third of arm to base of fingers with forearm at right angle to arm. Fair result.

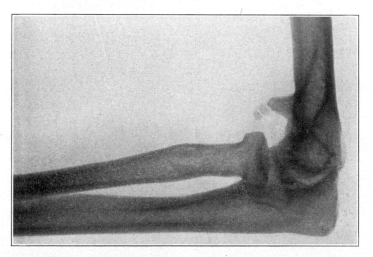

Fig. 636.—Myositis ossificans following old fracture of the lower end of the humerus and dislocation of the head of the radius. Treated by removal of the excess bone and then reduction and fixation of the head of the radius with a strip of fascia. Good result.

In other words, if the dislocation is complicated by a fracture of the head of the radius, the dislocation should be reduced by manipulation and then the fracture of the head of the radius should be treated by simple immobilization in acute flexion or open operation as indicated according to the principles laid down in the section on fractures of the head and neck of the radius.

An exception to the above rule is fracture of the olecranon because it is not wise to immobilize a fresh dislocation at the elbow in less than 90 degrees flexion. Consequently, if immobilization of the reduced elbow at a right angle causes separation of the fragments of the olecranon the latter should be sutured firmly together by open operation and then the elbow can be immobilized at a right angle or a few degrees less.

The period of immobilization is somewhat longer in dislocations which are accompanied by fractures.

Production of New Bone Around the Elbow (Figs. 635 and 636). (Myositis Ossificans, Ossifying Hematoma, and Exuberant Callus).—For some as yet unknown reason an abnormal production of new bone is more liable to occur after injuries to the elbow, and especially after dislocations, than it is after injuries in any other region. This is partly due to the fact that the periosteum is often stripped from the bones in elbow injuries, but this also happens elsewhere and consequently does not explain the peculiar susceptibility of this joint.

These complications are especially liable to occur after severe injuries in strong muscular individuals that are accompanied by considerable damage to the soft parts, are followed by much swelling, and are rare after mild injuries.

Myositis Ossificans is the formation of bone in muscle. The type which occurs after trauma is limited to the injured region and is often called local or traumatic myositis ossificans. The bone is laid down in the muscle substance and fibrous tissues and tends to make its first appearance as minute spicules of bone which lie parallel with the muscle fibers. These then coalesce to form a solid mass of bone. In the elbow the most frequent site is in the lower portion of the brachialis anticus muscle, but the bone may be laid down in the lateral ligaments or muscles adjacent to them, or, in fact, anywhere around the joint.

Ossifying Hematoma is the organization and ossification of a hematoma and is usually subperiosteal in location.

Exuberant Callus is the production of excessive callus at the site of an injury to bone. The injury may be a fracture, a stripping up of the periosteum, or the avulsion of a ligament or tendon.

Diagnosis.—New bone formation around the elbow is to be suspected if the area remains unusually tender for an unusually long time, if the restoration of motion is abnormally slow, and if active or passive motion causes an abnormal amount of pain. The early diagnosis can be made only by the x-ray, and if a simple dislocation is not free from tenderness and pain and quite freely movable six weeks after the accident, an x-ray picture should be taken in order to determine whether or not abnormal bone formation is occurring.

Treatment.—The ideal treatment would be prevention, but we know of no way in which the condition can be prevented. It either happens or it does not, regardless of the treatment. We believe, however, that in certain cases early or too strenuous active and passive motion aggravates the condition.

Once the process has begun, all authors are agreed that the treatment is rest of the involved joint. This rest should be complete, continuous, and of long duration. The reason for rest is that attempts to restore motion irritate the involved tissues and the irritation stimulates new bone formation. Consequently, as soon as myositis ossificans is diagnosed, the elbow should be placed in the best functional position for the patient (usually at an angle of about 135 degrees, and occasionally at an angle of about 70 degrees depending upon his occupation, with the forearm in the midposition as regards pronation and supination), and a well-fitting plaster cast should be applied from the upper arm to the base of the fingers. This immobilization should be continued for six weeks, or more if necessary, until the local tenderness has disappeared and the new bone formation has ceased, as can be determined by frequent x-rays.

Some patients will object to this prolonged immobilization, but the surgeon should not compromise, since the complication is a serious one and may result in complete ankylosis at the elbow, even with the best of care, and the degree of ankylosis is almost certain to be increased by too early attempts to restore motion.

Under prolonged rest the new bone formation not only ceases, but a considerable portion or even all of the abnormal bone may be resorbed. Some surgeons use diathermy or some other form of local heat in attempts to hasten this resorption, but we believe that the uninterrupted rest is more important. In a recent case of one of the authors (J. A. K.) the blood calcium was 11.2 milligrams per 100 c.c. of serum. This is a little high and suggests that a low calcium diet might be of value in these cases.

After the tendency to new bone formation has ceased, guarded attempts to restore motion should be made. These should consist of graded active exercises, gentle massage, and local heat. But passive motion should not be used, and above all the elbow should not be manipulated.

When the entire process has completely quieted down if there is a permanent bone block at the elbow the offending bone should be removed by operation. The dissection should be sharp and clean and especial care should be taken not to damage tissues or strip up the periosteum. The type of operation will depend upon the location of the bone, and it should not be attempted by any except a skillful surgeon.

Anterior Dislocation at the Elbow

Occurrence and Mechanism.—Anterior dislocation at the elbow is a very rare lesion and in about a third of the recorded cases the dislocation has been complicated by a fracture of the olecranon. The probable cause is a fall or blow on the point of the flexed elbow.

Pathology.—There is extensive tearing of ligaments and the olecranon rests on the anterior surface of the lower end of the humerus, and the head of the radius is anterior to and above the external condyle.

Diagnosis.—The elbow is supported in a position of almost complete extension, and is immobilized in this position by muscle spasm. On palpation the rounded condyles of the humerus can be palpated beneath the skin at the point of the elbow, the olecranon will be found to be absent from its normal position, and the axis of the shaft of the ulna crosses the humerus above the condyles.

Treatment of Anterior Dislocation at the Elbow.—The treatment is immediate reduction under adequate local or general anesthesia. When muscular relaxation has been obtained, the arm should be fixed by an assistant and the surgeon should grasp the injured forearm with both hands and make traction in the line of the arm. While the traction is maintained with one hand, the other pushes the upper end of the forearm backward and downward causing the olecranon to slip back around the lower end of the humerus. When the reduction is complete, the elbow should be immobilized for three or four weeks at an angle of about 135 degrees in a plaster cast or posterior mold. At the end of this time active motion should be started and the arm carried in a sling.

Lateral Dislocation of Both Bones of the Forearm at the Elbow

These are rare injuries in which the forearm bones may be displaced either outward or inward on the humerus. They may result from direct violence, wrenching of the forearm or falls upon the hand.

Inward Dislocation at the Elbow

Pathology.—In this rare injury the upper ends of the bones of the forearm are shifted directly inward on the humerus and the amount of displacement varies in different instances. It is said that the dislocation is always incomplete and the typical lesion is one in which the sigmoid of the ulna lies mesial to the mesial condyle of the humerus and the head of the radius rests upon the trochlea or may be below, or in front of, or behind it. In other instances the orbicular ligament is torn and the head of the radius remains in contact with the capitellum. The lateral ligaments are torn.

Diagnosis.—Unless it is limited by great swelling, motion of the forearm is fairly free in all directions, but very painful. On inspection the elbow is broadened and the axis of the forearm is shifted inward. The diagnosis is made by the abnormalities in the bony landmarks. The external condyle is unusually prominent and the sigmoid lies mesial to the internal condyle and usually embraces it. The triceps tendon can be traced upward and outward from the prominent olecranon which lies behind the internal condyle.

Treatment of Inward Dislocation at the Elbow.—When muscular relaxation has been secured by the anesthetic, the arm is immobilized by an assistant. The surgeon then grasps the wrist with one hand and makes moderate traction on the almost completely extended forearm. Simultaneously with the traction he manipulates the region of the elbow with his other hand, pushing the upper end of the ulna downward and outward. In most instances reduction is not difficult. Occasionally, however, the manipulation may result in the conversion of an inward into a posterior dislocation. If this occurs, the posterior dislocation should then be reduced as described above.

After reduction, the elbow is immobilized in a posterior plaster mold or plaster cast in as much flexion as the swelling permits and supported with a sling. The immobilization should be continued for three weeks. At the end of this time the plaster can be removed and the forearm supported in a Jones sling. The sling should be lengthened daily and active motion begun. In order not to lose flexion, the patient must flex the forearm fully each day. The sling can be discarded as soon as the patient is comfortable without it.

Outward Dislocation at the Elbow

Pathology.—The dislocation may be incomplete or complete. In the incomplete type the sigmoid rests upon the lateral part of the trochlea or capitellum and the coronoid remains in front of the lower end of the humerus while

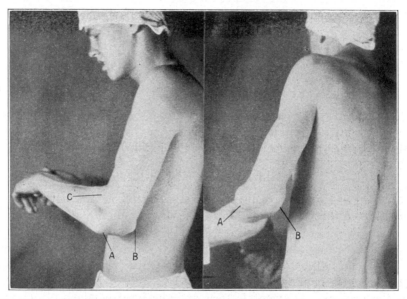

Fig. 637.—External lateral dislocation of the elbow. *A*, Olecranon; *B*, internal epicondyle; *C*, head of the radius.

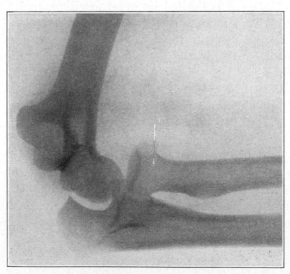

Fig. 638.—X-ray of preceding case. Treated by manipulative reduction and posterior plaster mold for two weeks.

the head of the radius is displaced outward and usually upward. In the complete type the sigmoid rests upon and grasps the lateral surface of the external condyle and the forearm is almost always rotated inward so that the head of the radius lies on a higher level than the olecranon. In both types the ligaments are torn.

Diagnosis.—The elbow is broadened and the forearm is usually pronated and shifted outward from the axis of the humerus. Motion at the elbow is free but painful. On palpation the internal condyle is unusually prominent and the skin is stretched over the sharp inner border of the trochlea. The olecranon is found behind or lateral to the external condyle and the head of the radius is unusually prominent, while the external condyle cannot be palpated. (Figs. 637, 638, and 640.)

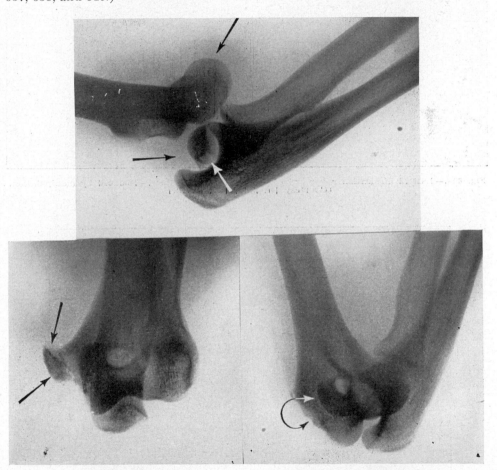

Fig. 639.—Posterior dislocation at the elbow with fracture of the internal epicondyle. After manipulative reduction it was necessary to suture the internal epicondyle in position with chromic catgut. The view at the right shows the epicondyle displaced anteriorly.

Treatment of Outward Dislocation at the Elbow.—Reduction is accomplished by traction and manipulation as follows: An assistant immobilizes the arm and the surgeon makes moderate traction on the almost completely extended forearm with one hand and with the other pushes the upper end of the

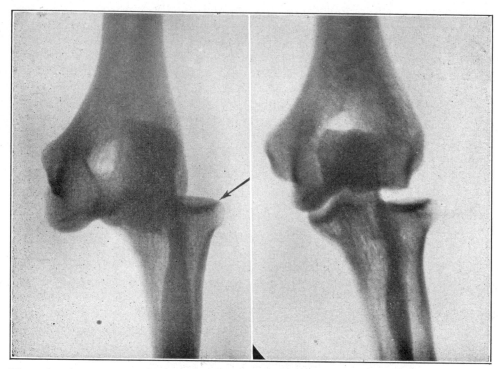

Fig. 640.—Lateral dislocation upper end of the radius at the elbow. Reduced by manipulation. (Courtesy Dr. John D. Sherrill.)

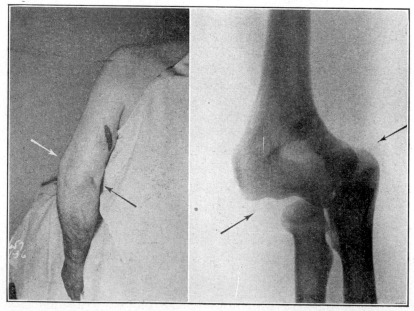

Fig. 641.—Mesial dislocation at the elbow, reduced by manipulation.

ulna downward and outward and backward to move it around the lower end of the humerus. As the ulna is moved outward, the forearm is supinated to bring the sigmoid against the trochlea and the head of the radius down against the capitellum. As the ligaments are torn, relatively little force is required, but it may be necessary to abduct or adduct the forearm to unlock the ulna and sort of work it outward.

As in the inward dislocation the manipulation for the reduction of an outward dislocation at the elbow may result in a posterior dislocation, because with extensive tearing of the ligaments the forearm tends to slip backward on the humerus. The posterior dislocation should then be reduced as described above.

When the reduction is complete, a posterior plaster mold or cast is applied with the forearm supinated and flexed as much as the swelling permits. This is left on for three weeks and then replaced by a Jones sling which is gradually lowered as motion is restored. The sling is worn until the patient is comfortable without it.

Divergent Dislocation at the Elbow

Divergent dislocation at the elbow is a rare injury in which both bones of the forearm are dislocated and spread apart in such a manner that the lower end of the humerus slips between them.

Pathology.—All of the ligaments of the elbow are torn, the orbicular ligament is ruptured, and the interosseous membrane is torn. As a rule the ulna slips up behind the humerus and the radius slips up in front (anteroposterior type). In extremely rare instances the ulna is displaced inward and the radius is displaced outward (lateral type).

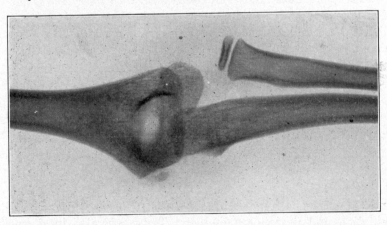

Fig. 642.—Dislocation of the head of the radius in a child. Manipulative reduction and immobilization in a posterior plaster mould with the elbow flexed.

Diagnosis.—The anteroposterior type resembles a posterior dislocation, but the head of the radius lies in the upper part of the cubital fossa and can usually be palpated there. The elbow is carried in almost complete extension and very little motion is permitted in any direction. In the lateral type, the elbow is markedly broadened and the widely separated olecranon and head of the radius can be palpated in their abnormal locations on either side of the lower end of the humerus.

Treatment of Divergent Dislocation at the Elbow.—In the anteroposterior type the ulna is first reduced by traction combined with backward pressure on the upper end of the ulna as in the ordinary posterior dislocation of both bones at the elbow. After the sigmoid has slipped over the trochlea the head of the radius should be pushed downward opposite the capitellum and the forearm slowly flexed and supinated to maintain reduction.

The lateral type of divergent dislocation can probably be easily reduced by direct traction on the extended forearm combined with downward pressure and followed by a squeezing together of the upper ends of the radius and ulna.

After reduction of either type the forearm should be immobilized in supination and as much flexion as the swelling permits by means of a posterior plaster mold or cast. The immobilization should be continued for three or four weeks and then the forearm should be supported in a Jones sling which can be lengthened as motion is restored.

Dislocation of the Radius Alone at the Elbow

This lesion is especially apt to occur in fractures of the shaft of the ulna with displacement, but may occur alone or in combination with fractures of the humerus, radius, or ulna near the elbow. The head of the radius may be displaced forward, outward, or backward.

Occurrence and Mechanism.—Outward and backward dislocations of the head of the radius are rare but forward dislocations are fairly common. The injury usually results from force transmitted upward through the shaft of the radius as in a fall upon the pronated hand. The direction of the dislocation is probably dependent upon torsion and lateral strain at the elbow, but the exact mechanism is poorly understood. It is probable that the predominance of anterior dislocation is due to the pull of the biceps muscle. The forward dislocation may also result from direct trauma to the upper end of the radius.

Pathology.—The head of the radius is absent from its normal position and displaced either anteriorly, lateral to, or behind the capitellum, as the case may be. Depending upon the type of the dislocation, the corresponding portion of the capsule of the elbow joint is torn and the orbicular ligament is usually ruptured, but the tear in this ligament may be incomplete.

The head of the radius may be fractured and the radial nerve, especially its posterior interosseous branch, may be stretched or even torn.

Diagnosis.—In all types of dislocation of the radius at the elbow the patient tends to carry the forearm in a position of pronation and slight flexion, and supination and flexion are limited. There are also local swelling and tenderness over the head of the radius and a variable amount of swelling of the elbow region, depending upon the effusion into the joint and the extravasation resulting from accompanying injuries at the elbow.

The differential diagnosis as to the type of dislocation is made by palpating the radial head in its abnormal position and unless there is an unusual amount of swelling, this can be done without difficulty. Gentle rotation of the forearm during the palpation aids in the identification of the head of the radius. At the examination the surgeon should determine whether or not the radial nerve has been injured by having the patient dorsiflex the wrist and extend the thumb and fingers and he should also make a rough sensory examination of the back of the wrist and hand.

Treatment of Dislocation of the Radius at the Elbow.—These dislocations are all reduced in about the same way. The pronated forearm is extended and slightly adducted and a moderate amount of traction is applied to the thumb or to the hand with the wrist forcibly deviated to the ulnar side. While the traction is maintained, the head of the radius is pushed back into its normal position and the forearm is then supinated and flexed. If the dislocation is forward, the head of the radius is pushed backward, if it is outward the head of the radius is pushed inward, and if the dislocation is backward it is pushed forward.

If supination and flexion are limited after the above manipulation, the reduction is not complete and should be attempted again.

After satisfactory reduction has been accomplished, the forearm should be placed in a position of full supination and acute flexion and immobilized in a posterior plaster mold. The plaster should be well molded around the upper end of the radius. The plaster should be worn for from two to three weeks and then the arm can be carried in a sling and motion resumed gradually. In certain cases the head of the radius can be pushed back in place, but it is not possible to maintain reduction. In these cases it is necessary to expose the head of the radius and fix it in its normal position, either by repairing the annular ligament and suturing the muscles over it or by tying it to the ulna with a strip of fascia lata.

Subluxation of the Head of the Radius in Young Children

Occurrence and Mechanism.—Subluxation of the head of the radius is sometimes called luxation by elongation, or Malgaigne's luxation. It is fairly common in young children, especially between the ages of two and four years and is extremely rare after the age of six years. The usual cause is forcible traction on the extended forearm, as when a child is being led by a nurse and is lifted by the arm or stumbles and throws his entire weight on the arm held by the nurse. However, we have seen the subluxation result from a fall to the floor, but it is possible that the child grasped a table or chair in falling and thus put traction on the forearm.

Pathology.—The pathology is not definitely known. The most plausible theory is that the cartilaginous head of the radius is pulled down through the annular ligament and held there by the contraction of the fibers which have been stretched over it.

Diagnosis of Subluxation of the Head of the Radius.—There may or may not be a history of forcible traction as described above, but this is not necessary, since the physical findings are characteristic. A child, usually between the ages of two and four years, complains of pain at the elbow and carries the forearm pronated and refuses to use it. Flexion and extension of the forearm are free but supination is sharply limited. Palpation is usually negative except for slight tenderness over the head of the radius, but there may be slight prominence of the head. The characteristic feature is the limitation of supination combined with free flexion and extension at the elbow. The roentgeno-gram is negative or shows slightly increased separation between the head of the radius and the capitellum.

Treatment of Subluxation of the Head of the Radius in Children.—The treatment is reduction by manipulation as follows: The surgeon grasps the affected elbow with one hand, with his thumb resting on the head of the radius. With the other hand he grasps the wrist, and holding the forearm in almost complete extension, supinates it. As the child's forearm is forcibly supinated, the surgeon makes moderate pressure on the head or neck of the radius with his thumb and pushes upward on the forearm. As a rule the manipulation requires relatively slight force and causes relatively little pain; no anesthetic is necessary.

As the child's forearm is supinated, a slight click can often be felt and the pain and limitation of movement disappear immediately. So easy is the reduction that frequently it occurs spontaneously or is accomplished accidentally by the parent or nurse.

Aftertreatment.—The forearm should be carried in flexion for a few days. This can be accomplished by a sling or Jones sling or bandage and adhesive dressing. The parent should be instructed to avoid hyperextension of the child's elbow or traction on the child's forearm for a few weeks.

Posterior Dislocation of the Ulna Alone at the Elbow

Occurrence and Mechanism.—These are very rare injuries because the upper end of the radius is so firmly bound to the ulna that it almost always travels with it. Occasionally, however, forcible hyperextension combined with adduction at the elbow may cause posterior dislocation of the ulna alone.

Pathology.—The ulna is dislocated backward and adducted (gunstock deformity) while the radius remains in situ. The internal lateral ligament is torn and the external is probably intact. The coronoid may be fractured.

Diagnosis.—The forearm is usually held in almost complete extension and a moderate adduction deformity is present. Flexion is markedly limited, but supination and pronation are free. The olecranon is prominent behind the elbow and its tip is displaced upward and outward. The condition resembles a posterior dislocation of both bones, but the head of the radius can be palpated in its normal position.

Treatment.—Treatment is reduction by manipulation and immobilization in flexion. Reduction is accomplished by hyperextension and abduction. As the hyperextended forearm is forced to the radial side, the gunstock deformity is corrected and the ulna slips back into place with relatively little difficulty. The elbow is immobilized in flexion, preferably in a posterior plaster mold or cast, and the after-treatment is the same as that described above in posterior dislocation of both bones of the forearm.

Anterior Dislocation of the Ulna Alone at the Elbow

This is an extremely rare injury which may result from a fall on the point of the flexed elbow as in Stimson's case. The tip of the olecranon lies in front of the trochlea and the head of the radius is in its normal position. In the recorded cases reduction was easily accomplished by adduction and forcible pronation, thus pushing the ulna back into position. The after-treatment would be immobilization at about 90 degrees flexion as described in anterior luxation of both bones of the forearm.

FRACTURES OF THE UPPER THIRD OF THE SHAFT OF THE ULNA WITH AND WITHOUT DISLOCATIONS OF THE HEAD OF THE RADIUS

Occurrence and Mechanism.—Fracture of the upper third of the shaft of the ulna is a rather uncommon lesion which results from direct violence to the posterior surface of the forearm just below the elbow; and, due to the

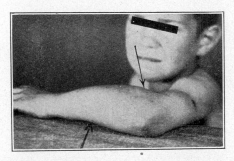

Fig. 643.—Fracture of the upper third of the ulna with anterior dislocation of the upper end of the radius. Treated by manipulative reduction and immobilization in anterior and posterior plaster molds with forearm in flexion slightly beyond a right angle at elbow. Good result.

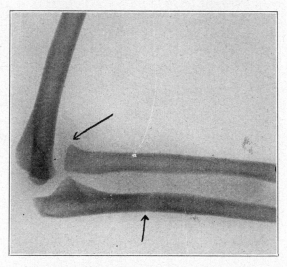

Fig. 644.—Roentgenogram of preceding case.

subcutaneous position of the bone, the fracture is often compound. The fracture line is usually roughly transverse, and the upper third of the shaft of the ulna tends to be bowed forward, thus rendering the posterior subcutaneous surface concave. In some instances there is complete separation of the fragments, the distal fragment being displaced anteriorly and slightly upward. These severe cases with anterior displacement are usually accompanied by anterior dislocation of the head of the radius.

Diagnosis.—If there is no displacement, the diagnosis depends upon the presence of point tenderness and swelling over the fracture line and pain here when cross or axial strain is put upon the shaft of the bone. Diagnosis should be confirmed by x-ray examination.

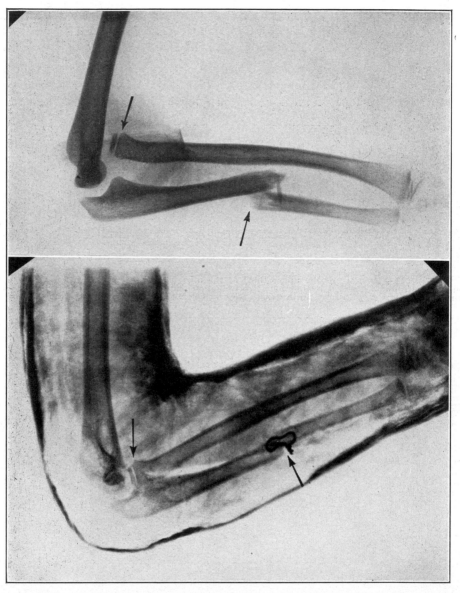

Fig. 645.—Monteggia fracture of the shaft of the ulna with anterior dislocation of the head of the radius. Reduced by open operation and the ulna fixed by a wire loop. Satisfactory result.

With displacement, the dorsal concavity is visible despite the swelling, and the deformity can be detected by palpation along the subcutaneous border of the bone (Figs. 643 and 644). Rotation of the forearm, or axial or cross strain on the ulna, causes pain at the site of the fracture and may demonstrate false motion and crepitus.

If there is overriding of the fragments or even marked anterior bowing of the ulna, the head of the radius is practically always dislocated (Figs. 643, 644, and 645), and the surgeon should always examine the head of the radius in fractures of the upper third of the ulna.

Treatment.—If these fractures are not accompanied by dislocation or fractures of the head of the radius, they should be treated just as is described in the consideration of simple fractures of the shaft of the ulna, but when the head of the radius is dislocated, this dislocation must be reduced and the fracture must be immobilized in a position of moderate flexion at the elbow in order to prevent recurrence of the dislocation. Consequently, the surgeon should first reduce the fracture of the ulna by direct pressure and traction as described below, and then press the head of the radius back into its normal position and supinate and flex the forearm until the head of the radius is quite stable, and immobilize it in this position. Usually it will be found that stability of the head of the radius can be obtained by placing the forearm in moderate supination and flexing the elbow to about 45 degrees, and it will be possible to obtain this position without causing displacement of the fragments of the ulna.

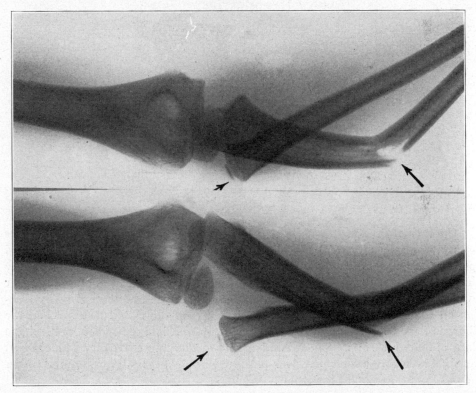

Fig. 646.—Monteggia fracture with marked deformity. Manipulative reduction and immobilization in a posterior plaster mould. Return of rotation of forearm was slow. Good result in four months.

If the head of the radius tends to slip forward after reduction, it must be exposed by operation and fixed in position by repair of the annular ligament or by a fascia loop.

The forearm should then be immobilized in this position either with short anterior and long posterior wooden splints incorporated in the plaster cast or with anterior and posterior plaster molds. The anterior splint must be pressed well down over the front of the elbow, but care should be taken to avoid obstruction to the circulation and the formation of pressure sores just below the bend of the elbow. The fracture should remain immobilized for from six to eight weeks. At the end of this time movement at the elbow and the wrist may be permitted and extension may be obtained. The patient should carry the arm in a sling until pain around the head of the radius has disappeared and should not attempt to pronate the forearm for at least four weeks after the injury, since this movement tends to bring the head of the radius forward and may reproduce the subluxation.

Watson-Jones has described an unusual flexion fracture of this type in which the ulna is bowed backward and the head of the radius is displaced backward. He states that it is readily reduced by full extension of the elbow and that the fragments lock in the reduced position. The extremity is then immobilized with the elbow in full extension in a long plaster cast for about eight weeks. We have not seen a fracture of this type.

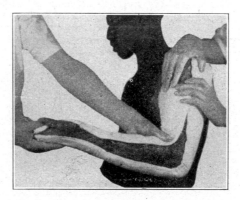

Fig. 647.—Application of anterior and posterior plaster molds for the treatment of fracture of the upper third of the ulna and dislocation of the head of the radius. The elbow is flexed to about 40 degrees from a right angle before the plaster sets.

Operative Treatment.—In fractures of the Monteggia type with severe deformity of the ulna and complete displacement of the head of the radius, open reduction and internal fixation may be necessary. The fracture of the ulna is exposed through a posterior incision and reduced by manipulation or leverage. Then, an attempt is made to reduce the head of the radius by traction on the flexed forearm and direct pressure on the radial head. Then the elbow is flexed and the anatomically reduced ulna is fixed with a metal bone plate and four screws. The wound is closed and the extremity immobilized for eight weeks in a long posterior plaster mold or a cylinder cast maintaining the position of flexion at the elbow.

REPAIR OF OLD MALUNITED FRACTURES AND UNREDUCED DISLOCATIONS OF THE ELBOW

Poor results with permanent impairment of function are more frequently seen after fractures and dislocations at the elbow than in any other region of the body. Many of these poor results are due to poor treatment; but in some instances with marked displacement and severe comminution of the joint surfaces, it is practically impossible to obtain a satisfactory result.

Not infrequently a patient with an old elbow injury with permanent impairment of function presents himself and demands relief. As a rule, relief can be obtained only by operative intervention, and this should not be undertaken lightly. Operative procedure will, of course, vary with the requirements of each individual case and must be decided upon after careful study of complete roentgenograms and analysis of the functional disability.

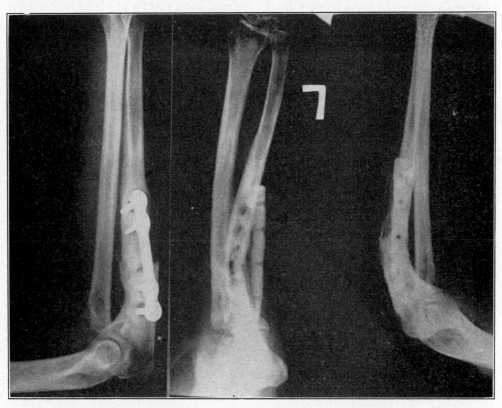

Fig. 648.—Monteggia fracture, one years duration, with nonunion and primary removal of the head of the radius. Union obtained by removal of plate and bone graft. Final result, considerable limitation of movement. (Courtesy Dr. Joseph Lembeck.)

Campbell* has laid down the following principles for the guidance of the surgeon in the reconstruction of these old traumatic elbows.

"1. Reconstruction of the normal contour and alignment of the elbow joint with especial reference to the carrying angle.

"2. An increased or normal motion. This is desirable, but stability and efficient function should not be sacrificed for the mere restoration of motion.

"3. Preservation of the condyles with their articular surfaces when possible and the securing of union between the detached condyles and the shaft in as nearly the normal relationship as possible.

*Campbell: Malunited Fractures and Unreduced Fractures about the elbow, J. A. M. A. 92: 122, 1929.

"4. Union and proper alignment, in T fractures, between the condyles themselves and between the condyles and the shaft.

"5. Excision of bony blocks or bridges that retard or prevent full motion. When the disability is due to an excess formation of callus or to a myositis ossificans, no operation should be attempted until ossification is complete."

In considering the reconstruction of these old elbows the surgeon should not ignore the factor of growth, and as a general rule in children every effort should be made to replace the bones in such a manner that normal growth will proceed, while in adults he may freely remove bone and bend his efforts toward the establishment of normal function. Arthroplasties should not be performed until growth has been completed.

Supracondylar Fractures

The most frequent type of malunion in these cases is one in which the posterior displacement of the lower fragment has not been reduced and the lower end of the proximal fragment projects into the cubital fossa and blocks flexion at the elbow. In these cases the simplest and most efficient operation is not to disturb the malunion, but to remove the offending distal end of the proximal fragment. This can be done through a lateral incision and a little more than enough bone must be removed to permit full flexion. Since no fracture has been created no splinting is necessary and exercises can be begun a few days after the operation.

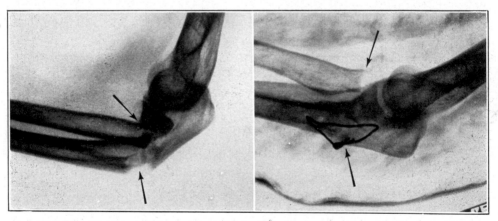

Fig. 649.—Fracture of the proximal third of the ulna and of the neck of the radius with flexion deformity. Head of the radius excised and ulna reduced and fixed with a stainless steel wire. Satisfactory result.

If in addition to the posterior displacement there is also some lateral displacement or angulation or deformity in rotation of the lower fragment, an osteotomy should be performed and the deformities corrected. Usually the osteotomy should be performed through the line of the old fracture. After the operation the arm must be immobilized and treated as a fresh supracondylar fracture of the extension type.

In the very rare cases of malunion with forward displacement of the lower fragment the deformity should be corrected after an osteotomy through the line of the fracture, and the extremity should be treated as a fresh supracondylar fracture of the flexion type or the offending bone may be removed from behind the elbow (Fig. 649).

Fractures of the External Condyle

In old fractures of the external condyle with malunion in children the surgeon should make every effort to replace the capitellum in its normal position and to fix it there either by sutures or beef bone screws, because if this is not done subsequent growth of the internal condyle may produce marked deformity. In adults it is usually better to remove the external condyle because it is difficult to get it back into its normal position and hold it there, and even if the capitellum could be correctly placed there is usually so much degeneration of the cartilage that its surface is no longer suitable for use as part of a joint. As the external condyle articulates only with the head of the radius, it has relatively little to do with flexion and extension at the elbow and a fairly serviceable and fairly stable joint may be obtained after it has been completely excised.

Fractures of the Internal Condyle

In fractures of the internal condyle with displacement the problem is more difficult because it is on the joint between the trochlea and the ulna that flexion and extension of the elbow depend. Consequently, in order that these motions may be restored this condyle must be replaced in approximately its normal position and in many instances it will probably be found that it will be wiser to leave the internal condyle in its abnormal position and restore alignment by osteotomy of the shaft and increase motion by the removal of the normal external condyle. Unless this is possible it will probably be necessary to more or less disregard the bony structures present and to perform an arthroplasty with whatever bone is left. In doing the arthroplasty the surgeon should not endeavor to restore the normal contours of the joint, but should endeavor to construct a simple hinge joint between the lower end of the humerus and the greater sigmoid of the ulna, and should not hesitate to remove sufficient bone so that with traction on the forearm there is a gap of approximately one-half inch between the bone ends and no limitation of motion in either flexion or extension.

Intercondylar or T Fractures

In these fractures especially where the condyles have been severely comminuted and there is ankylosis with marked deformity, it will usually be necessary and advisable to perform an arthroplasty from the mass of fused bone which is left. (Figs. 650 and 651.)

Fractures and Dislocations of the Head and Neck of the Radius

These injuries have been discussed under the treatment of the acute cases, but in old malunited complicated fractures at the elbow it is not infrequently found that fractures of the head of the radius are one of the chief causes of disability, and if this is true, the head and neck should be excised in order to restore motion of the forearm. This may be done at a separate operation or may be done simultaneously with the operation for the restoration of flexion and extension at the elbow. When the head of the radius is dislocated forward and has been out of position for some weeks it does little or no good to reduce the dislocation and attempt to maintain reduction. Consequently, an

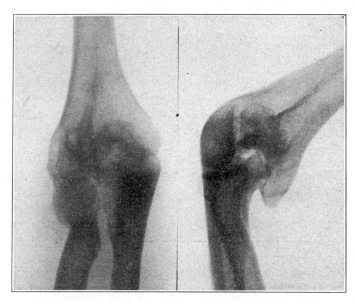

Fig. 650.—Old comminuted fracture of the elbow with malunion.

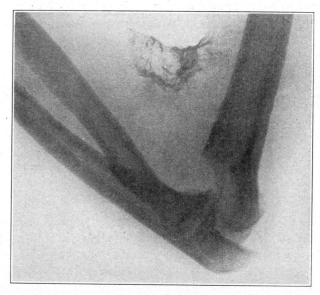

Fig. 651.—Same case as shown in Fig. 623, after plastic operation on bones. Result, almost normal motion; painless, stable joint.

open reduction should be performed and the radius should be reduced and retained in its normal position by a loop of fascia which is passed around the neck of the radius and through a small drill hole in the adjacent portion of the shaft of the ulna.

Old Posterior Dislocations of Both Bones at the Elbow

If the dislocation has existed longer than ten days the surgeon should be very careful in attempting to reduce it by manipulation as such attempts may result in crushing fractures of the condyles of the humerus or irreparable damage to the soft tissues around the joint. If the dislocation has existed more than three weeks, it is usually unsafe to attempt reduction by manipulation, and an open operation should be performed.

The following operation devised by J. S. Speed offers the expectation of a useful elbow unless the bones have been out of place so long that the cartilage covering the articular surface has undergone fibrosis. This usually does not occur until two months or longer after the injury.

Speed's Method for the Reduction of Old Dislocation at the Elbow*

"The incision is made over the posterior surface of the elbow beginning in the midline about 4 inches above the tip of the olecranon and extending down to just above the tip of the olecranon, where it turns outward over the external condyle of the head of the humerus and the head of the radius for about 2 inches down the forearm. The skin flaps are dissected back, completely exposing the tendinous insertion of the triceps muscle and the posterior surface of the elbow joint. The ulnar nerve is next located, dissected up from its bed along the groove of the internal condyle and retracted out of danger. The tendon of the triceps muscle is dissected out from its upper end and turned down and left attached to the olecranon. An incision is next made directly in the midline through the fibers of the triceps muscle down to the humerus extending from 3 inches up the shaft down to the reflexion of the joint capsule around the articular surfaces. Subperiosteally all of the muscular attachments over the lower end of the humerus are stripped free. When the attachment of the joint capsule is reached, it is necessary to divide this with a knife or scissors. Some difficulty may be encountered in freeing the tissues around the internal condyle and along the anterior surface of the humerus just above the joint, but it is essential that they all be loosened and that the lower end of the humerus be completely mobilized. This difficulty will be greatly lessened if the incision has previously been extended down over the radius exposing the head and a small portion of the shaft. Considerable callus is often formed over the posterior surface of the humerus around the olecranon fossa as a result of the stripping up of the periosteum at the original injury. This callus with the scar tissue in the olecranon fossa and incisura similunaris is next thoroughly removed.

"When the lower end of the humerus has been completely mobilized and the capitellum and the head of the radius have been exposed, one is ready to carry out the first step in the reduction. Simply twisting the forearm with gentle pressure over the capitellum causes the head of the radius to glide forward over the capitellum into the normal position. If this is not easily accomplished further dissection will render the maneuver possible without unnecessary force. The surgeon should avoid injury to the cartilage by levering or skid-

*South. M. J. 18: 193, 1925.

ding the head of the radius forward. After the radius is reduced the coronoid is slipped forward over the trochlea to complete the reduction. The joint is then carried through the full range of motion to ascertain that there is no obstruction. The periosteum and muscles are next closed along the posterior surface of the humerus, fascia is closed over the head of the radius, and the tendon of the triceps is sutured back into its normal position. The arm is placed in a posterior splint and the elbow flexed at a right angle.''

DIFFERENTIAL DIAGNOSIS OF FRACTURES AND DISLOCATIONS AT THE ELBOW

It is usually possible to decide from the history and the extent of the disability whether or not there is a serious injury at the elbow. If the patient can accurately flex and extend the elbow and supinate and pronate the forearm fully, there is probably no fracture or dislocation. A good deal can be learned about the extent and character of the injury from the location and amount of swelling and whether or not any gross deformity is present. Of course the surgeon should learn all that he can from the history and inspection, but the final diagnosis should be made by palpation and manipulation, and confirmed by the x-ray.

Palpation should be begun by identifying the three cardinal bony landmarks at the elbow. These are the internal and external epicondyles of the humerus and the tip of the olecranon. After they have been definitely identified, the surgeon should note whether or not they occupy their normal relationship to one another and whether or not they are displaced in relation to the shaft of the humerus.

As was stated in the section on examination of the elbow, the internal and external epicondyles of the humerus are at approximately the same level. With the elbow extended the tip of the olecranon lies about the middle of the line joining the two condyles, and with the elbow flexed to 90 degrees the tip of the olecranon occupies a position directly distal to the middle of the transverse interepicondylar line, and if lines are drawn between the epicondyles and from each epicondyle to the olecranon these three lines form an isosceles triangle.

The three cardinal bony landmarks are so important in diagnosis that depending upon their relations to one another and to the line of the shaft of the humerus the traumatic lesions at the elbow may be divided into three groups as follows:

1. The three cardinal bony landmarks are not normal in their relation to one another.

2. The three cardinal bony landmarks are normal in their relation to one another, but are not normal in their relation to the shaft of the humerus.

3. The three cardinal landmarks are normal in their relation to one another and to the shaft of the humerus.

After the surgeon has definitely identified the three cardinal bony landmarks of the elbow, he should decide whether or not they are normal in their relations to one another and to the shaft of the humerus. In deciding these very important points it is often helpful to compare the injured elbow with its normal fellow.

1. If the three cardinal bony landmarks are not normal, there is either a dislocation at the elbow or a fracture of the lower end of the humerus or of the olecranon with displacement.

If the tip of the olecranon is displaced backward or upward one of the following lesions is present:

1. *Posterior Dislocation of Both Bones at the Elbow.* (Common.) The elbow is fixed by muscle spasm and the head of the radius and the inner border of the sigmoid can be palpated behind the condyles. If the coronoid is broken it may be possible to pull the forearm forward with relatively little force, but the dislocation tends to recur when the traction is released.

If the head of the radius is not palpable behind the external condyle there is probably a fracture of the neck of the radius or very rarely a dislocation of the ulna alone.

2. *Intercondyloid Fracture or Epiphyseal Separation.* (Uncommon): False motion is present and the sigmoid can be felt to contain the internal condyle.

3. *Fracture of the Olecranon.* (Common): Tenderness and swelling over the olecranon with a palpable sulcus between the fragments and abnormal mobility of the detached fragment. There is loss of power in extension.

If the tip of the olecranon is displaced laterally or mesially, there is a rare *External* or *Internal Dislocation at the Elbow.*

If the tip of the olecranon is displaced forward in front of the humerus, there is a very rare *Anterior Dislocation at the Elbow.*

If the *Internal Condyle and Epicondyle and the Tip of the Olecranon* are displaced upward and there is false motion at the elbow, there is a rare *Fracture of the Internal Condyle.*

If the *Internal Epicondyle* is tender and displaced (usually downward and forward) there is a rather rare *Fracture of the Internal Epicondyle.*

If the *External Condyle and Epicondyle* are displaced or abnormal in contour and false motion is present there is a rather rare *Fracture of the External Condyle.*

If the *External Epicondyle* is tender and displaced downward there is a rare *Fracture of the External Epicondyle.*

1. If the elbow is broadened and the epicondyles are abnormally far apart and can be squeezed together or moved independently, there is an *Intercondylar* or *T Fracture of the Humerus.* In this rather common lesion the three cardinal bony landmarks may also be abnormal in their relation to the line of the shaft of the humerus.

2. If the three bony landmarks are normal in their relations to one another but are abnormal in their relations to the axis of the shaft of the humerus, there is a *Supracondylar Fracture of the Humerus.* In the common **Extension Type** the epicondyles and olecranon are displaced backward and in the rare **Flexion Type** they are displaced forward from the line of the shaft of the humerus. The diagnosis can be confirmed by demonstrating false motion of the lower fragment.

3. If the three cardinal bony landmarks are normal in their relations to one another and to the shaft of the humerus, any one or more of the fractures mentioned in the two preceding sections may be present without demonstrable displacement; and while the location of the tenderness and the disability may lead one to suspect the nature of the lesion, the diagnosis should be confirmed by the x-ray. The same is true of all of the following lesions except dislocation or subluxation of the head of the radius and fracture of the upper portion of the shaft of the olecranon with displacement, where the diagnosis can usually be made by palpation.

If the *Head of the Radius* can be palpated in its normal position and there is local swelling and tenderness with pain on rotation of the forearm, there is probably a *Fracture of the Head or Neck of the Radius.* These lesions are rather common.

If the *Head of the Radius* can be palpated in an abnormal position, there is a *Dislocation of the Head of the Radius,* and the character of the dislocation is determined by the location of the radial head. The anterior dislocation is rather common.

Sharp limitation of supination with pain and tenderness over the head of the radius in a small child points to the rather common *Subluxation of the Head of the Radius.*

Deformity (usually anterior bowing) of the upper third of the shaft of the ulna denotes a rare fracture in this region and the lesion is usually accompanied by an anterior dislocation of the head of the radius.

Fracture of the Coronoid may be suspected if there is moderate swelling and acute tenderness over the front of the elbow and acute pain at this point on passive flexion or on attempts to flex the forearm against resistance. This lesion is uncommon.

A rare intraarticular fracture of the *Capitellum* may be suspected in a patient presenting symptoms of a foreign body in the joint and no demonstrable lesion.

Sprain at the elbow is unusual, but a history of a moderate injury with moderate swelling and disability and moderate tenderness and a negative roentgenogram may be diagnosed as a sprain.

As was stated above, in most instances the diagnosis of elbow injuries should, when possible, be confirmed by the x-ray before treatment is instituted, and it is even more important to check the result of the reduction of a fracture or dislocation by the x-ray.

CHAPTER XIX

FRACTURES OF THE FOREARM

SURGICAL ANATOMY

The Shaft of the Ulna.—The ulna may be considered as the direct continuation of the humerus and its shaft, which is practically straight, is thick and strong in its upper portion, and gradually diminishes in size in its lower portion. The posterior border of the ulna is subcutaneous throughout its entire length and is easily palpated. The shaft is roughly triangular on cross-section and presents an interosseous crest for the attachment of the interosseous membrane. The anterior and posterior surfaces are roughened for the attachment of the flexor and extensor muscles of the forearm. The shaft is narrowed in its upper third by the bicipital fossa which lies opposite the bicipital tuberosity on the radius and this constitutes an area of weakness in the upper portion of the bone.

The Shaft of the Radius.—The radius may be considered as a continuation upward of the hand. It is thicker below and gradually decreases in diameter and becomes more cylindrical in contour in its upper half. The shaft is bowed laterally to enable it to rotate around the ulna and is covered by the muscles of the forearm in its upper half, but is practically subcutaneous on its dorsal and lateral aspects in its lower half. The bicipital tuberosity which serves as a point of attachment for the biceps tendon is an oval prominence which is located on the mesial surface about 2 cm. below the head of the radius.

The Interosseous Membrane is a strong fibrous membrane which stretches from the inner border of the radius to the outer border of the ulna and completely closes the space between the two bones with the exception of a small triangular area at the upper end which serves for the passage of the posterior interosseous vessels. It divides the forearm into anterior and posterior compartments. The great majority of the fibers of the interosseous membrane pass upward and outward from the outer border of the ulna to the inner border of the radius and are so arranged that they remain tense in all positions of rotation of the forearm. It is thus seen that the slope of the fibers is such that force received on the hand and transmitted upward through the shaft of the radius is gradually distributed through the interosseous membrane to the shaft of the ulna.

At its upper border the interosseous membrane is reinforced by the oblique ligament. The fibers of this ligament lie at right angles to those of the interosseous membrane passing downward and outward from the ulna to the radius and tend to resist traction forces which would otherwise pull the radius downward. The oblique ligament also resists extreme supination of the forearm.

Movements of the Bones of the Forearm.—Movement of the forearm on the arm is largely controlled by the ulna which may be considered as the continuation downward of the humerus, and movement of the hand on the forearm is largely controlled by the radius which may be considered as a continuation upward of the hand, while supination and pronation of the forearm are accomplished by rotation of the radius around the ulna. The rotation occurs at the superior and inferior radio-ulnar articulations and the normal range of movement is about 160 degrees. The axis on which the forearm and hand rotate passes through the center of the head of the radius above and through the styloid process of the ulna and the ring finger below.

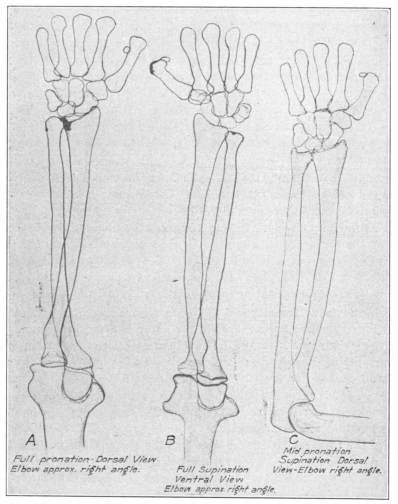

Fig. 652.—Drawing showing bones of the forearm and carpal and metacarpal bones in (*A*) pronation, (*B*) supination, and (*C*) midposition. (Sketches made from roentgenogram shown in Fig. 653.)

In full supination the shafts of the bones are widely separated and are approximately parallel, while in pronation the curved shaft of the radius crosses that of the ulna at the junction of the middle and upper thirds, and the bones are closely approximated at this point. The interosseous space is widest when the forearm is in the midposition and narrowest when the forearm is fully pronated. (Figs. 652 and 653.)

Muscles of the Forearm.—The muscles of the forearm may be divided into the flexors and pronators which lie on the anterior and mesial aspects, and the extensors and supinators which lie on the posterior and lateral aspects.

The flexors of the fingers and wrist may be divided into superficial and deep groups. The superficial flexors arise mainly from the internal condyle of the humerus and pass downward and outward to the wrist and hand. The deep flexors arise from the anterior surface of the radius and ulna and from the interosseous membrane and pass directly downward. The median nerve supplies all of the flexors of the forearm except the flexor carpi ulnaris and the ulnar half of the flexor profundus digitorum which are supplied by the ulnar nerve.

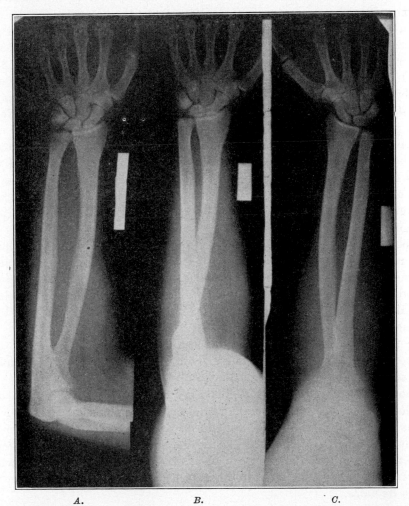

A.   B.   C.

Fig. 653.—Roentgenograms showing the bones of a normal forearm in (A) midposition. (B) full pronation, and (C) full supination. Elbow at approximately a right angle.

The pronators are two in number: (1) The *pronator radii teres* takes its origin with that of the superficial flexor group from the inner condyle of the humerus and from the coronoid process of the ulna and passes downward and outward to end in a flat tendon which winds around the shaft of the radius to be inserted into the middle of its outer surface. (2) The *pronator quadratus* is a flat muscle which passes transversely across the lower fourth of the forearm between the anterior surfaces of the radius and ulna. Both pronators are supplied by the median nerve.

The extensors of the wrist and fingers arise from the external condyle of the humerus and from the upper half of the posterior surface of the radius and ulna and interosseous membrane and pass downward to the wrist and hand.

The supinators are three in number. (1) With the forearm in a position of flexion the biceps, by virtue of its insertion into the bicipital tubercle on the inner surface of the shaft of the radius, is the most powerful supinator of the forearm. (2) The supinator brevis arises from the lateral condyle of the humerus and the upper portion of the posterior surface of the ulna and passes downward and outward to wind around the neck and upper portion of the shaft of the radius and be inserted into its lateral and posterior surfaces. (3) The supinator longus (brachioradialis) arises from the external supracondylar ridge of the humerus and passes down the lateral border of the forearm to be inserted into the styloid of the radius. It acts as a supinator when the forearm is in a position of full pronation and as a pronator when the forearm is in a position of full supination. The biceps is supplied by the musculocutaneous nerve, and the supinator brevis and longus are supplied by the radial nerve.

In fractures all of the muscles of the forearm tend to pull the distal fragments of the bones upward. In addition to this the pronator radii teres, the pronator quadratus, and the supinator brevis tend to pull the two bones toward one another, thus obliterating the interosseous space.

The supinator longus, by virtue of its attachment into the styloid process of the radius, tends to tilt this bone so that the proximal end of its distal fragment moves inward toward the ulna and the abductor and extensor muscles of the thumb, by virtue of their winding around the lower portion of the shaft of the radius, tend to squeeze the distal fragment of the radius inward toward the ulna.

In fractures involving the shaft of the radius above the insertion of the pronator teres, the proximal fragment tends to be supinated by the supinator brevis and the biceps and flexed on the arm by the biceps.

Blood Vessels and Nerves of the Forearm.—With the exception of the posterior interosseous branch of the radial nerve and the small posterior interosseous artery, all of the important vessels and nerves of the forearm lie in the anterior fascial compartment. The radial and ulnar arteries arise from the bifurcation of the brachial artery in front of the elbow and course downward in the forearm, each lying close to the anterior surface of the bone from which it takes its name.

The median nerve enters the forearm between the two heads of the pronator teres muscle and passes downward along the middle of the forearm between the superficial and deep flexor muscles.

The ulnar nerve enters the forearm between the humeral and ulnar origins over the flexor carpi ulnaris muscle and passes downward between this muscle and the flexor profundus digitorum in close relation to the ulnar artery.

In the lower third of the arm the radial nerve lies between the supinator longus and brachialis anticus muscles and in front of the elbow divides into superficial and deep terminal branches. The superficial branch is cutaneous and passes down the lateral surface of the forearm lying beneath the supinator longus muscle. The deep branch constitutes the posterior interosseous nerve and is entirely muscular and articular in its distribution. It passes backward, outward, and downward, winding around the lateral aspect of the upper portion of the shaft of the radius in the substance of the supinator brevis muscle to reach the posterior fascial compartment where it passes downward to supply all of the extensor muscles of the forearm.

EXAMINATION OF THE FOREARM

The forearm should be inspected for swelling and deformity, and the patient should be asked to move it in flexion, extension, pronation, and supination in order to determine the amount of the disability. The surgeon should then gently palpate the ulna and the radius to determine whether or not point tenderness and deformity are present. Palpation is most satisfactory if it is done with the fingers while the injured extremity rests on a table or pillow or is supported by an assistant (Fig. 654). It is difficult to palpate an extremity and support it at the same time. If there is an obvious deformity it may be possible by palpation to determine the position of the fragments.

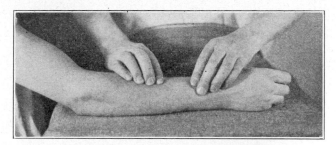

Fig 654.—Method of palpating the shaft of the radius in examination of the forearm.

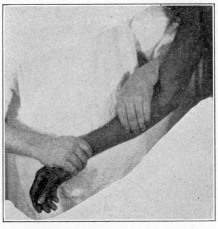

Fig. 655.—Method of testing for false motion in suspected fractures of both bones of the forearm. The movement should be very slight and gentle traction should be maintained during the manipulation.

If doubt exists as to whether or not there is a complete fracture of both bones, the forearm may then be tested for false motion, but especial care should be taken not to cause displacement of the fragments. A safe method is to grasp the forearm firmly with both hands as in Fig. 655, and while slight traction is maintained gently move the lower end of the forearm up and down on the upper end which is immobilized by the upper hand. Crepitus should not be sought, as it is unnecessary for the diagnosis and attempts to obtain it may cause displacement which will be difficult to correct.

In complete fractures of a single bone it may be possible to obtain false motion by grasping the shaft of the involved bone above and below the fracture and gently moving the fragments in opposite directions, but this, too, should be done with caution as it may cause displacement of the fragments.

The integrity of the shaft of the radius can be tested by supporting the elbow with one hand with the thumb pressed firmly against the head of the radius and then gently rotating the forearm with the other hand. If the head of the radius does not rotate with the shaft, there is a complete fracture of the shaft. If the head of the radius rotates with the shaft, the radius may be intact, or it may be incompletely broken, or it may be completely fractured and its ends interlocked.

The head of the radius should be examined carefully in isolated fractures of the shaft of the ulna in order to determine whether or not it is displaced or broken, and the inferior radio-ulnar joint should be examined in isolated fractures of the shaft of the radius in order to determine whether or not it is disrupted.

In doubtful cases without displacement, local pain at the site of the fracture may be produced by gently squeezing the two bones together or by making axial pressure on the forearm while the elbow is fixed, or by rotating the forearm. In rare instances an x-ray may be necessary for the diagnosis, and should be secured before attempting to reduce fractures with displacement.

FRACTURES OF THE SHAFT OF THE ULNA ALONE

Occurrence and Mechanism.—These fractures are rather frequent and are practically always due to direct violence as from a blow in putting the forearm over the head for protection or in falls upon the flexed and pronated forearm. The reason that isolated ulnar fractures do not occur from indirect violence, such as falls upon the hand, is that the force is transmitted upward through the radius, and it would be necessary for the radius to be broken or dislocated before sufficient force to cause a fracture could be transmitted to the ulna. Torsion fractures of the forearm are very rare. Due to the fact that the ulna is subcutaneous throughout its length and also that the isolated fractures of this bone are the result of direct violence, they are frequently compound.

Pathology.—The shaft of the ulna is most frequently broken in its lower half, where it is relatively slender, but may be broken at any point. When the fracture lies in the upper third of the shaft it usually involves the narrow area at the site of the bicipital fossa which lies opposite the bicipital tuberosity on the radius.

The fracture line may be transverse, oblique, spiral, or comminuted and the displacement is usually the direct result of a continuation of the fracturing force rather than of muscle pull, and in a considerable percentage of these injuries there is little or no displacement of the fragments. The brachialis anticus tends to draw the upper fragment forward in flexion, but this pull is

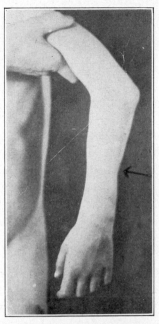

Fig. 656.—Typical deformity in fracture of the shaft of the ulna alone from direct violence.

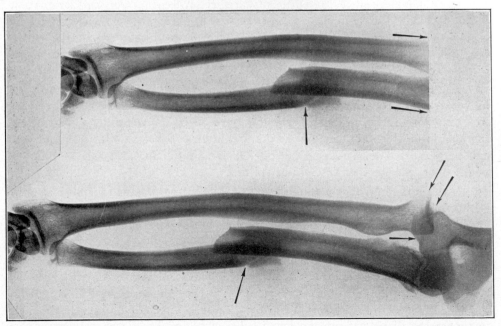

Fig. 657.—Fracture of the ulna. First x-ray, above, did not show any other lesion. Second x-ray, below, showed dislocation of head of radius. When fractures of ulna overlap, the radius must be fractured or dislocated either at the proximal or distal ends. Similar problems can occur with fractures of the tibia.

balanced by the triceps which tends to extend the forearm. The pronator quadratus tends to pull the lower fragment in toward the radius but this muscle is relatively weak. With the radius intact and not displaced, very little overlapping of the fractured ends is possible and the interosseous membrane prevents displacement away from the intact radius. Not infrequently the head of the radius is fractured or displaced.

Diagnosis.—As the shaft of the ulna is subcutaneous, the diagnosis is, as a rule, easily made from the history of the injury and the local swelling, tenderness, and deformity (Fig. 656). Unless the fracture is incomplete, it is usually possible to demonstrate false motion by grasping the two fragments between the fingers and thumb and moving them laterally upon one another. In doubtful cases in which there is no displacement and in which false motion cannot be demonstrated, squeezing the bones of the forearm together causes pain at the site of the fracture even when no pressure is made upon this point. Passive pronation and supination of the hand also elicit local pain, as do attempts to carry out these movements or to extend the elbow against resistance. The surgeon should examine the head of the radius in these injuries to make sure that it is not dislocated or fractured (Fig. 657).

Treatment

1. Cases in Which There Is Practically No Displacement.—In these injuries all that is necessary is to immobilize the extremity. This is most conveniently and comfortably done by applying a posterior plaster mold which extends from the middle of the arm down to the base of the fingers. The arm should be immobilized in the midposition as regards pronation and supination with the elbow flexed about 90 degrees. In applying the posterior mold or cast with the forearm in the midposition the surgeon should pad the entire length of the shaft of the ulna with a thin strip of felt or with an extra amount of sheet cotton.

The elbow and wrist should be immobilized in the first dressing because movements in pronation and supination put strain upon the site of the fracture and cause pain and disability and may result in delayed union. This dressing should be worn about three weeks and at the end of this time the patient can be permitted to use the hand and elbow and the forearm can be splinted with a short plaster cast or mold or splint.

If the surgeon prefers, a board or metal splint or plaster cast may be substituted for the posterior plaster mold suggested above. However, in applying circular bandages around a splint or in applying a plaster cast, care should be taken that the bandage does not squeeze the bones of the forearm together.

2. Fractures With Displacement.—Unless there is a fracture or dislocation of the radius, the displacement will be largely lateral and there will be relatively little overlapping of the fragments. Usually the fractured ends will be displaced forward and inward toward the radius (Figs. 656 and 658). In such instances the displacement can usually be corrected by direct pressure upon the fragments. The patient should have a general or adequate local anesthetic and the forearm should be supported in a position of supination and flexion by an assistant. Then the surgeon, by direct pressure with his thumbs, should force both fragments posteriorly until he has converted the deformity into a posterior bowing of the bone. When this has been accomplished it will usually be possible to get the fingers between the radius and the ulna and force the two bones apart, thus correcting the inward displacement and restoring the width of the interosseous space. After this has been accomplished the posterior bowing can be gradually corrected by direct pressure. If the fragments are overlapped, the posterior bowing, if carried far enough, will usually result in springing them by one another and getting them end on. If this is not successful, the assistant should make traction on the flexed and supinated forearm and force the hand into a position of lateral deviation in order to exert as much traction as possible upon the shaft of the ulna. This maneuver should be carried out by the assistant while the surgeon forces the fragments backward and produces the posterior bowing at the site of the fracture. If the proximal fragment is displaced anteriorly, the forearm should be fully pronated and immobilized in pronation.

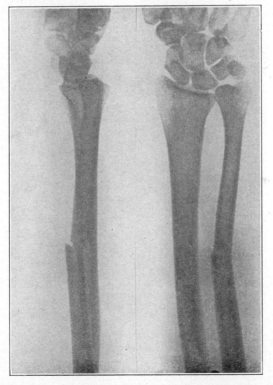

Fig. 658.—Fracture of the shaft of the ulna with angulation. Treated by manipulative correction of the deformity (ether anesthesia) and immobilization in a posterior plaster mold to arm and forearm and hand (right angle at elbow) for six weeks. Sling to forearm for two weeks. Good result.

These maneuvers, if properly carried out, will accomplish reduction in most cases. However, if they are not successful, the surgeon should then try the subcutaneous lever of Thompson. A small Steinmann pin is thrust through the skin and with fluoroscopic control is guided between the fragments and they are pried apart and permitted to settle back into a satisfactory position. If this is not successful, an open operation may be necessary.

Immobilization.—After the displacement has been corrected, the forearm should be flexed about 90 degrees and placed in the midposition between pronation and supination and a straight wood splint slightly wider than the forearm at its widest part and long enough to reach from the posterior surface of the elbow to the bases of the fingers should be strapped to the dorsal surface of the hand, wrist, and forearm and lateral surface of the elbow with adhesive. A short wood splint of equal width should then be strapped on the volar surface of the forearm directly opposite the site of the fracture.

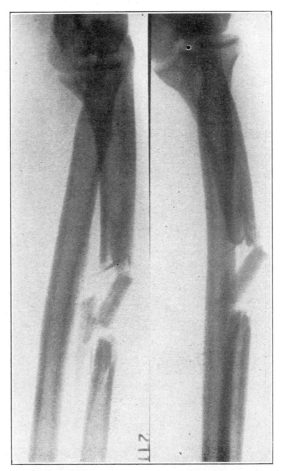

Fig. 659.—Compound comminuted fracture of the shaft of the ulna treated by conservative débridement with sulfonamide locally and closure of the wound and skeletal traction to the forearm with aid of lateral traction frame for four weeks, then immobilization in anterior and posterior plaster molds extending from the middle of the arm to the wrist for three weeks and a circular cast for five weeks with good result. As the large fragments retained their periosteal attachments, they were not removed.

The splints should be cut and padded with sheet cotton before the reduction is begun. The long dorsal splint maintains the alignment of the forearm and the short volar splint presses the soft tissues in between the bones and tends to keep the bones apart and maintain the width of the interosseous space. The volar splint need be only about 4 inches long or it may extend from the bend of the elbow to the fold of the wrist. The splints should be strapped on with broad strips of adhesive with moderate pressure, but not tightly enough to constrict the fingers.

After the splints have been applied, they should be incorporated in a light plaster cast extending from the middle of the arm to the finger tips.

After the reduction and application of the splints anteroposterior and lateral x-rays should be taken. If the fragments are not in good position, another attempt at reduction should be made. If the reduction is satisfactory the dressing should remain in place for from four to six weeks depending upon the age of the patient and the severity of the fracture. At the end of this time it should be removed and the solidity of the union tested. If the union seems quite solid, a short plaster mold or cast or wood or metal splint should be applied and the patient may begin to move the elbow and wrist. If the union is not solid, the complete dressing should be reapplied and continued as long as necessary.

The shaft of the ulna unites rather slowly and after complete fractures with displacement, it is a good plan for the patient to wear some form of splint at least eight weeks if a child and ten weeks if an adult.

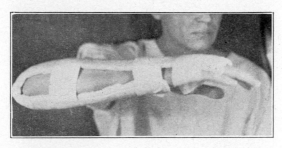

Fig. 660.—The so-called sugar tong plaster made of a single long molded plaster slab. Used in the treatment of fractures of the shaft of the radius or ulna or of both bones in which immobilization at the elbow is not necessary as regards flexion and extension, but where rotation of the forearm is not desired. This splint is not to be used if there is a tendency for the fragments to become misplaced. (See Figs. 676, 677 and 678.)

Stiffness of the fingers should be avoided by having the patient move them on the day after the reduction and continue to exercise them several times daily during the period of immobilization.

Operative Reduction of Fractures of the Shaft of the Ulna Alone.—Under careful asepsis a small incision should be made in the skin directly over the site of the fracture. The incision should be carried down to the bone, and after the soft tissues have been retracted, the ends of the bones should be levered into end to end apposition and pulled outward to restore the width of the interosseous space. As a rule no internal fixation will be necessary and the wound can be closed in layers and the posterior plaster mold or splint applied and the fracture treated as though it had not been operated upon. If the reduction is unstable the ends can be tied together with chromic catgut passed through drill holes in each fragment.

After operation a very thin dressing should be placed over the wound because thick dressings will tend to displace the fragments inward again.

FRACTURES OF THE SHAFT OF THE RADIUS ALONE

Occurrence and Mechanism.—Isolated fractures of the shaft of the radius are relatively rare because the hard compact shaft is considerably stronger than the lower cancellous end of the bone. However, these fractures may result from direct violence such as a blow upon the radial side of the arm, or from indirect violence such as a fall upon the hand in which the force has not been sufficient to cause a fracture of both bones. The shaft may be broken at any level, but the fractures usually occur in the exposed middle and lower thirds rather than in the upper third which is fairly well covered with muscles.

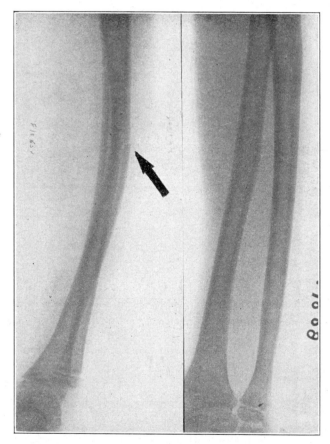

Fig. 661.—Greenstick fracture of the shaft of the radius with posterior bowing. This is rare as the bones are usually bowed toward the flexor surface of the forearm. Treated by manipulative correction of the deformity and immobilization in sugar tong splint for six weeks. Good result.

Pathology of Fractures of the Shaft of the Radius Alone.—The fracture line is usually roughly transverse but may be oblique or comminuted and in the lower portion the fractures are apt to be compound. In children the fractures of the shaft are often incomplete, those of the shaft proper being of the greenstick type (Fig. 661) while those near the lower end tend to be of the infraction type.

As contrasted with the ulna, the displacement of the fragments in fractures of the shaft of the radius depends largely upon the pull of the muscles rather than upon the fracturing force and in consequence varies with the level at which the fracture occurs. Also, displacement of the fragments is much more frequent than is the case in fractures of the ulna because the radius is the movable bone of the forearm and its ends are readily displaced during rotation around the ulna.

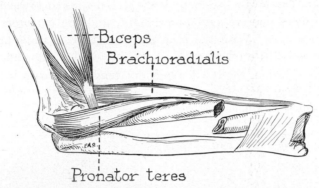

Fig. 662.—Drawing to show effect of muscle pull on fractures of the shaft of the radius below the insertion of the pronator teres.

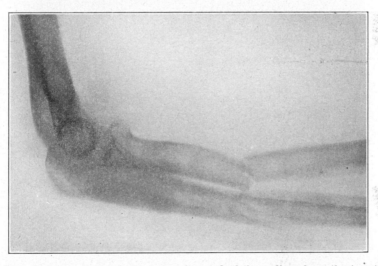

Fig. 663.—Fracture of the shaft of the ulna and of the radius above the insertion of the pronator teres muscle. Treated by manipulative reduction and immobilization with anterior and posterior plaster molds with the forearm moderately flexed and fully supinated. Good result.

The character of the displacement depends upon whether the fracture occurs above or below the insertion of the pronator teres muscle. In fractures above the insertion of the pronator teres—that is in the upper half of the shaft and below the bicipital tubercle, the upper fragment is supinated by the supinator brevis and the biceps and drawn forward (flexed) by the biceps while the lower fragment is pronated by the pronator teres and the pronator quadratus and is drawn inward toward the shaft of the ulna by the above two muscles, and by the supinator longus and the extensors and abductors of the thumb. The pronator teres also tends to draw the lower fragment forward; but with the ulna intact and the inferior radio-ulnar articulations intact, there is little tendency to overlapping of the fragments.

In fractures below the insertion of the pronator teres, that is, in the lower half of the shaft, the upper fragment is displaced forward by the biceps, and forward and inward by the pronator teres, but tends to remain in the neutral position as regards rotation because the tendency to supination by the biceps and supinator brevis is counteracted by the tendency to pronation by the pronator teres. The lower fragment is displaced inward toward the ulna by the pronator quadratus, the supinator longus, and the extensors and the abductors of the thumb. With the ulna and the inferior radio-ulnar articulation intact, there is little tendency to overriding of the fragments. (Fig. 635.)

As regards rotation, the lower fragment tends to remain in a position to pronation, but it may be supinated by the hand as it tends to follow the hand in all movements of rotation.

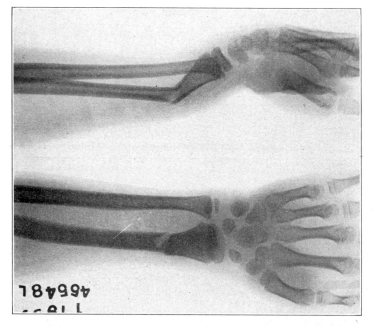

Fig. 664.—Fracture of the shaft of the radius with anterior bowing of the lower fragment.

Diagnosis of Fractures of the Shaft of the Radius Alone.—The patient tends to carry the forearm in flexion and pronation and there is complete loss of active supination. There is moderate swelling and tenderness over the site of the fracture, and in fractures in the lower half of the bone with displacement it is usually possible to detect the abnormality in the contour by palpation; but in fractures in the upper half, the muscles over the bone make palpation more difficult.

In fractures of the lower half of the shaft it may be possible to grasp the fragments between the thumb and fingers and move them laterally upon one another and thus demonstrate false motion and crepitus, but crepitus is, of course, not obtained in the complete fractures with wide separation of the fragments.

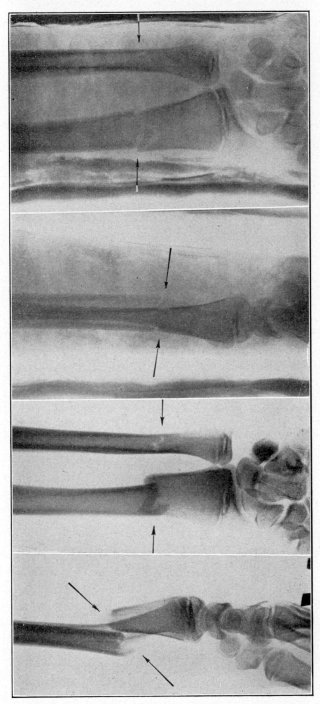

Fig. 665.—Fracture of both bones of the forearm, lower fourth, with radius displaced. Reduced by manipulation and immobilized in a plaster cast with board splints to the flexor and extensor surfaces of the forearm.

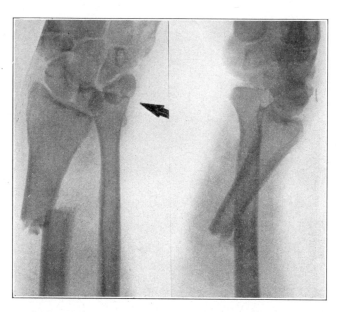

Fig. 666.—Fracture of the shaft of the radius with anterior and lateral displacement of the lower fragment and forward displacement of the lower end of the ulna. Treated by manipulative reduction of both lesions and then immobilized in anterior and posterior wood splints incorporated in a plaster cast. Good result.

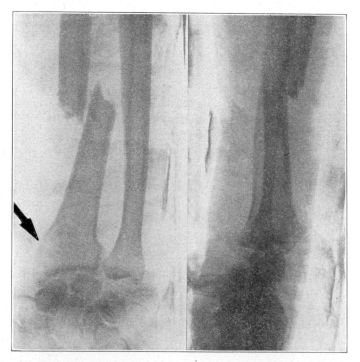

Fig. 667.—Fracture of the shaft of the radius below the insertion of the pronator teres. Treated by open reduction and fixation with chromic catgut with anterior and posterior splints incorporated in a plaster cast for eight weeks. There is also a fracture of the lateral margin of the lower end of the radius (styloid). Good result.

A pathognomonic sign of fracture of the shaft of the radius is the demonstration that the head of the bone does not rotate with the lower end when the hand is supinated and pronated. However, the fact that the head does rotate with the shaft is no evidence that a fracture is not present because the fragments may be interlocked.

In fractures of the shaft of the radius with displacement the surgeon should always examine the inferior radio-ulnar joint, as this may be disrupted and the lower end of the ulna may be dislocated (Fig. 666).

In fractures without separation in which the diagnosis is difficult, local pain at the site of the fracture can be produced by squeezing the bones of the forearm together or by abducting the hand or by gently rotating the hand, but the surgeon should be careful in performing these maneuvers as he should endeavor to make the diagnosis without causing displacement of the fragments.

In incomplete fractures in children, the x-ray may be necessary to clear up the diagnosis.

Treatment

The treatment depends upon the site of the fracture.

1. **The Treatment of Fractures of the Shaft of the Radius Above the Insertion of the Pronator Teres.**—In these fractures the proximal fragment which cannot be controlled by the surgeon is supinated and flexed by the action of the muscles. Consequently the distal fragment, the movements of which can be controlled by the surgeon, should be placed in this position and the forearm should be immobilized in flexion and supination. If there is no displacement of the fragments, all that is necessary is to supinate the forearm and flex the elbow to about 90 degrees and apply a posterior wooden splint or plaster mold extending from the middle of the arm to the base of the fingers. The splint should be incorporated in a light plaster cast.

In a complete fracture in adults this dressing should be worn at least six weeks because fractures of the shaft of the radius are relatively slow in healing. At the end of this time the long posterior splint or mold can be removed and the movements of the forearm and firmness of the union can be tested and x-rayed. If union appears quite firm, the patient can be permitted to begin to move the wrist and elbow, and the forearm can be splinted for about two weeks longer with a light plaster mold or board splint.

If the surgeon prefers, the immobilization can be accomplished with a plaster cast or a plaster cast applied over board splints as described under fractures of the ulna; but care should be taken in applying circular dressings that the bones of the forearm are not squeezed together by the bandage.

In fractures with displacement the displacement should be reduced; this can usually be accomplished in the following manner:

Under general or adequate local anesthesia the elbow should be flexed to a right angle and the forearm fully supinated and the fragments at the site of the fracture should be forced directly backward to produce a posterior bowing. When this has been accomplished, the surgeon should endeavor to force the fragments away from the ulna by pressure in the interosseous space and lateral pressure on the prominent ends of the fragments and then the posterior bowing can be corrected by gentle pressure. If there is no overriding of the fragments it will usually be possible to correct the deformity in this manner.

In fractures with overriding of the fragments traction on the radius is necessary and this traction must be very strong because it is difficult to affect the radius with the ulna intact. This may be obtained by having the arm fixed by a sling or bandage fastened to some immovable object while traction is made by an assistant who exerts most of his power on the thumb and holds the hand in a position of ulnar deviation while the traction is applied. In order that he may get a firm grip on the hand and thumb, it is often advisable to apply adhesive tape to these parts. The traction is applied with the forearm flexed and supinated and during the application of the traction the surgeon should carry out the manipulations described in the preceding paragraph and in this manner it will usually be possible to obtain reduction.

Immobilization.—After reduction the elbow should be flexed to about 60 degrees and supinated and a wooden splint well padded with sheet cotton slightly wider than the widest part of the forearm and long enough to extend from the tip of the olecranon to the base of the fingers should be applied to the dorsal surface and strapped on with adhesive. Then a short wood splint well padded of equal width should be strapped firmly to the volar surface of the forearm directly over the fracture. Care must be taken not to constrict the circulation at the elbow. These splints should be incorporated in a light plaster cast which should be worn from six to eight weeks or longer if necessary until the union is quite firm. (Figs. 682 and 683.)

Stiffness of the fingers should be avoided by having the patient begin to move them on the day after the fracture and continue to exercise them several times daily as long as the cast is worn.

2. **Treatment of Fractures of the Shaft of the Radius Below the Insertion of the Pronator Teres.**—In these fractures the forearm should be immobilized in the midposition as regards rotation and with the elbow flexed about 90 degrees.

In fractures without displacement all that is necessary is to apply anterior and posterior plaster molds from the middle of the arm to the base of the fingers with the forearm in the midposition as regards rotation and the elbow flexed about 90 degrees.

If one prefers, anterior and posterior wooden or metal splints or a plaster cast may be used in place of the mold, but care should be taken to avoid constricting the forearm by the bandage and squeezing the bones together.

In complete fractures the immobilization should be continued for at least six weeks. At the end of this time the anterior and posterior molds can be removed and the stability of the fracture tested and an x-ray taken. If it is fairly firm, the patient may be permitted to use the elbow and wrist, and the forearm can be splinted by a short plaster mold, splint, or cast. This should be continued from two to four weeks longer, at the end of which time union should be firm and support should no longer be needed.

In fractures with displacement with or without overriding, the reduction is accomplished in exactly the same manner as described above except that the manipulations are carried out with the elbow flexed at 90 degrees and the forearm in the midposition as regards pronation and supination. If there is dislocation at the inferior radio-ulnar joint this must be carefully reduced and immobilized.

After reduction the fracture should be immobilized with the elbow flexed to 90 degrees and the forearm in the midposition as regards rotation for eight to ten weeks. The long dorsal and short volar wooden splints incorporated in a light plaster cast extending from the middle of the arm to the base of the fingers as was described in the treatment of fractures of the ulna alone, should be used until the union is quite firm and should then be replaced by a short cast or splint which permits motion at the elbow and wrist. In three instances in which manipulation failed, one of us (J. A. K.) has used the subcutaneous pin of J. E. M. Thompson and levered the fragments into position.

Open Reduction of Fractures of the Shaft of the Radius Alone.—If the surgeon is unable to accomplish reduction from manipulation, open reduction should be resorted to (Fig. 667). The operation is a simple one; all that is necessary is to make a small incision directly over the bone, retracting the muscles and tendons, pull the bones outward and lever them in end to end apposition and correct alignment and close the wound in layers without drainage. After the wound is closed, long posterior and short anterior wood splints and a plaster cast should be applied and the fracture treated as described above, just as though no operation had been performed. If the fracture line is oblique and the fragments unstable after reduction, they may be tied together with chromic catgut, or stainless steel wire.

FRACTURES OF BOTH BONES OF THE FOREARM

Occurrence and Mechanism.—These fractures are fairly frequent, especially in children, and are usually the result of falls upon the outstretched hand, but they may be the result of direct violence as a blow on the forearm or

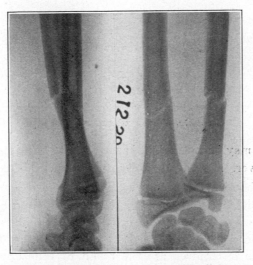

Fig. 668.—Fracture of both bones of the forearm with slight anterior bowing. No manipulation necessary. Treated by anterior and posterior wooden splints incorporated in a plaster cast, with good result.

a fall upon the surface of the forearm. They are occasionally caused by bending forces or by getting the forearm caught lengthwise between two approaching objects.

Pathology.—Most of the fractures occur in the lower half of the bones and are rather rare in the upper half. In those the result of direct violence the bones tend to be broken at approximately the same level (Fig. 668) while in those due to indirect violence they are often broken at different levels and the fracture of the ulna is usually at a lower level than is that of the radius.

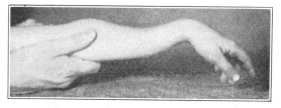

Fig. 669.—Typical deformity with anterior bowing in greenstick fracture of both bones of the forearm in a child.

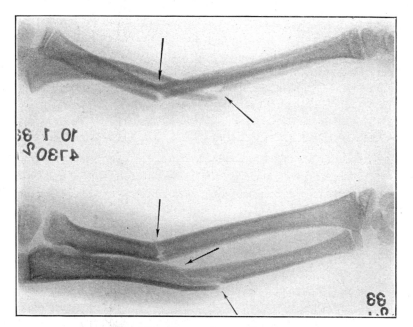

Fig. 670.—X-ray of preceding case.

The fractures may be incomplete, complete, or multiple, and the fracture lines may be transverse, oblique, spiral, or comminuted. Impaction is rare.

Because these bones are relatively subcutaneous and the fractures are often caused by direct violence, they are frequently compound and may be accompanied by extensive destruction of the soft tissues. In children the fractures are frequently incomplete and of the greenstick or infraction type. Most of the greenstick fractures in children are the result of falls upon the palm of the hand, and the tendency is for the force to produce an anterior bowing of both bones (Fig. 669). Occasionally the patient falls on the back of the hand and the bones are bowed posteriorly.

The displacement is partly determined by the direction of the fracturing force and partly by the action of the muscles. The fracturing force may produce angulation in any direction or push either the lower or upper fragments in any direction with the radius and ulna in approximately their normal relation to one another; but when the bones are completely fractured, the muscles

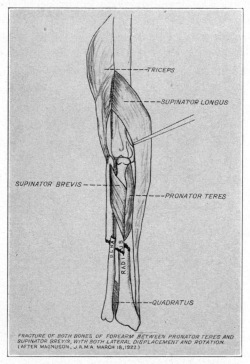

Fig. 671.—Drawing to show displacement in fracture of both bones of the forearm below the insertion of the pronator teres. (After Magnuson: J. A. M. A. March 18, 1922.)

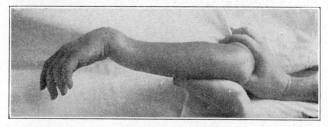

Fig. 672.—Typical fixed deformity in greenstick fracture of both bones of the forearm in a child.

of the forearm exert a decided influence upon them in certain directions and thus are an important factor in the final displacement. The interosseous membrane always remains intact and prevents divergence of the bones. The final displacement in fractures with complete separation of the fragments is largely dependent upon whether the fracture line lies above or below the insertion of the pronator teres just as was described in fractures of the radius alone.

In fractures above the insertion of the pronator teres, the **proximal fragment of the radius is flexed** by the biceps and supinated by **the biceps and** supinator brevis muscles, while the distal fragments of both bones **are approximated** by the pronator quadratus and that of the radius is tilted in toward the ulna by the supinator longus and the extensors and abductors of the thumb.

In fractures of both bones below the insertion of the pronator teres the upper fragment of the radius tends to remain in the neutral position **as regards** rotation because the pronator teres counteracts the supinating **action of** the supinator brevis and biceps and it is drawn inward toward the **ulna** by the pronator teres and slightly flexed by the biceps while the distal **fragments** of both bones are drawn toward one another by the pronator **teres,** supinator longus, and extensors and abductors of the thumb.   (Fig. 671.)

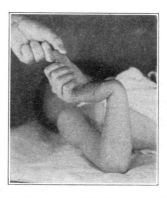

Fig. 673.—Fracture of both bones of the forearm with marked deformity.

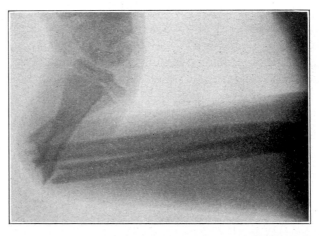

Fig. 674.—Roentgenogram of preceding case. Treated by manipulative reduction and immobilized in anteroposterior wooden splints incorporated in a plaster cast. Good result.

In fractures at any level in which the fragments are displaced **upon one** another all of the muscles of the forearm tend to draw the lower **fragments** upward and cause shortening and overlapping of the bones. Whether **or not** the fragments lie anterior or posterior or lateral to one another is **largely** determined by the fracturing force and by gravity.

Diagnosis.—The diagnosis of complete fractures of both bones of the forearm is obvious. There is complete disability with swelling, tenderness, and deformity at the site of the fracture and false motion can be demonstrated (Figs. 673 and 674). If there is no deformity or shortening and no displacement of the fragments, the diagnosis can be made from the disability, local pain, tenderness, and swelling and the surgeon should be very careful in manipulating such cases as manipulation may result in displacement; it is much easier to get the bones off than to get them back in place again.

In incomplete fractures in children there may be marked posterior or anterior bowing of both bones and the severe angulation deformity tends to be fixed (Fig. 672) or there may be no deformity and the diagnosis must be made from the pain, disability, swelling, and local tenderness over both bones, but should be confirmed by the x-ray.

In cases with or without displacement it is usually advisable to obtain an x-ray in order to ascertain the exact nature of the lesion before attempting treatment because these are among the most difficult of all fractures to treat successfully and the surgeon should know exactly what he is dealing with in order that he may adopt appropriate measures.

Treatment

Cases Without Displacement.—In these injuries which comprise a considerable percentage of the fractures of both bones of the forearm the surgeon should be careful not to cause displacement of the fragments by his manipulations. All that is necessary is to immobilize the forearm in the midposition as regards rotation, with the elbow in a position of 90 degrees flexion over a period of from six to eight weeks, depending upon the age of the patient (Fig. 675). In all of these fractures, however, we feel that it is important that the elbow and lower half of the arm be included in the immobilization in order that rotation may be controlled.

The method of immobilization which we have found most satisfactory in these cases is as follows: A posterior wooden splint slightly wider than the forearm at its widest part and long enough to extend from the posterior surface of the elbow to the first joints of the fingers is padded with sheet cotton and strapped to the forearm with adhesive (Fig. 676A). An anterior wooden splint of equal width and long enough to extend from the point of the elbow and to the fold of the wrist is then strapped to the volar surface (Fig. 676B). These splints are applied tightly enough so that they hold the forearm firmly, but can be compressed upon one another with moderate pressure to the extent that the adhesive strapping will be loosened. The extremity from the middle of the arm down to the ends of the splints is then covered with sheet cotton and the whole is incorporated in a plaster cast. (Figs. 677 and 678.) The object of the wooden splints, and especially the posterior splint, is to correct and maintain the alignment of the forearm, while the moderate pressure exerted by the two splints tends to force the soft parts between the bones and thus maintain the width of the interosseous space.

This type of dressing we find is much more efficient than the splints alone and is much more safely applied than is a plaster mold or cast, since there is practically no tendency for the fragments to be displaced during the application of the dressing as is apt to occur if one attempts to apply a circular plaster cast. Also the circular cast, if applied to the arm without the previous application of a splint, tends to squeeze the bones together and obliterate the inter osseous space.

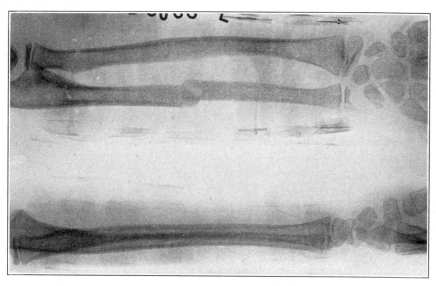

Fig. 675.—Fracture of both bones of the forearm with slight displacement of the ulna. No correction necessary. Treated by plaster cast. Good result.

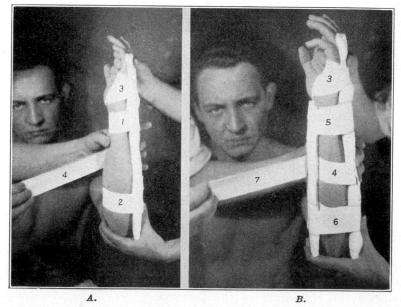

A.   B.

Fig. 676.—A, Application of the long posterior padded wooden splint after reduction of fractures of both bones of the forearm. The splint extends from the middle phalanges of the fingers to a point beyond the elbow; the elbow at a right angle.

B, Application of the long padded anterior wooden splint after reduction of fractures of both bones of the forearm. This splint extends from the bend in the wrist to a point beyond the elbow. Extending these splints beyond the elbow prevents rotation of the forearm.

If one objects to the wooden splints under the cast a dressing similar to the above may be applied by substituting a plaster mold for the wooden splints. The plaster mold should be long enough to reach from the first joints of the fingers along the extensor surface of the forearm around the elbow and down to cover the palm. In some clinics this is called a sugar tong plaster. It should then be incorporated in a plaster cast which includes the lower half of the arm as otherwise flexion and extension of the elbow would not be controlled. (Figs. 727 and 728.)

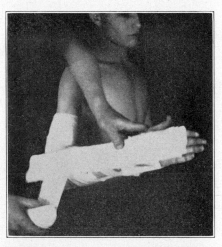

Fig. 677.—Application of sheet cotton to the arm and wooden splints in the treatment of fractures of both bones of the forearm. The elbow must be included in these cases because no rotation should take place.

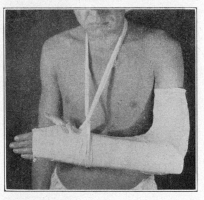

Fig. 678.—The arm, elbow, and splints incorporated in a plaster cast in the treatment of fractures of both bones of the forearm.

This dressing lacks the compression of the soft part between the splints; this we believe is very important in preventing a narrowing of the interosseous space.

Fractures of Both Bones of the Forearm With Angulation But No Displacement.—In these fractures the angulation should be corrected by slow, steady pressure. A simple method is to lay the forearm on a firm table or board with the convexity of the deformity upward and then by direct

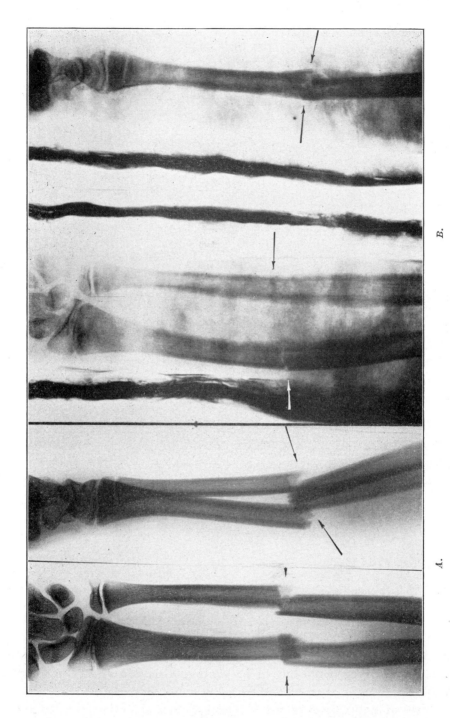

A.

B.

Fig. 679.—*A*, A transverse fracture of the radius and ulna, middle third, with overlapping of fragments. *B*, Anatomical restoration of the displaced fragments following closed reduction with the anteroposterior wooden splints applied and incorporated in circular plaster cast as described. Excellent functional and anatomical result.

pressure over the convexity straighten the bones. Then the wrist is lifted
up from the table or board a short distance while the bones above the fracture are held against it in order to slightly overcorrect the deformity. Another
method is to have the arm fixed by an assistant or by a strap around the
lower portion of the arm, and then the elbow should be flexed to 90 degrees
and maintained in a position of almost full supination, and an assistant should

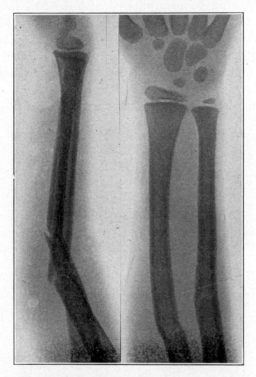

Fig. 680.—Fracture of both bones of the forearm above the insertion of the pronator teres
with deformity, but no displacement. Treated by correction of the deformity and immobilization in anterior and posterior board splints incorporated in a plaster cast with good result.
Great care was taken not to cause displacement during application of the cast.

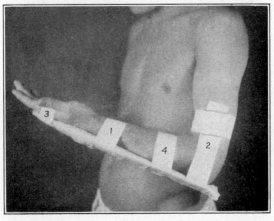

Fig. 681.—Method of applying a posterior board splint to the dorsal surface of the forearm for the treatment of fractures of the shaft of the radius above the insertion of the pronator teres.

make slow, steady traction on the wrist. The surgeon is then free to use both hands in correcting the deformity. In most instances the deformity will be an anterior bowing with some narrowing of the interosseous space. This tendency of the interosseous space to be narrowed can usually be corrected by the surgeon pressing firmly with the fingers and thumbs of both hands between the two bones and thus gradually forcing them apart by the pressure of the soft tissues (Fig. 680). If the fracture of the radius is in the upper half of the bone, the forearm should be manipulated and dressed in a position of full supination. If the fracture of the radius is in the lower half of the shaft of the bone, the manipulation should be conducted with the forearm in a position of moderate supination and the dressing should be applied with the forearm in the midposition exactly as was described above under fractures without displacement. In these fractures we think it is especially important that the wooden splints be used beneath the plaster cast. (Figs. 676, 677, and 678.)

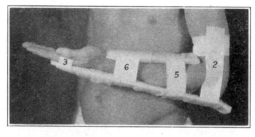

Fig. 682.—Application of short anterior board splint to make compression between the fragments in fractures of the shaft of the radius above the insertion of the pronator teres.

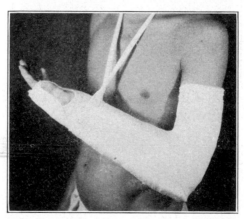

Fig. 683.—Incorporation of the two preceding splints in a plaster cast with the elbow fully supinated and flexed slightly beyond a right angle in treatment of fractures of the shaft of the radius above the insertion of the pronator teres.

In cases in which the fracture in the radius is in the upper half of the shaft the forearm should be immobilized in a position of full supination with the elbow flexed to at least 90 degrees. This is best done by applying a well-padded posterior wooden splint to the dorsum of the flexed and supinated forearm as illustrated in Fig. 681. Then a shorter well-padded anterior wooden splint should be applied as illustrated in Fig. 682. Care must be taken that the upper end of this splint is not too close to the fold at the elbow and does not cause undue pressure at this point. The lower end of the splint may reach to the base of the fingers or it may only reach to the fold of the wrist.

These splints should be applied tightly enough to exert moderate pressure on the soft parts and thus tend to force the bones apart, but not so tightly that they will cause undue pressure, ischemic paralysis, and contracture of the muscles.

After these splints have been applied, the arm and forearm should be covered with sheet cotton and incorporated in a plaster cast as illustrated in Fig. 683.

If the surgeon objects to the wooden splints in these fractures, anterior and posterior plaster molds may be applied. These should then be incorporated in a light plaster cast or they may be immobilized in a gauze bandage and adhesive. In applying the anterior plaster mold, care should be taken that no undue pressure is exerted at the fold of the elbow.

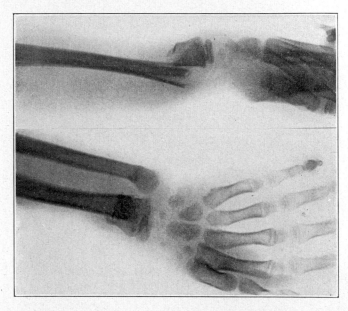

Fig. 684.—Typical low fracture of both bones of the forearm with complete displacement in a child. Treated by manipulative reduction and anterior and posterior wooden splints incorporated in a plaster cast.

Treatment of Fractures of Both Bones of the Forearm With Complete Displacement of the Fragments.—These are rightly considered among the most difficult of all fractures to treat. If the fractures are relatively transverse and the contour of the fractured ends is such that the surgeon feels that when properly reduced they will remain reduced, he should make a serious effort to obtain reduction by manipulative methods before he resorts to open operation, and if the manipulation described below is carefully followed out, it will usually be possible to obtain a satisfactory reduction. (Figs. 684 and 686.)

One reason so many competent surgeons fail so frequently in their attempts at the reduction of these fractures is that they use the method of angulation and attempt to engage the fragments of one bone and then use this

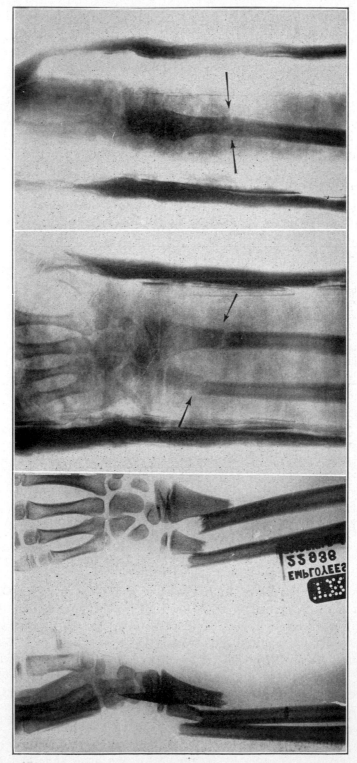

Fig. 685.—Fracture of both bones of the forearm in the lower third. Manipulation unsuccessful. Reduced by operation and the fragments fixed with chromic catgut and immobilized in a plaster-of-Paris cast over board splints.

bone as a lever on which to rock the other fragments into place. This method occasionally succeeds, but much more frequently it fails, and it should be abandoned.

The secret of reducing these fractures is to ignore the presence of two bones and reduce the fracture by the method of traction exactly as though only one bone existed in the forearm. In order to do this a great amount of force which can be perfectly controlled is necessary. (Figs. 689, 690, and 691.)

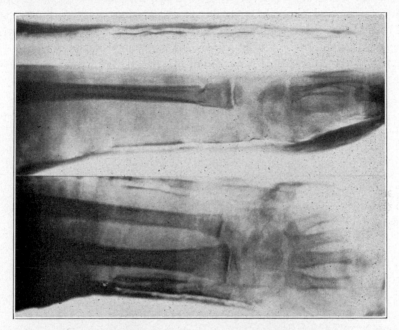

Fig. 686.—Anteroposterior and lateral view of the case shown in Fig. 684 after closed reduction, showing the effect of the posterior wooden splint in maintaining the alignment of the fragments.

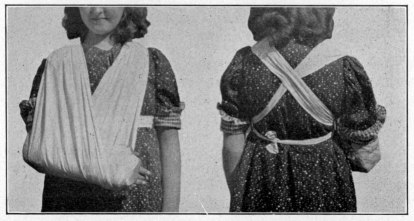

Fig. 687.—Method of arranging a sling by extending the ends of a long sling around the chest to take the weight off the back of the neck.

When adequate local or general anesthesia has been obtained, the elbow should be flexed to a right angle and the front of the arm above the elbow protected by a felt pad and then immobilized by a broad, strong strap which is fixed to the table or a door handle or some other unyielding object. This is for countertraction. It is frequently possible for a strong assistant to hold the arm, but this is not so satisfactory because he is always liable to let it slip at a critical moment. The fingers and thumb should then be strapped with adhesive tape in order that the assistant who makes traction on the hand may get a good grip. The forearm is then placed in a position of moderate to full supination, depending upon whether the fracture in the radius is below or above the insertion of the pronator teres, and the elbow is flexed to 90 degrees. A husky assistant should then secure a firm grip upon the hand and fingers and make slow, steady, and powerful traction in the long axis of the bones of the forearm. One of us (J. A. K.) uses the Soutter traction apparatus for traction and counter-traction and has found it satisfactory.

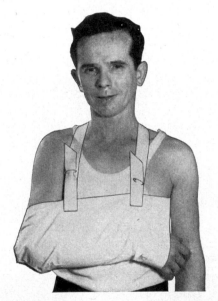

Fig. 688.—Zimmer arm sling. (Courtesy Zimmer Manufacturing Co.)

While the traction is maintained, the surgeon should manipulate the fragments with his fingers and thumb and endeavor to press the bones into line and to increase the width of the interosseous space by making firm pressure over the soft parts between the two bones. As a rule, if the traction is strong enough the ends of the fractured bones will slip by one another and tend to engage without assistance on the part of the surgeon and his main effort should be directed toward pressing the bones apart and increasing the width of the interosseous space.

When the surgeon feels that adequate reduction has been obtained, the forearm should be placed in the desired position depending upon the type of fracture; and the anterior or posterior wooden splints as described above should be applied and strapped on with adhesive. Then these should be incorporated in a plaster cast and the traction gently released and the plaster cast extended to the middle of the arm. If the fracture of the radius is above the insertion of the pronator teres, this dressing should be applied with the forearm in a position of full supination. If it is below the pronator teres the dressing should be applied with the forearm in the midposition. If the surgeon prefers, plaster molds may be used instead of the wood splints, but if they are used it is well to use the two small wood cylinders (about one-half inch in diameter and two inches long) over the molds to press the bones apart. Then the molds and the wood cylinders are incorporated in a light plaster cast which extends from the upper arm to the knuckles.

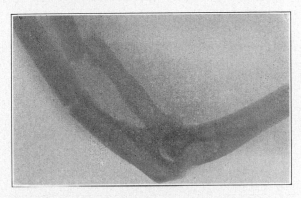

Fig 689.—Fracture of both bones of the forearm above the insertion of the pronator teres. Treated by closed manipulative reduction and immobilization in anterior and posterior wooden splints incorporated in plaster cast.

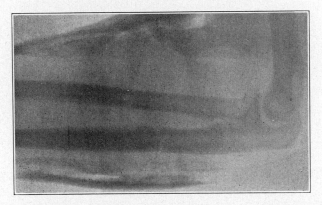

Fig. 690.—Same as preceding showing result obtained by closed manipulative reduction.

If the fractures are oblique or the bones are comminuted so that the ends will be unstable and tend to slip by one another after a satisfactory reduction, this can be prevented by placing Kirschner wires through the fragments and incorporating these wires in the plaster cast. The proximal wire should pass through the ulna just below the elbow and the distal wire should pass through the radius and the ulna about one inch above the wrist joint. When placing the distal wire the bones should be in the position in which it is expected to immobilize them after the reduction. After the plaster has set the ends of the wires should be fixed by clamps to prevent bending, which leads to displacement and movement of the wires, which may lead to infection.

The position obtained should be checked by anteroposterior and lateral x-rays, and if the reduction has not been successful another attempt may be made before resorting to open operation, but repeated manipulations may injure the soft tissues and are not to be undertaken unless there is some definite indication that another attempt may accomplish satisfactory reduction. At the second attempt a sterile subcutaneous lever or pin should be at hand and this should be used after the method of J. E. M. Thompson by pushing it through the skin and getting its end between the two fragments and levering them apart and then end on under the fluoroscope. In this way an open reduction may be avoided.

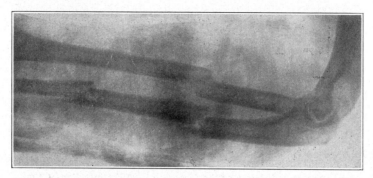

Fig. 691.—Multiple fracture of both bones of the forearm. Treated by manipulative reduction and immobilization in anterior and posterior board splints incorporated in a plaster cast, forearm in midpronation and supination. Good result.

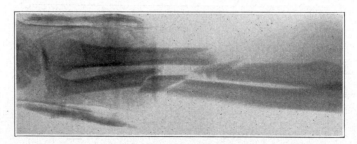

Fig. 692.—Compound comminuted fracture of both bones of the forearm. Treated by débridement and closure; then, suspension and traction, and later immobilized in anteroposterior wooden splints to forearm incorporated in a plaster cast for five weeks; sugar tong molded splint for three weeks. Good result in seventeen weeks.

Treatment of Fractures of Both Bones of the Forearm by Traction.—In fractures of both bones of the forearm in which there is comminution of one or both bones (Fig. 692), or in which there is a long oblique fracture line which will not remain in position even when reduced, it may not be possible to maintain a satisfactory position in the cast after the reduction. If the surgeon does not choose to use the Kirschner wires in the cast to maintain the position of the fragments after reduction, these fractures may be treated by traction; our experience has been that this traction is best applied with the patient in bed. By use of Conwell's lateral traction frame the traction bands are applied to the forearm, and the forearm is suspended. The arm down to the elbow is then bound firmly to the arm board of the lateral traction frame. This is most comfortably and successfully done if the arm and the board are included in a plaster cast which is moderately padded with sheet cotton. The cast should extend down to the fold of the elbow but should not make undue pressure upon the muscles of the forearm. For the first twenty-four hours about 10 to 12 pounds of traction should be applied to the forearm. At the end of this time roentgenograms, by means of portable apparatus, should be made in the anteroposterior and lateral direction in order to determine the position of the fragments. If the position is satisfactory a long wooden splint should be strapped to the dorsal surface of the forearm to immobilize the fragments and the weight can be reduced 6 to 10 pounds. If there is overriding of the fragments, the weight on the forearm should be increased, depending upon the muscular development of the individual.

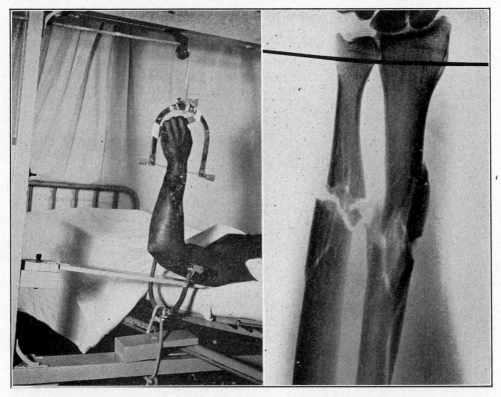

Fig. 693.—Compound comminuted fracture of both bones of the forearm. Treated by débridement and skeletal traction and countertraction for eighteen days; then immobilized in a plaster-of-Paris cast with good result.

If full length has been obtained and lateral displacement or narrowing of the interosseous space exists, an attempt should be made to correct this by manipulation. The traction is not disturbed. The surgeon manipulates the fragments as described above, and endeavors to align them, and by pressure on the soft parts between the bones, to force the bones apart and restore the width of the interosseous space. After the manipulation, well-padded long posterior and short anterior board splints are applied to maintain the pressure on the soft parts and keep the bones apart.

In fractures in which the radius is broken above the insertion of the pronator teres, the forearm should be immobilized in a position of full supination.

In fractures in which the radius is broken below the pronator teres, the forearm should be immobilized in the midposition. The lower end of the wooden splint should be strapped to the plaster cast around the arm and the arm board by adhesive tape. This fixing of the splints to the arm board controls the rotation of the forearm.

In compound fractures in which injuries to the soft parts make it impracticable to apply adhesive traction to the skin of the forearm, skeletal traction should be used. This is best obtained by a small rustless steel wire which is passed through both bones of the forearm at a point about one inch above the wrist joint. This wire is less painful and more satisfactory than the adhesive traction.

We believe that especially in the comminuted type of fracture much better results can be obtained with one of the methods described above than by an open operation. Some surgeons are able to obtain good results in these comminuted fractures of both bones of the forearm by means of an ambulatory traction splint such as that designed by Cleary.

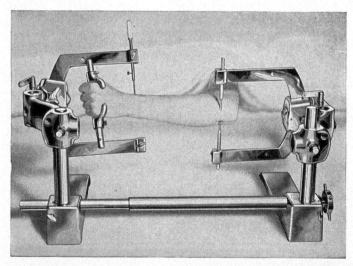

Fig. 694.—Zimmer fracture reduction apparatus applied to forearm. (Courtesy Zimmer Manufacturing Company.)

Operative Treatment of Fractures of Both Bones of the Forearm.—The question of whether or not the surgeon should institute operative treatment in fractures of both bones of the forearm is often a difficult one to decide, and the frequency with which it is done will vary considerably with the surgeon. If the fractures through the bones are of such contour that the ends will remain in place if they can be engaged, at least two serious attempts at reduction by manipulation should be made before operative treatment is decided upon, and we recommend that the method of reduction as described above be carried out. If this is unsuccessful, the surgeon must then decide whether or not he will use traction or operative treatment. In most instances it will be found that traction with rest in bed and immobilization of the extremity as described above will give a good result. This is particularly true in girls in whom the operative scar is to be avoided if possible.

Another point that must be taken into consideration is the fact that in children there is a marked tendency to the gradual spontaneous correction of apparently severe deformities after fractures of both bones of the forearm, and that a result which may seem relatively poor at the time of the reduction, often gives practically a perfect functional and anatomical result within two years or so. This was demonstrated by Bagley in a review of 200 cases, most of which were treated conservatively.

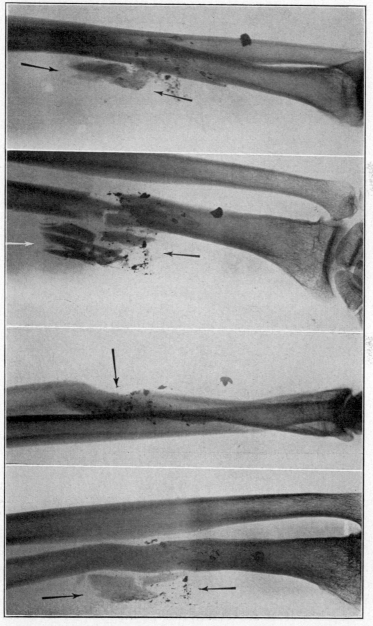

Fig. 695.—Gunshot fracture of the radius. Treated by immobilization in a plaster cast without débridement. After union was obtained the large loose fragment was removed.

In adults in whom reduction has not been possible and in whom it seems probable that by exposure and reduction the surgeon will be able to fix the fragments in good position, operative treatment is indicated (Figs. 696 and 697). This, of course, rules out the simple comminuted fractures as in these instances it is not possible to immobilize the fragments even after they are exposed. Consequently they should be treated by the traction method.

The operation should be the simplest possible, and it should be constantly borne in mind by the surgeon that the most important feature of the operation is to avoid displacement of the fragments after the wounds are closed.

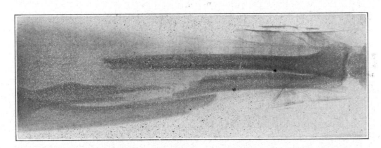

Fig. 696.—Comminuted fracture of both bones of the forearm in which traction failed to effect reduction. Treated by operation and suture of the fragments with chromic catgut, with good result. Immobilized by anterior and posterior wooden splints and circular plaster for ten weeks. Molded sugar tong plaster three weeks.

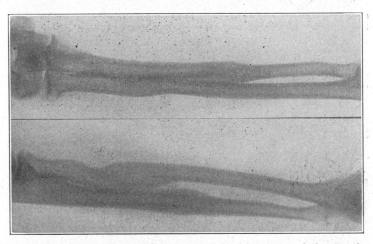

Fig. 697.—Result obtained in the preceding case. Function was good despite the narrowing of the interosseous space. No cross union. Good results in sixteen weeks.

Technic of the Operative Reduction of Fractures of Both Bones of the Forearm.—Two incisions are better than one. It is possible to perform operative reduction through a single incision, but it is considerably more difficult, causes more trauma to the tissues, and the bones are more liable to be displaced afterward. Consequently, longitudinal incisions are made on the ulnar and radial sides on the forearm directly over the sites of the fractures in the respective bones. These incisions are carried down to the bones by retracting the muscles, and the bones are levered into position. If the fractures are such that they are fairly stable after reduction is secured, no internal fixation is necessary.

If the obliquity of the fractures is such that they are unstable then it will be necessary to fix them by some method of internal splinting. Personally, we have never used steel or bone plates, but have simply drilled small holes through the bones and tied them together with chromic catgut or kangaroo tendon, or stainless steel wire.

After both bones have been reduced and immobilized, it is our custom for the surgeon to then support the extremity in the desired position—that is, flexion at the elbow of 90 degrees and in the midposition of rotation for fractures in which the shaft of the radius is broken below the insertion of the pronator teres and in moderate or full supination in fractures of the upper half of the shaft of the radius. From this stage on the important part of the operation is holding the forearm. Consequently, the surgeon should do this himself and have his assistant close both wounds. Neither wound should be closed until both bones are reduced and stable.

After the wounds have been closed in layers, the anterior and posterior splints and plaster cast should be applied as described above after manipulative reduction of fractures of both bones.

Aftertreatment in Fractures of Both Bones of the Forearm.—A good many of the poor results seen after fractures of both bones of the forearm are due to the fact that the belief is fairly common among the members of the medical profession that these bones unite quickly because they are small in diameter. This is not true. The shaft of the radius in an adult is a hard, compact bone and takes from 10 to 12 weeks to become solid, and short periods of immobilization are apt to result in deformity, malunion, or non-union at the site of the fracture. Consequently, after a complete fracture of both bones of the forearm we believe that the complete immobilization including the elbow and the wrist should be continued for at least 5 to 6 weeks in children and at least 6 to 8 weeks in adults. At the end of this time the original dressings and splints can be removed and the surgeon should test the stability of the fragments. If the callus is tender and the bones seem to be relatively unstable, he should re-apply the complete dressing for from 1 to 2 weeks or longer. At the end of this time the dressing should be removed and the forearm again tested. It is, of course, a good plan to obtain x-ray pictures at this time, but the surgeon should not depend upon the x-ray findings for his decision as to whether or not it is safe to decrease the amount of immobilization, since the x-ray shows only the amount of calcium laid down. While this is helpful, it is not the important factor.

When the union seems to be fairly stable, it is advisable to discontinue the immobilization at the elbow and at the wrist, and to apply a short cylindrical plaster cast or short anterior and posterior wooden splints to the forearm, thus allowing the patient a considerable amount of freedom and use of the extremity, but at the same time protecting the shafts of the bones from bending forces and from direct trauma. As a rule this short protective dressing should be worn from 2 to 4 weeks, but the patient can use the forearm and the hand during that time.

From the very beginning of treatment, it is advisable to have the patient exercise the fingers and thumb several times a day in order that stiffness of these members may be avoided. This can be done because the dressing on the flexor surface is never extended beyond the palmar crease.

When the final dressing is removed, the patient can be allowed to progressively use the extremity to the limit of toleration and, as a rule, no further physiotherapy is necessary.

Complications of Fractures of the Shafts of the Bones of the Forearm

The most frequent complication of these injuries is that the fractures are often compounded. When the compounding is indirect; that is, when the skin is broken from within outward by the extrusion of the ends of one or both bones, some surgeons are inclined to treat the wound as a simple fracture, but we believe that unless the wound is a very simple one and unless there is no possibility of the bone ends having been soiled, they should be exposed by operative incision and cleared of débris. It has been our experience to expose these bones after these injuries and find the marrow canal filled with dirt where the bone had been driven into the ground.

When the compounding is direct, as in injuries due to direct violence, it is nearly always necessary to perform a débridement as described in the section on compound fractures. In either instance after the operation the fracture should be treated as described under simple fractures of both bones.

If the fracture can be reduced and rendered stable, it should be treated by immobilization in a plaster cast and one or two windows, if necessary, should be cut in this cast in order to afford dressing of the wound. If the fractures are comminuted and cannot be rendered stable, the fractures should be treated by traction as described above. If the injuries to the soft parts are such that it is difficult or impossible to apply adequate adhesive traction to the skin, the injury should be treated by skeletal traction in recumbency. This is best applied by passing a small rustless steel wire through the shafts of the radius and ulna about one inch above the wrist joint. The pin, when properly inserted, is practically painless and rarely ever causes any difficulty on account of infection and should be left in place until union is solid enough to permit its removal and the substitution of the splint and plaster dressing.

The nerves and blood vessels are rarely damaged in fractures of the forearm unless there is a very extensive injury to the soft tissues at the time of the fracture.

Volkmann's ischemic paralysis occurs all too frequently in these cases, and it may be the result of tight circular plaster casts which not only tend to cause lateral displacement of the fragments by pressing them together, but also tend to obstruct the circulation or, by attempts on the part of the surgeon to reduce the fracture by pressure with board splints. It should be reiterated that the purpose of the anterior and posterior splints is not to cause reduction of the fractures, but the reduction must be obtained by manipulation and that the splints are applied with enough compression of the soft parts between the bones to hold them apart rather than to force them apart. If the splints are applied too tightly they do cause obstruction to the circulation, and after they have been applied, the circulation should be carefully watched for at least twenty-four hours after the reduction. This condition has been described in detail in the section on elbow injuries.

Late Complications or Nonunion or Fibrous Union, Rotation or Angulation Deformities and Synostosis.—Nonunion in these instances is due to (1) too short a period of immobilization after the injury; (2) imperfect reduction, usually with the interposition of soft parts between the fragments, and (3) loss of substance. Most of these cases can be prevented by proper treatment as described above.

Deformities are due to incomplete reduction, or inefficient traction, or too short periods of immobilization after reduction. They, too, are usually preventable.

Synostosis, or the bony union between the radius and the ulna is due to the tendency of the bone ends to be drawn together with the consequent narrowing of the interosseous space. This can, of course, be avoided if the fractures can be properly reduced and the fragments maintained in good position. (Figs. 112 and 113.)

Treatment of Late Complications of Fractures of the Shafts of the Radius and Ulna.—*Nonunion* should be treated by operation. The ends of the fragments should be exposed and freshened. They can be fixed by an autogenous graft, either the so-called onlay graft fixed with metal screws or an intramedullary peg. It is difficult to use inlay grafts in these small bones. In addition we place small osteoperiosteal grafts or bone shavings in the space between the bone ends, and drill numerous small holes in the ends of the fragments.

2. Deformity should be treated by osteotomy and correction.

3. Synostoses should be treated by osteotomy to correct the deformity and careful dissection of the union between the radius and ulna and the interposition of fat or fascia or muscle tissue between the bones to prevent its recurrence.

After any of the above operative procedures the forearm should be immobilized in the long posterior and short anterior wood splints incorporated in a plaster cast as described above.

CHAPTER XX

INJURIES IN THE REGION OF THE WRIST AND HAND

SURGICAL ANATOMY

The Distal Portion of the Radius.—In fracture literature the distal one and one-half or two inches of the bones of the forearm may be considered as belonging to the region of the wrist. In its lower portion the shaft of the radius expands to form a broad base for articulation with the carpals. This is roughly quadrilateral on cross-section and cancellous in structure and presents anterior, posterior, internal, external, and inferior surfaces. The transition zone between the dense cortex of the shaft and the cancellous lower portion is a point of least resistance in the radius and is frequently the site of fracture.

The posterior surface of the lower portion of the radius is slightly convex and is grooved by the extensor tendons. The anterior surface is deeply concave from above downward and is crossed by the pronator quadratus muscle. The lateral surface is prolonged downward to terminate in the prominent rather blunt styloid process which is on a distinctly lower level than the styloid of the ulna and gives attachment to the supinator longus muscle. The inner surface is rather narrow and at its lower portion presents the sigmoid cavity of the radius for articulation with the head of the ulna.

The inferior surface is almost entirely articular and is directed downward, forward, and inward. Its slightly concave articular portion is divided into outer and inner facets which articulate with the scaphoid and semilunar bones, respectively. Its inner portion is separated from the sigmoid cavity by a roughened area which serves as a point of attachment for the triangular fibrocartilage.

The lower end of the radius develops from a single center which appears at the end of the second year and forms an epiphysis which includes the entire lower end of the bone and unites with the shaft about the nineteenth year.

The Distal Portion of the Ulna.—The lower portion of the shaft of the ulna is cylindrical in shape and terminates in an enlarged head and a styloid process. The head projects forward and outward and presents a lateral articular facet which courses around the bone, making about two-thirds of a circle. This facet is for articulation with the lower end of the radius and enables the radius to swing around the ulna. The inferior surface of the head does not enter into the formation of the wrist joint, but articulates with the triangular fibrocartilage. The styloid process is a prolongation of the lateral surface and extends down beyond the head of the bone, from which it is separated by a rather deep groove. The lower epiphysis of the ulna includes the head and the styloid process.

Ossification of the lower epiphysis of the ulna begins about the fifth year and it fuses to the shaft about the nineteenth year.

The Inferior Radio-Ulnar Joint.—When viewed from the front the inferior radio-ulnar joint is an L-shaped cavity, the vertical limb of which lies between the lower end of the ulna and the sigmoid cavity on the mesial surface of the radius, and the horizontal limb lies between the lower end of the ulna and the triangular fibrocartilage. This cartilage is attached by its base to the inferior surface of the radius and by its apex to the deep surface of the styloid of the ulna and with the fibrous bands which reinforce it forms the main bond of union between the lower ends of the radius and ulna. This joint permits the radius to rotate around the ulna through an arc of about 140 degrees, the hand and the fibrocartilage moving with the radius.

The Hand

The hand is composed of the carpus, or wrist, the metacarpal bones, and the phalanges.

The Carpal Bones.—(Figs. 698 and 699.) The carpal bones are arranged in two rows of four bones each. The upper row from without inward consists of the scaphoid, semilunar, cuneiform, and pisiform. The lower row consists of the trapezium, trapezoid, os magnum, and unciform. The three outer bones of the upper row are bound together by strong ligaments to form an egg-shaped articular surface for the lower end of the radius and the triangular fibrocartilage. The inferior surfaces of these bones form a deep cavity which receives the head of the os magnum and the unciform. The pisiform is practically a sesamoid bone in the tendon of the flexor carpi ulnaris.

The four bones of the lower row are bound together by transverse ligaments and the upper surfaces of the unciform and the head of the os magnum project upward to fit into the cavity formed by the three outer bones of the first row, while the trapezium and trapezoid articulate above with the scaphoid. The inferior surface of the united bones of the second row is slightly convex for articulation with the metacarpals. The assembled carpal bones are deeply concave on the volar surface for the passage of the flexor tendons and are slightly convex on the dorsal surface. From the surgical standpoint the important bones of the carpus are the scaphoid, which is rather frequently fractured across its middle, and the semilunar, which may be dislocated either forward or backward.

The Wrist Joint.—Since the two rows of carpal bones move as units we may consider the hand as being united to the forearm by three joints—the radiocarpal joint, the intercarpal joint, and the carpometacarpal joint.

The Radiocarpal Joint is the articulation between the radius and the triangular fibrocartilage above and the scaphoid, semilunar, and cuneiform below. The joint cavity is convex upward in both its lateral and anteroposterior diameters and elongated in its lateral diameter. With the hand in the midposition, the radius articulates with the scaphoid and the semilunar while the cuneiform articulates with the triangular fibrocartilage. In adduction the scaphoid moves partly out from beneath the radius and the cuneiform moves outward so that more of its surface lies beneath the fibrocartilage, and in abduction these bones move in the opposite direction so that almost all of the scaphoid lies beneath the radius and the semilunar lies beneath the fibro-cartilage, while the cuneiform moves almost entirely out of the joint.

The Midcarpal Joint is the joint between the first and second rows of carpal bones and is irregularly S-shaped in the anteroposterior direction. The inner portion is strongly convex upward and is formed by the head of the os magnum and unciform being received into the deep cup-shaped cavity formed by the distal surfaces of the first row of carpal bones while the lateral portion is slightly concave upward and is formed by the articulation of the scaphoid above with the trapezium and trapezoid below.

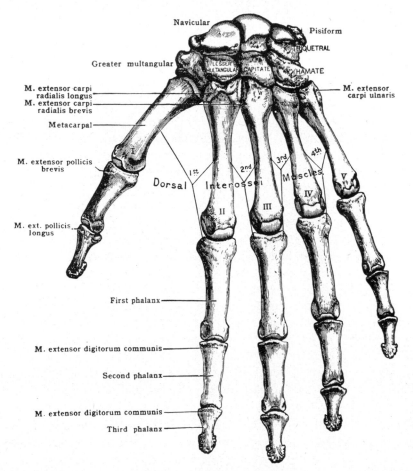

Fig. 698.—Bones of the left hand. Dorsal surface. (From Morris: Human Anatomy, P. Blakiston's Son & Co., Inc., Publisher.)

The Carpometacarpal Joints.—The four metacarpal bones of the fingers articulate with one another by lateral facets and with the distal surface of the second row of carpal bones by an irregularly transverse carpometacarpal joint. The metacarpal bone of the thumb articulates with the trapezium by a saddle-shaped joint which has a separate synovial cavity.

Ligaments of the Wrist.—The bones of the first row of carpals and of the second row of carpals are firmly bound together by anterior and posterior transverse ligaments. The same is true of the five metacarpal bones and relatively little motion is permitted between the bones of each row upon one another. In addition to the transverse ligaments there is a general capsular ligament which stretches from the lower end of the radius and ulna to the bases of the metacarpals and this is reinforced by numerous fibrous bands which are especially prominent on its anterior surface. On either side the capsular ligament is reinforced by lateral fibrous bands which may be considered the internal and external lateral ligaments of the wrist. The synovial cavities of the midcarpal and carpometacarpal joints communicate with one another but that between the first metacarpal and trapezium is separate. There is also a separate cavity for the articulation between the radius and the first row of carpal bones.

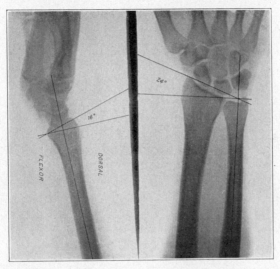

Fig. 699.—X-ray picture of a normal wrist and hand, lateral and anteroposterior views. Note that the lower articular surface of the radius faces inward and forward as well as downward.

Motions at the Wrist.—By means of the three transverse joints between the hand and the forearm bones, motion occurs in every direction except rotation. Adduction and abduction occur almost entirely at the radiocarpal joint. Flexion and extension occur largely at the radiocarpal joint, but there is also some motion in these directions at the midcarpal joint and at the carpometacarpal joint. Circumduction occurs almost entirely at the wrist, but the carpometacarpal joints add their quota of motion in flexion and extension. The metacarpal bone of the thumb has a separate articulation which is saddle-shaped and permits of motion in every direction including a small amount of rotation as in opposing the thumb to the fingers.

The Metacarpal Bones.—The five metacarpal bones radiate downward from the second row of carpals to form the hand. They are slender bones with an enlarged proximal extremity or base and a thickened, rounded head which articulates with the first phalanx of the corresponding finger or thumb. Their proximal extremities present small articular facets where adjacent bones come in contact and are firmly bound together by transverse ligaments. Their dorsal and volar surfaces are rough for the attachment of the ligaments of the wrist and of all of the flexor and extensor muscles of the wrist and of the wrist and hand. The distal extremities of the four inner metacarpal bones are loosely bound to one another by the transverse metacarpal ligament.

The Phalanges are short pipe bones with enlarged slightly concave proximal extremities, or bases, and rounded distal extremities, or tips. There are three phalanges for each finger and two for the thumb.

Metacarpophalangeal and Interphalangeal Joints are all simple hinge joints which permit only flexion and extension. In flexion the base of the distal bone glides under the head of the proximal bone and the knuckles of the hand and of the fingers are the heads of the proximal bones.

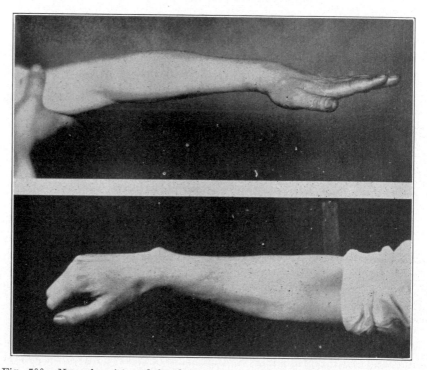

Fig. 700.—Normal wrist and hand viewed from the lateral aspect. Note the normal downward tilt at the wrist.

Fig. 701.—Pronated wrist and hand viewed from the lateral aspect and above. Note the prominence of the head of the ulna.

EXTENSION AND COMPRESSION FRACTURES OF THE LOWER END OF THE RADIUS (COLLES' FRACTURES)

Occurrence.—Next to fractures of the fingers and ribs and possibly to fractures of the clavicle, these extension and compression fractures of the lower end of the radius are the most frequent of all fractures. Because of their frequency and because of the impairment of function in the hand and wrist which frequently follows these injuries they are of great importance economically and every physician or surgeon who treats fractures at all should know thoroughly how to handle them.

These injuries are relatively rare in children but they are so frequent in adults that any patient who has suffered a fall upon the hand or has been kicked by the back-firing of an automobile and who has tenderness over the lower end of the radius and impairment of function in the hand may be considered to have a fracture of the lower end of the radius until it has been proved otherwise. And this is especially true if the patient is beyond middle life.

Mechanism.—Most of these fractures are due to falls upon the palm of the hand, but occasionally they result from a kick received while cranking an automobile. The automobile injuries are not so frequent as they were some years ago because most automobiles are now equipped with self-starters, but many commercial vehicles are still cranked by hand, and as most of us know self-starters sometimes do not work.

Much has been written about the mechanics of these injuries, and the question as to whether the fracture is the result of compression of the radius in its long axis or of hyperextension at the wrist has been argued pro and con. As a matter of fact the lesion is the resultant of several forces and the exact ratio and directions of these forces vary considerably in different cases, as anyone who has ever watched another person fall and attempt to catch his body weight upon the hands must realize. In such an accident the pronated hand meets the ground with the muscles tensed to receive the body weight, and the degree of extension at the wrist varies with the angle of the forearm to the ground at the time of the impact.

When the palm of the hand strikes the ground, force is transmitted directly upward through the carpal bones to the lower end of the radius. There is also a variable amount of shearing force or cross strain which tends to force the lower end of the radius directly backward and a certain amount of hyperextension at the wrist which tends to rotate the lower end of the radius in the direction of hyperextension; and in addition to the above there is a variable amount of torsion as the patient tends to forcibly pronate the forearm at the instant of the impact and there may be more or less lateral strain due to the inclination of the forearm to the ground at the instant of the impact.

From what has been said above it is obvious that attempts to attribute these injuries to force in only one direction are futile and that the important thing is that the pronated hand is jammed upward and backward against the radius with sufficient force to break it, and in many instances to cause a variable amount of displacement of the lower fragment.

Pathology of Compression and Extension Fractures of the Lower End of the Radius.—1. *Incomplete Fractures of the Lower End of the Radius* are more frequent in children and are generally of the infraction type with buckling of the thin posterior cortex of the radius rather than of the greenstick variety. In most instances there is practically no displacement, but the lower end of the bone may be bent backward to a variable degree and this may be accompanied by a similar fracture and deformity in the lower portion of the shaft of the ulna.

In adults the lower end of the radius may occasionally be broken in its long axis, the fissure beginning at the articular margin and extending up the shaft for a variable distance, or more rarely there may be an oblique or transverse fracture which does not extend completely across the bone. There is, of course, no displacement in any of these incomplete fractures in adults, and there is as a rule relatively little swelling or damage to the soft tissues.

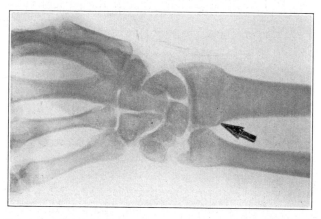

Fig. 702.—Extension and compression fracture of the lower end of the radius with no displacement. Treated by immobilization in a sugar tong molded plaster splint for three weeks; then a short posterior molded plaster splint to hand, wrist and forearm for one week. Good results and union in five weeks.

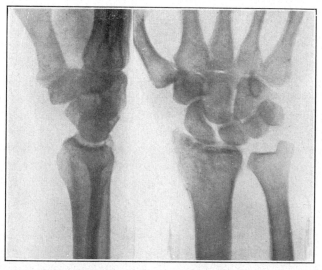

Fig. 703.—Extension and compression fracture of the lower end of the radius with slight hyperextension of the distal fragment and comminution of the articular surface. Treated by manipulative reduction under local anesthesia and immobilization with ulna deviation and circular cast from the middle third of arm down to the base of the fingers. Good result.

2. *Complete Fractures Through the Lower End of the Radius Without Displacement* are fairly frequent, especially in older people, and are usually the result of relatively slight trauma. The fracture line tends to be roughly transverse or slightly oblique, sloping upward and backward and the fracture is subperiosteal in nature (Fig. 702). There is relatively little damage to the soft tissues.

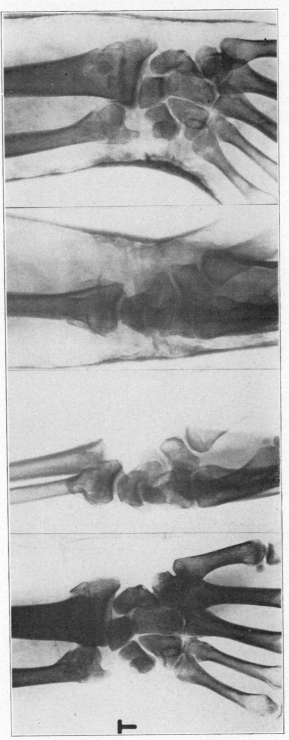

Fig. 704.—A typical Colles with fracture of distal end of ulna before and after reduction under local anesthesia. This amount of flexion of the hand at the wrist is maintained for about ten days; then, a new cast is applied in straight position.

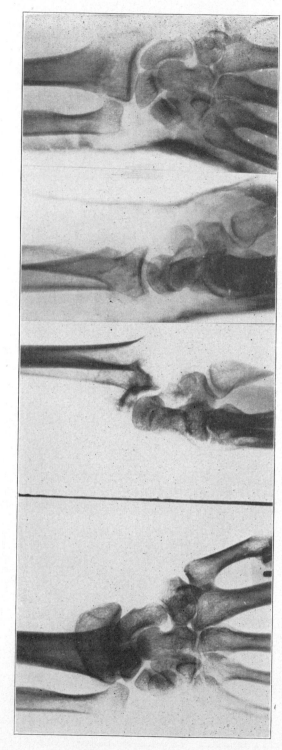

Fig. 705.—Severe Colles fracture with complete displacement, before and after reduction under local anesthesia.

3. *Complete Fractures Through the Lower End of the Radius with Displacement* comprise the great majority of the fractures at the wrist and are loosely called Colles' fractures by the medical profession, although the lesion described by Colles was a transverse fracture 4 c.m. above the articular margin with posterior and upward displacement of the lower fragment. The true Colles' fracture is quite rare, as in most instances the fracture line is from one-half to three-quarters of an inch above the articular margin and may run transversely across the bone or slope upward and backward or upward, backward, and outward or upward, backward, and inward. In a considerable percentage of the cases there is more or less comminution of the lower fragment and this is especially true in patients beyond middle life where it is often broken into several fragments and one or more of the fracture lines may involve the articular surface. (Fig. 705.)

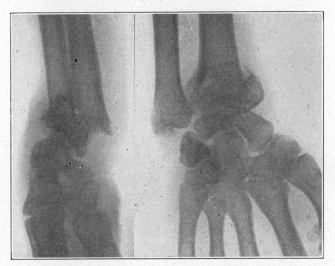

Fig. 706.—Roentgenogram showing extension and compression fracture of lower end of the radius.

The typical displacement is one in which the lower or distal fragment moves upward and backward on the shaft and is also hyperextended so that its articular surface instead of facing downward and forward, faces directly downward or even downward and backward. In addition to the above, the lower fragment may be abducted; that is, tilted toward the radial side and supinated; that is, rotated outward on the shaft.

Impaction, or at least entanglement, of the fractured ends is the rule in these fractures with displacement because the lower fragment is so broad that it does not clear the lower end of the upper fragment, but is impaled upon it by the cortical bone of the shaft being driven into the relatively soft cancellous bone of the lower fragment.

In addition to the displacement there is often actual compression of the cancellous bone. This may be so severe that there is practically a loss of substance and so extensive that even after a perfect reduction the lower fragment tends to slip upward because the radius has been shortened by the compression and there is nothing to hold the lower fragment down in its normal position. (Figs. 707 and 708.)

While the above is the classical displacement which causes the typical silver fork deformity, to be described below, it is by no means the only displacement which occurs in compression and extension fractures of the lower end of the radius. In many instances there is little or no backward displacement of the lower fragment and it may be driven directly upward, the bone being crushed in its long axis or hyperextended (tilted backward) or abducted (tilted outward), and either of these two last may be combined with displacement upward. It should be noted that any degree of displacement may occur.

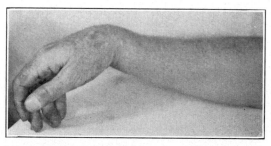

Fig. 707.—Extension and compression fracture of the lower end of the radius with moderate silver fork deformty.

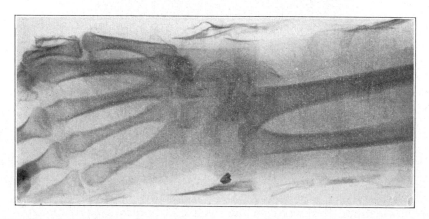

Fig. 708.—X-ray picture of preceding case. Treated by open reduction after two attempts at closed reduction had failed. Immobilization in anteroposterior board splints and sheet cotton and plaster cast extending from middle third of arm to middle phalanges of fingers with forearm in midsupination and pronation for four weeks; then sugar tong plaster splint two weeks. Fair functional results in twelve weeks.

In addition to the fracture of the radius, the styloid process of the ulna may be pulled off (Fig. 709), or the triangular fibrocartilage may be displaced, or the inferior radio-ulnar joint may be disrupted and the head of the ulna may be displaced anteriorly (Fig. 710).

In these fractures of the lower end of the radius with displacement there is usually a large amount of extravasation of blood and swelling of the soft tissues which begins very quickly, and the swelling may involve the hand and fingers and the entire forearm. The lower end of the upper fragment projects on the volar surface of the wrist beneath the flexor tendons and median nerve and may damage these structures. The hand, of course, is displaced with the lower fragment as are the extensor tendons which pass over it and the sensory branch of the radial nerve; this may be damaged. The periosteum may be torn or it may remain intact. The ligaments of the wrist joint are not, as a rule, injured. In rare instances the carpal scaphoid may be broken or the semilunar may be dislocated.

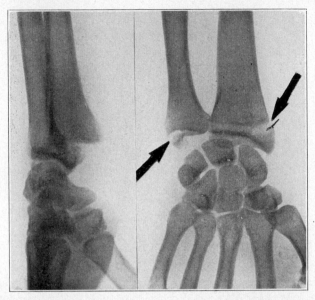

Fig. 709.—Extension and compression fracture of the lower end of the radius with moderate displacement. There is also a fracture of the styloid process of the ulna. Treated by reduction under general anesthetic and immobilized in sugar tong plaster molded splint, with circular plaster cast around the splint for sixteen days; then only the posterior part of the cast for a week.

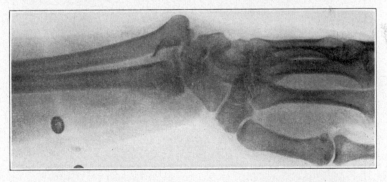

Fig. 710.—Comminuted fracture of the lower end of the radius with dislocation of the lower end of the ulna. Treated by manipulative reduction and immobilization with wooden splints and circular cast from lower third of arm to base of fingers. Good result. Limited rotation of the forearm in such type case is frequently encountered.

In rare instances the fracture in the radius may be accompanied by a complete fracture through the lower fourth of the shaft of the ulna or separation of the lower epiphysis and when this occurs the lower fragment of the ulna tends to be displaced backward and upward with that of the radius.

4. *Separation of the Lower Epiphysis of the Radius.*—In children and adolescents the fracture is apt to occur at the epiphyseal line, and the lower

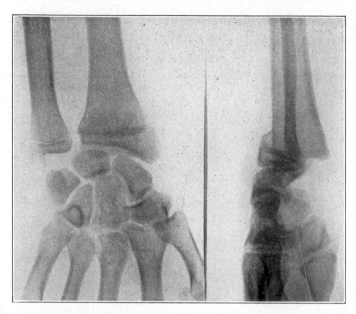

Fig. 711.—Epiphyseal separation of the lower end of the radius with fracture of the ulnar styloid. Treated by manipulative reduction and immobilization on a posterior wooden splint extending from the base of the fingers to the upper third of forearm with sheet cotton padding and a circular plaster cast. Good result.

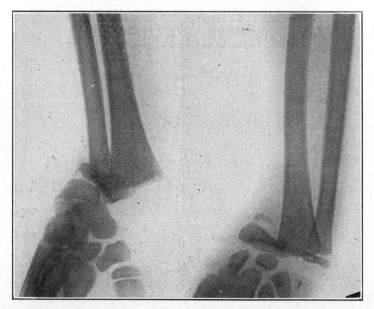

Fig. 712.—Epiphyseal separation of the lower end of the radius with marked posterior and lateral displacement. Treated by manipulative reduction and immobilization in a posterior padded wooden splint and circular cast from upper third of arm to the base of the fingers for three weeks; then posterior wooden splint for two weeks. Good result. In this type of case a guarded prognosis concerning retardation of bone growth should always be given.

epiphysis tends to be displaced in exactly the same manner as does the **lower** fragment in adults (Figs. 711 and 712). Not infrequently a portion of the cortex of the lower end of the shaft of the diaphysis is broken off and displaced with the epiphysis. In these epiphyseal injuries the epiphysis may be simply loosened and not displaced or it may be displaced upward and backward to any degree as is true of the lower fragment in adults. In any epiphyseal injury the epiphyseal cartilage plate may be damaged to such a degree that growth is interfered with. (Fig. 713.) Rarely the epiphysis may be fractured in a vertical plane, either with or without displacement.

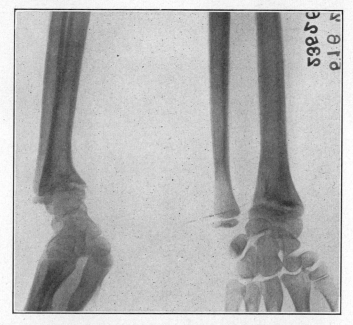

Fig. 713.—Old epiphyseal separation at the lower end of the radius in which growth was retarded after reduction. Perfect anatomical reduction accomplished and retained until union took place. Retardation of bone growth first noticed about two years following injury. (This is not the same case as shown in Fig. 712.)

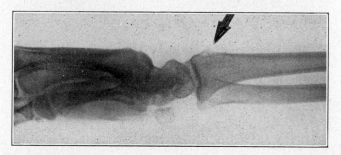

Fig. 714.—Posterior marginal fracture of the lower end of the radius (Barton's fracture). Treated by immobilization in dorsiflexion in circular plaster cast and later in anterior plaster cock-up molded splint. Good result.

5. *Fractures of the Posterior Articular Margin of the Radius. (Barton's Fracture.)*—Occasionally in these compression and extension injuries the **main** mass of the bone remains intact, but the prominent posterior margin is broken off and tends to be displaced upward and backward (Fig. 714). With this

displacement there is a subluxation at the wrist and this is really a fracture dislocation at the wrist, as the carpal bones tend to be displaced upward and backward with the detached marginal fragment.

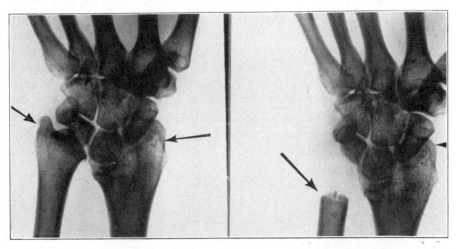

Fig. 715.—An old epiphyseal injury of the radius with arrested growth of the radius resulting in disability. Improvement by resection of the distal portion of the ulna. (Darrach's operation.)

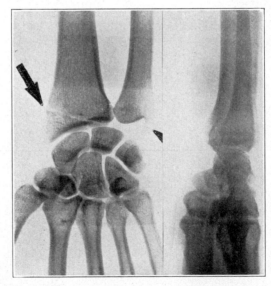

Fig. 716.—Fracture of both styloids, radius and ulna. Treated by immobilization in a sugar tong plaster splint with the hand in the neutral position for four weeks. Flexor part of the splint was cut away at end of two weeks. Good result. Prolonged immobilization is necessary on account of a fracture of the ulnar styloid.

6. *Oblique Fractures of the Lateral Articular Border and Fractures of the Styloid of the Radius* are quite common and are sometimes called chauffeur fractures because they are frequently received while cranking an automobile. It is probable that they are the result of force which is directed upward and outward and is received on the adducted hand. As a rule the fracture line begins near the middle of the articular surface and courses obliquely upward and outward to emerge on the lateral border of the bone about one-half an

inch above the tip of the styloid. This fracture is important because it involves the articular surface. (Fig. 716.)

Diagnosis of Extension and Compression Fractures of the Lower End of the Radius.—1. *Fractures without Displacement* are relatively frequent and are often diagnosed and treated as sprain of the wrist. Clinically the diagnosis can usually be made by the presence of moderate or marked swelling and point tenderness over the lower portion of the radius and disability of the hand (Fig. 717). When these symptoms are present after a compression or hyperextension injury at the wrist, the burden of proof is on the person who says that the lower end of the radius is not broken. By careful palpation the line of the fracture may be roughly determined by tracing the course of the acute point tenderness. It is important to distinguish between tenderness over the radius and tenderness over the wrist joint and to rule out displacement by comparing the level of the radial styloid with that of the other wrist. In a child the tenderness is apt to follow the course of the epiphyseal line. In fractures of the radial styloid the tenderness is most marked over the lateral surface of the bone, and pain may be produced by slight pressure on the tip of the styloid. As elsewhere, the diagnosis of a fracture without displacement should be confirmed by the x-ray.

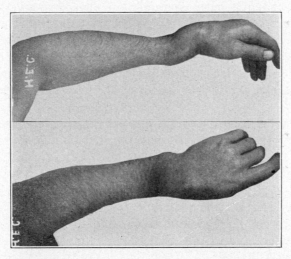

Fig. 717.—Extension and compression fracture of the lower end of the radius with considerable displacement. Note the silver fork deformity when viewed from the side and the radial deviation when viewed from the dorsal aspect.

2. *Incomplete Fractures with Deformity* are nearly always of the infraction type and occur only in children. They are really fractures of the shaft of the radius in which the fracture line lies unusually close to the lower end of the bone. The deformity is a backward bending of the lower end of the bone, and unless it is very slight, it is easily visible. In cases with slight deformity, this may be obscured by the moderate swelling which occurs over the infracted posterior cortex, but it can be demonstrated by palpating the lateral border of the radius. In other respects the clinical picture resembles that of the fractures without displacement.

3. *Fractures with Displacement.*—Marked swelling of the forearm, wrist, hand, and fingers may appear within a few hours after the injury, the skin often becoming tense and glossy and the hand slightly cyanotic. The patient maintains the hand in a position of pronation and may be unable to move the hand or fingers. The extensive swelling may obscure the deformity even with considerable displacement and in such instances it is difficult to determine the character of the displacement without an x-ray picture.

In the typical case with backward displacement of the lower fragment, the wrist when viewed from the side presents the characteristic silver fork deformity. This classical deformity is due to the pushing backward and hyperextension of the lower end of the radius and the flexion of the hand on the wrist. The result is a rather abrupt dorsal prominence which is more marked on the radial side and a gently rounded volar prominence which tends to be at a slightly higher level. The volar prominence is due to the lower end of the proximal fragment which pushes the flexor tendons forward. As stated above the silver fork deformity may be obscured by the swelling, or it may not be present, since there may be considerable upward displacement with practically no backward displacement.

Viewed from the dorsal aspect the wrist is broadened and the hand is deviated to the radial side (Figs. 718, 719, and 720). This abduction or radial deviation of the hand is more characteristic than the silver fork deformity and is the result of the shortening of the radius while the ulna remains intact. It is always present unless the shaft of the ulna is broken or the radioulnar joint is disrupted and the lower end of the radius is pushed directly upward on the radius. In these latter cases the radial deviation may or may not be present. The normal dorsal prominence of the head of the ulna is diminished or absent.

Viewed from the volar aspect the head of the ulna is unusually prominent, the folds of the wrist are deepened and the thenar eminence is displaced upward.

If the patient be asked to move the hand and wrist it will be found that the degree of disability varies greatly in different cases and a young man may be able to flex and extend the wrist and fingers while in an old person with marked swelling there may be practically complete paralysis of the hand. As a rule flexion is more limited than extension. Supination is practically always absent or markedly limited.

Palpation will practically always enable the surgeon to make the diagnosis of fracture of the lower end of the radius with displacement. In the beginning the tips of the radial and ulnar styloids should be definitely located. In the normal wrist the tip of the radial styloid is on a slightly lower level than that of the ulna and the normal relationship of the styloids in the given patient should be determined by palpating the other wrist. If there is upward displacement and the ulna is intact, the styloid of the radius will be unusually high and may be on a level with or even higher than that of the ulna. If there is posterior displacement or hyperextension of the lower fragment, the radial styloid will be displaced backward and the normal anterior curve of the volar surface of the lower end of the radius will be flattened or even reversed. This

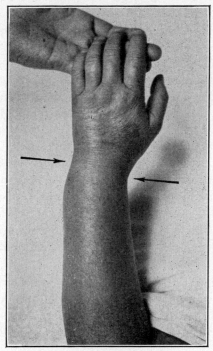

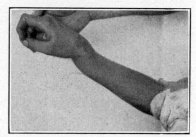

Fig. 718.   Fig. 719.

Fig. 718.—Extension and compression fracture of the lower end of the radius with considerable swelling and radial deviation.

Fig. 719.—Compound extension and compression fracture of the lower end of the radius.

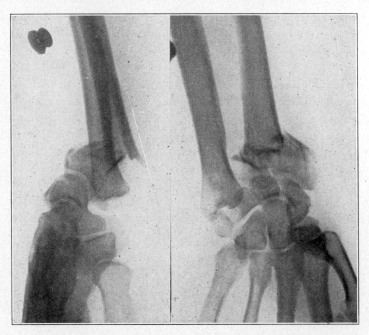

Fig. 720.—Roentgenogram of preceding case.

can be detected by palpating along the anterolateral border, and it may be possible to palpate the sharp lower end of the upper fragment beneath the flexor tendons and the upper end of the distal fragment beneath the extensor tendons.

With relatively little swelling and a cooperative patient, it may be possible to trace the line of the fracture around the radius by point tenderness, but this is out of the question in a markedly swollen wrist with a sensitive and nervous patient. The head of the ulna will be unusually prominent on the volar surface and often appears to be, and may be, dislocated. Acute tenderness over the ulnar styloid suggests a fracture of this process and it may be possible to detect an abnormality in its contour. Point tenderness over the lower portion of the ulnar shaft suggests a fracture here, and deformity and false motion make the diagnosis of a fracture of both bones of the forearm near the wrist.

When possible a roentgenogram should be taken before reduction is attempted, since it is very helpful to know the exact character of the fracture and displacement.

4. *Separation of the Lower Radial Epiphysis* is to be suspected in compression and hyperextension injuries of the lower end of the radius in children and adolescents. The diagnosis is similar to that of fractures in this region and the physical findings are similar except that the line of tenderness is nearer the lower end of the bone.

5. *Fracture of the Posterior Articular Margin of the Lower End of the Radius.*—In this rather rare injury the detached posterior margin remains attached to the carpus and may or may not be displaced. When it is not displaced, the symptoms are similar to those of an ordinary extension fracture through the lower end of the radius except that the swelling is less marked and may be limited to the dorsum of the wrist. The point tenderness is limited to the dorsum of the wrist and lies very close to the joint line.

In fractures of the posterior margin of the radius with displacement the carpal bones are displaced backward and upward with the detached fragment, and the lesion is really a fracture dislocation or subluxation at the radiocarpal joint. The silver fork deformity is present as in the typical extension and compression fracture of the lower end of the radius, but the posterior and anterior prominences are on a slightly lower level and the radial styloid is intact and in its normal position. Furthermore, the normal anterior curve of the volar surface of the lower end of the radius is not disturbed. The lesion can be differentiated from the rare simple posterior dislocation by palpating the detached fragment as different from the smooth rounded proximal surface of the first row of carpal bones.

In many cases the exact diagnosis of a posterior marginal fracture can be made only by the x-ray.

6. *Oblique Fracture of the Lateral Articular Border and Radial Styloid.*—These fractures are rather common and the detached fragment may or may not be displaced. When the styloid is not displaced, the clinical picture resembles that of an extension fracture of the lower end of the radius without

displacement with the exceptions that the swelling is most marked over the base of the styloid and that the line of point tenderness crosses the base of the styloid. Furthermore, supination of the forearm may be possible.

In fractures of the base of the styloid with displacement the wrist is broadened and the hand is abducted, but the silver fork deformity is not present and supination may be possible, since the radioulnar articulation is not disturbed. On palpation the radial styloid is displaced upward and outward and occasionally backward, and the point tenderness is limited to the base of the styloid while the normal anterior curve of the volar surface of the radius may be disturbed.

Complications of Fractures of the Lower End of the Radius

These fractures are rarely compound and this makes the lower end of the radius an exception to the general rule that fractures in bones which are practically subcutaneous are frequently compound. Occasionally, however, with severe violence the lower end of the upper fragment may be thrust through the skin or the radioulnar articulation may be disrupted and the lower end of the ulna driven through the skin (Figs. 719 and 720). Here, as elsewhere, the fractures due to direct violence are apt to be compound.

Fracture of the carpal scaphoid or semilunar or dislocation of the semilunar bone may be present in addition to the fracture of the radius. The fractures of the styloid and rarely of the lower portion of the shaft of the ulna and the dislocation of the ulna with disruption of the radioulnar joint are regarded as part of the typical radius fracture and not as complications.

The blood vessels are rarely injured.

Nerve Injuries.—A rather frequent complication is injury to the sensory branch of the radial nerve which supplies the dorsum of the thumb and the radial side of the hand. This nerve is stretched over the displaced lower fragment and may even be torn. Usually, however, the paresthesia and anesthesia in its area of distribution incident to the nerve injury clear up within a few weeks after the reduction and require no special treatment. Very rarely with marked displacement the median nerve may be injured by the lower end of the upper fragment.

Late Complications.—Unfortunately late complications occur all too frequently. Pain at the ulnar styloid due to nonunion or malunion of this process is a rather frequent and often troublesome late complication and may even require excision of the loose fragment.

The most frequent late complication is pain and limited motion at the wrist and at the inferior radioulnar joint. This may be due to true traumatic arthritis or to incomplete reduction, and we wish to emphasize the fact that complete reduction is essential. This is especially true in old people if one is to expect a good result.

A rather rare, but very interesting, late complication is a spontaneous rupture of the tendon of the extensor pollicis longus muscle. This occurs some months or even years after the injury and is due to fraying of the tendon by friction over the ridge of bone which is frequently left across the dorsum of the radius at the site of the fracture.

In epiphyseal separations at the lower end of the radius one occasionally finds that the subsequent growth of the bone either does not occur or occurs in an abnormal manner and that in consequence the patient may suffer considerable deformity of the hand and wrist. This cessation or abnormality in growth may occur even in the presence of apparently perfect anatomical reduction of the separated epiphysis and in treating these cases the surgeon should warn the parent of the possibility of later growth disturbances even though he may have obtained perfectly satisfactory reduction of the displaced epiphysis.

Treatment of Extension and Compression Fractures of the Lower End of the Radius

1. **Fractures Without Displacement.**—The important thing about these fractures is to be sure that there is no displacement; and for this reason all such fractures should be x-rayed when possible and the surgeon must make sure that the lower fragment is not hyperextended or telescoped on the shaft (pushed upward). A displacement is important and should be corrected if possible provided the general condition permits. Consequently, we feel that if the surgeon has the slightest doubt as to whether or not reduction should be attempted he should attempt to reduce the displacement. These fractures involve two joints and severe disability of the hand may follow even a slight displacement, although this is not always the case. Consequently the surgeon should treat them aggressively and he should constantly be on his guard against leaving well enough alone. In the aged or debilitated, of course, the general condition is to be given first consideration, but it is very embarrassing to have such a patient complain of pain at the inferior radio-ulnar joint for months and years after the surgeon has decided to let the fracture heal with slight upward displacement.

If the fragments are in good position, all that is necessary is to immobilize the wrist for three to four weeks in a short circular plaster-of-Paris cast or in anterior and posterior plaster molds, or sugar tong plaster mold, or wooden splints, and follow this with a leather wrist band or adhesive strapping until the patient is comfortable without it.

The splint or cast should be applied with the wrist and hand and forearm in the midposition as regards rotation, and the wrist in the midposition as regards flexion and extension with some adduction (ulnar deviation) of the hand at the wrist. The short wooden splint when used should be the exact width of the normal wrist and forearm and long enough to extend from the elbow along the extensor surface of the forearm to the base of the fingers. It should be cut out over the styloid process of the ulna, padded with sheet cotton and strapped to the forearm and hand and wrist. Plaster molds or casts when used should extend from the upper portion of the forearm to the bases of the fingers and should be applied with the hand and wrist and forearm in the neutral position; that is, with the forearm in the midposition as regards rotation and the hand in midflexion and extension with slight adduction at the wrist. (Fig. 731.)

The patient should begin to exercise the fingers as soon as the plaster is set and should be encouraged to use the hand in dressing, eating, etc., and should not be permitted to wear a sling longer than a week, since this tends to encourage lack of use with resultant stiffness of the joints of the upper extremity.

Treatment of Fractures of the Lower End of the Radius With Displacement.—The displacement of the lower end of the radius must be reduced and the fragments must be replaced in approximately their normal anatomical relation if one is to expect a good functioning wrist, and this is especially true in patients over forty years of age.

The route which the distal fragment must be forced to travel depends, of course, upon the displacement, but in the typical case it must be pulled downward until the radial styloid is at its normal level, pushed toward the volar surface of the forearm until the posterior displacement has been corrected, forced into flexion until backward tilting has been overcome and the articular surface faces forward as well as downward, and in certain cases it must be twisted in the direction of pronation until the normal dorsal prominence of the lower end of the ulna is restored and pushed inward until the radial deviation is corrected.

There are, in the main, two methods by which this reduction may be accomplished. In one, and this is the most popular, the lower fragment is levered into place and in the other the fragments are separated by strong traction and the lower fragment is pressed or molded into place. One of us (H. E. C.) favors the leverage method, while the other (J. A. K.) favors the traction and molding method. As a matter of fact, frequently in strong muscular individuals with considerable displacement both leverage and traction are brought into play.

It cannot be too strongly emphasized that the reduction should be done as soon as possible after the injury. Not only can the reduction be done with more ease and precision if it is done before the swelling becomes extensive, but early reduction tends to seal off the ends of the bones and prevent the great swelling which is prone to occur in these injuries and which we believe tends to damage the soft parts and prolong the disability.

Anesthesia.—Certain very skillful surgeons are able to reduce these fractures of the lower end of the radius by a quick manipulation without an anesthetic, but we do not advise this method. We do not attempt the reduction without adequate local or general anesthesia. Satisfactory local anesthesia and muscle relaxation can be obtained by injecting 1 per cent novocaine around the fracture as illustrated in the section on anesthesia.

Reduction by Leverage.—(Fig. 721.) In this method the wrist is first strongly hyperextended with traction and countertraction until the impaction or entanglement of the fragments is loosened. It is then strongly flexed in order to bring the lower fragment downward and forward. During the flexion the surgeon makes more or less traction on the distal fragment and presses it downward with the thumbs or with the hypothenar eminence and maintains countertraction on the forearm with the other hand. It is carried out as follows: The forearm is immobilized by an assistant, the surgeon grasps the patient's wrist just distal to the point of fracture with one hand and the lower end of the patient's forearm with his other hand. The method of "shaking hands with the patient" is not efficient, as the movements must take place at the site of the fracture, and if the hand is used as a lever to manipulate the lower fragment most of the motion will occur at the wrist joint and in the carpal joints, while the lower fragment will be affected relatively little.

The distal fragment is first manipulated into a position of marked hyperextension using enough force to loosen the impaction or entanglement. (See Fig. 721A.)

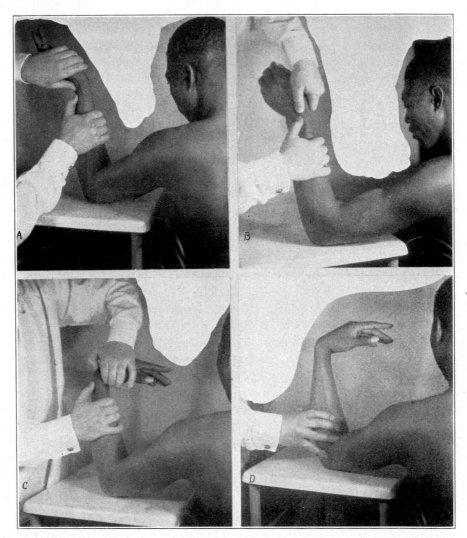

Fig. 721.—Manipulative reduction of compression and extension fractures of the lower end of the radius.

A. Forcible hyperextension and traction of the wrist producing an increased deformity of the fracture and countertraction on the patient's forearm combined with direct pressure of the operator's thumbs on the proximal and distal fragments.

B. With continued traction and countertraction and adduction of the hand at the wrist, flexion of the hand at the wrist joint with continued pressure on the fragments by the operator's thumbs is carried out.

C. The flexion when commenced should be rather sudden while traction and countertraction on the forearm and pressure over the fragments are continued. Note that the index finger of the operator's left hand is firmly pressing against the lower end of the proximal fragment. Countertraction by an assistant on the upper third of the forearm is effective during all the above procedures. This was left out of the pictures to show more detail of the operator's maneuvers.

D. Test for adequate reduction. The hand drops into a position of normal flexion at the wrist.

In obtaining the hyperextension the surgeon's thumbs are placed over the dorsal surfaces of the ends of the fragments and as the distal fragment is hyperextended the surgeon's thumbs are approximated and tend to force the distal fragment down. Then, exerting strong traction on the wrist and the distal fragment, and countertraction on the forearm, the hand and wrist are swept downward and to the ulnar side into flexion and ulnar deviation and at the same time pressure is made on the dorsal surface of the displaced lower fragment by the surgeon's thumbs in order to press it back into place (Fig. 721, *A, B, C*). The marked flexion (90 degrees) obtained by this maneuver tends to push the lower fragment back into place and restore the normal anterior concavity of the lower end of the radius, and if the reduction is adequate, the hand tends to drop into normal flexion.

Traction Method.—The arm is flexed at the elbow, a pad is placed over the flexor surface of the arm, and a strap or band is passed around it and fixed to the table or some other immovable object. The surgeon then grasps the patient's wrist and thumb with both hands and exerts slow steady traction combined with hyperextension to break up the impaction. An assistant can then maintain the traction or the traction may be exerted by the assistant from the beginning. When the fragments have been pulled by one another, the hand is strongly pronated and adducted and moderately flexed by the assistant while the surgeon, with the heel of one hand, presses the distal fragment first forward and then to the ulnar side while the other hand presses backward to restore the normal volar concavity of the lower portion of the shaft of the radius.

If the reduction appears satisfactory, moderate traction is continued and with the hand maintained in a position of full pronation, moderate flexion, and strong ulnar deviation, a short plaster cast is applied. This is a skin-tight plaster, or there may be a little padding around the wrist, and it extends from the upper forearm to the metacarpal heads. It is molded around the wrist by pressure while the plaster is setting and is then cut out in the palm to permit full flexion of the fingers. In instances where swelling is to be expected, the cast is split along the dorsum or extended well down over the fingers. After four or five days the plaster over the fingers is removed to permit full flexion of the fingers, and exercise and use of the fingers is insisted upon. In most instances the original cast is left on for six weeks. If moderate flexion at the wrist has been necessary to maintain reduction, the cast is changed at the end of two weeks and a new one applied with the wrist in the neutral position.

Criteria of Complete Reduction.—One of the most difficult things about the treatment of these fractures is for the surgeon to be satisfied when complete reduction has been accomplished. The following points are valuable aids in deciding this question: (1) When reduction is complete, unless there is very great swelling, the wrist can be easily flexed to the normal degree for the patient as can be determined by comparing with the uninjured wrist. (See Fig. 721, *D*.) (2) By palpation it will be found that the styloid process of the radius is now below that of the ulna and occupies approximately the same relation to it as does that of the normal radius to the normal ulna on the other side. (3) The normal anterior concavity of the volar surface of the lower end of the radius is restored. This can be determined by careful palpation. (4) The normal, slightly convex contour of the dorsal surface of the lower end of the radius has been restored. (5) The head of the ulna is no longer unusually prominent on the volar surface of the wrist and the abnormal broadening of the wrist has been corrected. (6) The silver fork and adduction deformities have disappeared.

Fixation.—There are a good many methods devised for the immobilization of these fractures. We believe that the most efficient method is to immobilize the hand with the wrist in full pronation, strong ulnar deviation, and moderate flexion, and we use a short plaster cast so cut out in the palm that full flexion of the fingers is possible. We rarely immobilize the elbow as we encourage our patients not only to exercise the fingers, but to use the hand as soon as possible.

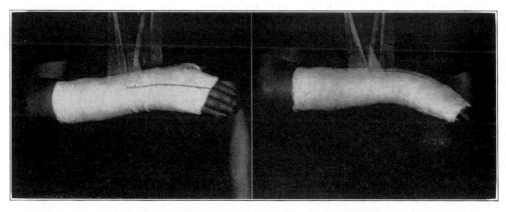

Fig. 722.—Prevention of swelling is very important in wrist fractures. The cast may be split along the dorsum or extended down over the proximal joints of the fingers. After four or five days it is removed back to the palmar crease to permit full flexion of the fingers.

Other methods of immobilization are: (1) A posterior padded board splint which is exactly the width of the normal wrist and forearm, which is cut out over the styloid process of the ulna and which is so cut that it holds the hand in a position of ulnar deviation, and extends from the base of the fingers along the posterior surface of the forearm to beyond the elbow joint. The details of this splint are shown in Figs. 723 and 724. In addition to this we frequently apply a short volar splint which is well padded with cotton, especially at a point opposite the lower end of the upper fragment and which reaches from the fold in the wrist to beyond the elbow. When the displacement has been completely reduced, these two splints are strapped on separately with adhesive and are then covered with sheet cotton and incorporated in a circular plaster cast extending from the middle of the arm to the base of the fingers. (2) Anterior (Fig. 725) and posterior molds or a molded sugar tong plaster cast (Fig. 727) are applied with a minimum amount of padding carefully molded around the lower end of the radius and ulna and elbow, and holding the hand in the same position. These plaster molds may or may not be incorporated in a plaster cast extending from the middle of the arm to the bases of the fingers.

Postoperative Roentgenograms.—As soon as possible after the reduction anteroposterior and lateral roentgenograms should be made in order to check the efficiency of the reduction. In studying these the surgeon should note particularly whether or not the radial styloid has been brought down to its normal position below the ulnar styloid and whether the articular surface of the radius faces downward and about 16 to 20 degrees forward as it should. If the

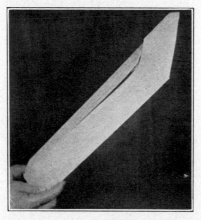

Fig. 723.—A method of making a posterior or extensor wooden splint to hold the hand in a position of ulnar deviation or adduction and immobilize the hand and wrist. The wide board is cut down from one side until it is the width of the normal wrist and forearm.

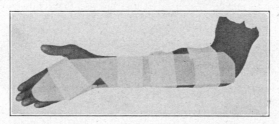

Fig. 724.—Showing the posterior wooden splint with a cut-out made for the ulna styloid cut away to adduct hand at the wrist. The splint is strapped to the dorsal surface of the forearm with adhesive. This type of splint is one of the types which are indicated in the severe comminuted fractures of the lower part of the radius when firm and fixed adduction of the hand at wrist is indicated. Padding has not been applied in order to show detail.

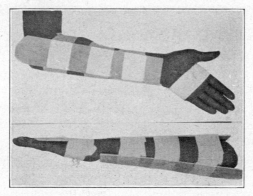

Fig. 725.—*A.*—Anterior or flexor wooden splint of the same width of the forearm and extending from beyond the elbow to the fold at the wrist, strapped to the flexor surface of the forearm. Padding left off to show detail.

B. Showing how the posterior alignment of the forearm is restored by the posterior wooden splint. No padding applied in order to show detail.

styloid is correct, the articular surface will also face inward about 20 to 25 degrees. He should also note the inferior radio-ulnar joint. If this articulation is not restored in approximately its normal relationship there is apt to be limitation of rotation and pain on rotation of the forearm.

If the position of the lower fragment is not satisfactory, another attempt at reduction should be made as soon as possible and if local anesthesia has been used this can be done immediately before the effect of the local anesthetic has worn off.

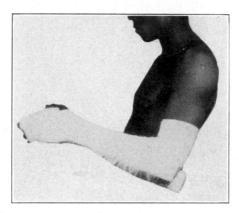

Fig. 726.—The splints are encased in sheet cotton which includes the lower part of the upper arm and down to middle phalanges of the fingers. This is covered with a plaster to complete the dressing. Forearm in midposition.

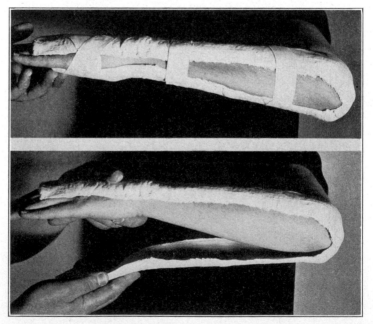

Fig. 727.—The so-called sugar tong plaster made from a single long plaster mold bound on with a gauze bandage. When dry it may be strapped on with adhesive. Useful in treating fractures of the lower end of the radius which are in good position and which do not have a tendency to displace.

Fig. 728.—At the end of two or three weeks the plaster may be cut from around the elbow, the anterior or flexor half discarded, and the posterior or extensor mold used as a retention splint which can be removed daily for exercises.

If the lower fragment is badly comminuted, a second x-ray picture should be made about ten days later in order to see whether or not any slipping has occurred.

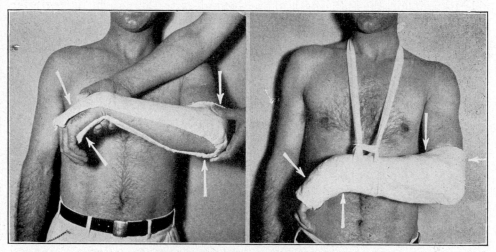

Fig. 729.—Immobilization in full flexion by means of plaster molds and covered with plaster for hyperextension fractures of the lower end of the radius. In comminuted fractures of the lower end of the radius the elbow should be fixed in most cases during the early stage. The flexed position should not be maintained more than two weeks. Then a new cast should be applied with the wrist in the neutral position.

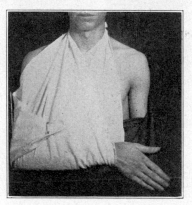

Fig. 730.—Shows how the hand and forearm should be worn in the sling in forearm fractures, especially lower end of the radius. Note that the edge of the sling extends only to the wrist and the hand drops into ulnar deviation.

The Cotton-Loder Position (Fig. 729).—This position, which is quite popular in this country, is one in which the wrist and hand are immobilized in a plaster cast or splint in a position of full flexion and ulnar deviation and full pronation at the wrist, the object being to pull the extensor tendons tightly across the dorsal surface of the displaced fragment and thus hold it in position. We rarely use this position because we feel that if it is maintained for any considerable length of time, it is very apt to cause permanent stiffness and especially permanent limitation of supination. However, occasionally in fractures in which there has been considerable comminution of the dorsal portion of the lower end of the radius and in which this amounts to a definite loss of substance so that the lower fragment tends to tilt backward when immobilized in a

straight position we immobilize the wrist in moderate flexion and full pronation and ulnar deviation, because we feel that by this method, owing to the
leverage exerted by the anterior portion of the cortex of the radius, we are
able to maintain the full length of the bone despite the gap in its posterior
portion.   At the same time we endeavor to get the hand into a better position
within a week or ten days after the reduction of the fracture and then immobilize
it in the short plaster cast in moderate flexion and with ulnar deviation as
described above.

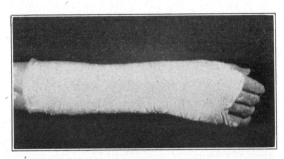

Fig. 731.—Circular plaster cast extending from upper third of forearm to the base of the
fingers and including the proximal phalanx of the thumb for treating fractures of the lower
end of the radius and ulna. A few days later the cast is trimmed to permit motion of the
fingers.

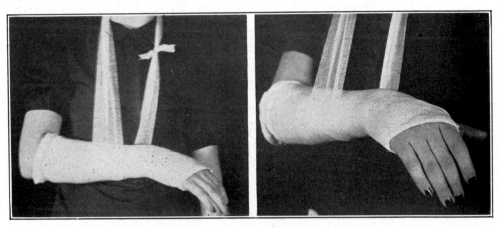

Fig. 732.—Type of plaster cast used for immobilization after reduction of typical Colles'
fracture, without comminution, at the wrist. This is cut out in the palm to permit flexion of
the fingers and thumb. Note slight flexion and adduction of hand at the wrist. The flexed
position should not be maintained more than two weeks. Then a new cast should be applied in
the neutral position.

**Aftertreatment of Extension and Compression Fractures of the Lower
End of the Radius.**—In the ordinary case we leave the original dressing on
for a period of from five to six weeks, but during this time we have the patient
continually exercise the fingers and thumb beginning as soon after the reduction as we can get him to do so. Close observation is to be carried out as
regards the circulation of the hand and forearm during the first forty-eight
hours. We advise the patient not to carry the forearm in a sling and encourage
him to use the hand as much as he can.

If marked swelling was present at the time of the reduction, a snug plaster
is applied at the end of two or three weeks.

With marked comminution and in older patients we leave the plaster on longer (six or seven weeks).

After the dressing has been removed and the patient begins to use the hand, we instruct him to soak the hand in hot water once or twice daily and to massage the wrist, forearm, and fingers, and in certain instances to practice definite exercises tending to increase the movements of the hand and wrist. This physiotherapy is not, as a rule, necessary in young patients, but is of considerable importance in old persons.

In cases complicated by fracture of the ulna styloid or by dislocation of the lower end of the ulna we prolong the period of immobilization about two weeks because we have found that these fractures and dislocations are slow to heal and may be the cause of prolonged pain and disability, and we have seen cases in which nonunion of the ulnar styloid occurred and was the cause of sufficient pain and disability to warrant removal of this process.

Treatment of Epiphyseal Separation of the Lower End of the Radius With Displacement.—This is treated in exactly the same way as are complete fractures in this region in adults. But we take especial pains to secure anatomical reduction because of the disturbance in growth which may follow. However, we do not believe in repeated manipulation in an attempt to secure an anatomical reduction, as this may injure the epiphyseal cartilage. Since reading Aikins'[*] article in which he shows that the deformity tends to be corrected by growth, we are more apt to be content with a fair reduction. It is to be remarked that even with great displacement and appalling deformity these epiphyseal displacements can usually be reduced with comparative ease. After reduction they tend to be stable and can be immobilized in the sugar tong plaster or short plaster or board splints in plaster for four or five weeks.

Treatment of Fractures of the Lateral Articular Border and the Radial Styloid

In a great many of these fractures there is no displacement, and all that is necessary is to immobilize the wrist and hand in a posterior wooden splint, anterior and posterior plaster molds, or in a light plaster cast as in fractures of the lower end of the radius without displacement.

In fractures in which the fragment is displaced, the displacement should be reduced by manipulation under general or local anesthesia and the method of reduction depends somewhat upon the displacement present. If the styloid process and the adjacent portion of the articular surface are displaced outward and upward, reduction can best be accomplished by ulnar deviation with strong traction on the thumb and wrist and pressure directly inward and downward upon the displaced fragment. If there is also posterior displacement, the same method is used except that the pressure is directed inward and toward the volar surface. When the reduction is complete, the normal contour of the bone should be restored as described under complete fractures of the lower end of the radius and the hand should drop into flexion without resistance. It is of considerable importance that these fractures be accurately reduced because they involve the articular surface of the radiocarpal joint.

---

[*]Aikins: J. Bone & Joint Surg., 1935, p. 302.

Immobilization.—After reduction the hand is best immobilized in a light plaster cast, molded snugly over the head of the radius and extending from the upper portion of the forearm to the base of the fingers. This plaster should be applied with the forearm in the midposition and with the hand in adduction (ulnar deviation). As there is no involvement of the inferior radioulnar joint in these fractures, it is not necessary to immobilize the elbow because, although movements of the forearm in rotation do tend to cause displacement of the fragments on account of the insertion of the supinator longus into the radial styloid, this can be prevented by molding the plaster around this region. This cast should be worn for from three to four weeks and then removed and adhesive strapping applied to the wrist for two weeks longer; or a bandage may be used and the patient instructed to soak the hand in hot water once or twice a day. The physiotherapy is more necessary in older patients. During the period when the cast is worn, the patient should use the hand in dressing and for eating and other light work and should be given definite exercises for the fingers. It is also wise to have the patient avoid carrying the arm in a sling, since this tends to increase the period of disability.

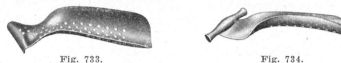

Fig. 733.   Fig. 734.

Fig. 733.—Zimmer special Colles splint. A useful emergency splint. (Courtesy Zimmer Manufacturing Co.)

Fig. 734.—Colles splint. (Courtesy Zimmer Manufacturing Co.)

Treatment of Fractures of the Posterior Articular Margin of the Lower End of the Radius (Barton's Fracture)

In these fractures there is, as a rule, little displacement, but there may be more or less tendency to subluxation at the radioulnar joint with a consequent upward and backward displacement of the detached fragment (Fig. 735). If there is displacement, it should be corrected by direct pressure over the fragment while the hand is maintained in a position of slight dorsiflexion. It is important to restore as nearly as possible the contour of the articular surface. This can be done by direct pressure on the displaced fragment and local or general anesthesia may be necessary.

After the fragment has been pressed back into place, a light circular plaster cast or molds extending from the upper portion of the forearm to the base of the fingers should be applied with the hand in slight dorsiflexion and in the midposition as regards rotation (Fig. 736). The plaster should be well molded over the site of the fracture in order to exert pressure upon this point and thus tend to hold the fragment in place. The reason for dorsiflexion is that if the wrist is not immobilized in dorsiflexion the first row of carpals tends to subluxate in a dorsal direction and thus cause displacement of the fragment. If there is much comminution of the lower end of the radius, the hand should be immobilized in the neutral position as regards flexion and extension rather than in the cock-up position (extension). The immobilization is continued for about two or three weeks; then a flexor or anterior plaster mold (Fig. 737) is used for two weeks, when bandage or adhesive strapping should be applied with an adhesive pad over the site of the fracture for a few days more.

After the dressing is removed, daily hot baths and exercises are prescribed.

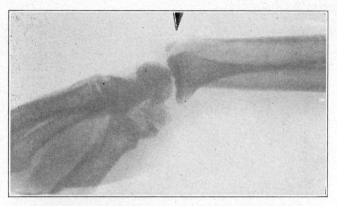

Fig. 735.—Posterior marginal fractures of the lower end of the radius (Barton's fracture). Treated by immobilization in the dorsiflexion in circular plaster cast and later in anterior plaster cock-up molded splint. Good result.

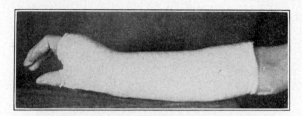

Fig. 736.—Plaster cast with wrist in dorsiflexion used in treating the Barton's fracture (posterior marginal fracture of the radius.)

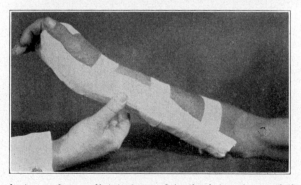

Fig. 737.—Molded plaster cock-up splint to be used in the later stages of the treatment of the Barton or the Smith fracture.

FLEXION AND COMPRESSION FRACTURES OF THE LOWER END OF THE RADIUS (SMITH'S FRACTURE)

Occurrence.—These fractures are frequently called Smith's fractures or Colles' fracture reversed. They are the result of falls or blows in which the force is received upon the dorsum of the flexed hand and wrist and is transmitted upward and forward to the lower end of the radius. These fractures are quite rare because most people in falling hyperextend the hand and receive the force upon the palm.

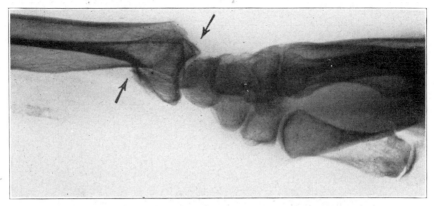

Fig. 738.—Flexion type (Smith's) fracture of the distal end of the radius. Reduced by forcible hyperextension and immobilized with the wrist in moderate extension. Good result.

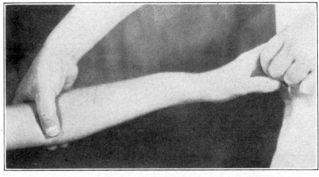

Fig. 739.—Flexion and compression fracture of the lower end of the radius (Smith's fracture) showing a mild degree of the typical garden spade deformity.

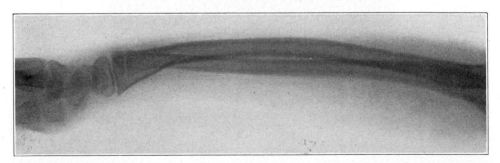

Fig. 740.—Roentgenogram of preceding case. Treated by closed manipulative reduction and immobilization with board splints incorporated in a plaster cast with good result.

Pathology of Flexion and Compression Fractures of the Lower End of the Radius.—The fracture line and displacement are similar to those of the extension type of fracture except that the lower fragment tends to be displaced forward and upward rather than backward and upward (Fig. 738). The fracture line usually takes an oblique course from below upward and forward through the lower cancellous portion of the radius and there may be more or less comminution in the lower fragment. There is rarely any involvement in the radioulnar joint, but this may be disrupted as with posterior displacement of the lower end of the ulna, or the ulnar styloid may be broken.

Diagnosis of Flexion and Compression Fractures of the Lower End of the Radius.—In cases with complete displacement the deformity is the opposite of the silver fork deformity of the classical extension fracture and has often been called the gardener's spade deformity (Figs. 739, 740, and 741). The swelling may be extensive and obscure the deformity. There is a dorsal prominence of the distal end of the upper fragment and a fullness of the wrist on the volar side due to the displaced distal fragment. In the silver fork deformity the dorsal prominence is more distal than the volar while in the gardener's spade deformity the volar prominence is the more distal. Point tenderness is usually present around the lower end of the radius at a variable distance above its lower margin and the radial styloid is displaced upward and forward and may be rotated in a direction of pronation. The lower end of the upper fragment can be palpated between the tendons on the dorsum of the wrist and it may be possible to palpate the upper and outer border of the lower fragment beneath the tendons on the volar surface of the wrist. The head of the ulna is unusually prominent on the dorsum of the wrist.

Treatment

Treatment of Flexion and Compression Fractures of the Lower End of the Radius Without Displacement.—In these fractures without displacement, which are rare, all that is necessary is to immobilize the wrist in the neutral position as regards flexion, extension, rotation, and supination. If desired, the hand may be placed in a position of adduction (ulnar deviation). For this position either the dorsal board splint, plaster molds, or the light plaster cast can be used, depending upon the surgeon's choice.

Treatment of Flexion and Compression Fractures of the Lower End of the Radius with Displacement.—In these fractures, just as in extension fractures, the displacement must be accurately reduced if one is to obtain a satisfactory wrist. The reduction must be accomplished under full anesthesia which may be either general or local, and as in the extension fracture, it may be accomplished by leverage or by traction and direct pressure. Usually in these fractures traction and direct pressure are rather more satisfactory than the leverage method. The traction method is exactly the same as was described under the extension fractures except that when the fragments are pulled apart the surgeon, with the heels of his hands and his fingers locked, presses the proximal fragment toward the volar surface and the distal fragment toward the dorsal surface, thus tending to reduce the displacement. In the manipulative method the surgeon first brings the wrist into a position of hyperflexion in order to disentangle the fragments or break up impaction if present and then with more or less traction forces the wrist upward and to the ulnar side in a movement of hyperextension and ulnar deviation. In other words, the manipulation is the reverse of the movements described for the reduction of the extension type of fractures.

The criteria for reduction of these fractures are exactly the same as are those for the reduction of the extension type of fractures except that here the wrist will usually go into full extension (dorsiflexion) without resistance when the reduction is complete. The immobilization is exactly the same as in the extension type; that is, the elbow, forearm and wrist should be immobilized in the neutral position as regards rotation with the wrist in the neutral position as regards flexion and extension and with the hand deviated to the ulnar side. This can be accomplished by either the plaster cast, plaster molds, or board splints incorporated in the plaster cast as described above under the treatment of the extension type and the after-treatment should be carried out in exactly the same manner.

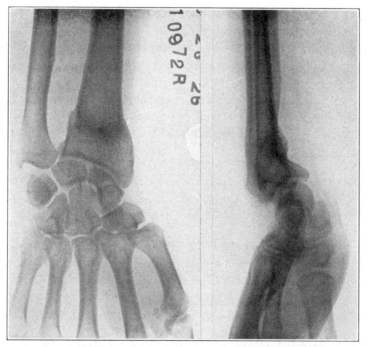

Fig. 741.—Old flexion and compression fracture of the radius (Smith's fracture) united with moderate deformity. The patient has limitation of dorsiflexion.

If the fragments are not stable in the neutral position the cast or plaster molds and cast should be applied with the forearm supinated and the hand in dorsiflexion and deviated to the ulnar side. The after-treatment is the same as for the extension type of fracture of the same degree.

FLEXION FRACTURES OF THE ANTERIOR ARTICULAR MARGIN OF THE RADIUS

This fracture, which is sometimes called reversed Barton's fracture, may result from a fall on the dorsum of the hand with hyperflexion of the wrist or the anterior margin may be torn off by forcible hyperextension of the wrist.

The fracture is a very rare one and may be accompanied by anterior luxation or subluxation of the carpus. Due to the fact that the detached portion of the anterior articular margin is usually small and is covered by the mass of flexor tendons, this fracture cannot as a rule be diagnosed definitely in the absence of the x-ray. It may be suspected in flexion injuries at the wrist in which there is localized tenderness of the volar surface of the lower end of the radius accompanied by considerable swelling and instability at the wrist joint with no tenderness on the dorsum of the wrist. The presence of an anterior dislocation of the carpus which can be easily reduced but which is unstable after reduction and tends to recur when the wrist is extended would point to the presence of a fracture of the anterior articular margin.

Treatment

These fractures as a rule can be treated without an anesthetic, simply by the application of a plaster cast extending from the upper portion of the forearm to the base of the fingers and applied with the hand in the midposition as regards rotation, abduction, and adduction, and with the hand moderately flexed (Fig. 742). The hand and wrist are placed in palmar flexion to prevent the forward luxation of the carpal bones on the radius, since this not only tends to produce an unstable wrist, but also tends to maintain displacement of the fragments. Immobilization should be continued for from five to six days, and the patient should be instructed to exercise and use the fingers. At the end of this period the plaster can be removed and the wrist brought up to the midposition as regards flexion and extension and immobilized in a circular plaster cast or plaster molds, or a padded posterior board splint. This is continued for two or three weeks, when it is removed and the wrist strapped with adhesive for two weeks longer.

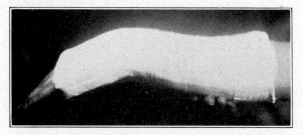

Fig. 742.—Plaster cast with wrist in moderate flexion as used in the treatment of anterior marginal fractures of the radius.

ISOLATED FRACTURES OF THE STYLOID OF THE ULNA

This is a rare fracture which may result from a fall on the ulnar side of the abducted hand, the styloid being torn off (sprain fracture). The detached fragment tends to be displaced downward and forward. As a rule there is relatively little swelling and disability, but there may be considerable pain. It is difficult to differentiate this injury from a sprain of the internal lateral ligament of the wrist unless it is possible to palpate the detached fragment. Consequently in question of doubt, an x-ray may be necessary for the diagnosis. There is point tenderness over the lower end of the ulna in both lesions.

Treatment of Isolated Fractures of the Styloid of the Ulna.—As a rule no anesthetic is necessary. The wrist should be immobilized with the hand in a position of ulnar deviation over a period of at least four weeks. This can be most comfortably accomplished by means of a light plaster cast which extends from the upper arm to the base of the fingers and is applied with the forearm in the neutral position as regards rotation and with the hand in the neutral position as regards flexion and extension, but deviated strongly to the ulnar side. If at the end of four weeks there is still rather definite tenderness and pain at the site of the lesion, the cast should be reapplied for two weeks longer. At the end of this time the detached fragment will usually be firmly united and no further immobilization is necessary although the patient should avoid straining the wrist in the position of abduction for a few weeks longer.

If union does not occur, and the styloid remains painful, the loose fragment should be removed. (Fig. 743.)

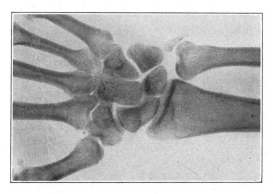

Fig 743.—Old fracture of the ulnar styloid with nonunion. Treated by excision. Pain relieved but wrist remained slightly weak.

FRACTURES AND DISLOCATIONS OF THE CARPAL BONES

Before the use of the x-ray became practically routine in the examination of wrist injuries both fractures and dislocations of the individual carpal bones were considered rare lesions, but in recent years the x-ray has shown us that these bones are quite frequently broken or dislocated and we have learned to diagnose the more common lesions by the history and physical examination and to confirm our diagnosis by the x-ray. The two more common lesions of the carpus are fracture of the scaphoid and dislocation of the semilunar.

FRACTURE OF THE CARPAL SCAPHOID (NAVICULAR)

Incidence.—This is the most common of the carpal injuries and is said to comprise about 0.5 per cent of all fractures. It is most often seen in young adults, especially males, but may occur in children or even in the aged as a rare injury. However, injuries which would tend to fracture the scaphoid usually cause epiphyseal separations or fractures of the bones of the forearm in children and fractures of the lower end of the radius in older adults.

Cause and Mechanism.—The carpal bones are interposed between the hand and the forearm and act as buffers when force is transmitted upward to the forearm. As was stated above, most of the force is received by the lower end of the radius and is transmitted to it through the scaphoid and semilunar bones. Consequently, most fractures of the carpal scaphoid are caused by indirect violence transmitted upward from the hand and the great majority are due to falls upon the hand. Very rarely the scaphoid may be broken by direct violence such as a blow upon the back or side of the wrist.

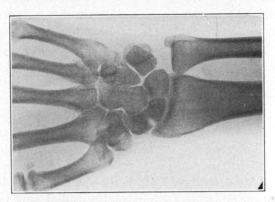

744.—Fracture of the scaphoid. Treated by immobilization in abduction in a circular plaster cast extending from upper third of the forearm to base of the fingers and including proximal phalanx of thumb for eight weeks. Good result.

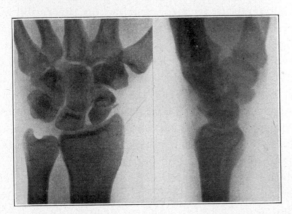

Fig. 745.—Fracture of the scaphoid treated as was preceding case. Good result.

The exact mechanism by which the scaphoid is broken has aroused considerable theoretical discussion and the question is still unsolved, largely because in sudden blows or falls upon the hand it is not possible for the patient to state the exact position of the hand when the blow was received. With the hand in dorsiflexion and deviated to the radial side, the scaphoid is locked against the articular surface of the radius; force transmitted upward reaches it through the head of the os magnum, and the narrow portion of the scaphoid is compressed between the head of the os magnum and the radius and may be broken.

The rare fractures of the tuberosity are avulsion or sprain fractures due to forcible adduction (ulnar deviation) of the wrist.

Pathology of Fracture of the Carpal Scaphoid.—In most cases the scaphoid is broken into two parts by an irregularly transverse fracture across the long axis of the bone near its middle. In cases where the fragments are unequal in size the lateral fragment tends to be larger. Occasionally the bone is comminuted. All of these fractures of the body of the scaphoid are intraarticular and as a rule there is practically no displacement. Occasionally, however, the lateral fragment may be displaced posteriorly or the mesial fragment may be displaced anteriorly, especially if the fracture of the scaphoid is accompanied by an anterior dislocation of the semilunar bone.

In the rare fractures of the tuberosity of the scaphoid, the fracture is largely or entirely extraarticular and the avulsed fragment retains its attachment to the lateral ligament of the wrist and may be displaced slightly outward and either upward or downward. (Fig. 745.)

A considerable percentage of the cases of fracture of the scaphoid are accompanied or complicated by other injuries in this region. The most frequent of these are dislocation of the semilunar, fracture of the semilunar, fracture of the lower end of the radius, or fracture of the radial or ulnar styloid.

Diagnosis of Fracture of the Carpal Scaphoid.—In a recent case there is considerable pain which is most acute on the radial side of the wrist. The patient tends to hold the wrist rigid with the hand pronated and is unable to grip with the hand. On inspection there is a variable amount of swelling of the wrist which tends to be more marked on the radial side and dorsum and may be limited to the region of the anatomical snuff box which is always obliterated. (Figs. 746 and 747.)

On palpation it will be found that the wrist presents no deformity other than the swelling and that the bony landmarks are in their normal relationships. The characteristic sign of fracture of the scaphoid is acute tenderness over the anatomical snuff box. This is the normally depressed area on the radial aspect of the wrist at the base of the thumb and is bounded behind by the tendon of the extensor longus pollicis and in front by the tendons of the extensor brevis and abductor longus pollicis.

On manipulation it will be found that all movements of the wrist are limited and cause pain, but that dorsiflexion and abduction (radial deviation) are especially limited and painful. Also axial pressure on the first, second, or third metacarpals or digits causes pain in the region of the scaphoid. In the rare fractures of the tuberosity of the scaphoid the pain on axial pressure may be absent.

The diagnosis should be confirmed by the x-ray, and it is well to mention that due to the forward tilt of the bone a transverse linear fracture may not show in the ordinary anteroposterior view, but may show in one taken with the wrist dorsiflexed or in the oblique position or with the back of the wrist against the film with the hand deviated to the ulnar side.

Treatment of Fracture of the Carpal Scaphoid.—The treatment is immobilization, immediate, complete, and prolonged. The most important point about fractures of the carpal scaphoid is early diagnosis and early immobilization. The cases with prolonged or permanent disability are usually those which have been diagnosed as sprains of the wrist and in which complete immobilization has not been used until some weeks after the injury.

Because the thumb must be immobilized we do not recommend the popular Commercial or Jones cock-up splint, but always use plaster of Paris. Here as elsewhere it may be reiterated that no splint fits like a properly applied plaster-of-Paris cast.

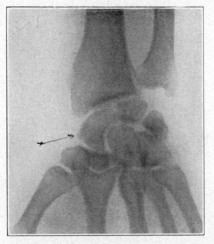

Fig. 746.—Slight fracture of the tubercle of the scaphoid treated by immobilization in a circular plaster cast for six weeks. Good result.

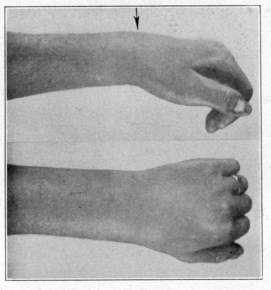

Fig. 747.—Fracture of the scaphoid. Typical deformity when viewed from the lateral and dorsal aspects.

No anesthetic is necessary. The hand and wrist are placed in the desired position and the plaster-of-Paris cast is applied as follows: A circular cast with little or no padding is snugly applied from the upper one-third of the forearm down to the base of the fingers including the thumb with the hand at the wrist moderately hyperextended and fully abducted; that is, deviated to the radial side. The thumb is fully abducted and extended as advised by Soto-Hall and Haldeman.* If the fragments are displaced, they should be reduced by strong traction and digital pressure before the cast is applied under local anesthesia.

If the hand and wrist were not swollen when the cast was applied, it is left on for at least seven or eight weeks or longer, according to the x-ray findings after this period. If it becomes loose because of subsidence of swelling or atrophy, or if it becomes softened or broken, it is removed and replaced by a new tight cast. At the end of six or eight weeks the cast is removed and x-ray pictures are made. If the scaphoid is united, the wrist is strapped with adhesive, and the patient is instructed to exercise and use the wrist and hand. If the scaphoid has not united, the cast is replaced for from two to four weeks, depending upon the appearance of the bone in the roentgenogram. New roentgenograms are made when the cast is next removed. By this method union can almost always be obtained, and the wrist will loosen up again after a few weeks of exercise and use.

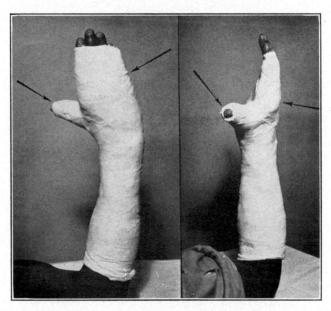

Fig. 748.—Immobilization of hand and wrist in abduction with thumb abducted and extended for fractures of the scaphoid. (After Soto-Hall and Haldeman.) (See also Fig. 751.)

Immobilization in the Functional Position.—The use of the above-described position with wide abduction and extension of the thumb may result in prolonged inability to flex and oppose the thumb. Consequently, we now immobilize the hand in the grasping or functional position with the wrist moderately dorsiflexed and deviated to the radial side. The thumb is opposed to the fingers and slightly flexed as though grasping a large ball. The case extends only to the palmar crease in the palm and permits full flexion of the fingers. It covers the entire thumb, except the tip, and slight movement of the terminal phalanx of the thumb

*Soto-Hall and Haldeman: J. Bone & Joint Surg., 1934, p. 822.

is permitted. This cast may be worn for months and the hand remain in excellent condition. In a fresh fracture of the wrist or proximal pole of the scaphoid the cast should remain on for eight weeks and should not be changed if this can be avoided. It is a mistake to remove the cast for x-rays before union can be expected.

Prognosis in Fractures of the Scaphoid.—If immobilization is begun soon after the injury and is continued over a period of seven or eight weeks, we believe that practically every case of fracture of the scaphoid will give good functional results and that most cases will obtain bony union. Occasionally, however, the fragments do not unite, but even in many of these cases with nonunion the functional result is good and the presence of nonunion does not seem to cause any disturbance. In old neglected cases, however, the prognosis is quite different. This is especially true with an avascular necrotic proximal fragment. We believe that this fragment should be excised relatively early before the necrotic fragment causes arthritis of the wrist.

OLD FRACTURES OF THE SCAPHOID

Occasionally one sees a patient in whom a wrist has remained tender, weak, and painful over a period of several months after an accident and more or less swelling may have persisted. On physical examination, in addition to the slight swelling on the outer and dorsal portions of the wrist, especially in the region of the anatomical snuff box, there will be a moderate amount of tenderness over the scaphoid, and limitation of motion, especially in extension and radial deviation. The grip is weakened, and the patient complains of a variable amount of pain both with and without motion. An x-ray will show an old fracture of the scaphoid with more or less rarefaction of the bone, failure of union, and a variable amount of absorption along the fracture line.

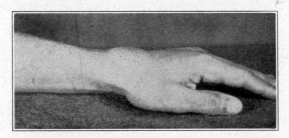

Fig. 749.—Fracture of the scaphoid with unusual amount of swelling viewed from the radial aspect.

In some cases the bone, instead of being rarefied, is more dense than the surrounding bones due to the fact that it has been deprived of its circulation while the surrounding bones have atrophied from disuse. Such a condition is known as Preiser's disease. (Fig. 752.)

Treatment of Old Fractures of the Scaphoid.—In these old cases with nonunion and absorption no treatment is indicated unless the patient complains of pain and disability at the wrist, but with these symptoms the usual treatment is to excise either one or both fragments. Some surgeons take out half of the bone while some take out all of it. We now remove only the proximal

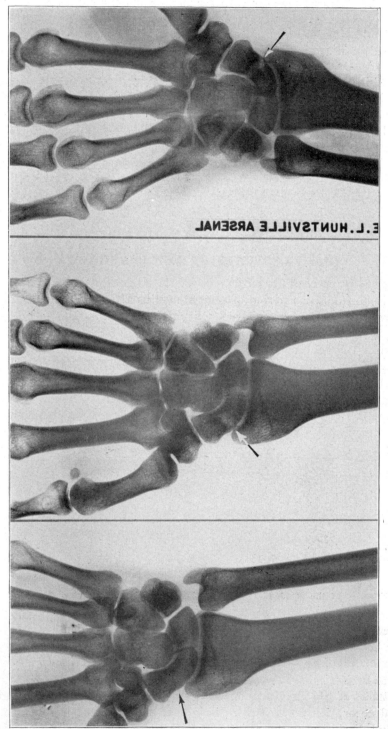

Fig. 750.—Fracture of the scaphoid barely seen in the figure at the left but easily seen in the middle and right figures, which were taken four and six weeks after the injury and show progressive rarefaction.

avascular fragment. If both fragments are living we prefer to attempt to secure union by a bone graft and prolonged immobilization. G. Murray and others have shown that if the fragments are in good or fair condition, union can usually be obtained by means of a small autogenous bone graft or peg which transfixes the lateral fragment and penetrates the mesial fragment. This is most easily placed by driving the graft in a drill hole made by a five-sixteenths-inch drill. The dorsum of the bone is exposed through the anatomical snuff box and the drill hole begins on the tuberosity and passes through the proximal fragment across the fracture line and into the distal fragment. Then a pin of cortical bone which will fit snugly in the hole is cut from the tibia and driven into the hole, thus pinning the two fragments together. Then a plaster cast is applied with the hand abducted and hyperextended.

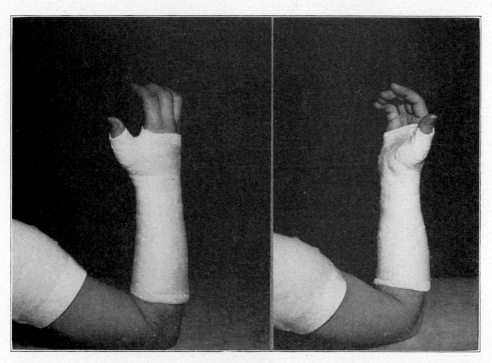

Fig. 751.—Fracture of the scaphoid immobilized in the functional or grasping position with the thumb opposed. This permits excellent function of the hand and is the method which one of us (J. A. K.) prefers.

Soto-Hall and Haldeman do not use a graft, but bore five or six small holes across the fracture line and report union in five out of seven cases operated upon by this method. After the operation the hand and wrist are immobilized in a plaster cast in dorsiflexion and abduction for eight weeks.

The objection to excision of the bone is that one does not obtain a normal wrist in such cases. The wrist continues to exhibit a certain amount of limitation of motion and weakness which may be sufficient to handicap the patient to a considerable degree. For this reason we have been impressed by the results recently shown by Boehler who seems to be able to obtain union of the scaphoid in many of these old neglected cases by the simple method of prolonged immobilization and not only obtains union but obtains a wrist which is apparently normal. His method is to apply a short plaster cast directly to

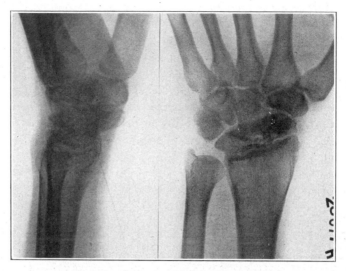

Fig. 752.—Old fracture of the scaphoid which was not immobilized showing destruction of the bone and Preiser's disease or scaphoid osteitis.

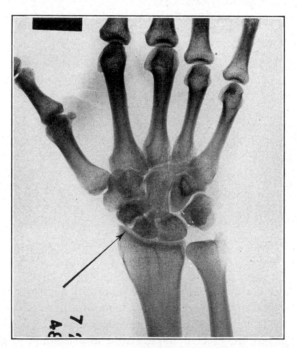

Fig. 753.—Old fracture of the scaphoid. Treated by multiple drilling with satisfactory union and function.

the skin with no padding beneath it and extend it from the base of the fingers to the upper portion of the forearm. This cast is applied with the hand in moderate hyperextension and slight radial deviation and includes the thumb.

It is replaced as often as necessary, but the period of immobilization lasts from six to eight months. During this time the patient uses the hand as much as he can with the plaster cast on. It seems quite probable that the patient could perform many gainful and useful tasks with this cast and might obtain a normal wrist under conditions which, with excision of the fractured bone, would result in a certain amount of permanent disability. For this reason we believe that when possible the conservative treatment should be given a thorough trial before excision is advised.

The progress of union is, of course, followed by x-rays and the immobilization is continued until the union is quite firm.

Operative Removal of the Scaphoid.—In those instances in which prolonged immobilization or bone grafting or drilling has failed, and in which the patient has considerable pain and disability, the scaphoid can be removed through a small incision on the dorsum of the wrist made directly lateral and parallel to the tendon of the extensor longus pollicis. This incision should be about two inches long, carried down to the bone, care being taken not to open the tendon sheaths, and the extensor longus tendon should be retracted mesially. The scaphoid is exposed by incising the ligaments and capsule over it and is removed in two pieces by sharp dissection, care being taken not to injure the adjacent cartilaginous surfaces, or only the avascular proximal fragment may be removed. After the operation, the ligament is sutured, the skin is closed, and an anterior plaster mold is applied extending from the tip of the fingers and thumb to the upper portion of the forearm and holding the hand in moderate dorsiflexion and slight radial deviation. This cast permits dressing of the wound without removal of the cast and should include the thumb and all of the fingers. The patient may begin to exercise the fingers immediately and by the end of the week the cast can be cut away down to the base of the fingers and thumb. At the end of ten days, active motion can be started at the wrist although the splint should be worn most of the time for a period of about three weeks.

After the wound has thoroughly healed, hot packs or baking may be instituted, but it is of great importance that the patient be given definite exercises to perform, and that he continue these for some months, although he may begin to use the wrist for light work within three weeks after the operation.

After the removal of the scaphoid, the patient may be expected to obtain a useful and painless wrist and hand, but they will be moderately weak and this will give him a certain amount of permanent disability; consequently, the bone graft is the operation of choice if the fragments are in good or fair condition.

If marked degenerative arthritis is present in the wrist, arthrodesis will give a stable, painless wrist and pronation and supination can be preserved. If the wrist joint is not badly damaged, arthrodesis of the proximal to the distal row of carpal bones is the operation of choice. One of us (H. E. C.) has, in several instances, removed the scaphoid and semilunar and even the whole proximal row of carpal bones in these cases with fairly good results. The other (J. A. K.) prefers an arthrodesis.

DISLOCATION OF THE CARPAL SEMILUNAR BONE
(OS LUNATUM)

Incidence and Mechanism.—Next to fractures of the scaphoid this is the most common carpal injury. Most of the dislocations of the semilunar bone are hyperextension and compression injuries and result from falls upon the hand. As the hand is forced into hyperextension the head of the os magnum tends to ride up on the dorsal surface of the semilunar and the dorsal ligaments between the two bones are ruptured. As the pressure is continued, the volar ligaments between the semilunar and the os magnum are ruptured and the semilunar is popped out into the space beneath the volar tendons.

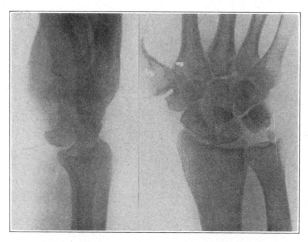

Fig. 754.—Dislocation of the semilunar carpal bone with fracture of the styloid process of the ulna. Treated by manipulative reduction and immobilization in slight flexion in a plaster cast. Good result.

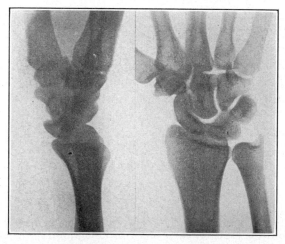

Fig. 755.—Dislocation of the semilunar carpal bone treated as preceding with good result.

In very rare instances the semilunar bone is dislocated backward beneath the extensor tendons on the dorsum of the wrist. These posterior dislocations are due to compression and hyperflexion injuries as in falls upon the dorsum of the hand.

Pathology.—As the semilunar is pushed forward into the space beneath the volar tendons all of its ligaments are torn except the anterior ligaments between it and the radius, and in very rare instances even these may be torn and it is completely detached (Fig. 756). With the anterior ligament intact the semilunar tends to rotate forward and upward to a variable degree (Figs. 754 and 755). In the average case the rotation is about 90 degrees and the dorsal surface of the semilunar faces downward. In rare cases the rotation may amount to 180 degrees and here the dorsal surface faces forward while the volar surface rests upon the volar surface of the lower end of the radius.

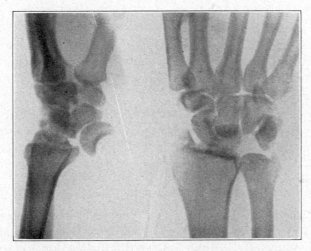

Fig. 756.—Complete dislocation of the semilunar, three weeks old, treated by operative removal of the bone with fair result. Closed manipulation was unsuccessful. There is also a fracture of the radial styloid. (Courtesy of Dr. I. P. Levi.)

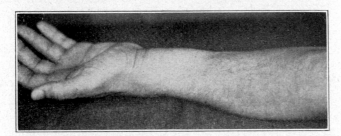

Fig. 757.—Typical deformity in dislocation of the semilunar bone.

Not infrequently dislocation of the semilunar is complicated by a fracture of the scaphoid, and in such cases the mesial fragment may be dislocated with the semilunar. Other frequent complications of semilunar dislocations are fractures of the styloid of the radius or ulna or of both. Not infrequently the median nerve is injured by the displaced semilunar.

In the dorsal dislocations the pathology is similar to that of the anterior dislocations except that the dorsal ligament between the semilunar and the radius remains intact and the bone rotates backward and upward to a variable degree, lifting some of the extensor tendons from the back of the wrist.

Diagnosis.—In an acute anterior dislocation the wrist is moderately swollen, especially on the volar surface and the patient maintains the hand in a position of slight flexion with the fingers moderately flexed (Fig. 757).

Palpation will reveal a tender depression on the dorsum of the wrist at the place usually occupied by the semilunar and a mass (the dislocated semilunar) can usually be felt deep in the volar surface beneath the flexor tendons. In an uncomplicated case the styloid processes will be found in their normal relationship and there will be no bony deformity at the wrist.

All motions of the wrist and hand will be limited and painful and passive extension of the wrist or fingers will elicit pain in the wrist. There may be intense pain in the hand from pressure on the median nerve.

In an old unreduced dislocation of the semilunar the symptoms are similar to those in the acute case except that the swelling is less and is limited to the volar surface of the wrist and movements of the wrist and hand are more free. But extension of the wrist and fingers is limited and painful and the grip is markedly weakened.

In the rare dorsal dislocations the swelling is more marked on the dorsum of the wrist and the dislocated semilunar can be palpated beneath the extensor tendons. Likewise the weakness, pain and limitation of motion are referable to pressure of the displaced semilunar on the extensor tendons.

Treatment

Anterior Displacement.—In an acute anterior displacement of the semilunar the treatment is immediate closed reduction by manipulation, if possible, and this is usually possible unless the dislocation has existed for two weeks or more.

The problem is to open up the socket and then push the semilunar back into place. The socket is opened by hyperextending the hand at the wrist and the semilunar is pushed into place by direct pressure with the thumbs and snapped home by acute flexion of the hand at the wrist. Anesthesia is necessary—either local or general. The latter is preferable.

Closed Method of Reduction of Anterior or Volar Semilunar Carpal Bone Dislocation.—(Figs. 758 and 759.) The operator grasps the distal third of the patient's forearm with one hand and makes firm pressure with his thumb on the flexor surface of the wrist over the dislocated semilunar bone. Now while the patient's forearm (upper third) is grasped by an assistant and strong countertraction is made, the operator grasps the patient's hand with his other hand, and while making strong traction, carries it into extreme dorsiflexion. The operator's thumbs over the semilunar continue to make strong pressure on this bone. Now, without relaxation of the traction, countertraction and strong pressure over the semilunar, the patient's wrist is suddenly manipulated into the position of acute flexion. A decided click is usually felt when reduction has been accomplished. The wrist usually stays flexed without difficulty when the semilunar has been successfully reduced.

It was formerly believed that great force was necessary to press the dislocated semilunar back in place, and for this reason we have in former years used the Thomas wrench or the broomstick method of Davis. We have abandoned these methods because we know that sufficient force may be exerted by the wrench or the broomstick to cause damage to the soft parts, especially the median nerve, and we also have learned that if a semilunar is completely rotated and bound to the anterior surface of the radius by adhesions great force will tend to crush it against the radius, but will not rotate it back to a position opposite its socket. Consequently, we believe that if the dislocation of the semilunar cannot be reduced by the thumbs, it is useless to try to exert more force with a wrench or a broomstick.

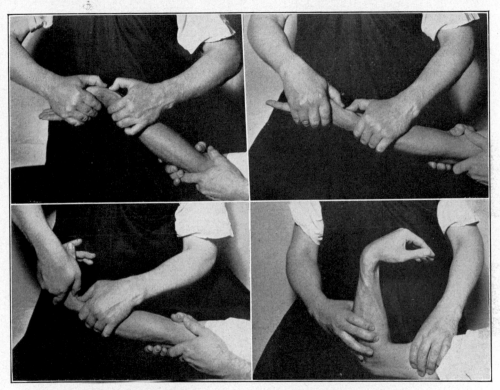

Fig. 758.—Manipulative reduction for anterior dislocation of the semilunar as described in the text. (Conwell: Ann. Surg. 1936.)

Aftertreatment.—When satisfactory reduction has been obtained, the hand and wrist should be immobilized for three or four days with a posterior plaster mold or cast, or a padded posterior wooden splint (Fig. 760) extending from the fingers along back of the forearm to the elbow with about 30 degrees of flexion of the hand at the wrist. After this period a padded posterior plaster mold or cast or a posterior wooden splint should be used with the hand in the straight or neutral position for one or two weeks (Fig. 761). During this time the patient should exercise the fingers daily. At the end of two or three weeks, in the uncomplicated case, the splint or support is removed, the wrist is strapped with adhesive or bandage, and the patient begins to use the hand for light work, but should avoid forcible hyperextension for three or four weeks longer. The adhesive strapping is continued for about two weeks, or until the patient is comfortable without it.

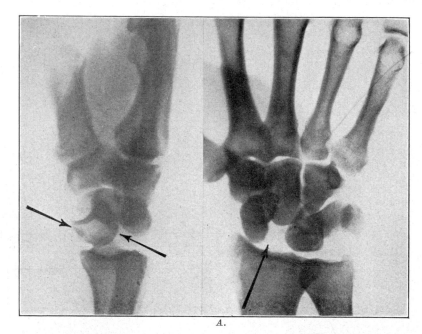

A.

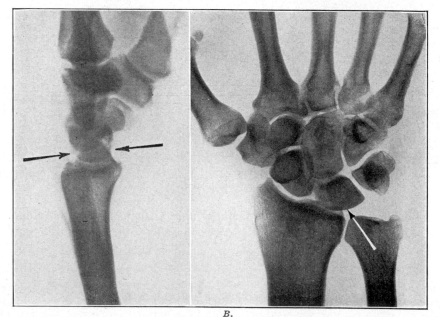

B.

Fig. 759 A and B.—Anterior dislocation of the semilunar before and after reduction.

Prognosis.—One of us (H. E. C.) has reduced twenty-one dislocated semilunar bones, four cases by the broomstick and seventeen cases by the single thumb method. These cases have been followed for from one and one-half to eight years. All returned to their original occupation in from five to ten weeks and all obtained useful wrists and hands although two had slight limitation of motion at the wrist. These cases had other complications, but Kienbock's disease did not develop in any of them. (Figs. 762, 763, and 764.) (Ann. Surg. 1936, p. 978.)

Operative Treatment of Dislocation of the Semilunar Bone.—In old cases or in fresh cases in which two or three attempts at reduction have failed, open operation is indicated and we believe that the operation of choice is open reduction and not removal of the semilunar bone unless the bone is obviously degenerated and its articular cartilage is largely destroyed.

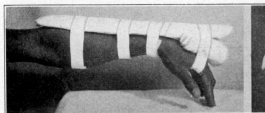 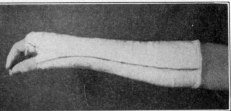

Fig. 760.   Fig. 761.

Fig. 760.—Padded posterior wooden splint with the pad over the dorsum of the hand to maintain flexion, used for the first three or four days in the postoperative treatment of dislocations of the semilunar carpal bone. This is covered with a bandage.

Fig. 761.—Plaster cast immobilizing the hand in the neutral position after reduction of a dislocated semilunar. The plaster is marked for bivalving if necessary.

Technic of Operation.—A straight incision two inches long is made on the volar surface of the wrist just to the ulnar side of the midline. This incision is carried down through the fascia and upper part of the annular ligament. The median nerve and flexor sublimis tendons are retracted to the radial side and the profundus tendons are separated or retracted to expose the displaced semilunar. This is easily identified and is cut loose from its adhesions and ligamentous attachments and removed or replaced in its socket if it is in good condition. In instances where the dislocation has been present for some weeks, the os magnum has slipped up and the space for the semilunar is decreased in size. This can be opened up by strong steady traction on the hand. The annular ligament, fascia, and skin are then sutured and the wrist is immobilized in an anterior plaster mold for two weeks. Exercise and movements of the wrist are begun at the end of the first week and continued as long as necessary.

At the end of two weeks the plaster is removed and the wrist is strapped with adhesive or bandage for two or three weeks longer.

Prognosis After Removal of the Semilunar Bone.—The patient should not be led to expect a normal wrist. Complete range of movement and freedom from pain may be expected unless traumatic arthritis has begun before the operation, but the patient will probably have some weakness in the hand and weakness of the wrist, especially in resisting compression and extension.

Treatment of Posterior Dislocation of the Semilunar Bone.—In the rare cases in which the semilunar bone is dislocated backward the treatment, in the cases which are seen within a week or ten days after the injury, is reduction by manipulation and this reduction is, as a rule, not difficult. It is car-

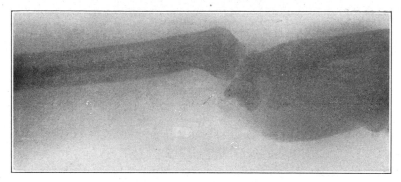

Fig. 762—Fracture of the scaphoid with dislocation of the semilunar. Treated by closed reduction of the semilunar and immobilization of the forearm and hand in padded posterior wooden splint with flexion of the hand at the wrist for three days and then a plaster cast in neutral position for eight weeks on account of the fractured scaphoid.

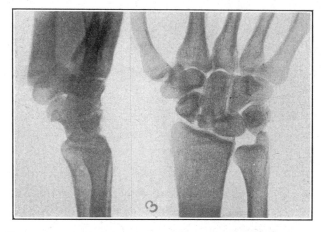

Fig. 763.—The same case as shown in Fig. 733, two years later. The semilunar appears normal. The scaphoid has not united, but the function of the hand is good. No pain or tenderness over scaphoid.

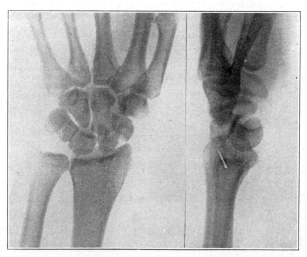

Fig. 764.—Dislocation of the semilunar and fracture of the scaphoid. The semilunar was reduced by the closed method. The scaphoid did not unite, but the patient has a practically normal hand and wrist. Treated in posterior padded wooden splint for three days, then in a circular plaster cast extending from the upper third of the forearm to base of the fingers with hand in adduction and midflexion and extension at the wrist for seven weeks.

ried out by a method similar to that used in the reduction of the anterior semilunar reduction except that the movements are reversed.

Closed Method of Reducing Posterior or Extensor Dislocation of the Semilunar Carpal Bone.—The operator grasps the patient's hand of the involved wrist and with his other hand grasps the lower third of the patient's forearm, making firm pressure with the thumb of this hand over the semilunar on the extensor surface of the wrist. The patient's forearm is grasped by an assistant and strong countertraction is made and the operator markedly flexes the hand at the wrist making strong traction on the hand and firm pressure over the semilunar with the thumb of the other hand. While this pressure and strong countertraction are being made, the operator suddenly hyperextends the hand at the wrist. Usually a definite "click" is felt when reduction is successful. The hand tends to stay in dorsiflexion when the semilunar has been reduced.

The after-treatment is a padded posterior wooden splint and a circular cast to the arm and forearm for from two to three weeks. The hand should be placed in slight extension at the wrist. The cast should be cut along one side immediately after the cast has set (Fig. 761). In these cases flexion of the wrist is liable to cause redislocation.

Treatment of Old Posterior Dislocations of the Semilunar.—In old unreduced dislocations the semilunar should be replaced, and this can be done through a small dorsal incision either directly over the bone or to one side. After the operation the hand should be immobilized on a molded anterior splint and then given active exercises and baking or hot soaks just as in the after-treatment of old anterior dislocations.

SPRAINS AT THE WRIST JOINT

Sprains at the wrist joint are not infrequent and probably outnumber all of the other carpal injuries. It is important for the surgeon to be sure that he is dealing with a simple sprain and with nothing else. For this reason all severe sprains at the wrist should be x-rayed in order to rule out fracture or dislocation in the vicinity.

Diagnosis of Sprains at the Wrist Joint.—After a compression, hyperextension, flexion, or torsion injury, the patient has severe acute pain which is generally distributed throughout the wrist; there may be complete inability to use the hand and there may be moderate swelling which involves the entire carpal region. Frequently there is tenderness entirely around the joint. At other times the tenderness tends to be localized over the dorsal or flexor surface or over one of the lateral ligaments. In some of these cases the clinical picture is very similar to that of a fracture of the scaphoid or a dislocation of the semilunar and it may be impossible to rule out such a lesion without an x-ray. Many of the permanent disabilities at the wrist are the result of an erroneous diagnosis of sprain when the patient was really suffering from some more severe carpal injury.

Treatment of Sprains at the Wrist Joint.—In the acute stage the pain can usually be relieved by immobilization. The method of obtaining this varies with the surgeon and with the circumstances. In some instances we

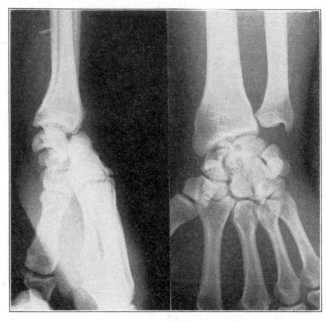

Fig. 765.—Midcarpal dislocation treated by manipulative reduction. Patient resumed work as a laborer twelve weeks later. (Courtesy Dr. Joseph Lembeck.)

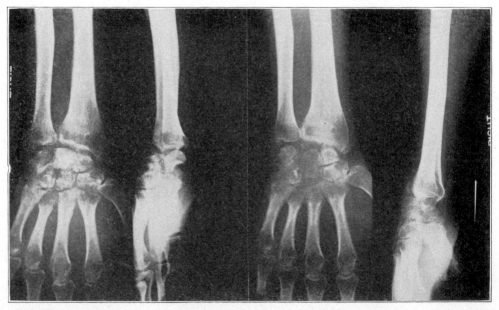

Fig. 766.—Midcarpal dislocation, three months' duration, with marked atrophy and median nerve pressure. Semilunar excised. Reduction incomplete. Final disability 30 per cent. (Courtesy Dr. Joseph Lembeck.)

use an anterior plaster mold; in other instances we apply a compression bandage of absorbent cotton to immobilize and compress the wrist and reduce the swelling.

In cases where the swelling is not great, we strap the wrist with adhesive. In any event the complete immobilization can be discontinued after a few days and the wrist supported with adhesive strapping which extends from the base of the fingers to the middle of the forearm. This is worn for a week or ten days and is then replaced by less extensive strapping with adhesive tape.

Prognosis is good and most of these cases are practically normal at the end of three or four weeks.

FRACTURES OF THE SEMILUNAR BONE

These are rare fractures which may result from compression injuries such as a fall upon the hand. It is believed that the semilunar is only fractured when the hand is in a position of adduction (ulnar deviation) when the force is applied as in this position the semilunar is swung outward under the articular surface of the radius and is thus compressed between the head of the os magnum and the radius.

Diagnosis.—The diagnosis is difficult and cannot be made with certainty in the absence of a positive x-ray. In a recent case the wrist is moderately swollen, the grip is weakened, and all movements are limited and painful, especially dorsiflexion. The swelling is apt to be more marked on the dorsum of the wrist, and there is point tenderness on the dorsum over the semilunar bone. Further evidence of fracture may be gained by placing the hand in slight ulnar deviation and pushing the middle finger upward. If this causes acute pain in the wrist at the site of the semilunar, the surgeon should suspect a fracture of this bone.

Treatment of Recent Fracture of the Semilunar Bone

After a recent fracture of the semilunar bone the hand and wrist should be immobilized in a short plaster cast from six to eight weeks. The hand is placed in a position of slight ulnar deviation and moderate dorsiflexion and the cast applied from the upper third of the forearm to the base of the fingers and the interphalangeal joint of the thumb. Some surgeons advise traction on the middle finger, but we cannot see that this does any particular good and it is certainly a nuisance to the patient as well as to the surgeon. The patient should not carry the hand in a sling but should exercise the fingers daily and use the hand as much as possible. After the cast is removed the patient gradually resumes the use of the hand.

Traumatic Osteitis or Malacia of the Semilunar Bone
(Kienböck's Disease)

This condition described by Kienböck is supposed to be traumatic in origin though it is freely admitted that the original injury may be so slight that it may result in relatively little disability and may not cause the man to stop work. It is also said that the osteitis may develop some months or even several years after the original injury. This naturally brings up the question as to whether the condition is really traumatic in origin and it also brings up

the question as to whether a workman who develops osteitis of the semilunar
is entitled to compensation. Apparently the condition may result from trauma,
but it may also occur without definite injury, or as an occupational condition from overuse, as in painters, or as in the case illustrated it may be due
to syphilis. It may affect any of the carpal bones. A similar condition in the
scaphoid is called Preiser's disease.

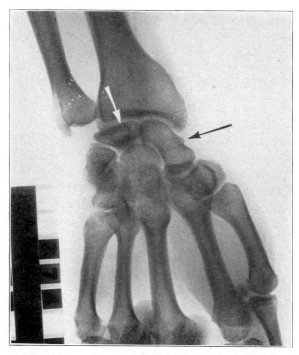

Fig. 767.—Necrosis of the semilunar (Kienböck's disease) with a healed fracture of the
scaphoid. Semilunar had to be removed before good function was obtained.

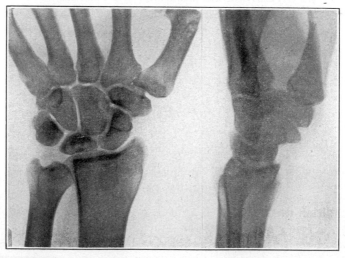

Fig. 768.—Osteitis of the semilunar, Kienböck's disease. No history of severe injury.
This patient had a positive Wassermann and his symptoms cleared up with antisyphilitic
treatment and fixation in circular plaster cast for three months.

Consequently, we feel that if a workman is to receive compensation for carpal osteitis a definite connection should be established between the development of the condition and some injury received while at work, or it should develop while the workman is engaged in some occupation which subjects the wrists to unusual strain.

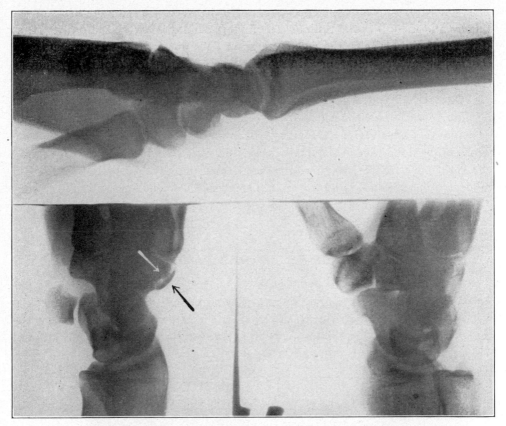

Fig. 769.—Sprain fracture of the os magnum which is visible only in one oblique view.

Diagnosis of Osteitis of the Semilunar Bone.—The symptoms are similar to those of a fresh fracture of the semilunar, though they are less marked in degree. The grip is weak, dorsiflexion at the wrist is moderately limited, and accompanied by pain, and there is a dull ache in the wrist which varies in degree from time to time and is apt to be increased after use. On physical examination there is apt to be a slight amount of swelling on the dorsum of the wrist, and pressure over the semilunar generally elicits tenderness. Pain at the semilunar can usually be elicited by pushing upward on the middle finger. The Wassermann should be determined.

The diagnosis is made by the x-ray. In a comparatively early case the x-ray shows an apparent condensation of the semilunar bone; it casts a shadow which is more dense than that of the other carpals. This may be due to atrophy of the other carpal bones or to increased density of the semilunar. In later cases the rarefaction or malacia of the semilunar makes its appearance and the x-ray shadow shows clear punched-out areas. Later still the bone may appear shriveled, shrunken, crumbled, or fragmented.

Treatment of Carpal Osteitis.—In early cases conservative treatment should be given a fair trial (about eight weeks). Conservative treatment consists of immobilization. Immobilization is conveniently obtained by a circular plaster cast extending from the upper third of the forearm to the bases of the fingers and including the thumb. The fingers should be exercised daily. If, at the end of eight weeks, the roentgenogram does not show improvement, or if the symptoms are not relieved, the abnormal semilunar should be removed. If improvement is noted, the conservative treatment should be continued.

Operative Treatment of Semilunar Osteitis.—In old cases with crumbling or fragmentation of the bone, or in comparatively early cases which do not respond to conservative treatment, the offending bone should be removed. This can be done through a small dorsal incision, care being taken to remove the right bone. After the wound is closed, the hand should be immobilized in moderate dorsiflexion in an anterior plaster mold or cock-up splint for about ten days. At the end of this time the mold or splint may be removed and baking and daily exercises begun.

INJURIES OF THE OTHER CARPAL BONES

In severe compression injuries or from direct trauma any of the other carpal bones may be fractured singly, or two or more of them may be broken simultaneously. These injuries are rare and can be diagnosed only by the x-ray which should always be made in severe carpal injuries. Figs. 770 and 771.)

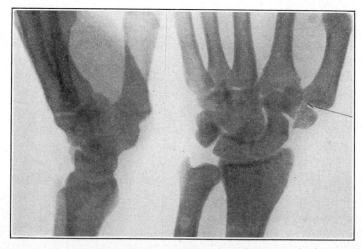

Fig. 770.—Fracture of the trapezium treated by traction and manipulation of the thumb and immobilization in a circular plaster cast with the thumb in a position of abduction and included in cast for a period of six weeks with good result.

Treatment.—Treatment of any of the fractures of the carpal bones consists of reduction by traction and direct pressure of any displaced fragments and immobilization in a short plaster cast or plaster mold for six or eight weeks, depending upon the severity of the injury just as was described in the treatment of fracture of the semilunar bone.

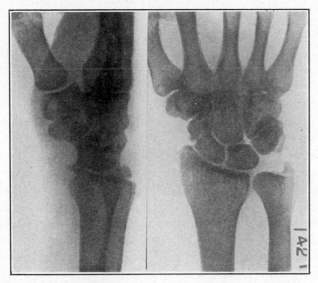

Fig. 771.—Fracture of the cuneiform (the scaphoid and the ulnar styloid). Treated by immobilization for eight weeks in a circular plaster cast. Good results.

DIFFERENTIAL DIAGNOSIS OF INJURIES IN THE REGION OF THE WRIST

For the purpose of differential diagnosis we shall consider the region of the wrist as including the lower two inches of the bones of the forearm, the carpals and the bases of the metacarpals.

The surgeon should obtain as accurate a history as possible, paying particular attention to the character of the injury and position of the wrist in extension or flexion when the injury was received. In recent injuries confirmatory evidence on this point may be obtained by inspection of the hand as abrasions or contusions on the palm suggest an extension injury while similar lesions on the dorsum suggest a flexion injury. The age of the patient should be considered because in children and adolescents the usual injuries are separation of the lower radial epiphysis or fractures of both bones of the forearm near the wrist, while in adults the usual injury is an extension and compression fracture of the lower end of the radius.

Both wrists should then be inspected, and any visible deformity or swelling in the injured wrist should be carefully noted. An obvious silver fork deformity denotes an extension type of injury with displacement and a garden spade deformity denotes a flexion type of injury with displacement, the apex of the curve being opposite the site of the lesion. Localized swelling suggests the location of the lesion. General extensive swelling suggests a severe injury.

The injured wrist should then be palpated carefully for deformity and tenderness. It is well to begin the palpation by definitely locating the radial and ulnar styloids. In the normal adult the tip of the styloid of the radius is about one-half inch lower than that of the ulna and nearer the volar surface of the wrist. The exact relations of the styloid processes of the patient should be determined by examining the opposite normal wrist.

If the radial styloid is displaced upward from its normal level below that of the ulna, there is a fracture of the lower end of the radius with displacement. If there is a silver fork deformity, with the styloid displaced backward, the normal anterior concavity of the lower end of the radius lessened, and disappearance of dorsal prominence of the head of the ulna, there is probably a typical extension and compression fracture of the lower end of the radius, or epiphyseal separation, if the patient is a child, with the typical displacement. The level of the fracture can be roughly determined by locating the line of point tenderness or palpating the ends of the fragments.

In rare instances the radial styloid is torn off and displaced backward and upward with the first row of carpal bones. In such cases palpation of the smooth rounded upper surface of these bones beneath the extensor tendons will suggest the diagnosis of radiocarpal dislocation with fracture of the radial styloid. Definite broadening of the wrist suggests comminution of the lower end of the radius or tearing of the inferior radioulnar ligaments. Tenderness over the ulnar styloid suggests a fracture here.

If the radial styloid is displaced upward and forward and a "garden spade deformity" is present, there is a flexion and compression fracture of the lower end of the radius.

If the styloid processes are normal in their relation to one another and a silver fork deformity is present there is an extension type of injury which may be: (1) Fracture of both bones of the forearm near the wrist with posterior displacement; (2) radiocarpal dislocation; (3) midcarpal dislocation; or (4) carpometacarpal dislocation. Palpation will reveal the site of the lesion.

Similar flexion types of injuries with anterior displacement and the garden spade deformity may occur, but are extremely rare.

If the styloids are at their normal level and there is no deformity, the diagnosis is more difficult and must be confirmed by the x-ray.

Point tenderness across the lower portion of the radius or ulna or of both bones suggests a fracture there without demonstrable displacement.

Point tenderness around the base of the radial styloid suggests a fracture of the lateral margin of the radius.

Isolated fractures of the tip of the radius or ulnar styloids are suggested by the local point tenderness.

Local swelling and tenderness in the anatomical snuff box with pain here on pressure transmitted upward through the index or middle finger suggest a fracture of the scaphoid, while similar pain and tenderness over the semilunar suggest a fracture of this bone.

Tenderness over the dorsal surface of the semilunar with swelling and tenderness beneath the flexor tendons and loss of power in flexion suggest an anterior dislocation of this bone. When the semilunar is dislocated backward, it can be palpated beneath the extensor tendons.

If there is simply slight or moderate swelling of the wrist and only moderate disability, and if none of the diagnostic signs mentioned above are present, the patient probably has a sprain of the wrist, but unless the injury is a very trivial one, the surgeon will do well to secure a roentgenogram before he makes a final diagnosis of sprain of the wrist.

FRACTURES OF THE METACARPALS

Occurrence and Mechanism.—These fractures are rather frequent and are of much greater importance than the size of the bones would indicate, since they involve the hand. Fractures of the metacarpals which are not properly treated may result in marked impairment of the function of the hand with resultant inability of a workingman to continue his occupation.

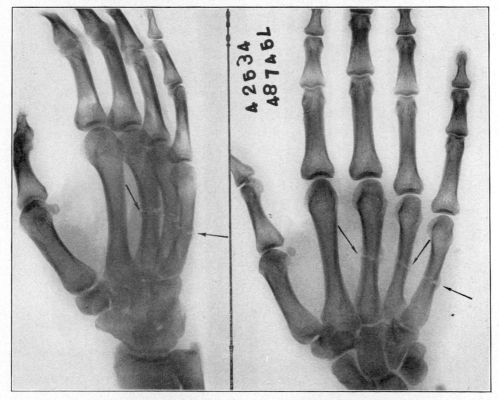

Fig. 772.—X-rays of transverse fractures through the middle thirds of the third, fourth, and fifth metacarpals. Treated in dorsal and volar plaster moulds for four weeks. Good result.

A high percentage of the fractures of the shafts of the metacarpals are the result of direct violence such as crushing injuries of the hand. Others result from indirect violence, the force being received on the knuckles, as in striking an object with the fist and this type occurs frequently in prize fighters.

Pathology.—As these are typical long bones, any of the types of fractures found in long bones may occur. In the fractures due to direct violence the shaft of the bone tends to be broken transversely and the displacement may be relatively slight or it may be considerable (Figs. 773, 774, and 775). In some instances the bone may be extensively comminuted. Many of these fractures are compound and the crushing injury which breaks the bone may break one, two, or even all of the metacarpals and may cause serious damage to the soft parts, especially the extensor tendons of the fingers.

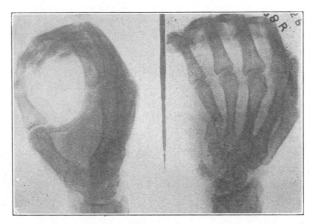

Fig. 773.—Fracture of the shaft of the fifth metacarpal. Good result obtained by open operation (local anesthesia) and immobilization on a posterior wooden splint. Closed manipulation and traction failed.

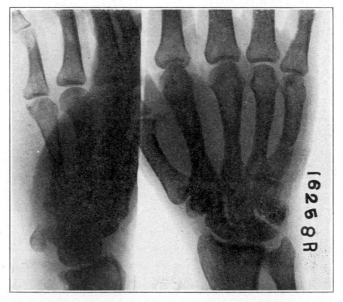

Fig. 774.—Roentgenogram of the preceding case after open operation. Fixation for one month in circular plaster cast from terminal phalanges to upper third of forearm. Chromic catgut through small drill holes in the fragments used for internal fixation.

The displacement depends partly upon the fracturing force and partly upon the muscle pull. If the broken ends remain in contact, the interosseus muscles tend to pull the metacarpal head forward into the palm and thus cause a posterior bowing at the site of the fracture. If the fractured ends do not remain in contact as in oblique or comminuted fractures or transverse fractures in which the fracturing force has displaced the fragments upon one another, the flexor and extensor muscles of the fingers tend to pull the distal fragment upward and cause shortening. In addition the distal fragment may be displaced laterally, mesially, anteriorly, or posteriorly, depending upon the fracturing force and is usually angulated in such a manner that the head of the bone tends to project in the palm of the hand.

In fractures due to direct violence the head of the bone may be driven directly upward and impacted upon the adjacent portion of the shaft (Figs. 776 and 778) or the distal portion of the shaft may be splintered or broken cleanly across or a long spiral fracture may occur. In all instances where there is displacement the head of the metacarpal tends to tilt forward into the palm.

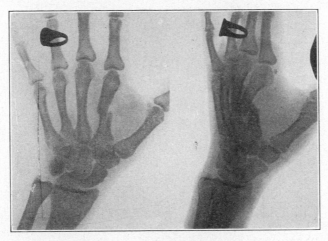

Fig. 775.—Fracture of the shaft of the first metacarpal. Treated by open reduction and a padded posterior wooden splint and circular plaster cast around splint with good result. Chromic catgut through small drill holes in fragments used for internal fixation. Local anesthesia used. Fixation one month.

Diagnosis.—The history of the injury and the presence of obvious damage to the soft parts will indicate whether one is dealing with an injury from direct or indirect violence. In either instance there is considerable disability of the hand and especially of the finger corresponding to the injured metacarpal. The swelling varies with the type of injury and in severe crushing injuries with multiple fractures the entire hand may be markedly swollen (Fig. 777) while in fractures from sharp direct blows or from indirect violence the swelling may be limited to the vicinity of the fracture (Fig. 778). This is particularly true of fractures near the head of the bone where the swelling tends to obliterate the outline of the knuckle.

If there is displacement with resultant shortening of the bone, the corresponding knuckle will be displaced upward and forward (Fig. 778). This displacement is best demonstrated by having the patient make a fist. When the fist is viewed from the dorsal aspect it will be seen that the knuckle (head) of the broken metacarpal is displaced upward out of the normal line of the knuckles, and when it is viewed from the side it will be seen that the knuckle has dropped downward (toward the palm) out of the normal line of the knuckles. These findings are pathognomonic of fracture of the metacarpal with displacement, but cannot always be demonstrated as the patient may be unable to make a fist or the swelling may obscure the displacement, or all of the metacarpals may be broken and all of the knuckles displaced upward and forward, thus maintaining the normal alignment.

On palpation point tenderness can be demonstrated over the site of the fracture, but in crushing injuries the tenderness may be general. The surgeon should then grasp the patient's injured hand with both hands and gently palpate each suspected metacarpal, squeezing it between his thumbs and fingers, and if there is a fracture with displacement it will generally be possible to detect the abnormality in outline and even to demonstrate false motion.

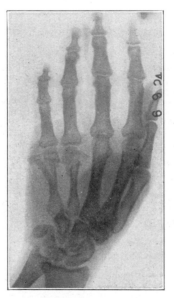

Fig. 776.—Compound impacted fractures near the heads of the fourth and fifth metacarpals. Treated by closed manipulation under local anesthesia to break up the impaction, and traction in a banjo splint. Good result.

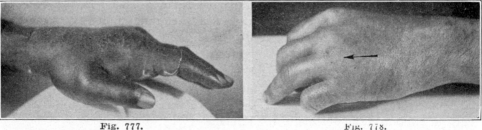

Fig. 777.   Fig. 778.

Fig. 777.—Severely contused hand with multiple fractures of the metacarpals and considerable damage to the soft parts. Treated on well-padded wooden splint with half wooden ball and wet dressings; and ten days later, a circular cast for three weeks. Good function.

Fig. 778.—Fracture of the hand of the fourth metacarpal. Note the obliteration of the knuckle and the swelling on the dorsum of the hand over the site of the fracture.

Finally he should grasp the patient's wrist and hand in one hand and the finger corresponding to the suspected metacarpal in the other and make gentle upward pressure on the extended finger, thus producing axial pressure on the metacarpal. In a fracture without displacement this will cause pain at the site of the fracture. In a fracture with displacement this pressure alternated with traction will cause telescoping of the finger. In case of doubt as to the exact displacement, an x-ray should be obtained.

Treatment of Fractures of the Four Inner Metacarpals.—In simple fractures without displacement all that is necessary is to immobilize the wrist, hand, and fingers until the broken bone or bones have united.

In fractures of the four inner metacarpals this can be done by means of a light wooden splint the width of the hand exclusive of the thumb and extending from the upper third of the forearm to the tips of the fingers. The splint is well padded with cotton and is strapped to the dorsum of the forearm, hand, and fingers with adhesive, the thumb and terminal joints of the fingers being left free.

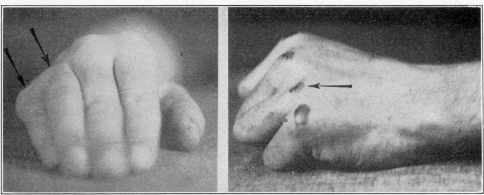

Fig. 779.   Fig. 780.

Fig. 779.—Old healed fracture (malposition) of the fourth and fifth metacarpal shafts. Note the obliteration of the knuckles.

Fig. 780.—Old healed fracture near the head of the fourth metacarpal. Note the loss of contour of the knuckle.

The dorsal splint is superior to a volar splint because it tends to prevent the dorsal bowing of the shaft and the volar displacement of the metacarpal head which tend to occur in these injuries and this dropping forward of the metacarpal head is the chief cause of disability in these fractures. As Magnuson[*] says, "One might as well carry a marble in the palm of the hand between the handle of a tool and the head of the bone as to have the head of the bone protrude like a marble under the pad in the palm of the hand, which is so essential to comfort in lifting or handling hard objects."

A posterior plaster mold or anterior and posterior plaster molds may be used in place of the wood splint. The splint should be left on for two or three weeks depending upon the fracture and the age of the patient and then should be replaced by a short dorsal or board splint extending from the middle of the forearm to the bases of the fingers. Movements of the thumbs and fingers should be begun immediately and these members should be exercised daily. With the long splint only the distal joints of the fingers can be used, but with the short splint they can be moved from the knuckles.

*Magnuson: J. A. M. A. **91**: 1339, 1928.

In compound fractures of the metacarpals the dorsal splint is not well tolerated and these are best treated in an anterior plaster mold which extends from the upper third of the forearm to the tips of the fingers and is applied with the hand in slight dorsiflexion and well molded in the palm of the hand and beneath the heads of the metacarpals.

At the end of a week the surgeon should cut the plaster away beneath the tips of the fingers and thumb and at the end of the second week it should be cut back to the proximal interphalangeal joints and at the third week back to the bases of the fingers. Cutting away of the plaster permits the patient to exercise the fingers; this should be insisted upon as it is extremely important in these compound injuries to prevent the extensive fibrosis of the hand which may come on quickly and result in marked limitation of the fingers and prolonged or even permanent disability.

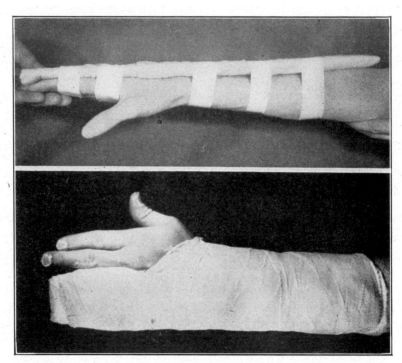

Fig. 781.—Immobilization on the dorsal splint encased in a plaster-of-Paris cast for fractures of the metacarpals.

In compound fractures with infection, where the surgeon wishes to use the Carrell-Dakin treatment or other moist dressings, the plaster mold is not practical because it soon becomes softened and here we use the wooden half ball or bandage or other pad placed upon a straight wood volar splint. This is not so efficient or comfortable as the plaster mold, but is the best that we can do under the circumstances. The apex of the ball or pad should be beneath the metacarpal heads and not beneath the center of the palm as is so often taught. Here, too, the fingers should be exercised daily to prevent fibrosis of the hand.

Fractures with Displacement.—In fractures with displacement, the displacement should be reduced and the reduction maintained if possible. However, as will be mentioned below, lateral displacement is of relatively little importance as compared with anteroposterior displacement.

Fractures with the ends in contact, in which the displacement is a simple posterior bowing, should be corrected by slow gradual pressure, care being taken not to disengage the fragments, and the hand should be immobilized on the posterior board splint or plaster mold as described above. If the fracture is compound, the anterior plaster mold or padded board splint should be used as described above. In impacted fractures near the head of the bone an anesthetic and considerable force may be necessary to correct the deformity.

In fractures with complete displacement, if the contour of the ends of the fragments is such that they will remain in place when reduced; that is, if they are roughly transverse, an attempt should be made to reduce the displacement by manipulation. This is done by strong traction on the corresponding finger with one hand while direct manipulation is performed by the fingers and thumb of the other hand. The patient's wrist should be immobilized by an assistant. Either local or general anesthesia may be used.

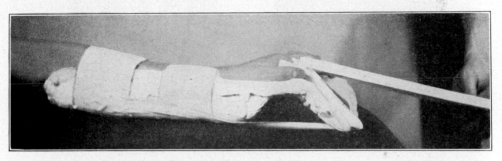

Fig. 782.—Method of obtaining immobilization and slight traction in fractures of the metacarpals by means of an anterior plaster mold in the cock-up position with adhesive strips running from the fingers and over the end of the splint. Useful in fractures involving the metacarpophalangeal articulation where some flexion of the fingers is desired and in severely contused hands where a circular cast is not indicated. The banjo splint is also useful in this type of injury.

The manipulation sounds simple and is, but not infrequently even a skilled surgeon will fail to obtain reduction and will be chagrined to find the fragments as far apart as ever (Figs. 773, 774, and 775). He is then confronted by the problem of whether to treat the fracture by open reduction or by traction. We advise open reduction under local anesthesia because, if it is not possible to obtain reduction by traction and manipulation, it is improbable that traction alone will accomplish it.

Treatment of Subcapital Fractures of the Metacarpals.—Under local anesthesia strong traction is made on the finger to break up the impaction. Then, the finger is flexed in the palm and axial pressure on the head of the first phalanx of the flexed finger presses the head of the metacarpal back into its normal position. Sheet cotton is placed between the skin surfaces and a thin felt strip over the metacarpal head, and the knuckle of the flexed finger and the closed fist or only two closed fingers and the hand are encased in a plaster cast. Pressure on the knuckle is maintained while the plaster is setting but care is taken not to cause a pressure sore by too much pressure, and pain over the knuckle demands removal of the plaster. The fixation is maintained for three or four weeks, until union is solid.

Open Reduction of Fractures of the Metacarpals.—Under strict asepsis the area is infiltrated with 1 per cent novocaine and a small longitudinal incision is made in the dorsum of the hand over the fracture. The bones are exposed by gently retracting the tendons, and the ends are pried or manipulated into place. If they tend to slip off, they are held by a single suture of chromic catgut which is passed through a small drill hole in each fragment. If the reduction is fairly stable, no internal fixation is used. The wound is then closed in layers and the anterior plaster mold, as described above, is applied and the fracture is treated as though no displacement had existed.

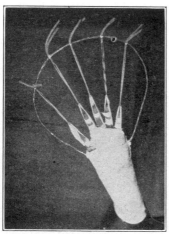
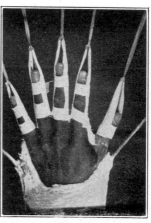

Fig. 783.   Fig. 784.

Fig. 783.—Banjo splint, which is made of wire fixed in a plaster-of-Paris cast, useful in fractures of the metacarpals and phalanges with overlapping of fragments and when marked soft structure involvement is present, with or without compound fractures of the metacarpals and phalanges.

Fig. 784.—Showing close-up of the application of adhesive to the fingers in the banjo splint. The adhesive should not be placed over the finger nails. In certain instances skeletal traction may be used. The authors prefer adhesive.

Treatment by Traction.—Comminuted or oblique fractures with displacement should be treated by traction and this may be obtained by rubber bands fastened to a loop of heavy silkworm gut passed through the pulp of the finger or by adhesive strips on the sides of the fingers as in Fig. 784. If the silkworm gut is used the loop should be held open by a small wood spreader. It is easily applied by transfixing the pulp with a straight needle threaded with the gut. Care should be taken not to put the adhesive over the nails, since continuous pressure on a finger nail causes pain. Where a considerable amount of traction is necessary the Mock's finger caliper for skeletal traction may be used, but this will rarely be necessary if traction is applied to all of the fingers as illustrated. We often apply traction to the adjacent fingers as well as to the one corresponding to the broken metacarpal.

In cases in which relatively little traction is needed, the banjo splint is not necessary. A long anterior plaster mold is applied with the hand in slight dorsiflexion, extending slightly beyond the tips of the fingers; long strips of adhesive are fastened to the traction straps on the fingers and carried over the end of the splint and fastened to its anterior surface (Fig. 782). These strips must be tightened or renewed as often as they become loose. A rubber band placed between them and the traction strips on the fingers makes them more efficient.

The Banjo Splint.—There are many varieties on the market and some of these are very elaborate. A serviceable and very stable one can be made by incorporating a loop of strong wire in a plaster cast which is applied to the forearm and hand. The cast must be applied with the hand in the cock-up position (45 degrees dorsiflexion) in order that countertraction may be obtained against the heel of the hand (Figs. 783 and 784). A narrow loop of wire is used for a single finger.

Traction is maintained for two or three weeks; then the straight dorsal splint or anterior plaster mold can be used and the fracture treated in the routine manner. During the period of traction, the fingers which do not correspond to the fractured metacarpal should be loosened and exercised daily.

FIBROSIS OF THE HAND

The prevention of fibrosis of the hand cannot be too strongly emphasized. It is especially likely to occur in infected wounds of the hand and is often ignored until all wounds have healed and the patient has a hand which is intact and approximately normal in contour, but is of relatively little use because it is stiff and practically lifeless.

Sometimes in infected hands it is impossible to prevent extensive fibrosis and bone atrophy, and often mild fibrosis occurs in hands which have been swollen and then immobilized for several weeks during the treatment of fractures of any of the bones of the upper extremity (Fig. 785). It is especially likely to occur in old persons or those with a tendency to arthritis (so-called rheumatic diathesis) and this is a real condition as industrial surgeons know to their sorrow, although one may search the textbooks in vain for a word about it.

Treatment

The natural impulse of the busy surgeon is to administer a general anesthetic and to forcibly manipulate the fingers and thumb into full flexion. This would be an easy and happy solution, but unfortunately it does not work. The fingers tend to become stiffer than ever after such treatment.

Mild cases with only moderate restriction of movement and weakness can be relieved by hot soaks or bakes followed by manipulation of the fingers and exercises in flexion and extension, abduction and adduction, and opposition of the thumb. The treatment should be repeated several times daily and can be done by the patient at home, but the surgeon should see that they are really done. A rubber ball makes a good thing to exercise the fingers against and should be carried in the pocket. As the motion increases a smaller ball can be used.

Severe cases with little or no movement are best treated with traction in a banjo splint of wire incorporated in a plaster cast as illustrated in the treatment of fractures of the metacarpals or phalanges. The wire is flexed a little more each day and the rubber traction bands are fastened with safety pins or hooks so that they can be loosened several times daily and the fingers manipulated or exercised. Motion at any given joint can be obtained by cutting the plaster off just proximal to the joint. Opposition of the thumb is obtained by swinging the traction band of the thumb across to the opposite side of the flexed wire ring. Progress will be slow and both surgeon and patient will be discouraged, but if the treatment is persisted in a surprisingly good result may be obtained.

Periods of traction should be alternated with periods of baking, manipulation, and exercise, during which time no splint should be worn. The traction periods should be from one to three weeks and the rest or physiotherapy periods about one week. In severe cases posterior capsulotomy or other plastic operations may be necessary.

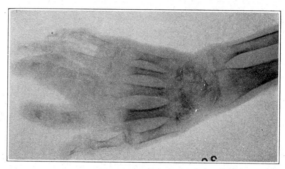

Fig. 785.—Marked fibrosis and bone atrophy affecting the entire hand and rendering it practically useless following prolonged immobilization for a compound infected fracture of the proximal phalanx of the middle finger. Union was obtained, but it would have been much better to have amputated the finger as the hand will never regain its usefulness.

FRACTURES OF THE FIRST METACARPAL OF THE THUMB

Fractures of the Base of the First Metacarpal of the Thumb.—This is not a rare injury and is usually due to axial compression as in striking a blow in which the force is received upon the end of the first phalanx of the thumb or to compression and hyperextension as in falls upon the abducted thumb.

Pathology of Fractures of the Base of the First Metacarpal of the Thumb.—Three types of fracture at the base of the first metacarpal are described: (1) An irregularly transverse or oblique fracture which does not involve the articular surface and is usually impacted. (2) An oblique articular fracture in which the fracture line runs upward and backward through the base of the thumb. This is called the stave of the thumb or the Bennett's fracture (Fig. 786). (3) Epiphyseal separation. The first metacarpal resembles the phalanges in that it has a single epiphysis which is located at its proximal extremity. In these epiphyseal separations a small portion of the diaphysis is usually detached with the epiphysis.

In all fractures of the base of the first metacarpal of the thumb the distal fragment tends to be drawn upward and backward, and there is a definite tendency to posterior and outward bowing as in fractures of the other metacarpals.

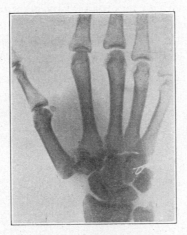

Fig. 786.—Fracture dislocation of the base of the first metacarpal (stave or Bennett's fracture) reduced by manipulation, and immobilized in abduction by a plaster-of-Paris splint around the thumb and wrist. Good result.

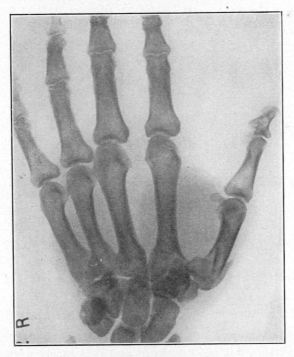

Fig. 787.—Fracture of the first metacarpal near the base. Treated by traction in a banjo splint. Good results.

Diagnosis of Fractures of the Base of the First Metacarpal of the Thumb.—The history of the typical injury with tenderness around the base of the metacarpal and in the anatomical snuff box leads one to suspect a fracture or a dislocation in this region. With both there is loss of power and pain on movement of the thumb. With a dislocation the proximal end of the metacarpal can usually be palpated in an abnormal position while with a fracture the deformity is less, unless there is complete displacement and with this lesion definite false motion can be obtained by manipulation. As much of the deformity may be obscured by the swelling, it is well to obtain x-rays of the lesions at the base of the thumb because failure to properly recognize and treat the injury may lead to marked disability of the hand.

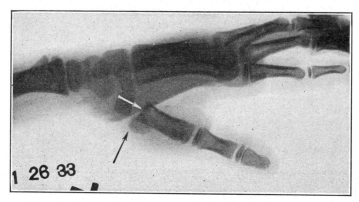

Fig. 788.—Epiphyseal separation at the base of the proximal phalanx of the thumb. Treated by open reduction.

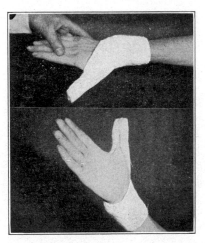

Fig. 789.—Type of molded plaster-of-Paris splint used for the treatment of fractures and fracture dislocations of and about the first metacarpal.

Treatment of Fractures of the Base of the First Metacarpal of the Thumb

These fractures must be treated with the thumb in a position of abduction. As a rule traction is not necessary and it is rarely necessary to manipulate these fractures extensively. In cases with considerable posterior bowing, it may be necessary to hyperabduct the thumb with traction while strong direct pressure is made upon the base of the metacarpal in order to correct the deformity. The same manipulation is used in the correction of fracture dislocations in this region.

The most convenient and efficient method of immobilizing the thumb is by a plaster cast (Fig. 789) or a posterior plaster splint which is fixed to the wrist and molded around the thumb. This dressing is far superior to any splint which has yet been devised for the treatment of these injuries. If plaster is not available, a large roller bandage can be placed between the thumb and the first finger, and the hand and the thumb can be strapped around this with adhesive plaster. This method gives a fair degree of immobilization in abduction, but is not so efficient as the light plaster cast which includes the tip of the thumb. These fractures should be completely immobilized for three weeks. At the end of this time the cast can be removed, the thumb strapped in a position of abduction with adhesive, and the patient allowed to begin to use the hand for light work. The strapping should be continued for two weeks more, when it can be removed and the patient permitted gradually to resume the full use of the hand. If properly treated, a normal hand may be expected.

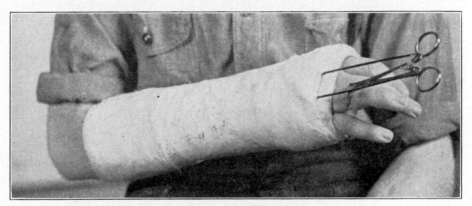

Fig. 790.—The use of a towel clip for skeletal traction in treating fractures of the metacarpals or phalanges. (Courtesy Drs. M. C. Cobey, H. C. Hansen, and M. H. Morris.)

If the thumb is not treated in a position of full abduction one may expect to have permanent limitation of abduction and a dislocation of the carpo-metacarpal joint which leads to traumatic arthritis in this region, weakness of the thumb, and disability of the hand. This condition may last for years, and it is extremely difficult to correct by surgical interference, since nothing less than an arthrodesis will relieve it and the results of this operation are usually worse than the original trouble. The same treatment applies to all three lesions in this location.

Traction may be necessary to maintain satisfactory position of the frag·ments. This can be accomplished by incorporating a wire loop in the plaster cast and attaching the traction to the projecting wire loop. Skin traction with adhesive or skeletal traction with a surgical needle wire clip or surgical towel clip may be used.

FRACTURES OF THE SHAFT OF THE FIRST METACARPAL

These injuries are quite unusual and are usually due to direct violence; for this reason they are apt to be comminuted or compounded. Because of the isolated position of the first metacarpal, the diagnosis is not difficult; in addition to the disability and pain and swelling, false motion can be demonstrated.

The treatment is more like that of a fracture of a phalanx than it is like that of a fracture of one of the inner metacarpals; the thumb should be immobilized in a position of opposition and abduction, and for this reason the fracture cannot be successfully treated on the straight board splint or even on the anterior plaster mold unless this is made unusually broad and is molded around the opposed and abducted thumb in such a manner that it immobilizes it in this position. The most convenient and efficient method of treating these fractures in which there is no displacement of fragments or in which the fragments remain engaged after they have been reduced is to apply a light plaster cast to the thumb and wrist just as was described in fractures of the base of the metacarpal, except that the thumb is immobilized in the grasping position; that is, opposition and abduction.

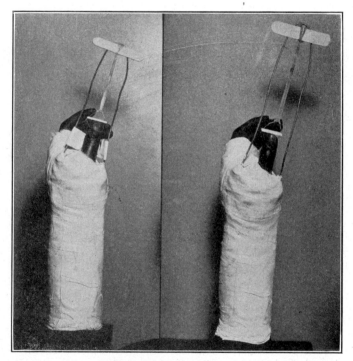

Fig. 791.—Wire traction (modified banjo splint) as applied for fractures of the bones of the thumb and at the base of the first metacarpal (Bennett's fracture) when traction is necessary to maintain position.

Another and much more popular method of treating these fractures is to place a wooden ball or a large roller bandage in the hand between the thumb and fingers and mold the hand around it and strap it with adhesive. With this treatment, a moderate amount of traction on the metacarpal and better opposition of the thumb can be obtained and in this respect this method is superior to the plaster cast in fractures which have a moderate tendency to displacement. In comminuted fractures in which there is a marked tendency to displacement, the best treatment is by traction on a banjo splint just as was described in treatment of similar fractures of the inner metacarpals. However, in fractures of the first metacarpal the wire of the splint must be bent in such a manner that the first metacarpal is immobilized in the grasping position when the traction is applied.

In all of these forms of treatment the original immobilization or traction should be continued for about three weeks. At the end of this time if union is fairly solid, the splint can be removed and the thumb can be strapped with adhesive two weeks longer. If union is not firm, the Davis ball or bandage roller should be applied for one or two weeks more, or as long as necessary. Fibrosis of the hand does not tend to occur so rapidly or as often in injuries of the thumb as it does in the injuries of the inner metacarpals.

FRACTURES OF THE PHALANGES

These are among the most frequent of all fractures and are among the most poorly treated of all fractures. Their frequency is largely due to the fact that the hand is more frequently placed in hazardous positions and more frequently receives abnormal violence than any other part of the body. The inefficient treatment which these fractures so frequently receive is largely due to the fact that they are considered minor injuries and relatively little attention is paid to them except by a few industrial surgeons who have learned by sad experience that these so-called minor injuries may lead to prolonged and even permanent disability with justifiable claims for compensation by the workman. As a rule fractures of the phalanges are very carefully treated by the industrial surgeons, but are more or less casually treated by general surgeons and general practitioners.

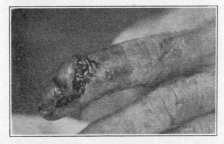

Fig. 792.—Compound fracture dislocation of terminal phalanx due to pressure injury. Treated by débridement, removal of the nail, suture of the extensor tendon, and primary suture and immobilization for two weeks on a straight padded splint tongue depressor with fair result. Disability of finger eight weeks.

Because these bones are quite superficial and the fractures are frequently the result of direct violence or crushing injuries, they are frequently compound (Fig. 792); and since each finger contains two interphalangeal joints in addition to the joint at its base, these joints are frequently involved in the fracture, and permanent limitation of motion is apt to result.

Pathology.—All of the types of fracture that occur in the long bones may occur in the phalanges. In compound crushing wounds, the tendons are often torn and the soft parts extensively damaged, while the bone may be extensively comminuted. On the other hand, the fracture may be simply a small chip from the articular surface or a transverse fracture of the shaft without displacement (Fig. 794). With complete fractures displacement of the fragments is the rule, although complete disengagement of the fragment ends is rather rare. The usual displacement is in the nature of an anterior bowing of the bone at the site of the fracture. This is just the opposite to that found

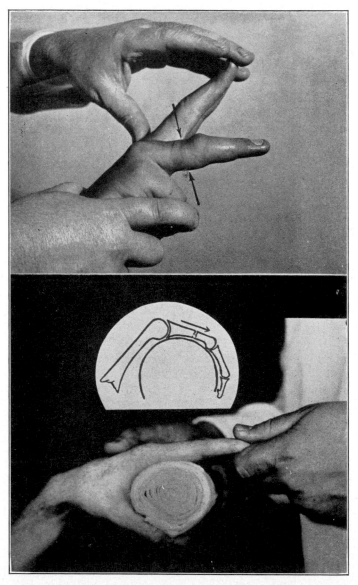

Fig. 793.—Fracture of the ring finger showing immobilization and reduction over a roller bandage.

in fractures of the metacarpal. This deformity causes a lump beneath the flexor tendons of the finger at the site of the fracture; and if the bones are permitted to heal in this position, marked disability of the finger will result.

Diagnosis.—The isolated and subcutaneous position of the bone usually makes the diagnosis of complete fractures obvious. Diagnosis can be made from the deformity where displacement is present or by the presence of false motion where the ends of the bones remain in contact (Fig. 798). The chip fractures which involve the joints and the crushing injuries of the distal phalanx cannot as a rule be diagnosed without the x-ray and anteroposterior and lateral views should be taken in all injuries of the fingers where fractures are suspected. This is particularly true of dislocations of the finger because these are frequently accompanied by chip fractures of the base of the distal phalanx.

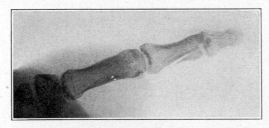

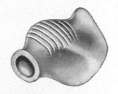

Fig. 794.   Fig. 795.

Fig. 794.—Fracture of the distal end of the proximal phalanx of right thumb and dislocation of the distal phalanx. (Baseball finger.) Reduced. Treated with slight flexion and traction (skeletal) with banjo splint for two weeks then a molded splint for a week then hot baths. Good result in six weeks.

Fig. 795.—Lytle metacarpal splint. (Courtesy Zimmer Manufacturing Co.)

Treatment

The treatment depends upon whether or not displacement is present and upon whether or not the fracture can be reduced and will tend to remain reduced. In simple fractures without displacement, in which there is no tendency for the bones to slip out of position or to bow anteriorly, all that is necessary is to immobilize the finger in a position of moderate flexion. This can be done with a small straight wooden splint which is so padded with three layers of felt so cut that when the finger is placed upon it the finger is moderately flexed. This is then strapped to the finger and to the palm of the hand with adhesive plaster. The most convenient splint is a throat stick or tongue depressor which has been padded with cotton (Fig. 799). There are numerous metal finger splints on the market which are equally efficient (Fig. 800), but no more so, and the surgeon rarely has one at hand unless he is in charge of an industrial clinic where such lesions are frequent.

Fractures with a tendency to displacement are best treated by traction or flexion or both; that is, traction in a position of flexion. If the displacement is a simple anterior bowing at the site of the fracture, this can be corrected by manipulation without an anesthetic and the finger flexed at both interphalangeal joints or at the metacarpophalangeal and proximal interphalangeal joints, depending upon whether the middle or the proximal phalanx is fractured, and bound in this position with strips of adhesive tape. Traction may be applied to the fingers in the following four ways: (1) By lateral strips of adhesive tape which are fastened to the fingers by circular bands of adhesive, as illustrated in the banjo splint. This is the most convenient and frequently used method, but cannot be used with satisfaction in

compound fractures. (2) By one or two small holes drilled through the finger
nail. Mock states that the finger nail will support traction to the amount of
eight ounces and that if the nail is not long enough, the skin can be pushed backward under local anesthetic until sufficient room is obtained to pass the small
silk ligatures through drill holes without danger of their pulling out. (3)
Boehler passes a loop of stainless steel wire through the pulp of the finger just
anterior to the tip of the distal phalanx. We have used heavy silkworm gut

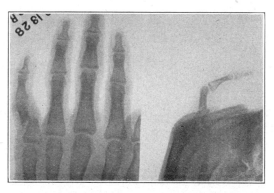

Fig. 796.—Fracture of the proximal phalanx of the little finger with typical deformity. Treated
by traction over a wooden ball splint with good result.

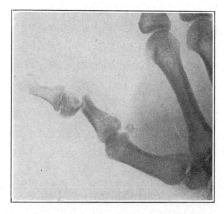

Fig. 797.—Fracture of the proximal phalanx of the thumb treated by traction on a padded
wooden ball splint with fair results. Disability nine weeks, fixation one month.

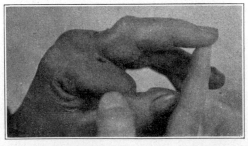

Fig. 798.—Fracture of the proximal phalanx of the middle finger showing the typical
deformity with anterior bowing. Treated by manipulative reduction and immobilization on a
circular bandage and adhesive traction. Fixation for three weeks, then daily hot baths. Good
result.

in the same manner and have found it efficient and painless. In using the silk-worm gut the pulp of the finger is dipped in tincture of iodine and infiltrated with novocaine and then transfixed with a straight needle which is threaded with the gut. The suture is pulled through the fingertip and tied in a loop about one inch in diameter. Traction is attached to the loop, and it is held open by a small wooden spreader. (4) Skeletal traction by means of the Mock finger caliper or a small stainless steel (Steinmann) pin passed through one of the phalanges or a towel clip.

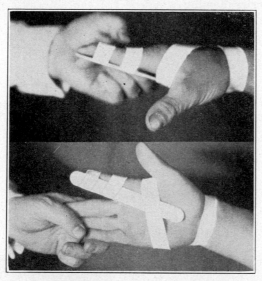

Fig. 799.—Application of tongue depressor for the immobilization of fractures of the phalanges in which the fragments tend to remain in place. Padding removed to show detail. Three layers of felt, so cut that they form a double inclined plane or convex surface, are placed between the finger and the splint in order to maintain flexion.

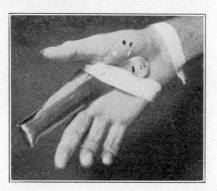

Fig. 800.—A commercial aluminum splint used in the treatment of simple fractures of the phalanges. Padding removed to show detail.

Finger Splints Permitting Traction.—The simplest finger splints are those in which the hand is molded around a large roller bandage or the wooden balls introduced by Dr. George G. Davis of Chicago (Fig. 801). These balls are some-what more stable than the bandage and consequently somewhat more efficient.

The method of application is similar in both instances. The traction strips are applied to the finger and the ball or roller bandage is strapped to the palm of the hand in such a position that the fingers and thumb grip it. Then the traction strips on the broken finger are pulled sufficiently taut to reduce the fracture, and the long strips of adhesive are carried around the ball or bandage and fastened above on the wrist (Fig. 802). The adhesive must not be allowed to press on the finger nails. The ball or bandage should be large enough to fit comfortably in the hand.

The advantage of this method is that it supplies traction and immobilization with the joints of the fingers in a position of moderate flexion and thus tends to overcome the anterior bowing which is the characteristic deformity in these fractures.

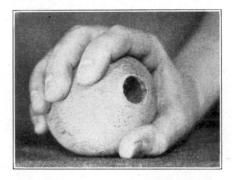

Fig. 801.—The Davis wooden ball useful in treatment of fractures of the phalanges. Different sized balls for adults and children.

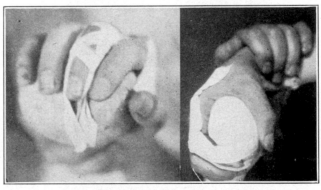

Fig. 802.—Traction on the fingers by means of adhesive tape stretched around the wooden ball (left) or around a plain gauze bandage (right).

A similar and very efficient method is that of Boehler who makes a straight splint of heavy iron wire so folded upon itself that the two sides are the width of the finger. This wire splint is padded with bandage and fixed in a plaster cast which includes the hand and wrist, the hand being immobilized in a position of dorsiflexion and the wire splint extending outward along the volar surface of the finger. When the plaster has hardened, the end of the broken finger is strapped to the wire splint with adhesive in the hyperextension position and with moderate traction; then by simple flexing of the wire, the finger, being on the convexity of the curve, is pulled outward and downward and the fracture is reduced and very efficiently immobilized.

Prolonged immobilization of fingers is to be avoided as it leads to permanent stiffness. Three weeks is usually ample.

COMPOUND FRACTURES OF THE FINGER

The above methods are not very efficient in the treatment of compound injuries of the fingers because frequent dressings may be necessary and the adhesive strapping will, of course, interfere with the keeping clean and healing

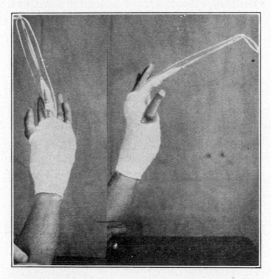

Fig. 803.—Simple wire traction splint for fracture of a single finger.

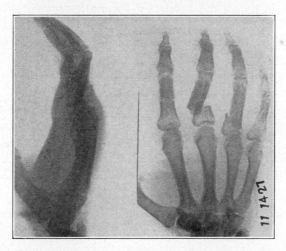

Fig. 804.—Multiple fractures of the phalanges treated by adhesive traction in a banjo splint for two weeks, afterward a molded plaster cock-up splint for twelve days. Hot baths daily after traction was removed.

of the wound. After the injury has been very carefully débrided and the wounds closed or left open, depending upon the condition, the modified banjo splint should be applied (Fig. 803). In treating finger fractures, it is not necessary to have the wide wire loop, but it is only necessary to immobilize the hand and wrist and obtain traction upon the given finger. The splint illustrated in Fig. 803 is quite efficient and serviceable.

Where two or more fingers have been broken, the wire loop can, of course, be made broader if necessary. The plaster cast is applied with the hand in a position of dorsiflexion and the wire extending out of the plaster parallel to the finger is so bent that traction can be made in a position of moderate flexion. Then either with adhesive strips, if the condition of the soft parts permits, or by means of small drill holes through the nail of the finger, or by a loop of heavy silkworm gut, or Boehler's stainless steel wire through the finger pulp, or by the Mock finger caliper, an elastic band is fixed to the finger and the end of the projecting wire. If the position is not satisfactory, it can be changed by changing the bend in the wire loop.

In severe injuries, the traction should be maintained for about three weeks. At the end of this time the wound will probably have healed and the fracture will be sufficiently united to permit treatment without traction and an ordinary throat stick can be applied, but in these compound fractures, especial care should be taken that the finger be exercised as soon as union is firm enough to permit it. Otherwise one may obtain a finger which is united with perfect alignment, but is stiff and practically useless.

FRACTURE DISLOCATIONS OF THE FINGERS AT THE INTERPHALANGEAL JOINTS

These apparently trivial injuries may be very troublesome because if the anterior lip of the base of the distal phalanx at the site of the dislocation is broken off there is a marked tendency for redislocation to occur when the finger is immobilized by means of a straight splint. For this reason these lesions should be reduced by traction and the finger strapped firmly on the Davis ball splint or on a large roller bandage in the hand, where it should be maintained in complete immobilization in slight flexion for at least three weeks. At the end of this time the dressing can be removed and the patient may begin very gently to use the finger. If the joint does not seem stable, however, the dressing should be reapplied immediately.

FRACTURES OF THE TERMINAL PHALANX OF THE FINGER OR SEVERE CONTUSION WITHOUT FRACTURE

These injuries warrant a special description because the pulp of the finger lies in a closed connective tissue sac which is waterproof and which, if not ruptured at the time of the fracture, may become distended with blood under pressure to such an extent that necrosis of the bone may occur. The very considerable importance of these fractures of the terminal phalanx is evident from the report by Hurley,* who in a series of 27 cases of chip fractures of the tip of the finger, which occurred in steel mill employees, found that one lost 196 days of work, 7 lost approximately 160 days each, and that 9 lost not more than 3 days each.

---

*Hurley: J. Indust. Hyg. 1: 85, 1919.

The important thing is whether or not there is an exit from the closed pulp sac of the finger tip for the hemorrhage incident to the fracture. If there is an exit the pain and swelling rapidly disappear and all that is necessary is to immobilize the finger in a straight wooden splint or in any one of the numerous metal splints on the market as there is rarely an important displacement of the fragment.

But if within a short time after the injury the throbbing, pain, swelling, and tenderness of the finger tip becomes progressively worse, and examination shows the tip of the finger to be under considerable tension and markedly cyanotic, the surgeon should take prompt measures to relieve the tension, as otherwise necrosis and later infection may develop. As a rule it is necessary in these severe cases to bore a hole in the nail over the hematoma or to make an incision into the side of the finger tip.

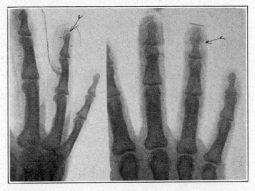

Fig. 805.—Chip fracture of the terminal phalanx of the ring finger. Treated by simple immobilization in a straight padded wooden splint along flexor surface of finger for four days. Removed daily and hot baths used. Good results in two weeks.

The hole in the nail may be made by boring a hole with the point of a sharp knife or by cutting through the nail with a very sharp knife and removing a very small triangular area. It requires no anesthetic. If the incision is to be made into the finger, it should be done with a sharp knife, under local anesthesia, on the lateral side parallel to the edge of the nail and some distance from it. It is preferable to soak the finger in full strength tincture of iodine before the incision is made as the thick skin is often dirty and difficult to cleanse. After the pressure has been relieved by the incision, the pain and swelling rapidly disappear and all that is necessary is to immobilize the finger in a straight wooden splint (usually for about ten to twelve days).

Occasionally in these chip fractures of the distal phalanx the finger remains tender. If such a condition persists and the x-ray shows nonunion with gradual absorption of the detached fragment, this should be removed by a small lateral incision and the wound closed without drainage. The removal of this fragment will usually result in complete cure with later regeneration of the phalanx from the periosteum which has been left.

Epiphyseal Separation of the Phalanges.—The phalanges possess single epiphyses which are located at the proximal end. In children and adolescents these epiphyses may be separated by the same injuries which cause fractures in adults.

The treatment of these epiphyseal separations with displacement is reduction by manipulation and traction and immobilization on a straight wooden splint as they rarely show tendency to displacement once they are reduced.

DROP OR MALLET FINGER (BASEBALL FINGER)

This is an avulsion of the extensor tendon from its insertion into the base of the terminal phalanx, and not infrequently a small sliver of bone is torn off with the tendon. It is usually due to sudden force striking the end of the extended finger and flexing it against the resistance of the taut extensor tendon. The rupture may occur with a subluxation or it may occur with no demonstrable displacement of the joint surfaces. On clinical examination the terminal phalanx is freely movable but is maintained in a flexed position and cannot be actively extended nor can the patient maintain it in extension when it is passively placed in this position. If the rupture of the tendon communicates with the joint cavity, there is little tendency for the tendon to heal without adequate and prolonged fixation or operative repair.

Treatment of Drop or Mallet Finger

As a rule in early cases operative interference is not necessary. All that is necessary is to maintain the finger in slight flexion at the proximal and hyperextension at the distal interphalangeal joints for a period of three or four weeks. This is most simply and easily accomplished by means of a small

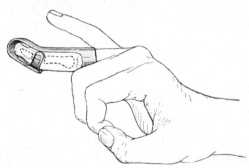

Fig. 806.—Lewin finger splint. (Courtesy Zimmer Manufacturing Company.)

plaster-of-Paris cast applied to the finger without padding. The hyperextension of the distal phalanx is maintained by direct pressure until the plaster has set. Or the Lewin finger splint may be used. In late cases operative repair may be attempted, but it will usually be found that the extensor tendon has become retracted and frayed and its end is difficult to identify and there is relatively little soft tissue to sew to at the site of its original insertion. However, in certain cases a perfect result may be obtained by a careful suture of the extensor tendon back to the tip of the terminal phalanx.

DISLOCATIONS AT THE WRIST AND IN THE HAND

With the exception of the metacarpophalangeal and the interphalangeal dislocations all of these injuries are rare.

Dislocations at the Inferior Radio-ulnar Joint

Occurrence and Mechanism.—With the exception of the dislocations of the distal end of the ulna which occur as complications of compression and extension fractures of the lower end of the radius, these lesions are very rare. However, occasionally the lower end of the ulna may be dislocated either forward or backward. The forward dislocation occurs as a rule as a complication of the extension type of fracture of the lower end of the radius, but may occur as an isolated injury from forcible hypersupination of the wrist. In like manner the dorsal dislocation is prone to occur in the rare flexion fractures of the lower end of the radius, but may occasionally occur as an isolated lesion from forcible hyperpronation at the wrist.

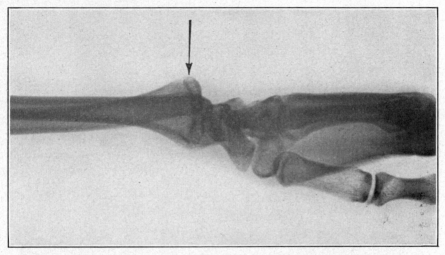

Fig. 807.—Posterior dislocation of the distal end of the ulna. Treated by manipulation and immobilization in full supination. If this is not successful, the lower end of the ulna may be resected. Also tunneling of the flexor carpi ulnaris through the lower end of the ulna has been used successfully.

It should be mentioned that in some individuals the inferior radio-ulnar joint is quite lax and that a considerable amount of movement is permitted. Consequently before dislocation of this joint is diagnosed the condition should be compared with that present in the opposite normal wrist. Also, there may be a chronic posterior subluxation of the head of the ulna which is thought to be due to some strain incurred in childhood, and this lesion is not accompanied by much disturbance of function although there may be some limitation of hyperextension and some weakness.

Diagnosis of Dislocations at the Inferior Radio-ulnar Joint.—A definite dislocation of the distal end of the ulna can as a rule be diagnosed without much difficulty. In the anterior dislocation the head of the ulna is unusually prominent on the volar surface of the wrist beneath the flexor tendons, and in the posterior dislocation it is unusually prominent on the dorsum; in both instances it is felt to be absent from its normal location. In both instances there is marked limitation of rotation of the wrist and pain on attempting these movements, with more or less swelling and tenderness over the head of the ulna and the adjacent portion of the wrist joint.

In addition to the anteroposterior displacement, there is usually definite narrowing of the wrist due to the fact that when it is dislocated the lower end of the ulna tends to be drawn outward or toward the midline of the wrist by the pronator quadratus and to rest upon the volar or dorsal surface of the radius as the case may be. Every case of traumatic ulnar luxation should be carefully examined to determine whether or not there is a complicating fracture of the radius or of the ulnar styloid.

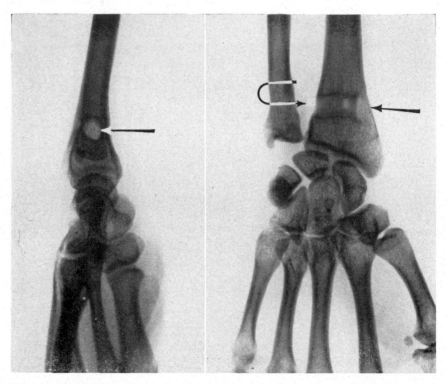

Fig. 808.—Results of case shown in Fig. 807 by use of fascia around the ulna extending through the radius with excellent results. (Eliason's technique, Ann. Surg. 96: 27, 1932.)

Treatment

In an acute case the dislocation should be reduced by traction and lateral deviation of the wrist with direct pressure with the surgeon's thumbs and manipulation of the head of the ulna, and for this an anesthetic may be necessary. After the reduction the wrist and the elbow should be immobilized in the neutral position as regards flexion and extension and rotation and with the hand deviated slightly to the ulnar side. This is best accomplished by a light plaster-of-Paris cast which extends from the middle of the arm to the bases of the fingers. This cast should be well molded around the head of the ulna and should be worn for four weeks. At the end of this time it may be removed and the wrist strapped with adhesive. The patient can now begin to cautiously rotate the forearm and flex and extend the wrist and use the hand, but should avoid forcible movements in rotation for at least two weeks longer, when the adhesive can be taken off and the patient can gradually resume normal function.

The dislocations of the lower end of the ulna which occur as complications fractures of the lower end of the radius with displacement are usually reduced when the fracture is reduced and require no special treatment.

In the chronic cases reduction and immobilization cannot be expected to result in cure, and it is necessary to operate and immobilize the ulna by means of a strip of fascia which can be passed through the lower end of the shaft of the ulna and radius. This is a rather difficult operation and should not be undertaken lightly.

A simpler and a satisfactory procedure is resection of the distal inch of the ulna (Darrach's operation).

Radiocarpal Dislocations

Dislocation at the radiocarpal joint is a rare injury, but may result from trauma such as usually causes extension or flexion fractures of the lower end of the radius. In most of the reported cases the dislocation is backward but very rarely it may be forward.

Pathology.—In the posterior dislocation the hand and carpals are displaced upward and backward and the first row of carpal bones rests upon the dorsum of the radius and ulna. In the great majority of cases there is a variable amount of fracturing of the lower end of the radius and ulna, usually a fracture of the posterior articular margin of the radius (Barton's fracture), but occasionally there is also a tearing off of both styloid processes. All of the ligaments around the radiocarpal joint are either ruptured or torn off with some of the adjacent bone, the extensor tendons are stripped up from the posterior surface of the radius, and the flexor tendons and nerves are stretched across the volar border of the lower ends of the radius and ulna and may be seriously injured. Occasionally the dislocation is compound.

Diagnosis of Radiocarpal Dislocations.—The deformity resembles the silver fork deformity of the typical hyperextension and compression fracture at the distal end of the radius except that the curves are at a slightly lower level. The level of deformities at the wrist is best determined by definitely locating the styloid processes. As in the fractures, there is complete disability and the great swelling may obscure the deformity. Unless the styloid processes of the radius and ulna have been torn off, they can be palpated in their normal positions and the rounded proximal surface of the first row of carpal bones can be palpated on the dorsum of the wrist beneath the extensor tendons. Due to the tearing of the ligaments the hand may be abducted or in the neutral position while the forearm is usually carried in a position of pronation.

Treatment.—The treatment is immediate reduction, because the tension on the vessels may seriously interfere with the circulation of the hand. Reduction is not, as a rule, difficult. All that is necessary is to make direct traction on the hand; pull it downward until the first row of carpal bones slips over or can be pressed forward over the lower end of the radius and back into their normal position. When this has been accomplished, the styloid process and posterior margin of the radius which may have been fractured should be molded back into place by firm pressure with the surgeon's fingers and thumbs and the wrist should be immobilized in anterior and posterior plaster molds or well-

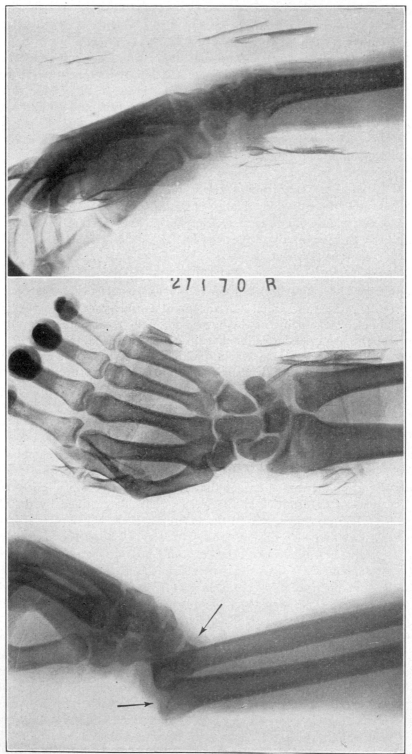

Fig. 809.—Severe fracture dislocation at the wrist. Treated by manipulative reduction and immobilization for six weeks in a plaster-of-Paris cast with good result.

padded anterior and posterior wooden splints with a circular plaster cast extending from the middle of the arm to the bases of the fingers. (See Forearm.)

In applying the cast, it is important that it should be split as soon as it has hardened in order to take care of swelling which may occur after the reduction.

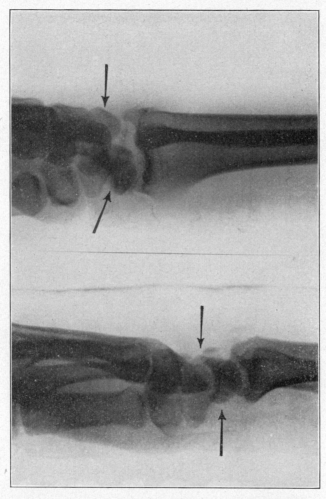

Fig. 810.—Midcarpal dislocations (recent injury). Results following closed reduction. Circular cast applied after anterior and posterior wooden splints had been applied to the hand and forearm. Good result. (Courtesy of Dr. Frank Wilson.)

The immobilization in midflexion and extension is necessary to prevent recurrence and this permits the torn ligaments and the avulsed fragments of bone to heal. This immobilization should be continued for four weeks, but the patient should be encouraged to move and exercise the fingers as soon as possible after the reduction. At the end of the four weeks' period the cast should be removed and the wrist and hand immobilized in an anterior plaster mold which extends from the upper portion of the forearm to the bases of the fingers and maintains the hand in dorsiflexion. This will permit more motion at the fingers, will permit rotation of the forearm, and can be removed if deemed

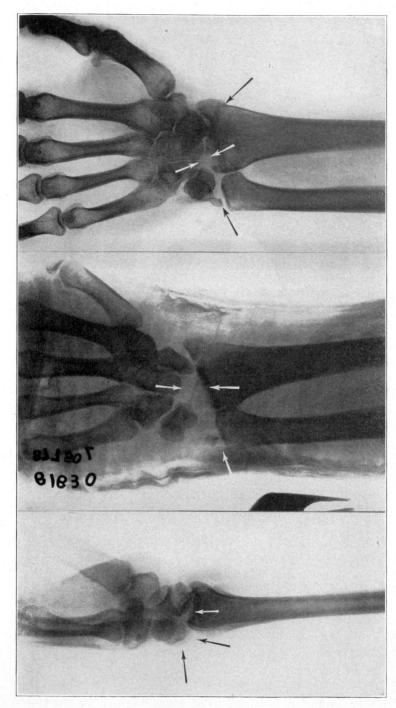

Fig. 811.—An old midcarpal dislocation of the wrist which necessitated removal of the semilunar, immediately after operation and one year later. It will be noted that there is also a fracture of the styloid process of the radius. Good anatomical result and good functional result one year later.

advisable for baking, massage, and guarded movements. It should be worn for from two to four weeks, depending upon the severity of the initial injury and the presence of fractures of the radius and ulna.

When the ligaments have healed and the bones have united this plaster splint can be removed and the wrist strapped with adhesive or bandage and the patient encouraged to begin to use the hand and gradually to resume normal function.

Anterior Dislocation at the Radiocarpal Joints

This very rare injury bears the same relation to the posterior dislocation as do the flexion fractures to the extension fractures of the lower end of the radius. It differs from the posterior dislocation in that the deformity resembles that of the gardener's spade characteristic of the flexion fractures with the curves at a slightly lower level, and the concave posterior margin of the lower ends of the radius and ulna can be palpated on the dorsum of the wrist beneath the flexor tendons.

Treatment of Anterior Dislocation at the Radiocarpal Joints.—As in the posterior dislocation, the treatment is immediate reduction by traction and backward pressure on the carpus, while the lower end of the radius is pressed forward. When reduction has been accomplished, the lower ends of the radius and ulna should be carefully molded by pressure if their contours are abnormal and the wrist should be incorporated in a plaster cast or mold which extends from the middle of the arm to the base of the fingers. The exact position of the hand must be determined by the surgeon after the reduction. If the reduction is fairly stable, the hand should be immobilized in the neutral position as regards flexion and extension and abduction and adduction, and the forearm should be in the neutral position as regards rotation. If it is not stable, and this will mean that there has been a fracture of the articular margin of the radius, it must be immobilized in sufficient palmar flexion to secure stability.

The after treatment is the same as in the dorsal dislocation.

Dislocation at the Midcarpal Joint

This is a very rare injury (almost always of the extension and compression type) in which the lesion occurs at the midcarpal joint and in which the distal row of carpal bones, or part thereof, is displaced backward upon the proximal row. The ligaments around this joint are all torn and there may be a variable amount of fracturing of the bones of the hand, wrist, and forearm.

Diagnosis.—The picture resembles that of the posterior dislocation at the radiocarpal joint except the deformity is on a slightly lower level, shortening of the wrist is more marked, and the volar prominence of the lower carpal bones can be palpated, while the round, rather narrow head of the os magnum can be palpated on the dorsum of the wrist. As a considerable percentage of these cases are incomplete, and as the extensive swelling tends to obscure the deformity, the diagnosis may be missed in the absence of a good x-ray picture which should, of course, be taken in all severe injuries about the wrist joint.

Treatment.—The treatment is immediate reduction which can usually be accomplished without great difficulty by traction with anterior and downward pressure on the dislocated second row of carpal bones. After the reduction has been completed and the normal contour of the carpus has been restored by molding the bones with the thumb and fingers, the hand should be immobilized

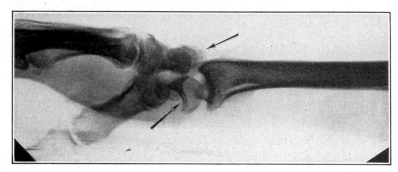

Fig. 812.—Posterior dislocation of the wrist at the midcarpal joint. Treated by manipulative reduction with satisfactory result. In old unreduced dislocations and certain unreducible recent dislocations of such type it is necessary to remove the proximal row of carpal bones. Some authorities prefer the removal of only the scaphoid and semilunar. We feel the former brings about better results. Such treatment, however, is rarely indicated, but is important when indicated.

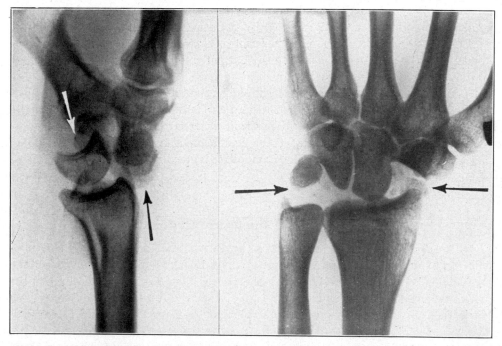

Fig. 813.—Old intracarpal dislocation which necessitated the removal of all the carpal bones of the proximal row. Patient developed a fairly good functional result.

in a circular plaster cast, well padded, extending from the upper portion of the forearm to the base of the fingers and this should maintain the hand in a position of midflexion and extension at the wrist. This cast should be worn for four or six weeks. At the end of this time the plaster or splint can be removed and the wrist strapped firmly with adhesive or bandage. This should be worn for two weeks. At the end of this time all dressings can be removed and the patient should begin to use the hand normally, but should avoid severe strain upon the wrist for at least two weeks longer, and should soak the hand in hot water and manipulate it daily.

In old dislocations of this type, open reduction is indicated and it may be necessary to remove the semilunar or even the proximal row of metacarpals in order to effect and maintain reduction.

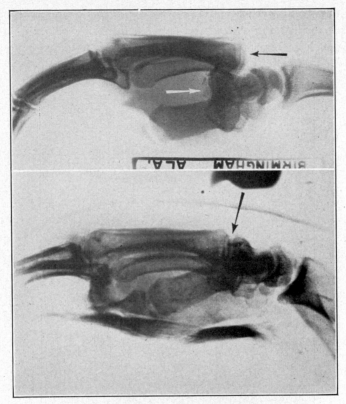

Fig. 814.—Posterior dislocation at the carpometacarpal joint. Open reduction and fixation in palmar flexion was necessary. Good functional result.

Carpometacarpal Dislocations

The most frequent of these rare injuries is the posterior dislocation of the first metacarpal bone, which will be considered separately. The four inner metacarpal bones are very rarely dislocated, usually en masse, but occasionally one or two of these bones may be dislocated upon the carpus. The dislocation is practically always backward and the prominent proximal ends of the dislocated bone or bones can be easily palpated on the dorsum of the wrist. Unless the swelling is very great, the diagnosis should not be difficult.

Treatment of Carpometacarpal Dislocations.—The treatment is reduction which should be accomplished without difficulty by traction on the finger of the involved bone aided by direct pressure downward and forward on the dislocated base of the bone or bones. After the reduction has been completed and the normal contour has been restored by pressure, the hand should be immobilized in anterior and posterior plaster molds or a posterior wooden splint well padded with a circular plaster-of-Paris cast which extends from the upper portion of the forearm to the middle of the fingers. This should be worn for three weeks. At the end of this time the fixation can be removed and the wrist strapped with adhesive and the patient can begin to use the hand.

Dislocation of the Metacarpal Bone of the Thumb

This injury results from violence which forces the metacarpal bone upward and backward, the most common cause being the striking of a blow with the fist in such a manner that the head of the metacarpal bone or thumb

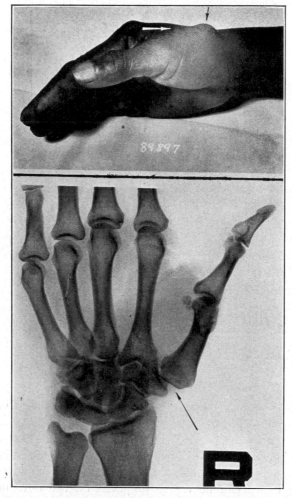

Fig. 815.—Dislocation of the base of the first metacarpal. Treated by manipulative reduction and immobilization in wide abduction in a plaster cast.

knuckle lands upon the opponent's skull. The dislocation may or may not be accompanied by fracture of the base of the metacarpal, the so-called Bennett's fracture. The posterior capsule of the joint is torn and the base of the first metacarpal rests upon the posterior surface of the trapezium.

Diagnosis.—In addition to the local swelling, the prominence of the dislocated base of the metacarpal is palpable and often visible in the region of the anatomical snuff box, the thumb is maintained in a position of moderate adduction and is completely disabled and shortened. Cotton notes that shortening of the thumb is most conveniently measured by noting the relation of the tips of the adducted thumbs to the first interphalangeal skin folds of the index fingers.

Treatment.—The treatment is reduction by traction on the abducted thumb and direct pressure upon the head of the metacarpal bone. As the thumb is pulled downward and outward, the head of the metacarpal is pressed forward and inward. When the reduction is complete, the thumb and wrist should be immobilized in a plaster cast which extends from the middle of the forearm to the bases of the fingers and out along the thumb to the tip and should be applied with the hand in a position of moderate dorsiflexion and with the thumb in a position of full abduction and extension. The plaster should be well molded around the base of the thumb and should be worn for about four weeks, for if it is removed too soon, a chronic subluxation at this joint may result. When the plaster has been removed, no further immobilization is necessary and the patient should begin gradually to resume the use of the hand.

Subluxation of the Metacarpal of the Thumb

This is a rather common condition which probably results from frequently repeated trauma or from weakness and debility. It continues to recur from time to time with slight injury or with no injury and may become chronic. The thumb is not shortened and there is little disability. The base of the first metacarpal is unusually prominent and may be tender.

Treatment.—In a recent case the result of a definite injury, the subluxation should be reduced. This can easily be done by pushing the head of the metacarpal downward and forward and the injury should then be treated in exactly the same manner as though a complete dislocation had occurred. In a chronic case if the patient wishes treatment, the plaster cast should be applied as in the recent case, and the thumb should be maintained in the position of extension and abduction over a period of at least four weeks. At the end of this time the patient should be given exercises in abduction and extension of the thumb and this may result in a complete cure. Operative intervention is rarely indicated.

DISLOCATIONS AT THE METACARPOPHALANGEAL JOINT

Posterior Dislocation of the Proximal Phalanx of the Thumb

This injury, which is practically always due to forcible hyperextension of the thumb, is rather frequent and deserves especial attention because of the difficulties presented by the periarticular tissues when reduction by the ordinary traction method is attempted.

Pathology.—Depending upon the position of the phalanx in relation to the metacarpal bone, the dislocation is usually described as being either first or second degree. In the first degree dislocation the phalanx is hyperextended and projects directly backward at right angles to the shaft of the metacarpal on the dorsal surface of which its cartilaginous base rests (Figs. 816, 817, and 818). In the second degree the distal phalanx is slightly flexed and the volar surface of its base rests upon the neck of the metacarpal. The second degree dislocation is usually the result of unsuccessful attempts at reduction by traction in which the phalanx has been pulled downward posterior to the metacarpal, but in which the dislocation has not been reduced.

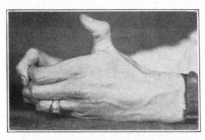

Fig. 816.—Typical incomplete dislocation at the metacarpophalangeal joint of the thumb seen from the dorsal aspect.

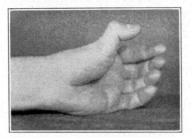

Fig. 817.—Typical incomplete dislocation of the metacarpophalangeal joint of the thumb seen from the palmar aspect.

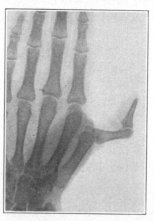

Fig. 818.—X-ray picture of incomplete dislocation at the metacarpophalangeal joint of the thumb.

In either type as the phalanx is hyperextended on the metacarpal the anterior and lateral ligaments and capsule of the joint are torn and the base of the phalanx is displaced backward and upward over the head of the metacarpal and comes to rest on its constricted neck or shaft, where it is held firmly by the tension of the tendons on either side while the head of the metacarpal projects forward between the two heads of the flexor brevis pollicis and in rare instances may project through the skin of the thenar eminence. Occasionally with extensive tearing of the soft parts, the base of the phalanx rests upon one side or even the anterior surface of the metacarpal.

Treatment.—Treatment is reduction and this should not be attempted by strong traction in the long axis of the thumb as the short flexor tendons of the thumb only grip the head of the metacarpal more tightly with traction, and sufficient traction to cause reduction may cause extensive tearing of these muscles. Reduction is usually difficult and a general anesthetic should be given.

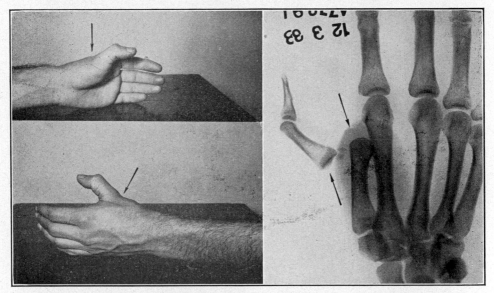

Fig. 819.—Complete dislocation at the metacarpophalangeal joint of the thumb. Reduced by closed reduction. Good results.

Reduction can be accomplished by hyperextension combined with traction and pushing forward of the base of the metacarpal, followed by flexion. This is best done by placing a bandage around the thumb as shown in Fig. 820 in order to get firm traction in the thumb. After the bandage has been looped around the thumb, it is wound around the surgeon's hand and then the patient's hand is immobilized by an assistant. By means of the bandage the thumb is pulled into a position of hyperextension, and with the traction maintained, the phalanx is gripped between the operator's thumb and index finger, and its base is pushed directly distalward to a position opposite the head of the metacarpal, when it is slowly flexed (Fig. 820). During flexion the displaced base slips over the head of the metacarpal. When reduction is complete, the thumb can be flexed normally at the metacarpophalangeal joint.

After reduction the thumb and wrist should be immobilized on a roller bandage (Fig. 821) in a short plaster-of-Paris cast extending from the middle of the forearm to the tip of the thumb and holding the thumb slightly flexed at the metacarpophalangeal joint. While the movements during reduction must be carried out with considerable force, the surgeon should never jerk the thumb or apply violent movements for fear of causing damage to the soft tissues. The immobilization in a plaster cast or plaster mold should be continued for two weeks. At the end of this time the plaster can be removed and the thumb strapped firmly with adhesive for two weeks longer when all dressing can be removed and the patient may begin to use the hand normally, but he should avoid forcible hyperextension of the thumb for some weeks to come.

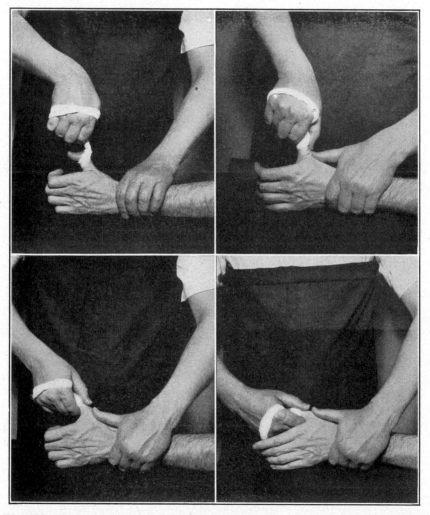

Fig. 820.—Upper left, method of grasping the thumb in reducing a dislocation at the first metacarpophalangeal joint; traction applied by means of a piece of gauze bandage looped around the thumb and wrapped around the operator's hand. Upper right, hyperextension of the thumb with pushing forward of the base of the first phalanx.

Lower left, traction and beginning flexion of the phalanx. Lower right, completing the reduction by flexion of the thumb. Strong countertraction is to be carried out in each of these maneuvers.

In cases of incomplete dislocation, the reduction is much less difficult and can be brought about by slight hyperextension and direct pressure on the displaced base of the phalanx and the period of immobilization can be shortened to two weeks.

Metacarpophalangeal Dislocations of the Fingers

These are rare injuries which are usually due to forcible hyperextension of the involved finger although occasionally the dislocation is anterior and is a result of force applied to the dorsum of the flexed finger. In either instance the base of the phalanx rests upon the neck of the metacarpal and the capsule of the joint is torn and stretched around the large metacarpal head. The finger is, of course, shortened, and whether the dislocation is backward or forward can be determined by palpation. Occasionally the dislocation is compounded by the projection of the metacarpal head through the skin.

Treatment of Metacarpophalangeal Dislocation of the Fingers.—Treatment is reduction and this can be accomplished by manipulations similar to those described in the reduction of posterior dislocation of the thumb except that the reduction is, as a rule, much less difficult and can be accomplished with only moderate traction on the finger, usually under local anesthesia. In a dorsal dislocation, the finger is slightly hyperextended and the base of the phalanx is pushed downward to a point opposite the metacarpal head and then slowly forced over it; the finger is then flexed, traction being maintained throughout the manipulation.

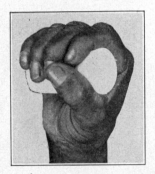

Fig. 821.—Another method of placing bandage in hand to maintain reduction after dislocation of the metacarpophalangeal joint of the thumb. The thumb and fingers are to be strapped around the bandage with adhesive tape. The plaster mold as shown in Fig. 763 can also be used to advantage.

In the rare anterior dislocations, reduction is accomplished in the same manner, except that the finger is first brought into a position of increased flexion, and after the base of the phalanx has been pushed downward, the finger is slowly extended.

After reduction the metacarpophalangeal joint should be immobilized for a period of from twelve to fourteen days depending upon the injury to the soft parts and this can be most simply accomplished by placing small straight splints over the dorsal and volar surfaces of the finger and hand, binding them in place with adhesive. The most convenient splints are tongue depressors which have been padded with cotton. At the end of twelve or fourteen days the splints are removed, and if the joint seems fairly stable, the patient can be permitted to go without further support and begin to use the hand, being careful to avoid strain or forcible movements in hyperextension or hyperflexion, depending upon whether the original injury was a posterior or anterior dislocation.

DISLOCATIONS AT THE INTERPHALANGEAL JOINTS OF THE FINGERS

These are rather frequent injuries resulting from force applied to the tips or sides of the fingers and may be the result of either hyperextension or direct violence. They may occur at either the middle or the terminal interphalangeal joints and the dislocated distal phalanx is usually displaced backward but may occasionally be forward or lateral to the proximal one.

Diagnosis.—The diagnosis would seem to offer no difficulty as the bones are so superficial that their abnormal positions can apparently be made out with ease (Figs. 822, 823, 824, and 826), but in the presence of considerable swelling it may be very difficult to determine whether or not one is dealing with a dislocation or a fracture dislocation, since not infrequently there is more or less chipping of the articular margin of one of the bones. This is especially apt to occur in the posterior dislocations where the prominent anterior margin of the base of the phalanx may be broken off. Consequently, when possible we advise that an x-ray be obtained in these dislocated fingers, although they are apparently very simple injuries.

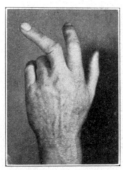

Fig. 822.

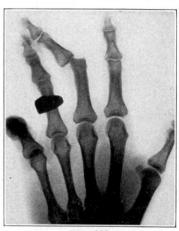

Fig. 823.

Fig. 822.—Photograph of a lateral dislocation of the middle finger at the articulation of the middle and proximal phalanges.

Fig. 823.—X-ray picture of case shown in Fig. 822. Treated by closed manipulative reduction and immobilization for ten days on a straight wooden splint (tongue depressor) with good results.

Treatment.—The dislocation should be reduced and this can as a rule be accomplished with little difficulty by direct traction in the line of the finger. In some instances in order to obtain a firm grip of the distal portion of the finger it is necessary to loop a bandage around the terminal phalanx and use this as a traction strap. As a rule no anesthetic is necessary. In a nervous or apprehensive patient, a little novocaine may be injected proximal to the dislocated joint. It is not always easy to determine when satisfactory reduction has been obtained as occasionally after apparently satisfactory reduction an x-ray will show that considerable lateral displacement persists. For this reason after the ends of the bones have been pulled by one another and the traction

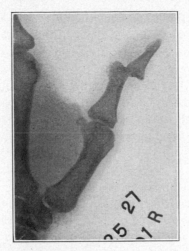

Fig. 824.—Compound dislocation at the terminal interphalangeal joint of the thumb. Treated by débridement (local anesthesia), manipulative reduction, and further débridement and surturing of a one-inch laceration. Immobilization for ten days by molded plaster splint shown in Fig. 789. Good result.

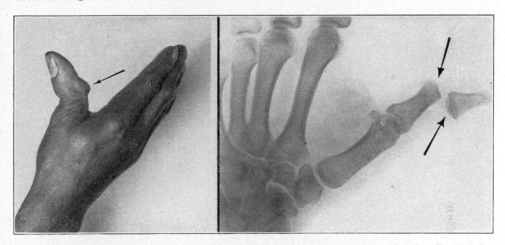

Fig. 825.—Compound dislocation of the terminal phalanx of the thumb. Treated by thorough débridement, reduction, primary closure of the wound, and splints, with good functional and anatomical results.

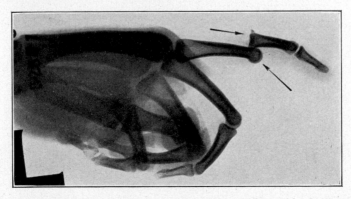

Fig. 826.—Dorsal dislocation of the second phalanx with a chip fracture at the base of the phalanx. Treated by manipulative reduction and immobilized in slight flexion over a bandage.

released the operator should squeeze the sides of the joint together and flex and extend the finger in order to test the stability of the reduction.

If there has been no fracture, all that is necessary after reduction is to immobilize the finger for a period of two weeks on a straight splint which can be made from a tongue depressor or a thin strip of aluminum. This should be padded with cotton and the finger should be strapped to it with adhesive in a position of almost complete extension. If redislocation or subluxation tends to occur in extension, the finger must be immobilized in a stable position which will usually be in slight flexion and this is best done around the wooden ball or a large bandage, as with this dressing one can obtain some traction on the finger.

In those dislocations which are stable after reduction, it is not necessary to immobilize the metacarpophalangeal joints. At the end of two weeks the splint may be removed and the patient may begin gently to use the finger. As a rule no further treatment is necessary; but if stiffness persists, the patient may soak the hand in hot water daily and massage and manipulate the fingers.

CHAPTER XXI

FRACTURES AND DISLOCATIONS OF THE PELVIS

ANATOMICAL CONSIDERATIONS

The pelvis is a strong, broad ring of bone which supports the spine and transmits the weight of the rest of the body to the lower extremities. It also supports and offers considerable protection to the abdominal and pelvic viscera and serves as points of attachment for muscles which move the lower extremities and trunk. It is composed of the two innominate bones which are united in front at the symphysis, and the sacrum which closes the ring behind and articulates with the innominate bones at the sacroiliac joints. (Fig. 827.)

The cavity of the pelvis is divided into an upper false and a lower true pelvis by a plane which passes through the promontory of the sacrum and above the top of the pubis. The false pelvis lies between the wings of the ilia and the true pelvis, and is surrounded by all of the bones of the pelvis. The prominent ridge of bone which lies between the true and false pelves is known as the brim of the pelvis.

The Innominate Bones.—Each innominate bone is composed of three separate bones which fuse in early life. The *ilium* forms the superior and posterior portion, the *pubis*, the anterior portion, the *ischium* forms the inferior portion, and the three bones unite at the acetabulum.

The ilium is composed of a body and an ala, or wing. The body forms part of the acetabulum and unites with the pubis and ischium in front and below and forms part of the great sacrosciatic notch behind. The alae, or wings, of the ilia form the sides of the false pelvis and their long curved superior borders are palpable throughout their length as the iliac crests; they terminate in front and behind in the anterior and posterior superior iliac spines. The inner surface of the ilium is divided by the iliopectineal line (brim of the pelvis) into a large concave upper portion, the iliac fossa, and a small roughened lower portion which presents an articular surface for the sacrum. The outer surface is lined for the origin of muscles.

The pubis consists of a body and two rami. The body unites with its fellow at the symphysis while the superior ramus extends outward to enter into the formation of the acetabulum and the inferior ramus passes downward to unite with the ascending ramus of the ischium.

The ischium consists of a body which enters into the formation of the acetabulum, a tuberosity which faces downward and supports the body weight when sitting, and a ramus which unites with the descending ramus of the pubis. The obturator foramen is the large oval opening between the ischium and the pubis.

The Sacrum is a large triangular bone which is composed of five fused and modified vertebrae. Its anterior concave surface forms the posterior wall of the pelvis and is perforated by four pairs of foramina for the passage of the anterior branches of the sacral nerves. Its posterior surface is roughened for the attachment of muscles and ligaments. The lateral masses present large

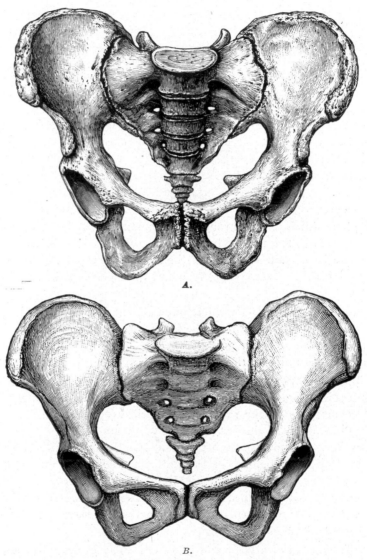

Fig. 827.—Pelvis as viewed from the front and above; A, male pelvis and B, female. (From Morris: Human Anatomy, P. Blakiston's Son & Co., Publisher.)

articular surfaces for articulation with the ilia. The sacrum is suspended by the sacroiliac ligaments between the two iliac bones and serves as a base of support for the presacral portion of the spine. It articulates above with the last lumbar vertebrae and below with the coccyx.

The Coccyx is a small triangular mass of four or five rudimentary vertebral bodies.

The Symphysis Pubis is a rudimentary joint which is strongly reinforced by dense transverse ligaments.

The Sacroiliac Joints are true joints, but the strong short ligaments which surround them permit very little motion. The planes of the joints are oblique from behind inward and forward and the cartilaginous surfaces are gently irregular. The posterior sacroiliac ligaments are very strong and resist the tendency of the body weight to force the sacrum downward and forward.

Mechanics of the Pelvis in Relation to Injury.—The pelvis is so formed that by the use of arches of strong bone it is enabled to support the body weight and resist shocks and blows on all sides. Morris has pointed out that the pelvis consists of two main arches and that the sacrum is the keystone of both of them. The femorosacral arch extends from the acetabula upward through the thick portions of the iliac bones to the sacrum to support the body weight in the erect position and the ischiosacral arch extends upward from the tuberosities through the bodies of the ischia and the thick portion of the ilia to the sacrum to support the body weight when sitting.

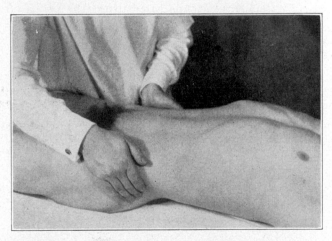

Fig. 828.—Method for examination in suspected fracture of the pelvis. The patient should not be turned over but should remain recumbent. By grasping the anterior superior spines and iliac crests it is possible by pressing the hands together to compress the pelvis, and by pressing them outward and downward to tend to spread the pelvis and thus detect fractures through the pelvic ring. Controlled, gradual pressure is necessary.

In addition to the two main arches there are two tie arches which prevent the main arches from spreading. The horizontal rami and bodies of the pubis support the femorosacral arch, and the united rami of the ischium and pubis support the ischiosacral arch. When an arch is subjected to strain the tie arches are usually broken before the main arches are affected. And clinically most fractures of the pelvic ring occur in the anterior portion (tie arches), and the posterior portion (main arches) is rarely broken without there being also a fracture of the anterior portion.

Examination of the Pelvis.—A patient with a fracture of the pelvis is usually lying on the back and may be in a condition of profound shock. Consequently it is not advisable to move him or subject him to manipulations which may be dangerous. The first thing to determine is how seriously the patient is injured and whether or not operation is indicated. In the presence of abdominal pain, the abdomen should be carefully examined for rigidity and dullness in the flanks and a leucocyte count should be made. Then the condition of the urinary tract should be determined, as will be noted below in the section on complications. Finally attention should be directed to the pelvis and this should be inspected for deformities and swelling, especially in the regions where the patient complains of pain. It should then be palpated gently for tenderness and deformities.

Finally the integrity of the pelvic ring should be tested. Without moving the patient this can be done by compressing the pelvis in the anteroposterior and lateral directions (Fig. 828). We usually use three maneuvers. (1) Placing the heels of both hands on the anterior superior spines of the ilia and pressing them directly downward and outward. If the ring is broken, very little pressure will be necessary to cause pain at the site of the fracture, as this maneuver tends to open up the ring. (2) Grasping one iliac crest lateral to the anterior superior spine with each hand and pulling or pressing them directly together. This maneuver tends to compress the pelvis laterally and in complete fractures of the pelvic ring very little pressure will be necessary to cause pain at the site of the fracture. (3) Direct downward pressure on the symphysis of the pubis. This maneuver is useful in those cases with fracture of the wing of the ilium where the lateral and anteroposterior compression cannot be depended upon on account of the tenderness incident to the iliac fracture. The pressure downward tends to spring the anterior ring inward, and as a rule relatively little pressure will be necessary to produce pain at the site of the fracture if the pelvic ring is broken.

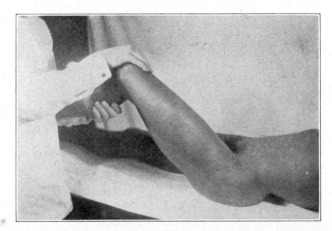

Fig. 829.—Method for determining fracture of the acetabulum. By pressing upward on the knee, pain is usually elicited in the hip if there is a fracture of the acetabulum.

Finally the integrity of the hip and acetabulum should be tested by measuring the distance between the anterior superior spine and the internal malleolus on each side, by manipulating the hip and by making upward pressure on the femur (Fig. 829). However, violent manipulations should be avoided, since they may do harm, and the final diagnosis is made by the x-ray.

FRACTURES AND DISLOCATIONS OF THE PELVIS

Incidence and Mechanism.—That fractures of the pelvis are not rare may be gathered from the fact that Noland and Conwell* report a series of 185 cases seen over a period of twelve years. Moreover they are becoming more frequent, since the automobile accounts for an ever increasing number of severe injuries. Many fractures of the pelvis are never diagnosed because they frequently occur in conjunction with other fatal injuries such as result from falls from a great height, mining, railroad, or automobile accidents, etc.

Most fractures of the pelvis are caused by direct trauma such as heavy blows or severe crushing injuries. When the force is applied in the antero-posterior direction, the front of the pelvic ring (one or both rami) usually breaks first, and then if the force continues to act the strong main arch is spread and the posterior portion of the ring is broken near the sacro-iliac joint and usually on the same side as the fracture of the anterior arch. With lateral force the same type of injury tends to occur, but the anterior ring is broken by being forced inward. In a fall upon the feet with the force acting from below upward the same sequence of fractures may occur.

Classification of Fractures of the Pelvis

As a result of its complex form and the fact that most of the fractures are caused by direct violence, many different types of fractures of the pelvis occur, and there are many classifications of these lesions in the literature. A very serviceable classification is the following:

    I. Fractures of Individual Bones Without a Break in the Continuity of the Pelvic Ring.

        1. Fractures of the wing of the ilium.

        2. Fractures of a single ramus of the pubis or ischium.

        3. Fractures of the anterior superior spine of the ilium.

        4. Fractures of the tuberosity of the ischium.

        5. Fractures of the sacrum.

        6. Fractures or dislocations of the coccyx.

    II. Single Breaks in the Pelvic Ring.

        1. Fractures through both rami.

        2. Separation at or fracture near the symphysis.

        3. Separation at or fracture near the sacroiliac joint.

    III. Double Breaks in the Pelvic Ring.

        1. Double vertical fracture of Malgaigne.

        2. Severe multiple fractures of the pelvis.

    IV. Fractures of the Acetabulum. (These will be considered in the section on injuries of the hip.)

While the classification includes practically all of the pelvic injuries, it is to be noted that in a rather high percentage of the fractures of the pelvis (about

---

*Noland and Conwell: Surg. Gynec. & Obst., February, 1933.

65 per cent) multiple lesions of the bones are present. The relative frequency of the various lesions is shown in the following table from Noland and Conwell's earlier paper.*

The X-ray in Fractures of the Pelvis.—Every case of severe injury in the region of the pelvis should be x-rayed. This is done because the lesions are frequently multiple and because much of the pelvis is so well covered by soft tissues that accurate diagnosis by physical examination is impossible.

ANATOMICAL CLASSIFICATION OF FRACTURES IN NOLAND AND CONWELL'S SERIES

	Left	Right	
Ala of ilium	20	6	
Crest of ilium	1	8	
Superior ramus of pubis	40	12	
Inferior ramus of pubis	3	1	
Inferior ramus of ischium	18	20	
Superior ramus of ischium	2	1	
Acetabulum	10	11	
Separation of symphysis			9
Definite sacroiliac separation			9
Isolated fracture of ischial tuberosity			2
Double vertical fracture of pelvis (Malgaigne)			8
Fracture of the sacrum with associated pelvic fracture			3

COMPLICATIONS OF FRACTURES OF THE PELVIS

The relatively high mortality in fractures of the pelvis (16 per cent in Noland and Conwell's series) is due to the complications and associated injuries which are so frequent in these lesions. In those cases that die within the first twenty-four hours after admission, death is usually caused by crushing injuries of the abdomen and pelvis with rupture of viscera and surgical shock or by fractures of the skull or chest. In these patients the fracture of the pelvis is of secondary importance.

In addition to the associated injuries which may or may not be fatal and cannot be considered complications of the pelvic fractures, injuries of the pelvic contents may occur, and the most frequent of these are ruptures of the bladder or urethra. So important and frequent (about 10 per cent) are these lesions of the urinary tract in fractures of the pelvis that the examination and diagnosis cannot be considered complete until the patient has voided clear urine or the condition of the urinary tract has been determined by catheterization.

Rare complications are injuries of the rectum, vagina, larger vessels, intestines or sacral or obturator nerves. In a considerable percentage of pelvic fractures in which there is no rupture of the bladder or of any other viscus, there is moderate abdominal rigidity and tenderness. This is believed to be due to a retroperitoneal hemorrhage.

Rupture of the Bladder

In rupture of the bladder the lesion is usually extraperitoneal, but may be intraperitoneal. In the extraperitoneal injuries the lesion is usually in the anterior wall near the neck of the bladder and may be caused by laceration by

*Conwell: J. A. M. A. 94: 174, 1930.

a displaced fragment of the ramus or by wide separation at the symphysis. In the intraperitoneal ruptures the lesion is usually in the posterior wall near the apex of the bladder and is the result of violence applied to the anterior abdominal wall, while the bladder is distended (Fig. 830).

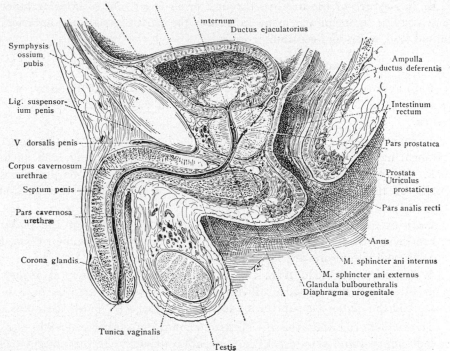

Fig. 830.—Sagittal section of male pelvis and contents. (From Morris: Human Anatomy, P. Blakiston's Son & Co., Publisher.)

Rupture of the Urethra

These injuries are usually the result of lateral crushing injuries in which the pelvic ring is broken and the rami are displaced inward. The urethra may be lacerated or compressed by the fragment or torn as a result of displacement of the triangular ligament, or it may be injured by direct violence to the perineum. The lesion may be a perforation, incomplete tear, or complete section of the urethra and is usually in the membranous portion, but may occur at any point.

Extravasation of Urine

1. In intraperitoneal rupture of the bladder the urine immediately escapes into the peritoneal cavity and the bladder collapses. The rapidity of escape of urine from the bladder depends on the size of the bladder wound.

2. In extraperitoneal rupture of the bladder the urine slowly escapes into the surrounding tissues and may pass up in the anterior abdominal wall between the transversalis fascia or down into the space between the bladder and the rectum in addition to infiltrating the loose tissue around the neck of the bladder.

3. In rupture of the posterior urethra the posterior layer of the triangular ligament is torn and the urine slowly escapes into the loose tissues around the neck of the bladder and may pass up or down as in extraperitoneal rupture of the bladder.

4. In rupture of the urethra through or in front of the anterior layer of the triangular ligament the urine infiltrates the perineum, groins, anterior abdominal wall, penis and scrotum or labia.

Diagnosis of Rupture of the Bladder or Urethra

Pain and distress in the lower abdomen with desire, but inability, to pass the urine should lead the surgeon to suspect a rupture of the bladder or urethra.

1. In intraperitoneal rupture of the bladder there are usually signs of peritoneal irritation with abdominal rigidity, nausea, vomiting, and surgical shock. It is to be pointed out, however, that these signs may be present with injuries of the abdominal viscera or kidneys or with large retroperitoneal hematoma.

2. In extraperitoneal rupture of the bladder or rupture of the posterior urethra there is usually swelling and tenderness in the suprapubic region, and the peritoneal symptoms are less prominent or absent.

3. A trickle of blood from the urethra is pathognomonic of injury to the urethra, and with rupture of the urethra the patient strains in vain to urinate and the distended painful bladder can be palpated above the pubis.

To complete the diagnosis the surgeon should determine when the bladder was last emptied and should ask the patient to urinate. If the patient passes clear urine, there is probably no injury to the urinary tract. If the patient passes a considerable amount of bloody urine, there is probably an injury of the kidney. If the patient is unable to urinate, a soft rubber catheter should be introduced into the urethra under strict aseptic precautions.

If the catheter passes easily into the bladder and normal clear urine is obtained, there is probably no serious injury to the urinary tract. If only a few drops of blood or blood-tinged urine are obtained, there is probably an intraperitoneal rupture of the bladder. If a moderate amount of blood-tinged urine is obtained, and especially if this can be increased by moderate suprapubic pressure, there is an extraperitoneal rupture of the bladder. In doubtful cases a cystogram may clear up the diagnosis.

If the catheter cannot be introduced into the bladder and is found to be stained with blood when it is withdrawn, there is a rupture of the urethra.

Treatment of Urinary Complications of Fractures of the Pelvis

These complications are so important and frequent that they take precedence over the fracture and demand immediate treatment.

1. **Treatment of Intraperitoneal Rupture of the Bladder.**—Immediate laparotomy should be performed and the tear in the bladder should be sutured in two layers and the bladder should be drained suprapubically with a mushroom or Pezzar catheter. Then the peritoneal cavity should be washed or

cleaned out with a large amount of normal salt solution or sponged out with plain gauze and the abdominal wound closed with a small wick or rubber tissue drain.

2. **Treatment of Extraperitoneal Rupture of the Bladder.**—The bladder should be exposed extraperitoneally through a median suprapubic incision. If the tear is easily accessible, it should be sutured in two layers and a suprapubic retention catheter introduced into the bladder. Then the skin wound should be closed and a small rubber tissue drain left in for a few days. The retention catheter should be continued for about two weeks and the bladder should be irrigated daily with boric acid solution.

3. **Treatment of Rupture of the Urethra.**—If a soft rubber catheter can be introduced, it should be left in place for about two weeks and the bladder irrigated daily with boric acid solution.

If the catheter cannot be introduced into the bladder, the urethra is probably severely injured, and operative intervention is necessary. Under general anesthetic or spinal anesthesia a rubber catheter is inserted in the penile portion of the urethra as far as it will go and then a midline incision is made in the perineum down to the rubber catheter exposing the rupture in the urethra. The proximal end of the ruptured urethra is picked up and another catheter is inserted into the bladder; this is drained and the catheter removed after making sure that no rupture of the bladder is present. The catheter in the penile portion of the urethra is then pushed up into the proximal end of the urethra, on into the bladder.

A rubber drain is placed deep down in the perineum to allow for drainage, and all of the structures of the perineum are sutured over the catheter. The rubber catheter should be held in place by adhesive applied around the catheter and penis (over the pendulous portion). This catheter should remain in until practically all drainage has ceased, averaging about two weeks or more, when it is removed. In the after-treatment close observation is to be carried out to prevent stricture of the urethra. Since this is one of the most troublesome complications in this type of case, it is prevented by repeated soundings with metal sounds.

In certain cases after the catheter has been passed through the penile portion of the urethra and the laceration in the deep perineum has been exposed, the ends of this rubber catheter are fixed together by a safety pin; a tube larger than the catheter is inserted into the proximal end of the urethra and into the bladder and sutured in place, where it is left for about ten days.

This tube is removed at the end of that time and the proximal end of the rubber catheter in the penile urethra is continued on into the bladder and held in place by adhesive around the catheter and the pendulous portion of the penis; the proximal end of the catheter must not be allowed to come out of the bladder for several days. Strictures of the urethra should be prevented, if possible, by sounding at frequent intervals.

So far as suprapubic cystotomies are concerned, we recommend that they be done after it is impossible to find either the proximal end of the urethra or the neck of the bladder after a fair trial has been carried out by the perineal route.

In these cases a suprapubic cystotomy should be performed. Through a perineal incision the two torn ends of the urethra should be located by means of sounds or catheters passed from the meatus and the bladder; a retention catheter should be introduced, and the perineal tissues sutured around it, no attempt being made to suture the urethra as such. The perineal wound is closed with a small tissue drain left in for two days. A cystotomy tube is left in ten days, and the retention catheter from three to four weeks, the bladder being irrigated daily with boric acid solution.

Rare Complications of Fractures of the Pelvis

Paralysis of the sciatic nerve occasionally occurs in fractures of the posterior pelvic ring (Fig. 831). The paralysis is usually temporary and clears up spontaneously although it may last for three or four weeks or may even be permanent. While it is present, foot drop should be prevented by a suitable support. Paralysis of the obturator nerve is a rare complication of fractures of the anterior pelvic ring. The paralysis usually clears up spontaneously and demands no special treatment.

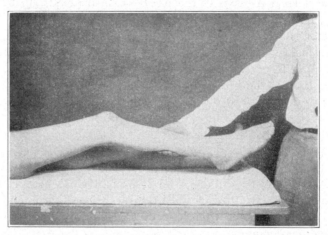

Fig. 831.—Sciatic paralysis with foot drop complicating a fracture of the pelvis. The paralysis cleared up after treatment of the fractured pelvis and with a splint to support the foot.

Rupture of the rectum or intestine gives rise to peritoneal symptoms, and demands immediate laparotomy. Rupture of large vessels may lead to fatal hemorrhage unless the vessel can be exposed and ligated.

Indications for Exploratory Laparotomy in Fractures of the Pelvis.—Evidence of an intraperitoneal rupture of the bladder as given above should be accepted as sufficient indication for an exploratory laparotomy. Even with the urinary tract intact, if the patient persistently complains of abdominal pain either constant or colicky in character, if there is rigidity of the abdomen, if there is evidence of severe hemorrhage with dullness in the flanks, and if there is an increasing leucocyte count, an exploratory laparotomy should be performed as soon as the patient's condition permits.

Edema and Thrombophlebitis.—Marked edema of one or both lower extremities may occur in severe fractures of the pelvis and is especially likely to occur in fractures of the posterior ring. The edema may persist over a period of months and be the cause of great disability.

Likewise, a definite thrombophlebitis with edema of one lower extremity may occur several weeks after the accident and may lead to prolonged disability following a relatively simple fracture of the pelvis. These conditions are probably the result of severe injury to the large veins in the pelvis.

Other major skeletal injuries such as dislocations of the hip, or fractures of the acetabulum or femur may occur and demand appropriate treatment.

Pregnancy and Fractures of the Pelvis.—It is the opinion of many obstetricians that the position of the fragments in fractures of the pelvis is of considerable importance as regards future pregnancies. It is true that if a woman has a very bad position in a pelvic fracture, it may constrict the pelvic outlet and interfere with delivery.

Despite the above, we believe that one should not adopt any unusual method in an effort to obtain perfect position of the fragments in a fractured pelvis in women in order to retain the normal pelvic outlet. In other words, fractures of the pelvis in women should be treated in the same manner as are similar fractures in men, and if necessary a cesarean operation can be performed should the occasion arise.

If a patient should receive a fracture of the pelvis during the first five months of pregnancy and not miscarry within the first few days following the injury, a therapeutic abortion might be advisable. On the other hand, if the fracture is received after the fifth month and the patient does not abort, she should be permitted to go on to term and the baby should be delivered by cesarean section if necessary.

FRACTURES OF INDIVIDUAL BONES WITHOUT A BREAK IN THE PELVIC RING

1. Fractures of the Wing of the Ilium

Fracture of the wing of the ilium is one of the most frequent of the fractures of the pelvis and is usually due to direct violence or lateral crushing injuries. The size of the separated fragment varies from a small chip of bone to a large mass of bone comprising over half of the entire wing of the ilium. In patients under twenty years of age a variable amount of the crest may be separated at the epiphyseal line. In most instances there is little or no tendency toward displacement of the fragment. The fracturing force tends to push the large fragments inward, but the muscles attached to their lateral surfaces pull them back into place again. (Fig. 832.)

Diagnosis of Fractures of the Wing of the Ilium.—With a history of a lateral crushing injury and severe direct trauma, and local pain, swelling, and tenderness over the side of the pelvis and no evidence of a break in the pelvic ring, the surgeon should suspect a fracture of the wing of the ilium. As a rule there will be no surgical shock, and the patient will not appear to be severely injured, but he will be unable to stand upon the leg on the affected side or to abduct it against resistance, and attempts to do so cause pain at the site of the fracture. It is rarely possible to palpate a deformity or to demonstrate false motion, but if the fracture includes the anterior superior spine, and if this is displaced upward (Duverney's fracture), the distance between the anterior superior spine and the internal malleolus will be increased. The diagnosis of fracture of the wing of the ilium should be confirmed by the x-ray.

Treatment of Fracture of the Wing of the Ilium.—The most important factor in the treatment of these fractures is rest in bed, and in many instances this is all that is necessary. Some patients are more comfortable on a fracture bed (a bed with boards between the springs and the mattress to prevent sagging); others are less so. As their presence seems to have no effect upon the fracture, we do not insist upon fracture boards in the bed. If the patient is more comfortable with pillows under the knees we let him have them. We see no necessity for placing these patients in a plaster cast and think that they are much more comfortable if permitted to move around in bed.

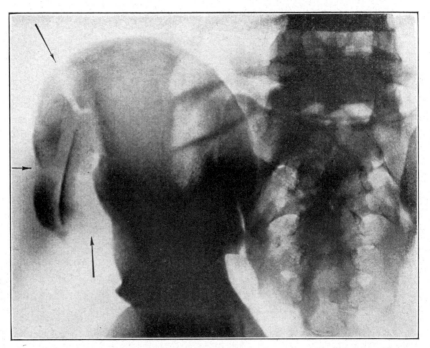

Fig. 832.—Comminuted fracture of the wing of the ilium. Treated by rest in bed with both hips flexed and a swathe around the pelvis. Good result.

During the first week or two many patients are more comfortable and feel more secure with a wide swathe of adhesive around the pelvis, and we usually apply such a swathe, being careful to keep it below the iliac crests.

Application of the Adhesive Swathe.—The patient is shaved and four strips of adhesive tape three inches wide and almost long enough to encircle the pelvis are cut. Then the patient is rolled on the sound side. Beginning as far on the sound side as possible and well down on the buttocks opposite the trochanter, the operator applies an adhesive strip, pulling it tightly across the back and carrying it around the front to the opposite side at about the level of the pubes. The second strip is applied over the first at a slightly higher level (Fig. 833). Then the patient is turned on the injured side and the other two strips are applied in the same manner, but in the opposite direction.

At the end of two or three weeks the adhesive swathe can be removed and a light canvas belt three inches wide can be fitted. This belt can be worn in bed or not, depending upon whether or not it makes the patient more comfortable, but it is made especially as an ambulatory support for the pelvis. At the end of four weeks the patient may begin to sit up, and in five weeks he may begin walking with a cane which is gradually discarded. The belt should be worn as long as the patient feels the need of it (three to six weeks). In small chip fractures all of the periods of time given above can be shortened.

The above may seem a rather casual method of treating these fractures, but it works, and the surgeon should remember that as there is little tendency to displacement of the fragments, all that he can do is to make the patient as comfortable as possible until the bones have united.

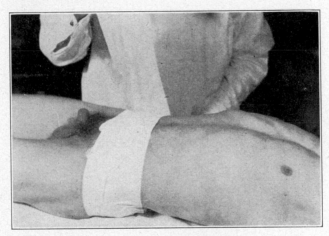

Fig. 833.—Application of adhesive swathes for simple fractures of the pelvis in which the continuity of the ring is not broken.

In fractures with displacement it is not, as a rule, possible to reduce the displacement, and the slight displacements which occur do not appear to have any effect upon the restoration of normal function in about ten weeks.

As a rule the less apparatus used the more comfortable the patient. A trapeze (monkey bar) is helpful at first to enable the patient to lift himself and move around in bed. This is especially true when it is necessary to use the bed pan. If a fracture bed which permits the mattress to be lowered is available it should be used, but the amount of pain incident to using the bed-pan is not as a rule sufficient to warrant placing the patient on a Bradford frame or in a pelvic sling.

2. Fractures of a Single Ramus of the Pubis or Ischium

Fractures of a single ramus of the pubis or ischium are usually due to direct violence from in front, but may be caused by lateral crushing injuries or falls. The pelvic ring is intact and consequently there is little displacement of the fragments and no tendency for them to become displaced later (Fig. 834).

Diagnosis of Fractures of a Single Ramus.—The history of the injury with local pain, swelling, and tenderness over the broken ramus leads the surgeon to suspect the diagnosis. Further evidence is gained if abduction or hyperextension of the thigh on the affected side causes acute pain at the site of the fracture (due to muscle pull on the broken ramus). The diagnosis should be confirmed by the x-ray (Fig. 834).

It should be remembered that these fractures may simulate breaks in the pelvic ring in that strong compression may elicit local pain (due to the spring in the intact ramus).

Treatment of Fractures of a Single Ramus.—The intact ramus acts as an efficient splint and all that is necessary is to make the patient comfortable in bed until the fracture has healed. Consequently we treat these fractures by rest in bed for three or four weeks and then activity is resumed gradually.

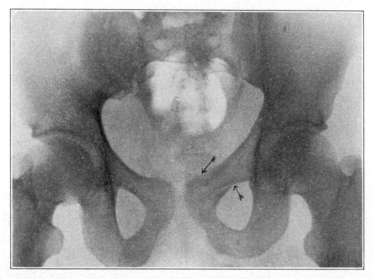

Fig. 834.—Fracture of the horizontal ramus of the pubis. Treated by adhesive swathe and rest in bed and sacroiliac belt during the ambulatory convalescence with good results.

FRACTURE OF THE ANTERIOR SUPERIOR SPINE

Fractures of the anterior superior spine are rare injuries which are usually the result of muscular violence as in running or jumping, the spine being pulled off by the tensor fascia femoris and sartorius muscles. There is local pain, swelling, and tenderness with pain on attempts to flex or abduct the thigh on the affected side and it may be possible to palpate the avulsed fragment which is displaced downward (Fig. 835). The diagnosis should be confirmed by the x-ray.

Treatment of Fractures of the Anterior Superior Spine.—Treatment is rest in bed with the thigh on the affected side in moderate flexion and abduction. This may be maintained with pillows or a splint. Sitting with the thighs

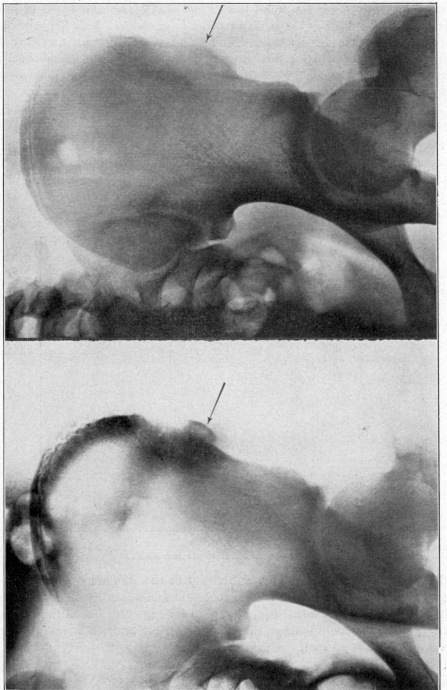

Fig. 835.—Avulsion of the anterior superior spine of the ilium due to muscle violence. Before and after treatment by rest in bed with the hip flexed in plaster spica. Good functional result. (Conwell and Alldredge: American Journal Surgery, 1936.)

abducted is the ideal position. The patient may be permitted to sit up as soon as he wishes. Immobilization is not necessary. The avulsed fragment usually unites at a slightly lower level and the patient may be up and about in four or five weeks. No disability is to be expected. One of us (J. A. K.) operated upon an acute fracture of this type. The relatively large fragment was drawn downward and backward by the gluteus medius, tensor fascia femoris, and sartorius. It was sutured in its normal position and the patient resumed his place on the track team the next season with no handicap.

FRACTURES OF THE TUBEROSITY OF THE ISCHIUM

Fracture of the tuberosity of the ischium is a very rare injury which may result from a fall in the sitting position. The diagnosis may be suspected from the history and the presence of local pain and tenderness with local pain when tension is put on the hamstrings, but should be confirmed by the x-ray. (Fig. 836.)

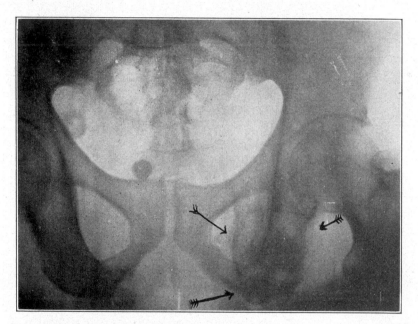

Fig. 836.—Isolated fracture of the tuberosity of the ischium. Treated by rest in bed with good results. Note abundant callus formation.

Treatment of Fractures of the Tuberosity of the Ischium consists simply of rest in bed until the patient is able to be up and about again (from four to six weeks). No permanent disability is to be expected, but sitting is frequently painful for months after the injury. An air cushion is useful when this complication is present.

TRANSVERSE FRACTURE OF THE SACRUM

The rare vertical fractures of the sacrum are fractures of the posterior ring and will be considered under the double fractures of the pelvic ring. The transverse fractures are usually due to direct violence from behind as in slipping on a step and landing on the sacrum on the edge of the step. These fractures are difficult to show in the x-ray and it is probable that many of them go undiagnosed. The fracture line tends to be roughly transverse at about the level of the lower end of the sacroiliac joints and the lower fragment may be displaced forward into the pelvis.

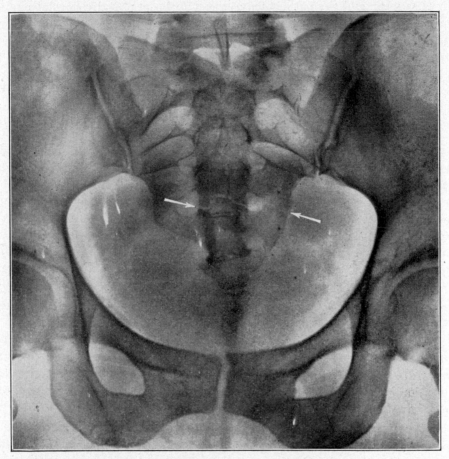

Fig. 837.—Transverse fracture of the sacrum without displacement. Treated by rest in bed with good result.

Diagnosis of Transverse Fracture of the Sacrum.—The history of the injury with pain, swelling and tenderness over the back of the sacrum and tenderness over the front of the sacrum on rectal examination leads one to suspect the diagnosis. Strain at the site of the fracture by local pressure on the lower part of the sacrum may elicit local pain at the site of the fracture or even demonstrate false motion. This is best done by alternate pressure with one finger in the rectum and the other hand on the back of the tip of the sacrum. With displacement a lateral x-ray will show the fracture, but the anteroposterior x-ray must be at exactly the proper angle or the fracture line may not be seen.

Treatment of Transverse Fracture of the Sacrum.—If there is much displacement a careful attempt should be made to push the lower fragment back into place with a finger in the rectum. As a rule, however, all that is necessary is to apply a tight cross strapping to the buttocks. The patient should remain in bed for from two to four weeks and then may be up and about, his activity being restricted by the amount of pain it causes. An inflated rubber ring (air cushion) to sit on affords a good deal of comfort in some cases. The symptoms gradually disappear and the patient may expect to be practically normal again in about six weeks. In some of our cases without displacement there has been so little disability that the patient did not go to bed at all and was quite comfortable in an ordinary corset and used a rubber ring in sitting.

FRACTURE AND DISLOCATION OF THE COCCYX AND COCCYGODYNIA

Injury of the coccyx is rather frequent and persistent pain may follow a direct trauma as a sitting down fall. Coccygodynia is the term used to describe a painful coccyx. It is usually caused by a direct injury, but it may appear gradually and without any known cause. Most of our cases have been in women. In cases from direct trauma there is exquisite pain and tenderness in the area over the coccyx. Rectal examination reveals tenderness over the anterior surface of the coccyx and may reveal a displacement or fracture, but this is rare. Bimanual manipulation of the coccyx which normally is quite movable causes pain. The roentgenogram is nearly always negative.

Treatment of Fracture and Dislocation of the Coccyx and Coccygodynia. —If there is a definite dislocation or fracture with displacement, this should be reduced by bimanual manipulation with a finger in the rectum.

As a rule there is no fracture or displacement and the inexperienced surgeon is at a loss to explain the severe pain of which the patient complains and so are we. It is probable that the acute traumatic cases are suffering from contusion of the coccygeal plexus or sacrococcygeal sprain, while the chronic cases have a mild arthritis at the sacrococcygeal joint.

Rest in bed for about a week is necessary for the acute cases. In some patients tight cross strapping of the buttocks lessens the pain while in others it aggravates the pain. If the strapping affords relief it should be continued about three or four weeks and the patient should avoid sitting on hard seats and should carry an inflated rubber ring around with him to sit upon. This should be continued until the symptoms disappear. A tight pelvic girdle which laces behind can be substituted for the adhesive strapping if the skin becomes irritated. In severe cases hot tub baths two or three times a day and daily warm enemata may be tried. Suppositories of opium and cocoa butter may be used for a short time in very severe cases.

Most of the cases clear up under the above treatment. In chronic cases postural exercises should be tried.

If after several weeks of conservative treatment the patient is still miserable whenever she sits down for more than a few minutes, the surgeon is justified in removing the coccyx. This is easily done through a small vertical incision directly over the bone. As the tip of the bone is quite deeply placed we have found that it facilitates the operation if its upper end is first separated from the sacrum and the coccyx then removed by sharp dissection. After the coccyx has been removed we excise the tip of the sacrum and are careful to leave a smooth rounded surface of bare bone. We then carefully restore the pelvic floor by suturing the muscles which were attached to the sides of the coccyx. In our limited experience this operation has given relief, but others report failure to relieve the symptoms. Removing the tip of the sacrum may be the deciding factor. In freeing the coccyx, especial care should be taken to avoid injury to the rectum.

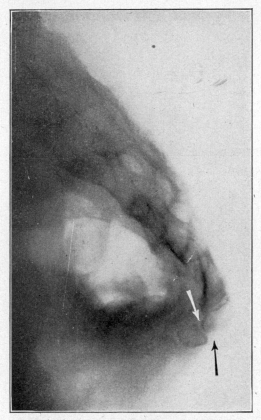

Fig. 838.—Old injury to the coccyx, painful over a period of a year. Treated by excision with relief of symptoms.

SINGLE FRACTURES OF THE RING OF THE PELVIS

1. Fractures of the Rami of the Pubis and Ischium

These complete fractures of the anterior pelvic ring (tie arch) are the most frequent of the fractures of the pelvis and are usually caused by crushing injuries, either in the lateral or anteroposterior direction. In the lateral crushing injuries the fragments tend to be displaced inward and override, but usually spring back to approximately their normal position. In the anteroposterior crushing injuries the pubis may be pushed backward or the pelvis may be spread, causing separation of the fragments. The fracture lines may be roughly transverse or oblique and in rare instances the bones may be com-minuted (Fig. 839). The fractures involve both rami and may lie at any point in each (Figs. 839, 840, and 841). The amount of displacement varies with the force, but is usually less than half an inch in any direction.

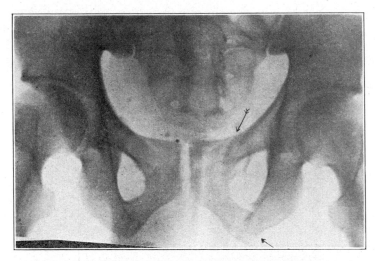

Fig. 839.—Fracture through the anterior ring involving pubic and ichial rami. Treated by hammock suspension and wooden spreader with traction to both extremities and sacroiliac belt during the ambulatory convalescent period. Good results.

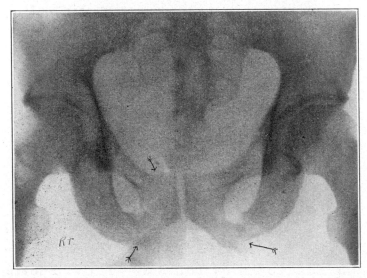

Fig. 840.—Fracture through both rami of the pubis on the right and through the ring of the ischium on the left. Treated by hammock suspension for five weeks and traction to both lower extremities. Good results. Sacroiliac belt used during the ambulatory convalescent period.

Diagnosis of Fractures of the Rami of the Pubis and Ischium.—Following a severe crushing injury or fall the patient is unable to walk or stand and may be in a condition of surgical shock. There is pain in the pubic and peri-neal regions and there may be local swelling and signs of trauma (abrasions, contusions, or lacerations). As a rule the patient will be unable to lift the leg on the affected side.

Palpation will reveal acute tenderness over the site of the fracture both in the horizontal and vertical rami, and if considerable displacement is present, it may be possible to detect the deformity. Compression of the pelvis both in the anteroposterior and lateral directions elicits pain at the sites of the fractures. The same type of pain can usually be elicited by gentle abduction of the thighs.

The details of the lesion should be determined by the x-ray and the condition of the bladder and urethra should be determined because lesions of the urinary tract are especially apt to occur in these lesions of the anterior ring.

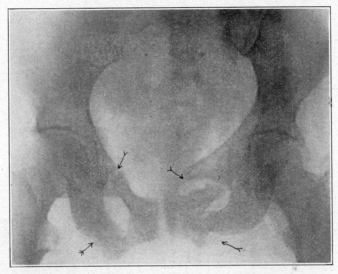

Fig. 841.—Double fracture of the anterior portion of the ring of the pelvis. There was an extraperitoneal rupture of the bladder. Treated by suprapubic drainage followed by suspension in a pelvic sling with a wooden spreader and traction to both lower extremities. Sacroiliac belt worn during the convalescent period. Good result. No attempt was made to approximate the displaced fragments. Excellent functional results obtained without any change in the position of bone fragments.

Treatment of Fractures of the Rami of the Pubis and Ischium.—If there is no displacement which demands reduction and if the patient is fairly comfortable lying in bed, these fractures are most comfortable by simple rest in bed. This is especially true if a fracture bed is available, as this eliminates the necessity of lifting the patient onto a bed pan. In certain instances an adhesive swathe around the pelvis makes the patient more comfortable. The same is true of pillows under the knees and of traction to one or both lower extremities.

Any bladder or urethral lesion or other serious complication demanding surgical interference should be attended to before treatment of the fracture of the pelvis is instituted.

A convenient and efficient suspension and traction method for the treatment of these fractures of the pelvic ring is that described by Noland and Conwell.*

*Noland and Conwell: J. A. M. A. 94: 174, 1930.

The patient is placed on a bed with fracture boards between the spring and the mattress, and the Conwell overhead pelvic suspension frame is attached to the bed (Figs. 842 and 843). (Any frame having a strong central longitudinal bar will answer.)

A hammock made of a strip of strong muslin six feet long and twenty-two inches wide is slipped under the patient in such a manner that it extends from the middle of the thighs to the dorsolumbar region. The ends of the muslin may be strongly sewn together, but it is more convenient to fasten them with webbing straps and buckles as shown in the figure. The weight is applied to the hammock through a wooden bar which prevents the muslin from wrinkling. The weight applied should about equal the weight included

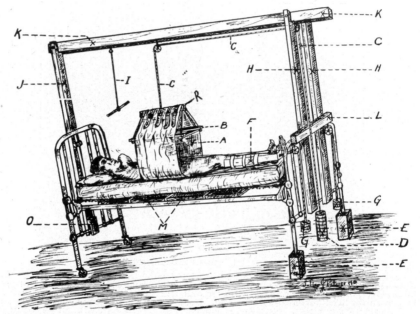

Fig. 842.—Overhead pelvic suspension frame with the muslin hammock and the wooden spreader: A, hammock, which is made of thick muslin, extending from the junction of the middle and upper third of thighs to the dorsolumbar region; average length, 6 feet; average width, 22 inches. B, wooden spreader, a rectangular affair made of one and one-half inch by one-half inch wood; every spreader should be made the width of each patient's pelvis; the length should extend 2 inches beyond the lateral borders of the hammock. C, main pull, which extends to top rail K, then along K, and then down to weights D, weights applied; the amount of the weight should be governed according to the weight of the area of the body where the hammock is applied; this amount averages about 35 to 45 pounds, or about one-fourth of the patient's weight; the amount of weight applied at D is one-fourth less pull than on the muslin hammock (A). E, the 12-inch wooden blocks applied to elevate the foot of the bed, thereby causing countertraction to the traction on the legs. F, adhesive plaster applied to the legs for the traction. G, weights applied to legs; these average from 4 to 8 pounds. H, two-foot uprights, 2 by 4 inch wooden pieces; these uprights steady the frame; their average height is 5 feet 10 inches. I, hand-hold for patient to shift himself around in bed. J, the head upright, a 2 by 4 inch wooden piece. The head and foot pieces should extend at least 3½ feet above the foot of the bed. K, the main cross wooden piece, 2 by 4 inches, with 2½ inch screw pulleys; this cross piece extends about 6 inches beyond the head and foot uprights; it is held in place at the head and foot with the aid of bolts and can be assembled easily; the length averages 8 ft. 5 inches. L, the cross foot piece with 2½ inch screw pulleys; these can be moved in or out according to the amount of adduction or abduction that is demanded at the hips. M, fracture boards, 2 by 10, which are applied underneath the patient to prevent sagging. O, attachment of foot and head pieces to bed. R, wooden piece (2 by 2 inches and the width of the muslin hammock about 22 inches), around which one end of the muslin hammock is looped; buckles (about five or six) are also sewed on this loop; the other end of the muslin hammock has webbing straps sewed on to correspond to these buckles, and the ends of the hammock are buckled over the wooden piece R; the small cords extending from each corner of the wooden spreader are attached to the piece R; these cords allow for the raising or lowering of the spreader. Besides being useful for treating fractures of the pelvis, this frame in certain cases is also adaptable for treating fractures of the neck and shaft of the femur. (Conwell: J. A. M. A. 94: 174, 1930.)

in the hammock (about a fourth of the body weight of the patient), and not enough to lift the patient off the bed.

In order to prevent too much lateral compression of the pelvis by the hammock, a rectangular wooden spreader the exact width of the patient's pelvis should be inserted in and tied to the hammock between the patient and the crosspiece. Elevating this spreader increases the lateral pressure on the pelvis.

When the bedpan is used, if the hammock is fitted with buckles, the two bottom ones can be unfastened and the hammock folded back. If the ends are sewn together, the hammock must be slipped up temporarily, or it can be cut back ten inches and laced on the lower edge; thus the lower ten inches can be folded up under the patient.

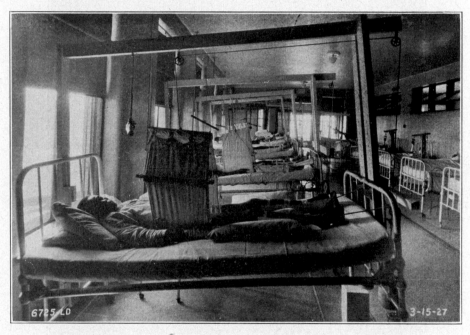

Fig. 843.—Series of pelvic frames in use. Note pillow under the knees.

Finally adhesive traction strips are applied to the legs (below the knees) and from five to eight pounds of weight are attached to each leg, and the foot of the bed is elevated in order that the body weight may serve as counter-traction. The legs are fixed in from 15 to 20 degrees of abduction and a pillow is placed under the knees to maintain slight flexion (traction with complete extension of the knees is painful). The leg traction relieves muscle spasm and makes the patient much more comfortable. It should be continued about three weeks and at the end of this time the patient should be given daily leg exercises to prevent muscle atrophy and limitation of abduction.

The patient should remain in the hammock from four to six weeks depending upon the severity of the fracture. At the end of this time all apparatus can be removed and he should be fitted with a supporting belt which can be strapped or laced tightly around the pelvis. We use a heavy canvas belt about three inches wide which is strapped around the pelvis just below the crests of the ilia. If the belt tends to slip up, it should be fitted with perineal straps to hold it in place.

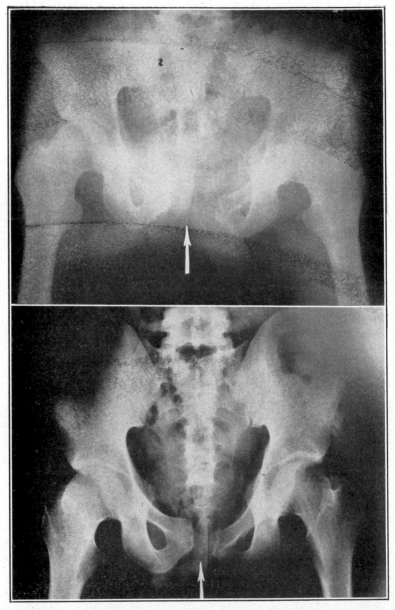

Fig. 844.—Separation of the symphysis pubis before and after improvement and following treatment by hammock suspension without spreader. Good function in spite of incomplete reduction.

After the belt is applied, the patient can move around in bed for from ten to fourteen days and then get up on crutches. The crutches are to be discarded as soon as he is able to get along without them (one to two weeks). Activity

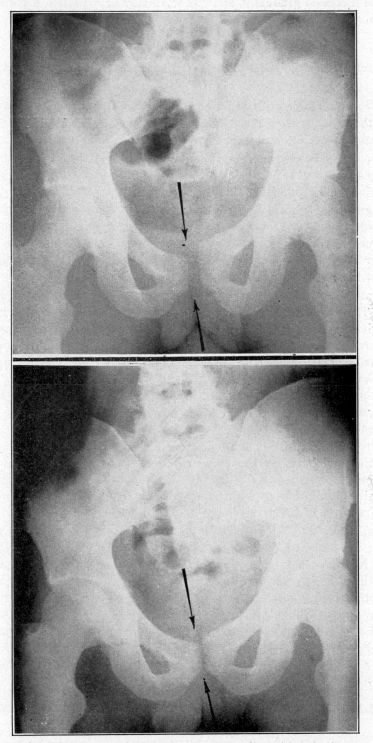

Fig. 845.—Separation of the symphysis pubis before and after improvement following treatment in a pelvic sling. Excellent functional result in spite of incomplete reduction.

should be increased gradually, and full work may be expected in from twelve to fourteen weeks, but he should continue to wear the belt for some weeks longer.

SEPARATIONS AT AND FRACTURES NEAR THE SYMPHYSIS OF THE PUBIS

These rather rare injuries may result during difficult labor from the pressure of the fetus or from force exerted by the obstetrician or they may result from anteroposterior or lateral compression or direct trauma to the pubes. The lesion may be a true separation or a roughly vertical fracture through the body of the pubis near the symphysis and there may be wide separation of the fragments (Fig. 844), and in severe injuries the rami may also be broken.

Diagnosis of Separations at and Fractures Near the Symphysis of the Pubis.—The symptoms and physical findings are similar to those described in fractures through the rami except that the pain and tenderness are localized over the symphysis and if there is wide separation of the fragments the sulcus at the pubis can be palpated by the examining finger.

Treatment of Separation of and Fractures Near the Symphysis of the Pubis.—These injuries are essentially fractures through the anterior part of the pelvic ring and the treatment is the same as that described above for fractures through the rami (hammock suspension and traction followed by a pelvic belt) except that more lateral compression is indicated and for this reason the spreader in the hammock should be made narrower than the pelvis or omitted entirely. The increased lateral compression is needed because in these injuries the pelvis tends to open in front and this tendency should be counteracted.

There is no indication for operating on these fractures and suturing or wiring the symphysis as the conservative treatment described above gives better results. It is especially true of the pelvis that good functional results are usually obtained even with poor anatomical position; hence, open reduction of fractures of the pelvis is not indicated.

Firm union is to be expected in from six to eight weeks and at the end of this time the patient may be gotten up with a sacroiliac belt. He may return to work in from ten to twelve weeks, but the patient should continue to wear the belt until he is comfortable without it. There is, of course, some stretching or other injury to the sacroiliac joints when the symphysis of the pubis is widely separated, but it has been our experience that with treatment as outlined above the patients recover without evidence of chronic sacroiliac strain or arthritis. This is the rule even in those cases in which complete reduction has not been obtained as in Fig. 844, in which there was no permanent disability.

DISPLACEMENTS AT OR FRACTURES NEAR THE SACROILIAC JOINTS

The so-called subluxations or strains of the sacroiliac joints which are believed to be the cause of certain cases of low back and sciatic nerve pain are considered in the section on the spine and will not be included here. In this section we shall discuss the definite displacements at the sacroiliac joints which are demonstrable by the x-ray and the vertical fractures through the ilium or sacrum near the joint. (Figs. 848 and 849.)

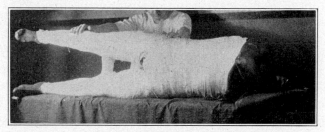

Fig. 846.—Double plaster-of-Paris spica jacket sometimes used in the treatment of fractures of the pelvis.

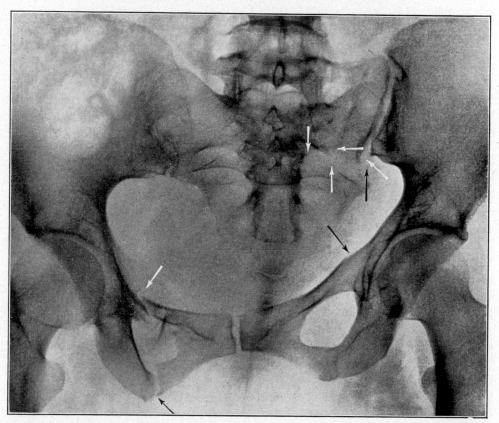

Fig. 847.—Comminuted fracture of the anterior ring of the pelvis and of the sacrum. Treated by hammock suspension with spreader. Good result.

These are isolated breaks through the posterior part of the pelvic ring and as was stated above they are quite rare because in nearly every instance where the strong posterior ring is broken there is also a fracture through the relatively weak anterior portion of the ring. However, occasionally with severe direct trauma from behind, or behind and laterally, the posterior ring

may be broken, while the anterior ring remains intact. The sacroiliac ligaments may be torn and the ilium displaced on the sacrum or there may be a
roughly vertical fracture through the adjacent portion of the ilium or sacrum.
The displacement is rarely more than half an inch.

Diagnosis of Displacements at or Fractures Near the Sacroiliac Joints.—
There is a history of severe trauma to the posterior portion of the pelvis, pain
and tenderness are present in the vicinity of the sacroiliac joint on the involved side, and the patient is unable to stand or even sit up or turn over in
bed. On compression of the pelvis in either the anteroposterior or lateral
direction the pain is elicited in the posterior portion of the pelvis on the affected side, and manipulation of the hip on the affected side causes the pain.
This is especially brought out when the thigh is flexed with the knee extended (straight leg raising). The diagnosis should be confirmed by the x-ray.

Treatment of Displacements at or Fractures Near the Sacroiliac Joints.—
If the x-ray shows a definite displacement of the ilium on the sacrum an
attempt should be made to reduce this. Conwell's method is as follows:

1. Under deep ether anesthesia a folded sheet is placed in the groin on
the uninvolved side and traction upward is made on the sheet while another
assistant makes traction downward on the leg on the injured side.

2. While traction is maintained, the surgeon grasps the crest of the ilium
on the injured side with both hands and presses it directly downward with
the heels of his hands. This pressure should be powerful but should be exerted in a slow and careful manner.

3. In certain cases where the ilium is rotated inward it should be rotated
outward by pressing backward, outward, and downward on the anterior superior spine of the ilium on the involved side while the traction is maintained
by the assistants. (Figs. 358, 359, and 360.)

In the isolated fractures through the posterior part of the pelvic ring the
displacement is usually slight and no reduction is indicated.

After the reduction of the sacroiliac displacement and in the isolated
fractures through the posterior part of the pelvic ring the treatment is exactly as was described above for fractures through the rami; suspension in the
canvas hammock with the spreader and traction to both legs in slight abduction, followed by a supporting belt.

These posterior injuries are a good deal more disabling than are those of
the anterior part of the pelvic ring and the suspension and traction should
be continued for from six to eight weeks and the patient should not be hurried
back to work, but should be given about from four to six months. It is to be noted
that considerable permanent disability may result even with apparently perfect reposition of the fragments and that complete functional recovery may
occur in the presence of definite displacement (Fig. 841).

DOUBLE FRACTURES THROUGH THE PELVIC RING (MALGAIGNE)

1. The Double Vertical Fracture of Malgaigne

The double vertical fracture of Malgaigne is not a rare injury. As a
matter of fact it is the lesion to be expected from severe compression of, or

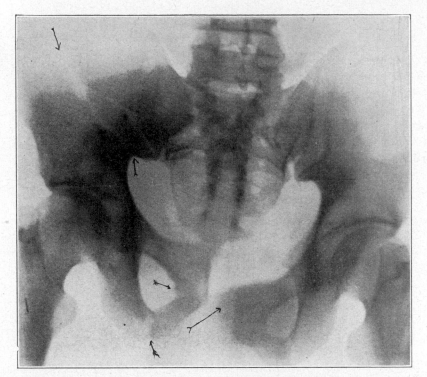

Fig. 848.—Double fracture of the pelvic ring. Separation of the symphysis and fracture through the posterior portion of the ilium with upward displacement. Treated by traction and hammock suspension, with wooden spreader. In bed nine weeks. Good results. Sacroiliac belt worn during convalescence.

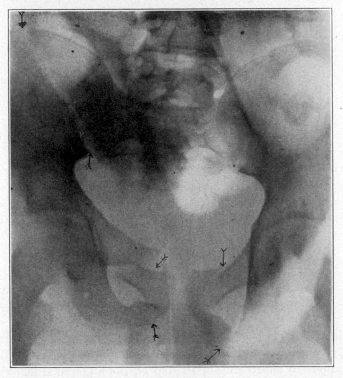

Fig. 849.—Double fracture of the anterior pelvic ring and fracture of the posterior ring. Treated by suspension and traction with wooden spreader. In bed for eight weeks. Good result. Sacroiliac belt worn during convalescence.

direct violence to, the pelvis. The anterior part of the ring (tie arch) is first broken and the continuation of the force breaks the posterior part of the ring (main arch). This injury is a combination of (1) a fracture through the rami, or (2) separation at or fracture near the symphysis, and (3) displacement at or fracture near the sacroiliac joint. As a result one side of the pelvis is completely separated (front and back) and tends to be displaced upward. (Figs. 848, 849, 850, and 851.)

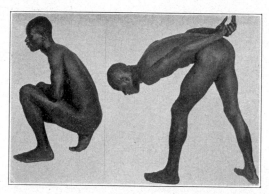

Fig. 850.—Functional result obtained in case shown in Fig. 849, one year following the injury.

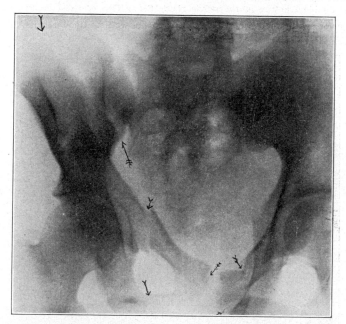

Fig. 851.—Double fracture of the anterior pelvic ring and fracture of the posterior ring. Treated by suspension pelvic hammock and wooden spreader and traction. In bed nine weeks. Good result. Sacroiliac belt worn during convalescence. This patient had an extraperitoneal rupture of the bladder which was treated by suprapubic drainage.

Diagnosis of Double Vertical Fracture of Malgaigne.—The pelvis is obviously severely injured and the deformity may be apparent either in the pelvis or as an apparent shortening of the leg on the affected side. The upward displacement can be measured by placing the legs in the same relative position and measuring the distance from the umbilicus to the internal malleoli. If the legs are of equal length, when measured from the anterior superior spines to the malleoli, and are unequal when measured from the umbilicus, then the pelvis on the short side is displaced upward. Care must be taken to place the legs exactly straight with the body while they are being measured, as abduction or adduction of the legs will produce apparent lengthening or shortening.

Compression of the pelvis in either the anteroposterior or lateral direction will produce pain in both the front and back of the pelvis, and false

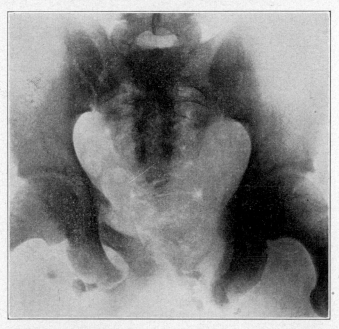

Fig. 852.—Multiple displaced fractures of the ischium and ilium with marked separation of the symphysis and a fracture of the right side of the sacrum. This patient had a rupture of the bladder and of the deep urethra, and was almost moribund on admission to the hospital. Besides the pelvic fracture the patient had very severe burns of the back, shoulders, and the abdomen. Suprapubic drainage was done. Very stormy convalescence. Treated by suspension and traction with wooden spreader in bed for eleven weeks. No improvement was made in the position of the displaced fragments. Sacroiliac belt worn during the convalescent period. (Noland and Conwell: J. A. M. A., Jan. 18, 1930.)

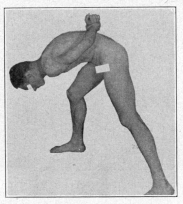

Fig. 853.—Showing the excellent functional result of the case shown in Fig. 852. This case is an excellent example that good position of the pelvic fragments is not always necessary for good functional results.

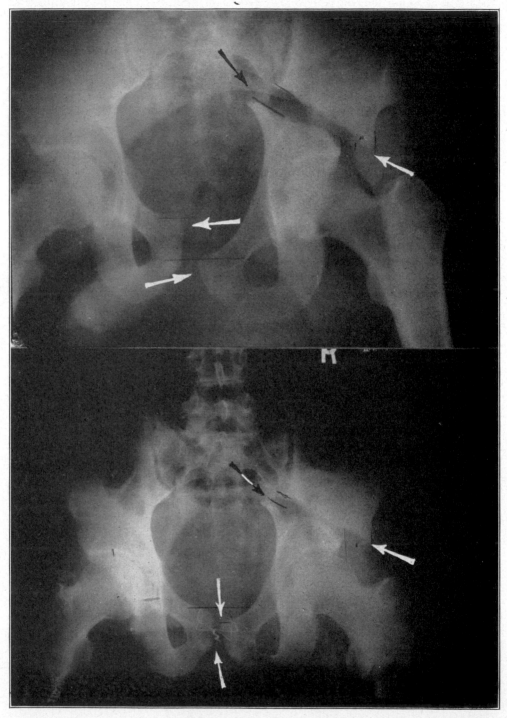

Fig. 854.—Unusual fracture-dislocation through the ilium with multiple fractures and dislocations through the symphysis and rami of the pubis. The fracture-dislocation of ilium was reduced by closed method after wiring the symphysis pubis. Continuous traction to lower extremities; later, bilateral plaster spica cast with fairly good functional result. (Courtesy Major Hugh Smith, United States Army.)

motion may be elicited, but this should not be sought for. The diagnosis should be confirmed by the x-ray.

Treatment of Double Vertical Fracture of the Pelvis.—The treatment is by the hammock suspension with spreader and traction method as described above for fractures of the rami except that in these fractures considerable more weight must be used on the leg on the injured side, as it is desirable to pull this side of the pelvis down into its normal position. We usually begin with twenty-five pounds on the side of the fracture and five pounds on the opposite leg. At the end of forty-eight hours the position of the fragments is checked by a portable x-ray. If it is satisfactory the traction on the injured side is reduced to fifteen pounds and a week later to ten pounds.

If the position is not satisfactory the twenty-five pounds is continued and new portable x-rays are made three days later. If the position is still poor and the patient's general condition is good we recommend that with the traction on, the patient be anesthetized and that an attempt be made to reduce the displacement by manipulations similar to those described for the displacements at the sacroiliac joints.

In these severe injuries the suspension and traction are continued for from eight to ten weeks and then the tight canvas supporting belt is applied. The disability usually lasts from four to eight months and there may be some permanent disability even with union in good position or there may be complete functional recovery with union in apparently poor position (Fig. 853).

Watson-Jones has shown that these fractures can be reduced by placing the patient in a position of lateral recumbency. The patient is placed on his sound side on a fracture table with the perineal post removed. The trochanter and ilium rest on the pelvic rest and the lower extremities are supported by an assistant. The crest of the injured ilium is pushed downward and inward until the displacement is corrected. This is checked with an x-ray. Usually no anesthetic is necessary. Then a double plaster-of-Paris spica is applied and the pelvic rest is cut out and the plaster is repaired. The plaster is left on for three months, and if it becomes loose, it is removed and a new plaster applied in the position of lateral recumbency. During this period the patient takes leg exercises and is encouraged to lie on his side.

Operative Reduction in Fractures of the Pelvis.—We mention this subject largely because we feel that operations for the reduction of displacement of fragments in fractures of the pelvis are rarely indicated. This is largely because these fractures tend to heal regardless of the displacement and because the disabilities which may result in these fractures are usually due to injuries to the soft parts and not to the malposition of the bone (Figs. 852 and 853). Furthermore, the operation is dangerous.

In very rare cases where a displaced fragment has injured the bladder or rectum an operation is indicated for the repair of the injured viscus and at the operation the offending fragment may be reduced or removed. Likewise, in an occasional case manipulation under an anesthetic may be indicated for the reduction of certain displacements, but as a rule the hammock suspension and traction as described above is adequate.

CHAPTER XXII

INJURIES IN THE REGION OF THE HIP

ANATOMICAL CONSIDERATIONS

The bones in this region are the acetabular portion of the innominate bone and the upper end of the femur.

The Acetabulum is a deep cuplike hemispherical cavity for the reception of the head of the femur which is formed by the union of the ilium, ischium and pubis. It is situated on the side of the pelvis at the summit of a bony ridge which divides the lateral surface of the pelvis into anterior and posterior planes. Its cavity faces outward, downward, and forward and is bounded by a thick uneven rim which serves for the attachment of the cotyloid ligament. This rim is interrupted below at the cotyloid notch which is converted into a foramen for the passage of vessels and nerves by the cotyloid ligament. The floor consists of a concave horseshoe-shaped articular portion which is covered by hyaline cartilage and a central fossa which lodges a mass of fat and gives attachment to the ligamentum teres.

The Upper End of the Femur consists of the head, neck, upper portion of the shaft, greater trochanter, and lesser trochanter.

The head of the femur forms a little more than a hemisphere and is directed upward, inward and a little forward to rest in the acetabulum. It is composed of quite dense cancellous bone and its smooth convex surface is covered with hyaline cartilage with the exception of an ovoid depression a little below and behind its center which serves for the attachment of the ligamentum teres.

The neck of the femur is a flattened pyramidal continuation of the shaft which is directed upward and inward at an angle of from 120 to 130 degrees to support the head. The angle tends to be smaller in the female to compensate for the extra width of the pelvis. An abnormal decrease in the angle which the neck forms with the shaft (bending down of the neck) is known as coxa vara and the deformity in which the angle is increased is known as coxa valga. The cortex of the neck is unusually thick and strong along the long, rather slender lower border and its interior is filled with cancellous bone which is strengthened near the base of the neck by a thick vertical plate of dense bone, the femoral spur.

The upper end of the shaft is expanded and cancellous in structure to become continuous with the base of the neck. The cortex of the inner surface is thickened and is continued upward as the thick lower border of the neck. The outer surface of the shaft is prolonged upward to form the lateral surface of the greater trochanter, but some of the deeper lamellae of the cortex curve inward beneath the trochanter to become continuous with the rounded superior border of the neck and these deeper lamellae form the true neck of the femur of Bigelow. The junction between the neck and the shaft is marked by the oblique anterior and posterior intertrochanteric lines.

The Greater Trochanter.—The greater trochanter is a broad flattened quadrilateral process of cancellous bone which projects upward from the junction of the superior border of the neck with the outer surface of the shaft. It serves as a point of insertion for some of the abductors and short rotators of the hip. The lesser trochanter is a conical process which projects from the posterior and inferior portion of the base of the neck at its junction with the shaft. It serves as a point of insertion for the iliopsoas muscle.

Ossification of the Upper End of the Femur.—At birth the upper end of the femur consists of a single plate of cartilage. During the latter half of the first year a center of ossification appears in the head and during the third year one appears in the greater trochanter. Ossification of the main cartilage plate proceeds upward from the shaft and during the fourth year the neck becomes ossified and the head and trochanter become separate epiphyses. A third center of ossification appears in the lesser trochanter at from eight to fifteen years. The head unites with the neck at about the eighteenth year and the trochanters unite with the shaft slightly later.

The Hip Joint.—(Fig. 855.) The hip is a ball and socket joint like the shoulder, but because of the greater depth of the socket and the great strength of the ligaments, the hip has a smaller range of motion and is much more stable. The acetabulum is further deepened by a thick marginal band of fibrous tissue, the cotyloid ligament, which spans the cotyloid notch and thus surrounds the head and aids in holding it in place by suction. The capsule arises from the margin of the acetabulum and the cotyloid ligament and extends downward around the neck like a sleeve to be attached to the region near the anterior intertrochanteric line in front and near the middle of the neck behind. The synovial membrane is reflected onto the neck from the capsular attachments and envelops it up to the margin of the articular cartilage.

The capsule is strengthened in front by the very strong iliofemoral or Y ligament which passes downward and outward from a point on the rim of the acetabulum just below the anterior inferior spine of the ilium to the anterior intertrochanteric line. In its distal portion this ligament splits and the divergent limbs of the Y are attached near the superior and inferior ends of the anterior intertrochanteric line. The posterior portion of the capsule is reinforced by the ischiofemoral or posterior Y ligament which arises from the ischiatic portion of the acetabulum and its superior limb extends outward to the digital fossa, while its inferior limb is inserted into the lower portion of the posterior intertrochanteric line.

The weak points in the capsule are between the divergent limbs of the Y ligaments and it is weaker behind than in front. The arrangement of the fibers of the anterior Y ligament is such that some of its fibers are tense in every movement of the hip except flexion. It thus acts as an important check ligament for extremes of motion.

The ligamentum teres is an intraarticular fibrous band which passes from the edges of the cotyloid notch to the depression in the head of the femur. It has little to do with the stability of the hip.

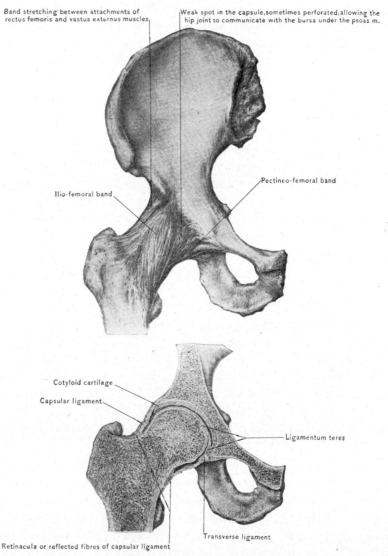

Fig. 855.—Anterior view and longitudinal section of the hip joint. (Deaver: Surgical Anatomy.)

Muscles of the Hip.—The strength and stability of the hip are increased by the large muscles which span the joint. In front the iliopsoas and rectus femoris lie close to the capsule and are the chief flexors of the hip. The short external rotators cross the capsule behind to reach the region of the great trochanter and nearer the surface the powerful gluteus maximus and the hamstrings add stability as well as serve as extensors of the hip. Abduction and internal rotation are accomplished by the gluteus medius and minimus which also aid in holding the head of the femur in the acetabulum and adduction is accomplished by the powerful adductor group.

Vessels and Nerves.—The blood supply to the head of the femur is in part derived by vessels which traverse the ligamentum teres, but these vessels may be relatively small and practically all of the blood to the head of the femur is obtained from the neck, and largely by vessels which course beneath the synovial membrane around the neck. Consequently, in fractures through the proximal portion of the neck with displacement and tearing of the periosteum, the blood supply to the head of the femur may be destroyed.

The femoral artery and vein lie directly over the head of the femur and are an important guide in palpation. The femoral nerve lies lateral to the artery and vein. The sciatic nerve crosses the neck behind, but is separated from the capsule by the short rotator muscles.

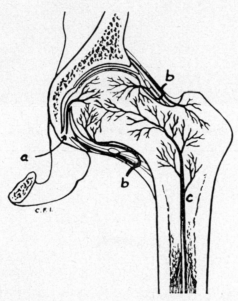

Fig. 856.—Schematic drawing showing the circulation of the head and neck of the femur. *A*, The artery of the ligamentum teres; *B*, the capsular arteries; and *C*, nutrient artery. (Courtesy of Dr. J. S. Speed.)

EXAMINATION OF THE HIP

The hip is so deeply seated that examination of the joint by inspection and palpation (Fig. 861) is unsatisfactory and we must derive much of our information from the position of the limb, the amount of motion permitted in the hip, and the relative positions of certain bony landmarks as determined by measurement.

The important points to be determined are: (1) Is the limb shortened? (2) Is the trochanter elevated? (3) Is the trochanter abnormally close to the midline of the pelvis?

1. **Method of Measuring the Length of the Lower Extremity.**—(Fig. 857.) In surgery the length of the lower extremity is usually considered to be the

distance between the anterior superior spine of the ilium and the tip of the internal malleolus. To determine this distance the anterior superior spine is located by palpation and one end of the tape is pressed firmly against its inferior surface just below the tip and the other end is stretched over the internal malleolus and the position of its tip is noted on the tape measure. A similar measurement is then made on the other side and it is important that the lower extremities be as nearly as possible in the same position in relation to the pelvis when the measurements are made because abduction, adduction, or flexion at the hip or flexion at the knee may change the distance between

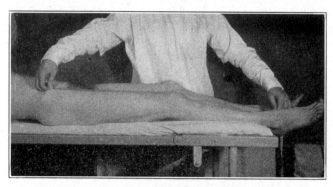

Fig. 857.—Examination of the hip joint. Method of measuring the distance from the anterior superior spine to the tip of the internal malleolus.

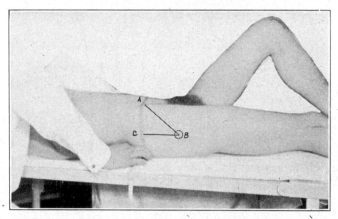

Fig. 858.—Method of determining the base of Bryant's triangle to show elevation of the trochanter. The length of the horizontal line, *BC,* is the base of the triangle, and this is decreased when the trochanter is elevated.

the anterior superior spine and the internal malleolus. For this reason measurement is unsatisfactory in the presence of fixed adduction deformity at the hip because the two extremities cannot be placed in the same position. It is also important that the same surgeon measure both sides, because different surgeons may vary as much as an inch in measuring the same limb, especially in a fat subject. The variation is largely the result of different methods of placing the tape against the anterior superior spine. Repeated measurements by the same surgeon on the same extremity will not vary more than a quarter of an inch.

Normally the two extremities do not differ more than a quarter of an inch in length, but occasionally a difference of half an inch is found in persons who are in other respects apparently normal.

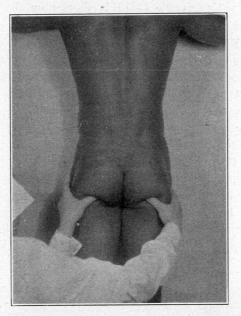

Fig. 859.—Palpation of the tuberosities of the ischia.

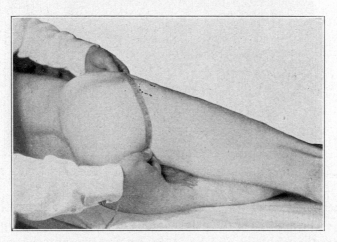

Fig. 860.—The Roser-Nélaton line: Anterior superior spine to the tuberosity of the ischium. Normally the tip of the trochanter is on or below this line.

Methods of Determining Whether or Not the Trochanter Is Elevated.—
1. **Bryant's Triangle.**—(Fig. 858.) With the patient lying upon the back the positions of the anterior superior spine (a) and the top of the great trochanter (b) are marked on the skin and a horizontal line is drawn through the point (b). Then a perpendicular line (a c) is dropped from the anterior superior spine to the table or bed. This intersects the horizontal line through the tro-

chanter at some point (*c*). The triangle is formed by the lines *a b c* and the important part of the triangle is its base (the line *b c*) and its length is carefully noted and compared with that of a similar triangle on the opposite side. If the base of Bryant's triangle (*b c*) is shorter on the injured side the trochanter on this side is elevated.

2. **The Roser-Nélaton Line.**—(Figs. 859 and 860.)   This is a line drawn from the tip of the anterior superior spine of the ilium to the most prominent portion of the tuberosity of the ischium.   It is most satisfactorily determined by having the patient lie upon the opposite side with the hips slightly flexed. The two points are then located and a tape measure is stretched around the hip from the spine to tuberosity, care being taken that it pursues a straight course on the skin and is not curved up or down.

Normally the tip of the trochanter lies just below (distal to) the Roser-Nélaton line.   If the trochanter is elevated its tip can be palpated on the line or above it.   This is not quite as accurate a measurement as is the base of Bryant's triangle, but it has the advantage that it fixes approximately the level at which the tip of the trochanter should be found regardless of the condition of the opposite hip, and is especially useful in bilateral lesions of the hips.

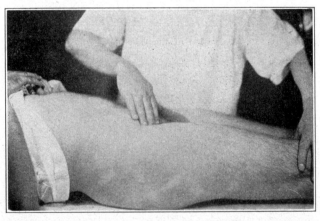

Fig. 861.—Examination of the hip, palpation of tenderness and swelling over Scarpa's triangle in fractures through the neck of the femur.

3. **Determination of the Distance of the Trochanter From the Midline of the Pelvis.**—The midline of the pelvis can be determined by dropping a perpendicular from the midpoint of a line between the two anterior superior spines. The point at which this line crosses the symphysis is marked on the skin, and the distance from this point to the trochanters can be measured with a tape or with a pair of large calipers.   In using a tape, it is advisable to measure to the posterior border of the trochanters as this is most easily palpated and it is important that the two extremities be in the same position as regards rotation.   If this distance is shortened on the affected side, the trochanter is displaced inward.

The final diagnosis and details of the lesion are made clear by the x-ray.

FRACTURES OF THE UPPER END OF THE FEMUR

Fractures of the Head of the Femur

Incidence and Pathology.—Not only is the head of the femur composed of unusually dense cancellous bone, but it lies deeply in the acetabulum and is protected from direct violence. Consequently fracture of the femoral head is a very rare injury, and when it does occur, it is usually as a complication of dislocation of the hip. Very rarely, however, the head of the femur may be broken without dislocation occurring.

The fracture line may be a linear crack extending down into the neck, or a marginal fragment may be detached or a small bit of bone may be pulled away by the ligamentum teres when the hip is dislocated.

Diagnosis.—The diagnosis can be made only by the x-ray or by arthrotomy. A fracture of the femoral head or of the rim of the acetabulum should be suspected if bony crepitus is encountered during the reduction of a dislocation at the hip.

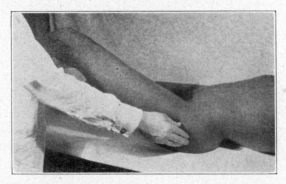

Fig. 862.—Examination of the hip. Manipulation to determine fracture of the acetabulum or telescoping of the femur with intermittent traction.

Likewise, if the hip remains stiff, sore, and painful after a severe trauma and there are no signs of a fracture of the neck of the femur, an x-ray may reveal a fracture of the head or of the acetabulum. Locking of the hip may result from a fracture of the head followed by the setting free of a loose fragment in the joint.

Treatment.—Simple cracks in the head of the femur require only a few days' immobilization in bed with traction followed by freedom from weight-bearing (crutches) until the pain disappears (from six to eight weeks).

Marginal fractures in which the separated fragment is not displaced demand immobilization, usually in abduction, in a plaster-of-Paris spica until the fracture has healed (from six to eight weeks). If the fragment is displaced, it should be removed by arthrotomy.

Separation of the Upper Femoral Epiphysis

This condition is sometimes called "epiphyseal" or "adolescent coxa vara." It is the result of a displacement of the head on the proximal end of the neck of the femur and is included in this book because many cases are definitely traumatic in nature.

Incidence.—The condition is almost limited to the adolescent period and is practically unknown in children under ten years of age. The majority of the cases occur in males between the ages of twelve and sixteen years, but the epiphysis may slip at any time up to twenty years or when it is firmly united to the neck by bone. About 15 per cent of the cases are bilateral. While slipping of the upper femoral epiphysis is not a common condition, it is the most frequent lesion of the hip in adolescence.

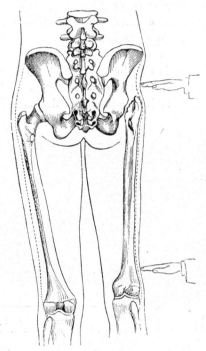

Fig. 863.—Drawing to show method of determining relaxation of the fascia. (After Allis. Hamilton: Fractures and Dislocations.)

Etiology.—Some of the cases are the result of severe trauma and probably occur in normal hips, but the majority of the cases give a history of a gradual onset with no injury or may date their symptoms from some mild injury such as would have no effect on a normal adolescent hip. Furthermore, the fact that about 15 per cent of the cases are bilateral is evidence that the condition is not purely traumatic and that in many cases there is some abnormal weakness in the attachment of the head to the neck of the femur. The cause of this weakness is unknown. Endocrine disturbances have been incriminated because some of the cases occur in the fat boys of the feminine habitus or in patients of the adolescent type of Mikulicz, but many of the cases occur in apparently normal adolescents. Key* has noted that the condition usually begins during a period of rapid growth and believes that the periosteum, which is the main bond of union between the head and the neck of the femur at this period, is stretched and weakened by the rapid growth.

*Key: J. Bone & Joint Surg. 8: 53, 1926.

Mechanism.—The majority of the cases are the result of a minor strain on the hip such as results when an individual steps into a hole when running or trips or stumbles and endeavors to save himself from falling. The epiphysis may be loosened by either a torsion strain or by force transmitted upward through the femur. In other cases the lesion is the result of a blow or fall on the trochanter. In some cases there is no history of injury and the epiphysis is gradually slipped down and back by the body weight.

Pathology.—The cases fall into two main groups: traumatic and non-traumatic types, but it is to be remembered that in many of the traumatic cases the epiphysis had begun to slip gradually some months before it was abruptly knocked off or twisted off by the injury.

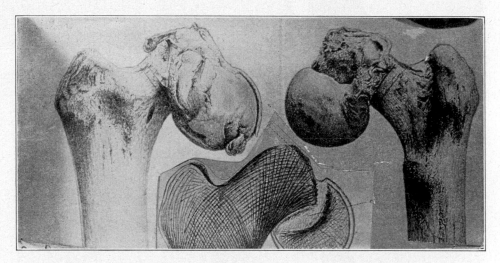

Fig. 864.—Sprengle's case of traumatic separation of the upper epiphysis of the femur. The specimen was removed three months after the accident.

Traumatic Type.—(Fig. 864.) In the acute case the head is usually attached to the neck by a strip of periosteum which is stripped up from the inferior and posterior surface of the neck. The ligamentum teres is not torn and the head remains in the acetabulum, but the neck of the femur is displaced upward and externally rotated so that the epiphyseal surface of the head is applied more or less closely to the posterior inferior portion of the end of the neck. Unless there is very severe trauma with wide separation of fragments the joint capsule is not ruptured and there is relatively little damage to the soft parts.

In the old unreduced traumatic cases the displaced head is firmly united to the posterior inferior surface of the neck and is more or less deformed and atrophied. The superior border of the end of the neck is rounded off and covered with fibrous tissue.

Nontraumatic Type.—(Fig. 865.) In the early case the head is still attached to the proximal end of the neck, but is displaced downward and backward to a variable degree. The displacement occurs gradually and continues to progress slowly over a period of from one to three years until the epiphyseal surface of the head rests upon the posteroinferior surface of the proximal portion of the neck. As the head remains in the acetabulum, the femur is adducted, flexed, and externally rotated on the head. The progress of the displacement may cease at any time. In this type the head is never entirely loosened from its attachment to the neck, and it is, of course, hopeless to attempt to restore it to its normal position by manipulation.

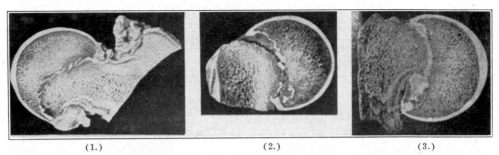

(1.)   (2.)   (3.)

Fig. 865.—Frangenheim's three specimens of epiphyseal separation. Duration (1) two months, (2) six months, (3) six weeks. One followed a fall on the hip. The other two were nontraumatic.

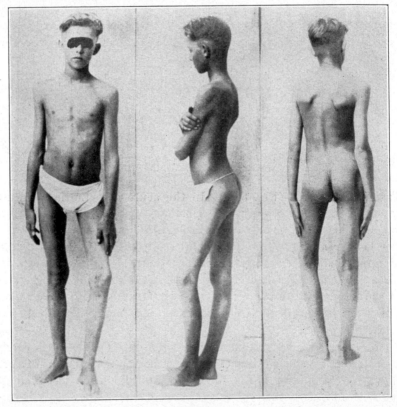

Fig. 866.—Three views showing the typical deformity of a case of epiphyseal coxa vara in a fourteen-year-old boy. Duration one year. (From Key, J. Bone and Joint Surg. 8: 53, 1926.)

In the old nontraumatic cases the pathologic picture is practically the same as that in the old traumatic epiphyseal separations.

Diagnosis of Epiphyseal Coxa Vara.—The most important point in the diagnosis is the age of the patient at the onset of the symptoms (Fig. 866).

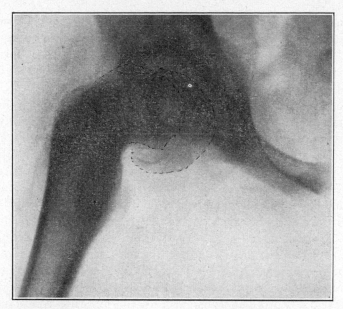

Fig. 867.—X-ray picture of hip of patient shown in previous illustration.

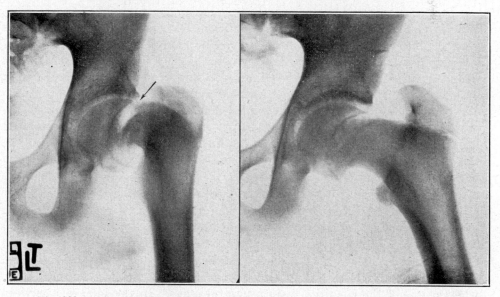

Fig. 868.—Acute dislocation of the capital epiphysis of the femur. Treated by manipulative reduction and immobilization in a plaster-of-Paris cast with good result. Immobilized twelve weeks and no weight bearing for six months.

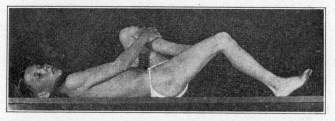

Fig. 869.—Method of demonstrating permanent flexion at the hip. This patient has permanent flexion of 35 degrees due to epiphyseal coxa vara of two years' duration.

Disability at the hip beginning in adolescence and especially between the ages of twelve and sixteen should be suspected of being due to an epiphyseal displacement. The acute traumatic cases resemble a fracture of the neck of the femur and the nontraumatic cases resemble a chronic arthritis and are often diagnosed tuberculosis.

Diagnosis of Acute Traumatic Type.—As was stated under the pathology, in this type there is a sudden complete separation of the epiphysis and the picture resembles that of a fracture through the neck of the femur. One usually obtains a history of injury or unusual strain upon the hip which may be mild in character such as a fall from a chair or stepping in a hole while running. The patient has a sudden pain in the hip which is followed by a complete inability to stand or actively to move the hip. On physical examination there is swelling in Scarpa's triangle, slight shortening (usually one-half to one inch) and the thigh assumes a position of external rotation and slight adduction. Active movements of the hip are impossible and passive movements cause severe pain and may elicit soft cartilaginous crepitus. The diagnosis is confirmed by the x-ray which shows the head in its socket and the neck displaced upward and shortened by the external rotation. (Figs. 870 and 871.)

Diagnosis of the Nontraumatic Type.—In the nontraumatic type the diagnosis is more difficult and is rarely made until some months or even years after the onset of symptoms. A characteristic history is one of gradually increasing pain and disability in the hip which is intermittent in character in that the patient has periods when the hip is almost normal, alternating with periods of several weeks in which the hip causes considerable pain and disability and may even result in confinement to bed. In most instances the onset of the condition and the onset of periods of pain are attributed to mild injuries. Pain may be in the hip, in the knee, or along the inner side of the thigh and many of these cases go along for months without consulting a physician.

From the above it is seen that the symptoms resemble those of an early tuberculosis of the hip and this is the diagnosis which is usually made. On physical examination the extremity is maintained in a position of external rotation with slight adduction and there is a variable amount of permanent flexion, or at least loss of extension. The degree of deformity depends upon the amount of displacement. Also the mobility of the hip depends upon whether or not the condition is in a painful stage. In the intervals between the painful stages the hip may be quite freely movable and painless except that internal rotation and abduction and extension are limited (Figs. 866 and 869). During a painful period the hip may be practically immobilized in a position of external rotation and flexion by muscle spasm. Measurement will reveal slight shortening and moderate atrophy of the muscles of the thigh and calf, the amount of displacement and the amount of atrophy depending upon the duration of the symptoms. The trochanter is found to be prominent and elevated above the Roser-Nélaton line and on palpation over the front of the joint one gets an impression of fullness as though the head and neck of the femur were enlarged.

The diagnosis should be confirmed by the x-ray, which shows the sickle-shaped head slipped downward and backward to a variable degree, but firmly attached to the neck of the femur. The posterior position of the head is more clearly seen in a lateral view of the hip taken with the thigh flexed to ninety degrees.

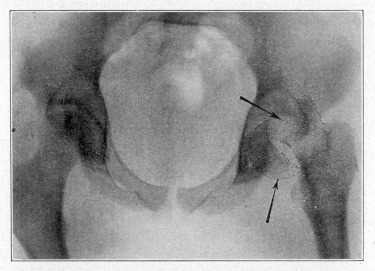

Fig. 870.—Complete traumatic separation and dislocation of the upper epiphysis of the femur. Open reduction and fixation with Smith-Petersen nail.

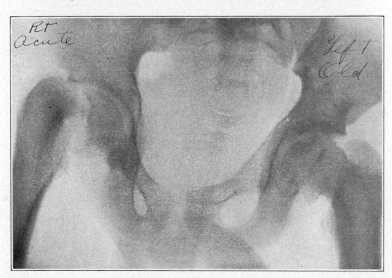

Fig. 871.—Bilateral traumatic separation of the upper epiphysis of the femur; right hip acute, left hip was separated two years before and was reduced by closed manipulation soon after the accident.

Prognosis.—In the traumatic type with complete separation of the head, if the deformity is not reduced the head will become united to the postero-inferior surface of the neck and the hip will be almost completely ankylosed in a position of external rotation, flexion, and adduction, and will be subject to frequent attacks of pain in later life. If reduction is obtained and maintained, an almost normal hip may be expected. (Fig. 871.)

In the static cases without treatment the prognosis is better, but the treatment is more difficult. In these cases the head is never free unless they be converted into the traumatic type, and it is impossible to correct the deformity without open operation. Furthermore, the displacement of the head tends to be progressive. In cases with only moderate displacement, if this is not reduced, there will be a slight amount of shortening and limitation of abduction and internal rotation and extension with the probability that the hip will develop traumatic arthritis and become painful in later life. In cases with more displacement, the same symptoms are exaggerated. In cases with very slight displacement or in which the displacement is reduced, an almost normal hip may be expected.

This injury usually results in the destruction of the epiphyseal line, but as it occurs in adolescence and as there is relatively little growth at the upper epiphysis of the femur after this period, the shortening is rarely of much importance. The chief cause of disability is the deformity of the head of the femur.

Treatment.—The treatment depends upon the type of case.

Treatment of the Acute Traumatic Separation of the Upper Epiphysis of the Femur.—In these cases the head is loose and the lower fragment is freely movable. Consequently, it is frequently possible by manipulation to obtain quite accurate reduction and to maintain this by immobilization in abduction. In other words, the treatment is similar to the abduction treatment in a fracture through the neck of the femur.

The patient, fully anesthetized, is placed on a fracture table, the hip is flexed to 90 degrees and by strong traction the shaft is pulled upward and while the upper thigh is pulled outward in line with the neck of the femur the hip is internally rotated and abducted and extended. When the reduction has been accomplished, the hip is immobilized in a large plaster spica in a position of full abduction and internal rotation and extension for twelve weeks. At the end of this time the plaster can be removed and the patient may be permitted to move around in bed, when he is measured for a Thomas caliper walking splint. The patient should remain in bed for from two to four weeks, then be got up on the splint and crutches. The crutches should be discarded as the patient is able to get along without them.

X-ray pictures are taken immediately after the reduction in order to be sure that accurate reduction has been accomplished and if it is not obtained it should be tried again, and if not obtained the second time, an open operation should be performed. Repeated x-ray pictures should be taken for at least two years after the injury, for some of these cases tend to slip again; if there is any tendency for this to occur, weight-bearing should be prohibited temporarily.

Dr. Paul Steel tells me that he is applying an abduction plaster cast as stated above and after a few days the patient is gotten up on crutches and encouraged to walk in the plaster. We have not tried this method, but believe that it should be used as the weight bearing tends to accelerate union and the cast can then be removed in eight to ten weeks and no further apparatus is needed.

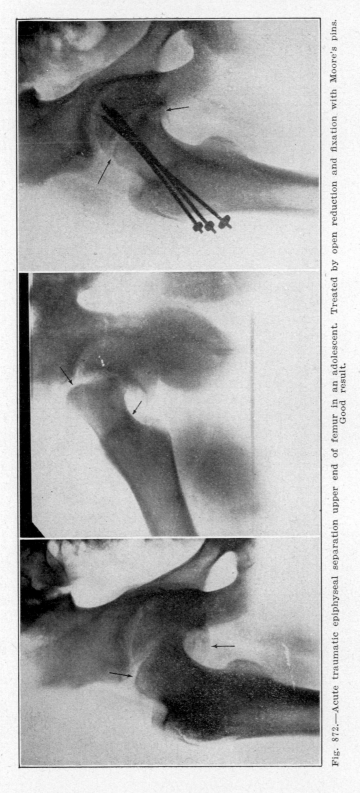

Fig. 872.—Acute traumatic epiphyseal separation upper end of femur in an adolescent. Treated by open reduction and fixation with Moore's pins. Good result.

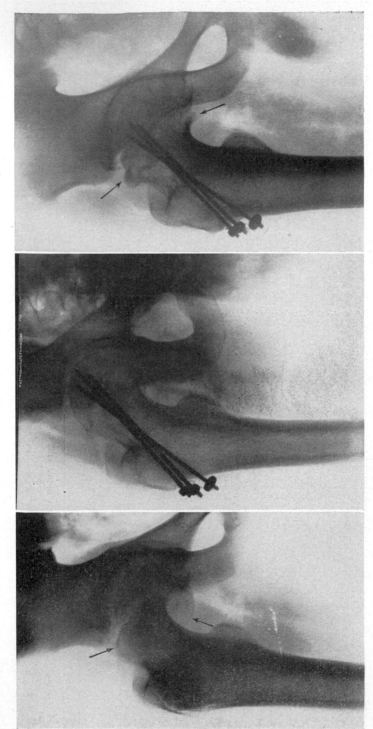

Fig. 873.—Traumatic epiphyseal separation of the upper end of the femur in an adolescent. Reduction was carried out with internal fixation by Moore pins. Three years later patient developed a definite aseptic necrosis of the head and neck of the femur with a painful hip.

Treatment of the Nontraumatic Type.—In the nontraumatic type attempts to reduce the displacement are useless as the head is not only firmly bound to the posteroinferior portion of the neck, but leverage by manipulation is such that the head is simply traumatized against the acetabular margin and definite injury to the cartilage covering the head results. Consequently, these patients should either be left alone and treated by simply giving them crutches to reduce weight-bearing, or an open operation may be performed and displacement accurately reduced and after excising an oblique wedge from the neck, the displacement is corrected and the head is fixed with a Smith-Petersen nail or Moore pins. One of us (J. A. K.) has performed this operation about a dozen or so times, and in two patients aseptic necrosis developed in the head of the femur. In the others the result was satisfactory. A subtrochanteric osteotomy is reported to improve the function of the hip, but one would not expect this operation to prevent the development of malum coxae senilis in adult life.

Steel also reports good results in these cases of gradual slipping by having the patients walk in an abduction plaster spica.

In old cases in adults with traumatic arthritis, the subtrochanteric osteotomy or the Smith-Petersen acetabuloplasty is to be considered.

Fractures of the Greater Trochanter

This rather rare injury may be either a fracture or an epiphyseal separation, depending upon the age of the patient. Most of the cases are due to direct injury such as a kick from a horse or a blow or fall on the trochanter, but occasionally the trochanter is pulled off by muscular action. In adults the separated fragment is apt to be more or less comminuted and varies in size from a small particle of bone to practically all of the trochanter, while in adolescents the separation usually occurs at the epiphyseal line and the entire trochanter is displaced upward. The displacement is, as a rule, slight and tends to be upward and inward toward the midline. (Fig. 874.)

Diagnosis of Fractures of the Greater Trochanter.—The diagnosis is largely made by the history of the injury with localized tenderness and swelling of the trochanteric region and it may be possible to palpate the loose fragment. As a rule the patient is able to bear weight upon the limb, but rotation and active abduction of the hip are painful and the patient experiences pain when the body weight is shifted to the affected leg. The x-ray confirms the diagnosis and gives an exact idea of the amount of displacement present.

The prognosis is good; full function may be expected from conservative treatment.

Treatment of Fractures of the Greater Trochanter.—As the loose fragment tends to be drawn upward and inward by the muscles which are attached to it, an effort should be made to approximate the base from which it has been separated to this loose fragment. This can usually be accomplished by fully abducting the limb. Consequently a plaster-of-Paris spica jacket either with the long single jacket by Whitman, or the double spica which includes both legs in full abduction, is applied. No anesthetic is necessary.

Aftertreatment of Fractures of the Greater Trochanter.—The patient should remain in the jacket for about four weeks, or until the separated fragment is again attached to the femur. At the end of this time the plaster can be removed and the patient may be allowed to move around in bed for a week or two longer and can be allowed up with a cane. No further treatment is necessary. The cane can be discarded as soon as the patient is able to bear full weight on the limb.

In old cases with permanent separation and weakness of the leg in abduction, it will be necessary to perform an open reduction and either suture or nail the loose fragment back in place.

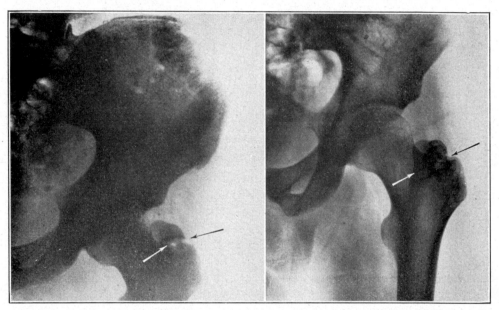

Fig. 874.—Fracture of the greater trochanter. Treated by immobilization in abduction and external rotation in a plaster-of-Paris cast, with good result.

Fractures of the Lesser Trochanter

Most of the cases of fractures of the lesser trochanter occur as complications of trochanteric fractures of the upper end of the femur in which there is more or less comminution of the fragments, and in these cases the lesser trochanter may be ignored, as its separation apparently does not affect the end-result. Occasionally, however, in adults the lesser trochanter is torn off by muscle action incident to hyperextension and abduction injuries at the hip, or in adolescents the apophysis of the trochanter may be separated (Fig. 875). The lesion is practically always the result of muscle violence and is due to unusual strain on the iliopsoas muscle which is attached to this prominence. The separated fragment usually involves the entire trochanter and tends to be drawn upward along the path of the iliopsoas tendon.

Diagnosis of Fractures of the Lesser Trochanter.—The diagnosis is made from the characteristic history of the injury followed by pain, tenderness, and swelling in the upper and inner aspects of the thigh and by weakness of the iliopsoas muscle, or pain when this muscle is passively stretched by hyperextending the hip. Ludloff's sign of fracture of the lesser trochanter: the patient in the sitting position is unable to flex the hip actively on the affected side because this motion is carried out by the iliopsoas muscle. The lesion is more frequent in adolescents than in adults. The diagnosis should be confirmed by the roentgenogram which should be taken in moderate external rotation; otherwise the lesser trochanter will be obscured by the shaft of the femur.

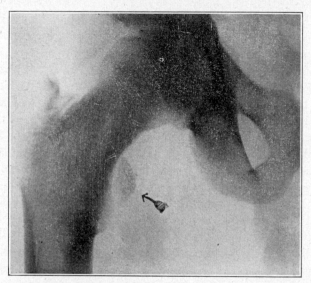

Fig. 875.—Avulsion of the lesser trochanter from muscular action. Treated by immobilization in flexion with good result. (Courtesy of Dr. A. H. Meyer.)

Treatment of Fractures of the Lesser Trochanter.—Since the avulsed fragment tends to be pulled upward by the iliopsoas muscle, the object of treatment is to bring the base on the inner and posterior surface of the shaft of the femur as close as possible to the displaced fragment. This can be accomplished by flexing the hip and rotating it slightly outward; consequently, a plaster spica extending from the middle of the leg to the middle of the abdomen should be applied with the hip in a position of slight external rotation and flexed 90 degrees. As soon as the cast is dry the patient is permitted to get up on crutches and may sleep in any position that affords comfort. The cast is worn for four or six weeks, and at the end of this time it can be discarded and the patient may begin to walk with a cane, or on crutches, if they are found to be necessary. No further treatment is indicated; a normal hip may be expected.

DISLOCATIONS AT THE HIP

Incidence.—Traumatic dislocations at the hip are quite rare and comprise only from 2 to 5 per cent of all dislocations, the exact percentage varying slightly in different series. This is in marked contrast to the shoulder where over 50 per cent of all dislocations occur. The hip and the shoulder are both ball and socket joints with a wide range of movement and subject to powerful leverage, but the hip is a much more stable joint. This stability is largely due to the comparatively great depth of the acetabulum and to the glenoid ligament which surrounds its margin and grasps the head of the femur slightly beyond its middle, thus making an air-tight socket into which the femoral head fits, and where it is held by suction. So strong is this suction that even with the ligaments and capsule severed considerable force is required to disarticulate the hip. Furthermore the ligaments of the hip are among the strongest in the body.

Due to the fact that great force is required to dislocate the hip, most of the cases occur in those who are subjected to great violence; namely, young adult males. In addition to the greater liability of young adult males to severe injury there are certain anatomical factors which render traumatic dislocation of the hip rare in early life and in the aged. In children a trauma which would tend to dislocate the hip results in a fracture of the shaft of the femur, in adolescents a similar injury causes epiphyseal separation, and in the aged it fractures the neck of the femur.*

Classification.—A line drawn from the anterior superior spine of the ilium to the tuberosity of the ischium (really the Roser-Nélaton line projected inward to the bone) bisects the acetabulum and divides the external surface of the pelvis into anterior and posterior portions. Due to the fact that this line represents the summit of a ridge from which the bony pelvis slopes forward or backward, as soon as the head of the femur is out of the acetabulum, it tends to slip forward or backward and comes to rest either in front of (below) or behind (above) the Roser-Nélaton line. Consequently dislocations at the hip may be divided into anterior and posterior dislocations.

Depending upon the final resting place of the head of the femur, the anterior dislocations are divided into high or pubic and low or obturator dislocations, while the posterior are divided into high or iliac and low or ischiadic dislocations.

The posterior dislocations are much more frequent and will be described first. Simultaneous dislocations are very rare, but may occur and one hip may be posterior and the other anterior. Compound dislocations at the hip are very rare and often fatal injuries.

Central, acetabular, or intrapelvic dislocations are those in which the head of the femur is driven inward through the floor of the acetabulum and comes to rest inside the pelvis. They will be described under "Fractures of the Acetabulum."

Posterior Dislocations at the Hip

Mechanism of Production.—In most dislocations of the hip the head of the femur is forced through the inferior relatively weak portion of the capsule, which lies between the anterior and posterior Y ligaments, and it is generally believed that the head is lifted out of its socket and pressed through the capsule by force applied to the femur in such a manner that it acts as the long arm of a lever while the anterior Y ligament or rim of the acetabulum acts as the fulcrum, and the head and neck of the femur act as the short arm.

*Key: South. M. J., 1924.

When the hip is in a position of adduction, flexion, and internal rotation, the Y ligament is tightened around the neck and if the internal rotation or adduction is forced, the head is lifted out of the acetabulum and presses upon the posterior and inferior portion of the capsule. If the force is continued, and especially if a backward thrust in line with the shaft is added, the head slips over the acetabular brim, ruptures the capsule, and moves back onto the dorsal surface of the pelvis, and a posterior dislocation is produced.

From the above it is evident that posterior dislocations may be produced by falls upon the feet or by crushing loads falling upon the patient's back or by any other force which approximates the knee and the pelvis and forces the flexed thigh into internal rotation and adduction. Predominance of direct thrust over leverage action tends to cause a fracture of the rim of the acetabulum.

With the hip flexed 90 degrees or more and in the neutral position or adducted or in any position as regards flexion, a strong backward thrust on the femur may snap the head out of the acetabulum or fracture its posterior rim and produce a posterior dislocation. Two ladies were riding in the back seat of an automobile which struck a tree. They were thrown forward, their knees striking the back of the front seat and each of them suffered a dislocation of one hip, and in one the posterior rim of the acetabulum was fractured.

Very rarely a posterior dislocation may result from forcible hyperabduction of the thigh. The tip of the great trochanter impinges on the border of the acetabulum and levers the head out of its socket and through the lower portion of the capsule. If the hip is internally rotated, the head slips backward and a posterior dislocation results. Likewise, internal rotation may convert an anterior into a posterior dislocation by causing the head to travel backward around the lower margin of the acetabulum.

Pathology.—As the head of the femur is nearly two inches in diameter it tears a large hole in the capsule when it is dislocated and causes considerable damage to the soft tissues in its path as it moves to its abnormal position. Consequently, traumatic dislocation at the hip is always a serious injury and may be accompanied by considerable shock.

The capsule is torn in its inferior and posterior portions and may be torn away from the acetabulum or femur, or a portion of the rim of the acetabulum may be avulsed or knocked off by the head. The ligamentum teres is usually torn at its attachment to the head, but may be ruptured or avulsed from the acetabulum. Bigelow has shown that in the classical types of posterior dislocation the Y ligament is always intact and that it is the tension on this ligament which maintains the femur in the position of flexion, adduction, and internal rotation. (Fig. 876.)

The short external rotator muscles are always damaged by the passage of the head and some of them may be ruptured, but the glutei are pushed out of the way and are not as a rule injured to any great extent. The head of the femur usually rests on the posterior surface of the ilium at about the level of a line joining the anterior superior spine with the upper border of the great sciatic notch. In the low or ischiadic dislocations the head rests upon the ischium posterior to and slightly below the acetabulum.

In the rare everted posterior dislocations the Y ligament is torn by the extreme violence, and gravity causes the extremity to roll outward so that the head is lifted away from the ilium and comes to rest in the tissues above the acetabulum and posterior to the anterior superior spine.

Diagnosis.—The characteristic point in the diagnosis of a posterior dislocation of the hip is that the hip is fixed in an abnormal position of flexion, adduction, and internal rotation.

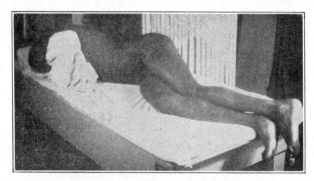

Fig. 876.—Characteristic deformity in a patient with a posterior dislocation at the left hip with the patient lying on his side.

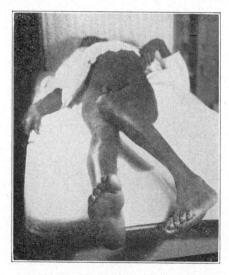

Fig. 877.—View with patient lying on his back.

There is usually a history of a severe injury followed by intense pain in the hip and the patient is unable to bear weight upon, or even to move, the affected thigh, but prefers to lie on the back with the knee of the affected side resting upon the opposite thigh.

On inspection the lower extremity on the affected side appears to be considerably shortened, but the shortening is largely the result of the flexion and adduction and is more apparent than real. The apparent shortening is usually from two to three inches, but the real shortening is rarely more than one inch. The trochanter on the affected side is unusually prominent and the gluteal fold is elevated and less pronounced than on the sound side. Due to the presence of the head of the femur and to the approximation of insertions to the origins of the gluteal muscles, the buttock on the affected side is unusually prominent.

Accurate measurement of the lengths of the lower extremities is impossible because the fixation of the dislocated hip in adduction and flexion makes it impossible for the surgeon to place the two extremities in the same relative position; consequently, the tape measure is not of much use in the diagnosis. Rough measurement, however, will usually disclose an actual shortening of about an inch, and what is of more importance, the tip of the trochanter will be found to lie above the Roser-Nélaton line (anterior superior spine to tuberosity of the ischium).

On palpation it will be found that the trochanter on the affected side is elevated and in thin subjects it may be possible to palpate the head of the femur in its abnormal position beneath the glutei, but in fat or muscular subjects this cannot be done with any degree of accuracy. On palpation over the front of the joint it is not possible to detect the empty socket because the iliopsoas and capsule are stretched over it, but the fingers do sink in deeper than on the sound side, and there is no feeling of increased resistance and fullness in Scarpa's triangle such as one finds in fractures of the neck of the femur.

Active motion is usually impossible and passive motion is painful, but it is usually possible to move the hip in flexion, adduction, and internal rotation, while extension, abduction, and external rotation are limited. The limitation of passive movement is somewhat elastic and suggests ligamentous and muscle tension rather than bony block. If flexion is also limited it is probable that the head has passed above one or more of the short external rotator muscles.

Most posterior dislocations at the hip are of the high or iliac type and the low or ischiadic type is rare. The diagnosis as given above applies to either type. The differential diagnosis is made by the degree of the deformity. In the low or ischiadic dislocations the flexion and adduction are greater. According to De Quervain ''an iliac dislocation exists if the patient, on lying down, is able to conceal the flexion by a compensatory lordosis of the lumbar spine, and bring his two legs into an approximately parallel position, and if on standing up he is able to touch the ground with his toes. On the other hand, a sciatic dislocation is present if the most extreme lumbar lordosis is unable to abolish the flexion, if the patient on lying down, places the thigh of the dislocated side on the healthy thigh, and if he is unable to touch the ground with his toes on standing up.''

Diagnosis of Everted Posterior Dislocation.—In this rare condition the clinical picture resembles that of a fracture of the neck of the femur as the thigh is rotated outward and the flexion and adduction deformity so characteristic of the usual posterior dislocation is absent. As the Y ligament is torn, the hip is quite freely movable and the shortening may reach two inches or more. The everted posterior dislocation can be differentiated from a fracture of the neck of the femur by the facts that in the dislocation there is decreased resistance instead of swelling in Scarpa's triangle and the head of the femur can be palpated above the acetabulum and posterior to the anterior superior spine and can be felt to move with the shaft when this is manipulated. An x-ray should be made when possible to rule out a possible fracture.

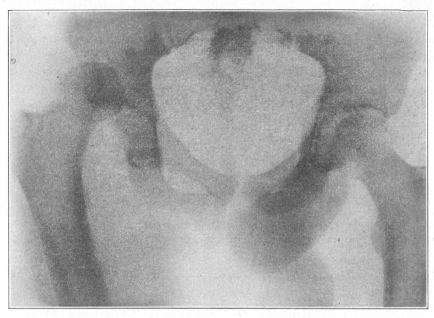

Fig. 878.—Traumatic posterior dislocation at the hip. Treated by manipulative reduction and bandaging knees together for two weeks. Walking in five weeks. Good result.

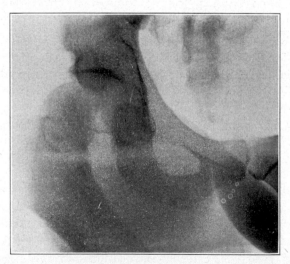

Fig. 879.—Traumatic dislocation at the hip and marked adduction showing very little upward displacement. Treated by manipulative reduction. Knees bandaged together for twelve days. Walking in five weeks. Good result.

Treatment.—(Figs. 878, 879, and 880.) The treatment is reduction. This should be done as soon as possible because delay renders the reduction more difficult. There are three methods in general use—Allis, Bigelow, and Stimson. All utilize the fact first emphasized by Bigelow in 1869 that in order to replace the posteriorly dislocated head of the femur in the acetabulum, the Y ligament, which is the chief obstacle to reduction, must be relaxed by increasing the deformity of flexion. The position of flexion also brings the head down to the posterior inferior border of the acetabulum near the rent in the capsule.

The methods of Allis and Bigelow are manipulative methods and should not be attempted without thorough relaxation by general or spinal anesthesia. The method of Stimson utilizes the weight of the extremity, and the reduction is aided by gravity; consequently, it is often successful with no more anesthetic than that obtained by a heavy dose of morphine.

In the ordinary case of posterior dislocation the method of choice is that of Allis because it causes less trauma and is less dangerous than that of Bigelow. When the Allis method fails to accomplish reduction Bigelow's method should be tried. Stimson's method is the gentlest of all, though slower and less spectacular than the others, as frequently the reduction is very gradual and the surgeon is robbed of the satisfaction of feeling and hearing the head of the femur "pop" back into its socket, by this sign knowing when reduction has been accomplished. It is the method of choice in feeble patients and where general anesthetic is contraindicated, and should be used more frequently as a routine procedure.

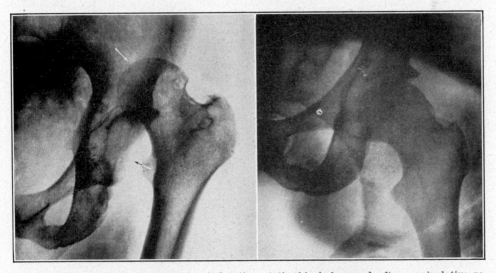

Fig. 880.—Typical traumatic posterior dislocation at the hip before and after manipulative reduction. Immobilized in a plaster-of-Paris cast with good result.

Allis Method of Reducing Posterior Dislocation of the Hip.—(Fig. 882.) In this method the head of the femur is lifted back into place by direct traction on the flexed thigh. It is performed as follows: The fully anesthetized patient is placed on the floor on his back and the pelvis is immobilized by strapping it to the floor or by having an assistant press downward on the anterior superior spines, or by the surgeon's stockinged foot on the anterior superior spine on the affected side. The surgeon then grasps the affected extremity and gently flexes the hip and the knee to about a right angle, maintaining the slight adduction and internal rotation. The flexed lower extremity

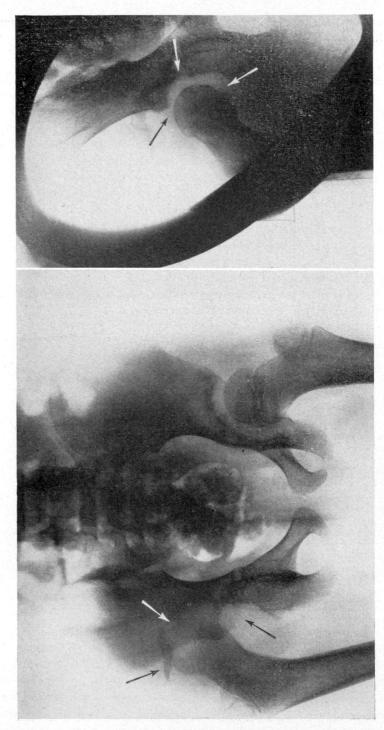

Fig. 881.—Fracture dislocation of a hip in a child with a fracture of the posterior rim of the acetabulum. Closed reduction carried out with anatomical results. The fragment of the posterior rim of the acetabulum was reduced. Good functional result following adhesive traction to the thigh and leg for eight weeks and a plaster spica cast to the hip for six weeks. Good results in six months.

is then lifted directly upward thus drawing the head up onto and over the rim of the acetabulum and through the rent in the capsule and permitting it to slip back into place. The thigh should then be gently lowered to the floor, not forcibly extended.

As a rule relatively little force will be necessary. If undue resistance is encountered in lifting the thigh the adduction and internal rotation should be increased to relax the capsule and disengage the head from the pelvis. If resistance is still encountered the thigh should be adducted and rotated slightly outward and then lifted as the head may be entangled with the sciatic nerve or some of the small rotator muscles. By adduction and gentle rotation the head can usually be freed and the reduction accomplished.

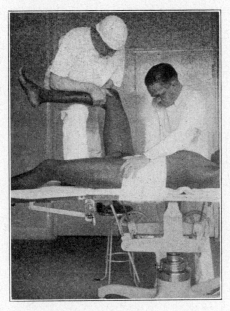

Fig. 882.—Photograph posed to show the Allis method of reduction in posterior dislocations of the hip.

The head may slip into the acetabulum as the thigh is lifted or as it is lowered to the position of extension. In some instances slight external rotation at the moment of extension will effect the reduction, or direct pressure on the head of the femur by an assistant may aid in forcing it over the rim of the acetabulum.

In high posterior dislocations the rent in the capsule is apt to be higher and consequently the thigh should be flexed only about 60 degrees in order to bring the head opposite the rent, when traction is applied in the line of the femur.

Bigelow's Circumduction Method for the Reduction of Posterior Dislocation at the Hip.—(Fig. 883.) This method relaxes the Y ligament by flexion of the hip and then uses it as a fulcrum to lever the head into the acetabulum. There are certain objections to the method because by the use of undue force the surgeon may rupture the Y ligament or damage the sciatic nerve or other soft tissues posterior to the hip. It is performed as follows: The fully anesthetized patient is placed on his back on the floor and the pelvis is immobilized by an assistant who presses downward on the anterior superior spines. The surgeon then grasps the affected extremity and flexes the adducted and internally rotated thigh on the abdomen. With the thigh in this position, traction is made on the thigh to lift the head to the rim of the acetabulum, and while the traction is maintained, the movement of circumduction is performed. In this maneuver the flexed thigh is swept outward and then downward into extension. As it is abducted, it is also externally rotated, and the head is levered over the acetabular rim. Traction must be maintained until the head slips into the acetabulum, and external rotation must not be performed on the adducted thigh, but is a part of the movement of circumduction (abduction and extension). Forcible abduction is to be avoided.

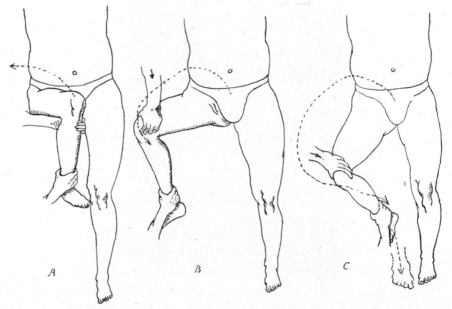

Fig. 883.—Drawings to show the Bigelow method of reducing posterior dislocation at the hip. *A, B,* and *C* are sketched from *Imperative Traumatic Surgery* by Forrester. (Paul B. Hoeber, Inc., Publisher.)

(*A*) The thigh is flexed at the hip, then with moderate traction it is slightly adducted.

(*B*) While the traction is continued, the maneuver of circumduction outward is carried out.

(*C*) The thigh is then extended.

Stimson's Gravity Method for the Reduction of Posterior Dislocation at the Hip.—(Fig. 884.) In this method the weight of the extremity is used to aid in the reduction. In other respects the mechanics of the method are practically the same as those of the Allis method. Stimson* wrote: "The patient is placed face downward on a table with his legs projecting so far beyond the edge that the injured thigh hangs directly downward while the surgeon grasps the ankle, the knee being flexed at a right angle. The other limb is held horizontal by an assistant. The weight of the limb now makes the needed traction in the desired direction, and the surgeon has only to wait for

*Stimson: Fractures and Dislocations, Philadelphia, 1910, Lea & Febiger.

the muscles to relax and the bone to resume its place without further effort on his part other than a slight rocking or rotation of the limb. Occasionally I have added the weight of a small sandbag at the knee or have added sudden slight pressure at the same point. It will often succeed without anesthesia and sometimes so quietly that there is no jar or sound indicating the return to place. In only two cases has it failed in my hands. Both were then reduced by traction in the axis of the partly flexed limb. I presume that in both the bone had left the socket at its upper posterior segment—'iliac' dislocation.'' The reason this method is not used more often is that most of us like to manipulate.

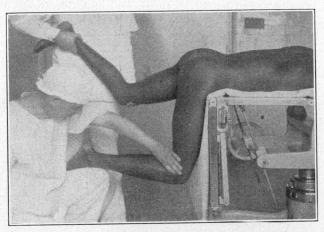

Fig. 884.—Photograph posed to show Stimson's method of reduction for posterior dislocation at the hip.

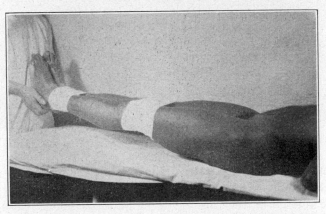

Fig. 885.—Method of bandaging the legs together in order to guard against recurrence after the reduction of a dislocation at the hip.

Aftertreatment of Posterior Dislocation at the Hip.—(Fig. 885.) In the uncomplicated case there is little tendency to recurrence after reduction and all that is necessary is to keep the patient recumbent and prevent adduction and flexion at the hip, since this position favors recurrence. For this reason the patient should be kept in bed with the knees moderately abducted and immobilized between sandbags. No traction is necessary. Some surgeons prefer to tie the knees together; this is a satisfactory method though less comfortable and secure than the abduction. It is to be noted, however, that this simple form of after treatment applies only to uncomplicated dislocations. If there is a fracture of the posterior rim of the acetabulum the hip should be immobilized by traction or a large plaster spica in a position of abduction and slight external rotation for eight weeks, if the position of the fragment is satisfactory after reduction. If it is not satisfactory, it should be exposed through a posterior incision and fixed with one or more nails or screws.

The immobilization is continued two weeks; then the patient should remain in bed another week without immobilization. At the end of the third week he is got up on crutches and permitted to bear some weight on the leg. The crutches are discarded as the strength and stability in the hip return.

The prognosis is good and a normal hip may be expected in about two months. Rarely aseptic necrosis of the head or in older patients a mild form of traumatic arthritis may develop, but these are rare in cases which have been reduced soon after the injury.

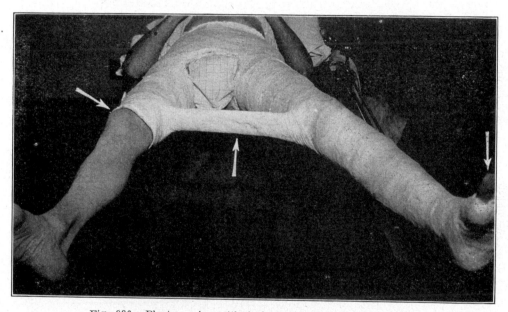

Fig. 886.—Plaster spica with inclusion of the opposite thigh.

Treatment of Everted Posterior Dislocations.—These are as a rule easily reduced by the direct traction (Allis) method, but because of the extensive tearing of the soft parts, they are apt to be quite unstable. Consequently the hip should be immobilized in a plaster spica in a position of abduction and slight internal rotation for four weeks to permit healing of the capsule. Then the cast should be removed and the patient should begin to move the hip daily, but should remain in bed two weeks longer, and then get up on crutches. Some permanent stiffness and weakness in the hip may result.

Anterior Dislocations at the Hip

Mechanism of Production.—The most important factor in the production of anterior dislocations is forcible abduction. In this movement the neck or trochanter impinges upon the rim of the acetabulum and the head of the femur is levered out of its socket and through the anterior capsule. In addition to the abduction forcible external rotation also tends to force the head forward through the capsule. If the abduction acts with the hip in a position of flexion, the head of the femur tends to move downward to the obturator foramen and if it acts with the hip extended the head tends to move upward to the pubic region.

These abduction injuries may result from falls on the feet or knees or crushing injuries received on the back or pelvis with the hip in a position of abduction. They are considerably less frequent than are the injuries which produce posterior dislocations.

Pathology of Anterior Dislocations at the Hip.—The capsule of the joint is ruptured in its anterior portion and usually in the lower anterior portion and near the rim of the acetabulum. After the head escapes, it may move downward or upward and usually comes to rest in the obturator foramen or on the body of the pubic bone. The Y ligament nearly always remains intact, and it is largely the tension on this ligament which maintains the thigh in the characteristic position of abduction and external rotation. These muscles which lie in the path of the head are stretched or torn and the adductors and obturator externus are especially liable to injury. When the head is widely displaced the ligaments and capsule are extensively torn and the hip is quite unstable.

In the low anterior dislocations the head usually rests in the obturator foramen. Variations of this classical obturator type are the perineal in which the Y ligament is partly torn and the head is pushed unusually far inward and projects in the perineum, and the infracotyloid in which the head moves to a position just below the acetabulum and rests on the body of the ischium.

In the high anterior dislocations the head usually rests on the body of the pubis. Variations of the pubic type are the suprapubic or intrapelvic in which the head has passed under or through Poupart's ligament and come to rest in the pelvis, the iliopectineal in which the head rests upon the horizontal ramus of the pubis near the ilium, and the supraglenoid or subspinous in which the head rests upon the ilium below the anterior superior spine and above the acetabulum.

Diagnosis.—In the typical anterior dislocations at the hip the thigh is maintained in a position of abduction and external rotation and may be in slight flexion or extension, and the head of the femur can be palpated and is often visible in its abnormal position. The lateral surface of the hip is flattened and the trochanter is displaced inward.

In the low anterior or obturator dislocations the abduction is marked and the limb appears to be lengthened and is maintained in slight flexion and external rotation. The apparent lengthening is due to the abduction and there is really about one inch actual lengthening of the limb. Palpation of the head is apt to be unsatisfactory because it is usually buried deep in the tissues. On manipulation the thigh can be moved in flexion, abduction, and external rotation, but adduction is sharply limited to a variable degree.

In the high anterior or pubic dislocations there may be little or no abduction, but the external rotation is marked, the hip is usually in a position of full extension, and the limb is slightly shortened. The displaced head is usually visible and easily palpable and the hip can be manipulated into external rotation and abduction, but internal rotation and adduction are sharply limited.

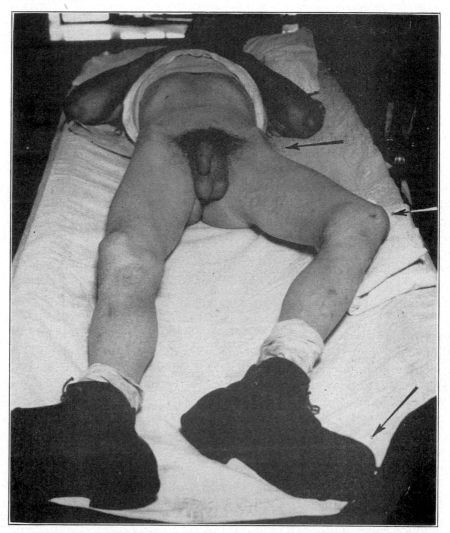

Fig. 887.—Characteristic deformity with anterior dislocation of left hip.

The variations from the classical types can usually be diagnosed by palpating the head of the femur in its abnormal position.

Treatment.—1. Low or Obturator Dislocations: Reduction is best accomplished by the method of Allis which releases the head and then pulls it back along the path which it traversed during the dislocation (Fig. 888 A and B). It is performed as follows: With the knee flexed to relax the hamstrings, the abduction is increased to about 90 degrees and the external rotation and flexion are slightly increased to lift the head of the femur away from the pelvis. Direct traction is made in the line of the femur to pull the head out to a point opposite the rent in the capsule. When this has been accomplished the thigh is gently rotated inward and adducted without relaxing the traction. This last maneuver slips the head over the rim of the acetabulum and into its socket. It may be aided by an assistant who presses upon the head of the femur and attempts to guide it into the acetabulum or who makes traction upward and outward by means of his hands or a sheet or towel around the upper thigh.

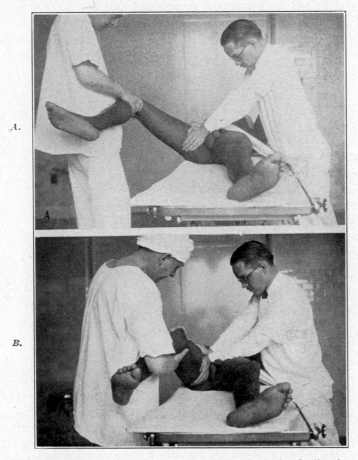

Fig. 888.—*A*, Photograph posed to show the Allis method of reduction in anterior dislocations at the hip. Traction and abduction of the thigh while an assistant makes pressure outward over the inner surface and upper third of thigh and groin.
B. Showing adduction and internal rotation.

In the perineal type the maneuver is the same except that the head must be drawn farther by outward traction. In the rare everted thyroid type with the trochanter resting in the acetabulum the hip should first be rotated inward to relax the capsule and cause the head to sink down near the acetabulum.

2. **High or Pubic Dislocations.**—These, too, are most safely reduced by releasing the head and pulling it back along the course which it passed during

the dislocation. Allis' method is to abduct and flex the thigh moderately and make traction in the line of the femur to draw the head down opposite the rent in the capsule, and then without relaxing the traction to internally rotate and adduct the hip. The head is slipped over the acetabular rim and into its socket during the last maneuver. During the reduction an assistant makes pressure on the head of the femur and attempts to push it back into place.

If the above maneuver fails, the internal circumduction method of Bigelow may be tried (Fig. 889), but it is rather dangerous and may result in a posterior dislocation. It is performed as follows: With the knee flexed, the thigh is abducted with traction downward and is then swung inward in flexion and adduction and internally rotated and then extended. The head should slip into its socket during the internal rotation and extension.

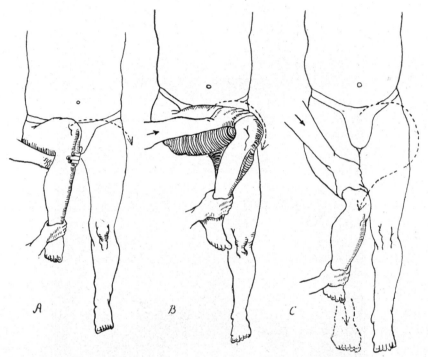

Fig. 889.—Drawings to illustrate the Bigelow method of reduction of anterior dislocations at the hip by circumduction. *A, B*, and *C* all were sketched from *Imperative Traumatic Surgery* by Forrester. (Paul B. Hoeber, Inc., Publisher.)

(*A*) With moderate traction upward the thigh is flexed and slightly abducted.

(*B*) While the traction is continued, the thigh is circumducted inward.

(*C*) The thigh is then extended.

If the head moves around the lower border of the acetabulum into a posterior position this can be reduced as described under "Posterior Dislocations at the Hip." The tendency to posterior displacement is lessened if traction is maintained while the hip is being internally rotated and extended.

Suprapubic or intrapelvic dislocations are first pulled down into the pubic position and then reduced as described above. The subspinous and iliopectineal types can often be reduced by direct traction combined with pressure on the head. If this fails, they are treated as are the pubic dislocations.

Treatment After Reduction of Anterior Dislocation.—Here, too, as in posterior dislocation there is little tendency for the hip to slip out once reduction has been accomplished, and all that is necessary is to keep the patient in bed about three weeks. As the dislocation occurred in abduction, it is advisable to tie the knees together and prevent abduction while the patient is in bed. At the end of three weeks the patient can be got up on crutches and a normal hip may be expected in about three months.

COMPLICATIONS OF DISLOCATION AT THE HIP

Fractures.—The most frequent complication is a fracture, usually of the rim of the acetabulum, but occasionally of the head of the femur. These fractures cannot as a rule be diagnosed except by the x-ray, and it is for this reason that an x-ray should, when possible, be made before reduction is attempted. The occurrence of bony crepitus during reduction suggests a fracture of the acetabular rim or femoral head and a tendency for the hip to dislocate after reduction suggests a fracture of the rim of the acetabulum.

When a fracture, either of the head or of the rim of the acetabulum is present, the dislocation should be reduced in the ordinary way and the thigh should be maintained in a position of abduction and the neutral position as regards rotation. An x-ray picture should be taken to determine the position of the fragment. If the fragment is in good position, a plaster cast should be applied and the hip maintained in abduction and the neutral position as regards rotation for from four to six weeks. (Fig. 895.)

If the fragment is not in good position an open operation is indicated and the surgeon should remove loose fragments of the head or remove small fragments of the rim of the acetabulum which lie in the joint. If these latter are large enough, they can be replaced and fixed by stainless steel or vitallium nails or screws.

After the operation, the hip should be immobilized in a plaster cast for from six to eight weeks. When the cast is removed, the patient should remain in bed about two weeks and then get up on crutches and gradually resume weight-bearing. The prognosis is, of course, not so good as in uncomplicated dislocations, but usually a good hip can be obtained.

Very rarely the neck or shaft of the femur is broken when the hip is dislocated. In these cases attention is apt to be centered on the fracture, and the dislocation may be missed. Attention is directed to the dislocation by the abnormal position of the upper fragment or by palpating the head in an abnormal position, or by the x-ray.

The treatment is reduction of the dislocation and then treatment of the fracture. The Allis or Stimson method of reduction should be used, and direct pressure on the head should play a prominent part in the reduction. If closed reduction fails, an open reduction is indicated.

Nerve Injuries.—The sciatic nerve may be contused by the head of the femur in posterior dislocations, or the head may slip under the nerve, and it

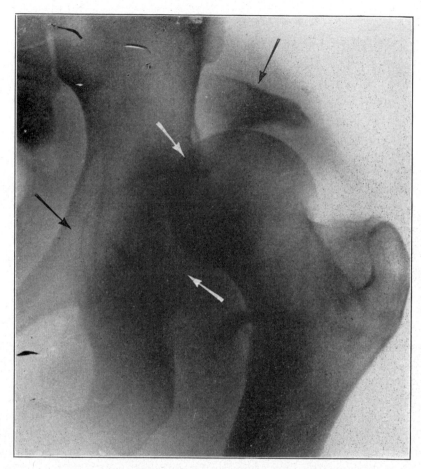

Fig. 890.—Posterior dislocation of the hip with a fracture of the posterior rim of the acetabulum. Treatment attempted by closed reduction, but posterior fragment of rim of acetabulum could not be reduced. Open reduction was carried out, fixation of femur with traction to lower end of femur for eight weeks, after which traction was removed and a plaster spica of the hip was applied for six weeks. Good result in four months.

may then be stretched over the femoral neck. These nerve injuries are rare and can be diagnosed by the pain, numbness, and paralysis in the sciatic distribution. In most of the reported cases the symptoms tend to clear up spontaneously after the reduction, but they may persist for several months.

Very rarely the sciatic may be picked up by the head of the femur in attempts to reduce a posterior dislocation by the circumduction method of Bigelow. When this occurs and the hip is reduced, the nerve is stretched over the front of the neck of the femur. The accident may be recognized by the fact that the taut nerve holds the thigh and leg slightly flexed, and attempts to extend the hip or straighten the knee are resisted by an elastic tension; when such attempts are made, the tense nerve can be palpated in the popliteal space.

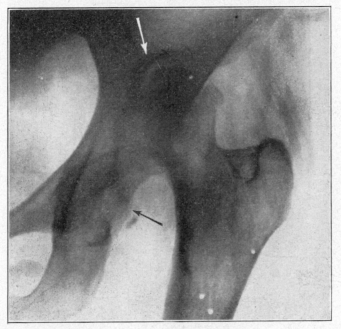

Fig. 891.—Fracture dislocation of the hip with a fracture through the posterior rim of the acetabulum, six months' duration. This case was supposedly reduced, but no traction or any follow-up was carried out, with the result as shown. Such type of case demands continuous traction following reduction and in many cases demands an open operation with a replacement and fixation of the fractured rim of the acetabulum.

The remedy is immediate redislocation and disentanglement of the nerve. Redislocation is accomplished by flexion, adduction, and internal rotation; a backward thrust may be necessary. The knee is then extended to tighten the nerve and the hip is strongly adducted to move the head out across the nerve and is then gently internally rotated and flexed and reduced by the Allis or Stimson method. If this is unsuccessful, it will be necessary to cut down on the nerve and pull it out of the way. The injury to the nerve may result in permanent paralysis.

Muscles and Vessels.—Muscle ruptures and tears occur in all hip luxations, but are rarely of any consequence and demand no special treatment.

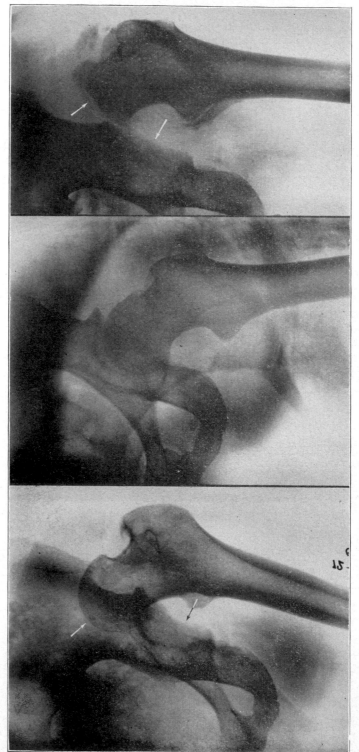

Fig. 892.—Dislocation of the hip followed by complete necrosis of the head of the femur, six months following. Treatment was carried out there-after by applying a vitallium cup with fairly good functional result.

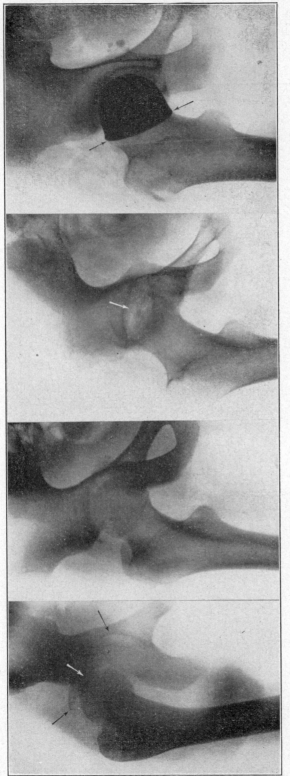

Fig. 893.—Fracture dislocation of the hip which was properly reduced, with necrosis of the head and femur six months later. Treated by application of Smith-Petersen vitallium femoral head cup. Fairly good result.

Very rarely in anterior luxations the femoral vessels may be ruptured and this demands immediate operation and ligation. Occasionally the obturator or femoral nerves are contused, but these nerve injuries usually clear up spontaneously.

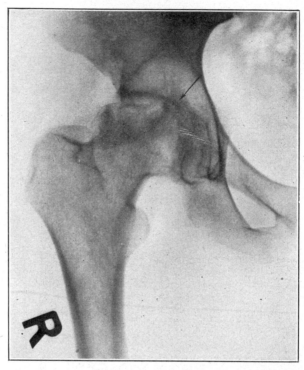

Fig. 894.—Aseptic necrosis of the head of the femur following traumatic dislocation. Hip was immobilized in traction for twelve weeks after manipulative reduction. Condition two years after the injury.

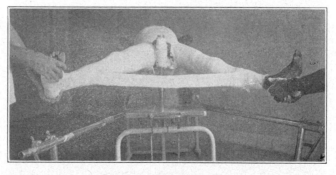

Fig. 895.—Photograph of a patient immobilized in a bilateral plaster-of-Paris spica of the hips. Used when treating certain cases after reduction of fracture dislocation at the hip when traction is not indicated.

Aseptic Necrosis of the Head of the Femur.—A late and very disabling complication of a dislocation of the hip is an aseptic necrosis of the head of the femur. This is due to interference with the blood supply to the head and results in a deformed head and chronic arthritis of the hip. An arthroplasty with Smith-Petersen's vitallium cup probably offers the best chance for a useful joint.

OLD DISLOCATIONS AT THE HIP

Other things being equal the difficulties encountered in the reduction of a traumatic dislocation vary directly with the length of time which has elapsed since the dislocation occurred. This is especially true of the hip, where the bones are large and the surrounding structures are very strong. A hip which has been out of place a week or ten days may be quite difficult to reduce, but up to six weeks after the original injury, reduction by manipulation may be expected to succeed.

In cases in which the dislocation has been present more than six weeks and in old cases of shorter duration, an effort should be made to pull the femur down with heavy traction before the reduction is attempted. The traction should be applied to the femur by means of a wire or a pin through the bone, and 80 pounds or more may be used. As a rule one or two weeks of such traction is all that is necessary to pull the head of the femur down to a position opposite the acetabulum.

In hips which have been dislocated six months or more, the traction should be followed by an open reduction. This is a difficult and hazardous operation and should be undertaken only by an experienced surgeon.

PATHOLOGIC DISLOCATIONS AT THE HIP

Pathologic dislocations at the hip are almost always posterior in type and are usually the result of one of three causes: (1) Infantile paralysis; (2) acute synovitis; and (3) chronic arthritis with destruction of the head or acetabulum. In infantile paralysis with strong adductors and flexors and weak abductors and extensors the hip may be dislocated and be thrown in or out at will. Here operative fixation is necessary.

The acute synovitis cases usually occur in the course of some severe infectious disease such as scarlet fever, typhoid fever, etc. With the capsule dis-

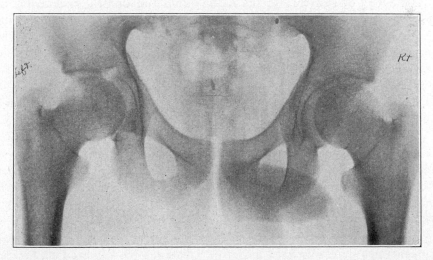

Fig. 896.—Bilateral fracture of the floor of the acetabulum. There was practically no displacement on the right, but slight displacement on the left. Treated by immobilization in double plaster-of-Paris spica for five weeks. Then adhesive traction for two weeks. Walking in ten weeks. Good result.

tended, the patient tends to maintain the thigh in a position of adduction, flexion, and internal rotation and the head slips out over the inferior portion of the posterior rim of the acetabulum. If seen early, these dislocations are easily reduced by traction and external rotation of the flexed thigh. They should be prevented by avoiding the position of flexion, adduction, and internal rotation, and as soon as symptoms develop in the hip, it should be immobilized by traction in a position of slight abduction.

The destructive cases are usually the result of tuberculosis or pyogenic arthritis, and are best treated by arthrodesis.

FRACTURE OF THE ACETABULUM AND CENTRAL DISLOCATION AT THE HIP

Fractures of the acetabulum are really fractures of the pelvis and are so classified in some textbooks, but we are including them among the hip injuries because the symptoms are chiefly those of a hip injury and the resultant disability affects the hip.

Incidence and Causation.—Fracture of the acetabulum was formerly considered a rare injury, but with increasing use of the x-rays the lesion is being diagnosed more frequently. This is especially true of the rather mild cases which are not accompanied by inward or central dislocation of the head of the femur.

The usual cause of the lesion is force applied to the great trochanter, thus driving the head of the femur inward against the floor of the acetabulum. It may result from a fall or blow on the trochanter or from a lateral crushing injury. In rare instances the acetabulum may be fractured indirectly by a fall upon the feet. Most of the cases occur in young or middle-aged adults as in old people and children the neck of the femur is the point of least resistance.

Pathology of Fracture of the Acetabulum and Central Dislocation at the Hip.—The fracture may involve either the rim or the floor of the acetabulum or both. Most of the fractures of the rim occur as complications of dislocations at the hip and have been mentioned as complications of those lesions. Occasionally, however, the rim may be broken and no dislocation follow. These rare fractures usually involve the upper and posterior part of the rim and one or more fragments of variable size may be broken off and slightly displaced.

In the fractures of the floor of the acetabulum the head of the femur may or may not be displaced inward, depending upon the severity of the fracturing force and the strength of the bones (Figs. 896, 897, and 898). In the simplest cases there are one or more fracture lines traversing the floor of the acetabulum and the fragments may or may not be appreciably displaced. The fracture lines may extend into the surrounding bone.

In the more severe cases the floor of the acetabulum is shattered and the fragments are driven inward a variable distance by the head of the femur; in extreme cases the entire head may project into the pelvis and the fragments of the floor of the acetabulum may be displaced inward or folded back around the neck of the femur and hinder reduction. In rare instances the fracture line follows or lies just outside of the rim of the acetabulum and the acetabulum is separated from the rest of the os innominatum (punched out en masse) and displaced inward.

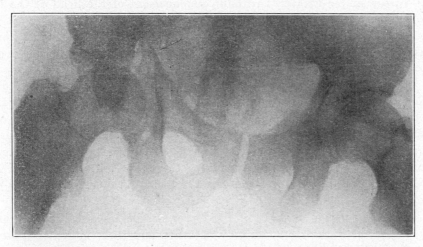

Fig. 897.—Fracture of the acetabulum with moderate inward displacement. Treated by closed reduction and immobilization in a bilateral plaster-of-Paris spica of the hips for eight weeks, adhesive traction for three weeks. Walking in five months. Good result.

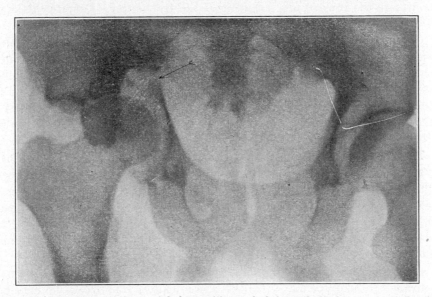

Fig. 898.—Fracture of the acetabulum with marked inward displacement of the femur. Treated by manipulative reduction and immobilization in a bilateral plaster-of-Paris spica of hips with adhesive to the leg and thigh for traction for five months. Adhesive traction three weeks. Walking in fourteen weeks. Fair result.

The pelvic fascia and iliopsoas muscle cover the inner surface of the pelvis opposite the floor of the acetabulum, and as the fracture occurs beneath these structures visceral and blood vessel injuries are rare complications, but both have been reported. In about 50 per cent of the reported cases of fracture of the acetabulum with central dislocation of the femur there were other fractures of the pelvis. Consequently these should always be looked for and the complications mentioned under fractures of the pelvis (especially bladder, urethra, and nerve) should be excluded before the diagnosis is complete.

Diagnosis of Fracture of the Acetabulum and Central Dislocation at the Hip.—In the simple fractures without displacement of the head of the femur the diagnosis is difficult and must be made or at least confirmed by the x-ray because there is no disturbance of any of the bony landmarks of the hip (Figs. 896, 898, and 899). The character of the injury with the presence of pain and disability in the hip and the absence of the signs of a fracture of the neck of the femur or of the pelvis suggest a fracture of the rim or floor of the acetabulum. The movements of the hip are free, but painful, and the patient may be able to walk on the limb. As in a fracture of the neck of the femur, there is usually some fullness and tenderness in Scarpa's triangle and pain is always elicited by pressure on the trochanter. The most important diagnostic point in fractures of the floor of the acetabulum is the palpation of a tender swelling opposite the floor of the acetabulum on rectal examination.

In cases in which the head of the femur has been driven into the pelvis, the trochanteric region is moderately flattened and there is actual shortening of the limb of from one-half to one and one-half inches. Careful measurement of the distance between the trochanter and the symphysis of the pubis will demonstrate the inward displacement of the trochanter. Despite the shortening, the tip of the trochanter will not be found to be above Nélaton's line.

On palpation the displacement of the trochanter will be perceptible, the tensor fascia lata will be relaxed, and there will be swelling and tenderness in Scarpa's triangle. Manipulation of the hip will usually elicit immediate crepitus and pain and the hip may be quite freely movable or locked in slight adduction or abduction and external or internal rotation. The displaced head of the femur can be palpated by rectal examination. The details of the lesion are best obtained from the x-ray before treatment is instituted.

Treatment of Fracture of the Rim of the Acetabulum Without Dislocation at the Hip.—In these cases there is as a rule relatively little displacement of the fragment and all that is necessary is to prevent weight-bearing until union is firm (about eight weeks). During the first three weeks the patient should be kept in bed and traction should be applied to the leg (about 10 pounds). The limb should not, as a rule, be abducted, since this tends to cause displacement of the fragment.

At the end of three weeks the traction should be removed and the patient encouraged to begin to move the hip; at the end of four weeks he may be got up on crutches or in a walking caliper splint. Weight-bearing without support should be begun gradually after eight or ten weeks.

If the fragment is large and so displaced that the fracture will result in a serious deformity of the acetabulum, a skillful surgeon should attempt open anatomical reduction and fix it in place with small bone or ivory pegs or screws.

Treatment of Fractures of the Floor of the Acetabulum Without Central Dislocation of the Hip.—These fractures, while apparently simple and requir-

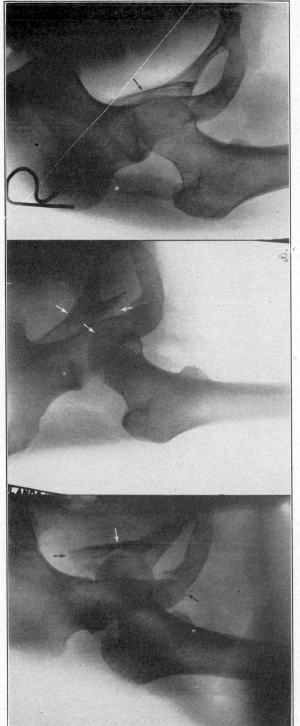

Fig. 899.—Fracture of the floor of the acetabulum with central dislocation at the hip. Treated by manipulative reduction, under general anesthesia and immobilized by traction for nine weeks, beginning weight-bearing in four months. Good result.

ing no treatment other than rest in bed, may be the cause of considerable disability on account of the development of traumatic arthritis. We believe, consequently, that they should be treated with a certain amount of respect.

No reduction is necessary, and we particularly wish to warn surgeons against the temptation to place the finger in the rectum and by direct pressure force the floor of the acetabulum outward in those cases where it has been forced inward to a variable degree. This apparently simple procedure is liable to result in perforation of the rectum with subsequent infection.

Routinely we treat these cases by traction in recumbency for four weeks.

The patient is placed on a fracture bed with a fracture frame having a strong central horizontal bar. A canvas pelvic sling is placed under the patient and this is suspended by a weight equal to about one-fourth the body weight of the patient. It is important that a spreader slightly wider than the pelvis be placed in the sling in order that lateral pressure on the trochanter be prevented, as this would tend to jam the head of the femur against the fractured area. Adhesive traction strips are placed on both legs, and about 10 pounds of weight are placed on the affected leg and 5 pounds on the sound leg. Finally, with the legs in a position of slight abduction, a large pillow is placed crosswise under the knees. J. A. K. does not use the sling.

The traction is continued for from four to six weeks depending upon the severity of the fracture. At the end of this time the traction and pelvic suspension sling are removed and the patient is given hip flexion and abduction exercises in bed. At the end of one or two weeks, the patient is got up on crutches and weight-bearing is permitted as tolerated. Normal function is to be expected in from three to four months.

These fractures may be treated by immobilization in wide abduction in a plaster-of-Paris hip spica with or without traction to the leg over a period of from four to eight weeks with good results. In order to prevent pressure of the head of the femur on the fractured floor of the acetabulum, adhesive traction is applied under the plaster.

Treatment of Fracture of the Acetabulum With Central Dislocation at the Hip.—In this lesion the head of the femur must be pulled out of the pelvis and held out by traction or wide abduction until the acetabular floor has reformed and weight-bearing can be resumed. From the x-ray and the physical examination the surgeon can usually determine whether or not a manipulative reduction will be necessary. If the head of the femur is displaced inward to such a degree that its widest part lies internal to the normal line of the floor of the acetabulum, manipulative reduction will be necessary. If the inward displacement is less, no manipulative reduction is indicated and the fracture should be treated by traction just as described above except that the foot of the bed should be raised and the traction on the affected leg should be 25 pounds at first and to this should be added lateral traction on the upper thigh of about 10 or 15 pounds so that the resultant parallelogram of forces will be traction in the line of the neck of the femur for eight weeks. At the end of forty-eight hours the longitudinal traction may be decreased to 15 pounds and the lateral traction to 8 pounds, and in about a week more these may be decreased to 10 and 5 pounds, respectively. The traction should be continued for eight weeks and then removed, when the patient is encouraged to exercise his legs and move his hips in bed for two weeks longer. Then he should be got up on crutches, which may be discarded as weight-bearing becomes painless.

Application of the Lateral Traction.—In order to apply lateral traction to the upper thigh a strip of adhesive tape six inches wide and about twenty inches long, depending upon the size of the thigh, is applied to the outer surface of the shaved thigh and carried over the front of the thigh and down between the thighs and then out over the side of the bed. The inner surface of the thigh is protected by a strip of saddler's felt slightly wider than the thigh and longer than the width of the adhesive strip. Tongue depressors or a piece of stiff cardboard or sole leather is applied to the inner surface of the adhesive between it and the felt to prevent it from wrinkling and cutting into the skin; the free end of the adhesive is folded over another spreader (four tongue depressors) and the traction is applied to this.

If the pull in internal rotation is not desired, both ends of the adhesive can be left long and fixed to the spreader to which the traction is applied.

The Well Leg Traction Splint.—If the head of the femur has been driven into the pelvis and is locked there, it cannot, as a rule, be pulled out by direct traction, but the hip should be manipulated under anesthesia and the femur pulled out by traction in line with the neck of the femur. Then some form of the well leg traction splint may be used, as is described under trochanteric fractures of the femur.

Manipulative Reduction of Central Dislocation at the Hip.—As a rule all that is necessary is strong traction in the line of the neck of the femur. With the patient fully anesthetized and the pelvis fixed to the table by an assistant or straps, one assistant applies traction downward on the leg while the surgeon in charge pulls directly outward on the upper thigh. He may use his hands, a towel, or a sheet around the thigh. If reduction is not easily accomplished, the assistant should gently rotate the hip outward and inward or flex and extend it while the outward traction is maintained.

In very difficult cases it may be necessary forcibly to abduct the thigh, thus prying the head out, using the pressure of the trochanter against the rim of the acetabulum as a fulcrum, but this is dangerous, since it may cause further fracture of the acetabulum.

After the reduction is accomplished, the patient should be treated as described above under "Central Dislocations in Which Reduction Is Not Necessary" and in many cases a good serviceable hip may be expected in about four months.

FRACTURES OF THE NECK OF THE FEMUR (HIP)

Classification.—From the practical standpoint of prognosis and treatment, fractures of the neck of the femur fall naturally into two groups: (1) Fractures through the narrow part of the neck; and (2) trochanteric fractures of the femur (Fig. 900). Many subdivisions of these two main types are to be found in the literature, but the elaborate classifications lead only to confusion and obscure the diagnosis and treatment.

The fractures through the narrow part of the neck include the intracapsular or subcapital and intermediate fractures of the neck, while the trochanteric fractures include the extracapsular or intertrochanteric and transtrochanteric fractures as well as those at the base of the neck. Either type may be impacted.

Incidence.—These fractures may occur at any age, but are primarily lesions of advanced life. In different series the average age of the patients varies from fifty to sixty years, the patients with the trochanteric type of fracture averaging from five to ten years older than those with the fractures through the narrow part of the neck.

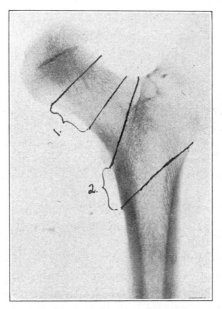

Fig. 900.—X-ray picture of a dried femur. (*1*) Location of fractures through the neck; (*2*) location of trochanteric fractures.

These fractures are very rare in children and young adults, fairly frequent in middle-aged adults, and frequent in the aged. They are slightly more frequent in women than in men.

Predisposing Causes.—The changes which occur in the femoral neck with advanced age are the most important predisposing cause of fractures in this region. These changes consist of a variable amount of absorption of the bony framework of the neck leading to rarefaction of the cancellous bone with replacement by fatty marrow and thinning of the cortex with resultant weakening of the structure. Whether or not this rarefaction is pathologic is a moot question. In many cases the rarefaction is especially pronounced in the neck of the femur and seems to be an increased local manifestation of the mild generalized osteoporosis which is regarded as a physiologic change incident to senility.

In addition to the local osteoporosis there is also a general loss of elasticity or brittleness of the bones which comes on with advancing years and renders the bones of old persons less tough and strong than are those of young adults.

A third factor is that the reflexes in old persons are less active and their muscles are more likely to be caught off guard with the result that sudden and unusual strains may be thrown upon the bones, or that old persons fall more frequently than do younger ones. It was formerly believed that the femoral neck was gradually bent downward with advancing age and that the resulting coxa vara predisposed to fracture, but this has been proved incorrect, since the neck of the femur has been found to maintain its normal oblique angle throughout life.

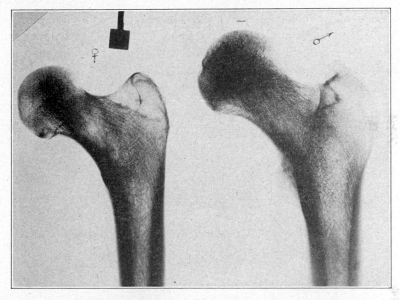

Fig. 901.—X-ray picture of two dried femurs. The one on the left is from a woman and the one on the right from a man. In the female note that the neck of the bone is considerably smaller and that the angle is nearer a right angle than in the male.

The greater frequency of these fractures in women is usually attributed to the fact that the angle between the neck of the femur and the shaft is nearer a right angle in women (Fig. 901). It is also to be remarked that the neck of the femur in women is on the average considerably smaller than in men (Fig. 902) and it is quite possible that the senile osteoporosis mentioned above is more common in women.

Direct Causes of Fractures of the Neck of the Femur.—In young and middle-aged persons fractures of the neck of the femur result only from severe violence, such as automobile accidents or falls from a height. In old persons they may result from very slight violence, such as a misstep or a sudden twist of the extremity or body, or while walking across the floor the patient may trip on a rug and endeavor to catch herself and thus throw the body weight suddenly on one leg. It is probable that in the majority of instances the fall is the result rather than the cause of the fracture. Because the patient falls toward the fractured side, it is usually stated that the fractures are the result of falls on the trochanter, the fracturing force being transmitted through the trochanter. And it is true that these fractures can be produced by blows on the trochanter, but such forces are more likely to crush the trochanter or fracture the acetabulum.

Sir Astley Cooper taught that the fractures through the neck were the result of axial torsion of the limb. "I was informed by a person who had sustained a fracture of this kind that being at her counter and suddenly turning to a drawer behind her, some projection in the floor caught her foot and preventing it turning with the body, the thigh bone became fractured," and that the trochanteric fractures were the result of force applied upward through the shaft of the femur: "Mary Clements, aet. 83½, when walking across her room, October 1, 1820, supported by a stick, which from the debility consequent upon old age, she was obliged to employ, unperceived by herself, placed the stick in a hole in the floor, by which her balance was lost, and tottering to recover herself from falling which she would have done but for those near her, she had as she supposed dislocated her thigh bone."[*] This latter patient did not fall, but she had a trochanteric fracture.

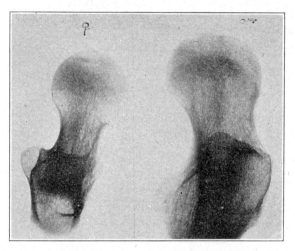

Fig. 902.—X-ray pictures of male and female femurs taken from above. Note the greater thickness of the neck in the male.

We believe that in the great majority of cases the mechanism will be found to be similar to those described above in the quotation from Sir Astley Cooper: fractures through the neck are due to axial torsion on the femur and trochanteric fractures are due to force transmitted upward through the shaft of the femur and tending to bend the neck downward.

Pathology of Fractures Through the Neck of the Femur.—In the great majority of cases the fracture line runs transversely or slightly obliquely across the neck at its narrowest portion (middle). Occasionally the fracture line lies nearer the head (subcapital). Rarely it traverses the thick basal portion of the neck. The fractures in which the neck is broken off from the shaft (fractures at the base of the neck) are here classified as trochanteric fractures.

*Stebbing, G. F.: Brit. J. Surg. 15: 201, 1928.

Due to the fact that the capsule of the joint extends downward over the front of the neck to the intertrochanteric line, and extends only a short distance on the posterior surface of the neck, these fractures are usually partly intracapsular and partly extracapsular; and depending upon the amount of displacement, the periosteum over the neck is torn to a variable degree and may be completely severed, or the two fragments may be united by a strip of periosteum usually on the posterior and inferior surfaces of the neck. This periosteal union between the two fragments is important, as it provides a means of blood supply to the proximal fragment which otherwise is dependent upon the minute vessels in the ligamentum teres. It has been shown that in the adult these vessels are insufficient to nourish the head.

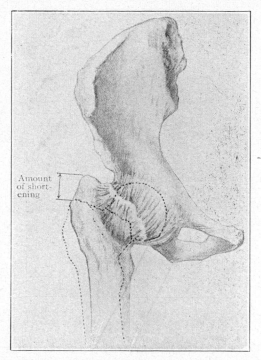

Fig. 903.—Intracapsular fracture of the neck of the femur showing the shortening. The dotted line represents the outline of the normal bone. (Davis: Applied Anatomy.)

Displacement in Fracture Through the Neck of the Femur.—The displacement is largely due to muscular action rather than to the fracturing force. The gluteal muscles, the iliopsoas, adductors, and the hamstrings all tend to pull the lower fragment upward and cause shortening of the extremity (Fig. 903). The iliopsoas tends to rotate the lower fragment outward. With the patient recumbent gravity causes the distal fragment to drop downward (backward), and the weight of the foot causes it to rotate outward; consequently the distal fragment tends to be displaced upward and backward and rotated outward. The amount of shortening varies from 0 to 1½ inches. or more, and the shortening may increase for some hours after the injury. In unusual cases with marked shortening this is due to the body weight at the time of the accident and in these cases there is considerable tearing of the soft parts.

No muscles are attached to the proximal fragment and the head remains in the acetabulum. It may be tilted forward into internal rotation by the outward rotation of the distal fragment, but it usually remains in the neutral position.

Impaction occurs in a relatively small percentage of fractures through the neck of the femur and these are believed to be due to strain or to force applied while the hip is in a position of abduction. In impacted fractures the head is in a valgus position and appears to be perched on top of the neck and the neck is slightly lengthened. The dense cortex of the neck is driven into the cancellous bone of the head and the impaction is, as a rule, quite firm.

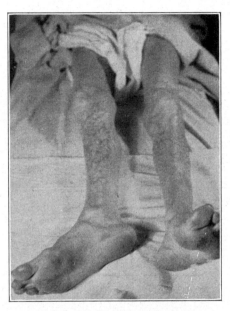

Fig. 904.—Typical deformity in a fracture of the neck of the femur. Note the external rotation and helpless attitude of the limb.

Pathology of Trochanteric Fractures of the Femur.—Since these fractures are usually the result of force transmitted upward through the shaft of the femur, the tendency is for the neck to be bent downward on the shaft into the varus position and the fracture line begins in the region of the great trochanter and passes inward and downward roughly parallel to the intertrochanteric lines to the region of the lesser trochanter. The fracture line may lie slightly proximal to the intertrochanteric line, thus separating the base of the neck from the shaft and leaving the intact trochanters attached to the shaft, but as a rule it involves the great trochanter and emerges on the inner border of the shaft just above the lesser trochanter. (Figs. 944 and 945.)

Many of these trochanteric fractures are comminuted and the upper cancellous portion of the shaft of the femur may be broken into several fragments. Not infrequently the lesser trochanter is detached and the shaft may be split. Very rarely the lesser trochanter remains attached to the proximal fragment.

In most of these trochanteric fractures, the fracture is for the most part extracapsular, but the fracture line may extend within the capsule at the point where it is reflected down over the anterior surface of the neck; consequently there is some tearing of the capsule.

Displacement in Trochanteric Fractures of the Femur.—The fracturing force tends to drive the distal fragment upward and this upward displacement is accentuated by the pull of the muscles passing from the pelvis to the distal fragment (gluteals, hamstrings, adductors, and iliopsoas). The proximal fragment is also pushed upward (abducted) by the fracturing force and by any muscles which may remain attached to it, and an increased angulation between the two fragments results. If the lesser trochanter is completely detached, it tends to be displaced upward and forward along the course of the iliopsoas tendon which is inserted into it. The upward displacement of the distal fragment may slowly increase some hours after the injury leading to increased shortening of the limb.

In addition to the upward displacement, the lower fragment tends to drop downward (backward) on account of gravity with the patient in the recumbent position and the weight of the foot tends to cause it to rotate outward. This outward rotation is aided by the iliopsoas if the lesser trochanter remains attached to the distal fragment.

In the rare cases where the lesser trochanter remains attached to the proximal fragment, this fragment is flexed.

Diagnosis of Fractures of the Upper End of the Femur.—This injury is so frequent in the aged that if an elderly person falls to the ground and is unable to rise and walk again, it may be assumed that he has a fracture of the neck of the femur until it is proved otherwise.

The classical symptoms are pain and disability at the hip, swelling over the joint, and some shortening and eversion of the limb. In old persons the posture and appearance are characteristic, and often the diagnosis of a fractured hip can be made at a glance (Fig. 904). The patient lies upon his back with the injured limb in a position of external rotation and slight abduction and the appearance is that of a flaccid paralysis of the extremity.

Disability.—This is as a rule complete and not only is the patient unable to support his weight on the limb, but he is unable to lift the heel on the injured side from the bed. However, many patients by contracting the hamstrings and flexing the knee are able slowly to slide the foot upward and raise the knee from the bed. Very rarely in incomplete or firmly impacted fractures the patient can raise the heel from the bed, or even walk on the extremity. The absence of complete disability in the hip, therefore, does not rule out the possibility of a fracture.

Shortening may be absent or so slight that it is not demonstrable by measurement, but in most cases there is from one-half inch to one inch of actual shortening of the extremity as measured from the anterior superior spine to the tip of the internal malleolus. Very rarely, with great displacement, the shortening may amount to two inches or more. The shortening is due partly to decrease in the angle of the neck of the femur and partly to overriding of the fragments.

Not only is the limb shortened but the trochanter is elevaтed above the Roser-Nélaton line and the base of Bryant's triangle is shortened (Fig. 905). The amount of elevation of thc trochanter is equal to the shortening.

The shortening is one of the most important diagnostic signs and should be measured accurately and recorded at the first examination. An increase in the shortening as determined by subsequent examinations indicates further displacement upward and is absolute evidence that the fracture is not impacted. It may indicate tearing of the periosteum or capsule or breaking up of a primary impaction.

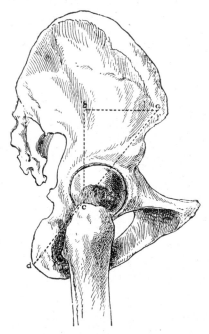

Fig. 905.—View of the lateral surface of the bones of the hip showing Roser-Nélaton line, *ad;* Bryant's triangle, *abc* (*bc* being its base); the iliotrochanteric line, *ac;* and the iliotrochanteric angle, *bac.* (Davis: Applied Anatomy.)

Pain.—The intensity and location of the pain vary in different types of fractures and in different individuals. Some persons suffer more than others with the same type of injury. The trochanteric fractures tend to cause more pain; this is usually localized in the trochanteric and gluteal regions. The fractures through the neck often cause relatively little pain unless the extremity is moved and the pain tends to be localized in the groin.

Swelling.—Some swelling is always present in fracture of the hip, and the upper thigh appears broadened and thickened. In trochanteric fractures the swelling usually involves the trochanteric and gluteal regions as well as the area over Scarpa's triangle, and the digital fossa behind the trochanter is obliterated. In fractures through the neck the swelling tends to be localized over the hip joint (Scarpa's triangle). A day or two after the injury ecchymosis may appear below Poupart's ligament or in the posterior thigh and buttock.

Tenderness is always present and is a very useful diagnostic sign, as in fractures through the neck, it is most acute over the front of the joint (Scarpa's triangle) (Fig. 861) and in trochanteric fractures it is most acute over the trochanteric region. Because of the deep-seated location of the fracture, it is, of course, impossible to elicit point tenderness and to thus identify the line of fracture.

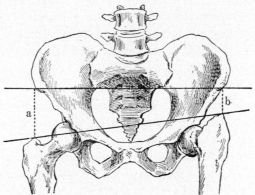

Fig. 906.—Showing elevation of the tip of the trochanter and shortening of Bryant's triangle in fracture of the neck of the femur; *a*, base on sound side; *b*, on fractured side. (Piersol: Human Anatomy.)

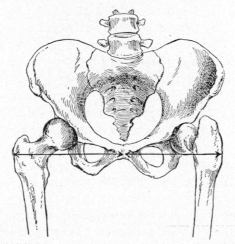

Fig. 907.—Morris' measurements to show the trochanter of the injured side nearer the median line in fracture of the neck of the femur. (Piersol: Human Anatomy.)

Allis' sign is a relaxation of the fascia, enabling the operator to press the fingers in more deeply over the trochanter on the injured side than on the sound side. It is caused by an abnormal looseness of the fascia lata between the iliac crest and the trochanter; this depends upon the shortening of the distance between the crest and the trochanter. The sign is not very reliable, since it is not present in cases with little shortening and it may be obscured by the swelling in trochanteric fractures.

False motion and crepitus should not be looked for aggressively, but in certain cases in which one wishes to determine the presence or absence of impaction, these signs may be noted during gentle manipulations of the hip

Violent manipulations should be avoided both because of the pain which they cause the patient and because they may result in displacement of the fragments and further stripping or tearing of the periosteum and other damage to soft parts.

The false motion usually described as pathognomonic of a fracture of the neck of the femur is the rotation of the trochanter, when the thigh is rotated, around an axis which is shorter than normal. This is true especially where the fragments are not impacted or entangled, since in these cases the trochanter rotates around the center of the shaft; however, efforts to demonstrate this point cause great pain and may do considerable damage; consequently we do not advise it.

Occasionally, however, we do demonstrate false motion by telescoping the hip. This is done by placing the thumb on the anterior superior spine and the tips of the fingers of the same hand on the trochanter while the other hand alternately makes slow traction and upward pressure on the thigh. If the fragments are loose, the trochanter can be moved up and down on the pelvis without producing much pain.

Impaction in Fractures of the Upper End of the Femur.—As a general rule the pain, swelling, disability, and shortening tend to be greater in the unimpacted fractures. In an unimpacted fracture the limb usually assumes a position of eversion and the patient is powerless to roll it in or even to move the leg around in bed. But if the fragments are entangled, the limb may be in the neutral position with the toes pointing straight up and the patient may be able to rotate the limb, move it about a bit, or even to flex the hip by flexing the knee and sliding the heel up on the bed. The above signs are those usually accepted as indicating impaction, but they are not reliable and it may be practically impossible by physical examination or x-ray to determine whether or not a fracture of the hip is impacted. This is especially true of cases without much shortening or eversion.

If there is impaction in eversion, the problem is less difficult because in such a case the eversion can be increased to an abnormal degree, and without pain, but the hip cannot be rotated inward without exerting enough force to break up the impaction. In an unimpacted everted fracture the limb can be rotated inward with relatively little force, though the manipulation may cause considerable pain to the patient.

If the x-ray shows the head in the valgus position, that is, on top of the neck, the fracture is usually impacted (Fig. 908).

Differential Diagnosis Between Fractures Through the Neck and Trochanteric Fractures.—Both types of fracture of the hip exhibit approximately the same amount of disability, pain, deformity, limitation of motion or false motion, and in many cases a roentgenogram is necessary to determine the type of fracture.

The location of the swelling and tenderness are of some help in deciding whether we are dealing with a fracture through the neck or a trochanteric fracture. In the fractures through the neck the swelling and tenderness are usually limited to the region over the front of the joint (Scarpa's triangle) while in trochanteric fractures the swelling and tenderness are more marked in the region around the trochanter.

The X-Ray in Hip Fractures.—The hip is so deeply seated that it is impossible to learn much about its condition by palpation, and as it is very important that we know as exactly as possible with what we are dealing before we give a prognosis and start our treatment, x-ray pictures should be made of every case of hip injury which results in pain and disability. Not only this, but often lateral x-ray pictures should also be made as it is only by means of views in two planes that the true relation of the fragments can be determined. In doubtful cases x-ray pictures of the uninjured hip should be made and the two hips compared. (Fig. 908.)

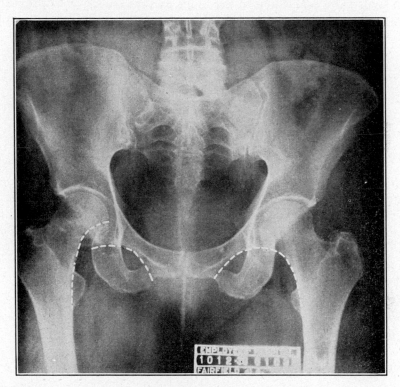

Fig. 908.—Impacted fracture of the neck of the femur showing Shenton's line which demonstrates the displacement.

Not only should the x-ray be used for diagnosis, but it should also be used at suitable intervals to check the results obtained by treatment. This is especially true of lateral views made with the cassette in the groin, as these are very important in determining whether or not accurate reduction has been obtained.

Prognosis in Hip Fractures.—Hip fractures are serious injuries, and from 10 to 20 per cent of the patients die. The high mortality is not due to any great tendency of hip injuries to produce surgical shock or to endanger life peculiarly, but is due to the fact that such a large proportion of these cases occur in old people who may be said to be nearing the end of life before the accident, and the hip injury with the resultant pain, discomfort, and confinement to bed are just enough to precipitate a not far distant death. Under these conditions the lesion will continue to carry a high mortality though adequate treatment and careful nursing may be expected to cut it down to perhaps 10 per cent. With proper treatment the comparatively young, robust patients will practically all live, but a considerable number of the old, decrepit patients will die.

In a few cases death results within a day or so from shock and exhaustion, and a few others die of cardiac failure, but in the majority of the fatal cases death is due to pneumonia, that ''friend of the aged'' which carries them off quickly and with relatively little pain. The pneumonia is largely the result of hypostatic congestion in the lungs and we endeavor to prevent it by such measures as having the patient sit up or lie on the face frequently.

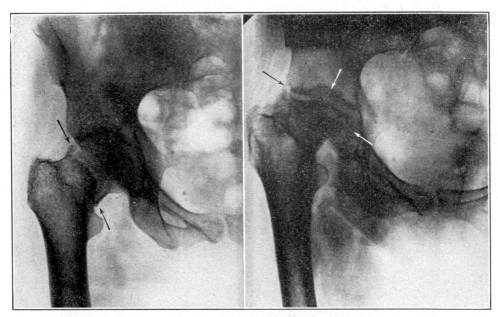

Fig. 909.—Fracture through the neck of the femur which was treated by Whitman's abduction method. Union obtained but aseptic necrosis of the head was present two years later.

As regards union, fractures through the neck will not unite unless properly treated, but if they are properly treated, bony union and a useful hip may be expected in from 40 to 60 per cent of the patients that do not die (Fig. 910.) Even with union there may be considerable disability from late absorption of the head. Most of the others will obtain fibrous union and a certain percentage of these will deserve operative measures for the relief of pain and instability, but a considerable number of them will obtain serviceable hips. The results to be expected by operative treatment will be considered later.

Practically all of the trochanteric fractures, and it is to be remembered that these include the fractures at the base of the neck, may be expected to

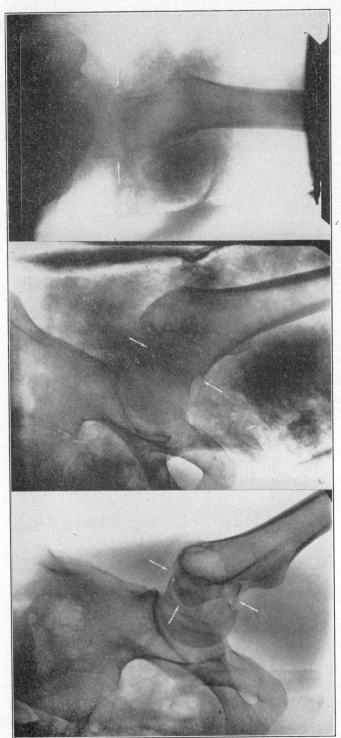

Fig. 910.—Fracture through the neck of the femur. Closed reduction by Whitman method and treated in a plaster cast; anteroposterior view and lateral view with excellent anatomical position. Good result.

unite by bony union if the patient survives. The problem in these fractures is not to obtain union, but to prevent deformity as most of them unite with a coxa vara deformity unless this is prevented by proper treatment.

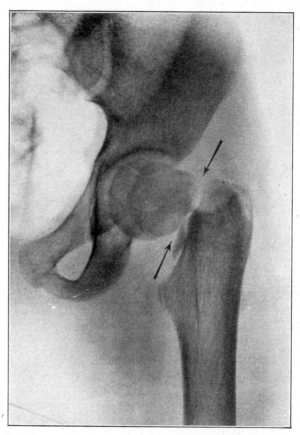

Fig. 911.—Fracture through the neck of the femur in a child. Treated by Whitman's abduction method with good result. (Courtesy Dr. John D. Sherrill.)

Treatment of Hip Fractures

The objects of treatment are first to save life and second to restore function to the hip. Since we have divided these fractures into those through the neck and trochanteric fractures, we shall consider the treatment under these two headings. Before we describe the treatment, however, we shall discuss briefly the question of hip fractures in the aged.

The Question of Treatment of Fractures of the Hip in Old Persons.— Since a large proportion of these fractures occur in old persons and since many of these patients are already the victims of constitutional diseases which render their tenure of life uncertain, it has been the custom in the past for the surgeon largely to ignore the fracture and to devote his energies to getting the patient up at the earliest possible moment in the hope of avoiding the terminal pneumonia which is so frequent in old people who are forced to lie in a position of dorsal decubitus for any great length of time. For this reason many of these patients have had no treatment for the fracture, but have been got up in a chair daily in spite of the great pain and exhaustion, while others have been left in bed with sandbags around the leg or Buck's extension and forced to sit up daily.

We believe that the above methods are wrong. Not only do they result in cripples (either from nonunion in fractures through the neck, or from malunion in trochanteric fractures), but they actually endanger the lives which they strive to save. The severe and almost constant pain which they inflict on these feeble old men and women leads to such a state of weakness and exhaustion that they readily fall victim to some infection (usually pneumonia) or die of exhaustion. Pain can be relieved by immobilization of the fracture; consequently these fractures should be reduced and immobilized as soon as possible after the injury. The fractures through the neck are best immobilized in a plaster cast, while either a cast or the Hodgen or Thomas splint is satisfactory for the trochanteric fractures.

It is objected that many of these patients are too feeble to stand the application of a cast. Our answer is that any patient who is too feeble to stand the application of a cast will certainly die unless the fracture is immobilized, and that one is often surprised at how well these patients do stand the cast treatment and how comfortable they are after it has been applied. Hypostatic congestion and resultant pneumonia are combated by turning them on the face twice daily or by getting them up in a chair daily as will be mentioned below.

Immediate Treatment and Transportation in Hip Fractures.—The patient's strength should be conserved in every way possible; for this reason it is important not to cause unnecessary pain by careless handling, and to relieve the pain by a full dose of morphine.

Most of these patients must be transported to a hospital for treatment; this should be done on a stretcher in an ambulance.

During transportation and until treatment is instituted the fracture can be partially immobilized by strapping or bandaging the two legs together and by applying a long Liston splint or strapping a board along the injured side. The board should extend from the axilla to the toes and should be padded and bound firmly to the chest, pelvis, knees, and ankles.

Definite treatment should be instituted as soon as possible after the injury. If it is necessary to wait a day or so Buck's extension with 15 pounds traction should be applied and the extremity should be immobilized with sandbags.

Treatment of Fractures Through the Neck of the Femur (Intracapsular Fractures of the Hip)

Internal fixation with a Smith-Petersen nail or the Moore pins or a lag screw or other types of nails or pins has largely supplanted the nonoperative or so-called conservative methods of treating fractures of the hip. This is because in skillful hands the operative methods decrease the mortality and increase the percentage of satisfactory results. However, if a surgeon who is familiar with the operative method is not available, the abduction method of Whitman is the method of choice. Consequently, we shall describe both methods.

The Treatment of Impacted Fractures.—If the fracture is firmly impacted, union may be expected to occur with the head in a position of valgus. In such cases no fixation other than rest in bed and freedom from weight bearing is necessary. This should be continued for from eight to ten weeks. At the end of this time the patient should be gotten up on crutches and weight bearing resumed gradually. If the hip is sensitive it may be immobilized by a plaster boot with a cross board fixed in the plaster to prevent rotation, by sand bags with a pillow under the knee or by light traction.

In young patients it is questionable whether or not the impaction should be broken up and the hip nailed, because one of us (J. A. K.) has seen osteoarthritis develop in hips within two years after impacted fractures had healed in the valgus position.

The Abduction Method of Whitman is the simplest routine method for the treatment of fractures of the hip.

The crux of the abduction method is that if a fracture through the neck of the femur is accurately reduced, immobilization of the extremity in a position of full abduction and internal rotation and extension jams the fractured surfaces together and maintains immobilization of the fracture.

That the above is true is obvious because by abduction and internal rotation the stump of the neck is swung inward toward the acetabulum on the Y ligament as a fulcrum, and the capsule of the hip is tightened around both fragments like a sleeve.

The joker in the abduction method is that in order to be successful the fracture must be reduced before the abduction is started, because abduction does not reduce the displacement, but locks the fragments in whatever position they may lie and renders further reduction impossible. This fact has not been sufficiently emphasized. On the contrary there is a quite general belief that the reduction is effected by the abduction, and many hips with the fragments in poor position have been forced into abduction, internal rotation, and extension and immobilized in a large plaster spica and consequently have failed to unite.

We do not believe that all fractures of the neck of the femur will unite if properly reduced and immobilized in abduction, but we do believe that improper reduction accounts for many of the failures.

Technic of the Abduction Method in Fractures Through the Neck of the Femur.—In order to treat a fracture of the hip by the abduction method the surgeon needs three and preferably four assistants and an anesthetist, a fracture table having a pelvic support (Hawley table), and an adequate supply of plaster-of-Paris bandages, felt and cotton padding.

The patient is placed upon the fracture table and anesthetized. Some surgeons use local anesthesia and some use spinal anesthesia. We usually use local anesthesia.

The perineal post is inserted and a long strip of saddler's felt 6 inches wide and ½ inch thick is placed beneath the patient extending from the tip of the sacrum up the spine as far as the plaster jacket is to go. The pa-

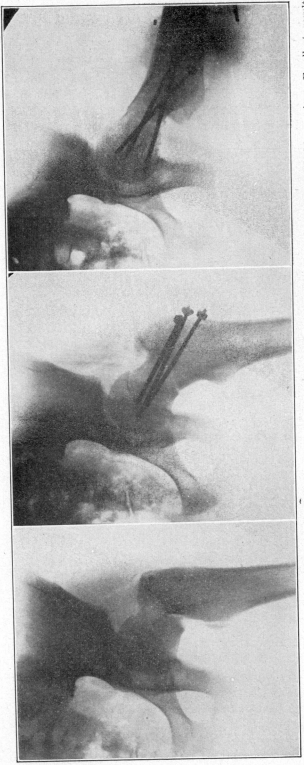

Fig. 912.—Fracture through the neck of the femur in a child treated by manipulative reduction and fixation with Moore pins. Excellent result. (Courtesy Dr. **John D. Sherrill.**)

tient is then pulled down against the perineal post and is ready for the manipulation which will effect the reduction.

We shall describe two methods of manipulation: Whitman's and Leadbetter's. In performing either manipulation the surgeon should realize that he is endeavoring to fit the end of the neck fragment against the end of the head fragment which lies loose in the acetabulum, and that the distal or neck fragment is displaced backward by gravity, upward by muscle pull, and is directed anteriorly (externally rotated) by gravity.

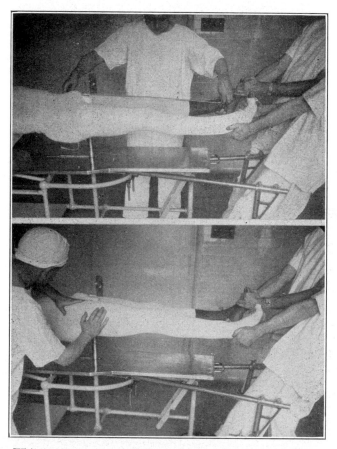

Fig. 913.—Whitman method of reducing fractures through the neck of the femur. Patient on a Hawley table. Manual traction pulling the legs down to equal length.

Fig. 914.—The surgeon lifting the trochanter while an assistant applies manual traction and rotates the limb inward.

Whitman's Manipulation.—1. By manual traction the injured extremity is pulled down until it is the same length as its fellow, thus reducing the upward displacement. During the traction the opposite leg is pulled on by an assistant to immobilize the pelvis. (Fig. 913.)

2. The upper thigh is lifted to the level of the sound thigh to reduce the posterior displacement. This is the point that is often neglected and it should be done by the surgeon himself as it is very important. We not only lift the upper thigh, but pull it laterally to enable the distal fragment to clear the proximal one (Fig. 914).

3. The limb is slowly rotated inward to a point slightly beyond the neutral position (Fig. 915).

4. Both limbs are slowly abducted to the limit permitted.

Traction sufficient to maintain full length of the limb is maintained throughout the procedure until the fragments are locked by the abduction when the traction may be discontinued and the hip merely supported in abduction, extension and internal rotation while the cast is applied (Fig. 917).

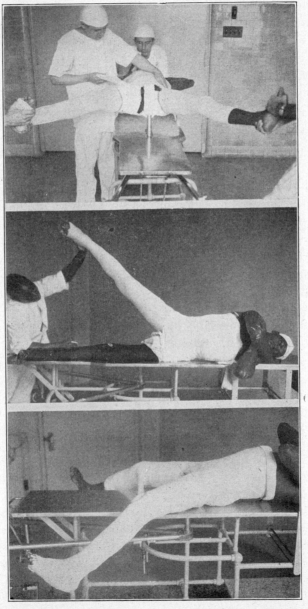

Fig. 915.—Abduction, internal rotation and slight extension of the fractured limb. Application of the plaster-of-Paris spica.

Fig. 916.—Patient with fracture of the neck of the femur in plaster-of-Paris single spica to show the abduction.

Fig. 917.—Patient with fracture of the neck of the femur in abduction in double spica of hips to show the hyperextension.

Leadbetter's Method.*—1. The pelvis is fixed by an assistant and under moderate traction the hip (with the knee flexed) is slowly flexed to 90 degrees to relax the capsule and muscles and then the slightly adducted thigh is lifted directly upward to correct the posterior displacement and shortening and is gently rotated inward (45 degrees) to engage the fragments. During this procedure it is sometimes helpful to have an assistant pull the upper thigh directly outward and thus clear the inner fragment and line the two fragments up by tension on the capsule. (Fig. 918.)

2. When the fragments are felt to be engaged, the hip should be circumducted into abduction and extension and the opposite thigh should be fully abducted. (Figs. 918 and 919.)

Test of Reduction.—A fracture of the hip reduced by either of the above methods should fulfill the following requirements:

1. Full abduction (equal to that on the sound side) can be obtained and maintained without undue force.

2. In a position of full abduction the hip should be stable as regards length; that is, no traction should be necessary to prevent the distal fragment from slipping upward (shortening recurring).

3. In a position of full abduction the hip should be stable as regards rotation; that is, no force should be necessary to prevent the extremity from rolling outward.

In other words, after a successful reduction the position of the abducted hip can be maintained by supporting the heel in the palm of the hand. This is Leadbetter's palm test, and unless the hip meets this test the reduction has not been successful and should be tried again.

The plaster cast should not be applied until the reduction is believed to be successful and meets Leadbetter's palm test.

Postoperative X-Rays.—In addition to the heel-palm test, it is well to check the position of the fragments by anteroposterior and lateral x-rays before the cast is applied. These should be made without changing the position of the patient if possible. In order to do this, a tunnel to carry the casette should be placed under the patient for the anteroposterior view and the lateral view may be made with the casette (preferably a curved one) in the groin or held against the trochanter and pelvis, the rays being so directed that they pass through the neck of the femur and onto the film.

Application of the Plaster Cast.—When the reduction is believed to be complete assistants support each leg in the position of full abduction and slight extension, and the leg on the injured side is rotated inward. With the patient in this position the fracture table is tripped or lowered, leaving the patient supported on the pelvic rest and pulled down snugly against the perineal post. The legs are held by assistants. The strip of felt to protect the sacrum and spine is under the patient. Then the body and extremity or both extremities are covered with a stockinet or a thin layer of sheet cotton. Thick cotton padding is to be avoided, as snugly fitting plaster casts give bet-

---

*Leadbetter, G. W.: J. Bone and Joint Surg. 15: 931, 1933.

ter fixation and are more comfortable. Finally, a triangular piece of felt is placed over each anterior superior spine and a strip of felt under the heel and tendo achillis.

The surgeon and another assistant, if available, should apply the plaster as smoothly and evenly as possible, avoiding indentations which would produce pressure later. If a proper spica bandage is applied around the hips, no reinforcements are necessary. In some cases, however, we place a wide plaster reinforcement front and back across the hip, extending from the abdomen down the thigh and incorporate this in the plaster. Particular care should be taken to mould the cast snugly around the trochanters and pelvis and to extend the plaster well inward behind to support the buttock, so that the patient will not sag out of it. The body cast and hip spica are applied first and then the plaster is continued down over the leg and foot being well moulded around the knee and foot.

Some surgeons flex the knee about 45 degrees in order to be sure of maintaining inward rotation. We fix the knee in extension, because difficulty may be experienced later in restoring full extension to the knee after the long period of immobilization. We have had no difficulty in maintaining inward rotation because we use very little padding on the knee and foot.

Wide plaster bandages (12 inches or more) greatly lessen the amount of labor involved in applying a large plaster spica.

Either a large single spica (Fig. 916) or a double spica (Fig. 917) may be used, as either type affords effective immobilization if it is properly applied. If the single spica is used, it must be the large spica jacket as has been emphasized by Whitman, and the plaster jacket must fit snugly around the pelvis and extend up to the arm pits. In order to apply this jacket successfully the head of the fracture table must be pulled well up and it may be necessary to support the back with metal strips extending from the pelvic rest to the head of the table. These can be pulled out after the plaster has set.

The single spica, which includes only the lower ribs, should not be used as it does not immobilize the hip.

If a double spica is used, the jacket part may be stopped at the lower third of the chest and the plaster should extend down the opposite lower extremity to the junction of the middle and lower thirds of the leg. Some surgeons place a wooden crossbar between the legs just below the knee in order to strengthen the cast and facilitate turning the patient (Fig. 917).

Every effort should be made to make the cast as comfortable and efficient as possible, since it should remain on the patient at least three months. The cast should be cut out around the perineum and buttocks to prevent soiling, but not cut out enough to lose fixation.

Care of the Patient in the Cast.—If the fracture is properly reduced and the cast is properly applied, the pain will be relieved and the patient will be comfortable.

In order to avoid hypostatic congestion of the lungs the patient must be turned on the face twice a day and should lie on the face from two to four hours after each turning. This will occasion some discomfort at first, but the patients soon get used to it and many of them stay on the face about half of the time. When on the face the exposed parts of the back should be rubbed with alcohol and powdered.

The patient must be fed by a nurse or attendant.

A fracture bed, that is, a bed with boards running lengthwise under the mattress to prevent sagging, should be used. A frame is placed over the bed

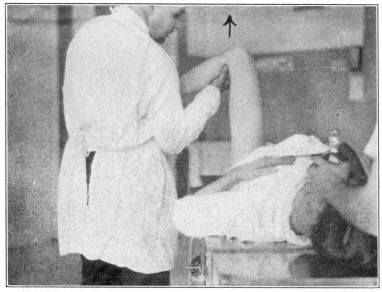

A.

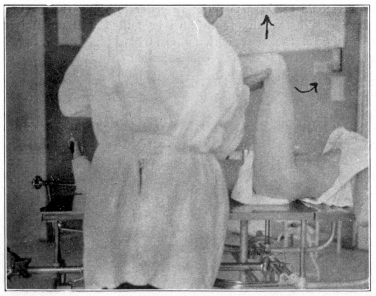

B.

Fig. 918.—Leadbetter's maneuver of the reduction of fracture through the neck of the femur.
A. Knee and hip flexed 90 degrees. Traction upward.
B. Internal rotation with traction and flexion maintained.

and a bar suspended from this so that the patient can grasp the bar and lift himself to change position or get on or off the bedpan.

The bed must be kept clean and dry. A wet bed not only leads to the development of pressure sores, but softens the cast and necessitates its removal and application of a new cast.

With a single spica the patient may be propped up in bed by letting the leg on the affected side hang over the side of the bed, or he may be got up in

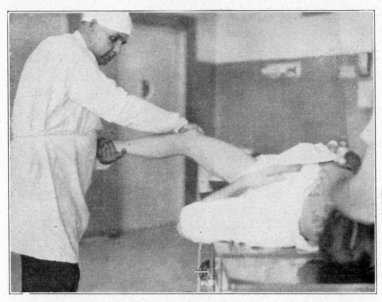

A.

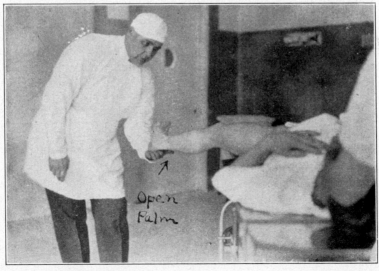

B.

Fig. 919.—A. Leg brought down in measured abduction and internal rotation. Reduction complete.

B. Heel palm test. Leg remains in abduction and internal rotation. Reduction complete. (Courtesy Dr. Guy Leadbetter.)

a chair daily, but this involves a lot of effort and the turning twice daily is all that is necessary to safeguard the general health.

The patient really has little or no pain, but may be uncomfortable on account of the confinement in the cast. Sedatives should be given sparingly and the nervousness should be combated by small doses of bromides.

The diet should include plenty of green vegetables and milk, and the bowels should be kept open. During the first week or two after the cast has hardened daily enemas should be given if necessary. After this time mineral oil or mineral oil and agar-agar should be used with mild cathartics when necessary.

Aftertreatment of Fractures Through the Neck of the Femur

As soon as the plaster is dry, an x-ray (anteroposterior and lateral) should be made to check the position of the fragments. If the position is not satisfactory the cast should be removed and a new attempt at reduction made as soon as the patient's general condition permits. The lateral view is very important and can be obtained with the curved cassette in the groin.* It is, of course, advisable to obtain these x-ray pictures before the cast is applied if conditions permit.

If the position is satisfactory the cast should remain on for three or four months and it should not be changed unless it becomes inefficient, because in changing the plaster beginning union may be broken up or position lost and a nonunion result. Casts become inefficient from being broken by improper handling or softened on account of inefficient nursing care.

If the plaster cast becomes inefficient it must, of course, be reinforced or removed and a new one applied; great care must be taken in lifting the patient out of the old cast and onto the fracture table because every possible movement of the hip should be avoided.

At the end of three or four months the plaster should be bivalved and the hip tested for union clinically and by the x-ray.

The best clinical test of union is to grasp the knee and make alternate gentle traction and upward pressure on the limb while the pelvis is fixed. If the extremity moves up and down on the pelvis (telescopes) there is no union and further immobilization is useless. If the hip feels solid (does not telescope) union is probably present.

If the hip telescopes, the x-ray will probably show marked absorption of the proximal end of the distal fragment and the case must be treated as a nonunion.

If the hip does not telescope and the x-ray shows some absorption of the neck and upward displacement of the distal fragment, nonunion is probable, but the patient should be treated expectantly; that is, permitted to lie in bed for two weeks longer, when new x-ray pictures should be made. If these show upward displacement of the distal fragment, nonunion is present. If the position of the fragments is unchanged, beginning union is probable and the patient should remain in bed at least another month, but the hip need not be immobilized.

*Leonard and George: Am. J. Roentgen. and Radium Therapy 28: 261, 1932.

If the hip feels solid, and the x-ray shows the fragments in good position with little or no absorption, union is probable and the patient is kept recumbent in bed without immobilization for another month; the hip, knee, and foot should be exercised daily. At the end of this time the patient is got up on crutches which should be used for from three to nine months or until the roentgenogram shows firm bony union. We give these fractures through the neck of the femur three or four months' immobilization in plaster and no

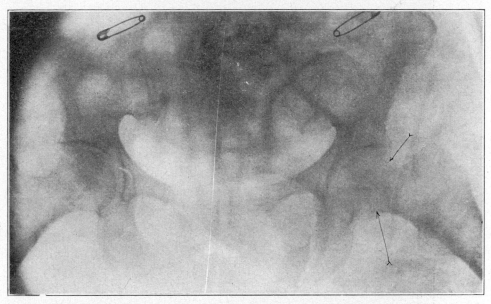

Fig. 920.—Fracture through the neck of the femur after apparently perfect reduction and artificial impaction by Cotton's method and immobilization in a double abduction plaster.

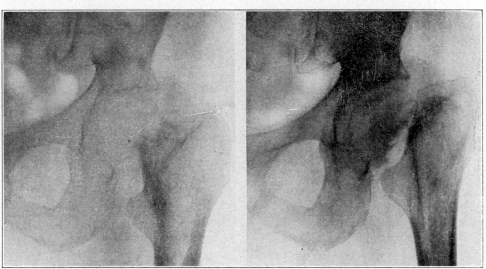

Fig. 921.   Fig. 922.

Fig. 921.—Same case as in Fig. 920, two months later, showing beginning absorption of the neck of the femur. Cast removed after absorption was noted.

Fig. 922.—Same case, three months after the artificial impaction showing complete absorption of the neck of the femur and nonunion.

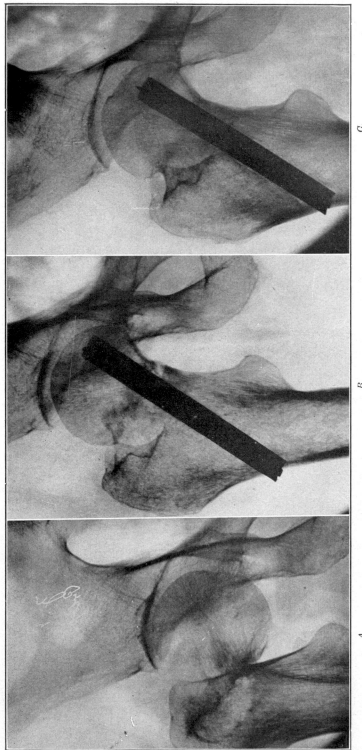

Fig. 923.—A, Fracture of the neck of the femur fixed by Smith-Petersen nail; B, one month and, C, thirteen months after operation. (Courtesy Dr. Smith-Petersen.)

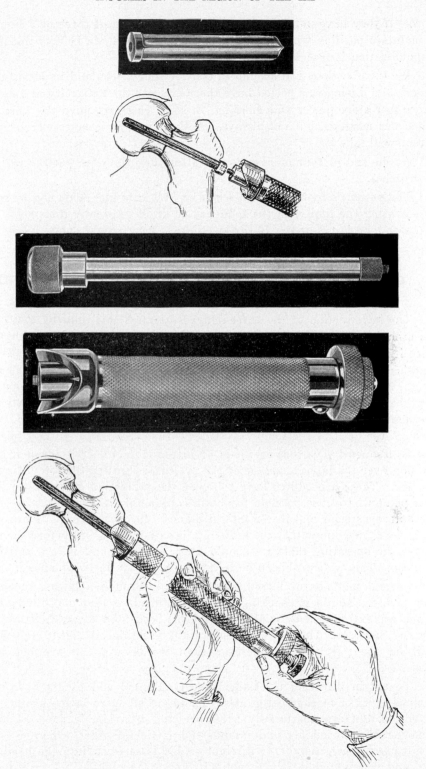

Fig. 924.—Smith-Petersen nail with combined extractor and impactor and White handle for guiding nail. (Courtesy Zimmer Manufacturing Company)

more. If they have not united sufficiently at the end of three or four months to maintain position while the patient is lying in bed, we believe that further immobilization is useless.

We then let them roll around in bed for four weeks and in doubtful cases longer, and during this period have them exercise the extremity and move the joints to restore power and motion. In some cases we have the knee baked and order massage, but not always. Active exercise is more effective if the patient will take it.

At the end of four or five months after the injury we get the patient up on crutches.

The patient's foot will swell when he first gets up. This can be relieved by elevating the limb, and the tendency to swell gradually disappears as the vascular tone is restored. If the swelling is very troublesome, it can be relieved by an elastic stocking or bandage.

OPERATIVE TREATMENT OF FRACTURES THROUGH THE NECK OF THE FEMUR

The introduction of the three-flanged stainless steel nail by Smith-Petersen stimulated interest in the operative treatment of fractures of the femur, since it is possible with this nail to hold two pieces of cancellous bone firmly together. In his earlier cases Smith-Petersen opened the hip by the antero-lateral route, reduced the hip, and inserted the nail under direct vision. This is probably the most accurate method, but it is too large an operation for the average surgeon to perform on the average patient who suffers a fracture through the neck of the femur.

Consequently, various methods of introducing the nail through a small incision over the lateral surface of the proximal third of the femur have been devised. These procedures have followed the perfection of our x-ray technic to a point where it is possible to obtain satisfactory views of the hip in both the anteroposterior and in the lateral planes. In other words, before we nail a hip we should know that the reduction is satisfactory and before the patient leaves the operating table we should know that the nail is in a satisfactory position. This we are able to do by means of x-rays in two planes.

Several methods of introducing the nail through a lateral incision are now in use. The least shocking but most difficult is that of "blind nailing" which was introduced by O'Meara* and has been used successfully by Thornton and Sandison. Our chief objection to blind nailing is that it requires more skill on the part of the operator than we believe the average surgeon possesses.

To aid in directing the nail, Wescott, Bunnel and others have devised various types of mechanical guides. These are effective in the hands of their inventors, but are not usually available, and if available must be used by someone who thoroughly understands the particular guide which he is using. White uses a long handle or director which is screwed into the head of the nail and which enables him to point it more accurately.

*O'Meara: New England J. Med. 212: 43, 1935.

Johanssen* and others have introduced and used a cannulated Smith-Petersen nail which is threaded on a Kirschner wire and driven home. This is probably the most popular method at present. Three or more Kirschner wires are drilled into the reduced hip and anteroposterior and lateral x-rays are then made and the nail is threaded on the wire which is most favorably located and driven home, and after the hip has been impacted the wire is pulled out. Our objections are that the nail may bind on the wire and force the wire into the pelvis or so bend it that its removal is difficult. A further objection is that, while the ordinary three-flanged nails cost from three to six dollars, the cannulated nails cost from nine to eleven dollars each.

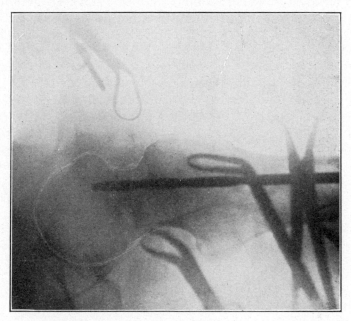

Fig. 925.—Lateral view of hip after reduction of fracture with three-sixteenths of an inch drill in place to be used as a guide for inserting nail.

One of us (J. A. K.†) has published a method which uses the standard Smith-Petersen nail and with an ordinary drill for a guide (Fig. 925). It requires no special instruments and we believe that it can be used by any surgeon who can successfully use any of the methods mentioned above. We will describe this method in detail with the suggestion that the surgeon use that method for which he has the necessary equipment at hand and which seems to him most likely to succeed in his hands. All methods are difficult and should not be undertaken lightly by the uninitiated.

Technic of the Procedure

Anesthesia.—We have used avertin or morphine and local anesthesia. The patient is given a relatively small dose of avertin (65 to 70 mgm. per kilo) or ¼ grain of morphine. About 10 c.c. of 1 per cent novocaine is then injected into the hip joint. The injection is made by inserting the needle ver-

---

*Johanssen: Acta. Orthop. Scandinav., 1932.
†Key, J. A.: Am. J. Surg., 1937.

tically to the surface at a point about 1 inch below Poupart's ligament and 1 inch lateral to the femoral artery. The needle can be felt to slip through the distended capsule and some sanguineous fluid can be aspirated when the point of the needle is in the joint. On two occasions it has been necessary to use gas during the reduction. One of us (H. E. C.) prefers spinal anesthesia or pentothal in most cases, preferably the latter.

Reduction.—The patient is then placed upon a fracture table and the sound limb is fixed to the traction apparatus in full abduction without undue tension and with just enough traction to hold the patient against the perineal post. The hip is then reduced by the Leadbetter method as follows: While an assistant fixes the pelvis by pressing downward upon the anterior superior spines, the surgeon flexes the hip and knee of the fractured leg to slightly beyond a right angle and, while maintaining it in a position of slight external rotation and slight abduction with moderate traction upward in the long axis of the femur, has a second assistant pull outward and downward on the upper portion of the thigh, thus tending to unlock the fragments and to stretch the capsule around them. The surgeon maintains the axial traction and circumducts the hip outward and downward, at the same time internally rotating it, thus bringing it downward to a position level with the table in moderate abduction and internally rotated to about 30°. Leadbetter's heel-palm test is then applied; that is, if the reduction has been successful it will be possible to maintain the limb in a position of internal rotation by simply resting the heel of the abducted leg on the surgeon's palm. If the reduction has not been successful, as soon as the foot is released, the extremity will roll outward into external rotation. If this occurs the reduction is repeated until the Leadbetter test is positive. The foot on the fractured side is then fixed to the traction apparatus of the table in a position of about 45° of internal rotation and moderate abduction, the abduction being maintained without undue tension and just enough traction being applied to hold the pelvis firmly against the perineal post.

First X-Ray.—At this point anteroposterior and lateral x-rays are taken. We have used the curved casette for the lateral x-rays. However, any method which gives a satisfactory lateral x-ray may be used, but we think it important that the patient not be moved again until the nail has been driven home. For the anteroposterior views a casette tunnel under the patient is useful.

Preparation of Patient and Local Anesthesia.—While the x-rays are being developed, the surgeon scrubs up and the operative field is prepared by an assistant and the patient is draped, and the skin and subcutaneous tissues down to include the periosteum over the lateral border of the femur from just above the trochanter downward a distance of about 8 inches are anesthetized with novocaine (1 per cent for the skin and ½ per cent for the deeper tissues and containing 3 drops adrenalin to the ounce). The first x-rays are developed by the time the surgeon is ready to begin the operation. Then, if the reduction is satisfactory, the operation is begun. If not, the reduction is repeated.

Operation.—An incision about 5 inches long is made over the lateral surface of the femur, the upper end of the incision being at about the tip of the trochanter and the incision extending straight downward along the lateral border of the thigh. This incision is carried down to the bone and through it the tip of the trochanter can be felt. Then, from the x-ray film the distance can be roughly measured on the outer border of the femur to reach a point from which a nail or drill inserted through the outer cortex, being directed parallel to the neck of the femur, will penetrate the center of the head. This point is about 1 inch below the base of the greater trochanter. The drill is then inserted at this point parallel with the table and directed upward at an angle corresponding roughly with that of the axis of the neck of the femur. We use an ordinary carpenter's hand drill and a $\frac{3}{16}$ of an inch twist drill 6 inches long. This is started just below where we think it should be, because our tendency is to put it a little high, and we give it just a little more angulation than we think is necessary, because our tendency is to put it too near a right angle with the shaft of the femur. The drill is inserted about 3 inches and is left in situ.

Second X-Rays.—The field is then covered with a sterile sheet and anteroposterior and lateral x-rays are again made. It is necessary to wait until these are developed before proceeding further.

Insertion of the Nail.—From the position of the drill the length of the nail desired for this particular hip is selected. It is, of course, not necessary that the drill penetrate to the cartilaginous margin of the head as due allowance can be made for any lack of penetration. Likewise, if the drill has been driven through the head into the acetabulum, as may occur, this can be allowed for. If the drill is in the correct position—that is, extends down the center of the neck, preferably just below its middle—it is pulled out, and it slips out easily with the fingers, and the nail is driven home along the drill hole. If, however, it is found that the drill is too high or too low or is pointed up or down toward the head or foot of the patient a little too much, or if it is pointed forward or backward a little too much, then the nail is not driven in parallel with the drill hole, but in such a direction that it will reach the vicinity of the center of the head of the femur.

If the surgeon has difficulty in fixing in his mind the direction of the drill during the slight interval when it is pulled out of the hole and the nail is started, then he should drive a nail or insert a small drill into the femur about an inch above or an inch below the drill while the drill is in situ as a guide while the Smith-Peterson nail is being driven parallel to this guide. If it has not been found to be in the desired position, then the guide acts as a line from which the correction can be made. It should be remembered that absolute mathematical accuracy in placing the nail is not necessary. All that is necessary is to get it through the neck and firmly into the head of the femur. After the nail has been driven home, the distal fragment is firmly impacted upon the head. For this the Smith-Petersen impactor is desirable, but if this is not at hand, a short length of $\frac{1}{2}$ inch metal pipe or the handle of a hammer or large chisel may be used.

Third X-Rays.—The field is again covered with a sheet and anteroposterior and lateral x-rays are made with the nail driven home and the fragments impacted. While these are being developed, the surgeon proceeds to close the wound, but asepsis is maintained until the final x-rays have been inspected, because if the final x-rays are not satisfactory, the wound can be opened and the nail extracted and reinserted if necessary. After the wound is closed and the dressing applied, the patient is placed in bed with a pillow under the knee.

The limb is not immobilized after the operation and the patient may sit up in bed immediately and up in a chair within two or three days. As soon as he is strong enough he may stand and bear some weight upon the leg or walk on crutches. These should be continued until at least three months after the operation and the nail should remain in for a year unless it gives trouble. If the nail does not give any trouble, there is no necessity for removing it at all.

A word should be said in regard to the reduction. It is not our belief that an anatomical reduction is necessary. We prefer a slight over-reduction of the fracture; that is, we would rather have the distal fragment displaced slightly downward so that the head tends to sit on the top of the neck, thus producing a slight coxa valga. This permits more thorough impaction than does an anatomical reduction and gives a better chance of union, because it tends to lessen the shearing force at the site of the fracture.

If the postoperative x-rays show the nail in only fairly good position (and this happens occasionally), we apply a rather light short abduction spica cast (extending to the lower thigh) and have the patient walk in this cast and use crutches for eight or ten weeks.

The Smith-Petersen-Johanssen Nail Technic.—In this method it is necessary to use the cannulated or Johanssen-Smith-Petersen nail. The hip is reduced as described above, only on an ordinary operating table, and with the knee flexed and the foot resting on a chair the moderately abducted leg is held in internal rotation by an assistant during the operation. The lateral x-rays are made with the tube on the opposite side of the table and the cassette is held against the side of the pelvis on the affected side.

The side of the femur is exposed as described above through a lateral incision. Three or four Kirschner wires are drilled into the femur, starting on the lateral surface one inch below the base of the trochanter, attempting to so direct them upward and inward that they will reach the center of the head of the femur.

New x-rays are made and from these the wire which most nearly approaches the center of the head is selected and the Johanssen-Smith-Petersen nail is threaded on this wire. The other wires are removed and the nail is driven home along the wire selected. Then this wire is removed, the fragments are impacted, final x-rays are made, and the wound is closed.

O'Meara's Method of Blind Nailing.—In this method the hip is reduced by the Leadbetter method, and after satisfactory x-rays in two planes have been obtained, the lateral surface of the femur is exposed through a lateral incision as described above and the Smith-Petersen nail of the proper length (the length having been determined from the x-rays of the sound hip) is started in the lateral surface of the shaft of the femur at a point about one inch below the base of the great trochanter and is directed upward and inward at an angle approximating that made by the neck with the shaft of the

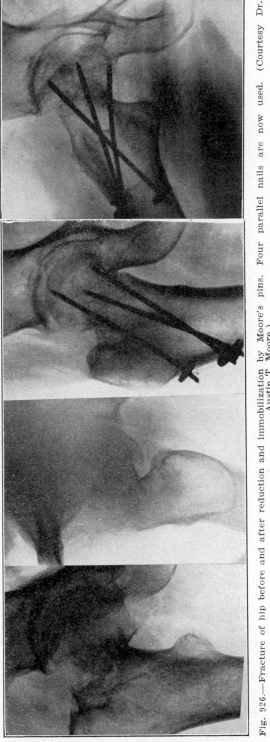

Fig. 926.—Fracture of hip before and after reduction and immobilization by Moore's pins. Four parallel nails are now used. (Courtesy Dr. Austin T. Moore.)

femur.   After the nail has been driven home the fragments are impacted
and x-rays in both the anteroposterior and lateral direction are made and the
wound is closed.   This is the simplest and the quickest method, provided the
surgeon has the requisite skill to drive the nail in the proper direction.

The use of the drill as a guide and the Johanssen method were devised
because considerable difficulty has been experienced by other surgeons in
directing the long nail so that it will become firmly fixed in the head of the
femur.   In place of the drill or wire we have inserted a long hypodermic

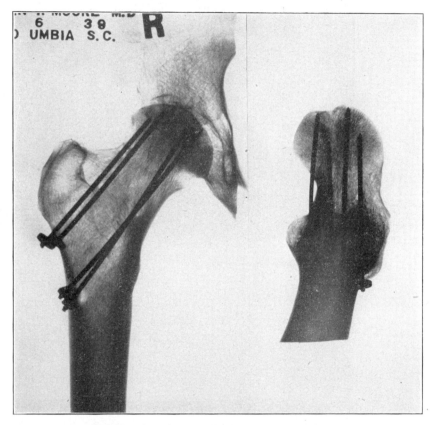

Fig. 927.—Properly placed nails according to Moore's present technique when using
Moore nails for treating fractures through the neck of the femur.   (Courtesy Dr. Austin
T. Moore.)

needle into the soft tissues, endeavoring to place it parallel with and anterior
to the neck of the femur, while Thornton and Sandison have placed a small
metal marker over the head of the femur and fastened it to the skin with adhesive before the post-reduction x-rays were made.   As stated above, other
surgeons have constructed mechanical guides to aid in directing the nail.   In
all of these methods after the nail is driven home the fragments are impacted
and then, if the final x-rays do not show satisfactory position of the nail, it
must be removed and reinserted.   It is extremely important that satisfactory
anteroposterior and lateral x-rays showing the nail in the head of the femur
be obtained before the patient is removed from the operating table.

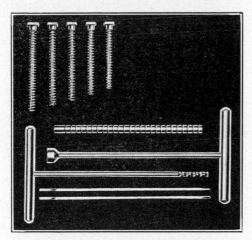

Fig. 928.—Instruments required for application of the lag screw. (See page 970.) (Courtesy Lorenzo, F. A.: Surg., Gynec., and Obst., July, 1941.)

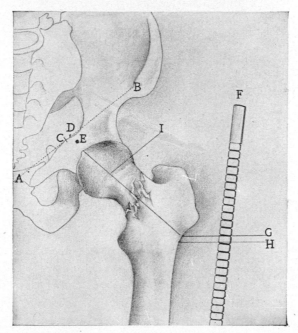

Fig. 929.—A to B is a line drawn from the symphysis pubis to the anterior superior spine of the ilium. This line is bisected at C ¼ inch externally from C toward B. One-quarter inch immediately below D, a dot is drawn which is E. This dot represents the middle of the head of the femur. The measuring rod F, marked by quarter inches, is in a plane parallel to the femur. G represents the point immediately below the great trochanter at the middle of the shaft of the femur for the introduction of the first Kirschner wire. H represents a point ½ inch below G. This point is for the introduction of the second Kirschner wire, to run parallel to the first wire. In order to get the proper length screw for the immobilization of the fracture, measurement is taken from the middle of the head of the femur—point G, immediately below the great trochanter, represented by line I. This measurement is superimposed upon the measuring rod and in this manner the number of quarter inches are counted on the marker, giving the correct measurement for the length of the screw necessary for the immobilization of the fracture. (Courtesy Lorenzo, F. A.: Surg., Gynec., and Obst., July, 1941.)

Austin T. Moore's Method.—One of us (H. E. C.) prefers the method of internal fixation by the use of four threaded pins as described by Dr. Austin T. Moore (Fig. 926). The modified technic is as follows:*

"The patient is placed on a fracture table with a cassette and proper padding beneath the patient. The fracture is reduced by the Whitman-Leadbetter technic. Radiographic checks are then made, always taking lateral and anteroposterior views. If reduction has been accomplished an incision about 4 inches long is made directly over the great trochanter, the four nails are driven in parallel to each other, and radiographic rechecks with the same technic as described above are carried out. If the nails are found to be properly applied, the distal fragment is impacted against the proximal fragment,

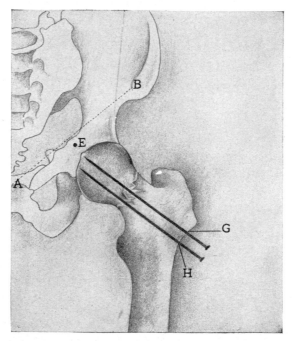

Fig. 930.—Two 3/32-inch Kirschner wires have been introduced in a parallel plane. G represents the wire in the center of the shaft of the head of the femur. H represents the second Kirschner wire which is 1/2 inch below the first Kirschner wire or G. These wires are introduced for stabilizing the fracture. G, the first Kirschner wire, or central wire, acts as a guide over which the screw is introduced. (Courtesy Lorenzo, F. A.: Surg., Gynec., and Obst., July, 1941.)

the nuts are then screwed up and the nails are gently tapped, a small wire is applied around the nails and the nails are then cut away near the nuts and the wound is closed. Nothing but a gauze-adhesive dressing is applied. The patient is allowed to move about in bed at will. It is insisted that he sit up in a semireclining position by the second day and he usually is out of bed in a wheel chair on the fourth or fifth day, and going home by the eighth or tenth day.

"No weight-bearing should be allowed until radiographic checks show a continuity of the bone and a disappearance of the fracture line which seldom takes place before three months following the operation. The usual radio-

*Conwell and Sherill: The Southern Surgeon 6: 194, 1937. Internal Fixation of Intracapsular Fractures of the Neck of the Femur.

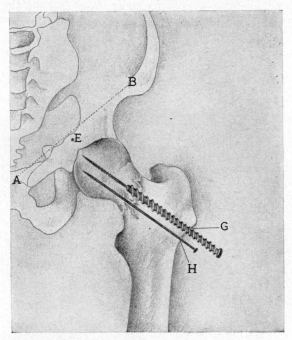

Fig. 931.—The two parallel Kirschner wires are in position and the screw is being introduced over the first Kirschner wire G. (Courtesy Lorenzo, F. A.: Surg., Gynec., and Obst., July, 1941.)

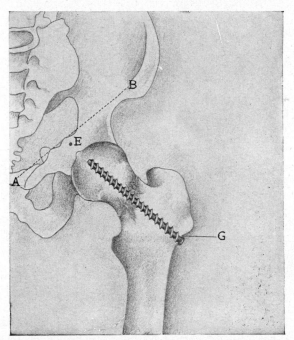

Fig. 932.—The screw is in position and the fragments are immobilized. The two parallel Kirschner wires, *G*, and *H*, have been withdrawn. (Courtesy Lorenzo, F. A.: Surg., Gynec., and Obst., July, 1941.)

graphic findings when union occurs in these cases is that there is a definite continuity of bone tissue and a disappearance of the fracture line. No external callus is present. Frequent radiographic checks should be made of the fracture following weight-bearing and the patient should be able to discard all supports within four or five months following internal fixation in the average fracture.''

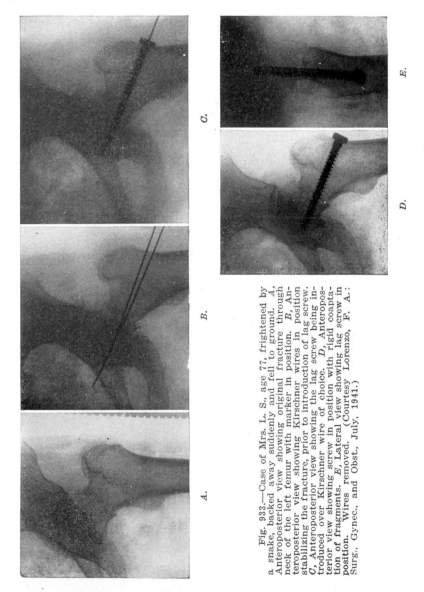

Fig. 933.—Case of Mrs. L. S., age 77, frightened by a snake, backed away suddenly and fell to ground. A, Anteroposterior view showing original fracture through neck of the left femur with marker in position. B, Anteroposterior view showing Kirschner wires in position stabilizing the fracture, prior to introduction of lag screw. C, Anteroposterior view showing the lag screw being introduced over Kirschner wire of choice. D, Anteroposterior view showing screw in position with rigid coaptation of fragments. E, Lateral view showing lag screw in position. Wires removed. (Courtesy Lorenzo, F. A.: Surg., Gynec., and Obst., July, 1941.)

Lag Screw for Internal Fixation of the Neck of the Femur.—Since the introduction of the Smith-Petersen nail, other methods of fixation have been devised. One of the most efficient of these is a lag screw of which several have been devised, both here and abroad. In this country the lag screws devised by Henderson and by Lorenzo are the most widely used. The lag screw (Figs. 928-

933) is inserted by the closed method over the heavy Kirschner wire ($\frac{3}{32}$ of an inch) just as is the Smith-Petersen nail, except that it is screwed rather than driven into the head of the femur. When properly inserted it holds the fragments firmly together.

With the use of local anesthesia and the lateral incision, the Smith-Petersen nail can be inserted with little shock and may be regarded as a conservative procedure, because it can be used on patients who are very poor operative risks and in whom the prognosis would be poor if they were immobilized in a large spica cast. As soon as the operation is finished, the patient may sit up in bed, and if it is desired, he may be got up in a chair or on crutches within a few days. Experience has shown that the nail is well tolerated by the tissues, and the danger of infection is no greater than in other surgical procedures.

The Open Treatment of Fracture of the Neck of the Femur

Open Reduction and Nailing.—This is the method originally used by Smith-Petersen, and he used his anterolateral approach. The technic has been simplified by Cubbins, Scuderi and Callahan and others who use a simpler incision. One of us (J. A. K.) prefers this method and usually performs the operation under local anesthesia.

The skin incision begins about an inch posterior to the anterior superior spine of the ilium and extends downward and backward to cross the midline of the thigh about three inches below the tip of the greater trochanter. The anterior border of the tensor fascia femoris is isolated and separated from the sartorius and the external circumflex vessels are ligated and cut. The lower portion of the tensor fascia femoris or, preferably, the iliotibial band just below the insertion of the muscle is cut across.

The dissection is then carried down through the deep fat to expose the anterior surface of the capsule of the hip joint. The fat is wiped off with gauze and the capsule is opened longitudinally and transversely to expose the fracture. The displacement is then reduced by traction and internal rotation and leverage if necessary. With reduction maintained by full internal rotation the vastus lateralis is split to expose the shaft of the femur below the base of the trochanter and a guide drill is started in this area and so directed that it will emerge through the center of the neck at the site of the fracture.

When the drill has been inserted to the proper depth the extremity is externally rotated to expose the point of the drill. If it is not in approximately the center of the neck its direction is changed to get it in the desired position.

The extremity is again internally rotated and with the fracture reduced a Smith-Petersen nail of suitable length is selected (about $\frac{1}{2}$ of an inch longer than the distance from the drill hole in the shaft to the rim of the acetabulum). The drill is then removed and the nail driven in the same direction. When the point of the nail has reached the line of the fracture the extremity is externally rotated and the point of the nail is inspected. If it is not in a satisfactory position its direction is changed accordingly.

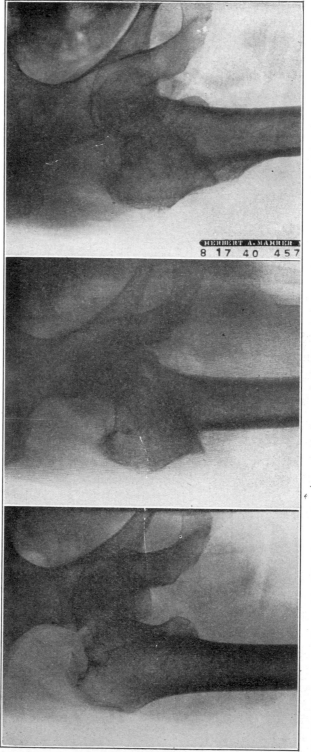

Fig. 934.—Fracture of the neck of the femur with nonunion. Treated by oblique osteotomy and immobilization in a plaster-of-Paris cast which was followed by union. (Courtesy Dr. Rudolph Reich, Cleveland.)

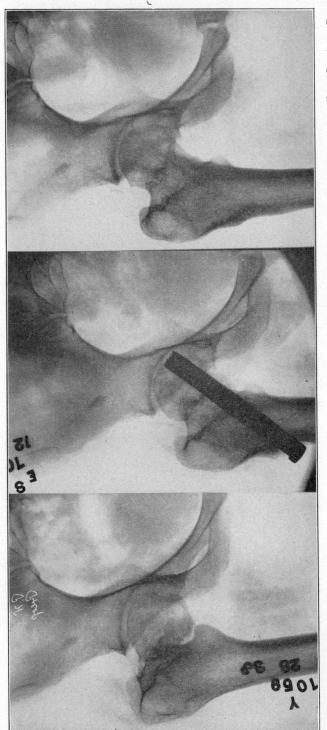

Fig. 935.—Nonunion of the neck of the femur, nineteen months' duration. Treated by application of Smith-Petersen nail. (Courtesy Dr. Smith-Petersen.)

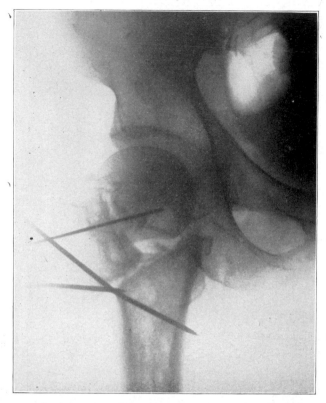

Fig. 936.—Old nonunion of hip treated by osteotomy and external skeletal fixation with small pins. Pins were removed at the end of four weeks.

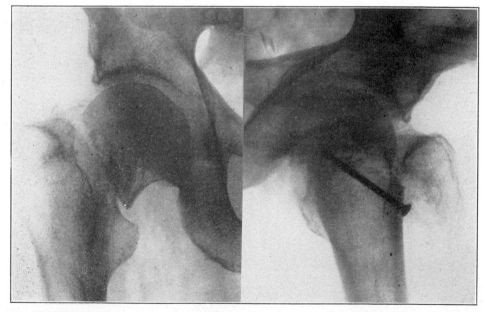

Fig. 937.—Old fracture of the hip with nonunion. Treated by modified Brackett operation.

The extremity is again internally rotated, the fracture is reduced accurately, the nail is driven home, and the fragments are impacted. The stability of the hip is then tested and anteroposterior and lateral x-rays are made. While these are being developed, the wound is closed.

If the x-rays do not show a satisfactory position of the nail, the wound is opened immediately and the position of the nail is changed.

Fibrous Union of the Neck of the Femur

In a considerable percentage of the cases of fracture through the neck of the femur in which bony union is not obtained the fragments become united by dense fibrous tissue which is strong enough to support the body weight. These hips are not normal, but many of them are relatively free from pain and quite stable, and the patients are able to walk a moderate amount with a crutch or with the use of a cane. Pain can be relieved temporarily by rest in bed or by rest in bed with moderate traction.

Operative Treatment of Nonunion of the Neck of the Femur

Nonunion of the neck of the femur is still a problem. If the head of the femur is viable, it should be left in the acetabulum and an attempt made to secure union by a Brackett operation or by a high oblique or McMurray osteotomy or by a Smith-Petersen nail and bone graft. If the head is dead a high oblique osteotomy may be performed or it should be removed and a Whitman or Colonna reconstruction performed. Usually the head is living and occasionally it is in such good condition that freshing of the surfaces and fixing with a Smith-Petersen nail may obtain union.

The High Oblique Osteotomy.—This has been used extensively by Reich (J. Bone & Joint Surg., January, 1941) in this country and his reports are very encouraging. The operation is similar to that used by McMurray (Brit. J. Surg., **22**: 716, 1935).

If there is marked coxa vara or upward displacement of the distal fragment, this is partly corrected by preliminary traction. Usually this is not necessary.

The patient is placed on a fracture table, and the legs are fixed by the foot supports, with the involved extremity in slight abduction and moderate internal rotation. The incision on the lateral surface of the thigh extends directly downward from the top of the trochanter for four or five inches. This incision is carried down to the side of the femur and a wire or drill is inserted to determine the site of the osteotomy. It is desired to section the femur obliquely just below the greater and above the lesser trochanter. The section extends upward and inward at an angle of from 20 to 30 degrees.

After the wire or drill has been inserted, an anteroposterior x-ray is taken to determine the position of the wire. Then, using this as a guide, the femur is cut across with a sharp thin osteotome. The section should be complete. The proximal end of the distal fragment is then pushed or levered inward about ½ of an inch and the extremity is abducted to about 30 degrees, and the wound is closed.

A plaster-of-Paris spica cast is then applied with the hip and knee in a position of slight flexion. Reich recommends that the spica be left on for from six to eight weeks and McMurray three months. The patient is then gotten up on crutches.

One of us (J. A. K.) has modified the above procedure by using two stainless steel screws to hold the fragments in position. The operation is done on an ordinary operating table, and the incision begins anterior to the top of the trochanter and extends down and back for four or five inches. This exposes the front and lateral side of the trochanteric region of the femur, and the space between the lesser trochanter and the neck of the femur is felt and marked by a blunt dissector. Then, using this as a guide, the oblique osteotomy is performed and the distal fragment is displaced inward and the limb abducted about 30 degrees.

This brings the tip of the proximal fragment down over the lateral side of the distal fragment, and it is fixed to the lateral cortex by a short stainless steel screw. A large (3½ inch) screw is then passed through the trochanter and fixed in the inner cortex of the distal fragment.

Plaster boots are then applied and united by a cross bar to maintain abduction and internal rotation. In from four to six weeks union is sufficiently firm to permit removal of the boots, and a week or so later the patient is gotten up on crutches.

The elimination of the spica cast permits the patient to sit up in bed and flex the knees and hips and the convalescence is shortened. In some instances a small triangle of bone is removed from the distal cut surface of the proximal fragment in order to facilitate the internal fixation.

The Schanz Osteotomy.—Gaenslen and Schumm have shown excellent results in cases of nonunion of the neck of the femur after performing a cuneiform osteotomy just below the great trochanter and abducting the distal fragment. The position of the fragments is controlled by a large spike screwed into each fragment and the ends of these spikes project through the wound and are fixed in a clamp. The hip is then immobilized in a plaster spica until union has occurred (eight to ten weeks). As soon as the hip is strong enough, the patient begins to bear weight on the extremity. The shearing force has now been changed to a push upward against the head and union occurs in about six months.

Reconstruction Operation With a Smith-Petersen Nail.—During the past few years one of us (J. A. K.) has been using an operation which has given good results in the few cases on which it has been tried. The anterolateral incision is used as described above and the greater trochanter is cut off as in the Whitman procedure. Then the lesser trochanter is cut off in order to mobilize the upper end of the femur. The pseudarthrosis is then cut across and the stump of the neck is turned out and all fibrous tissue is removed down to bleeding bone. The fibrous tissue is then removed from the head of the femur and this is slightly cupped, as in the Brackett procedure, and the stump of the neck is fitted into the head and fixed firmly with a short Smith-Petersen nail. The head is placed slightly on top of the neck. Then the greater trochanter is reattached to the shaft at a lower level. The patient is put to bed with the limb in abduction in a Thomas splint for four weeks and then got up on crutches.

Where there is a fairly long neck, the trochanter is not detached, and in some instances an autogenous tibial graft is inserted below and parallel to the nail.

Postoperatively the limb is fixed in abduction and internal rotation by plaster boots fixed to a crossbar. This permits the patient to sit up and is more comfortable than a plaster spica cast.

Immobilization is continued for from four to eight weeks or more, depending upon how well the nail has gripped the fragments.

The Whitman Reconstruction Operation for Nonunion of the Neck of the Femur can be performed more easily and quickly and with less shock to the patient than can the nailing or pegging operation, and the after-treatment is greatly shortened. These factors are not true as regards osteotomy of the femur. Consequently, it is especially useful in older patients. Its main objection is that the hip may be expected to be quite stiff and not entirely free from pain. However, in the majority of cases a very serviceable hip can be obtained. (Figs. 938 and 939.)

The operation is performed as follows: We use the anterolateral incision as described under the Smith-Petersen operation; that is, an anterior incision which begins at the anterior superior spine, is carried down about six inches, and then swung outward and backward for about two inches across the iliotibial band, and from the upper end an incision is carried backward along the crest of the ilium for about four or five inches. These incisions are carried down to the bone, the tensor fascia femoris tendon is severed from its origin on the ilium, and the anterior portion of the gluteal muscles are raised from the ilium with a periosteal elevator, and the entire flap is retracted outward, thus exposing the upper end of the femur and the hip joint. At this point we cut across the base of the great trochanter. We then open the capsule of the hip by a T incision, the capsule being cut longitudinally with a cross incision parallel to the rim of the acetabulum. This exposes the fracture and the head of the femur.

The head of the femur is then removed. This is facilitated by cutting the ligamentum teres and slipping a large gouge behind the head and prying it outward as the limb is externally rotated. After the head is removed the proximal end of the neck is rounded off and if the neck is completely absorbed the proximal end of the shaft is rounded off, the capsule being stripped up, so that the end of the neck or shaft can be placed in the acetabulum as the limb is abducted. When the upper end of the femur is thus prepared it is placed in the acetabulum and the limb is fully abducted and rotated slightly inward. The flap is then retracted to expose the lateral surface of the shaft of the femur.

Two small holes are bored in the trochanter and this is then pulled downward on the shaft as far as the gluteal muscles will permit it to come with the limb in a position of abduction and the point on the shaft is noted. A horse-shoe-shaped incision is then made in the periosteum on the shaft of the femur and the periosteal flap is turned down. Beneath this two small holes are bored in the shaft of the femur at the same level and a heavy chromic catgut or wire suture is placed through these holes and through the separated trochanter. This is then sutured down against the shaft and the flap of periosteum is sutured over the trochanter.

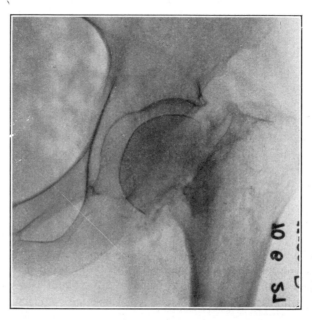

Fig. 938.—Nonunion of the neck of the femur with a dead head.

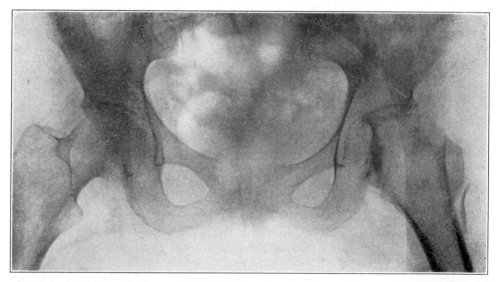

Fig. 939.—Same hip as shown in Fig. 938, after Whitman reconstruction operation. Two years after operation this patient's hip was stable and painless and had a moderate range of movement.

The hip is now inspected to see that the proximal end of the distal fragment is in the acetabulum, and the capsule is closed snugly over it and without changing the position of the extremity the wound is closed in layers and a large plaster-of-Paris spica jacket is applied to hold the limb in the position of abduction.

Colonna dissects the muscle attachments from the great trochanter, removes the head and any stump of the neck which may be left, inserts the tip of the trochanter into the acetabulum, and reattaches the abductor muscles at a lower level onto the shaft of the femur.

Aftertreatment.—As soon as the plaster is dry x-ray pictures are taken through the plaster to be sure that the upper end of the femur is still resting in the acetabulum. If it is not, the plaster should be removed and an attempt be made to manipulate the femur into its proper place. It may even be necessary to reopen the hip.

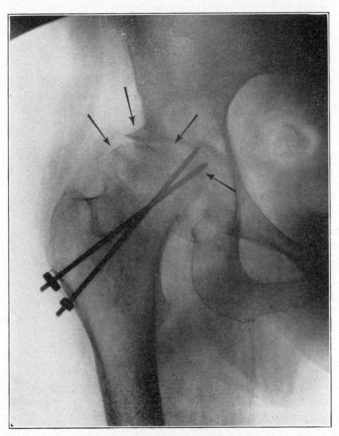

Fig. 940.—Late results of a fracture through the neck of the femur with necrosis of the head of the femur two years later. Originally this patient had a fracture through the middle third of the neck of the femur which was properly reduced and four Moore nails were applied with good union. A necrosis of the head of the femur developed which necessitated the removal of two of the nails and later the remaining two. Fair result.

If the position is satisfactory, the plaster cast is left on for four weeks. At the end of this time the cast is removed, the limb is placed in a Thomas splint with from five to ten pounds of traction, the patient is permitted to move the hip and knee daily, but the abduction position is maintained. This active and passive movement of the leg is kept up in bed over a period of from two to four weeks. The patient is then got up on crutches which are gradually discarded as soon as the hip is stable.

As was stated above, this operation does not result in a perfect hip, but if it is properly performed, the result is far better than that obtained by fibrous union.

Aseptic Necrosis of the Head of the Femur.—A late and very disabling complication of fractures through the neck of the femur is aseptic necrosis of the femoral head. This is believed to be due to a disturbance in the blood supply of the proximal fragment which occurred at the time of the injury. This loss of the blood supply causes death of that portion of the bone which was deprived of its nutrition. If union occurs, the dead bone is gradually absorbed and replaced by living bone (creeping replacement). This occurs several months or even a year or more after the injury. During this process the head of the femur may become softened and deformed or may disintegrate to a variable degree.

This deformity and disintegration of the head appears to be aggravated by weight bearing. The result is a hip which is painful on weight bearing and in which the range of movement is limited. Recent papers by John Wilson (J. Bone & Joint Surg. **22**: 53, 1940) and Brandon Carrell and W. B. Carrell (Ibid. **23**: 225, 1941) indicate that aseptic necrosis is much more apt to occur in fractures through the neck of the femur in children and adolescents than in adults.

Treatment.—The subsequent course of patients with fractures of the neck of the femur should be followed by the surgeon, and at the first sign of pain or stiffness or increasing disability new x-rays should be made and activity and weight-bearing restricted.

If the x-rays show areas of rarefaction in the head of the femur and areas of apparently increased density (necrotic bone in an atrophic head), weight bearing should be prohibited, and if union is firm, the nail should be removed.

If the head collapses and becomes markedly deformed, an arthroplasty with Smith-Petersen's vitallium cup offers the best chance for a useful joint.

Treatment of Trochanteric Fractures of the Femur

The problem in the treatment of these fractures is not to obtain union, because practically all of them unite by almost any form of treatment, but to prevent malunion with a coxa vara deformity (Figs. 944 and 945). Consequently in contrast to the fractures through the neck of the femur the trochanteric fractures can be treated either by immobilization or by traction, depending upon the choice of the surgeon. Just as in the neck fractures, however, these injuries tend to occur in old people and the first duty of the surgeon is to save the life of the patient. For this reason many of these cases have been permitted to go without treatment.

We believe, however, that the mortality is greater without treatment than if the fracture is immobilized by traction or by means of a plaster cast. Consequently, we feel that the fracture should be actively treated, not only in order to obtain a perfect result, but also in order to make the patient more comfortable.

It is to be noted that patients with trochanteric fractures of the femur are on the average about five years older than are patients with fractures through the neck of the femur. Also, the trochanteric fracture is accompanied by more pain and surgical shock. Consequently, the mortality in trochanteric fractures is much higher than is that in fractures through the neck of the femur.

Because of the high mortality we have discontinued immobilization of trochanteric fractures in a plaster-of-Paris spica with or without traction, as advised in former editions, and in our own practice no longer use traction in bed with the Thomas or Hodgen splints. We usually use internal fixation with a nail with a plate attached or well-leg fixation with a splint or cast.

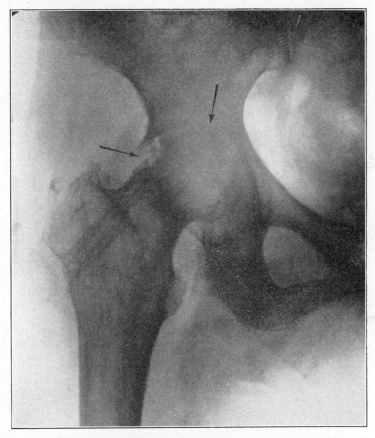

Fig. 941.—Old fracture through the neck of the femur which was properly reduced and fixed with Moore nails and good union, but developed a degenerative change of the head of the femur three years later with an aseptic necrosis. This is the type of complication which happens in a small percentage of cases even though properly reduced and properly fixed by internal fixation soon after injury.

We operate upon an increasing percentage of our trochanteric fractures and fix the fragments with a Neufeld nail or with the Moore or Blount blade plate. Others we treat with one of the well-leg traction splints or with well-leg fixation after manipulative reduction under a brief general anesthetic.

The Internal Fixation of Trochanteric Fractures.—The difficulty in nailing trochanteric fractures is that the proximal end of the distal fragment may be comminuted by the original injury or may be split by the surgeon attempting to drive the nail through the lateral cortex of the femur. Finally, the grip of the nail or of the pins or lag screw on the distal fragment is much less secure than is that when a fracture through the neck of the femur is nailed. This has been partly obviated by fixing a plate to the head of the nail, and the plate is fixed to the shaft of the femur.

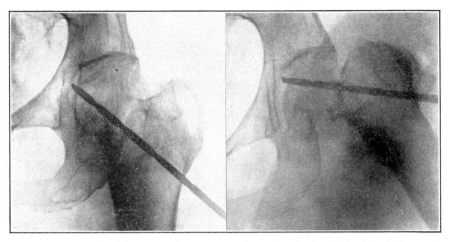

Fig. 942.—Trochanteric fracture, anteroposterior and lateral views, showing the guiding drill in position.

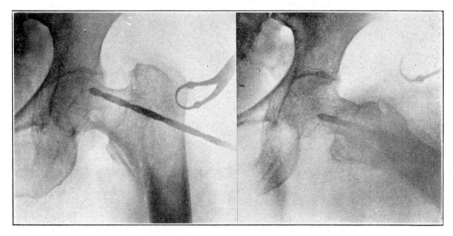

Fig. 943.—Trochanteric fracture incompletely reduced, with guiding drill in position. Drill is too high.

Viewed from the standpoint of the operative procedure, trochanteric fractures fall into three groups:

1. Fractures through the base of the neck or trochanteric region with little or no visible comminution or displacement. These require no manipulative reduction and can be nailed or pinned blindly or by whatever method the surgeon chooses, and the operation can be done through the straight lateral incision. These are treated as are fractures through the neck of the femur, except that the novocain is placed around the fracture and not in the hip joint and a chan-

nel is cut through the lateral cortex for the nail, and the fragments are impacted very gently. The final position of the nail is checked by anteroposterior and lateral x-rays taken before the wound is closed and developed while the wound is being sutured.

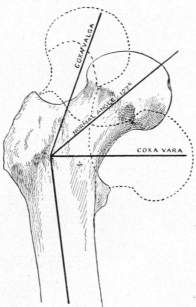

Fig. 944.—Normal angle of head and neck of the femur to the shaft of the femur with the alteration in position in coxa valga and coxa vara shown by dotted lines. (Davis: *Applied Anatomy.*)

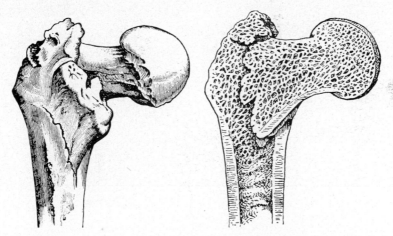

Fig. 945.—Impacted extracapsular trochanteric fracture of the neck of the femur. (Von Bergman: *System of Surgery*, after Lossen.)

2. The usual trochanteric fracture with considerable separation and comminution, but with the lateral cortex of the shaft of the femur intact up to or beyond a point about in line with the superior surface of the neck of the femur. After manipulative reduction these are nailed through a lateral incision or by direct exposure through an oblique incision as is described below, using a nail with a plate attached (Thornton, Moore, Blount or Neufeld).

3. Fractures involving the lateral cortex of the femur below the level of the line through the superior surface of the neck of the femur. These are really subtrochanteric fractures and can be fixed with a nail with a long plate attached.

Unless the patient is in a condition of shock, the operation is performed as soon after the patient is admitted to the hospital as possible. Before the patient is removed from bed, 20 to 30 c.c. of 1 per cent solution of novocain is injected into the hematoma at the site of the fracture. This can be done by directing the needle downward and inward on the anterolateral surface of the thigh at the level of the fracture and aiming at the line of the fracture as determined by the x-ray. When the needle is in the hematoma, blood can be drawn back into the syringe. Then the patient is placed on a fracture table with a tunnel under him to facilitate placing the carrier for the x-ray films under the hip. The entire limb is painted with tincture of merthiolate or iodine and the foot is fixed to the traction apparatus.

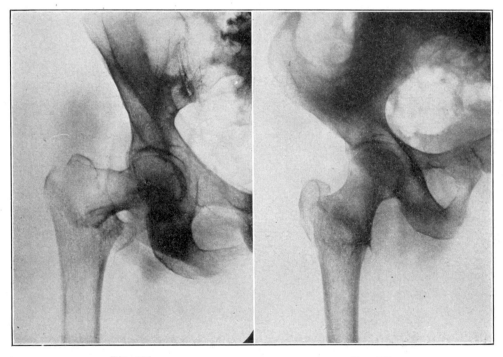

Fig. 946.   Fig. 947.

Fig. 946.—Trochanteric fracture with moderate displacement.
Fig. 947.—Same as Fig. 946 five days after well-leg fixation.

The skin is infiltrated in the line of the incision with 1 per cent novocain which contains three drops of adrenalin to the ounce. Then the deeper tissues are infiltrated with 0.5 per cent novocain which also contains three drops of adrenalin to the ounce. After the skin and deeper tissues have been infiltrated with novocain, the extremity is rotated inward to about 30 degrees beyond the mid-position. If the fragments are displaced, mechanical traction is made on the extremity, and then it is rotated inward about 30 degrees and abducted about 30 degrees. The limb is maintained in this position until the nail has been driven home into the head of the femur. The lateral x-rays are taken with a curved cassette or by elevating the opposite extremity.

The straight lateral incision begins on the lateral surface of the thigh opposite the tip of the trochanter and extends downward for about ten inches. It is carried down through the deep fascia to expose the lateral surface of the trochanter and the vastus lateralis muscle. This muscle is split in its upper five inches, and its origin is cut from the side of the trochanter to expose the lateral surface of the femur below the trochanter.

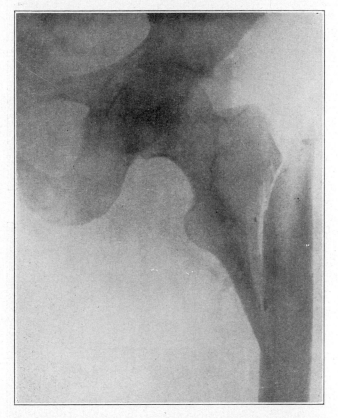

Fig. 948.—Trochanteric fracture of the femur with lesser trochanter attached to upper fragment. Treated by reduction under an anesthetic, abduction adhesive traction with leg and thigh in Thomas splint and Pearson knee flexion for ten weeks. Walking in caliper splint four weeks later. Good result. Patient resumed work in five and one-half months.

The anterior surface of the trochanteric region and the base of the neck now can be palpated, and it is possible to determine roughly the accuracy of the reduction and the position of the neck and head of the femur. If the reduction is not satisfactory, the limb can be manipulated again while the surgeon's finger palpates the line of the fracture. It is to be noted that the smaller fragments and the lesser trochanter are ignored and that one attempts only to restore the two major fragments to a satisfactory functional position.

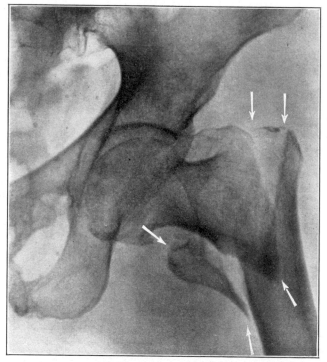

A.

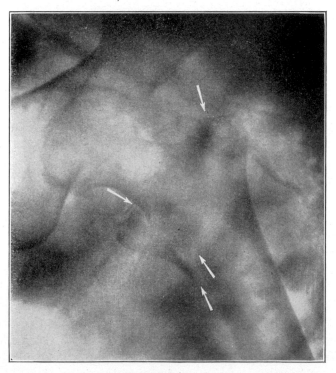

B.

Fig. 949.—Trochanteric fracture before and after reduction treated by skeletal traction through lower end of the femur for eight weeks and a short plaster spica cast for four weeks. (H. E. C. prefers this type treatment in such cases.)

At a point as low down on the lateral surface of the shaft as is consistent with passing the nail through the neck of the femur, a $\frac{3}{16}$ of an inch drill is inserted for a distance of about 3 inches. This point is about 1 inch below the base of the trochanter and the drill is directed upward and inward toward the center of the head, as determined by palpation and the preoperative x-rays. If reduction by traction has been necessary, due allowance for this is made in directing the drill. The direction of the drill in the anteroposterior plane is controlled by keeping the drill horizontal, since the long axis of the neck of the femur lies approximately in the horizontal plane when the foot is rotated inward about 30 degrees.

With the drill point in place and binding the two major fragments together, anteroposterior and lateral x-rays now are made. While these films are being developed, the drill is removed and the exact length of the drill point which has entered the bone is noted, as this will aid in determining the length of nail to be used in this case. Now, with a small thin osteotome, two channels are cut for the flanges of the Neufeld nail. This cutting of the channels must be done carefully and gently; otherwise, one may split the cortex. When completed they should permit driving the nail with relatively little resistance. After the channels have been completed, the drill is reinserted and with this size drill no difficulty is encountered in pushing it back into the hole in the head, if the extremity has not been moved while it was out.

If the x-rays show the drill to be pointing in the proper direction, it is withdrawn and a Neufeld nail or blade plate of the proper length is driven home into the head of the femur, directing it as nearly as possible in the line taken by the drill. If the surgeon has difficulty in keeping this line in mind while the nail is being substituted for the drill, a small drill can be placed in the shaft about $\frac{1}{2}$ of an inch from and parallel to the drill which is directed toward the head of the femur, and this can then be used as a guide in directing the nail. The length of nail desired is determined by adding the distance of the tip of the drill from the articular surface of the head, as seen in the x-rays, to the length of the drill which penetrated the bone.

If the position of the drill is not satisfactory, then the nail is started in the drill hole with the two channels for the flanges of the nail cut around it and is not driven in the direction taken by the drill, but is tilted up or down or forward or backward as much as necessary to direct it toward the center of the head of the femur and is then driven home. The fragments are then impacted very gently and anteroposterior and lateral x-rays are made. The plate attached to the nail or blade is clamped against the shaft of the femur and fixed to the shaft with screws. The wound is closed without drainage, and if the position of the nail is found to be satisfactory, no external fixation is necessary.

If the final x-rays show that the nail is not fixed firmly in the head of the femur, the wound is opened immediately and the nail is withdrawn and driven in again in the corrected direction.

Reduction and Well-Leg Fixation.—A method which one of us (J. A. K.) has been using for several years may be termed reduction and well-leg fixation.

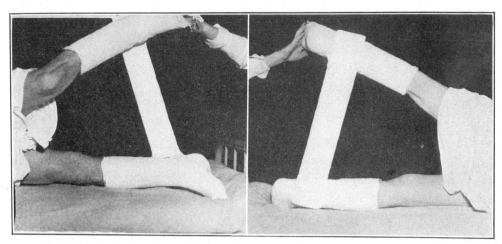

Fig. 950.—Plaster boots united by crossbar to immobilize the hip in abduction and internal rotation as used after nailing of intertrochanteric fractures in which adequate fixation has not been obtained.

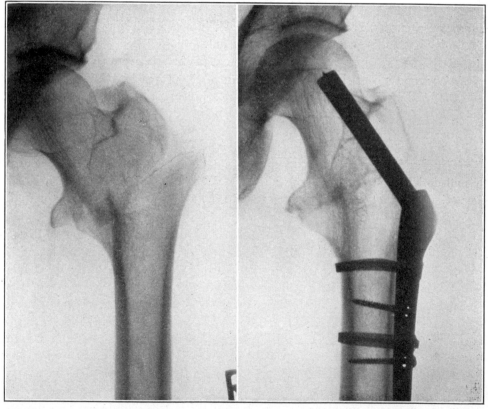

Fig. 951 A.—Trochanteric fracture fixed by open reduction and a Smith Petersen nail with bone plate attached.   (Courtesy Dr. Lawson Thornton, Atlanta, Ga.)

It is a modification of the well-leg traction method, but has the advantage that the fixation is more rigid and the patients appear to be more comfortable and can be turned on the face with greater ease if this is necessary. Also, the only apparatus required is two boards, one two feet and the other three feet long. The method is as follows (Fig. 959) :

Under local anesthesia a Kirschner wire or Steinman pin is drilled through the lower third of the tibia on the side of the fracture. Well-padded plaster casts are then applied to each leg. On the side of the fracture the plaster boot extends only to the middle of the leg, because if it stops at the upper third of the leg it may cause pressure on the peroneal nerve where it winds around the fibula. One of us (J. A. K.) has seen three instances from well-leg traction. Or it should extend above the knee.

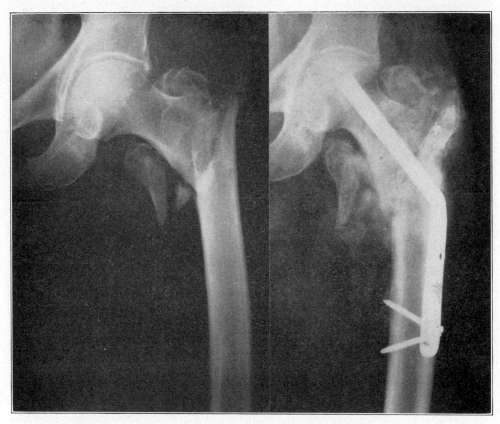

Fig. 951 B.—Shows comminuted fracture intertrochanteric of the femur with displacement. Neufeld nail applied with an abundant callus formation. (Courtesy Dr. Taylor, Neufeld, and Pelka.)

On the well leg the sole and lateral side of the foot are padded with felt over the sheet cotton and the plaster extends to the upper third of the thigh and is applied with the foot dorsiflexed and everted and with the hip adducted.

As soon as the plasters have set the fracture is reduced and fixed by anchoring the abducted injured extremity to the adducted normal extremity. For this a brief general anesthetic is desirable, but local anesthesia may be used. When local anesthesia is used, the novocain should be injected into the hematoma at the beginning of the procedure before the casts are applied. When general anesthesia is used it is not started until after the plasters have set.

The reduction is accomplished by manual traction, abduction, and internal rotation of the fractured extremity. This is maintained while the sound extremity is adducted and a board two feet long and about three inches wide is bound to the lower portions of the two casts with plaster-of-Paris bandages, and a similar board three feet long is fixed to the lower part of the injured leg and back of the thigh of the well leg.

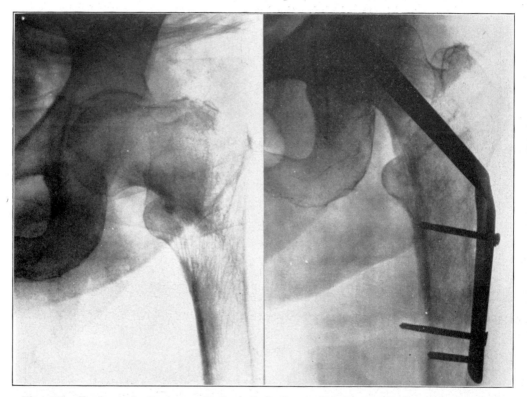

Fig. 952.—Trochanteric fracture with typical displacement before and after reduction with traction and internal rotation and fixation with a Neufeld nail.

The two boards act like the frame of a garden gate and maintain the position of adduction of the sound leg and abduction of the fractured extremity.

This cast is left on for from eight to twelve weeks, depending upon the type of fracture.

Treatment of Trochanteric Fractures of the Femur by Means of the Well-Leg Traction Splint.—The use of the well leg for countertraction is a principle which has been used by Hoke for many years and later by Jones, but the popularization of the method and the construction of a satisfactory splint

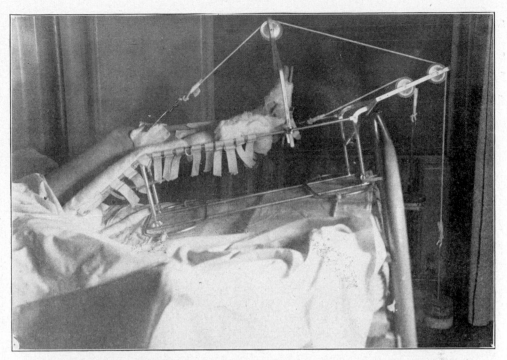

Fig. 953.—Trochanteric fracture of the femur under treatment with skeletal traction and Boehler-Braun splint. Excellent method for treating these cases where operative reduction and internal fixations are contraindicated. (Courtesy Dr. Joseph Lembeck.)

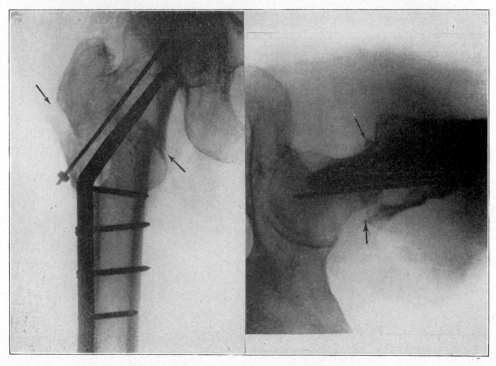

Fig. 954.—Blount blade plate internal fixation for an intertrochanteric fracture of the femur. (Courtesy Dr. W. B. Blount.)

for the purpose are the work of Roger Anderson. There are now several types of splints on the market which are modifications of Roger Anderson's splint.

The splint is fixed to the sound leg by means of a well-padded plaster cast which extends well above the knee and is applied with the hip adducted,

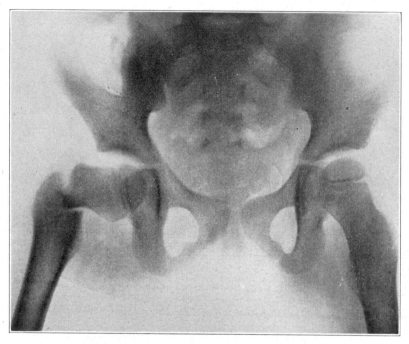

Fig. 955 *A.*—Trochanteric fracture of the femur in a boy eight years old. (Courtesy Dr. J. D. Sherrill.)

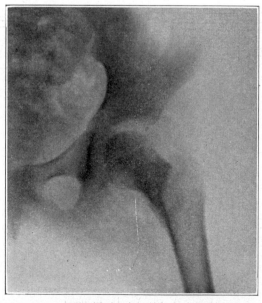

Fig. 955 *B.*—Same case as shown in Fig. 955 *A* after reduction by manipulation and immobilization in a plaster spica for sixteen weeks. Good union and good functional results.

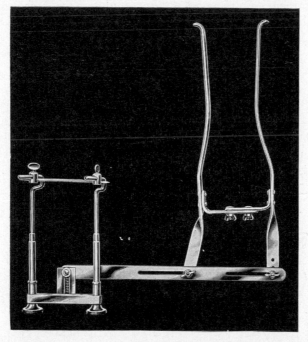

Fig. 956.—Well-leg traction splint. (Courtesy Zimmer Manufacturing Company.)

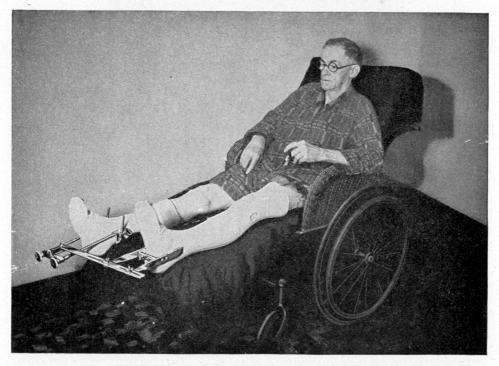

Fig. 957.—Well-leg traction splint as applied for trochanteric fracture, right.

the knee straight, and the foot at a right angle. Then a Kirschner wire or pin is drilled through the lower fourth of the tibia of the injured limb and this is encased in a plaster boot. The free arm of the splint is then attached to the wire or pin by means of a stirrup, and as the screw adjustment is tightened, pressure is made upward on the well leg and traction is made on the injured leg. This pressure and pull are transmitted to the pelvis, and the well leg is adducted while the injured leg is abducted. Rotation is controlled by a set screw on the stirrup for the injured leg. This apparatus will pull down and internally rotate the distal fragment and maintain a satisfactory position. We like it because the patient can be sent home in the splint and needs no great amount of nursing care.

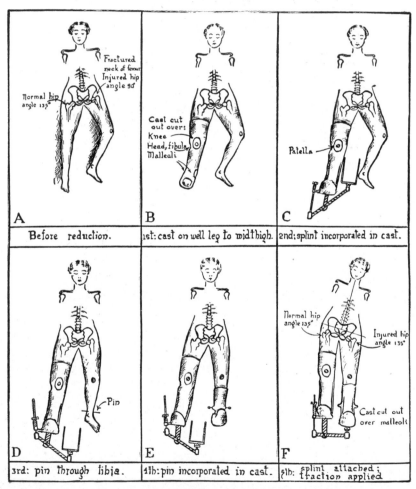

Fig. 958.—Steps in standard routine application of well-leg countertraction splint. (Courtesy Zimmer Manufacturing Co.)

When union is firm, the splint is removed and the patient is got up on crutches as with other types of treatment of these fractures.

In applying the cast to the well leg, the sole of the foot and the malleoli should be well padded with felt and the cast should not extend too high on the inner side of the thigh. Our only complication in the use of this method has been a thrombosis in the veins of the well leg which was apparently due to pressure on the inner side of the leg.

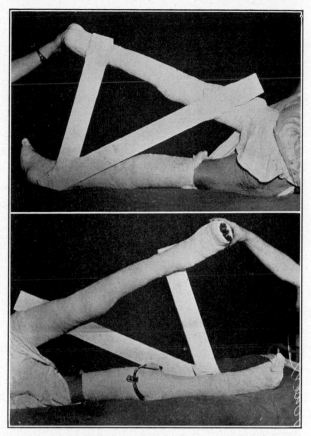

Fig. 959.—Well-leg fixation after manipulative reduction of a trochanteric fracture of the right femur.

Bradford Frames and Fracture Beds in the Treatment of Fractures of the Pelvis and Femur.—The question as to whether or not the patient is more comfortable on a Bradford frame is frequently difficult to decide. There is no doubt that the Bradford frame enables the patient to use the bedpan with less discomfort. On the other hand, with a patient in a Thomas splint or a plaster spica or a Hodgen splint, it is extremely difficult to keep him at the proper level on the frame, the frames quickly become soiled and are as a rule quite uncomfortable and tend to cause rather than prevent bed sores and to restrict the activity of the patient. Consequently we rarely use the Bradford frame in the treatment of these patients. If a special fracture bed with a mattress which can be lowered to leave the patient suspended on straps is available, this is an advantage and should be used, and in most hospitals such beds are now available.

CHAPTER XXIII

FRACTURES OF THE SHAFT OF THE FEMUR

ANATOMICAL CONSIDERATIONS

The Shaft of the Femur is a long cylinder of heavy compact bone which is roughly cylindrical on cross section throughout most of its extent. At either extremity the cortex is thinned, the large marrow cavity is filled with cancellous bone, and the bone is enlarged and somewhat quadrilateral on cross section. The linea aspera is an elevated ridge which extends along the posterior border of the shaft and serves for the attachment of muscles. Above it is continuous with the intertrochanteric lines and below it divides to be continuous with the supracondylar ridges.

The femoral shaft is not straight, but is bowed forward and outward. In treating fractures of the shaft of the femur it is important that this normal anterolateral bowing be preserved, otherwise the line of weight-bearing will be disturbed and the knee and hip joints will not function properly.

The Fascia of the Thigh.—The muscles of the thigh are encased in a strong sheath of dense fibrous tissue, the fascia lata, which is continuous below with the deep fascia of the leg and above is attached to Poupart's ligament in front and extends up on to the gluteal region behind. On the lateral surface of the thigh the fascia lata is unusually thick and this thickened portion which is called the "iliotibial band" receives the insertion of the tensor fascia femoris and serves as the tendon of this muscle.

From the deep surface of the fascia lata bands of fibrous tissue project inward to the femur and separate the muscles of the thigh from one another. The more important of these are the internal and external intermuscular septa which divide the thigh into anterior and posterior compartments. The anterior compartment contains the quadriceps femoris muscle and the posterior compartment contains the hamstrings and adductors. The internal intermuscular septum in its deep portion forms the floor of Hunter's canal which contains the femoral vessels and nerves.

The Thigh Muscles.—Most of the muscles in the thigh are divided into extensors and flexors of the knee and the adductors which act on the thigh.

The extensor group composed of the rectus femoris, vastus internus and externus and crureus muscles occupies the anterior portion of the thigh and the muscles fuse into a common tendon which is inserted into the tubercle and upper end of the tibia, the patella being a sesamoid bone in the tendon. They arise almost entirely from the shaft of the femur, and their principal action is to extend the leg on the thigh. Flexion of the thigh is largely accomplished by the iliopsoas muscle.

The extensor group, usually called the hamstrings, includes the biceps, semimembranosus, and semitendinosus. They arise from the ischium and the biceps is inserted into the head of the fibula, while the other two form the inner hamstrings and are inserted into the mesial surface of the upper end of the tibia. They flex the leg on the thigh and extend the thigh on the hip. The flexion of the leg is aided by the gastrocnemius and the extension of the hip is aided by the gluteus maximus.

The Adductors.—These muscles make up the mass on the upper and inner aspect of the thigh. They arise from the ischiopubic ramus and spread out fan-like to be inserted into the femur as far down as the adductor tubercle on the internal condyle. Their action is to adduct the thigh on the pelvis. Abduction of the thigh is largely accomplished by the gluteus medius which is inserted into the great trochanter.

Vessels and Nerves.—The femoral artery begins beneath Poupart's ligament as a continuation of the external iliac and passes downward and inward through Scarpa's triangle and Hunter's canal to the junction of the middle and lower thirds of the thigh, where it turns backward, lying close to the femur and passes through the insertion of the adductor magnus muscle to reach the popliteal space, where it terminates in the popliteal artery. As it is separated from the bone by muscle and fibrous tissue the femoral artery is rarely injured in fractures of the femur, but the popliteal artery is not so well protected and occasionally it is injured in supracondylar fractures.

The femoral veins and nerve accompany the artery. The sciatic nerve enters the posterior compartment of the thigh at a point beneath the junction of the inner and middle thirds of a line between the tuberosity of the ischium and the great trochanter and passes directly downward to the middle of the popliteal space. It lies beneath the hamstrings and is separated from the bone only by loose areolar tissue, and is occasionally injured in fractures of the femur.

FRACTURES OF THE SHAFT OF THE FEMUR

Fractures of the shaft of the femur are one of the most important conditions with which the fracture surgeon has to deal. The lesion is important because it is one of the most frequent of the major injuries and because the primary injury may be accompanied by severe shock and danger to life; if the fracture is not skillfully treated over a prolonged period, it may result in considerable permanent disability.

Incidence and Causes.—In normal bones these fractures are always the result of great violence and many of them are accounted for by falls from a height, automobile, or railroad accidents, or by severe industrial accidents. They may be due to direct or indirect violence and are more frequent in those who lead an active outdoor life and are exposed to the hazards of severe injuries. The majority of the cases occur in young adult males and in children.

Pathology.—The femur being a typical long bone, the fracture may be of any of the varieties found in long bones; but in the great majority of the cases the fracture line is roughly transverse or short or long oblique, or spiral.

Comminution is fairly frequent, especially in the cases due to direct violence, and the fracture may be multiple.

Due to the fact that great force is necessary to break the femur, many of these fractures are accompanied by severe damage to the soft parts and a considerable percentage of them are compound either from within from the projection of one of the fragments through the skin or from without from the lacerations produced by the force which caused the fracture.

The shaft of the femur may be broken in any part of its length, but the majority of the fractures occur in the middle third of the bone, partly because this includes the apex of the normal anterolateral bowing of the shaft, and partly because this seems to be the part most frequently subjected to severe direct violence.

Displacement.—As in any other long bone the original displacement of the fragments in fracture of the femur is largely the result of the fracturing force, and the final position is largely dependent upon the pull of attached muscles and the effect of gravity upon the limb.

In fractures of the shaft of the femur complete displacement with over-riding of the fragments and shortening of the limb is the rule, though very rarely the ends may remain engaged and simple angulation occur. In practically all cases, there is a tendency for the proximal fragment to rotate outward on account of gravity and the pull of the external rotator muscles and the normal anterolateral bowing of the shaft is lost because of the solution of continuity in the bone.

Due to the fact that the muscle pull varies in fractures at different levels we shall describe the type of displacement which is characteristic of fractures in the upper, middle, and lower thirds of the shaft of the femur, but it must be pointed out that the characteristic displacement is not always present, and that in any given fracture the displacement may be quite different from that usually expected as a result of muscle pull.

In all fractures of the shaft of the femur rotation of the distal fragment is determined by the position of the leg and this usually rolls outward from gravity.

Displacement in Fractures of the Upper Third of the Shaft of the Femur. —Here the short proximal fragment is usually in a position of flexion, abduction, and external rotation. The flexion is due to the iliopsoas muscle; the abduction, to the gluteus medius; and the external rotation, to the short rotators and to gravity, as with the patient lying upon the back the trochanter and shaft tend to fall backward in the position of external rotation. The flexion and abduction tend to vary inversely with the length of the proximal fragment and are greatest in the subtrochanteric fractures with a short upper fragment. (Figs. 960 and 961.)

The lower fragment is drawn upward, inward, and backward by the hamstrings and adductors and falls backward from gravity. Thus the tendency is for the fragments to override and angulate outward and forward with the proximal end of the distal fragment lying behind and mesial to the proximal fragment.

Displacement in Fractures of the Middle Third of the Shaft of the Femur.—Here the displacement is less constant than in fractures near the ends of the bone and the fragments may be in almost any relation to one another. The lower fragment is practically always drawn upward by the muscles which span the fracture, and there is a variable amount of overriding

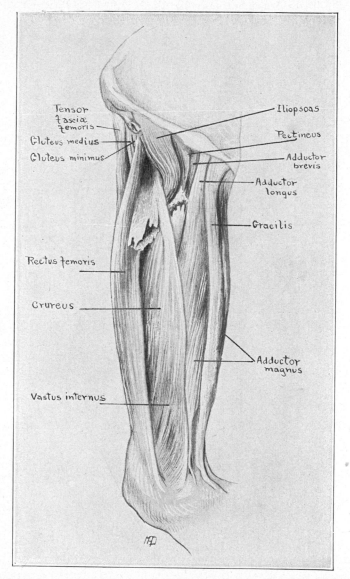

Fig. 960.—Fracture of the femur at the junction of the upper and middle thirds. The upper fragment is displaced forward and outward. (Nifong: *The Hodgen Wire Cradle Extension Suspension Splint,* The C. V. Mosby Company, Publishers.)

of the fragments. The next most constant displacement is flexion of the proximal fragment and a dropping back of the distal fragment so that it tends to lie behind the lower end of the proximal fragment, but this relation may be reversed. There is no rule as regards lateral displacement except that in fractures in the upper half of the middle third the proximal fragment tends to be abducted and in fractures in the lower half it tends to be adducted, but this is not constant.   (Figs. 961 and 967.)

Displacement in Fractures of the Lower Third of the Shaft of the Femur. —In these fractures the muscle pull has little to do with the lateral displacement and the lower fragment may be displaced either inward or outward or

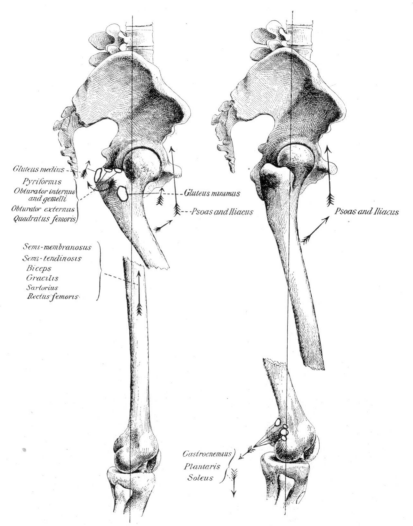

Gluteus medius
Pyriformis
Obturator internus and gemelli
Obturator externus
Quadratus femoris

Gluteus minimus

Psoas and Iliacus

Psoas and Iliacus

Semi-membranosus
Semi-tendinosis
Biceps
Gracilis
Sartorius
Rectus femoris

Gastrocnemius
Plantaris
Soleus

Fig. 961.—Showing the usual displacements of the fragments in fractures of the upper and middle thirds of the femur.   (Deaver: *Surgical Anatomy.*)

lie near the midline.   In addition to the tendency of the muscles which span the fracture to draw the lower fragment upward, the chief deforming factor is the gastrocnemius muscle which arises from the posterior surface of the distal fragment and tends to flex it upon the leg, thus tipping the proximal end of the distal fragment back into the popliteal space where it may damage vessels and nerves.   Thus the distal fragment tends to lie behind the proximal one.   (Fig. 962.)

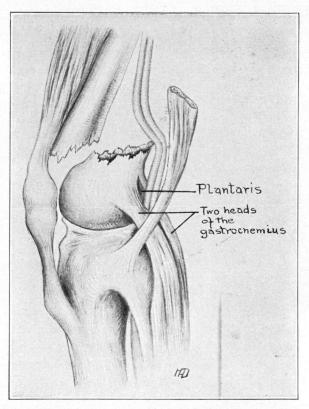

Fig. 962.—Supracondylar fracture of the femur. The distal fragment is displaced back-ward into the popliteal space by the gastrocnemius, and the vessels are stretched over its sharp edge. (Nifong: *The Hodgen Wire Cradle Extension Suspension Splint,* The C. V. Mosby Company, Publishers.)

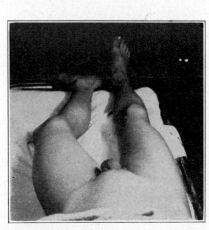

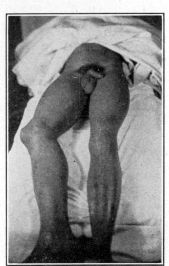

Fig. 963.   Fig. 964.

Fig. 963.—Photograph of a patient with a fresh fracture of the left femur, middle third, seen from above.

Fig. 964.—Photograph of a patient with fracture of the right femur, middle third seen from below.

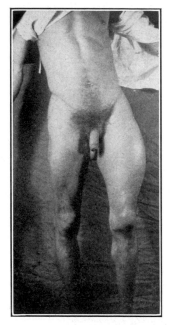

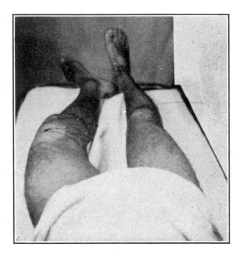

Fig. 965.   Fig. 966.

Fig. 965.—Large hematoma of left thigh caused by a kick by a mule. The swelling suggests a fracture of the femur, but the bone is not broken.

Fig. 966.—Compound (gunshot wound) comminuted fracture of the left femur.

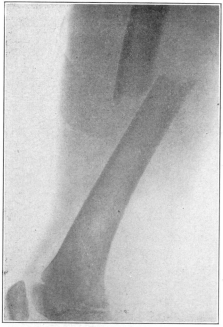

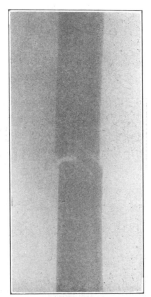

Fig. 967.   Fig. 968.

Fig. 967.—Short oblique transverse fracture of the shaft of the femur, middle third showing the usual posterior displacement of the lower fragment. Treated by closed reduction, then traction with a Kirschner wire through the upper end of the tibia with the extremity in a Thomas splint then plaster cast. Good result; patient walked in three and one-half months, and had full function in six and one-half months.

Fig. 968.—Same case as shown in Fig. 967, after the displacement had been reduced by traction.

Diagnosis.—The history of the injury with the resultant disability, shortening, and distortion of the limb render the diagnosis self-evident in the average case. Figs. 963, 964, 965, and 966.) The shortening varies from a fraction of an inch to four or five inches. Fracture of the neck can be ruled out by noting that the tip of the trochanter is at its normal level.

The general condition of the patient should be noted and be considered, and great care should be taken not to add to whatever shock is present by inflicting unnecessary pain or damage to soft parts in attempts to make a very exact diagnosis of the lesion present. After it has been determined that the femur is broken, the patient should be looked over for other injuries and then made comfortable and let alone until proper treatment can be instituted.

The circumference of the thigh is always increased, partly by the effusion of blood and partly by the thickening of the muscles incident to the shortening. In the typical case the patient lies upon his back with the fractured limb completely everted, and the swollen thigh has lost its normal anterolateral bow and may present an angular deformity.

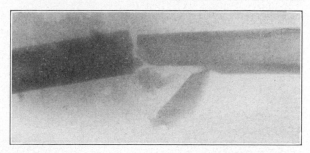

Fig. 969.—Severely traumatized thigh with a comminuted fracture, middle third of femur. The displacement has been reduced and the shortening slightly overcorrected by skeletal traction in a Thomas splint and Conwell's overhead femur frame. The loose fragments were ignored. Severe soft structure damage prevented open reduction and replacement of same. Good union. Good result.

Crepitus should not be sought, and except in very thin subjects seen soon after the injury it is useless to attempt to locate the ends of the fragments and determine the character of the displacement by palpation, since the bone is too well covered by the soft parts and obscured by the swelling.

The level of the fracture can be roughly determined by noting the level of greatest tenderness and by noting the level at which false motion occurs. False motion is best demonstrated by making traction on and gently raising the foot and leg and moving it from side to side while one hand rests upon the thigh. In this manner the level of the fracture can be demonstrated with very little pain to the patient or danger of injury to the soft parts. The other method of grasping the trochanter in one hand and rotating the leg with the other to determine whether or not the trochanter rotates with the leg is quite painful and rarely necessary.

Finally a roentgenogram should be obtained as it is important to know the exact level and nature of the fracture. This is especially true if one expects to reduce the fracture by manipulation and immobilize it. If one expects to treat the fracture by traction, however, there is no reason why the

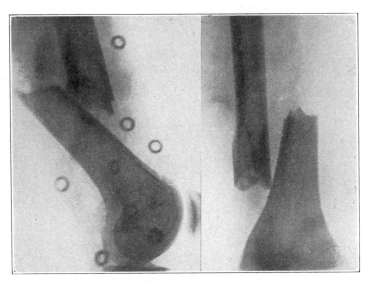

Fig. 970.—Fracture in the lower third of the femur showing the typical posterior and lateral displacement of the lower fragment. Treated by skeletal traction (Kirschner wire through upper end of the tibia) and Conwell's overhead extension frame, and Thomas splint with Pearson knee flexion apparatus. Good result.

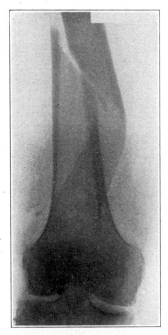

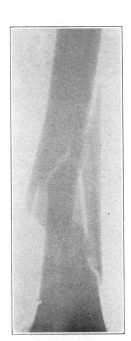

Fig. 971. Fig. 972.

Fig. 971.—Spiral fracture, lower third of the femur. Treated by skeletal traction (with Kirschner wire) in a Thomas splint on overhead wooden frame. Good result. Perfect position was not obtained in this case. Good alignment—no shortening. Excellent functional result.

Fig. 972.—Comminuted fracture at the junction of the lower and the middle third of the femur. Treated by skeletal traction in a Thomas splint with overhead frame with good result.

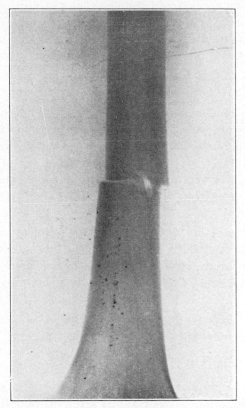

Fig. 973.—Simple transverse fracture of the junction of the middle and the lower thirds of femur, right, with very slight displacement. No reduction indicated. Treated by double plaster spica for eight weeks, unilateral spica for four weeks. Good result in five and one-half months.

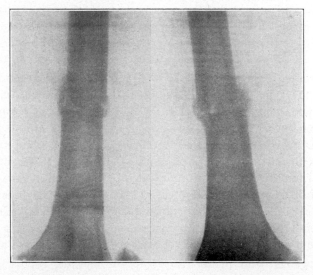

Fig. 974.—Lateral and anteroposterior views of preceding case three months following injury.

traction should not be applied and the fracture put up in a splint; the roent-genogram can be taken the next day. This latter course expedites the treatment, saves the patient a good deal of pain, and does not affect the end-result, because it is the later roentgenograms which govern the details of the treatment.

Complications

Other than the tendency of these fractures to be comminuted or compound, complications are rare. Very rarely, however, the femoral or popliteal vessels or sciatic or peroneal nerves may be injured. These accidents are most apt to occur in fractures of the lower third from the tipping back of the distal fragment and may result in paralysis or even gangrene of the limb. Consequently, the sensation of the foot should be tested and the condition of the circulation noted.

Injury of the knee joint with effusion and ligamentous or even cartilage injury occurs rather frequently and should be looked for, as it may cause considerable trouble later. It should also be remembered that the entire extremity has been subjected to severe strain and may be broken in two or more places.

The late complications of delayed union, nonunion, malunion, and stiffness of the knee will be mentioned under treatment.

Treatment

The methods of treatment are: (1) manipulative reduction with immobilization; (2) reduction by continuous traction; and (3) operative reduction with or without internal splinting.

Choice of Method

We see no reason why a patient with a fresh fracture of the shaft of the femur, which is not compound, should be subjected to the dangers incident to an operative reduction; consequently, we do not recommend operative treatment until conservative treatment has been tried and has failed.

The choice between manipulative reduction and treatment by traction depends upon the type of fracture and upon the surgeon, who should use that method with which he is most skillful. In those cases of simple transverse fracture of the femur in good position, or of ordinary simple oblique fracture of the femur when there is no tendency for the fragments to override, when there is no compound wound, and when the soft structures are not too severely traumatized, no manipulation or traction is necessary; the limb may be immobilized in a plaster spica. If displacement is present, however, this must be corrected either by manipulation or traction. Some surgeons who are especially skillful at reducing fractures of long bones by manipulation use this method routinely and report excellent results. (Campbell.)

Other surgeons who prefer the traction method report equally good results.[*]

---

*Conwell: Fractures of the Femur—Treatment and Results Attained by Traction and Suspension, A Report of 110 Cases, Surg. Gynec. and Obst. 40: 112-118, January, 1925.

The manipulative method has a certain advantage in that once the femur is reduced and immobilized in a plaster cast, the fracture requires relatively little attention. The traction method has the advantages that often no anesthetic is required and that the limb can be constantly observed. It has the disadvantage that it must be constantly under the observation of the surgeon, who should inspect it daily until consolidation has begun.

Other things being equal, fractures which are approximately transverse are most easily treated by the manipulative method because it is a relatively simple procedure to get the ends of the bones engaged and they tend to be stable once the fracture is reduced. Long oblique and comminuted fractures, on the other hand, are most easily treated by the traction method, because it is difficult to get the ends engaged, and there is a tendency for the bones to slip after they are engaged. Furthermore, in the oblique fractures there is relatively little tendency to the lateral or anteroposterior displacement which is especially troublesome in the treatment of the transverse fractures by the traction method.

Immediate Immobilization and Transportation of Fractures of the Shaft of the Femur

As fractures of the shaft of the femur should be transported to and treated in a hospital, and as these severe injuries are often accompanied by surgical shock which is increased by the pain and tissue damage incident to movement of the limb, it is important that the limb be immobilized and the pain relieved as soon as possible after the injury.

The pain should be relieved by a full dose of morphine given if possible before the patient is moved.

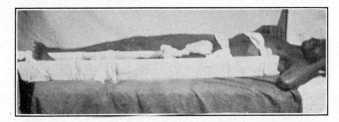

Fig. 975.—Emergency dressing for fracture of the femur when a Thomas splint is not available.

Immobilization is most satisfactorily obtained by means of a Thomas ring splint if this is available. The splint is applied as follows: Without removing the clothing or shoe the limb is gently straightened and traction is applied while the splint is slipped up over the limb and against the tuberosity of the ischium.

The traction is applied to the foot either by means of a double clove hitch around the well-padded ankle or over the shoe or a nail or rope passed through the shoe beneath the arch of the foot. The leg is then pulled down firmly and the splint pushed upward and the traction rope is tied to the end of the splint. More traction may be obtained by using two traction ropes, passing them in opposite directions around the side bars of the splint, then tying them over the end and twisting them with a short stick between them. Slings are then placed under the thigh and leg to support the limb.

The Thomas splint is rarely available and some immobilization can be obtained by tying the knees and ankles together and placing a pillow under the knees, thus using the opposite leg as a splint. Or with a long board bound to the side of the patient a long Liston side splint may be improvised as described under fractures of the neck of the femur. (Fig. 975.)

In the hospital, with the patient on a stretcher, a pillow under the knee and a weight of from five to ten pounds suspended from the foot makes the patient a lot more comfortable while waiting for the x-ray examination, etc.

Treatment of Fractures of the Shaft of the Femur by Manipulative Reduction and Immobilization

There are two methods by which fractures of a long bone can be reduced by manipulation. One is the method of angulation and the other is the method of direct traction and lateral pressure. The surgeon should, of course, choose the method at which he is most skillful. If one method does not succeed, he may try the other.

In the execution of either method the patient is placed on a fracture table with a pelvic rest and perineal post, and a long strip of felt is placed under him before the reduction is attempted. When the surgeon is sure that plenty of plaster bandages, felt and stockinet or sheet cotton for padding are at hand, the patient is anesthetized, preferably with gas and ether, and the manipulative reduction is carried out, with the patient on the table and in a position ready for the application of a plaster cast as soon as the fracture is reduced.

Some surgeons use a fluoroscope, but we have never felt the need of it, finding that the reduction is more easily carried out in the light where full view of the extremity and freedom of movement is permitted. In either method the general principle should be remembered that any fracture of a long bone is most easily reduced if the muscles are relaxed by semiflexing the joints on either side of the fracture. For this reason the manipulation should be carried out with the hip and knee in a position of about 45 degrees flexion.

Reduction by Angulation.—The patient is pulled down firmly against the perineal post and both feet are fixed to the foot extension pieces (Figs. 976 and 977) or held by assistants (Fig. 978). The injured limb is then suspended or supported at the level of the knee in such a position that the hip and knee are flexed about 45 degrees. This can be done by placing a felt pad over the popliteal space and hanging the knee from the thigh suspension arm attached to the perineal post of the fracture table or by a rest under the knee. Moderate traction is then applied to both legs by means of the foot extension apparatus and the surgeon grasps the thigh at the level of the fracture and lifts it directly forward, thus angulating the fragments forward and causing the ends to slip by one another and engage. If the ends do not engage when they are lifted forward, they are gently moved from side to side until they do engage.

When the fragments are felt to be engaged, the angulation is corrected and the stability of the reduction is tested by pushing upward on the knee. If the fragments are felt to slip by one another the reduction must be done over again. If the fragments are found to be quite stable, the extremity is measured to be sure that the length is correct, and if there is more than one-half inch shortening, the reduction should be done over (Fig. 979). If there is less than one-half inch shortening and the limb is stable to upward pressure, the reduction may be considered satisfactory and the plaster cast should be applied with the knee and hip in a position of about 20 degrees of flexion and supported in such a manner that the normal anterolateral bowing of the femur is maintained.

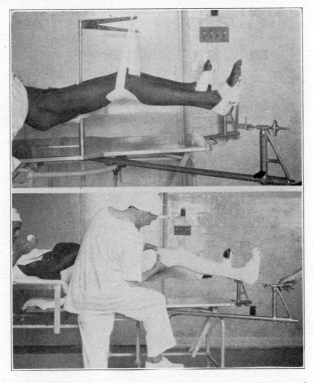

Fig. 976.—Manipulative reduction of a fracture of the femur by manual traction, counter-traction, and manipulation. Patient on fracture table with leg and thigh supported and sus-pended preliminary to manipulative reduction. This is the position to be attained after the re-duction when the plaster cast is being applied.

Fig. 977.—The surgeon angulates the fragments while an assistant increases the traction on the leg.

It is advisable for the surgeon to support the limb at the site of the fracture in order to maintain the normal anterior bow of the femur, while the main weight of the limb is taken by the knee support, and let his assistants apply the plaster-of-Paris spica. The spica should extend from the umbilicus to the toes. (Fig. 981.) If the knee is supported by a sling hung from the thigh support, the sling should not be permanently included in the plaster, as it may cause a severe pressure sore in the popliteal space. Before the plaster cast is completed, the sling should be loosened, the plaster cut out over it, the sling removed, and the defect in the plaster repaired. Relatively little padding need be used. We usually use stockinet and a thin layer of sheet cotton around the trunk and the extremity, the sacral pad of felt which has been placed under the patient before reduction has been attempted, one small triangular felt pad over each anterior superior spine, and a long narrow felt pad under the heel and tendo Achilles. We endeavor to maintain the position of the limb until the plaster has set. Portable fluoroscopic examination can be made after attempting reduction and before applying the cast, if facilities of a portable fluoroscope are present.

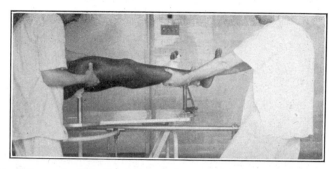

Fig. 978.—Manipulative reduction of a fracture of the shaft of the femur by manual traction, countertraction, and manipulation.

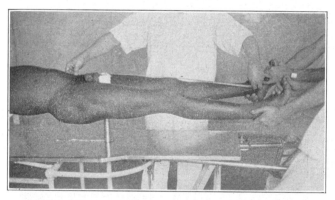

Fig. 979.—Measurement in order to determine whether or not normal length has been obtained.

Instead of the fracture table, the traction may be applied manually by the surgeon himself or a strong assistant or mechanically by the Soutter apparatus.

As soon as the plaster is dry, anteroposterior and lateral x-ray pictures should be taken in order to check the position. If this is satisfactory the patient is let alone and another roentgenogram is taken at the end of ten days. If the position is still satisfactory the plaster is left on for a period of from eight to twelve weeks. At the end of this time the plaster is bivalved, the anterior portion is removed, and the stability of the union is tested. Clinically if it is quite solid the plaster is removed, an x-ray picture is taken, and if the callus appears good and the position is satisfactory, the patient is permitted to lie in bed for from two to four weeks and begin to move the knee and hip while the knee is supported on a pillow. At the end of this time the patient is got up either on crutches or on a Thomas walking caliper splint. One of us (H. E. C.) frequently uses crutches and a long lateral plaster-of-Paris splint. The other (J. A. K.) uses only crutches. The splint must fit accurately; otherwise deformity may occur. The crutches are discarded as soon as union seems to be firm enough to bear weight—usually about four to five months after the injury.

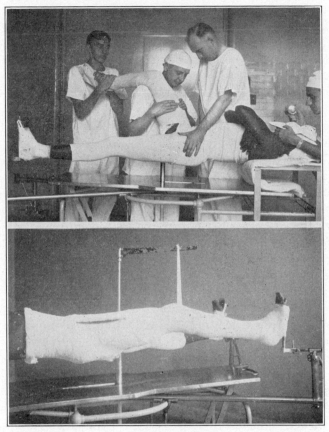

Fig. 980.—Reduction of a fracture of the shaft of the femur by direct traction with the knee and hip flexed with countertraction against the pelvis by an assistant. The flexed knee is held over the surgeon's shoulder and the foot against the surgeon's back by an assistant.

Fig. 981.—Plaster-of-Paris spica applied after reduction of a fracture of the right femur by manipulation.

The position should be checked by physical and x-ray examination at intervals of a week or ten days in order to be sure that bowing of the femur is not occurring during the convalescent period. Should bowing occur, the patient is put back to bed and the bowing corrected either by manipulation under an anesthetic or by traction. We have found traction a very efficient method of correcting the deformity while the callus is soft. After the deformity is corrected, traction is maintained until the union seems to be firm and the patient is got up as before.

If when the first x-ray is taken after the reduction, the position is not satisfactory, the cast should be removed and the surgeon may either attempt a new reduction or treat the patient by traction. If the position has been satisfactory as shown in the first x-ray picture, but if deformity has occurred when the second x-ray picture is taken, the surgeon may do one of two things: If the deformity is a lateral or anteroposterior angulation, this must be corrected as it is most important to obtain normal alignment if normal function is to be expected. As a matter of fact, angulation of the fragments results in much more disability than does a small amount of shortening. However, if the ends of the fragments are engaged the plaster should be left on for two weeks. At the end of this time union should be fairly firm, but the callus will be soft enough to admit of correction of the deformity by cutting and wedging the plaster cast. On the other hand, if complete displacement with overriding of the fragments has occurred, the plaster should be removed and the shortening should be corrected immediately, either by traction or manipulation or open operation.

Reduction of Fractures of the Femur by Direct Traction.—If direct traction is to be used, considerable more force in traction is necessary for the reduction. We have found the following an efficient way of applying this force to the femur. The patient is placed on the fracture table and anesthetized as described above. Then the surgeon lifts the fractured leg and places the flexed knee over his shoulder so that the foot and leg of the patient is hanging down the surgeon's back. An assistant should hold the foot against the surgeon's back, and another assistant should immobilize the pelvis by holding it firmly down on the pelvic rest. The surgeon makes traction on the femur by simply lifting upward; thus the traction is made with his back and he has both hands free to manipulate the thigh (Fig. 980). In this manner a great deal of force can be applied and the femur can be pulled down to well beyond its original length. The reduction is accomplished by pulling the femur down and pressing inward or forward or backward on the fragments as may be necessary, then relaxing the traction momentarily. This maneuver is repeated until, when the traction is relaxed, the fragments are felt to engage. The stability of the reduction is tested by pressing upward on the knee. If this does not result in shortening, the ends of the fragments are firmly engaged. A more generally used method is to fix both feet to the foot pieces and apply mechanical traction to the extremity until full length is obtained. The fracture is then manipulated and traction maintained until the cast has set.

When a stable reduction has been accomplished in this manner and the extremity has been measured to see whether the length is satisfactory, the cast should be applied and the treatment carried out just as described in the section on reduction by angulation (Fig. 981).

Treatment of Fracture of the Shaft of the Femur by Traction.—We shall describe the four following methods for the treatment of fractures of the shaft of the femur by traction: (1) The skeletal and skin traction and the Thomas splint; (2) the Russell method; (3) the Hodgen splint; and (4) the Hoke traction apparatus. The surgeon should use that method with which he is most familiar and for which he has the proper equipment. Any of the above methods may be expected to give satisfactory results provided they are properly carried out, and none of them may be expected to give satisfactory results unless the traction is properly applied and the position of the femur and the efficiency of the traction are checked by daily examination and attention to details.

Fracture Bed and Frame.—Any patient with fracture of the shaft of the femur that is to be treated by traction should be placed on a fracture bed; that is, either a special fracture bed or a bed which does not sag in the middle or which has boards placed between the mattress and the spring and an overhead frame strong enough to bear the weight of the patient and to which the leg can be suspended or traction applied. There are dozens of different frames designed by various surgeons and most of these are quite efficient. The surgeon must, of course, use the one which he has at hand. Perhaps the most popular is the ordinary Balkan frame. The Conwell frame is illustrated in Fig. 994 and is a very good frame and easily made. More elaborate frames are made by instrument houses and the same is true of fracture beds, some of which are made in such a manner that the mattress may be lowered and the patient suspended on the frame for nursing care.

It is of some advantage to have the frame attached to the bed and the bed on wheels so that it can be moved out on the porch if such is available, for these patients must remain in bed over a considerable period of time and change of scene is often grateful to them.

In addition to the fracture bed and frame there must be at hand the Thomas or Hodgen splint, if such is to be used, with an adequate supply of slings, ropes, pulleys and weights.

Treatment of Fracture of the Shaft of the Femur by the Thomas Splint

Having the material at hand the surgeon must first decide whether or not traction is to be applied to the skin or to the bone itself. Skeletal traction has four advantages: (1) it is more efficient; (2) it is more comfortable to the patient and it is more reliable, as it does not slip; (3) it permits free movement of the knee; and (4) it permits frequent inspection of and free access to the thigh in case of compound wounds or for any other purpose. Skeletal traction has the disadvantage that an anesthetic, either local or general, is necessary for its application and that there is always a certain danger of infection. This danger, however, is relatively slight if the wire pin is applied under rigid aseptic conditions and is negligible if wire traction is used.

Skeletal traction is especially indicated in supracondylar fractures of the femur and in compound fractures with extensive wounds, and in fractures in very muscular individuals in whom a large amount of weight may be necessary to overcome the shortening.

Skin traction is indicated in older patients and those with weak musculature, and in children.

It will be noted that we use the Thomas splint for suspension and immobilization of the extremity and apply running traction. We use intrinsic traction for transportation in the Thomas splint, but do not recommend it for bed treatment, since, if efficient traction is maintained, the patients complain of the pressure of the ring.

Application of Skin Traction.—Skin traction may be applied by means of ordinary adhesive tape or by mole skin adhesive or by glue. Mole skin is the best, but is rarely available. We usually use ordinary adhesive. Glue tends to harden and cause blisters under the traction which are quite uncomfortable to the patient and may necessitate the removal of traction.

In applying skin traction, the leg should be shaved and washed with ether and alcohol and the surgeon should bear in mind the fact that the traction which he is applying must lie smooth on the leg and must be so bound on that it will resist a force of from ten to twenty-five pounds over a period of from four to six weeks. For this reason the adhesive strips should be applied carefully and smoothly, should be fixed firmly by spiral strips, and then covered with a firm gauze bandage which in turn should be wrapped generously with adhesive in order that the dressing will remain undisturbed as long as possible. One of the most frequent errors in the treatment of fractures by skin traction is that the traction is carelessly applied and consequently it must be renewed frequently with resultant damage to the skin, disturbance of the position of the fragments, and a tendency to delayed union and deformity.

The traction is applied as follows: After the extremity has been shaved and washed off with alcohol, adhesive is applied on either side of the limb from a point about two inches above the fracture or as high as possible on the thigh to beyond the heel. The adhesive should be three or four inches wide, depending upon the size of the leg and either one long or two shorter strips may be used. If the single strip is used its middle should be passed over a wood or metal spreader slightly wider than the ankle and the inner surfaces opposite the ankle should be covered with adhesive to prevent the strips from sticking to the ankle. (Figs. 982 and 983.)

If the double strips are used one end of each of these is folded over obliquely so that the lower end of each strip forms a strap about an inch wide. When the adhesive is applied to the leg the edges are cut obliquely from above downward so that the adhesive may lie flat on the leg, especially in the region just below the knee.

Four oblique strips of adhesive of about the same length are prepared and these are wound around the leg in a spiral direction. We start at the bottom, placing the first strip across the front of the ankle, then proceed spirally upward around the leg and thigh. The second strip starts from the front of the ankle, going in the opposite direction. The third and fourth strips are spiraled from the back running in opposite directions. When these spiral strips have been applied, a few turns of sheet cotton are made around the ankle, then two strips of adhesive about four inches long and an inch and one-half wide are applied from before backward, then from behind forward in a circular direction around the ankle at the level of the malleoli in order to hold the lower portion of the traction strips down against the leg.

The entire leg and thigh, as far upward as the traction strips extend, is then firmly bandaged with a gauze bandage in the figure-of-eight manner, making neat herring bones on the front of the leg (Fig. 983). This bandage is then fastened by several spiral strips of adhesive and by wide circular strips at the ankle and at the upper end, the upper strip overlapping the skin for about an inch. In this way we have applied an adhesive traction which will last several weeks and under ordinary circumstances need not be changed until fairly firm union has been obtained. We now use a woven elastic bandage over the adhesive.

During the application of the adhesive and bandage two assistants are needed to support the leg, one to lift the foot and make traction upon it, and the other to support the knee and thigh at the site of the fracture. The adhesive should be applied with the knee flexed about twenty degrees.

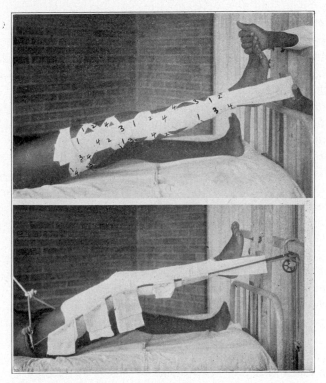

Fig. 982.—Adhesive traction strips applied to the leg with spiral adhesive bands, ready to be covered by a gauze bandage.

Fig. 983.—Treatment of a fracture of the shaft of the femur, by means of adhesive traction, suspended in a Thomas splint.

Some surgeons apply the adhesive to the thigh and to the leg separately. We do not believe that this is a very efficient method, as it is impossible to get adequate traction on the thigh by means of short adhesive strips. The main traction, unless it is applied directly to the end of the femur, must come from the leg because by pulling on the leg we are pulling on the muscles which span the fracture and are inserted into the tibia. By pulling on the thigh we are pulling on the skin and fascia which is fastened to the pelvis, and the traction has little effect on the muscles which we are attempting to stretch.

Likewise, some surgeons feel that traction applied to the leg puts an unusual strain on the knee. This is not true, because the muscles which we are stretching are the quadriceps and hamstrings which are inserted into the tibia, and relatively little traction is applied to the lower fragment of the femur. Consequently, even with great force the traction is expended upon the leg rather than upon the femur. It is for this reason that the hinged knee piece is not needed on the Thomas splint if adhesive traction is to be used. The surgeon should realize that if he is going to use adhesive traction, he must sacrifice motion at the knee during the time when the traction is applied. Motion at the knee cannot be obtained unless skeletal traction is used. Otherwise the efficiency of the traction will be sacrificed.

Application of the Thomas Splint.—The ordinary straight Thomas splint or the Blake modification in which there is only a half ring of the size suitable for the patient has been procured before the application of the adhesive is started. After the adhesive is on, the splint is applied. The surgeon places his arm through the ring of the splint, grasps the patient's foot, and then slips the splint up over the arm and foot without releasing the foot. Before being applied, the splint should be flexed about twenty degrees at a point opposite the patient's knee.

The splint should be placed firmly up against the tuberosity of the ischium and the supporting slings tightened under the thigh and leg. The slings under the thigh should be pulled tightly enough to restore the normal anterior bow of the femur which can be judged by examination of the thigh on the opposite side. A rather thick cotton pad should be placed under the knee and also under the site of the fracture; this tends to make the patient more comfortable. The slings should be of such material that they do not wrinkle; otherwise they tend to slip up on the bars of the splint and cut into the patient's skin.

The end of the splint should be bound firmly to the foot of the bed at such an elevation that the thigh is flexed about twenty-five or thirty degrees. The traction ropes should then be fastened to the spreader or to the free ends of the adhesive traction strips, and a spreader about four inches wide should be inserted to prevent lateral pressure of the traction strips on the malleoli. (Fig. 983.)

There are a great many ways of fastening the ropes to the adhesive strips. Some surgeons use a spreader with buckles; this is an efficient method. Others use one with large buttons; this is not efficient, because the buttonholes in the adhesive tend to tear, usually in the middle of the night, with resultant loss of position and considerable discomfort to the patient. Unless a spreader with good, strong buckles is at hand, we advise tying the strips to the rope in a knot which will not slip. Probably the most satisfactory knot is that known as the back wall: The adhesive strip is folded back on itself and the traction rope is run through the loop; it circles the loop twice and then is pulled through and pulled tight. The square and granny knots between the loop and the adhesive usually slip.

A pulley is then fastened to the fracture frame or foot of the bed, the traction rope is passed through the pulley, and the weights are attached. With skin traction it is usually better to use ten pounds traction for the first three or four hours until the adhesive has had a chance to set. At the end of this time the weight may be increased as much as is deemed necessary. We believe in using a lot of weight in the beginning in order to pull the fracture down and overcome the shortening as soon as possible before it has become set. For this reason we apply twenty to twenty-five pounds on skin traction for the first twenty-four or forty-eight hours. At the end of this time the limb is carefully measured or checked by means of a portable x-ray machine, and it is usually found that full length has been obtained. In certain cases the full amount (twenty to twenty-five pounds) of traction is applied immediately, and the patient is anesthetized in bed in order to secure muscle relaxation. An effort is made to obtain immediate reduction of the displacement by the traction plus any necessary manipulation.

After the initial traction weight has been applied, a rope should be attached to the ring of the Thomas splint and run upward and outward toward the head of the bed and a weight of about five or more pounds should be attached to this rope in order to hold the ring of the splint snugly up against the tuberosity of the ischium. A short, wide strip of adhesive should then be applied smoothly to the sole of the foot. This should be cut at the sides in order to make the adhesive lie flat and should be covered with a gauze bandage or circular adhesive strips. The free end of this strip should be wrapped around a throat stick in order to keep it from wrinkling; a small rope fastened to this should be run over a pulley attached to the overhead frame carrying one or two pounds of weight. This prevents foot drop and takes a part of the weight of the leg off the slings. (The foot piece attached to the splint is not practical where running traction is used.) A trapeze should be slung over the patient in order that he may raise himself with his hands.

Finally the foot of the bed should be elevated from ten to fourteen inches, depending upon the weight attached to the traction rope, in order that the patient's body weight may act as countertraction.

After-Treatment of Fracture of the Femur Treated by Adhesive Traction with the Thomas Splint.—At the end of twenty-four hours, the limb should be carefully measured to determine whether or not full length has been obtained. At the end of forty-eight hours it should be measured again and lateral and anteroposterior x-ray pictures should be taken to determine the position of the fragments. If the full length has been obtained, eight to ten pounds of the weight may be removed, leaving from ten to fifteen pounds traction, depending upon the musculature of the individual. From this time on the patient and apparatus should be seen frequently by the surgeon in charge.

The points particularly to be noted are: (1) that the traction is continuous; that is, that the ropes are not too long and the weights do not rest on the bed or floor; (2) that the adhesive is not beginning to tear or slip; (3) that none of the pulleys are fouled so that the rope is locked in the pulley; (4) that the slings remain in place and that the normal anterior bowing of the femur is maintained; (5) that the patient remains comfortable and is kept clean and dry and has his back rubbed twice a day with alcohol, and powdered.

At the end of the first week roentgenograms should be taken again in order to check the position of the fragments. There may be (1) underextension, (2) overextension, (3) lateral displacement. If the fragments have not been pulled down to sufficient length, it is, of course, necessary to add more weight and see that the traction ropes run free. This will rarely happen as usually with heavy traction during the first forty-eight hours the length will have been obtained. Rather frequently the shortening is overcorrected and the bones are pulled by one another. This must be carefully guarded against, since it may lead to delayed union. When it happens the weight must be taken off, sometimes until only five pounds are left on and even then the overcorrection may persist for several days and may even be permanent and the surgeon may not be able to push the lower fragment up again until it is in contact with the proximal one on account of intervening callus. This, of course, leads to delayed union. Consequently the limb should be examined daily and overextension carefully guarded against.

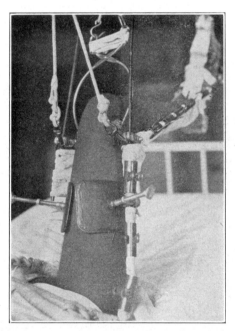

Fig. 984.—Pressure pads arranged for the correction of lateral displacement of the fragments. These must be used with great caution.

Lateral or anteroposterior displacement or angulation can sometimes be corrected by shifting the slings under the patient, by moving the splint in abduction or adduction, or up or down as indicated in order to bring the lower fragment in line with the upper, or by means of pressure pads, after the Pearson type (Fig. 984). These are screw pads which are attached to the splint and exert any desired amount of pressure in any direction. When they are used care must be taken not to let too much pressure be exerted or pressure sores will result.

After the first week the patient may sit up or be propped up in bed at will. X-ray pictures should be taken at the end of three weeks by means of portable apparatus, and at the end of eight weeks they should be taken again and the solidity of union should be tested clinically. If the position is satisfactory and union seems quite solid, the splint may be removed, traction may be placed on the lower leg. With a pillow under the thigh and knee, the patient may move around in bed with about ten pounds traction (Buck's extension) on the leg. During this time the patient should move the knee and ankle daily in order to restore muscle strength. This should be continued for one or two weeks, when the traction may be removed entirely and the

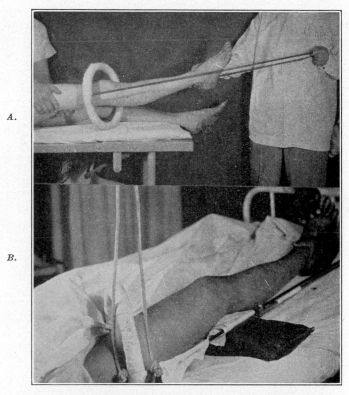

Fig. 985.—*A.* Method of holding leg while applying a Thomas splint. *B.* Leg in Thomas splint ready for the application of wire traction.

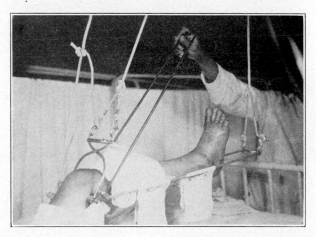

Fig. 986.—Calipers in place; leg and thigh being suspended. Also showing Thomas splint with Pearson knee flexion attachment.

patient remain in bed for another week. At the end of this time he may be fitted with a Thomas caliper walking splint or with a lateral plaster-of-Paris splint and then got up on crutches. The crutches are to be used from four to six weeks, when, if union is quite firm, they may be discarded. The same is true of the caliper walking splint. One of us (J. A. K.) rarely uses a splint, but gets the patient up on crutches without any other support.

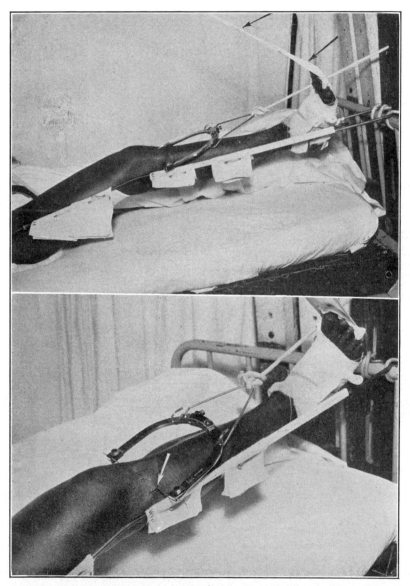

Fig. 987.—Kirschner wire through upper fourth of tibia as applied for traction in fractures of the lower half and lower end of the shaft of the femur.

Application of Skeletal Traction.—Skeletal traction is especially indicated in fractures of the lower third of the femur where it is necessary that the fracture be treated with the knee in a position of flexion in order to preserve alignment of the fragments. It should also be used in fractures of the middle and upper thirds in patients who have very large and powerful muscles, and in compound fractures or fractures with severe damage to the soft tissues, and in those simple fractures in which skin traction has failed.

Either a Kirschner wire or a Steinman pin may be used and the pin or wire may pass through the tibia or through the femur. We routinely use the wire through the upper third of the tibia, selecting a point about one inch distal to the tubercle and at about one-half inch posterior to the crest. In the femur the wire is passed through the condyles one-half inch anterior and one-half inch proximal to the adductor tubercle.

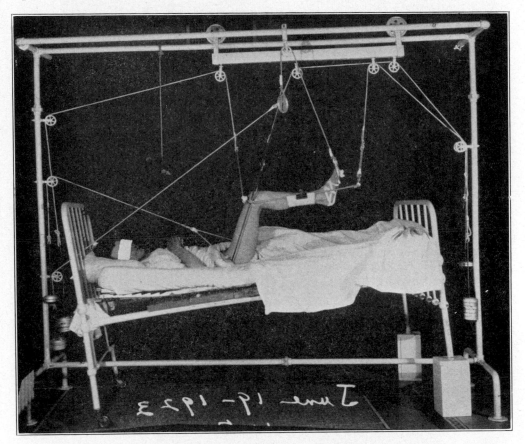

Fig. 988.—The traction has been applied and the Thomas splint is suspended with the thigh flexed at an angle of about 60 degrees, the leg resting in the movable knee piece. The muslin strips have been removed to show detail.

The site is selected and the skin is painted with the skin antiseptic, and 1 per cent novocain is injected into the skin and deeper tissues, including the periosteum. Then the Kirschner wire is pushed directly through the skin without a preliminary stab incision and is drilled through the bone and out through the skin on the opposite side of the leg. Care is taken to place the wire at right angles to the long axis of the leg. If a large pin is used, a small stab incision in the skin is advisable.

Sterile dressings are now slipped over the ends of the wire or pins and fixed to the skin. The Thomas splint is slipped on and the extremity is suspended in the splint.

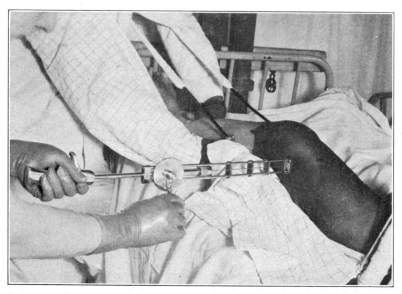

Fig. 989.—Application of Kirschner wire to femur. Leg and thigh in a Thomas splint with Pearson knee flexion attachment.

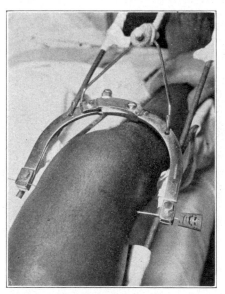

Fig. 990.—Kirschner wire through a femur held taut by the bow or spreader with traction applied. (De Puy bow.)

The splint is now fastened to the foot of the bed or frame and the caliper is applied to the wire or pin. The foot of the bed is elevated and the traction rope is tied to the caliper, and the weights are hung to the rope.

The traction rope is attached to the caliper or to the clamp which holds the pin and is carried upward and toward the foot of the bed in line with the Thomas splint and over a pulley on the overhead frame and through a second pulley at the foot of the bed so that the weights hang over the foot of the bed. About twenty-five pounds of weight should be used for the first day or two until full length of the femur has been obtained.

As in adhesive traction, the length of the limb should be carefully controlled and the limb should be inspected daily and frequent roentgenograms should be taken in order to guard against overlengthening. The knee should be moved about two inches daily so that the knee moves from about ninety degrees flexion to a position of approximately full extension about once in ten days. It should then be gradually flexed again. This amount of movement can be carried out and no disturbance of the fragments will result. In other respects the after-care is just the same as that advised above in the treatment of fractures of the femur by adhesive traction.

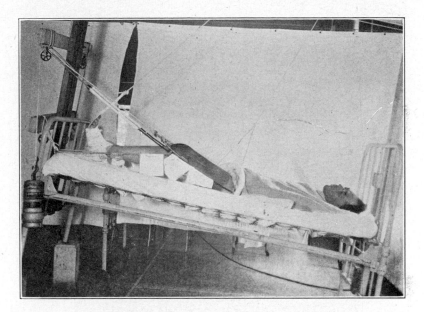

Fig. 991.—Use of Kirschner wire in the treatment of a fracture of the femur.

The skeletal traction should remain on for from three to five weeks or until union is fairly solid. One reason that skeletal traction has come into ill repute in the hands of some physicians is that it is kept in the bone too long with resultant pain, low grade osteomyelitis, etc. The skeletal traction should be removed as soon as the soft structures have healed and when sufficient union has taken place in the bone to prevent malposition. At the end of this time the skeletal traction may be removed and adhesive traction on the thigh is used with the leg and thigh in the Thomas splint with the Pearson knee flexion apparatus (Fig. 988). Gradually the leg is extended at the knee until full extension is accomplished, the extremity and the splint (Thomas) being brought gradually down to a horizontal plane just a few inches above the bed; then adhesive traction to the leg is applied for three or four weeks and the traction on the thigh is discontinued. When good union is present a

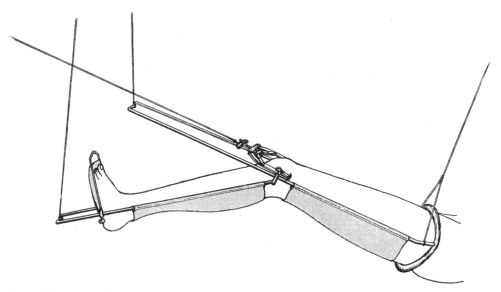

Fig. 992.—Application of Thomas leg splint with Pearson attachment.   (Courtesy Zimmer Manufacturing Co.)

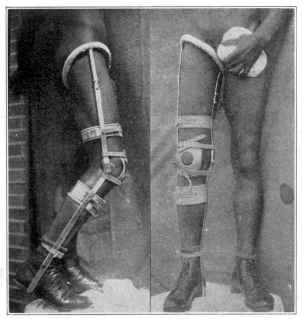

Fig. 993.—Walking caliper splint with Thomas ring used in the convalescent treatment of fractures of the shaft of the femur.

walking caliper (Fig. 993) or the molded plaster splint is applied. This can be discontinued about five or six months following injury, or earlier. The walking caliper can be worn to light work if necessary.

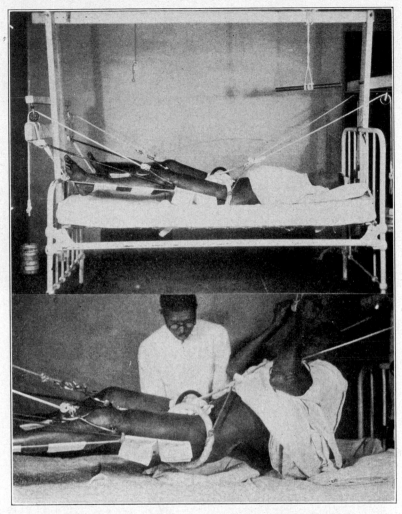

Fig. 994.—Skeletal traction used in bilateral fractures of the femur. Conwell's overhead pelvic femur frame is being used. Note the patient is able to lift himself in bed.

Treatment of Fractures of the Femur by the Russell Method

We have used this method occasionally and find it satisfactory in selected cases. The method requires a spreader with a pulley attached and a special frame with two pulleys at the foot of the bed in order that the traction rope may pass through it twice. A very convenient apparatus is illustrated in Fig. 996. The principle of the method is that the muscles are kept in balance and as a result relatively little traction is needed to overcome the shortening and deformity. It will be noted that the same rope suspends the leg at the knee and makes traction on the leg at the foot and that the amount of traction is approximately double the amount of suspension.

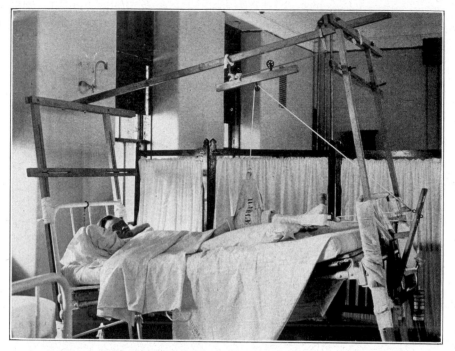

Fig. 995.—Treatment of fracture of the shaft of the femur by the Russell method.   (Courtesy Dr. John F. Connors, New York City.)

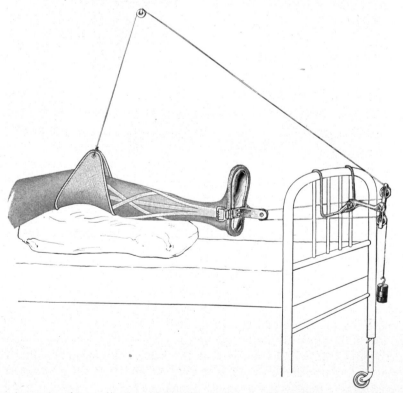

Fig. 996.—Apparatus for application of Russell traction in the treatment of fractures of the shaft of the femur.   (Courtesy of Zimmer Manufacturing Company.)

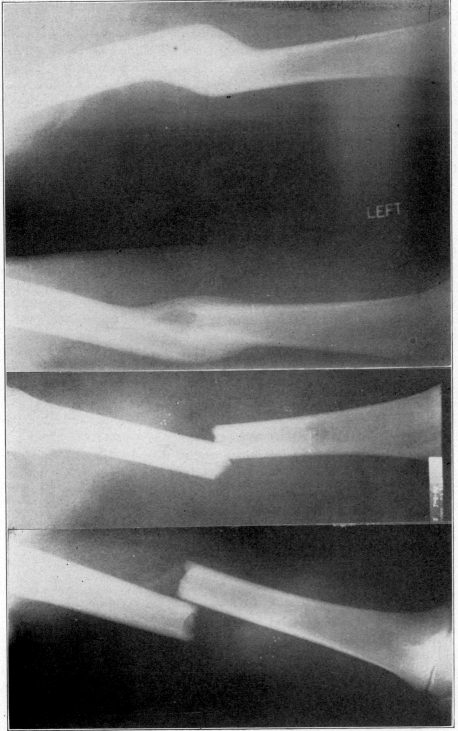

Fig. 997.—Fracture of the femur in a boy fourteen years of age. Treated with Russell traction for seven weeks; then, plaster cast for five weeks. Union with three-eighths of an inch shortening. Good functional result. (Courtesy Dr. Joseph Lembeck.)

The application of the method is best illustrated by referring to Fig. 995. Adhesive traction strips with the spreader are fastened on the leg extending from the ankle to the knee as described above under the application of traction strips. The knee is then suspended by means of a large turkish bath towel or other large wide sling to which a suspension rope is attached. This rope is directed upward and toward the foot of the bed at an angle of about thirty degrees with the vertical and passes over a pulley in the overhead frame and then down through a pulley in the frame attached to the foot of the bed, back through the pulley attached to the spreader to which the skin traction strips are fixed, and back again to the foot of the bed and over a pulley; and here the weights are suspended.

Because there is a double pull from the foot piece to the foot of the bed, the traction is equal to approximately double the amount of weight while the traction upward is equal approximately to the amount of weight used. in this way there is a parallelogram of forces acting in the line of the shaft of the femur. Russell states that from eight to ten pounds of weight is all that is necessary in the average adult femur and that full length should be obtained in about twenty-four hours. If full length is not obtained in two or three days he suspects muscular interposition, and the necessity for an open reduction to disentangle the ends of the fragments from the muscles arises.

The thigh is supported by means of a large pillow which is pushed up under it. The apparatus should be so arranged that the knee is flexed about thirty degrees, and the foot should just clear the mattress of the bed. In some clinics the thigh is supported by a wide band to which from five to ten pounds of weight is attached, the amount depending upon the size of the leg, enough weight being used to restore the normal anterior bowing to the femur.

The aftertreatment is exactly the same as that described in the treatment with the Thomas splint and skin traction. The foot should be supported by a strip of adhesive to which from one to two pounds weight is attached, and the patient should be provided with a trapeze in order that he may move himself about in bed. The foot of the bed should, of course, be elevated from ten to fourteen inches.

Treatment of Compound Fractures of the Shaft of the Femur

Compound fractures of the shaft of the femur may present a very serious problem because of the extensive tissue damage and shock which are apt to be present. There is also constant danger of infection which in the thigh may be serious. This danger of infection prohibits the use of the immediate manipulative reduction and incorporation in a plaster cast and makes it imperative that the fracture be treated by traction in order that the thigh may be observed and adequate drainage afforded to any infection which may arise.

The question as to whether or not débridement is to be done in every case must be decided by the surgeon. Campbell* believes that débridement causes

---

*Campbell, W. C.: Surg. Gynec. and Obst., November, 1924.

further damage to the tissues and finds that 75 per cent of compound fractures in civil practice do not become infected. He cleans out the wound with iodine and then applies a sterile hot dressing of ½ to 1 per cent carbolic acid solution and places the limb in a Thomas splint with traction. If no infection has occurred at the end of ten days, the fracture is reduced by the manipulative method and immobilized in a plaster cast.

We are convinced that a débridement, if properly done, not only does not cause increased trauma to the tissues, but removes devitalized tissue, and for this reason we believe that with the exception of certain gunshot wounds, these fractures should be débrided (Fig. 1002). When the case is seen early we treat these fractures by débridement and primary closure, with a rubber drain for forty-eight hours, and traction in a Thomas splint usually with skeletal traction (Figs. 998, 1000, and 1001). If the patient is seen late and the wound is obviously infected, we insure drainage and use the Dakin technic or Orr method as described in the section on the treatment of compound fractures.

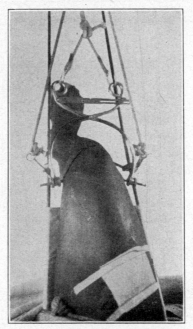

Fig. 998.—Compound fracture of the femur treated by skeletal traction. Note the freedom of access to the thigh.

In the treatment of compound fractures of the femur which have become infected it should be emphasized that it is important that the fracture be immobilized in a Thomas splint as completely as possible by bandages which surround both the thigh and the splint, and also that the knee be kept as close to the bed as possible in order that the tendency of the pus to travel along the fascial spaces toward the hip be minimized. We have seen compound fractures of the femur which, when treated with hip flexion of forty-five degrees, develop large pockets of pus in the upper thigh and these gravity abscesses may go unrecognized for a considerable period of time.

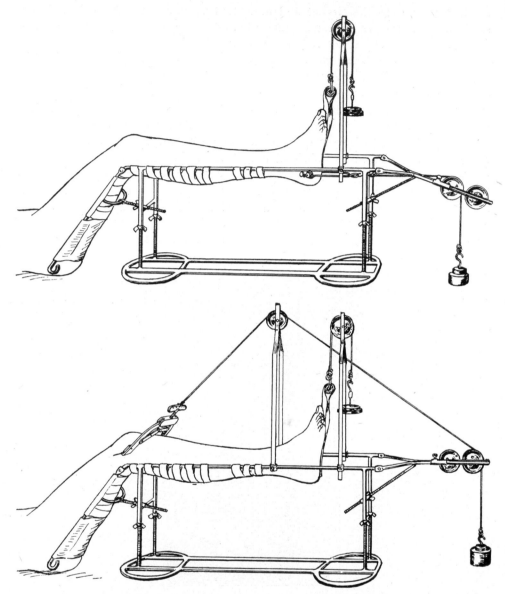

Fig. 999.—Zimmer modification of Boehler-Braun splint; useful for fractures of the shaft of the femur or of the leg. (Courtesy Zimmer Manufacturing Co.)

Treatment of Fractures of the Shaft of the Femur by Open Reduction

In the past we have operated on fractures of the shaft of the femur only as a last resort and after conservative treatment had failed. Since we have been implanting sulfonamide powder in our clean operative wounds, we have much less fear of infection and resort to open operation and internal fixation earlier and more frequently than in the past. Many surgeons, on the other hand, use open reduction and internal fixation routinely in the treatment of these fractures and report excellent results. One important point is that the surgeon should watch his cases carefully and not wait several months before resorting to open

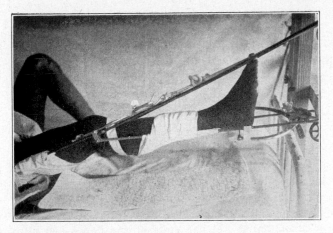

Fig. 1000.—Skeletal traction being used in fractures of both the femur and the leg. Traction on the leg is made by a pin through the os calcis, using overhead pelvic femur frame. In shaft fractures involving the upper two-thirds of the tibia and fibula, skeletal traction can be applied through the lower end of the tibia.

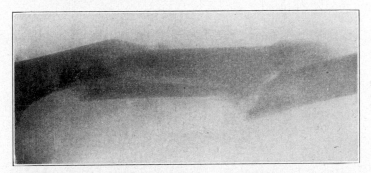

Fig. 1001.—Compound double fracture of the femur with beginning union. Treated by skeletal traction with Thomas splint and Pearson knee flexion attachment.

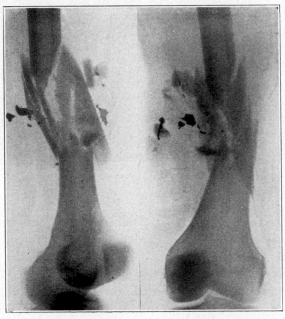

Fig. 1002.—Compound comminuted fracture of the femur from a pistol wound. Treated by skeletal traction without débridement. Good result.

reduction in those cases which he is unable to reduce by manipulation or traction, because in many of these cases muscle or fascia is interposed between the fragments, and this must be removed before union can occur. Consequently, unless the position is satisfactory and there are signs of beginning union he should do the operation within a few weeks after the injury and thus shorten the period of disability.

Technic of the Operation.—A longitudinal incision about six inches long is made on the anterolateral surface of the thigh and carried down to the bone, retracting the rectus and splitting the crureus muscle to expose the site of the fracture. The fracture is then reduced by angulation or leverage or traction as indicated. If the ends of the bones are quite stable after reduction and do not tend to be displaced, no internal fixation is necessary. On the other hand, if there is a tendency for the fragments to slip, some internal fixation should be used.

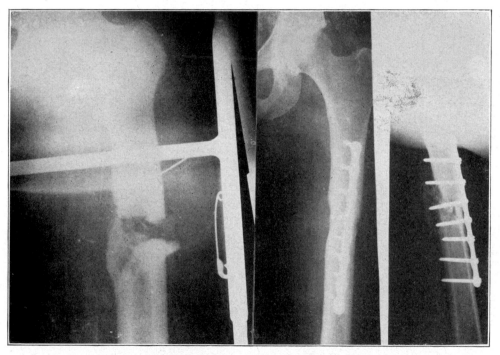

Fig. 1003.—Fracture of the femur treated by skeletal traction through tibial tubercle on Boehler-Braun splint without successful reduction. Stainless steel plate three weeks later and solid union in eleven months. (Courtesy Dr. Joseph Lembeck.)

The popular types of internal fixation are steel plates, Parham bands, wire, and kangaroo tendon or heavy chromic catgut. It should be remembered that the internal fixation is not supposed to maintain the alignment and position of the femur, but is merely supposed to hold the ends of the bones in contact while immobilization is secured by external splintage. We prefer either the stainless steel or vitallium plates and screws. The methods and indications for the use of these materials are given in the section on the "Operative Treatment of Fractures."

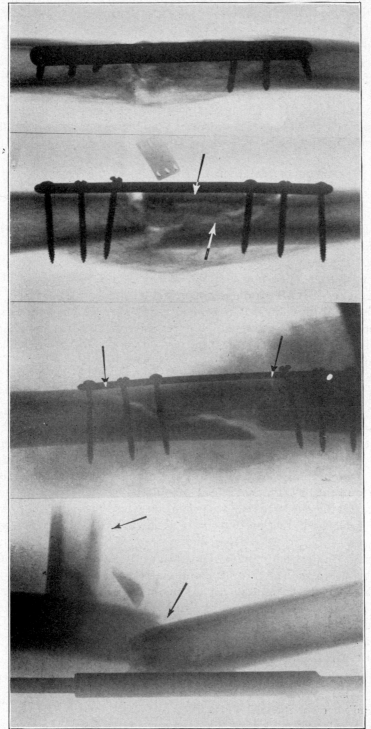

Fig. 1004.—Severe comminuted fracture through the middle third of the femur. Skeletal traction failed. Open reduction and internal fixation. Good result.

After the fragments have been united by a plate or catgut or other material, sulfonamide powder is implanted in the wound and it is closed, care being taken to preserve proper alignment of the limb, and the fracture is immobilized either in a large plaster spica as described under the "Treatment of Fractures of the Shaft of the Femur by Manipulative Reduction" or it can be immobilized by suspension and traction by the application of a Thomas splint with a moderate amount of traction. In either case the aftertreatment is exactly as is that described under the "Treatment of Simple Fractures by either Manipulation or Traction."

Treatment of Malunion in Fractures of the Femur

Fractures of the femur which have become united in poor position offer a very serious problem and treatment should only be undertaken by an especially skillful bone surgeon. The first thing to be decided is whether or not it is safe to treat the fracture. If the fracture has been compounded and infected there is always the danger of infection lighting up again either after manipulation or open operation and the danger is just as great in the case of manipulation as it is after an open operation.

If there are open wounds it is probably better to do an open operation, chisel the bones apart, remove dead bone, reduce the fracture if possible, and treat in a plaster cast or by traction, and use either the Dakin or Orr method of treatment for osteomyelitis.

If there has been a wound with open infection, at least six months should pass before the fracture is manipulated or an attempt made to correct the malunion. If the fracture has been a simple fracture, or if it has been infected and six months have passed since there has been any evidence of activity of the infection, the surgeon is justified in attempting to correct the malposition which may be either shortening or angulation. Unless the shortening is more than one-half inch and unless the angulation is sufficient to cause real disability to the patient, the fracture should be let alone, because not only must the patient be subjected to a serious operative procedure followed by a period of prolonged traction, but there is always the danger of resultant nonunion.

Old cases with firm bony union demand open operation as it is useless to attempt to break up the fracture by manipulation, but in recent cases (up to three months in children and up to six months in adults) the surgeon is justified in attempting to break up the malunion by manipulation and then treat the fracture by skeletal traction.

The best series of cases treated in this manner has been reported by L. C. Abbott.* His method is as follows:

"A forty-eight-hour preparation of the skin of the thigh and leg is a preliminary to manipulation. To avoid strain on the knee joint, padded board splints, extending from the site of fracture to the sole of the foot, are firmly bandaged to the lateral and posterior surfaces of the limb. Control of the upper fragment is secured by taking a hitch with padded rope just above the fracture. Under nitrous oxide anesthesia, with an assistant controlling the

---

*Abbott, L. C.: Arch. Surg., September, 1924.

upper fragment by means of the rope, the operator quickly refractures by forcibly increasing the deformity. The fragments are further disengaged by internal and external rotations as well as by traction applied to the lower fragment. Often lengthening of an inch or more can be obtained at this time. A Thomas splint with knee flexion piece attached is then applied, forcing the ring against the tuberosity of the ischium. The thigh and calf are supported by flannel bands fastened to the uprights of the splints.''

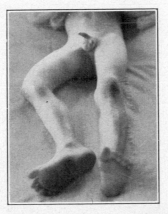

Fig. 1005.—Child with fracture of the shaft of the femur, middle and upper third.

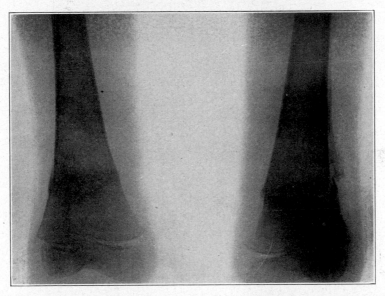

Fig. 1006.—Bilateral incomplete fracture of the shaft of the femur in a child. Treated in plaster. Good result.

After the fracture has been broken up, skeletal traction must be used to obtain reduction. For this reason either a wire or pin through the lower end of the femur or calipers should be applied and from thirty to forty pounds weight attached. The fracture is then treated as described under the "Treatment of Fractures by Skeletal Traction by the Thomas Splint" except that it is usually necessary to keep the heavy weight on for a longer period.

Fractures of the Shaft of the Femur in Infants and Children

The pathology and diagnosis of fractures of the shaft of the femur in infants and children are practically the same as in similar lesions in adults (Fig. 1005) except that one occasionally sees greenstick or subperiosteal fractures without displacement, such as the bilateral case illustrated in Fig. 1006.

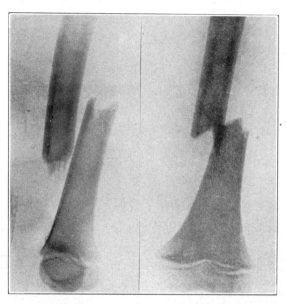

Fig. 1007.—Fracture of the shaft of the middle and lower thirds of the femur in a child showing typical displacements.

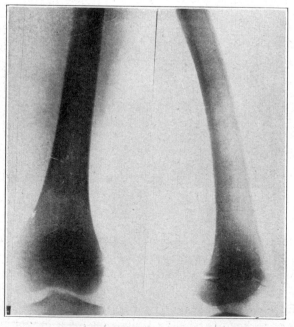

Fig. 1008.—Same as preceding after treatment by manipulative reduction and immobilization in a plaster-of-Paris cast.

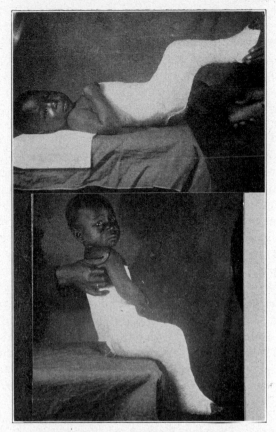

Fig. 1009.—Plaster-of-Paris spica used in the immobilization of fractures of the shaft of the femur in infants and small children up to one and one-half or two years of age, after reduction.

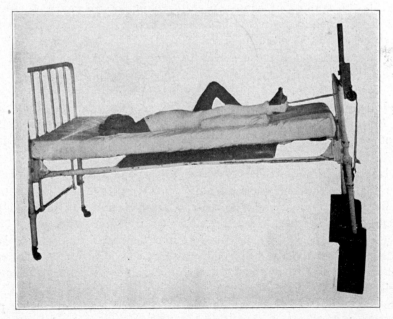

Fig. 1010.—Traction combined with plaster-of-Paris immobilization, treatment of fracture of the shaft of the femur in a child. This treatment is best for those patients past the age of six or eight where the fragments cannot be held in place by a plaster cast without traction.

The treatment is based upon the same principles as is that in adults except that in infants and young children it is possible to place the leg in extension and apply traction with the hips at ninety degrees flexion because the hamstrings are so lax. For this reason the Bryant's method, which will be described later, is probably the most efficient method of treatment.

In transverse fractures the fracture can usually be reduced by manipulation and a plaster cast can be applied with the hip and knee flexed as illustrated in Figs. 1007 and 1008, or it may be applied with the leg in the extended position. The flexed position is particularly useful in infants, as it permits much better and easier alignment of the fragments (Fig. 1008). In certain cases a plaster spica is applied over traction strips to the leg as illustrated in Fig. 1010. It should also be mentioned that skeletal traction is rarely ever necessary in children, except in cases of early malunion where it is necessary to apply a large amount of traction in order to correct shortening which has been present for some time or in cases of severe compound comminuted fractures where amputation would probably have to be done otherwise or where the soft structures are so severely injured that it would not be possible to apply adhesive traction. When skeletal traction is used it should be applied by means of a wire or pin through the lower portion of the shaft of the femur or proximal third of the tibia as calipers may slip and pull off the lower epiphysis. Open reduction is rarely indicated in children and a shortening of one-half of an inch will usually be corrected by growth, but correct alignment is as important as it is in adults.

The Bryant Vertical Traction Method of Treatment of Fractures of the Shaft of the Femur in Infants and Children

This is the method of choice in children under six years of age. After the age of six to eight years the hamstrings begin to tighten up and the vertical method cannot be used so successfully.

For the treatment it is necessary to have a frame over the crib. There are numerous types of frames in use in various hospitals. A very satisfactory one is that illustrated in Fig. 1011. Adhesive traction strips with a spreader attached are applied to both legs; then the ropes extending from these are passed through pulleys which are located directly over the hip joints, and sufficient weight is attached to these pulleys just to counterbalance the body weight of the child.

In larger children it is also advisable to suspend a trapeze from the frame in order that the child may use his hands in lifting himself. In children who do not lie quietly in bed, and who tend to twist around and thus displace the fragments, the two thighs can be strapped together with wide bands of adhesive and the pelvis can be fixed to the bed by a canvas restrainer as illustrated in Figs. 1012 and 1013. Some surgeons also put traction strips on the feet in order to prevent foot drop, but we have not found this necessary although they are shown in Fig. 1011.

The position of the fragment should be checked by x-ray (using portable apparatus), and the vertical traction should be maintained until union is quite firm—six to eight weeks. At the end of this time in young children all

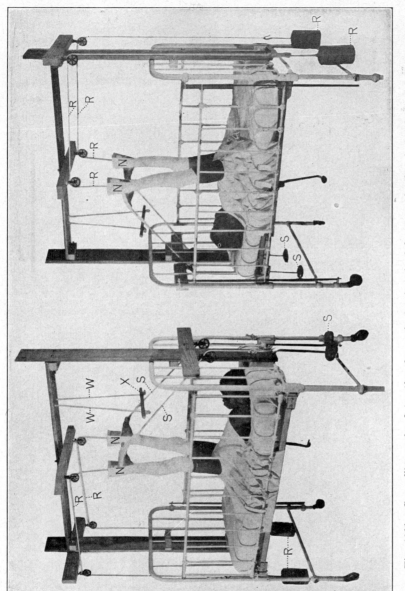

Fig. 1011.—Conwell's overhead traction frame in treatment of fractures in the shaft of the femur in children showing the ease with which the frame can be adjusted; when, if desired, the main traction can be placed at the foot of bed and the traction on soles of feet remain at the head of frame. This is not often necessary, and is not as desirable as when the weights (R-R) are at the head of the bed. Also showing how the frame can be lowered or raised depending on the size of the child; i.e., the length of the child's legs. (Conwell: J. Bone and Joint Surgery, July, 1929.)

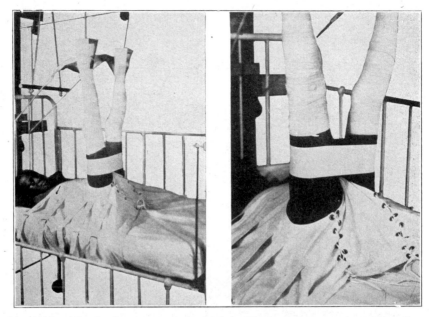

Fig. 1012.—Adhesive band around the thighs and canvas apron to immobilize the patient during the treatment by vertical traction. Close-up views of the retractor, showing application of adhesive around the thighs, which is used sometimes where there is too much external displacement of either proximal or distal fragments. This procedure is very successful for improving the alignment in certain cases. It is necessary to use this only during the first few days, because after a few days of prolonged traction the fragments remain in position without difficulty, and, with the rapid formation of callus, this aids also in keeping the fragments in alignment. (Conwell: J. Bone and Joint Surgery, July, 1929.)

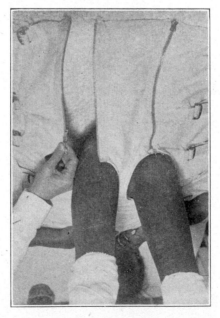

Fig. 1013.—The muslin retractor with zippers. Note that zippers separate completely, enabling lower part of muslin retractor to be removed entirely from around buttocks and upper part of thighs. (Conwell: J. Bone and Joint Surg., October, 1933.)

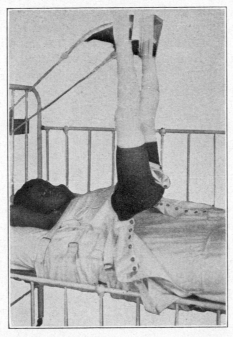

Fig. 1014.—View showing the ease of removal of the lower part of the muslin retractor for patient to use bedpan or any other necessary toilet. Also note that the traction across patient's lower abdomen is still in place. (Conwell: J. Bone and Joint Surg., July, 1929.)

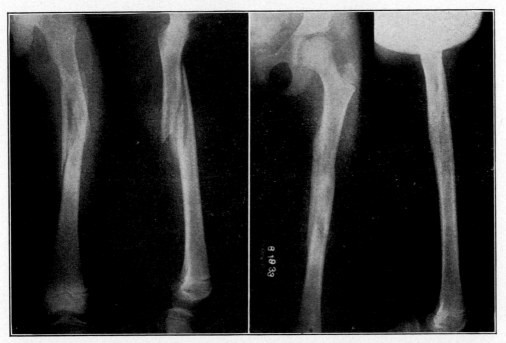

Fig. 1015.—Fracture of the shaft of the femur. Treated by adhesive traction showing satisfactory union and position.

traction can be removed. The slightly older children may be left in Buck's extension from one to two weeks longer. At the end of this time if union is solid they can be got up with lateral plaster molds or a Thomas walking caliper splint which should be worn for from four to eight weeks, or until there is no longer any danger of bending from callus. If it is not possible to obtain reduction with traction or manipulation, open reduction should be performed as described under ''Treatment of Fractures of the Femur in the Adult.''

The Prognosis in Fractures of the Shaft of the Femur in Children.—The prognosis is better in children than in adults because even with a moderate amount of shortening—one-half to one inch—there is a tendency for the shortening to be corrected spontaneously by growth. Likewise, mild errors in alignment tend to be corrected by growth. On the other hand, one occasionally sees a small amount of overgrowth after a fracture in a child and the injured extremity may become slightly longer than the normal one.

We have found that seldom is it necessary to do open reduction in fractures of the femur shaft in children except in the very marked neglected overlapping fragments which traction cannot improve. An overlapping of an inch in fracture of the femur in children is seldom an indication for open reduction. Such cases if treated conservatively will in most instances develop a compensatory lengthening. However, every effort possible should be carried out to bring about good approximation of the fragments by the closed manipulation or traction method.

CHAPTER XXIV

INJURIES IN THE REGION OF THE KNEE JOINT

SURGICAL ANATOMY

The Lower End of the Femur.—In its lower portion the femur is expanded and cancellous in structure and terminates in two condyles which articulate with the patella in front and the tibia below. The condyles are convex from before backward and project posteriorly beyond the line of the shaft. Anteriorly the two condyles fuse to form the floor of a shallow groove for the patella and below and behind they are rounded to articulate with the tibia, and the rounded surfaces are separated by the intercondylar notch. The lateral surfaces are flattened and roughened for the attachment of ligaments. The adductor tubercle which serves as the point of attachment of the adductor magnus muscle is situated in the posterior and superior portion of the flattened mesial surface of the condyle.

The Upper End of the Tibia.—The expanded upper end of the tibia is cancellous in structure, and roughly ovoid on cross-section. It consists of two tuberosities which project beyond the line of the shaft behind and here they are separated by the popliteal notch. The superior surface of each tuberosity presents a shallow concavity for articulation with the corresponding condyle of the femur and these two articular facets are separated by a roughened area for the attachment of the crucial ligaments. The spine of the tibia projects from this roughened area and terminates in two peaks with a shallow groove between them. The borders of the tuberosities are roughened for the attachment of ligaments, and the posterior border of the lateral tuberosity presents a small articular facet for articulation with the head of the fibula. The tibial tubercle is an eminence on the anterior surface of the bone which serves for the attachment of the patellar ligament.

The Patella is a lozenge-shaped bone which lies in the quadriceps tendon and affords leverage for extending the leg on the thigh. Being a sesamoid bone, it is not covered by periosteum, but its anterior and lateral surfaces are covered by fibers of the quadriceps tendon, while its posterior surface is articular and presents two shallow lateral depressions and a median ridge to conform to the anterior surface of the lower end of the femur on which it glides. The main mass of the quadriceps tendon is inserted into the upper end of the patella and the patellar ligament is attached to its lower end.

Ossification.—The lower end of the femur and the upper end of the tibia each develop from a single center which is usually present at birth and unites with the shaft about the twenty-first year.

The patella is cartilaginous at birth and a center of ossification appears during the fourth year and gradually enlarges until the entire bone is ossified.

The Knee Joint is a hinge joint between the lower end of the femur and the upper end of the tibia, the structure of which is rendered unusually complex by the presence of the semilunar cartilages and crucial and alar ligaments in the joint cavity (Figs. 1016, 1017, and 1018). It is the largest and one of the strongest joints in the body. Its great strength is evidenced by the fact that although it is subject to great strain, dislocations at the knee are very rare injuries. The stability of the knee joint is due to the strong ligaments in and around the joint rather than to the conformation of the bones.

The articular cavity is prolonged upward on the front of the femur for a distance of four or five inches as the suprapatellar bursa and is prolonged upward on the posterior surface and sides of the femur for a short distance above the borders of the condyles.

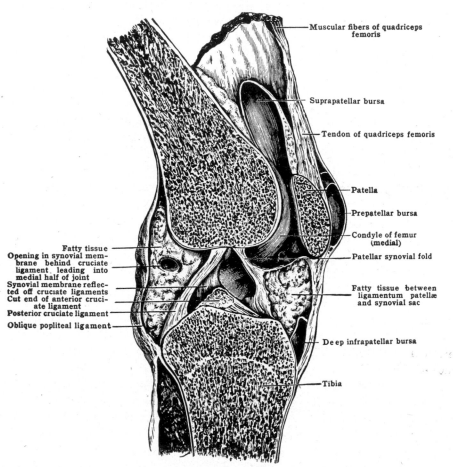

Fig. 1016.—Sagittal section through the knee joint. (From Morris: *Human Anatomy*, P. Blakiston's Son & Co., Inc., Publisher.)

The Capsule.—The fibrous capsule is attached above to the lateral surfaces of the condyles and to the posterior surface of the shaft of the femur, and below it is attached to the borders of the condyles of the tibia and to the upper end of the fibula. In front the capsule merges with the quadriceps tendon and its lateral expansions on either side of the patella and is attached to the margins of the patella. The front of the knee is covered by the quadriceps tendon, the patella, and the patellar ligament. On the sides the capsule is reinforced by the internal and external lateral ligaments and posteriorly it is reinforced by the popliteal and gastrocnemius muscles and a strong fibrous band (ligament of Winslow) which passes outward from the semi-membranosus tendon.

The Crucial Ligaments.—(Figs. 1017 and 1018.) Much of the stability of the knee depends upon the integrity of the crucial ligaments. These are two strong fibrous bands extending from the intercondylar fossa of the femur to the roughened interarticular area on the superior surface of the tibia.

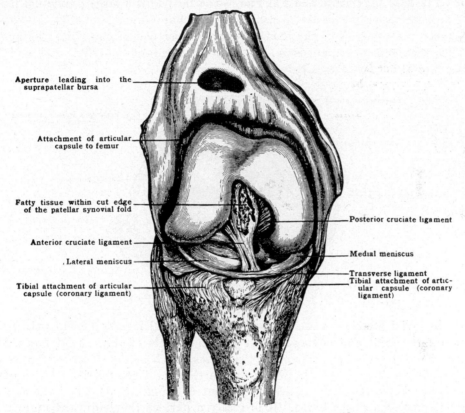

Fig. 1017.—View of the knee joint with capsule removed and the patella turned down to show the crucial ligaments. (From Morris: *Human Anatomy*, P. Blakiston's Son & Co., Inc., Publisher.)

The anterior crucial ligament is attached above to the posterior portion of the inner surface of the lateral condyle and extends obliquely downward, forward, and inward to be attached to the roughened area in front of the spine of the tibia. It is taut when the knee is extended and prevents hyper-extension at the knee and instability of the tibia on the femur when the knee is extended.

The posterior crucial ligament is attached above to the anterior portion of the outer surface of the internal condyle and passes downward, outward, and backward behind the anterior crucial to be inserted into the roughened area behind the spine of the tibia. It is taut when the knee is flexed and prevents instability of the tibia on the femur in this position.

The Semilunar Cartilages.—(Figs. 1017 and 1018.) These are two crescent-shaped pieces of fibrocartilage which are interposed between the condyles of the femur and those of the tibia. The ends of the semilunar cartilages are firmly attached to the tibia and they follow this bone in all movements of the knee joint. Their thick outer borders blend with the capsule of the joint and their thin edges project into the articular cavity and fill the space caused by the condyles of the femur being more sharply curved than are those of the tibia. The internal semilunar is C shaped and the external is broader and forms almost a complete circle.

The Alar Ligaments and Fat Pad.—The fat pad is a large pyramidal mass of adipose tissue which lies beneath the patellar tendon and fills the space between the condyles of the femur and the upper end of the tibia. Its apex, called the ligamentum mucosum, is attached to the intercondylar notch and its free lateral borders are called the alar ligaments.

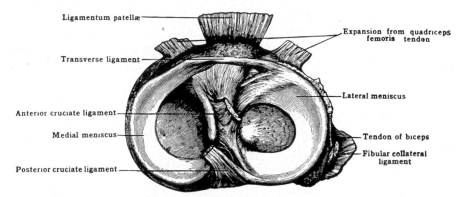

Fig. 1018.—Upper surface of the tibia showing semilunar cartilages in position. (From Morris: *Human Anatomy*, P. Blakiston's Son & Co., Inc., Publisher.)

Synovial Membrane and Bursae.—The synovial membrane lines the capsule of the joint and covers the fat pad and parts of the crucial ligaments and the intraarticular portions of the bones which are not covered by cartilage. It does not cover the semilunar cartilages. That portion of the joint cavity which extends upward on the front of the femur is called the suprapatellar or quadriceps bursa. It is really a part of the joint, although it is developed as a separate cavity. The deep infrapatellar bursa lies between the patellar tendon and the upper border of the tibia. There is a small bursa beneath the inner head of the gastrocnemius and this may communicate with the joint. The prepatellar bursa lies between the patella and the skin.

Movements at the Knee.—The chief movements are flexion and extension and these are accomplished by a gliding of the tibia and semilunar cartilages over the condyles of the femur. The patella glides up and down on the trochlear surface of the femur, being pulled up beyond the articular surface in extension and resting on the lower surface of the external condyle with only its inner border touching the internal condyle when the knee is fully flexed. In complete extension there is a slight amount of external rotation of the leg and in semiflexion the ligaments are relaxed and a slight amount of rotation is possible, but this is mainly passive.

Vessels and Nerves.—The popliteal artery and vein and internal and external popliteal nerves lie in the fat tissue which fills the popliteal space. The external popliteal nerve passes downward and outward beneath the tendon of the biceps to wind around the upper end of the shaft of the fibula. In this latter position the nerve is subcutaneous and is susceptible to injury.

SUPRACONDYLAR FRACTURES OF THE LOWER END OF THE FEMUR AND INTERCONDYLAR OR T FRACTURES OF THE FEMUR

As in fractures of the shaft of the femur most of the supracondylar fractures result from falls from a height, the patient landing either on the foot or on the knee, but they may also result from direct violence or torsion injuries.

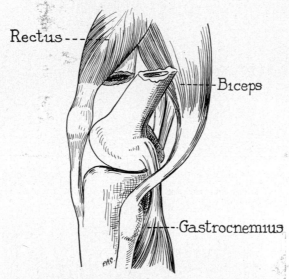

Fig. 1019.—Sketch showing usual displacement of fragments in lower third of femur.

In the intercondylar or T fractures the end of the proximal fragment is driven into the distal fragment and splits the condyles apart. These fractures are rather uncommon, but are very important because of the difficulties encountered in controlling the short lower fragment and because of the severe and permanent disability which may result if successful reduction is not obtained.

Pathology.—The fracture line across the shaft tends to be roughly transverse, or slightly oblique from before backward (Fig. 1019), and in the intercondylar type the fracture through the shaft is complicated by a vertical split in the lower end of the femur which ends below in the intercondylar fossa and results in a separation of the condyles. Many of these fractures, however, do not run true to form, and the fracture through the shaft of the femur may be a long oblique fracture while the supracondylar region of the femur may be extensively comminuted (Fig. 1022). This shattering of the supracondylar region is especially apt to occur in falls from a height. Fortunately other than the splitting apart of the condyles the articular portion of the bone is rarely involved in the fracture. This is due to the fact that the convex condyles are more dense than the bone above them.

In children and in atrophic bones these fractures may be impacted. When this occurs, the proximal fragment is driven into the cancellous bone in the lower end of the femur. In most instances the fracture line communicates with the knee joint, and this may be widely opened and filled with blood. Even in cases in which there is no obvious tearing of the joint capsule the knee joint is usually filled with blood; this frequently results in chronic thickening of the synovial membrane with later difficulty in the restoration of motion in the joint.

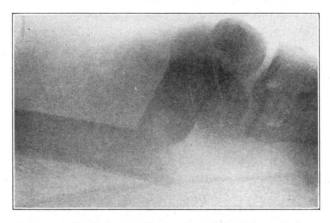

Fig. 1020.—Fracture of the lower third of femur with backward displacement of the distal fragment. This is an ideal type for skeletal traction. Treated by skeletal traction (Kirschner wire through distal fragment) for six weeks, by adhesive traction for three weeks, and walking caliper for three months.

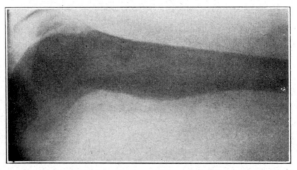

Fig. 1021.—Showing union six months later, in the same case.

Displacement.—In rare instances supracondylar and dicondylar fractures occur with little or no displacement, but as a rule there is complete separation of the fractured ends, and the short distal fragment is tipped backward so that its proximal end projects into the popliteal space. This tipping backward of the distal fragment is due to the pull of the two heads of the gastrocnemius muscle which arise from the posterior surface of the femur just above the condyles.

In addition to the posterior displacement of the distal fragment there is also more or less upward displacement with overriding of the fragments and in injuries due to a fall from a height the distal end of the upper fragment may be driven downward into the knee joint and may rest against the patella or project through the skin. There is also apt to be some lateral displacement of the lower fragment; this is usually inward on account of the pull of the adductor magnus which is inserted in the adductor tubercle.

In intercondylar fractures there may or may not be separation of the condyles. In some instances the fracture is merely a line between them, while in others they may be widely separated and the distal end of the proximal fragment may rest between the two condyles so that one is tipped backward more than the other, thus causing additional incongruity of the surfaces of the joint. Very rarely the classical picture is reversed and the short distal fragment is displaced forward and pulled upward on the anterior surface of the distal end of the proximal fragment, while the proximal fragment projects into the popliteal space.

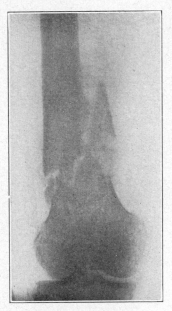

Fig. 1022.—Severely comminuted T fracture of the femur. Treated by skeletal traction and suspension by means of a pin through the upper end of the tibia with good result.

Diagnosis.—The diagnosis of a fracture through the lower end of the femur is not difficult, but it may be practically impossible to determine from physical examination whether or not there is also a fracture between the condyles. Consequently these fractures should be x-rayed when possible before treatment is instituted. There is a history of a severe injury followed by complete disability, and on inspection there is marked swelling in the lower half of the thigh and there may be a variable amount of visible deformity.

Measurement will disclose a variable amount of shortening of the extremity and palpation will reveal the presence of excess fluid in the knee joint and a rather definite line of point tenderness in the supracondylar region which extends entirely around the femur. In addition to the tenderness it is also possible to palpate the ends of the fragments beneath the quadriceps tendon and in the popliteal space. Even with the knee joint distended with fluid the patella choc may not be present because the patella may rest upon the distal end of the upper fragment or the flexed position of the knee may hold it down against the condyles.

Intercondylar fractures can be detected if there is considerable separation of the fragments because the marked broadening of the lower end of the femur is visible and palpable, and unless the distal fragment rests between the condyles, the two condyles can be squeezed back together by lateral pressure.

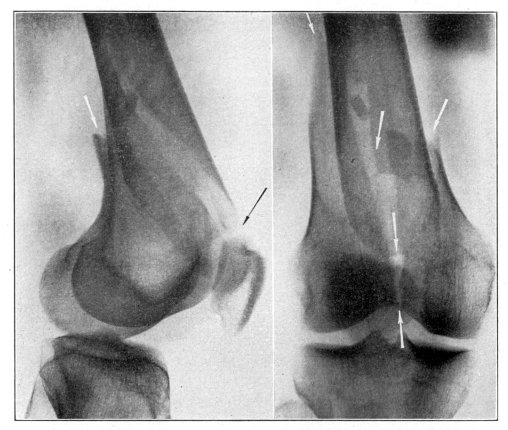

Fig. 1023.—Supracondylar T fracture of the femur.

Manipulation is to be avoided in these fractures because of the possibility of causing injury to the popliteal vessels and nerves, but when there is little or no displacement and the signs mentioned above are questionable, one is justified in demonstrating false motion. This can be done most safely and definitely by grasping the ankle in one hand and the femur above the fracture with the other and slowly moving the leg from side to side. If an unimpacted fracture is present, false motion will occur at the site of the fracture.

Complications of Fractures of the Lower End of the Femur.—The examination should not be completed without determining the condition of the circulation in the leg and whether or not the sensory and motor nerves are intact because with the lower fragment projecting into the popliteal space the popliteal vessels and nerves are frequently injured and may be completely torn across.

Rupture of the popliteal artery or vein will be evidenced by a large hematoma in the popliteal space, and this necessitates immediate operation and ligation of the torn vessel. When the artery is ruptured the vein and artery should both be ligated. These vascular injuries may necessitate amputation, as the collateral circulation at this level is very poor. The nerve should be treated by support to prevent stretching of the paralyzed muscles, and the patient will usually recover within the course of a few months.

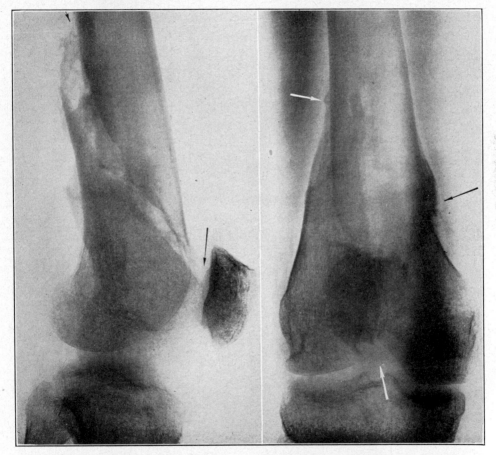

Fig. 1024.—Same patient after treatment by skeletal traction through the upper fourth of the tibia. Good functional results.

Treatment of Supracondylar and Intercondylar Fractures of the Lower End of the Femur

The treatment of supracondylar fractures in which there is no line of fracture between the condyles is similar to that described above for fractures of the shaft of the femur, and, depending upon the individual surgeon and upon the contour of the fracture, these fractures may be treated by immediate manipulative reduction and immobilization or by traction.

The intercondylar or T fractures should always be treated by traction and on rare occasions require an open reduction.

Aspiration of the Knee.—In these fractures the knee joint is practically always distended with blood; this should be removed by aspiration with a relatively small sterile needle. If the fracture is reduced by manipulation, the joint should be aspirated before the cast is applied. If the fracture is treated by traction the knee should be aspirated immediately after the traction has been applied and the aspiration should be repeated the next day if necessary.

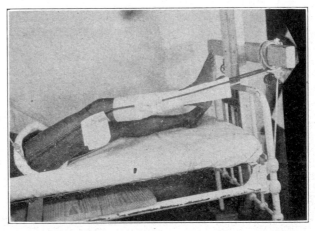

Fig. 1025.—Skin traction applied to the leg used in the treatment of supracondylar fractures in which there is very little displacement and in which only slight flexion at the knee is necessary. This type of traction is frequently used in fractures of the upper end of the tibia, tibial spine, and contusions without fracture.

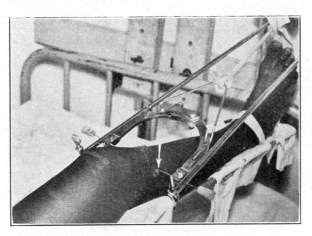

Fig. 1026.—Kirschner wire as applied to the upper fourth of the tibia for traction in the treatment of fractures of the lower half of the femur.

Manipulative Reduction.—When the fracture line is roughly transverse, it is relatively easy to reduce these fractures because the bones are quite superficial. Reduction is accomplished as described above in reduction of fractures of the shaft of the femur by direct traction in the line of the flexed femur with the knee flexed about 45 degrees. While the traction is applied, the fragments should be pulled down so that they no longer overlap and then molded by anterolateral and posterior pressure over the ends of the fragments until approximately anatomical reduction is obtained. Then the traction is released, permitting the fragments to engage.

The reduction should be performed with the patient under local, general or spinal anesthesia and while lying on a fracture table and prepared for the application of a plaster-of-Paris spica. When the reduction appears to be satisfactory, the surgeon should hold the fractured limb and his assistants should apply the plaster-of-Paris spica from the waistline to the base of the toes. The fractured limb should be immobilized with the thigh and knee flexed about 45 degrees.

Treatment by Traction.—With the exception of cases with practically no displacement (Fig. 1025) we treat these fractures by means of skeletal traction because it is necessary that the traction be applied with the knee in a position of flexion, and it is not possible to exert adequate traction in the line of the shaft of the femur on the lower fragment by means of adhesive. The skeletal traction may be applied by means of calipers to the condyles of the femur or by means of a wire or pin through the condyles of the femur or by means of a wire or pin through the upper third of the shaft of the tibia. In dicondylar fractures and in supracondylar fractures in which the fracture line lies very close to the joint, we prefer to apply the traction by means of a wire through the tibia (Fig. 1026).

Application of the Wire or Pin Through the Tibia.—The patient is anesthetized, a Thomas splint is slipped over the leg and pillows are placed under the knee. The skin over the upper end of the tibia is painted with iodine and pulled upward, and a small incision is made on the lateral border of the leg one-half inch below the tibial tubercle and one-half inch posterior to the crest of the tibia. The wire drill is inserted through the incision, drilled through the bone, and out the other side of the leg. When it reaches the skin on the other side, the skin is pulled upward and incised, and the drill is pushed through. The pin wounds are then dressed with gauze, the leg is slung in the Thomas splint, which is bent at the level of the joint from 20 to 30 degrees, and from 20 to 25 pounds or more of traction applied to the pin in the tibia, depending upon the musculature of the patient. After the traction is on and while the patient is still anesthetized, the fragments are manipulated in an effort to correct the displacement.

At the end of twenty-four hours anteroposterior and lateral x-ray pictures are taken, and if the position is satisfactory, about six or eight pounds of traction are removed. If the shortening has not been corrected, the heavy traction should be continued. If the shortening has been corrected and the fragments are not in good position, they should again be manipulated with the patient anesthetized and the leg in the splint.

In cases of dicondylar fracture, it is very important that the condyles be squeezed together and that a tipping backward of one condyle be corrected. This can be done by means of the operator's hands, frequently without an anesthetic. With wide separation it may be necessary to apply a clamp. Scudder has recommended that the ordinary carpenter's clamp be used to squeeze the fragments together. The sides of the condyles are padded with felt and the clamp is tightened. As soon as the desired amount of compression is obtained, the clamp is quickly removed to avoid necrosis of the soft tissues. If the condyles tend to separate after they have been compressed laterally, coaptation splints may be applied on either side of the knee and strapped together with adhesive just as was recommended for the treatment of T fractures of the humerus.

With this method it should rarely be necessary to perform an open reduction on these fractures, and this should not be done until traction and manipulation under traction with lateral compression have failed, because even when open reduction is performed, it is extremely difficult to maintain reduction after it has been obtained. If, however, the surgeon is unable to reduce the displacement by manipulation and to maintain it by traction and lateral compression, an open reduction should be done because marked disability at the knee may follow unless approximately anatomical reposition of the condyles is accomplished.

When an open reduction becomes necessary the leg should be given forty-eight hours' skin preparation and the fracture site exposed through a long lateral incision. The displacements should then be reduced and the fragments maintained in position with the application of as little foreign material as necessary. In some instances chromic catgut will be sufficient. In others bone screws, wire, or bolts may be used. Plates are not very useful in this region because it is difficult to adapt a plate to the contour of the bone and because it is unwise to place a plate so close to the knee joint.

After open reduction and fixation the leg should be immobilized in a plaster-of-Paris cast.

Aftertreatment.—The immobilization in a plaster cast or traction in a Thomas splint should be continued over a period of from six to eight weeks, depending upon the age of the patient and the rapidity with which the fracture consolidates. In cases in which skeletal traction has been used this should be removed as soon as sufficient consolidation has occurred to prevent displacement (about four to six weeks) and adhesive traction should be applied to the leg until union is firm (two to four weeks longer) (Fig. 1025). During this period nothing can be done in the way of restoring motion in the knee joint, but the patient should be told to contract the quadriceps muscle numerous times each day and thus keep the patella free. When the immobilization is discontinued, graded exercises, heat, and massage may be used to restore extension and flexion at the knee. As soon as extension has been obtained, the patient may be fitted with a Thomas caliper walking splint, the use of which should be continued until union is firm, about two months; that is, about four months after the injury.

The stiffness which remains in the knee will, in most instances, disappear gradually. If, at the end of six months after the fracture has consolidated, there is still marked limitation of motion in the knee, and if the amount of motion is not increasing, the surgeon should make some attempt to restore motion. The methods used are traction, manipulation, and quadriceps lengthening.

Traction is effective in mild cases. If the limitation is in extension, the extremity is placed in a straight Thomas splint and adhesive traction is applied to the leg while pressure by means of a bandage over a large cotton pad is applied to the anterior surface of the thigh. If the limitation is in flexion, the Thomas splint is bent at the knee and countertraction is applied by means of a wide sling under the lower third of the thigh. Or the splint may be eliminated and the thigh elevated by means of the sling while Buck's extension is applied to the leg. In the latter type a rope should run from the sling so that the patient by pulling on it may elevate the thigh and thus increase the flexion at the knee and exercise the extremity.

In cases in which traction has failed or in which traction is not deemed advisable, the surgeon may anesthetize the patient and manipulate the knee joint. This manipulation of the knee joint appears to be a very simple thing, but is really quite a dangerous procedure. If too much force is used, the patella may be fractured; if it is done before the fracture is firmly consolidated, the femur may be refractured; and if it is done in the presence of marked bone atrophy, the ends of the bones may be crushed. There are cases on record in which the patients have died of fat embolism following manipulation of atrophic knees. With the bones in good condition, however, and the fracture firmly united, manipulation can be attempted and the surgeon should not hesitate to apply a good deal of force.

After manipulation the knee is fixed in flexion or extension, depending upon which motion has been increased. Fixation should be continued for a few days and then active and passive exercises begun in order to maintain the motion.

Quadriceps Lengthening.—In rare instances it is found impossible to restore motion by traction or manipulation and this is usually due to the fact that the quadriceps tendon is involved in the scar or in the callus at the site of the fracture. When this has occurred motion at the knee should be restored by freeing up and lengthening the quadriceps tendon. This is best done by the method of Bennett who exposes the tendon through an anterior incision, cuts a tongue about six inches long from its lower portion, the lower end of this tongue remaining attached to the patella, and then flexes the knee. In order to obtain flexion in the knee, it may be necessary to divide the adhesions in the upper part of the quadriceps bursa and to open the knee joint widely. When the desired amount of flexion is obtained, the tongue is sutured back in place with the knee flexed and the upper portion of the tendon from which it was removed is sutured together and the wound is closed. The leg is immobilized in flexion for two weeks and at the end of this time active and passive motion are started.

FRACTURES OF A SINGLE CONDYLE OF THE FEMUR

These are rare injuries which may result from direct violence, such as a blow on the side of the knee or getting the knee caught and crushed between two approaching objects, or they may occur from indirect violence, such as falls upon the feet or torsion injuries of the leg.

Pathology.—The fracture line may be vertical (Fig. 1027) or roughly transverse, breaking the lower end of the condyle off or very rarely the condyle may be split in the frontal plane, thus separating its prominent posterior portion, or the condyle may be shattered or a small portion of the lateral surface of the condyle may be torn off with the lateral ligament. These last are classed as sprain fractures and result from adduction or abduction

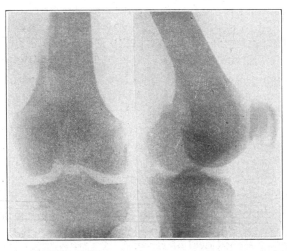

Fig. 1027.—Vertical fracture through a single condyle of the femur with marked effusion of the knee joint. Treated by Kirschner wire through the upper end of the tibia with the knee slightly flexed. After aspiration of the knee, the fragmnts were compressed laterally.

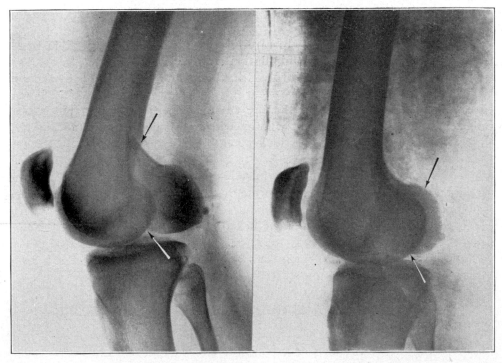

Fig. 1028.—Fracture with backward displacement of the external condyle, lower end of femur. Anatomical result following open reduction. Good result.

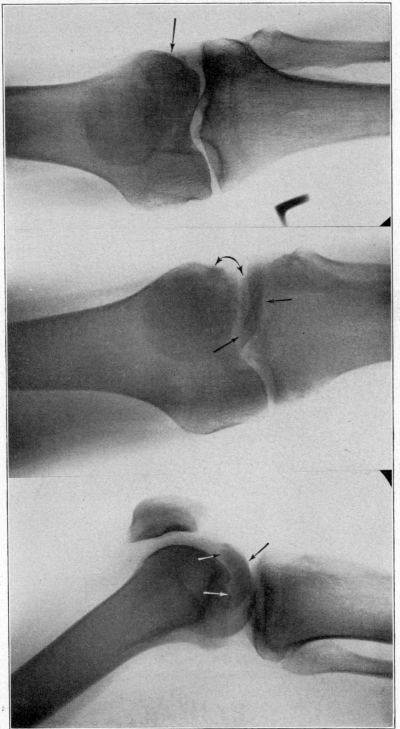

Fig. 1029.—Fracture of the external condyle, lower end of femur. Treated by removal of the completely detached fragment with excellent functional result.

injuries in which, instead of the lateral ligament being torn, its osseous insertion is avulsed. Displacement is not as a rule very marked because the ligamentous attachments tend to maintain the fragments in position and the tibia usually maintains its normal position in relation to the intact condyle. However, occasionally the fractured condyle may be slipped upward or downward in instances where the entire condyle is separated from the rest of the femur and in instances where the end or posterior portion of the condyle is broken off this may be moderately rotated or displaced within the knee joint. In the sprain fractures the avulsed fragment tends to be displaced downward. The knee joint is always involved and is filled with blood.

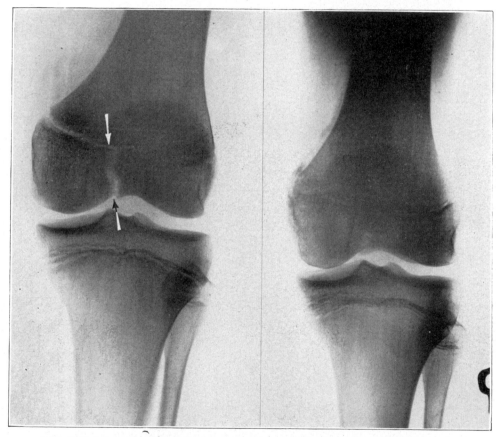

Fig. 1030.—An unusual fracture through the lower epiphysis of the femur in a child fourteen years old. No reduction necessary. Treated by fixation in a cast. Good functional result.

Diagnosis of Fracture of a Single Condyle of the Femur.—The diagnosis is not easy and an x-ray picture is usually necessary in order to determine the exact nature of the injury. There is a history of a severe trauma, the region of the knee is swollen and the joint is distended with fluid. There is no shortening and if false motion is present, it is due to a pushing up of the condyle, in which case the false motion is toward the side of the lesion; or to a tearing loose of the lateral ligament, in which case the false motion is away from the side of the lesion.

On palpation there is local tenderness over the fracture and there may be general tenderness around the knee. It is rarely possible to palpate the separated fragment or to detect abnormalities in the contours of the bone by palpation. With displacement of an intraarticular fragment there may be blocking of motion at the knee joint.

Treatment of Fracture of a Single Condyle of the Femur

Treatment depends a good deal upon the type of fracture and the displacement, and in planning the treatment the fact should be uppermost in the surgeon's mind that in intraarticular fractures anatomic reduction is necessary and the completely loose fragments in the joint must be removed. Where a complete condyle has been broken off and displaced upward it can usually be reduced by traction and a small amount of manipulation with lateral pressure which should be performed after the traction has been applied. Traction tends to reduce the fragment because the lateral ligaments are attached to the loose piece. The knee should be aspirated before reduction is attempted.

If the fragment has been rotated or slipped posteriorly, the manipulation may be combined with flexion and extension at the knee or with abduction or adduction at the knee in order to obtain reduction.

After reduction has been obtained, either by traction or manipulation, it is necessary that the fracture be immobilized over a sufficient period of time to permit healing. This can be done either in traction or in a plaster-of-Paris spica. If a plaster-of-Paris cast is used, the knee should be aspirated before it is applied and the cast should fit snugly around the knee and should extend from around the waist and pelvis to the toes. If the Thomas splint and traction are used, adhesive traction with about ten pounds or more of weight is necessary. The immobilization in a plaster-of-Paris cast or traction should be continued over a period of about four or five weeks. At the end of this time the patient may begin to move the knee, but should abstain from weight-bearing for from five to eight weeks longer, depending upon the type of injury. A molded posterior plaster splint can be used for ten days or two weeks after the spica or traction is removed.

If a satisfactory reduction (approximately anatomical reposition of the fragment) cannot be obtained by manipulation, the fracture should be operated upon and the fragment reduced and fixed with screws or wires. If a portion of the articular surface is loose in the joint, this should be removed.

Treatment of Sprain Fractures at the Knee.—In these injuries the effusion into the knee joint should be removed by aspiration and the area over the fracture should be compressed by cross strapping of adhesive plus an elastic bandage which is applied over felt pads. (Fig. 1075.) In severe injuries the knee should be immobilized over a period of about four weeks. This immobilization should be in a position of slight flexion and may be obtained by immobilization in a plaster-of-Paris cast or by traction in a Thomas splint. At the end of this time the patient may begin to walk, but he should wear an elastic knee cap or elastic bandage around the knee and should have the corresponding border of the heel elevated one-fourth of an inch. The elevated heel should be continued for at least eight weeks. The knee cap can be discarded as soon as the knee feels stable. Dry or moist heat should be used during the convalescence.

PELLEGRINI-STIEDA DISEASE

This term is applied to calcification of the internal lateral ligament of the knee. It may appear some weeks after an injury (sprain of this ligament) and it is probable that some osteogenic tissue is avulsed and lays down bone in the ligament. The area over the mesial side of the internal condyle is tender, and tension on the ligament causes pain. The flake of bone, which varies in size, is seen in the x-ray (Fig. 1031).

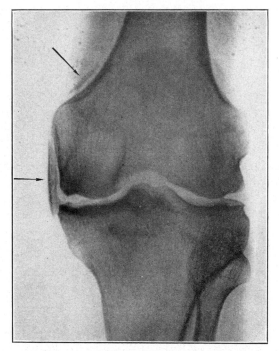

Fig. 1031.—Pellegrini-Steida disease due to an old injury to the internal lateral ligament. Treated by operative removal of the new bone with good result.

Treatment is conservative or operative. If the extremity is encased in a cylinder plaster cast and the patient given crutches for four weeks, the symptoms may subside and the knee cause no further trouble. If the symptoms reappear with use, the bone should be excised and the ligament repaired.

SEPARATION OF THE LOWER EPIPHYSIS OF THE FEMUR

This is a rare injury which may occur at any time up to twenty years of age, but is most frequent in boys between the ages of eight and fourteen. It was formerly called the wagon wheel fracture because the majority of the cases occurred by boys getting their leg caught in the spokes of a revolving wagon wheel. Most of the cases occur as a result of hyperextension and torsion injuries at the knee, but very rarely the epiphysis may be knocked off by direct violence. With forcible hyperextension the strong posterior ligaments and the origins of the gastrocnemius muscles which are largely attached to the epiphysis tear the epiphysis off the diaphysis and carry it forward.

Pathology.—In the majority of the cases the lower epiphysis is displaced forward and upward and rests on the lower end of the shaft between it and the patella (Fig. 1032). The separation may be incomplete and the epiphysis may be only partly displaced (Fig. 1035). In rare instances due to direct violence the epiphysis may be displaced laterally or posteriorly into the popliteal space. There is, of course, marked involvement of the knee joint as the fracture is intraarticular and there may be more or less stripping up of the periosteum. The displacement may be compound and there may be severe damage to the popliteal vessels and nerves.

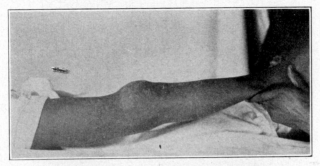

Fig. 1032.—Epiphyseal separation of the lower end of the femur with anterior displacement.

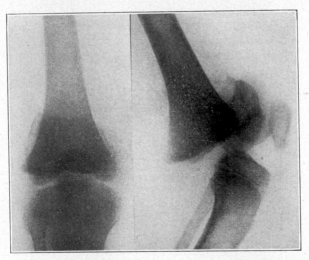

Fig. 1033.—Anteroposterior and lateral views of preceding case.

Diagnosis of Separation of the Lower Epiphysis of the Femur.—In a severe injury at the knee with marked evident pathology and the signs of a fracture through the lower end of the femur in a patient below the age of twenty years, the surgeon should suspect an epiphyseal separation at the lower end of the femur.

On inspection the region of the knee is markedly swollen, especially in its anteroposterior diameter, and there may be obvious deformity of the leg

(Fig. 1032).   On measurement there is usually about an inch of shortening. On palpation it is usually possible to feel the lower end of the diaphysis beneath the skin in the popliteal space, and it may be possible to palpate the condyles of the femur anterior to the adductor tubercle on the lower end of the diaphysis.   In order to locate this tubercle, it is advisable to place the legs parallel and at right angles to the pelvis and first determine the level of the tubercle in the sound leg.   In an epiphyseal separation at the lower end of the femur the level of this tubercle is not altered, but in a supracondylar fracture, it is usually displaced upward.   Gentle manipulation of the leg will reveal abnormal mobility at the knee joint in all directions.

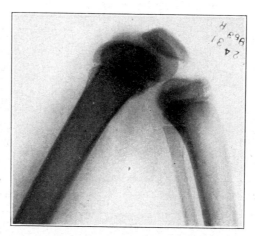

Fig. 1034.—Result obtained in the preceding case by means of manipulative reduction and fixation in a plaster cast with leg flexed at knee to about 35 degrees.   Good result.

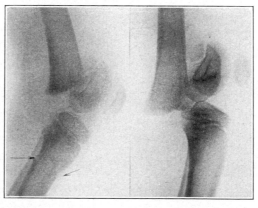

Fig. 1035.—Epiphyseal separation of the lower end of the femur with complete and another with incomplete displacement and fracture through the upper third of the tibia.   (Courtesy of Dr. W. J. Patterson.)

Complications.—The same complications are apt to occur in these epiphyseal separations as in supracondylar fractures.   These are compression or rupture of the popliteal vessels by the diaphysis or injury to the popliteal nerves.   Absence of pulsation in the posterior tibial and dorsalis pedis vessels or marked coldness or cyanosis in the leg or foot call for immediate reduction, as delay may result in gangrene of the leg. In case of rupture of the blood vessel, immediate operation is necessary.

Treatment of Separation of the Lower Epiphysis of the Femur

The treatment is reduction, which should be done as soon after the injury as possible and can usually be accomplished by manipulation. Reduction of incomplete dislocations is usually possible by simple traction on the moderately flexed knee, combined with lateral or anteroposterior pressure on the epiphysis as indicated in the roentgenogram. With complete dislocations the knee and femur should be flexed about 45 degrees, and under strong traction the displaced epiphysis should be pulled down over the lower end of the diaphysis, and as it moves down the knee should be flexed to 90 degrees or more in order to bring the epiphysis back into its normal position. By means of this maneuver practically all of the recent anterior displacements can be reduced.

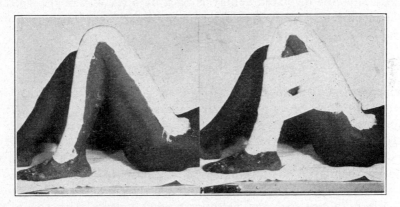

Fig. 1036.—Anterior plaster mold with the knee in flexion, used in the treatment after reduction of a lower epiphyseal separation of the femur. On the right the skin of the popliteal space is protected by padding and the plaster mold is reinforced by adhesive. A circular bandage of sheet cotton and gauze around the plaster and lower extremity is usually necessary before applying the adhesive.

In posterior displacements, of course, the epiphysis must be pushed forward after it has been brought down to the proper level by traction, and the knee must be extended in order to mold it into place. Anatomic reduction should be aimed at; otherwise deformity and disability at the knee may result.

After anatomic reduction has been obtained, the extremity should be immobilized in a plaster-of-Paris mold (Fig. 1036) or cast with the knee in moderately acute flexion. When the extremity is immobilized in a cast with the knee flexed, the popliteal space should be well padded and the circulation in the foot should be watched. This immobilization should be continued for a period of from three to four weeks. At the end of this time the plaster cast may be removed and the patient may begin to move the knee. At the end of six weeks he may be got up on crutches. With accurate reposition and fairly early immobilization, a practically normal knee may be expected in five or six months. However, as in other epiphyseal injuries even after perfect reduction there may be some interference with growth, and the parents should be warned of this.

Treatment of Irreducible and Old Unreduced Epiphyseal Separations at the Lower End of the Femur.—Although these injuries are quite rare, a considerable percentage of them are permitted to go for some weeks or months without reduction, and these cases must be reduced by open operation, because the displaced epiphysis becomes firmly united to the anterior surface of the femur. Likewise an occasional acute case is seen in which reduction by manipulation fails. The operation should be performed under a tourniquet. Probably the least traumatizing and most reliable method is that of Cochrane who makes long anterior and posterior incisions. Through his posterior incision he exposes the popliteal vessels and nerves, gets them out of the way, and is enabled to see the lower end of the shaft of the femur. Through the anterior incision he exposes the displaced epiphysis which he separates from the shaft with a chisel if necessary and then by manipulation or the use of a bone skid slips the displaced epiphysis back onto the end of the shaft and it is then immobilized in moderate flexion in a plaster cast. At the end of three weeks, active motion is started.

FRACTURES OF THE PATELLA

Incidence and Cause.—Due to the exposed position of the bone and to the fact that it is subject to great leverage, fractures of the patella are rather frequent in adults, but are rare in children and adolescents. Most of the cases are due to indirect violence, the mechanism being a snapping of the patella over the condyles of the femur when force is applied to the extremity with the leg semiflexed on the thigh. In this position the patella lies at the highest point on the condyles of the femur and is subjected to the tension of the quadriceps above and the patellar tendon below. Consequently with sudden strain the bone is apt to be broken transversely in its lower half. This sudden strain may result from jumping or from falls from a height or even in running or stumbling. Many of the cases resulting from falls are believed to be the result of direct violence, but as a matter of fact the patella is broken before the knee hits the ground, and in falls on the knee the patella is rarely injured unless the patient falls forward on the face because ordinarily if the patient's knees strike the ground the impact is received by the tibial tubercle and not by the patella. Cases resulting from direct violence are usually due to kicks or blows on the kneecap rather than to falls.

Pathology of Fractures of the Patella.—Most fractures of the patella communicate with the knee joint. Consequently there is bleeding into the joint and it becomes distended with fluid (Fig. 1037). In addition there is a variable amount of bleeding into the subcutaneous tissues over the site of the fracture and the prepatellar bursa may become distended with blood. In cases due to indirect violence the patella is usually broken transversely in the lower half of the bone and in addition to the main transverse fracture, there may be a small amount of comminution (Figs. 1038 and 1039). As the force is such that the bone fragments tend to be pulled apart, there is a variable amount of tearing of the lateral expansions of the quadriceps tendon and of the anterior portion of the capsule of the knee joint. When the patella is widely separated (Fig. 1040) the tear in the anterior capsule may extend far

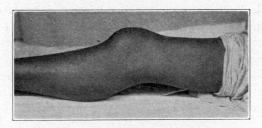

Fig. 1037.—Acute fracture of the left patella. Note the swelling of the knee joint and the dome-like swelling over the patella.

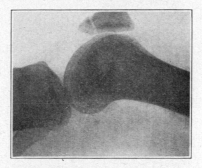

Fig. 1038.—Simple transverse fracture through the patella with practically no displacement. Treated conservatively by immobilization in a plaster-of-Paris cast for six weeks after aspiration of the knee. Good result.

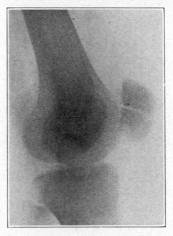

Fig. 1039.—Transverse fracture through the patella from indirect violence with slight separation, treated by open operation with kangaroo suture of the aponeurosis with good results. Circular cast for two weeks.

out on either side almost to the region of the lateral ligaments. With little or no separation of the fragments, the tear in the quadriceps tendon may be relatively slight. In addition to the tear in the lateral expansions the fibers of the quadriceps which pass over the front to the patella are also torn and shreds of these fibers tend to drop down between the fragments and thus are a factor in the prevention of union by bone.

In fractures due to direct violence there is, as a rule, relatively little separation of the fragments and no tearing of the capsule of the knee joint unless force has been applied to the leg after the patella is broken (Fig. 1041). The fracture is apt to be broken into several pieces and the lines may run in any direction. Very rarely there is a single longitudinal fracture of the bone or it may be split in the frontal plane. Due to the subcutaneous position of the bone these fractures by direct violence are apt to be compound and as practically all fractures of the patella open into the knee joint, this is opened in compound fractures.

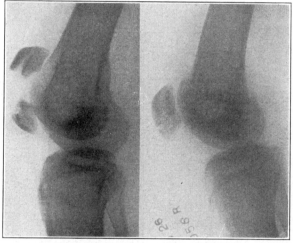

Fig. 1040.   Fig. 1041.

Fig. 1040.—Typical fracture of the patella from indirect violence with considerable separation of the fragments. Treated by open reduction and wiring of the fragments with good result. Disability ten weeks.

Fig. 1041.—Irregular fracture through the patella due to direct violence with practically no separation of the fragments. Treated conservatively by immobilization and circular cast for five weeks with good results.

In all fractures of the patella the tendency is for the upper fragment to be drawn upward by the quadriceps muscle. The amount of displacement varies with the amount of tearing of the lateral aponeurosis and this is proportional to the force causing the fracture and to the continuation of force after the fracture has occurred. In cases with no tearing of the aponeurosis, there is practically no displacement for the fibers are able to withstand the power of the quadriceps muscle, but with wide tearing of the aponeurosis, the upper fragment may be displaced upward from one to two inches and in the course of time may be drawn further upward so that in old untreated cases the displacement may be as much as three inches. It should be remembered that the lower fragment is anchored to the tibia by the patellar ligament and that there is no tendency for this to be displaced either upward or downward, but it may be tilted forward (Fig. 1040). There is little tendency toward a lateral displacement of the fragments. In comminuted fractures loose fragments of the patella may be displaced into the knee joint.

Diagnosis of Fractures of the Patella.—The diagnosis can usually be made from the history and resultant disability and physical examination, but occasionally in fractures from direct violence or in fractures from indirect violence in which there is little or no displacement of the fragments an x-ray picture is necessary. One usually obtains a history of either a fall with sharp pain in the kneecap or a direct blow upon the bone followed by complete inability to bear weight on the leg or to actively extend the knee. On physical examination the region of the knee is markedly swollen and the joint is found to be distended with fluid while the ligaments are not injured. The swelling of the knee is rather characteristic in that it tends to be symmetrical and dome-like with the region of greatest swelling over the region of the patella (Fig. 1037) as contrasted with synovitis in which the greatest swelling is above and on either side of the patella. The cause of the swelling directly over the bone is the extravasation of blood into the tissues at the site of the fracture. The knee is not, as a rule, very tense or painful because as tension in the joint increases, the fluid escapes into the surrounding tissues through the tear in the capsule.

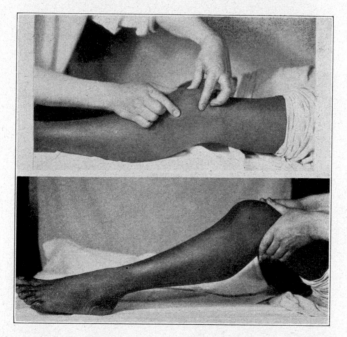

Fig. 1042.—Method of obtaining crepitation in fractures of the patella by pushing the fragments together.

Fig. 1043.—Characteristic inability to lift the leg against gravity in an acute fracture of the patella.

On palpation it is possible to grasp the patella and in the case of a transverse fracture with separation of the fragments, it is usually possible to palpate the sulcus between the fractures and thus determine roughly the amount of separation (Fig. 1042). It is also possible to demonstrate false motion in the patella by moving the two fragments independently from side to side, but no crepitus can be demonstrated unless the superior fragment can be pulled down until it touches the inferior one, and this, of course, is not necessary for the diagnosis. With separation of the fragments there is usually complete loss of power actively to extend the knee and attempts to do so cause pain (Fig. 1043). If the aponeurosis is not torn, it is possible in some cases for the patient actively to extend the knee if the thigh is also extended. This is known as Dreyer's test.

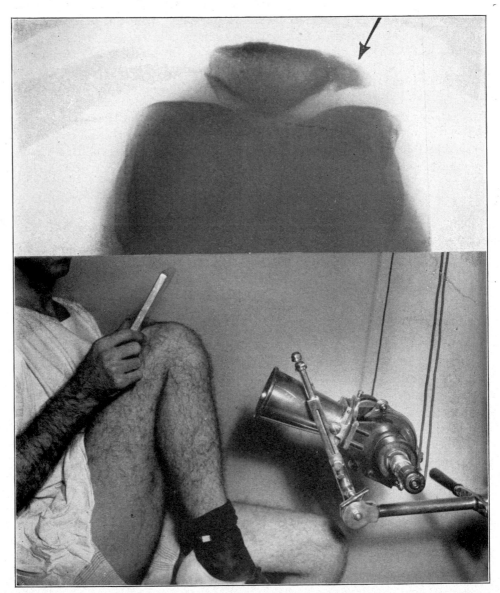

Fig. 1044.—Lateral fracture of the patella and method of obtaining an x-ray of this bone in the vertical plane.

In fractures from direct violence and also in those from indirect violence, in which there is practically no separation of the fragments, the diagnosis is more difficult. In these cases the knee joint is distended with fluid as noted above, but the distention resembles that of an acute synovitis with the most prominent part of the swelling above and lateral to the patella except for the small boggy area directly over the site of the bone which is due to the local extravasation of blood in the tissues. On palpation the patella is tender, appears to be normal in size, and false motion and deformity are not as a rule demonstrable. The patient may be able actively to extend the leg on the thigh or to raise the heel from the bed with the knee extended, but this motion causes considerable pain. In these fractures without demonstrable displacement an x-ray picture is usually necessary for the diagnosis, and the fracture may not show up in the lateral and anteroposterior views, and in rare longitudinal fractures a vertical view with the knee acutely flexed may be necessary.

Treatment of Fractures of the Patella

The object of treatment in these fractures is to bring the fragments into apposition and to immobilize them until they have united. In cases in which the aponeurosis is torn, it should be repaired. The treatment may be either conservative or operative, depending upon the type of fracture present. Conservative treatment should be used in those cases in which there is no separation of the fragments, and in these fractures firm bony union and a good functional result may be expected to follow from such treatment. (Figs. 1038 and 1041.)

Operative treatment should be used in those fractures in which the fragments are separated, even if this be only a quarter of an inch. Doubtful cases should be operated upon. (Fig. 1039.) Very rarely bony union and a good functional result may be obtained in these cases by conservative treatment, but it is not the rule, and most of the cases of this type of fracture which are treated by conservative methods obtain fibrous union with a weak knee which tends to develop arthritic changes after a few years.

Conservative Treatment.—The leg should be fully extended at the knee and the excess fluid in the knee joint should be aspirated under aseptic conditions. In aspirating the knee, all that is necessary is to have a sterile needle and syringe, ether, alcohol, and 7 per cent tincture of iodine. A small spot on the skin lateral or mesial to, and slightly above, the patella is washed with alcohol and ether and painted with the iodine, and the needle is inserted through this area into the joint. One of us (H. E. C.) believes that the surgeon should scrub up and wear gloves. The other (J. A. K.) does not because there is no need for him to touch the needle or the skin through which the needle passes.

After the fluid has been removed from the joint, an effort should be made to immobilize the patella by means of strips of adhesive. Strips about eighteen inches long and an inch wide are applied obliquely above and below the bone in such a manner that when the strips above are pulled taut, they tend to pull the upper fragment downward, while those below tend to pull the lower fragment upward.

After the adhesive has been applied, the extension at the knee should be continued, and the knee should be immobilized in either a plaster-of-Paris cast (Fig. 1046), a posterior plaster mold, a long wooden splint (Fig. 1045), or a

Cabot posterior wire splint. Personally we prefer the plaster-of-Paris cast and bivalve the cast if there is much swelling. We keep the patient in bed for the first week or ten days with the leg elevated. If the fluid reappears in the knee we aspirate it again.

The strapping with adhesive and the period of immobilization should be continued over a period of four weeks. At the end of this time the patient may begin to exercise the knee. In the beginning this should be done by having the patient simply pull up the patella by tightening the quadriceps muscle. A few days later he can begin to flex the knee slightly, and at the end of a week he may begin to lift the heel from the bed with the knee extended. During the sixth week he may gradually increase the flexion to a right angle or more, and at the end of the sixth week, the patient may be got up on crutches, but while he is walking around, he should keep the knee immobilized in the straight position. This should be continued for about two weeks, when the splint holding the knee straight may be discarded entirely and the patient may begin to bear weight on the leg. Instead of the crutches, a Thomas caliper walking splint may be used.

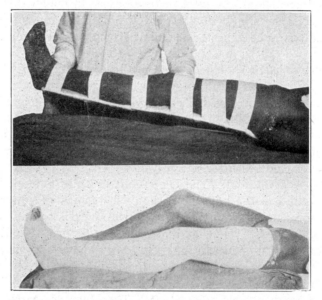

Fig. 1045.—Emergency first aid dressing for fractures of the patella. Merely a posterior wooden splint padded and strapped on with adhesive. Also useful in ligamentous injuries of the knee joint. This splint soon becomes loose and uncomfortable.

Fig. 1046.—Plaster-of-Paris cast used in the nonoperative and sometimes in the post-operative treatment of fractures of the patella. This cast may or may not be bivalved.

With severe fractures the program must be continued for a somewhat longer time and the resumption of weight-bearing must be done gradually as the patella is probably refractured more often than any other bone (Fig. 1048). It is to be noted that the refracture does not always occur in the line of the original fracture. This is due to the fact that the bone undergoes considerable atrophy during prolonged immobilization and becomes weakened.

Operative Treatment.—Operative treatment is indicated in those fractures of the patella in which there is definite separation of the fragments

(Figs. 1049 and 1052), and in all doubtful cases. The operative treatment should not be undertaken unless the patient is in a hospital where the surgeon is confident of his asepsis; it is much better to treat one of these fractures by conservative means and obtain fibrous union than it is to infect the knee joint with the possibility of amputation or death from infection. Under proper conditions, however, these fractures should be treated by open operation.

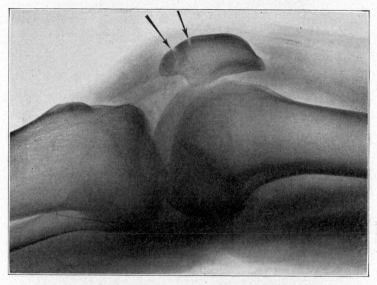

Fig. 1047.—Incomplete double fracture of the distal third of the patella. Treated by immobilization in a long plaster cast for four weeks, then, gradual resumption of function.

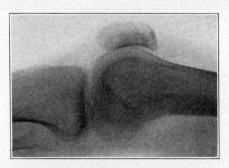

Fig. 1048.—Healed fracture of the patella showing marked atrophy of the bone and explaining the tendency to refracture.

Time of Operation.—The time of the operation depends upon the condition of the skin. If the skin is intact and there are no lacerations or evidences of infection around the knee, the patella can be sutured immediately or a forty-eight-hour skin preparation may be used. On the first day the skin from the groin to the ankle is shaved, scrubbed with green soap, washed with alcohol, and a sterile dressing is applied. On the second day the scrubbing with soap and water and washing with alcohol are repeated and another sterile dressing is applied. On the third day the patient is ready for the operation.

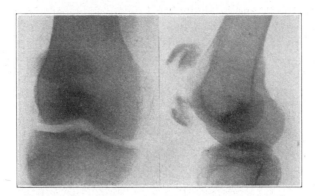

Fig. 1049.—Fracture of the patella due to indirect violence followed by separation of the fragments. Treated by operation and wiring of the fragments.

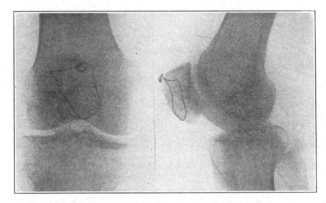

Fig. 1050.—Same case, postoperative.

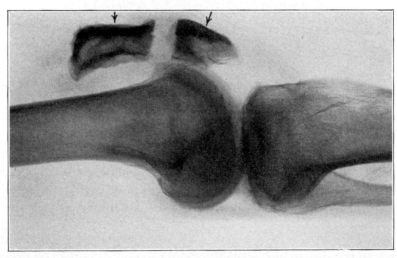

Fig. 1051.—Fracture of a hypertrophied patella. This patient had received a previous
fracture with the result of the overgrowth of patella. The patella was trimmed down to
normal size and wired. It was not considered advisable to remove the patella. Good function.

Operative Suture of the Patella.—The operation may be performed with or without a tourniquet as the surgeon chooses. The patella is exposed either through a long median incision or an inverted U incision, the skin flap being reflected upward (Fig. 1053). J. A. K. prefers the U incision with its base over the patellar ligament. The longitudinal incision which H. E. C. prefers is about six inches long, its center being over the fracture, and it is carried directly down

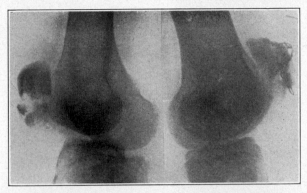

Fig. 1052.—Comminuted fracture of the patella caused by direct violence. Treated by operation with wiring of the fragments. Early motion. Good results. Disability ten weeks.

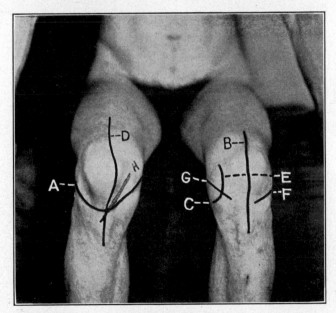

Fig. 1053.—Various incisions for operations on the knee joint.

to the quadriceps tendon, bone, and patellar ligament. The skin and subcutaneous tissue are reflected to expose the patella and the rent in the lateral aponeurosis on either side. By retracting the skin, the lateral margins of this tear can be exposed. Any excess blood is wiped out of the knee joint with clean gauze and any lose fragments of bone are removed. The patella is then inspected, and a decision is made as to whether the fragments are to be wired together or part or all of the patella is to be removed. With two large fragments the operation

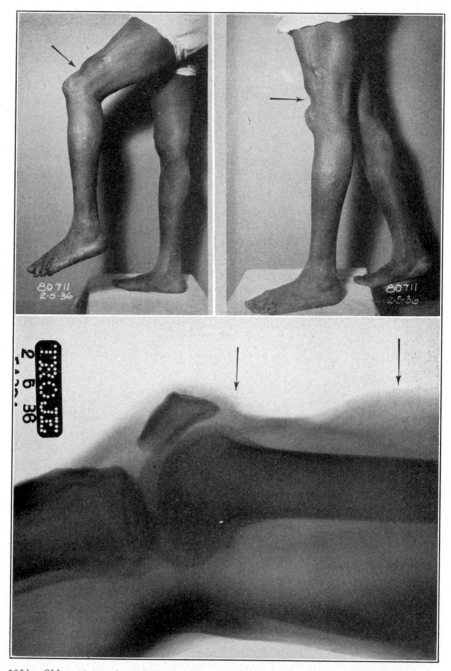

Fig. 1054.—Old rupture of quadriceps tendon showing loss of function. Treated by operative repair with fascia lata with good result.

of choice is to wire them together. With one large and one or more smaller (usually distal) fragments it is advisable to remove the smaller fragments and suture the patellar ligament or quadriceps tendon directly to the large fragment, as advocated by Thomson. If the patella is extensively comminuted, it is advisable to excise the entire patella. We seldom find this advisable or necessary. After the operation on the bone is completed, the aponeurosis is repaired with mattress sutures of silk or chromic catgut. Sulfonamide powder is sprinkled in the joint cavity and over the wound surfaces before it is closed.

We wire the fragments together with rather heavy stainless steel wire which is passed through holes through the substance of each fragment or through the larger and around the smaller fragment, care being taken to keep well away from the articular surface. In wiring the patella the bone is wired first and the aponeurosis is sutured afterward, because the wire holds the fragments so firmly that the aponeurosis can then be sutured with very little tension. This method admits of early motion and all splints are removed and movements of the knee are begun on the eighth or tenth day. With the heavy wire there is little danger of refracture, and the period of convalescence is shortened.

The drill holes through the fragments may be vertical or transverse, depending upon the contour of the fragments and the exposure. Heavy chromic catgut may be used instead of the wire.

The knee is immobilized in a large cylinder cast for about ten days, until the wound is healed. Then, the cast is removed and exercises are instituted gradually.

Old Fractures of the Patella.—As was stated above in old fractures of the patella, there is a tendency to progressive upward displacement of the upper proximal fragment with the resultant wide separation of the fragments. This may be so great that it is impossible to draw them down. However, if the patient experiences great weakness and disability on account of the injury an attempt should be made to repair the fracture. This can be done by an operation similar to that described above in fresh fractures of the patella except that it may be necessary to lengthen the quadriceps tendon by the V method in order to get the superior fragment down and place a wire around or through the fragments in order to maintain the fragments in apposition. It is, of course, understood that at the time of operation the ends of the fragments should be excised until approximately normal bone is reached and that the tear in the lateral aponeurosis should be repaired. The after-treatment is the same as that described after the conservative treatment of fracture of the patella.

RUPTURE OF THE PATELLAR LIGAMENT

Rupture of the patellar ligament is a rather rare injury which is produced by the same type of violence that causes transverse fractures of the patella, the difference being that occasionally the patella remains intact and the ligament is torn across or a small fragment of bone may be avulsed from the lower end of the patella (Fig. 1055). The ruptures are usually complete and the tear in the tissues may extend outward on either side for a variable distance. The injury may or may not communicate with the synovial cavity of the knee joint, and if it does communicate, there is a variable amount of bleeding into the joint and the knee is distended with fluid.

Diagnosis of Rupture of the Patellar Ligament.—The history and physical signs are similar to those present in a fracture of the patella from indirect violence. The patient is unable to extend the leg on the thigh and there is localized pain, tenderness, and swelling over the front of the knee. On palpation the knee may be distended with fluid, and there is a subcutaneous swelling at the site of the rupture in the ligament which is situated below the patella, while the patella itself which is displaced upward, appears to be intact, and is not tender. It is usually possible to palpate a definite depression in the tissues below the patella. (Fig. 1055.)

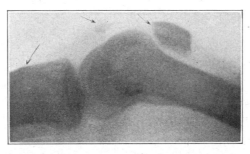

Fig. 1055.—Rupture of the patellar ligament with avulsion of the fragment from the tibial tubercle, sutured with kangaroo tendon through drill holes in the tibia circular cast, bivalved. Later a circular nonbivalved for five weeks. Good result.

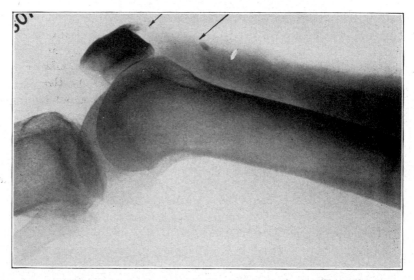

Fig. 1056.—Rupture of the quadriceps extensor tendon from its attachment to the patella; soft structure x-ray technique used. Physical examination was as diagnostic as the x-ray and should be in most instances.

Treatment of Rupture of the Patellar Ligament

Treatment is suture which should be done as soon as convenient after the accident in order that further upward displacement of the patella may be avoided. The torn tendon is exposed through a longitudinal incision and the ends are united with mattress sutures of heavy chromic catgut or fascia lata. If the tear extends out into the tissues on either side of the tendon, these also should be sutured. If the tendon is torn away from the lower end of the patella or from the tibia or if a small fragment is torn off with the tendon, it is necessary to resuture the tendon to the bone. This can be done by boring two or three small holes through the bone. If the knee joint is distended with blood, this should be removed at the time of the operation.

After the operation the limb should be immobilized in a plaster-of-Paris cast which extends from the upper thigh to the toes, and this immobilization should be continued for about six weeks. At the end of this time the patient may begin to exercise the limb and after two weeks he may be got up on crutches or may walk with a plaster cast or knee cage which prevents flexion at the knee. Two weeks later this may be discontinued and a flannel bandage or an elastic knee cap may be substituted. This should be worn for about a month, or until the patient no longer feels the need of it.

RUPTURE OF THE QUADRICEPS TENDON

Rupture of the quadriceps tendon (Fig. 1054) is another rare injury which is analogous to fracture of the patella by indirect violence in which the quadriceps tendon is torn across or pulled away from its attachment to the upper end of the patella. The rupture may be complete or incomplete, may occur at any point in the tendon, or a small bit of the upper end of the patella may be pulled off from the body of the bone.

Diagnosis of Rupture of the Quadriceps Tendon.—The history and physical findings are similar to those present in a fracture of the patella due to indirect violence, and there is localized pain, tenderness, and swelling over the site of the tear in the tendon, with inability to extend the leg on the thigh. With incomplete rupture it may be possible for the patient actively to extend the leg, but the movement is weak and is accompanied by pain. On palpation, with complete rupture, the patella is intact and in its normal position; there is tenderness over the tendon above it, and it may be possible to palpate a sulcus across the torn tendon. The knee joint is usually distended with fluid.

Treatment of Rupture of the Quadriceps Tendon

If the rupture is incomplete, complete restoration of power and function may be expected by conservative treatment, but if the rupture is complete, the torn tendon should be sutured. Otherwise permanent weakness and disability will result. In incomplete ruptures all that is necessary is to immobilize the knee in extension over a period of from three to five weeks. This can be done in a plaster cast or in a posterior wooden splint. At the end of this time the patient may begin to exercise the quadriceps and gradually to use the knee.

In a complete rupture of the quadriceps tendon the tendon should be exposed by a median longitudinal incision and the ends should be sutured by mattress sutures of heavy chromic catgut or fascia lata. After the tendon is sutured, and the wound is closed, the knee should be immobilized for from four to six weeks in a plaster-of-Paris cast. At the end of this time the patient may begin to exercise the quadriceps tendon and to practice flexion of the knee. About a week later the patient can be got up on crutches or with a support to prevent flexion at the knee. This should be continued for about two weeks, when all support may be discarded and the patient may gradually increase his activity.

DISLOCATION OF THE PATELLA

Types of Dislocations of the Patella.—In most cases of dislocations of the patella, the kneecap is displaced outward and comes to rest on the lateral condyle; this type of injury may result from an acute trauma or may be recurrent and result from very minor strains. In rare instances as the result of direct violence the patella may be dislocated inward or it may be rotated upon its long axis (vertical dislocation) in such a manner that one of its lateral borders or even its anterior surface is engaged between the condyles of the femur. (Figs. 1057 and 1059.)

OUTWARD TRAUMATIC DISLOCATION OF THE PATELLA

Mechanism and Pathology.—This is usually the result of direct trauma which forces the patella outward over the lateral border of the condyle. Very rarely an acute dislocation may result from forcible contraction of the quadriceps muscle. The dislocation may be complete or incomplete. In the incomplete dislocation the patella rides on the edge of the condyle, and in the complete dislocation, it slips over the edge of the condyle and rests upon its lateral surface and may be more or less rotated. In addition to the displacement, there is a variable amount of injury to the joint capsule on the inner side of the patella. With incomplete dislocation this injury is relatively slight, but with complete dislocation there may be a wide vertical tear in the mesial portion of the inner aponeurosis of the knee. As a result of the injury to the capsule, there is a hemorrhage into the joint with resultant hemarthrosis.

Diagnosis of Acute Dislocation of the Patella.—There is a history of a fall or of a blow on the kneecap followed by a complete loss of function in the leg with pain and swelling in the knee. On inspection it is usually possible to see the patella in its abnormal position and to note the flattening of the anterior surface of the knee. Palpation reveals the absence of the patella from its normal position, and the smooth edges of the condyles can be felt beneath the skin and subcutaneous tissues while the patella can be palpated in its abnormal position. In early cases it may be possible to palpate the tear on the inner side of the capsule.

Treatment of Acute Dislocation of the Patella

Treatment is immediate reduction followed by aspiration of the knee and immobilization. The patella can be reduced by fully extending the knee and forcing the patella back over the border of the condyle and into its normal position by direct pressure over the bone. As a rule no anesthetic is necessary. If, after reduction, the knee joint is distended with fluid, this should be removed by aspiration. While the fluid is in the joint it may be possible by palpation to detect a vertical tear in the inner side of the capsule. After the joint has been aspirated the knee should be immobilized in a position of full extension over a period of two or three weeks. This can be done in a posterior splint or plaster-of-Paris cast, and at the end of this time an elastic bandage or knee cap can be fitted and the patient can gradually begin to walk on the leg.

In cases with obvious severe damage to the inner side of the capsule, if conditions are at hand for doing good, clean surgery, the skin may be given a forty-eight hour preparation, the rent in the capsule exposed by a mesial vertical incision and the capsule sutured. After the capsule is sutured, the case should be treated as described above. The capsule is sutured to prevent recurrence.

RARE DISLOCATIONS OF THE PATELLA

In the rare inward dislocations, the symptoms, physical signs, and treatment are similar to those described above for the outward dislocations, the only difference being that the patella is dislocated onto the border of the inner condyle and must be moved outward in order to accomplish reduction.

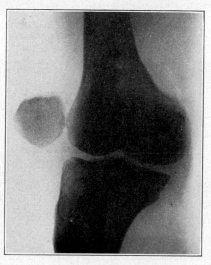

Fig. 1057.—Rotary dislocation of the patella in which the articular surface faces outward, while the inner border rests between the condyles of the femur. Reduced by manipulation under anesthesia, with good results. Ten days' fixation in a bivalved circular cast.

In the rotary dislocations, the patella rests between the condyles of the femur either on its edge (Figs. 1057 and 1059) or turned upside down. There is complete disability at the knee and considerable pain. It is usually possible to detect the direction of the rotation by noting the dimpling in the skin as the skin over the subcutaneous surface of the patella is loosely attached to it and tends to follow it during rotation. Consequently if the patella is resting upon its lateral edge, there is dimpling of the skin lateral to the patella. An indication of the direction of the rotation may also be obtained by carefully palpating the quadriceps tendon, since with the patella resting on its lateral edge the inner border of the tendon should be prominent.

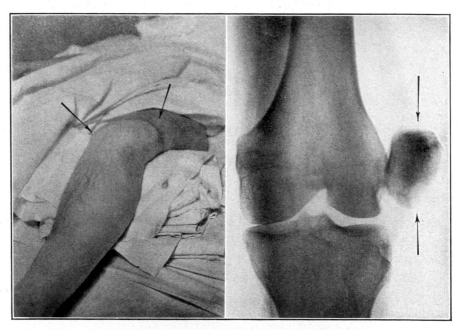

Fig. 1058.—Traumatic lateral dislocation of the patella. Reduced by manipulation; cast for two weeks; then quadriceps exercises.

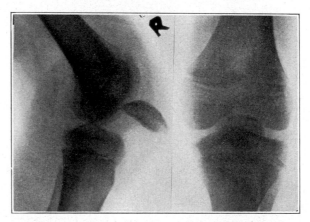

Fig. 1059.—Vertical dislocation of the patella. Reduced under anesthesia. No disability.

Treatment

The treatment is reduction; the knee should be fully extended and an effort made by direct pressure to reduce the rotation. It is helpful to relax the quadriceps muscle by flexing the thigh and then push downward on the patella. In cases of complete rotation, reduction by manipulation may not be possible, and it may be necessary to perform an open reduction. If this is done and if there is a rent in the capsule this should be sutured at the time of the open reduction.

Aftertreatment.—If the patella has simply been turned upon its edge, all that is necessary is to aspirate the knee, apply an elastic cap or bandage and keep the patient in bed for a few days. As soon as the soreness disappears, he may begin to walk.

RECURRENT DISLOCATIONS OF THE PATELLA

Most of the recurrent cases begin in childhood and occur in females, and the individuals who are thus afflicted usually present certain abnormalities which predispose to the dislocation. These abnormalities are (1) knock knee deformity; (2) flattening of the ridge of the external condyle of the femur; (3) unusual length of the patellar ligament; and (4) attachment of the patellar ligament lateral to the midline of the leg.

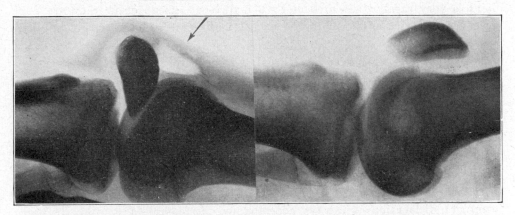

Fig. 1060.—Vertical dislocation of the patella, superior border, extending into the knee joint. It was necessary to do open reduction in this case with good anatomical reduction with prolonged convalescent period. Good functional result. (Courtesy Dr. Charles Wilson.)

Diagnosis of Recurrent Dislocation of the Patella.—If a careful history is taken, one will usually find that the primary dislocation occurred in childhood as a result of muscular violence rather than direct trauma. In some cases the patella tends to be dislocated quite frequently, while in others it is dislocated only once or twice a year or even less frequently. Each dislocation results in a fall with more or less pain and is followed by an effusion into the knee joint and temporary disability. The symptoms are less in those cases in which the dislocation occurs at frequent intervals. In many instances the patient has learned to reduce the dislocation herself or to instruct a layman to do so and in aggravated cases the patient may be able to produce the dislocation at will.

Prognosis.—After a single traumatic dislocation, if the patella is reduced and the knee is immobilized over a period of three weeks, a normal knee may be expected. The recurrent dislocations, however, do not yield to conservative treatment, and the dislocation may be expected to recur unless recurrence is prevented by some operative measures.

Operative Treatment of Recurrent Dislocation of the Patella

Types of Operations.—Numerous types of operations have been suggested and performed, and most of these may be expected to result in a cure of the condition. Operations on the bone include osteotomy of the femur for correction of knock knee, osteotomy of the external condyle with elevation of the condyle, and transplantation inward of the tibial tubercle with the patellar ligament, which is attached to it. We prefer the method of Hitchcock, who splits the patellar ligament and removes the inner half of the tibial tubercle with the inner half of the ligament and transplants this thick rectangle of bone downward and inward into a defect cut for it adjacent to the inner border of the tibia and as far down as the plug of bone can be pulled without undue tension.

DISLOCATIONS AT THE KNEE

Due to the great strength of the ligaments which surround the knee, this joint is very rarely dislocated and when dislocations do occur they are due to severe injuries either in the nature of a direct trauma or strain applied through leverage.

Types.—The tibia may be dislocated anteriorly (Fig. 1061), posteriorly, internally, or externally (Fig. 1062) or it may be rotated upon the femur. Any of the above dislocations may be complete or incomplete, and a large percentage of them are associated with fractures of the upper end of the tibia. The anterior dislocation is the most frequent type, and this results from violent hyperextension at the knee while the posterior dislocation is the result of force applied to the front of the leg near the knee. Lateral dislocations may result from abduction or adduction strains or from direct violence.

Pathology.—Due to the fact that the bones at the knee are very broad, complete dislocation is always accompanied by complete rupture of both crucials, internal and external lateral and posterior ligaments, and in addition there may be damage to the hamstrings and the popliteal vessels and nerves. As a result of injury to the popliteal vessels, gangrene may supervene and necessitate amputation, or paralysis may result from the nerve injury. As the joint is quite superficial, the injury may be compound, and as was stated above it is often complicated by fractures of the upper end of the tibia.

Diagnosis of Dislocations at the Knee.—Due to the subcutaneous location and large size of the bones, the deformity is obvious in a complete dislocation at the knee and the diagnosis not only of a dislocation, but also of the type of dislocation can usually be made by inspection alone. In an incomplete dislocation, the swelling may obscure the deformity and make the diagnosis more difficult, but palpation of the margins of the condyles of the femur and tibia will disclose the abnormal positions of the bones of the leg in relation to the femur. In either type the crucial and lateral ligaments are ruptured, and gentle manipulation will disclose abnormal mobility at the knee. A roentgenogram is necessary to rule out fractures of the condyles or tibial spines, and should be taken when possible. The condition of the circulation and nerve supply in the foot and leg should be determined at the first examination.

Treatment of Dislocations at the Knee

The treatment is reduction and this should be done as soon as possible after the accident. Due to the fact that there is extensive tearing of all of the ligaments of the knee joint, reduction can usually be accomplished with relative ease after relaxation of the muscles has been obtained by an anesthetic. All that is necessary is to have an assistant make traction on the leg while

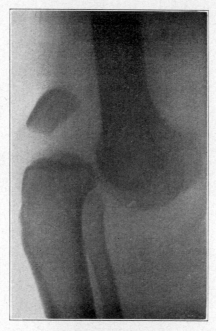

Fig. 1061.—Anterior dislocation at the knee joint treated by manipulative reduction with five weeks' immobilization in bivalved plaster cast. Good result.

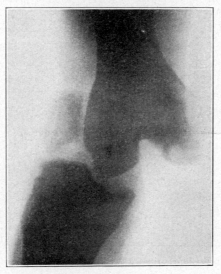

Fig. 1062.—Incomplete rotary dislocation at the knee joint. Treated by manipulation with one week of immobilization in a bivalved cast and six weeks in a circular cast. Good result in three months.

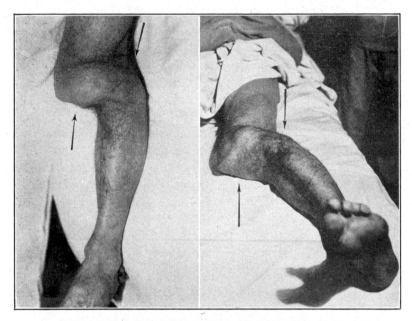

Fig. 1063.—Lateral dislocation of the knee reduced by manipulation.

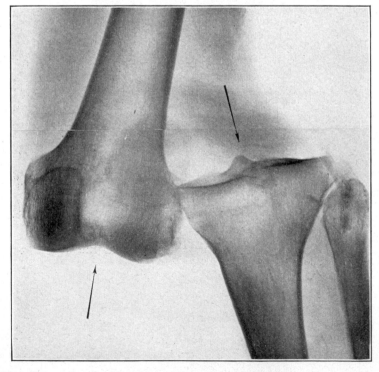

Fig. 1064.—X-ray of preceding case. (Conwell and Alldredge: J. A. M. A., 1936.)

countertraction is made on the thigh, and the surgeon, by direct pressure on the bones, pushes or pulls the tibia back into place. If this is not successful in an anterior dislocation the leg may be hyperextended and then by direct pressure on the upper end of the tibia, it may be engaged upon the condyles and then reduced as the knee is flexed. This method, however, may result in damage to the popliteal vessels and nerves and should not be tried until simple traction with direct pressure on the bone ends has failed.

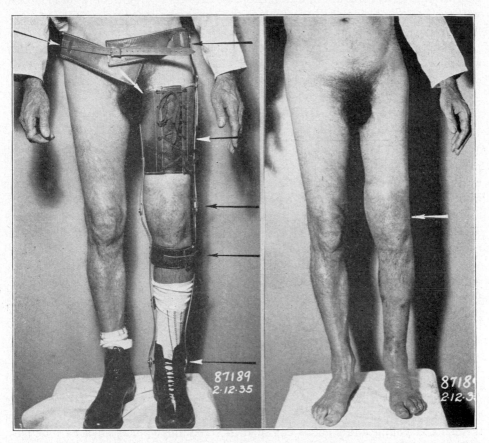

Fig. 1065.—Type of long leg brace used in convalescent period of preceding case. Good alignment with good functional result.

Aftertreatment.—After the dislocation has been reduced, the knee should be aspirated to remove the excess fluid and the extremity should be immobilized with the knee in a position of about 15 to 20 degrees of flexion in a plaster-of-Paris cast which extends from the groin to the toes. When the original cast is applied, this should be bivalved immediately and strapped on or the patient should be put to bed with the leg elevated and the circulation in the toes carefully watched. If the toes become cyanotic, the cast should be bivalved and if there is marked swelling of the knee this should be aspirated again. This treatment should be continued until the swelling has disappeared when a new tight-fitting plaster should be applied.

Since the crucials and lateral ligaments are torn, this immobilization should be continued for at least eight to twelve weeks as advised below in injuries to the crucial ligaments. At the end of this time the cast should be removed and the stability of the knee tested. If the knee is not quite stable, the cast should be reapplied and immobilization should be continued. At the end of three or four months the patient may be given a knee cage and got up on crutches. The crutches may be gradually discarded as power and function at the knee return. Manipulation at the knee should be avoided, as it will tend to create instability which will be more harmful than will the benefit accruing from the extra movement which may be gained.

We do not advise open operation in these cases, as the ligamentous damage is so extensive that there is little chance of operative repair, and the chance is not worth the risks incident to the operation.

INTERNAL DERANGEMENTS OF THE KNEE

The term "Internal Derangement of the Knee Joint" was first used by William Hay in 1784. He used it to include any alteration in the joint which prevented the condyles of the femur from moving truly in the hollow formed by the semilunar cartilages and depressions of the tibia. At the present time we use the term to include those conditions which interfere mechanically with the function of the joint, while the femur, tibia, patella, and capsule are intact. Exceptions to this rule are that injuries to the lateral ligaments and to the tibial spine are usually classed as internal derangements of the knee

The principal causes of internal derangement of the knee are: (1) sprain or rupture of the lateral ligaments; (2) injuries of the semilunar cartilages; (3) ruptures of the crucial ligaments; (4) loose bodies including hypertrophied synovial fringes; (5) fractures of the tibial spine; and (6) hypertrophy of the infrapatellar fat pad.

SPRAINS AND SPRAIN FRACTURES OF THE KNEE JOINT
(INJURY OF THE LATERAL LIGAMENTS)

Incidence and Mechanism.—Despite the fact that the knee is one of the strongest joints in the body, injuries of the lateral ligaments are relatively frequent in young adult males engaged in strenuous sports, such as foot ball, or in hazardous occupations, such as mining. The injury to the ligament may occur from a direct cross strain on the extended limb such as results from a kick or blow on the side of the leg or thigh, but more frequently it results from a sudden torsion strain on the partly flexed knee such as occurs in lifting or in a fall with the feet widely separated. The internal lateral ligament is injured much more frequently than is the external.

Recurrent sprains of the knee are frequent because the injury to the lateral ligament is considered a minor affair and the patient, either an athlete or a workman, is often treated vigorously by physiotherapy for a few days and then got back in the game or on the job at the earliest possible moment, while the torn or stretched ligament is not given an opportunity to heal. Many of these patients carry a weak knee through life, and a minor twist or strain is followed by pain and effusion into the joint.

Pathology.—The lateral ligaments of the knee are really thickened portions of the joint capsule and an injury to the ligament is accompanied by capsular and synovial damage and is nearly always followed by effusion into the joint. The ligament and adjacent portions of the capsule may be torn across or merely stretched with diffuse tearing of the fibers. In some cases the ligament is torn from its attachment to either the femur or tibia, and a small piece of bone is avulsed with it. These sprain fractures may be difficult to diagnose; consequently, all severely sprained knees should be x-rayed in order to exclude them because they require a longer period of immobilization than do the simple sprains.

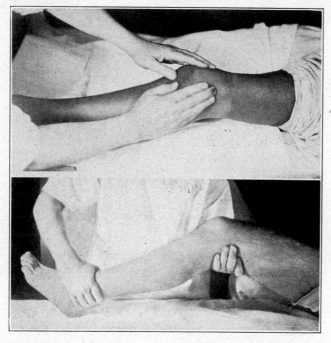

Fig. 1066.—Examination of the knee joint. Method of palpation of the knee in order to determine the presence of excess fluid in the joint. As pressure is made on the quadriceps pouch, the patella is floated upward on the condyles and ballottement can be detected by pressing it down with the fingers.

Fig. 1067.—Methods of testing the integrity of the lateral ligaments by swinging the leg from side to side or rotating it.

The semilunar cartilages are frequently injured in these sprains of the knee because they are intimately bound to the lateral ligaments.

Diagnosis of Sprain at the Knee.—There is a history of a severe strain or direct injury to the knee followed by pain at the site of the lesion or all through the joint and a variable amount of disability. In a mild case the patient may be able to move the knee actively or walk with a limp, but movement and weight-bearing are painful. In a severe injury there is complete disability and the knee is unstable.

On physical examination there is a variable amount of local swelling over the torn lateral ligament, and the knee is distended with fluid (Fig. 1066). The patella floats and the normal contour of the joint is obliterated by the swelling. In uncomplicated cases the tenderness is limited to the area over the torn ligament which is well back on the side of the knee. Flexion is painful and is limited by the effusion in the joint, but unless the semilunars are injured, extension is free. Lateral mobility is usually increased and may be markedly so in complete tears of the ligaments. (Figs. 1068, 1069, 1070.) The increase in lateral mobility is away from the side of the lesion; that is, with a tear of the internal lateral ligament the leg can be moved outward (abducted) on the thigh to an abnormal degree. This is usually painful at the limit of the

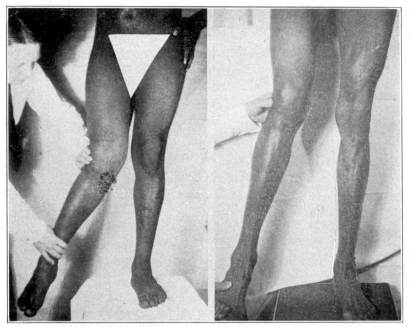

Fig. 1068.   Fig. 1069.

Fig. 1068.—Severe rupture of the internal lateral ligament showing abnormal mobility of the leg outward. Treated by immobilization in a plaster-of-Paris cast for eight weeks, metal knee brace for seven weeks with good result.

Fig. 1069.—Moderate rupture internal lateral ligament of right knee. Treated as above with good result.

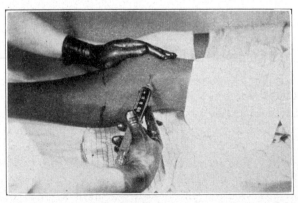

Fig. 1070.—Aspiration of the knee joint with the removal of excess fluid after ligamentous injury or fracture. Note that pressure is being made against the knee with the left hand in order to localize the fluid at the needle point, while aspiration is being carried out with the right hand. This procedure is usually useful in the later stages of aspiration, preventing the necessity of moving the needle about unnecessarily in the knee joint.

motion. If the crucial ligaments are not injured, the stability of the joint in the anteroposterior plane is not impaired.

In a sprain fracture tenderness is most acute over the involved osseous attachment of the ligament and it may be possible to palpate the avulsed piece of bone. In cases where this injury is suspected, the fracture should be ruled out or confirmed by an x-ray picture.

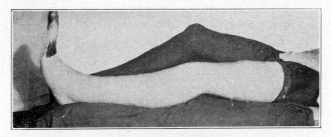

Fig. 1071.—Plaster-of-Paris cast for the treatment of severe ligamentous injuries at the knee in a position of slight flexion at the knee.

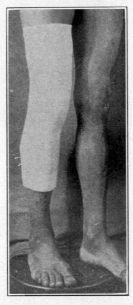

Fig. 1072.—Short plaster for mild ligamentous injuries at the knee.

Treatment of Sprain of the Knee.—The effusion in the joint is largely blood and this should be removed by aspiration (Fig. 1070) because the blood acts as a mild irritant and may cause synovial thickening and delayed restoration of motion in the joint. After the aspiration, the joint should be immobilized in order to give the torn ligament a chance to heal.

Aspiration of the Knee.—The joint may be entered laterally or mesially to the patella or just above and laterally or mesially to this bone. A point on the skin is selected and painted with strong (7 per cent) tincture of iodine. An area 2 cm. in diameter is all that is necessary. A sterile needle on a sterile syringe is then thrust into the joint, and the fluid is withdrawn until no more can be obtained. In removing the last few cubic centimeters, it is helpful to have an assistant compress the posterior and lateral aspects of the joint. Fresh blood will flow through a small needle (21 gauge) and to use a large trocar invites infection. No anesthetic is necessary unless the patient is hypersensitive, when the tissues at the site of the aspiration may be infiltrated with 1 per cent novocaine. (Fig. 1070.)

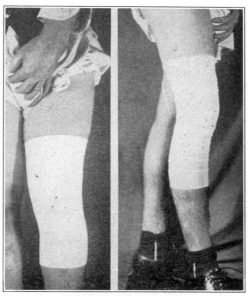

Fig. 1073.   Fig. 1074.

Fig. 1073.—Elastic knee cap for moderate support during convalescence from ligamentous injuries.

Fig. 1074.—Elastic bandage applied to the knee after mild sprains and contusions and as moderate support after ligamentous injuries.

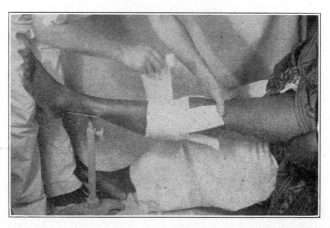

Fig. 1075.—The amount of support given by the bandage can be increased by incorporating three strips of felt.

Immobilization.—The degree and duration of the immobilization vary directly with the severity of the injury. In mild cases all that is necessary is to apply a pressure dressing or an elastic bandage and prohibit weight-bearing for a few days until the soreness has disappeared. Then the patient may be permitted to walk with a cane which can be discarded as the knee returns to normal.

In severe cases the knee should be immobilized over a period of at least four weeks and in sprain fractures six or eight weeks' immobilization is advisable. One of us (J. A. K.) prefers a plaster-of-Paris cast which is applied with the knee in a position of slight flexion with the leg drawn toward the side of the torn ligament. Very little padding is used and the cast is bivalved as soon as the plaster has set. The other (H. E. C.) prefers immobilization with adhesive traction to the leg in a Thomas splint for from seven to ten days; then a circular plaster cast for from six to eight weeks. (Fig. 1071.)

In moderately severe cases the period of immobilization can be shortened to two weeks. After the splint or plaster cast has been removed, the knee should be supported by an elastic bandage (Fig. 1074) or elastic knee cap (Fig. 1073) or an adhesive dressing and when the patient begins to bear weight on the leg the inner or outer border of the heel should be elevated one-fourth of an inch in order to take the strain off the injured ligament. The shoe with the elevated heel should be worn for several weeks, or until the knee is apparently normal again. During the convalescent period exercises to strengthen the quadriceps and hamstrings are useful. The walking caliper is used in some cases, but is rarely necessary.

In very severe injuries the torn ligament may be repaired early by open operation.

INJURIES TO THE INTERNAL SEMILUNAR CARTILAGE

These are the most frequent types of internal derangement of the knee joint and like the sprains of the knee most of the cases occur in young men who are engaged in strenuous athletics or heavy manual labor.

Mechanism.—The majority of the lesions of the internal semilunar cartilage are due to sudden forcible internal rotation of the femur on the slightly flexed and fixed tibia. The movement is usually combined with a variable amount of abduction at the knee which tends to open up the inner side of the joint and stretch or tear the internal lateral ligament. The cartilage is drawn inward and nipped between the condyles and torn as the movement progresses. The most frequent injury is a longitudinal split in the cartilage in which the inner portion is torn from the outer margin, but remains attached at both ends. This is called the bucket handle tear and this detached portion may slip into the middle of the joint and lie between the condyles. In addition to the primary tear, one or even more secondary tears may occur. In other instances the posterior, or more rarely, the anterior horn is torn across or loosened near its end and slips into the joint. These tears may be the result of direct violence.

Occasionally the cartilage is broken across near its middle or its middle portion is torn loose from the lateral ligament and the middle third of the edge of the cartilage being caught between the bones, a longitudinal or bucket handle type of fracture is produced. More rarely the posterior horn is torn loose and this is believed to be the result of external rotation of the femur on the fixed tibia followed by flexion which nips and tears the cartilage.

Pathology.—In tearing of the posterior or anterior horn the loosened portion hangs free in the joint and may become hypertrophied or frayed from repeated injury. In the bucket handle type the torn edge may slip over the condyle and remain in the intercondylar notch. The transverse or oblique fractures occur opposite the attachment to the internal lateral ligament. Very rarely an abnormally loose cartilage may give rise to symptoms. The injury to the cartilage may be accompanied by an injury to the internal lateral or crucial ligaments. Torn or loosened cartilages heal with difficulty and the edges may hypertrophy, and then after a period of many years the cartilage may almost completely disappear, only a few shreds remaining.

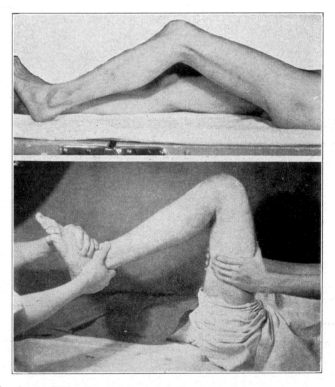

Fig. 1076.—Acute dislocation of the internal semilunar cartilage. The effusion into the joint has not yet appeared. Extension of the knee is limited.

Fig. 1077.—Manipulation of the knee for the reduction of a dislocated semilunar cartilage by traction on the leg with countertraction on the thigh followed by extension of the leg.

In addition to the semilunar cartilage injury, the displaced cartilage may cause contusion and gradual erosion of the articular cartilage, and the slow development of hypertrophic arthritis in the knee.

Diagnosis of Acute Injury of the Semilunar Cartilage.—It is usually possible to obtain a definite history of the manner in which the accident occurred and as this is an important factor in the diagnosis, it should always be done when possible. A characteristic history is that a man made a sudden turn while running and as his weight was thrown upon the abducted and flexed knee, the joint suddenly gave way and he fell to the ground with resultant severe pain over the inner side of the knee and has not been able to completely extend the leg since.

If this patient is seen immediately after the accident, there is acute tenderness, usually over the anterior portion of the semilunar cartilage and active motion at the knee is painful, while passive motion is fairly free except that extension is limited by from ten to thirty degrees (Fig. 1076). Within a few hours swelling develops as a result of bleeding and effusion into the joint, and the normal contour of the knee is obscured. As a rule, floating of the patella cannot be demonstrated because it is not possible to extend the knee. Localized swelling may develop over the anterior portion of the internal semilunar cartilage.

On manipulation it is found that flexion of the joint is fairly free and painless except as limited by the swelling, but that the knee cannot be extended. This pain is deep in the knee and the limitation of extension is somewhat elastic in character. This limitation of extension is the most characteristic sign and in an acutely injured knee is almost pathognomonic of a dislocation of the semilunar cartilage. It may not be present if the cartilage is merely torn and not dislocated and in the rare lesions of the posterior portion of the cartilage extension may be free and flexion may be limited. In these cases tenderness and pain are localized posterior to the internal lateral ligament. If the lateral ligaments are intact, there is no excess lateral mobility at the knee, but it should be recalled that injury to the internal semilunar cartilage is often accompanied by injury to the internal lateral ligament and in these cases the leg can be abducted on the thigh to an unusual degree. If the crucial ligaments are intact, the stability of the joint in the anteroposterior plane is not impaired.

In cases in which the locking in extension is not present, the diagnosis may be very difficult and can occasionally be cleared up by an x-ray picture which is taken after air has been injected into the knee joint. By this procedure the fracture in the cartilage may be visible. Without the air injection the x-ray picture is negative as there is no bone injury and the cartilage does not show in the picture. The main reason for taking x-ray pictures of these knees is to rule out fractures, especially of the tibial spine.

Diagnosis of Recurrent Dislocation of the Internal Semilunar Cartilage. —In recurrent cases the symptoms are not so severe and the locking is often transient in character or the patient may have learned to reduce the semilunar cartilage himself or to supervise its reduction by a layman. The severity of the symptoms tends to decrease with the frequency of the dislocation. Some of these chronic cases in which the cartilage slips out very frequently develop chronic synovitis with persistent excess fluid in the joint and a variable amount of hypertrophic arthritis. In these cases the history is the most important factor in the diagnosis and it is always possible to obtain the history of an original injury with a variable amount of disability afterward. In most of the recurrent cases the period of disability following a cartilage dislocation is not long, but in an occasional case it tends to lengthen and the dislocations appear to become more severe as the injury is repeated.

If the patient is seen in the interval between attacks, there may be no physical signs upon which the surgeon can base his diagnosis, and it must depend almost entirely upon the characteristic history of the knee giving way and locking. On physical examination the diagnosis is rendered more certain if any or all of the following signs are present: (1) An abnormal depression or protrusion over the anterior horn of the internal semilunar cartilage; (2) tenderness in this area; this is best elicited by firm pressure continued while the knee is extended; (3) excess lateral mobility of the knee; (4) lack of complete extension of the knee; (5) chronic synovitis; (6) atrophy of the thigh; (7) pain elicited by sharply rotating the flexed and dependent leg outward on the thigh; (8) pain elicited by forcible hyperextension or flexion or adduction or abduction of the leg on the thigh; and (9) a slight palpable "click" at the posterior part of the cartilage when the fully flexed knee is slowly extended.

Treatment of Acute Injury to the Semilunar Cartilage

If the patient is seen soon after the accident with a swollen, acutely painful knee, a diagnosis may not be possible unless the knee is locked in flexion. The treatment should be conservative. If the swelling is marked the knee should be aspirated and as much of the blood removed as possible. If the knee is locked an effort may be made to reduce the dislocation, but this has not been successful in our hands in acute cases with locking. The knee is partially immobilized with elastic bandages or a large pressure dressing and the patient is given crutches. Hot fomentations are applied several times a day. In many instances the locking will disappear in a day or so. In others, attempts may be made to reduce the displacement, but these should not be too violent, as further damage to the knee is to be avoided.

Reduction of Dislocation of the Semilunar Cartilage.—In reducing an internal semilunar cartilage in the right knee in a patient without an anesthetic the patient is placed on his back on a table or bed, the surgeon stands at his right, grasps the patient's ankle with his right hand and the upper third of the leg with his left hand and tells the patient that he wants him to assist in the reduction by kicking violently when told to do so. The surgeon then flexes and extends the knee three or four times and then pulls it forcibly out in extension at the same time telling the patient to kick. As the knee is extended the surgeon pushes inward with his left hand on the upper third of the leg in order to open up the inner side of the knee joint and also rotates the leg outward on the femur in order to unlock the displaced cartilage. As the knee is extended, the loosened cartilage slips back into place. The patient feels sharp pain at the instant the knee is extended, but this is only momentary. If the first attempt at reduction is not successful, a second or third attempt should not be made.

If the above maneuver fails, the displaced cartilage can sometimes be reduced by forcibly flexing the knee while the surgeon's forearm is in the popliteal space. Flexing the leg against the forearm tends to push the upper end of the tibia forward and may dislodge the cartilage. The knee is then slowly extended. The sign of reduction is free and complete extension at the knee without pain to the patient. A third method is acute flexion of the knee. (Fig. 1078.)

Aftertreatment.—In the case of a primary injury if the surgeon believes that there is a fair chance that the cartilage will heal the knee should be immobilized in a plaster cast over a period of three or four weeks. If there is much effusion into the joint, it should be removed by aspiration before the cast is applied. The cast should fit snugly and extend from the upper thigh to the toes. The patient may be up on crutches at will while in the cast, but should not attempt weight-bearing. At the end of three or four weeks the cast should be removed and the knee immobilized by means of an elastic knee cap or an elastic bandage, and the inner border of the heel of the shoe on the affected side should be elevated one-fourth of an inch.

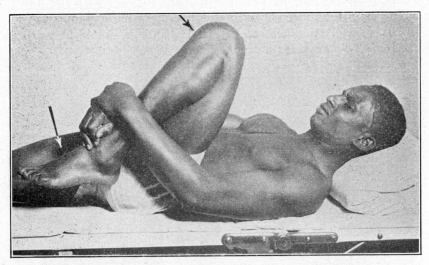

Fig. 1078.—Barnett Owen's method for the reduction of a displaced semilunar cartilage.

One of us (J. A. K.) does not have much faith in the ability of the cartilage to heal and treats these patients symptomatically with rest and hot fomentations to the knee, elastic bandages or a kneecap rest and quadriceps exercises.

If the cartilage gives trouble enough to warrant the operation it is removed at a later date.

Recurrent Cases.—It is questionable when a lesion of the semilunar cartilage may be termed recurrent and demand radical treatment. The decision depends somewhat on the patient's occupation, upon the frequency of the recurrence, and upon the amount of disability incurred. Strictly speaking any semilunar which has been out more than once is a recurrent case. On the other hand, one occasionally sees a case in which the semilunar has slipped two or three times over a period of several years and in which the knee is normal between times. In such a case if the patient is not engaged in a hazardous occupation, the knee can bt treated conservatively. On the other hand, if the patient is engaged in a hazardous occupation, the semilunar should be removed, as it may slip out at an awkward time and put the patient's life in danger. At present we feel that walking on the streets is a hazardous occupation, because if the semilunar should slip out while the patient is on the street he might be run over by an automobile; consequently, we operate a little more frequently than we did some years ago.

In many older patients symptoms suggesting a mild semilunar cartilage injury are relieved by heat, rest, support and quadriceps exercises.

Treatment

Treatment of these cases is operative removal of the torn or displaced cartilage. Any other treatment is merely palliative, but if the patient does not want to be operated upon, or if there is any contraindication for the operation, recurrences can be rendered less frequent or sometimes prevented over a long period by having the patient learn to walk with the toes in and wear a shoe with the inner border of the heel elevated one-fourth of an inch (Fig. 1079). An elastic knee cap or elastic bandage should be worn around the knee for a few weeks or until the synovitis subsides.

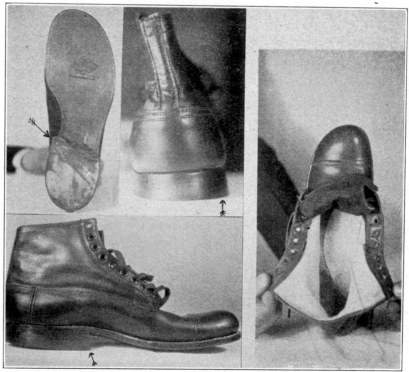

Fig. 1079.   Fig. 1080.

Fig. 1079.—Shoe with Thomas heel. The inner border of the heel is extended forward about one inch and is elevated one-fourth of an inch at the front and three-sixteenths of an inch at the back.

Fig. 1080.—Hard felt arch or sponge rubber support glued in the shoe.

Technic for Removal of the Internal Semilunar Cartilage.—A twenty-four hour preoperative preparation of the skin should be insisted upon. The patient is placed on the table in such a manner that the feet hang over the foot of the table with the knees flexed 90 degrees. A better exposure is obtained if a large sandbag is placed crosswise beneath the knee, thus giving slightly more flexion. The patient is draped in such a manner that the leg and foot on the affected side are free and can be manipulated. The operation is done without a tourniquet and may be done under general or local anesthesia.

The joint is opened by a straight incision which begins over the mesial condyle of the femur about an inch above the joint line and about an inch mesial to the patella and passes downward and inward toward the tibial tubercle for about two inches. If necessary this incision can be extended upward or downward. This incision is carried directly into the joint above and below the semilunar cartilage. Bleeding vessels are clamped and ligated before the synovial membrane is opened. In cutting through the subcutaneous tissue (superficial fascia) an attempt is made to identify and preserve the patellar branch of the saphenous nerve which may cross the incision.

The cartilage cannot be adequately inspected through this or any other incision without removal. Consequently, the surgeon should proceed to remove the cartilage immediately. The edges of the wound are retracted and the anterior pole of the cartilage lateral to the incision is cut free from the fibrous capsule and pulled out into the wound. The mesial edge of the wound is then retracted inward and the anterior pole of the cartilage is grasped with strong-toothed forceps and dissected free from the joint capsule on the mesial side of the joint. With a deep, narrow retractor and a small knife (stab blade or blade curved on the flat) the dissection can be carried well back into the posterior compartment of the knee.

When the cartilage is freed as far back as possible, its anterior portion is grasped by the heavy-toothed forceps and pulled outward across the joint so that it is delivered into the intercondylar notch. In doing this it is torn from a part of its posterior attachment. It is then pulled forward between the condyles and cut off as far back as possible.

Not infrequently in cases where full extension is not possible or is painful before the operation the surgeon will encounter a bucket handle tear with the torn cartilage lying in the intercondylar notch. In such instances the anterior portion is dissected from its attachment and the cartilage is pulled forward and cut off as far back as possible. Then, the mesial portion of the joint is inspected and any projecting tags of cartilage are removed. Unless the narrow rim of cartilage which is left seems likely to interfere with joint movement, it is not disturbed.

Occasionally it will be found that the cartilage is torn across in its posterior half or it may be torn in attempting to deliver it into the intercondylar notch. In such instances it is not possible to remove the posterior portion through the anterior incision and a second vertical incision should be made opposite the posteromesial aspect of the joint and the posterior portion of the cartilage is removed through this incision.

After the cartilage is satisfactorily removed the fat pad is pulled forward and the crucial ligaments and anterior portion of the external semilunar cartilage are inspected. In a considerable number of cases the anterior crucial ligament will be found to be relaxed or torn and rarely it will be seen that the external cartilage is injured. No attempt is made to repair the damaged crucial ligament, but any tags of fibrous tissue are excised. If the external cartilage is injured it is exposed and excised through an anterolateral incision.

The leg is straightened and the joint is closed with interrupted sutures in four layers—synovial tissue, aponeurosis, subcutaneous tissue and skin—and a pressure dressing is applied.

Aftertreatment.—The patient should remain in bed for four to ten days, but may begin to move the knee and exercise the quadriceps on the fourth day. At the end of six days the sutures are removed and the patient should begin seriously to exercise the knee in order to restore power in the quadriceps and flexion at the joint. At this time he may be got up with a cane and this may be discarded gradually as power returns. Within four weeks after the operation the average patient will be walking with little or no limp or pain.

INJURY TO THE EXTERNAL SEMILUNAR CARTILAGE

The external semilunar cartilage is subject to the same types of injury as the internal semilunar cartilage, but is injured only about one-tenth as often as is the internal. The mechanism of the injury is usually an adduction and inversion wrench of the leg or a direct blow upon the cartilage which may drive it into the joint where it becomes caught between the bones and is torn. The lesions in the cartilage resemble those described above in the internal cartilage in that either end of the cartilage may be torn loose, it may be split longitudinally with a bucket handle type of fracture, or rarely it may be fractured transversely near the middle. The symptoms and physical signs are practically identical with those described above in injuries to the internal semilunar cartilage except that the local pain and tenderness are in the outer side of the knee in the region of the external cartilage.

As in the lesions of the internal cartilage both acute and recurrent or chronic types of derangement occur.

The treatment in injuries of the external semilunar cartilage is exactly the same as in injuries of the internal except that when the knee is manipulated in order to reduce an acute dislocation the tibia should be abducted and rotated inward on the femur in order to loosen the displaced cartilage from between the condyles and in operating to remove the cartilage, the incision should be lateral to the patella and curved inward and downward.

The aftertreatment is just the same and the prognosis is the same. When both cartilages are injured, they are best removed through two small straight incisions, as these incisions heal more quickly and leave less permanent disability than do the extensive midpatellar or curved incisions which are necessary to expose both cartilages through one incision.

Cysts of the Semilunar Cartilages.—Occasionally after an injury to a semilunar cartilage a multilocular cyst develops in the cartilage and the cartilage increases in size until it interferes with movement of the joint and causes pain (Fig. 1081). These cysts are more frequent in the external semilunar cartilage. The treatment is excision of the cartilage preferably with the cysts intact. This is best done through a straight lateral incision with incisions into the joint anterior and posterior to the lateral ligament. The

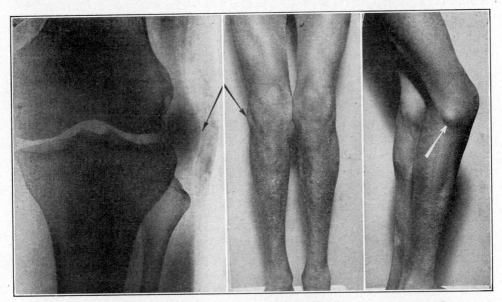

Fig. 1081.—Cyst of external semilunar cartilage of the knee. Treated by excision and removal of the cartilage. Good result.

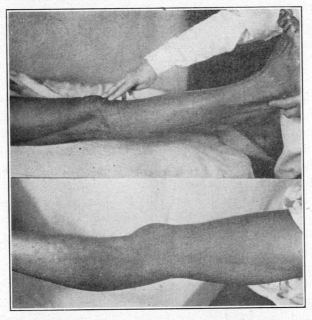

Fig. 1082.—Two cases of rupture of the anterior crucial ligaments. Note the hyperextension at the knee with dropping backward of the tibia.

cartilage is freed in its anterior portion; then, delivered through the incision behind the ligament and it is excised in one piece.

Prognosis in Lesions of the Semilunar Cartilage.—The prognosis varies with the type of case and with the treatment. Since it is not possible to determine the extent of the lesion without exposing the entire cartilage, the prognosis should be guarded. In an acute case where the injury is in an area with a blood supply and which is completely reduced and immobilized over a period of at least four weeks in a plaster-of-Paris cast, it is possible that the torn cartilage will heal and that a normal knee will result. In acute cases which are not treated in this manner, it is probable that the lesion will recur and that the condition will become chronic and demand operative removal of the cartilage. After the cartilage is removed, if the knee is normal in other respects, if it is not unduly traumatized at the time of the operation, and if no infection should intervene, one should expect a practically normal knee within from six to eight weeks. If there are lesions, such as tears of the crucial ligaments, relaxation of the lateral ligaments, or hypertrophic arthritis in the joint, a normal knee cannot be obtained, but one may expect to relieve the tendency of the knee to lock and also remove a causative factor in the arthritis.

INJURIES OF THE CRUCIAL LIGAMENTS

Incidence and Mechanism.—Because of their great strength and their protected location near the center of the knee joint, the crucial ligaments are rarely injured. But their integrity is so important to the stability and function of the knee that injuries of these ligaments may be followed by grave permanent disability which in some cases it is impossible to repair. Consequently injuries of the crucial ligaments should be regarded as serious injuries and should be treated with great care.

The anterior crucial is injured more frequently than the posterior. The anterior crucial is taut when the knee is fully extended and prevents hyperextension at the knee and slipping forward of the tibia on the femur with the knee in a position of extension. When the internal lateral ligament has been divided, the anterior crucial also prevents abduction and external rotation of the tibia on the femur. Consequently the anterior crucial ligament may be injured by forcible hyperextension at the knee or by forcible abduction and external rotation of the leg. In the abduction and external rotation injuries, the internal lateral ligament is first ruptured and the internal semilunar cartilage may be torn or dislocated.

The posterior crucial ligament is taut when the knee is flexed and prevents the flexed tibia from slipping upward on the femur (Fig. 1083). It can be stretched or torn by forcible flexion of the knee or by driving the flexed tibia upward and backward on the femur. The posterior crucial, however, is rarely injured alone. Both crucials may be injured by temporary or permanent dislocations of the tibia on the femur in any direction. (Fig. 1084.)

Pathology of Injuries to the Crucial Ligaments.—The injured crucial ligament may be stretched or torn across at any point or it may be avulsed with its bony attachment from the femur or the tibia. When the posterior crucial is injured, the anterior crucial is usually injured also. These injuries to the crucials are often accompanied by injuries to the lateral ligaments and semilunar cartilages.

Diagnosis of Injuries to the Crucial Ligaments.—There is a history of a severe wrench or direct trauma to the region of the knee followed by marked pain and disability and a sense of instability in the knee.

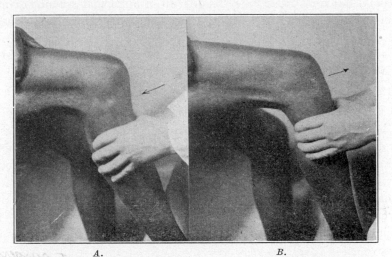

A.   *B.*

Fig. 1083.—Rupture of posterior crucial ligament. Note that the flexed tibia has slipped upward on the femur (*A*) and can be pulled down to its normal position (*B*), but slips back when the traction is released.

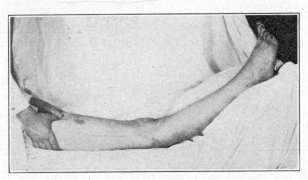

Fig. 1084.—Laceration of anterior and posterior crucial ligaments with chip fracture of the upper end of the tibia. Treated by arthrotomy and suture of the crucial ligaments and immobilization in a plaster cast for three months, then in a knee cap. Fair result, knee unstable. Metal knee brace with lock joint being worn.

In a recent case the region of the knee is swollen and the joint is distended with excess fluid. There is usually tenderness over the anterior fat pad and in the popliteal space. If the internal lateral ligament and semilunar cartilage are injured there is tenderness over these structures.

The important point is that the knee is unstable in the anteroposterior plane, and in the absence of a fracture this lack of stability is pathognomonic of crucial ligament injury.

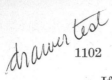

If the knee can be hyperextended or if, with the knee flexed, the tibia can be moved forward on the femur, the anterior crucial is stretched, torn, or avulsed from one of its attachments (Fig. 1082).

With the knee flexed, if the tibia can be moved backward on the femur, the posterior crucial is injured (Fig. 1083).

If both of the above forms of false motion can be elicited, then both crucials are injured (Fig. 1084).

Crucial ligament injury also results in an abnormal amount of motion in rotation at the knee and if the lateral ligaments are injured abnormal lateral mobility is present (Fig. 1085).

A roentgenogram should always be taken to rule out bone injury and to determine whether or not a ligamentous attachment has been torn off (Fig. 1086).

In an old case the patient complains of weakness and of a sense of insecurity in the knee and may state that in walking he feels the bones slip on one another. On physical examination there may or may not be effusion into the joint, but the lack of stability and false motion in the anteroposterior plane as mentioned above are present. In addition there is usually some abnormal lateral mobility and rotation, and if the condition has existed for some years, there is a variable amount of traumatic (hypertrophic) arthritis in the joint. These cases also should be examined by x-ray to rule out bone pathology.

Treatment of Injuries of the Crucial Ligaments.—The treatment of an acute injury to the crucial ligaments is immobilization—complete, prolonged, and uninterrupted. The natural inclination is to open the knee and suture the ligament, but experience has shown that this is rarely successful, and that frequently a stable painless knee may be obtained by conservative treatment if this is begun soon after the injury.

In a fresh case the excess fluid should be removed by aspiration of the joint and the knee should be immobilized in a position of moderate flexion in a plaster cast which is applied over a minimum of padding and extends from the groin to the toes. The knee is immobilized in a position of moderate flexion (20 to 30 degrees) because in this position both crucial and both lateral ligaments are relaxed.

As soon as the plaster is set, the patient should be put to bed with the knee elevated. If swelling causes pain or circulatory disturbance in the toes, the plaster cast must be bivalved and strapped together again, and if indicated, the aspiration of the knee should be repeated. Then in a week or ten days after the swelling has disappeared, a new skin-tight plaster cast of the same type should be applied.

The immobilization should be continued for two months, but the patient may be up on crutches during much of this time if the cast is snug. During this period the patient should practice straight leg raising and quadriceps tension in order to preserve the power in this muscle. At the end of two months the cast is removed and the patient begins to exercise his leg in flexion

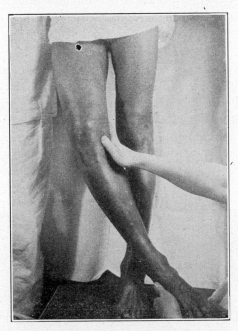

Fig. 1085.—Rupture of the posterior crucial and external lateral ligaments with avulsion of the upper end of the fibula. Treated by suture of ligaments and of fibula and immobilization in a plaster cast for ten weeks. Metal knee brace worn for nine weeks. Good result.

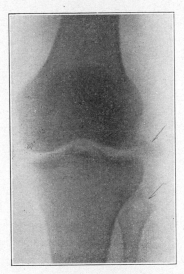

Fig. 1086.—Roentgenogram of preceding case. Note the upward displacement of the upper end of the fibula.

and extension and the quadriceps exercises are increased and weight-bearing is encouraged, at first with crutches or a cane and then without support. An Ace bandage may be applied to the foot and leg if the swelling is troublesome and hot fomentations may be applied to the knee in order to hasten the return of motion.

If the lateral ligaments are satisfactory, a patient may have an almost normal knee if he will develop his quadriceps muscle. One of us (J. A. K.) has never attempted to repair a torn crucial, nor has he advised such an operation. He has repaired the internal lateral ligament on several occasions in unstable knees and secured useful extremities by developing the quadriceps. Torn cartilages are removed if they cause disability. Nor has he ever used a knee cage. This encourages muscle atrophy and this increases instability and disability.

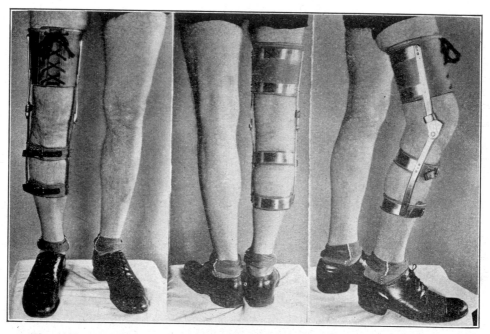

Fig. 1087.—Knee cage used in the treatment of crucial ligamentous injuries or severe lateral ligamentous injuries. In the very severe ligamental injuries of the knee joint the brace should extend down to the shoe.

The Knee Cage.—The knee cage (Fig. 1087) consists of two lateral side bars which are hinged at the knee and are united by four curved metal cross pieces, two above and two below the knee. The cross pieces are curved to fit the thigh and leg and are padded with felt and covered with leather. The cage is then fitted with thigh and leg straps, a patellar cap for the front of the knee, and a wide soft strap for the popliteal space. It is important to have two metal cross pieces above and two below the knee, and with marked instability a caliper splint may be advisable (Fig. 1087).

The knee cage should be worn for from four to six months. At the end of this time it may be discarded and an elastic knee cap may be worn for two or three months, when all support may be discarded. The patient should be taught to walk with the toes in and to bear the weight on the outer border of the foot. In order to encourage this, the inner border of the heel of both shoes should be elevated one-fourth of an inch.

It will be objected that this long period of complete immobilization will lead to muscle atrophy and stiffness of the knee and ankle. Of course it will; but we are dealing with a serious injury and are endeavoring to stiffen an unstable knee by rest. After the patient begins to walk, the knee and ankle will gradually loosen up and if the knee is stable, the muscles will be restored to their normal tone. The restoration of motion in the joints and of power in the muscles can be hastened by active exercises, but manipulation of the knee should be avoided.

Old cases with unstable knees should be fitted with a knee cage for a year. If at the end of this time they are no better, an attempt may be made to replace the torn ligaments by the operation of Hey Groves or of Cubbins or of Gallie and Le Mesurier. But these are formidable operations and should be attempted only by a skilled surgeon and with the understanding that permanent benefit is only problematical.

INJURIES OF THE TIBIAL SPINE

The spine of the tibia is a roughened elevated area which is surmounted by internal and external tubercles. Robert Jones and Allyn Smith* classify injury to the tibial spine as follows: (1) Avulsion of the tibial spine or of its internal tubercle; (2) fracture of the external tubercle of the spine; (3) injury of the spine combined with a fracture of a tuberosity of the tibia.

Mechanism and Pathology.—An avulsion of the tibial spine or of its internal tubercle is really a lesion of a crucial ligament, usually the anterior crucial, and will not be considered here as this lesion has been described in the preceding section.

Fracture of the external tubercle of the tibial spine is said to be produced by the sharp inner margin of the external condyle of the femur when the leg is rotated outward and is driven backward and flexed upon the femur. In order for this injury to occur, the internal lateral ligament must be stretched or torn. In this injury there is no lesion of the crucial ligaments; the tip of the tubercle is simply knocked off by the condyle.

Injury to the spine combined with fracture of a tuberosity of the tibia is usually a crush fracture such as is produced by severe direct violence or by a fall from a height, and these lesions will be considered under fractures of the upper end of the tibia. In this section we shall consider only the fracture of the external tubercle of the spine without crucial ligament injury and without other fractures of the upper end of the tibia.

Diagnosis.—There is a history of an abduction and flexion strain upon the knee joint which is accompanied by severe pain in the knee and is followed by pain, swelling, and effusion into the joint and a variable amount of dis-

*Jones, Robert, and Smith, Allyn: Brit. J. Surg. 1: 70, 1913.

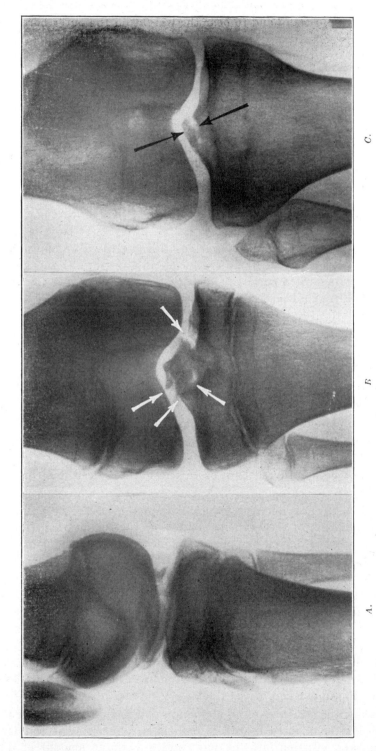

Fig. 1088.—*A*, Fracture of tibial spine with displacement of one fragment. Open reduction not considered advisable. Treated with circular cast for two months and long leg brace for two months thereafter. Good function.

B, Fracture of tibial spines in a child. Treated by full extension of the leg at the knee joint in a circular cast for six weeks. Felt pad and Ace bandage for six weeks. Good result.

C, Fracture of tibial spine in an adult with practically no displacement. Treated in a circular cast for six weeks. No weight-bearing for two months. An Ace bandage and felt pad followed the cast for two months. Good function.

ability. If the crucial ligaments are intact, there is no abnormal mobility in the anteroposterior plane, and if the lateral ligaments are intact, there is no abnormal mobility in the lateral plane. It should be remembered that the lateral ligaments, semilunar cartilages, and crucial ligaments may be injured along with the spine and when present the injury to the spine is obscured by the symptoms of the above lesions.

The most important diagnostic sign of injury to the tibial spine is firm bony block which limits extension at the knee. This limitation of extension is slightly different from the elastic block which is characteristic of the displaced semilunar cartilage and the pain caused by attempts to extend the knee is not localized over the cartilage, but is felt beneath the patellar tendon. A positive diagnosis can be made only by the x-ray. In old neglected cases the bony block and limitation of extension persist and the knee is the object of recurrent effusion into the joint.

Treatment of Isolated Fracture of the Tibial Spine

It is usually possible by manipulating the knee in flexion and rotating the leg from one side to the other and by then extending it while pressure is made over the patellar tendon and fat pad to dislodge the separated portion of the spine from between the condyles of the tibia and femur and to obtain full extension at the knee. When this has been accomplished, the knee should be immobilized in a plaster cast in a position of full extension over a period of four weeks. At the end of this time the cast should be removed and the patient may begin to exercise the knee joint and to tighten up the quadriceps muscle to restore power there. At the end of another week the patient may be got up on crutches, but he should continue to exercise the knee daily. The crutches can be discarded as soon as the patient is comfortable without them.

If the displaced fragment cannot be reduced, and if full extension at the knee cannot be obtained, the joint should be opened and the detached fragment should be removed. In operating upon a knee joint for acute injuries to the tibial spine, it is advisable to wait a few days after the accident in order that a forty-eight-hour preparation of the skin may be made. At the end of this time the knee is opened by an incision on the mesial side of the patella five or six inches long. This incision is carried directly into the joint. The retraction of the edges of this incision and the fat pad will usually reveal the loose fragment. If necessary, the incision may be enlarged upward and the patella can be displaced outward.

On two occasions one of us (J. A. K.) has opened acutely injured knees and tied the avulsed tibial spines back in place once with fine stainless steel wire and once with silk passed through two holes drilled from the tubercle to emerge in the defect left by the avulsed spine. Both patients have good knees two years later and we believe that this is the method of choice when the diagnosis is made early.

In cases which have been reduced and treated conservatively if it is found that there is a block to motion after the immobilization is discontinued, then the spine should be removed by operation just as described above. The postoperative treatment is the application of a pressure bandage for a period of about two weeks. At the end of this time the skin sutures having been removed, the patient may begin to take exercises and can be got up on crutches. The crutches can be discarded gradually at the end of about four weeks. If there is no ligamentous injury to the knee, a normal knee may be expected.

LOOSE BODIES IN THE KNEE JOINT

Fischer* classifies loose bodies in the knee joint as follows: (1) Loose bodies composed of unorganized fibrin; (2) loose bodies composed of connective tissue other than bone and cartilage; (3) loose bodies composed of bone

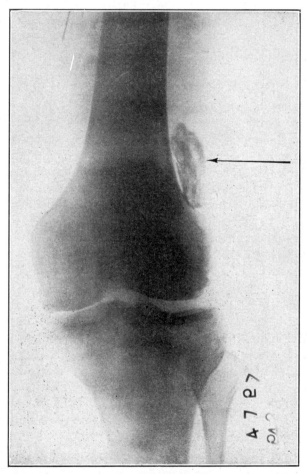

Fig. 1089.—Joint mouse or loose body in the quadriceps pouch following an injury. Treated by removal of the loose body with good result.

and cartilage. In this book we are concerned only with those loose bodies which are the result of injury, and these may be single or multiple and are usually composed of cartilage and a variable amount of the underlying bone which has been detached from the articular surface of one of the bones entering into the joint.

*Fischer, A. G. T.: Internal Derangement of the Knee Joint, Lewis, London, 1924.

Koenig has given the name "osteochondritis dissecans" to the process by which the loose body is detached and believes that the condition is due to a dissecting inflammation with resulting necrosis. At the present time we still use the term "osteochondritis dissecans," but find that most of the cases give a history of a definite injury with direct trauma on the condyle and in some instances the injury is followed almost immediately by the symptoms of a loose body in the joint. Consequently we believe that these osteocartilaginous loose bodies or joint mice are traumatic in origin although a period of several weeks or months may elapse between the injury and the beginning of the symptoms. After it has become free in the joint the loose body may continue to grow or it may become fragmented and the pieces may grow or it may become adherent to the synovial membrane.

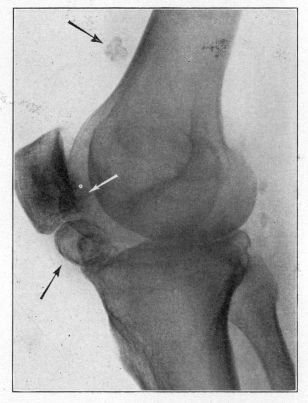

Fig. 1090.—Loose bodies in the knee joint. Treated by excision. Good result.

Diagnosis of Loose Bodies in the Knee Joint.—Momentary locking of the joint with sudden severe pain is the characteristic sign of a loose body in the joint. As a rule the locking disappears spontaneously or can be relieved by some movement which the patient has learned and it may or may not be followed by a mild transient synovitis. In some instances the locking is accompanied by a palpable protrusion at the joint line and the patient may find it necessary to push this inward in order to relax the joint. In other cases a large loose body may be palpable beneath the skin and subcutaneous tissue. These large loose bodies tend to be localized in the quadriceps bursa. If the loose body becomes adherent to the capsule, the symptoms of locking tend to disappear. The diagnosis should be confirmed by the x-ray because loose bodies are frequently multiple, and it is advisable when operating upon them to remove all that are present.

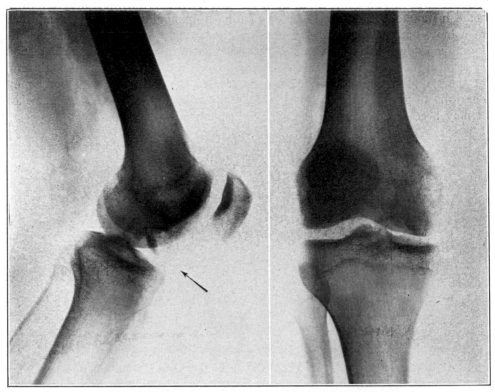

Fig. 1091.—Large joint mouse or loose body in the knee joint which followed an injury, apparently broken off from the external condyle. Treated by removal with good result.

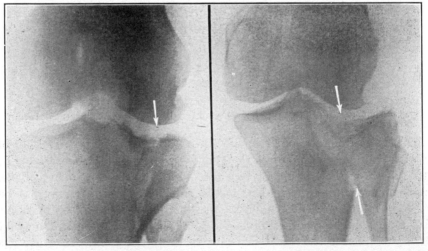

Fig. 1092.—Fracture of the external condyle in which weight-bearing was permitted too early as seen on the right. Later, open operation with elevation of condyle and bone chips under it gave only a fair result.

Treatment of Loose Bodies in the Knee Joint

Treatment is removal by arthrotomy. The operation should be preceded by a forty-eight-hour preparation of the skin and should be performed under a tourniquet. For loose bodies in the anterior portion of the joint a long incision beginning about three inches above the superior margin of the patella

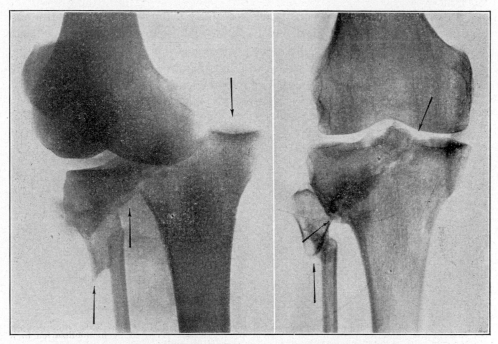

Fig. 1093.—Severe fracture of the external condyle of the tibia and of the shaft of the fibula with displacement. Treated by manipulation and skeletal traction to the lower third of the leg with good functional result.

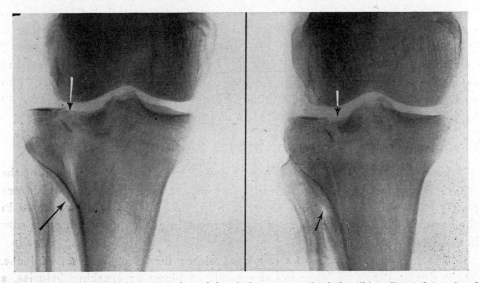

Fig. 1094.—Fracture of the external condyle of the upper end of the tibia. Treated by closed manipulation and reduction with anatomical result. Good function.

and extending along the mesial side of the patella down to the tibial tubercle should be carried down into the joint. The patella should then be displaced laterally over the end of the condyle and the anterior portion of the joint can be thoroughly inspected and any loose bodies removed. The advantage of this incision is that the patella is not split, and prolonged immobilization is not necessary.

In osteochondritis dissecans there is usually a depressed area in the end of the condyle which marks the place from which the loose body has been detached. This area is lined by connective tissue. At the operation for the removal of the loose body we excise the margins and base of this area in the hope that the cavity will become filled from beneath.

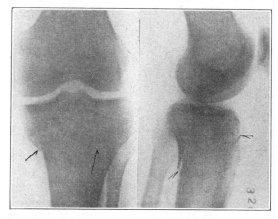

Fig. 1095.—Compression fracture through the upper end of the tibia. This fracture does not involve the joint. Consequently traction is not necessary. Treated by immobilization in a plaster cast with slight flexion at the knee. Ten weeks' disability.

Loose bodies in the posterior portion of the joint may be removed through the popliteal incision of Brackett and Osgood which is carried directly downward through the popliteal space and into the joint cavity, or by the lateral incisions of Henderson which are made posterior to the lateral ligaments and carried into the joint cavity. After the operation a mild pressure dressing should be applied and the patient ordered not to use the knee for about two weeks. At the end of this time he may be got up on crutches and gradually begin to bear weight upon the knee. A normal knee may be expected.

FRACTURES OF THE UPPER END OF THE TIBIA

Incidence and Mechanism.—The expanded cancellous proximal end of the adult tibia overhangs the shaft on either side, and its lateral margins are poorly supported from below. Consequently, this is a point of weakness in the bone, and fractures here are fairly frequent in adults, although quite rare in children.

The fractures may be the result of either direct or indirect violence. Those due to direct violence are the result of blows or crushing injuries, a not uncommon type being the result of being hit just below the knee by an

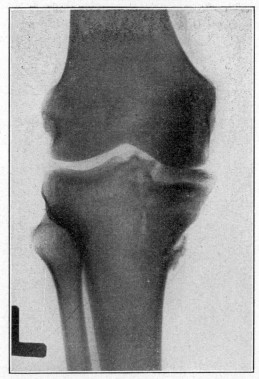

Fig. 1096.—Fracture of internal condyle of tibia with slight displacement. Immobilized in cast ten weeks, then gradual weight-bearing with metal brace. Good result in four months.

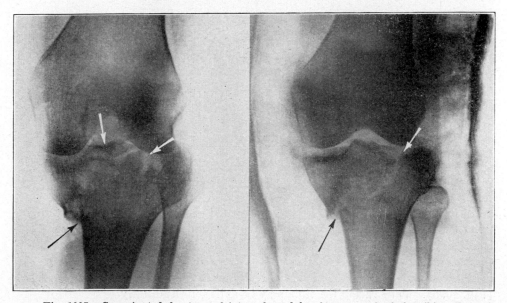

Fig. 1097.—Comminuted fracture of internal condyle of upper end of the tibia. Treated by manipulative reduction and lateral manual compression and a circular cast with good anatomical result. Good function in six months. Cast remained on leg three months and then a long leg brace applied. Weight-bearing was not allowed until four months following injury.

automobile bumper. The fractures in the upper end of the tibia from indirect violence may be crushing injuries caused by falls on the feet or avulsion injuries caused by abduction or adduction of the leg.

Pathology.—The fractures vary from a crack in one condyle of the tibia without displacement to a transverse fracture of both bones of the leg just below the knee with vertical splitting and severe comminution of the proximal fragment with disorganization of the knee joint. A fairly common type is one in which a small triangular section of the margin of one condyle has been split off and displaced downward and impacted. Such a fracture results from

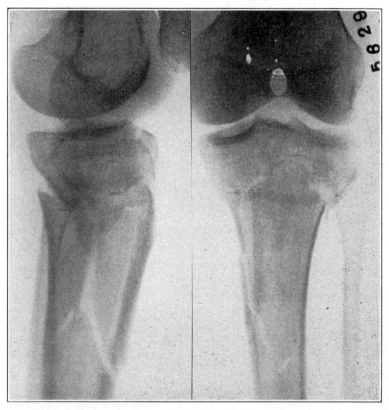

Fig. 1098.—Compound comminuted T-fracture through the upper end of the tibia with anterior bowing. Treated by traction (Kirschner wire through lower end of tibia) in full extension, for four weeks. Circular cast five weeks. Weight-bearing within three months with metal brace. Good result in five months.

a fall on the feet, the leg being bowed outward or inward as the margin of the tibial condyle is crushed. With more severe trauma of the same type the fragment may be larger, or both condyles may be split and separated from the shaft and driven downward, thus creating an inverted V or Y fracture. In these severe fractures of the tibia, the fibula is usually broken in its upper third (Fig. 1098). Very rarely the tibia may be split longitudinally.

Abduction or adduction injuries may result in a crushing down of the margin of the tibial condyle on the side toward which the leg is bent or in the avulsion and pulling upward of a fragment of the condyle on the other side (sprain fracture).

Injuries from direct violence may result in fairly simple transverse fractures of one or both bones or in almost explosive comminution of the upper end of the tibia. A considerable percentage of the fractures from direct violence are compound.

Displacement of the fragments is not as a rule marked, but relatively slight displacements may be of considerable importance when they involve the articular surface. Whenever the fracture line extends into the joint, and this includes most of the cases, the knee becomes distended with blood. In addition to the injury to the tibia there may be a variable amount of injury to the lateral and crucial ligaments of the knee, and there may be subluxation or even dislocation at this joint.

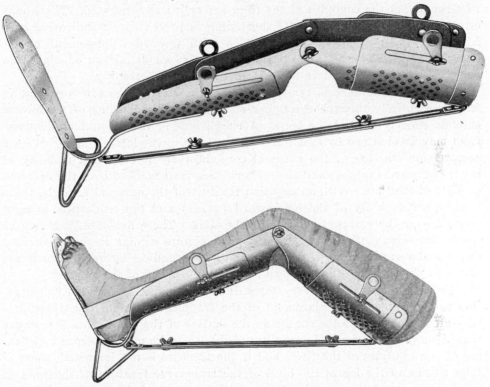

Fig. 1099.—Adjustable leg splint and adjustable leg splint applied; useful emergency splint for any leg and foot injury. (Courtesy Zimmer Manufacturing Co.)

Diagnosis of Fractures of the Upper End of the Tibia.—The diagnosis of these fractures may be very difficult because all of them are close to the joint, and many of them are incomplete fractures in that the continuity of the shaft of the bone is not interrupted. Consequently, wherever a fracture of the upper end of the tibia is suspected, anteroposterior and lateral x-ray pictures should be taken in order that minor fractures may be detected and because it is important to determine as nearly as possible the exact nature of the fracture before treatment is instituted and this cannot be done without an x-ray examination.

There is a history of a severe injury to the knee followed by pain and disability. The disability is usually complete in that the patient is not only not able to bear weight upon the leg, but he is also unable to move the joint voluntarily, although passive movement may be fairly free. In an acute case there is a variable amount of effusion into the knee and swelling which may be general or may be localized to the region directly over the fracture. In addition to the swelling there may be a variable amount of deformity.

With a compression fracture of the external condyle, the leg is usually in a varus or knock knee position and with an avulsion fracture of this condyle the leg may be in a valgus or bowleg position. There may or may not be a deformity of the leg in rotation, depending upon whether or not the fracture extends completely through the shaft of the tibia. Likewise there may or may not be a broadening of the region below the knee, depending upon whether or not the condyles of the tibia are split and separated. There may or may not be a shortening. If shortening is present, it is indicative of a fracture through the shaft of the tibia with upward displacement of the lower fragment. This upward displacement is, as a rule, absent or slight. In fractures of a single condyle there is, of course, no shortening.

On palpation there is tenderness over the site of the fracture and in fractures entirely through the upper end of the tibia the line of tenderness extends entirely around the bone. A rough idea of the amount of displacement may be obtained by manipulating the knee in the lateral plane. With a compression fracture of the external condyle, there is abnormal mobility of the leg outward (valgus) and the tenderness is most marked over the external condyle of the tibia. With an avulsion fracture of the external condyle, there is abnormal mobility of the leg inward (varus) and the tenderness is most marked over the external condyle of the tibia. These avulsion fractures or sprain fractures of the knee give a clinical picture similar to that described above under ruptures and sprains of the corresponding lateral ligament except that the tenderness is localized over the upper end of the tibia.

Unless the case is seen very early, it is not, as a rule, possible by palpation to determine the displacement of the fragments because the tissues are edematous and obscure the change in the outline of the bone. In a T fracture with definite separation it is usually possible to make out a definite broadening of the condyles of the tibia, and if the fracture is not impacted, there is false motion of the leg at the level of the transverse fracture of the tibia in all directions and it may be possible to demonstrate independent motion of the condyles of the tibia by squeezing them together or gently moving one of them backward and forward while the other is held firmly.

In many of these fractures of the upper end of the tibia there is also a fracture of the upper portion of the fibula. The presence of a fracture of the fibula should be suspected if there is localized pain and tenderness over the upper end of this bone and if pain can be produced in this area by squeezing the tibia and fibula together in the middle of the leg.

Prognosis of Fractures of the Upper End of the Tibia.—With the exception of sprain fractures with considerable separation of the avulsed fragment, these fractures tend to unite rather rapidly because they are through cancellous bone, but the prognosis as regards restoration of normal function of the knee joint is poor in any except the avulsion fractures because the fracture line enters the joint surface, and there is, as a rule, displacement downward of one or of both condyles and perhaps separation of one or both condyles or of the separated fragment, with the production of incongruity in the joint surfaces. And as the knee is a large weight-bearing joint, this incongruity, if allowed to persist, tends to lead to the development of traumatic arthritis. Even in fractures in which there is practically no displacement of the fragments traumatic arthritis may develop. On the other hand, we have seen fractures of the upper end of the tibia in which considerable displacement has been allowed to persist and in which a very useful painless knee was obtained.

In compound fractures the prognosis is especially grave because the fracture communicates with the knee joint, and if infection occurs the knee joint is liable to be involved. We are also more apt to treat these fractures conservatively than by débridement on account of the danger of carrying infection into the knee joint.

Consequently in simple fractures, the prognosis is good as regards union and alignment, but should be guarded as regards function of the knee. In compound fractures, the prognosis is grave.

Treatment

Treatment of Fractures of the Upper End of the Tibia.—The treatment of fractures at the upper end of the tibia with involvement of the knee joint depends primarily upon the type of fracture.

Treatment of Sprain Fractures of the Upper End of the Tibia.—In an avulsion or sprain fracture the knee should be immobilized in a plaster-of-Paris cast, the plaster being applied with the knee in a position of slight flexion and the leg drawn to the side of the injury in order to relax the lateral ligament. If effusion is present, we aspirate the knee at the beginning of the treatment.

In other words, treatment of avulsion fractures is the same as described above under injuries of the lateral ligaments.

Treatment of Compression or T Fractures Without Displacement.—If the displacement is not sufficient to interfere with the function of the knee joint or to disturb the alignment of the leg, all that is necessary is to aspirate the blood from the knee joint and to immobilize the extremity in a plaster-of-Paris cast which extends from the upper thigh to the toes. The cast is applied with the knee slightly flexed and is left on for from four to eight weeks, depending upon the extent of the fracture. While the cast is on, the patient may be up on crutches, and he should practice straight leg raising and quadriceps exercises. After the cast is removed, the patient is instructed in exercising the extremity and may be up on crutches, but he does not bear weight upon the leg until about a month later, when weight-bearing is resumed gradually.

Treatment of Fractures of One Condyle With Displacement.—The displaced bone may consist of one large or of many fragments, and the displacement may be outward or downward or both. The displacement should be reduced and the normal contour of the upper end of the tibia should be restored if possible.

The excess blood from the knee joint is removed by aspiration, and under general anesthesia the limb is strongly flexed laterally to the opposite side against a fulcrum (the perineal post of a fracture table is useful) which is applied at the level of the knee. With a fracture of the external condyle the leg is adducted on the femur, and with one of the internal condyles the leg is abducted.

The adduction or abduction of the leg on the femur is then maintained, and the condyles of the tibia are strongly compressed with a large carpenter's clamp or with a Boehler's vice. The compression should be applied and released quickly; otherwise, necrosis of the skin may ensue.

Still maintaining the position of adduction or abduction of the extended knee, a plaster-of-Paris cast is applied from the upper thigh to the toes.

A few days later x-rays of the knee in two planes are made, and if the position of the fragments is satisfactory, the cast is left on for eight weeks. During this period the patient practices tensing of the quadriceps and straight leg raising exercises and may be up on crutches, but he should not bear weight on the leg.

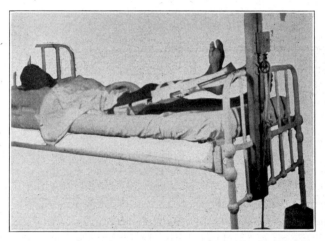

Fig. 1100.—Method of applying skin traction for fractures of the upper end of the tibia. Thomas splint is fixed to the foot of the bed and traction goes over a pulley attached to the foot piece.

After the cast is removed, the patient continues the above and adds exercises to restore flexion of the knee and motion at the ankle, but he should not bear weight for at least a month. When the bone is quite solid, weight-bearing is begun gradually.

Treatment by Traction and Manipulation.—Either skeletal traction through the lower end of the tibia or the os calcis or skin traction is useful in many of these fractures of a single condyle. This is especially true of those in which the joint is extensively involved and the knee is not stable.

The fracture is manipulated and the leg supported in a Thomas or other splint and the traction applied. Then, the condyle is molded back into position by lateral pressure after the leg is in the splint and the traction is acting. This pressure can be applied manually or with a vise or clamp.

The position should be checked by a portable x-ray. The traction (eight to fifteen pounds) should be continued for from four to eight weeks and may be followed by a cast for a few weeks or by restricted activity and exercise without weight-bearing until the proximal end of the tibia is well consolidated.

The judicious use of traction and lateral compression, which may be repeated if necessary, may avert an operative reduction and yield a better knee, because the results of operative treatment of these fractures are none too good.

Operative Treatment.—If the fragments are comminuted and the displacements are marked, it is not unusual to find that the position after manipulation is not satisfactory and traction plus further manipulation and lateral compression or operation is indicated.

The difficulty is to maintain the position of the fragments after the operation. This is best done by following the method of Dr. James A. Dickson, who operates through a large window in the cast which maintains the adduction or abduction of the limb. The cast is reinforced if necessary, and the window over the fractured condyle extends from the lower third of the thigh to the middle of the leg.

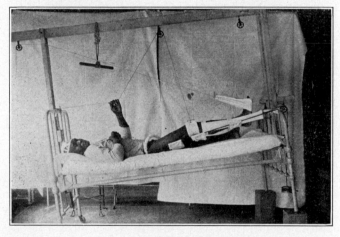

Fig. 1101.—Method of exercising knee and ankle with sling under knee or over foot while traction is applied to the leg.

The skin is prepared in the usual way and the area draped and the fracture is exposed through a longitudinal incision which lies well anterior to the lateral ligament of the knee. The knee joint is opened and inspected. If the semilunar cartilage is torn or displaced, it is removed. (In two recent cases one of us (J. A. K.) found the external cartilage torn and displaced downward between the fragments of the tibia.) The fragments of the articular surface of the tibia are then pushed up and inward to restore the weight-bearing surface. If necessary, bone chips are cut from the tibia below the fracture to fill in the dead space and hold the fragments up in position. If the large lateral fragment tends to spring outward, it is held in position by one or two long thin stainless steel wire nails placed obliquely. These may be left in place or project from the wound to be removed later. When a satisfactory joint surface is obtained, the wound is sprinkled with sulfonamide powder and closed. The cast is still in position and so protects the limb that there is little tendency to displacement. The after-treatment is similar to that described above.

Treatment of Fractures of Both Condyles of the Tibia.—These fractures are best treated by traction which may or may not be combined with compression. One of us (H. E. C.) uses a Thomas splint and the other (J. A. K.) passes a traction wire through the lower fourth of the tibia and then attempts to reduce the fracture by traction and lateral compression with a clamp or vice and applies a cast from the midthigh to the toes with the knee straight. The traction (ten to fifteen pounds) is applied to the wire and the foot of the bed is elevated.

This is continued for four weeks. Then a snug nonweight-bearing cast is applied for from four to eight weeks longer, and the patient may be on crutches. The aftertreatment is similar to that used for a fracture of a single condyle.

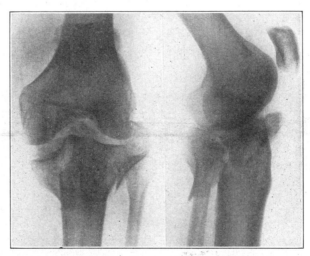

Fig. 1102.—Very severe compression fracture of the upper end of the tibia. Treated by open operation. Fair result. Flexion to 90 degrees.

Fusion of the Knee.—In severe fractures through the upper end of the tibia or through the condyles of the femur in which efforts to obtain anatomic reposition of the fragments have failed and in which the mechanics of the joint are disorganized the operation of fusion of the knee should be seriously considered. This operation, if successful, and it is almost always successful in traumatic cases which have not yet been infected, will give the patient a leg which is painless and useful, and will enable him to walk with a relatively slight limp. The knee should be ankylosed in about ten or fifteen degrees of flexion.

SEPARATION OF THE UPPER EPIPHYSIS OF THE TIBIA

Separation of the upper epiphysis of the tibia is one of the rarest of the epiphyseal separations because the epiphysis is so narrow and broad. Most of the recorded cases have occurred between the ages of three and ten years, and the usual displacement of the epiphysis is forward and lateral.

Diagnosis of Separation of the Upper Epiphysis of the Tibia.—With complete displacement there is obvious deformity, with disability and marked swelling at the knee joint, and there may be injury to the popliteal vessels and nerves. With incomplete displacement, the deformity of the bone may be obscured by the swelling and an x-ray may be necessary for the diagnosis.

Treatment of Separation of the Upper Epiphysis of the Tibia

Treatment is immediate reduction and immobilization in a plaster-of-Paris cast. In a recent case reduction should be possible by manipulation. This can usually be accomplished under general anesthesia by strong traction in the line of the shaft of the femur with the knee and hip flexed about 45 degrees to relax the muscles. As the shaft is pulled down beyond the epiphysis by an assistant, the surgeon, by lateral pressure with the heels of his hands, attempts to restore the normal contour of the bone. After satisfactory reduction has been accomplished, the limb should be immobilized in a position of moderate flexion in a plaster cast over a period of three weeks. Weight-bearing may be resumed in from six to eight weeks. In cases in which there is a splitting apart of the epiphysis with separation of the condyles it is advisable after reduction to treat the case in a Thomas splint in traction in a manner similar to that described above in the treatment of fractures of the upper end of the tibia.

AVULSION OF THE TIBIAL TUBERCLE

Avulsion of the tibial tubercle is a rare injury and is often confused with Osgood-Schlatter's disease, which is a much more common condition. In an avulsion of the tibial tubercle the signs, symptoms, and disability are those

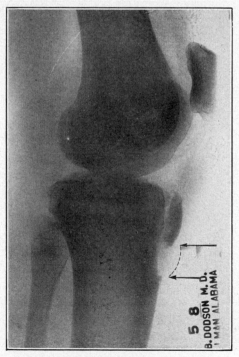

Fig. 1103.—Traumatic fracture and displacement of the tibial tubercle. Treated by open operation and fixation with good result. (Courtesy of Dr. John D. Sherrill.)

of a rupture of the patellar ligament, the only difference being that instead of the ligament being ruptured, its osseous attachment is pulled off and the tenderness and swelling are localized over the tibial tubercle. With the detachment of a large piece of bone it is possible by palpation to identify the avulsed fragment which tends to be displaced upward, especially if the knee is flexed.

Treatment of Avulsion of the Tibial Tubercle

With definite avulsion the treatment is replacement and suture of the displaced fragment by means of an open operation. This should be done after

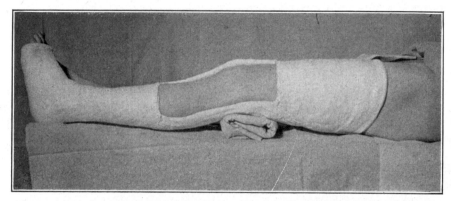

Fig. 1104.—Fracture of the lateral condyle of the tibia in plaster cast with window cut for operation. (Courtesy of Dr. J. A. Dickson.)

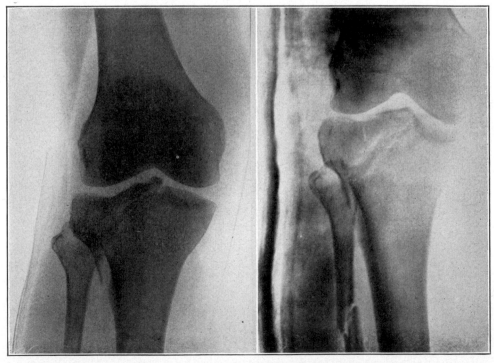

Fig. 1105.—Depressed fracture of the lateral condyle of the tibia before and after treatment by Dr. Dickson's method.

a forty-eight-hour preparation of the skin and can be done through a rather short anterior longitudinal incision. The separated fragment of bone is exposed and with the knee straight, it is pulled down into its normal position and sutured with chromic catgut. Under ordinary circumstances it will not be necessary to use any rigid material to hold the epiphyses in place, and it may not be necessary even to drill holes through the bone as there is enough fibrous tissue around the tubercle to permit firm suturing with chromic cat-gut. After the operation, the knee is immobilized for eight weeks in a plaster cast.

OSGOOD-SCHLATTER'S DISEASE

Osgood-Schlatter's disease is a condition of unknown etiology which occurs in adolescents, usually in boys of about the age of from twelve to fifteen years, and in which x-ray examination shows what appears to be a partial avulsion of the tibial tubercle (Fig. 1106). Whether or not the disease is traumatic in origin is doubtful as many of the cases are bilateral and there is evidently some factor other than trauma involved. There is a possibility

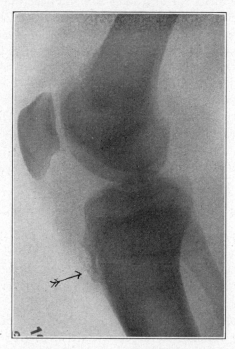

Fig. 1106.—Osgood-Schlatter's disease of the tibial tubercle.

that it is due to a low grade infection and one of us (J. A. K.) has succeeded in growing diphtheroid bacilli from an operated case, but these may have been contaminations. At any rate, the condition is one which in spite of conservative treatment may persist over a period of from a few months to two or three years.

Diagnosis of Osgood-Schlatter's Disease.—The patient complains of swelling and tenderness of the tibial tubercle and the pain at this point after strenuous exercises or after kneeling or bumping the tubercle. On physical examination motion at the knee is free, the tubercle is moderately swollen and tender. The roentgenogram shows irregularity and hypertrophy of the tubercle and there may be islets of bone in the cartilage which resemble an incomplete separation.

Treatment

Conservative Treatment of Osgood-Schlatter's Disease.—If the condition is acutely painful, the surgeon is justified in putting the patient to bed and immobilizing the knee in a plaster cast or with adhesive strapping until the pain has disappeared. The average patient will be able to get along with relatively little pain, and is quite comfortable with an elastic bandage around the knee. This is worn only when the knee is especially tender or for sports. The condition tends to last for from six months to three years and then the tenderness disappears, but the tubercle may remain larger than normal.

Operative Treatment.—Operative treatment usually affords prompt relief of symptoms as soon as the operative wound is healed (about three weeks). An incision about an inch long is made over the tubercle and carried down to the bone and a series of holes is drilled through the tubercle and into the underlying bone; three vertical rows of three holes each with a one-eighth inch drill is a good plan. Sulfonamide powder is sprinkled into the wound, and it is closed and a firm bandage is applied. The patient may begin walking in about two weeks and relief may be expected as soon as the tenderness has disappeared. The operation is reserved for the more severe cases which do not yield to conservative treatment and for those patients who wish to engage in athletics. We prefer the drilling to the prolonged fixation in a plaster cast.

One of us (J. A. K.) has seen four adult patients with loose pieces of bone beneath the patellar ligament. It is believed that these were old Osgood-Schlatter's disease that healed without complete fusion.

Isolated Fractures of the Upper End of the Fibula

The majority of the fractures of the upper end of the fibula occur with fractures of the tibia either at the upper end or in the shaft of the bone, but occasionally as a result of direct violence the head or neck of the fibula may be broken. The fracture line may be oblique or transverse and there is relatively little tendency to displacement of the fragments.

Diagnosis of Isolated Fractures of the Upper End of the Fibula.—There is a history of direct violence to the outer side of the leg just below the knee followed by pain, swelling, and tenderness in this area and more or less pain upon weight-bearing, although as a rule the patient is able to walk without support. The tenderness may be the result of contusion of the tissues or of a fracture, but if pain can be produced in the traumatized area by squeezing the tibia and fibula together in the middle of the leg or rotating the foot while the knee is fixed by flexion, there is probably a fracture of the fibula. Further confirmation of the diagnosis may be gained by having the patient flex the leg against resistance. If the fibula is broken in its upper portion, this causes pain because the biceps femoris is attached to the upper end of the fibula. The diagnosis should be confirmed by x-ray examination.

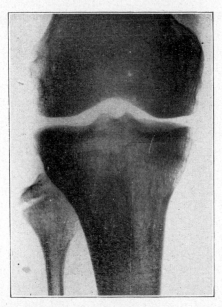

Fig. 1107.—Isolated fracture of upper end of fibula. Circular cast for four weeks. Gradual weight-bearing thereafter with Ace bandage and felt pad. Good result in eight weeks.

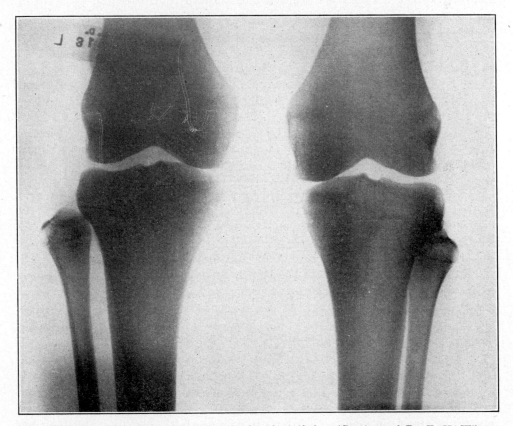

Fig. 1108.—Traumatic dislocation of proximal end of fibula. (Courtesy of Dr. E. H. Wilson, Columbus, Ohio.)

Treatment of Isolated Fractures of the Upper End of the Fibula

Since there is little tendency to displacement, no reduction is necessary and many cases get along comfortably and without pain with no treatment whatever except freedom from weight-bearing. This can be accomplished by giving the patient crutches. If the patient has considerable pain, this can be relieved by the application of a plaster cast which immobilizes the leg in a position of slight flexion. The plaster should extend from the midthigh to the base of the toes and should fit snugly around the knee joint. This should be continued over a period of four weeks. At the end of this time the plaster may be removed, and the patient may begin to walk on the leg at the end of six weeks, when there will probably be no further trouble.

In fractures of the upper end of the fibula, the surgeon should always be careful to notice whether or not there is an injury to the peroneal nerve. In some instances this nerve is injured by being contused or crushed as it curves around the neck of the bone, and in others it is injured by being caught in the callus. In the latter type the paralysis comes on gradually some weeks after the accident. With peroneal nerve injuries the foot should be supported in a position of dorsiflexion in order to put the peroneal, anterior tibial, and extensor muscles at rest. If improvement is not evident within two months, the nerve should be exposed and sutured or freed from pressure of the surrounding structures if necessary.

Very rarely in a fracture through the head of the fibula the proximal fragment to which the biceps femoris muscle is attached is displaced upward and backward. These cases should be treated with the knee in a position of moderately acute flexion in an attempt to immobilize the loose fragment close to its normal position. If, after immobilization in flexion has been done, the x-ray shows the loose fragment still drawn upward and backward, an open operation should be performed and it should be sutured back into its normal position. After the operation, the extremity should be immobilized in a plaster cast with the knee flexed to a right angle.

DISLOCATION OF THE UPPER END OF THE FIBULA

These are rare injuries which may result from direct violence on the bone or as a result of leverage in connection with a fracture lower down in the tibia. The dislocation may be backward, forward, outward, or upward.

Diagnosis of Dislocation of the Upper End of the Fibula.—The diagnosis is not difficult as the bone is subcutaneous, and if the surgeon's attention is drawn to the region, the diagnosis is obvious from inspection and palpation.

Treatment of Dislocation of the Upper End of the Fibula

The treatment is reduction and in most cases this can be accomplished by direct manual pressure on the displaced bone combined with strong inversion of the foot. In the case illustrated Wilson strapped the foot in eversion and the head of the fibula stayed in place. If this fails attempt should be made to reduce the dislocation, strap it in place with adhesive, and then immobilize the leg in a plaster-of-Paris cast (midthigh to base of toes) with the knee in a position of flexion in order to relax the biceps tendon. In applying the adhesive under a cast, care must be taken that the peroneal nerve is not compressed; otherwise paralysis may result. If, after the immobilization, the x-ray picture shows that the upper end of the fibula is in its normal position, the cast should be worn for a period of from four to six weeks. At the end of this time it may be removed, the fibula strapped with adhesive and the patient may begin to use the leg.

If, after the cast has been applied, the roentgenogram shows that displacement persists, it is necessary to perform an open operation and suture the fibula back into its normal position. This can be done by means of chromic catgut. Some surgeons arthrodese the superior tibiofibular joint, but we do not believe that this is necessary.

CHAPTER XXV

FRACTURES OF THE SHAFTS OF THE TIBIA AND FIBULA

SURGICAL ANATOMY

The Shaft of the Tibia.—The shaft of the tibia is a long tube of heavy bone which is abruptly broadened at its upper end to support the condyles and is moderately expanded at its lower end to rest on the astragalus (Fig. 1109). The extremities are cancellous in structure and here the cortex is thin, but the main portion of the shaft is composed of thick compact bone. In its upper portion the shaft is triangular on cross section and in its lower third it becomes more rounded or roughly quadrilateral on cross section and is considerably narrowed. Consequently the lower third is the weakest point in the shaft and it is here that the majority of the fractures occur.

The shaft of the tibia is usually described as presenting three borders and three surfaces. The anterior border or crest is sharp in its upper two-thirds and is subcutaneous throughout its length. It begins above lateral to the tubercle and extends downward to the front of the internal malleolus. The internal border is more rounded and can be palpated throughout its length. The external border is sharp for the attachment of the interosseous membrane. It is covered by muscles and cannot be palpated. The mesial surface is subcutaneous throughout its extent. The posterior and lateral surfaces are covered by muscle. The high percentage of compound injuries among fractures of the tibia is largely due to the fact that the anterior and mesial borders and mesial surface are subcutaneous. (Fig. 1109.)

The Shaft of the Fibula.—The shaft of the fibula is a slender column of dense cortical bone which contains a narrow medullary cavity. It terminates above in an expanded head which presents a rounded articular facet for the external tuberosity of the tibia and a short styloid process which is palpable. Below the shaft is expanded and terminates in the external malleolus. The inner border of the shaft gives attachment to the interosseus membrane and its outer borders to the external intermuscular septa.

The Interosseous Membrane.—This is a strong sheet of fibrous tissue which closes the space between the tibia and fibula except at its upper end where there is a small opening for the passage of the anterior tibial vessels. In fractures it prevents a separation of the bones unless it is extensively torn. As the majority of its fibers run downward and outward the interosseous membrane serves to distribute indirect violence acting on the tibia to the fibula.

Function of the Tibia and Fibula.—The tibia transmits practically all of the body weight from the femur to the astragalus and is the weight-bearing

1128

bone of the leg. The main functions of the fibula are to serve as an attachment for muscles and to preserve the integrity of the ankle joint. In an adult its upper half may be excised without disturbing the function of the leg. The fibula also tends to support the tibia, and if the tibia alone is fractured, it splints the broken bone and prevents marked displacement.

Muscles of the Leg.—The muscles of the leg are divided into four groups, each of which is contained in a separate fascial compartment. The extensor group consisting of the tibialis anticus, extensor longus digitorum, and extensor longus hallucis, lies on the front of the leg, and the abductor group, consisting of the peroneus longus and brevis, is lateral to the extensor group, but lies anterior to the external intermuscular septum. The calf or triceps surae group consisting of the soleus, gastrocnemius and plantaris occupies the posterior compartment and beneath this group and separated from it by an intermuscular septum is the deep flexor group which consists of the tibialis posticus, flexor longus digitorum and flexor longus hallucis.

None of these muscles exert cross strains on the tibia and fibula and when these bones are broken none of them tend to cause serious displacement, other than to draw the lower fragments upward.

Blood Vessels and Nerves.—The anterior and posterior tibial and peroneal arteries are the main blood vessels of the leg. The anterior tibial is one of the terminal branches of the popliteal artery and passes forward through the opening in the interosseous membrane to reach the anterior compartment where it passes downward on the interosseous membrane to terminate in the dorsalis pedis artery. The posterior tibial is the direct continuation of the popliteal artery. It passes downward in the space between the deep flexor muscles and the calf muscles to terminate in the plantar arteries. The peroneal arises from the proximal portion of the posterior tibial and passes downward in close relation to the posterior surface of the fibula.

The extensor and abductor muscles are supplied by the anterior tibial and peroneal nerves which are the terminal branches of the external popliteal. This nerve winds around the upper portion of the shaft of the fibula to reach the anterior compartment of the leg, and where it passes over the bone, the nerve is subcutaneous and is exposed to injury by direct trauma or by pressure from casts or splints or slings.

The calf and flexor muscles are supplied by branches of the internal popliteal and its terminal branch, the posterior tibial nerve. The posterior tibial nerve follows the course of the posterior tibial artery to terminate in the plantar nerves. It is well covered by muscles and is rarely injured.

ISOLATED FRACTURES OF THE SHAFT OF THE TIBIA

Isolated fractures of the shaft of the tibia are not particularly rare, especially in children where, due to the elasticity of the fibula, the tibia is frequently broken while the fibula remains intact. They may occur as a result either of direct or indirect violence, and the fracture line may be roughly

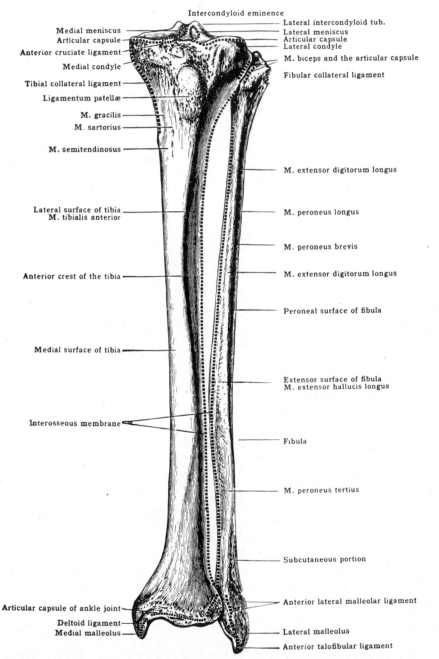

Fig. 1109.—The left tibia and fibula, anterior view. (Morris: *Human Anatomy*, P. Blakiston's Son & Co., Inc., Publisher.)

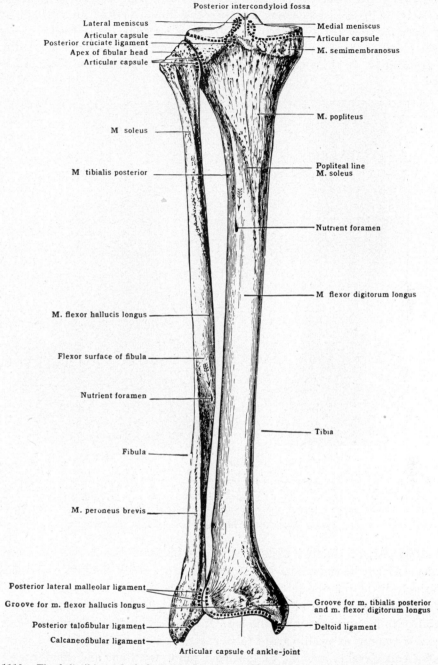

Fig. 1110.—The left tibia and fibula, posterior view. (Morris: *Human Anatomy*, P. Blakiston's Son & Co., Inc., Publisher.)

transverse (Fig. 1111), oblique (Fig. 1112) or spiral. In cases due to direct violence, the fracture may be comminuted (Fig. 1113) or even compound. There is relatively little displacement because the fibula acts as an efficient splint and permits very little shortening. In rare instances as a result of severe direct violence there may be complete displacement with slight overriding of the fragments. In these cases the distal fragment tends to be displaced backward.

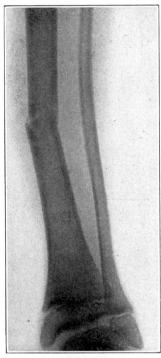

Fig. 1111.

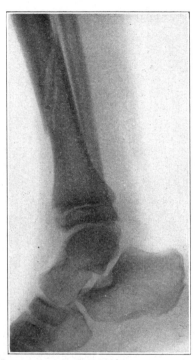
Fig. 1112.

Fig. 1111.—Fracture of the tibia alone in a child. There is some deformity due to bending of the fibula. Treated by correction of the lateral deformity and immobilization in a plaster-of-Paris cast extending from the toes to the upper one-third of the thigh. Good results. Seldom does much displacement take place when tibia or fibula alone is fractured.

Fig. 1112.—Oblique fracture of the tibia alone with practically no displacement in a child. This fracture did not show in the anteroposterior view. Treated by immobilization in a plaster-of-Paris cast, for four weeks. Weight-bearing eight weeks with good result.

Diagnosis of Isolated Fractures of the Shaft of the Tibia.—In fractures of the shaft of the tibia alone the leg is not appreciably shortened and there is relatively little definite deformity. There is a history of an injury either of a fall upon the feet or of a direct blow upon the leg followed by pain and inability to bear weight upon the leg. In the region of the fracture there is a variable amount of swelling and tenderness. It is to be remembered, however, that a considerable amount of localized pain, swelling, and tenderness may follow a contusion on the leg in which the bone is not broken. On palpation the tenderness can be quite definitely localized over the line of fracture because the bone is subcutaneous. Further evidence of fracture is the production of pain at the site of the fracture by squeezing the leg bones together or by rotating the foot while the knee is immobilized, or by pushing upward on the foot. In the presence of a fracture of one bone in the leg each of these maneuvers tends to produce pain at the site of the fracture. In severe injuries there may be a variable amount of anteroposterior displacement of the fragments and in such cases the irregularity in the contour of the bone can be palpated. In unusual cases where the fracture is relatively transverse or subperiosteal, it may be possible for the patient to walk upon the leg without support or with a cane, but weight-bearing causes pain at the site of the fracture.

The diagnosis of incomplete fractures and fractures without displacement should be confirmed by the x-ray.

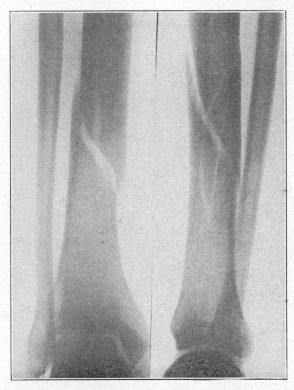

Fig. 1113.—Comminuted fracture of the tibia alone in an adult. No reduction necessary. Treated by immobilization in a plaster-of-Paris cast five weeks, weight-bearing eight weeks with good result in eleven weeks. Displacement seldom takes place when an individual bone of the leg is fractured.

Treatment of Isolated Fractures of the Shaft of the Tibia.—The treatment depends upon whether or not displacement has occurred. In the great majority of these fractures practically no displacement occurs. There is consequently no indication for reduction of the fracture, and all that is necessary is to immobilize the leg for comfort and prevent weight-bearing. Immobilization is most satisfactorily obtained by the application of a light plaster-of-Paris cast which extends from the midthigh to the toes. The cast should be applied with about 10-15° flexion at the knee. As soon as the plaster is dry, the patient is allowed crutches. At the end of from four to six weeks the plaster may be removed, x-ray pictures taken, and if sufficient callus is present weight-bearing may be gradually commenced. If the surgeon is skillful in the use of plaster, the skin tight plaster of Boehler with the walking iron may be applied and the patient may begin to bear weight upon the leg as soon as the plaster is dry.

In cases with definite displacement, the fracture should be reduced and for this an anesthetic, either local or general, is necessary. Reduction is accomplished by having an assistant make traction and abduction on the foot, while the surgeon by manual pressure molds the ends of the bones back into good functional position as described in fractures of both bones of the leg.

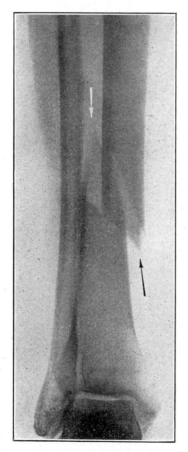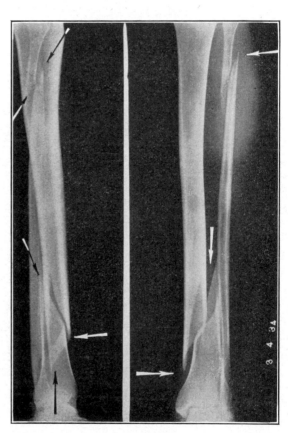

Fig. 1114.—Spiral fracture of the tibia. Note overlapping of tibia. First x-ray showed no fracture of the fibula, but complete x-ray of leg at right showed fracture in the upper third of the fibula.

If this fails, Thompson's subcutaneous lever or pin may be used to lever the fragments into position.

In the rare cases with complete displacement it is usually possible to reduce the displacement by pressing the proximal end of the lower fragment forward and inward. If this is not successful an open reduction is indicated. With the fracture exposed the fragments can be pried into place and frequently no internal fixation is necessary. The after-treatment is the same as for simple fractures of the tibia alone.

FRACTURES OF THE SHAFT OF THE FIBULA UNASSOCIATED WITH INJURY OF THE ANKLE JOINT

Incidence.—Most of the isolated fractures of the shaft of the fibula occur as a result of leverage action in injuries of the ankle joint, and these will be considered in the section on injuries of the ankle. Occasionally, however, the shaft of the fibula is broken by direct violence acting on the lateral side of the leg. The fracture tends to be roughly transverse at the level where the violence acts, and there is relatively little tendency to displacement. Shortening does not occur because the bone is splinted by the tibia. These injuries do not tend to be compound.

Diagnosis.—There is a history of direct injury to the leg followed by pain on weight-bearing, but not by inability to bear weight on the leg. On physical examination local tenderness is present over the site of the fracture and pain may be elicited here by pressing the tibia and fibula together or by rotating the ankle while the knee is flexed. False motion and crepitus cannot as a rule be demonstrated.

Treatment

As the displacement is slight, reduction is rarely necessary and treatment consists of immobilizing the leg in a light plaster-of-Paris cast which extends from the midthigh to the toes. The cast is applied with from ten to fifteen degrees of flexion at the knee. This plaster should be worn for about three weeks when it may be removed and replaced by a plaster legging which extends from the malleoli to the tuberosities of the tibia. This splints the leg, tends to limit lateral motion at the ankle, permits weight-bearing, and enables the patient to walk with a crutch or cane. This is worn for from two to four weeks and at the end of this time it may be discarded and the patient may begin to walk without support.

In certain cases where the patient is able to bear weight with little pain, all that is necessary is a cross strapping of adhesive over the area of the fracture in order to produce a certain amount of immobilization, and the patient may be permitted to walk with a cane. In cases where there is displacement of one or more fragments inward, reduction can usually be accomplished by traction on and inversion of the foot while the knee is flexed. The reduction may be assisted by manual pressure on the fragment which is displaced outward. The after-treatment is similar to that described above. The prognosis is good even without reduction.

When there is marked displacement or a tendency to cross union, and when closed reduction is impossible, open reduction should be done.

FRACTURES OF BOTH BONES OF THE LEG

Incidence and Etiology.—Fractures of both bones of the leg are among the most frequent of the serious traumatic injuries and for this reason the subject is of considerable importance. The injury may occur at any period of life, but the cases are most frequent in young adult males who lead an active outdoor life or are engaged in hazardous occupations. The fracture may be due to either direct or indirect violence. The cases from indirect violence may be due to falls from a height, the patient landing on the feet, or to torsion injuries in which either the foot or the thigh is fixed while the other end of the bone is twisted.

Types of Fracture.—Fractures of both bones of the leg differ from other fractures of long bones in that a large percentage of the cases are compound. The tendency of these fractures to be compound is due to the subcutaneous position of the tibia. In fractures from direct violence the laceration of the soft parts is due to the direct trauma, and there is a variable amount of destruction of the tissues. In fractures from indirect violence the sharp end of the upper fragment tends to be thrust through the skin by the body weight or by a continuation of the fracturing force.

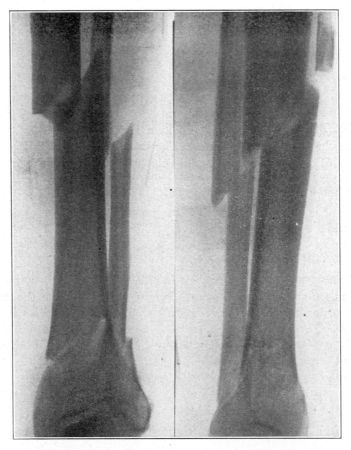

Fig. 1115.—Double fracture of both bones of the leg with a small puncture wound on the lower third of the leg with very little displacement. Puncture wound painted with iodine, displacement reduced by manipulation under an anesthetic, and a plaster-of-Paris cast applied for seven weeks. Weight-bearing twelve weeks. Good results in fifteen weeks.

In fractures due to direct violence both bones tend to be broken at approximately the same level and the fracture in the tibia is frequently comminuted, or double (Fig. 1115), the most common type of fracture being one in which a rather large triangular fragment is broken out of the bone on the side on which the violence was received; that is, toward the side away from which the bone is bowed. In fractures caused by indirect violence the tibia tends to be broken in its weakest portion; that is, at about the junction of the middle and lower thirds, while the fibula is broken at a higher level, usually the junction of the middle and upper thirds (Fig. 1114). In these fractures due to indirect violence the fracture line tends to be oblique or spiral, but may be transverse or comminuted, especially in severe injuries.

Displacement.—Due to the fact that the muscles of the leg and thigh exert no particular cross strain on the fragments, there is no constant type of displacement in these fractures other than the tendency of the lower fragment to be drawn upward whenever the ends of the fragments are not engaged. This overriding of the fragments with shortening of the leg varies from one-half to two or more inches and is present in practically all of the spiral, long oblique, and comminuted fractures, and in the short oblique or roughly transverse fractures in which the ends of the bones have slipped by one another. As a rule the amount of upward displacement is relatively slight immediately after the injury, but in the course of a few hours it tends to increase as a result of swelling and muscle spasm.

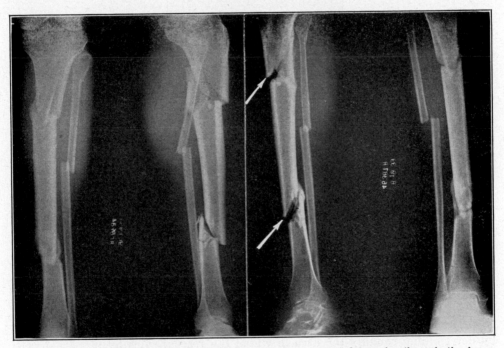

Fig. 1116.—Double fracture of the tibia and fibula. Treated by wire through the lower one-fourth of the tibia and upper one-fourth of the tibia, and circular cast from the midthigh to the toes with good result in eight months.

Displacements in the lateral or anteroposterior plane are largely the result of the fracturing force, of gravity, or of manipulation. The distal end of the proximal fragment, however, tends to occupy a position anterior and lateral to the proximal end of the distal fragment. This is due to the insertion of the quadriceps muscle into the tibial tubercle, and this muscle tends to pull the proximal fragment forward into a position of extension while gravity causes the distal fragment to drop backward. In addition to the above the distal fragment tends to be rotated outward by gravity because the foot tends to roll outward. Unless the interosseous membrane is widely torn, there is no tendency for the bones to be abnormally separated, but with extensive tearing of the interosseous membrane the tibia and fibula may be widely separated (Fig. 1117). Occasionally the ends of the fragments of the tibia and fibula lie close to one another and synostosis may occur in healing.

Diagnosis.—As these fractures are nearly always complete, the diagnosis rarely presents any difficulty. In the average case there is obvious shortening and angulation of the leg or rotation of the foot is present and the deformity alone is sufficient for the diagnosis. If there is no demonstrable deformity, the diagnosis can usually be made by eliciting abnormal mobility.

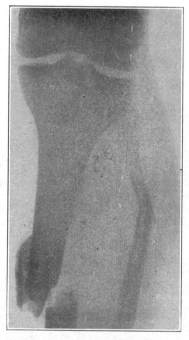

Fig. 1117.—Compound comminuted fracture with extensive tearing of the interosseous membrane. Note the wide separation of the tibia and fibula. Treated by traction with a Kirschner wire through the lower fourth of the tibia and fibula, after débridement and later immobilization in a plaster-of-Paris cast. Good result. Eight months' disability.

The demonstration of abnormal mobility can be carried out with relatively little pain or danger of further injury to the soft parts. It is best done by determining roughly the area in which the fracture lies by palpation and then while the upper portion of the leg is steadied with one hand the surgeon gently lifts the foot from the table or moves it from side to side (Fig. 1118). If there is a fracture with displacement the leg will bend at the site of the fracture. In fractures of both bones in which the periosteum is intact as sometimes occurs in children, the leg does not bend, and here the diagnosis rests upon the demonstration of point tenderness over both the tibia and fibula and should be confirmed by x-ray examination.

In addition to the diagnosis of a fracture, the surgeon should attempt to determine the character of the displacement; this can be done roughly by physical examination. The amount of shortening is determined by measuring the distance from the inner or outer condyle of the tibia to the tip of the internal or external malleolus and comparing it with that of the opposite leg. The rotation is determined by aligning the foot with the knee. Lateral and anteroposterior displacement of the fragments can be determined roughly by palpating the crest and inner border of the tibia. In spite of the fact that swelling occurs with unusual rapidity after these fractures and tends to be excessive it is usually possible by careful palpation to make out the subcutaneous position of the tibia and arrive at the relative positions of the fragments.

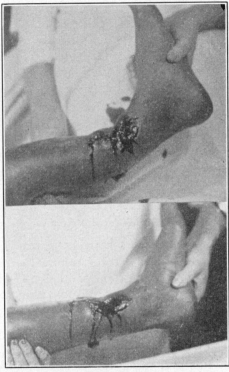
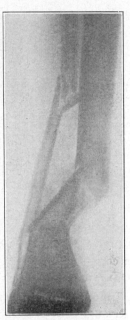

Fig. 1118.   Fig. 1119.

Fig. 1118.—Compound fracture of both bones of the leg with severe soft tissue damage. Treated by débridement, Dakin's solution, and drainage with Dakin's tube, and traction with Steinman pin through the heel. Good result. Note the ease with which the deformity can be corrected.

Fig. 1119.—Roentgenogram of preceding case.

In cases with severe compound injuries it is important to determine the state of the circulation and nerve supply in the foot.

Complications.—The most frequent and serious complication of these fractures is that they tend to be compound and there may be extensive destruction of the soft parts and foreign material may be driven into the leg by the fracturing force or the end of the upper fragment may be thrust out through the skin and grossly contaminated with dirt (Fig. 1120). Occasionally the anterior and posterior tibial arteries are compressed or torn, and the circulation of the foot may be impaired. This is especially true when the posterior tibial is involved and gangrene may result. The nerves are not often injured in these fractures but with severe compound wounds any of the soft tissues may be damaged.

Prognosis.—In uncomplicated cases in which no displacement has occurred or in which approximately anatomic reduction has been accomplished, union may be expected in from six to eight weeks and full weight-bearing in from twelve to sixteen weeks. In cases with extensive comminution or gross displacement which has been imperfectly reduced, union may be delayed and it is to be remembered that one of the most frequent sites of nonunion is at the junction of the middle and lower thirds of the tibia.

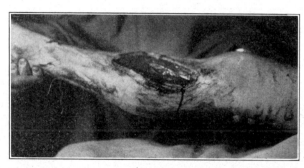

Fig. 1120.—Compound comminuted fracture of the upper third of the leg with severe damage to the soft parts. Treated by débridement and traction with a Kirschner wire through the lower fourth of the tibia for three weeks, followed by immobilization in a plaster-of-Paris cast. Good result. Six and one-half months' disability.

Treatment of Fractures of Both Bones of the Leg

In the order of their importance the objects of treatment in fractures of both bones of the leg are: (1) to secure union; (2) to restore the normal alignment of the leg; (3) to restore the normal length of the leg; (4) to prevent equinus; and (5) to secure anatomic reposition of the fragments.

In compound fractures we are also concerned with saving the life of the patient, saving the leg, and preventing infection.

1. Union.—Since delayed union and nonunion are very common in fractures through the junction of the middle and lower thirds of the tibia, the treatment of these fractures should be so directed that the bones are given every possible chance to unite. In a fresh fracture we believe that the most important single factor in securing union is absolute immobilization, and we believe that one of the most frequent causes of nonunion in these fractures is incomplete immobilization or repeated change in the position of the fragments while union is in progress. For this reason we make it a practice whenever possible to immobilize these fractures in a plaster-of-Paris cast which extends from the upper thigh to the toes. When this is not practicable from the beginning we treat the fracture by traction in a Thomas splint and then apply the cast treatment as soon as traction is no longer necessary.

2. Restoration of Normal Alignment of the Leg.—In order that the knee and ankle may continue to function normally, it is important that the normal alignment of the leg be restored. If there is a lateral bowing either inward or outward, the foot is thrown into the varus or valgus position and both the lateral ligaments of the knee and the ligaments of the foot and ankle are strained with weight-bearing (Fig. 1121). Consequently, in addition to the unsightliness of malunited fracture, if the normal alignment is not restored, we may expect later pain and disability with strain of the knee and ankle with eventual development of traumatic arthritis in one or both of these joints.

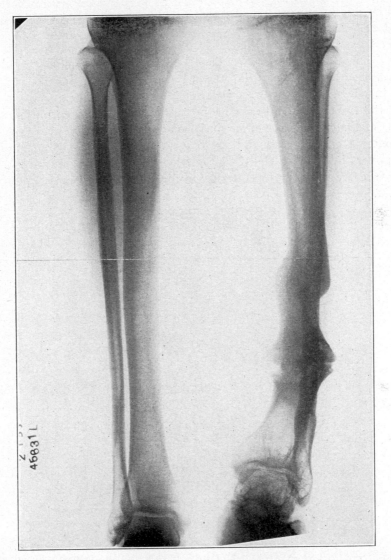

Fig. 1121.—Old fracture of the tibia and fibula of right leg united with outward bowing.

Likewise, if the normal alignment in the anteroposterior plane is not restored we may expect strain on the ankle and knee in addition to the unsightliness of the leg. The most common deformity is a posterior bowing or sagging of the tibia and with this deformity the knee must be in a position of slight flexion when the patient stands upright; otherwise the foot is thrust forward.

Likewise, if the bones are permitted to unite with the foot in a position of outward rotation, the patient walks with the foot in the flat foot position, and in addition to the abnormal strain which this produces on the foot, there is also chronic strain on the internal lateral ligament of the knee.

In immobilizing these fractures it is important first to correct the rotation (usually external), then correct the lateral deviation, and finally to prevent posterior bowing at the site of the fracture. In order to do this, the foot should be rotated inward or outward, depending upon the rotation deformity present and traction is made upon the foot so that a line drawn from the hip joint and passing downward through the middle of the patella will pass between the first and second toes (Fig. 1122). If the tibia is straight and the foot is so rotated that this line passes between the first and second toes, the leg is in correct alignment as regards lateral deviation and rotation. The site of the fracture should now be supported by pressure from beneath until the line of the crest of the tibia conforms with that of the other leg. This is practically a straight line, but in cases with considerable swelling of the tissues over the crest of the tibia the leg must be bowed upward at the site of the fracture in order to compensate for the swelling and thus straighten the tibia.

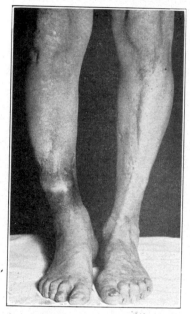

Fig. 1122.—Clinical case showing the malalignment of the right leg. Same case as shown in the preceding figure.

3. **Restoration of Normal Length.**—In the oblique, spiral, or comminuted fracture this is not so important as is ordinarily supposed and is rarely the cause of disability in fractures of the leg. We believe that if the position is good as regards rotation and alignment, a shortening of one-half an inch or less may be ignored. Of course if this can be corrected without endangering the position, it should be done, but rather than lose the alignment and run the risk of nonunion by frequent changes of position we are content to obtain union in

these fractures with not more than one-half an inch of shortening. If the shortening is more than one-half an inch, an attempt should be made to correct it regardless of the other factors mentioned above.

4. **Prevention of Equinus.**—A very frequent cause of prolongation of disability after fracture of the leg is equinus deformity of the foot. This is because the normal tendency, when traction is made upon the foot, is to pull the forefoot downward, relax the tendo achillis and immobilize it in this position. Whenever it can be done without throwing the fragments out of position, we believe the foot should be immobilized in a position of slight dorsiflexion; that is, dorsiflexed slightly more than a right angle. Occasionally, however, we find that whenever the foot is dorsiflexed a posterior bowing at the site of the fracture is produced and in these instances the correct position of the foot must be sacrificed temporarily, and it is advisable to immobilize the foot in the equinus position until union has been obtained and then gradually to stretch it up into dorsiflexion.

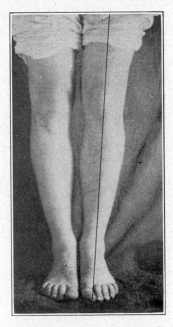

Fig. 1123.—Normal alignment of the leg. Vertical line through the middle of the patella passes over middle of the ankle and between the first and second toes.

Anatomical Reduction is the least important of the considerations mentioned, and in reducing a fracture of both bones of the leg if the alignment and length are satisfactory and if one-third of the cross-section of the ends of the tibial fragments are in apposition, we consider the reduction satisfactory. For cosmetic reasons (in order to give the patient a smooth contour) we endeavor to get the tibial fragments as nearly "end on" as possible, but we do not resort to frequent manipulations and jeopardize union in order to do this. We ignore the fibula almost entirely.

Compound Fractures.—Many of these compound fractures of the leg are severe injuries and the patient is in shock and there is danger either of death or of losing the limb. Consequently our first concern is to save the life of the patient. Alarming hemorrhage should be controlled by a tourniquet applied immediately. It should be remembered that the tourniquet should not be left on more than two hours. Otherwise gangrene of the leg may occur. Shock should be combated by morphine, heat, and transfusion if necessary. It is of great importance to immobilize the leg to prevent further damage to the soft tissues. On account of the danger of infection it is necessary that treatment be instituted as soon as possible after the injury and that every effort be made to save the leg and prevent infection. (Figs. 1118 and 1120.) The method of treating compound fractures is described in Chapter VII.

Emergency Pillow Splint for Fractures of Both Bones of the Leg.—In these fractures it is important to immobilize the fragments as soon as possible after the injury. This should be done during the interim between the injury and the application of specific treatment of the fracture. The tendency of the foot to roll outward and dangle whenever the patient is moved causes increased damage to the soft parts as well as pain and shock to the patient. For this reason the fracture should be splinted as soon as possible after the accident. The most universally obtainable, and at the same time efficient, method of splinting these fractures is by means of the well-known pillow splint. The materials required are an ordinary feather pillow, three board splints the length of the pillow, and straps, strings, or bandages to tie the splints around the leg.

Application of the Pillow Splint.—The leg is placed on the pillow with the heel about six inches from the end of the pillow. While traction is made on the foot with the rotation corrected, the pillow is folded up on either side of the leg and pinned tightly with safety pins. Then with one splint on either side and one behind the leg these are tied tightly around the leg and pillow. Finally the end of the pillow is folded over the foot and pinned as tightly as possible, thus immobilizing the foot in the corrected position.

If a pillow is not available lateral and posterior board splints can be padded and tied around the leg.

Classification of Fractures of Both Bones of the Leg as Regards Treatment

According to the treatment necessary, fractures of both bones of the leg may be divided into the following groups:

1. Simple fractures with practically no displacement.
2. Simple fractures which can be reduced by manipulation.
3. Simple fractures in which reduction cannot be maintained without traction or skeletal fixation.
4. Compound fractures with puncture wounds.
5. Compound fractures with moderate damage to the soft tissues.
6. Compound fractures with extensive damage to the soft tissues.
7. Compound fractures in which there is active infection.

1. **Simple Fractures of Both Bones of the Leg with no Displacement.**— These fractures are more frequent in children than in adults. They may be subperiosteal in character with no displacement or they may be transverse, spiral, oblique, or mild comminuted fractures in children or adults with slight

displacement and slight shortening. If the shortening is not over one-fourth of an inch and if the position of the fragments as regards rotation and alignment is good, an attempt to improve the slight amount of shortening or to secure anatomical reposition of the fragments should not be made, since not infrequently such attempts result in making the position worse rather than better. Furthermore, the position of the fragments of the fibula may be disregarded. All that is necessary is to secure good union, good alignment, and relatively little or no shortening in the tibia. The fibula will take care of itself.

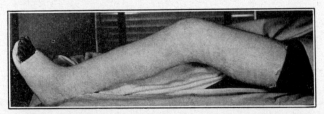

Fig. 1124.—Cylindrical plaster cast from the upper thigh to the toes applied with the knee moderately flexed. Used in treatment of fractures of both bones of the leg. Note the extension of cast to the flexor surface of toes, preventing contracture of toes.

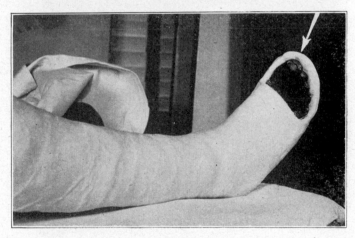

Fig. 1125.—Cylinder plaster cast.

In these fractures no anesthetic is necessary and the surgeon should simply correct any slight rotation deformity which may exist and then support the leg in a position of correct alignment and immobilize it and prevent weight-bearing until union is solid.

Immobilization is most comfortably, conveniently, and efficiently secured by means of a well-fitting plaster-of-Paris cast which extends from the upper thigh to the toes. The cast is applied with 10 to 15 degrees of flexion at the knee (Fig. 1124). If this is applied immediately after the accident and the patient is then put to bed with the leg elevated, extensive swelling will not occur. However, the toes should be watched and if they become cyanotic and cold, or if the patient complains of great pain, the cast should be split down one side or bivalved and strapped on again if necessary. Many surgeons bivalve their plasters immediately and strap them on again, but this reduces

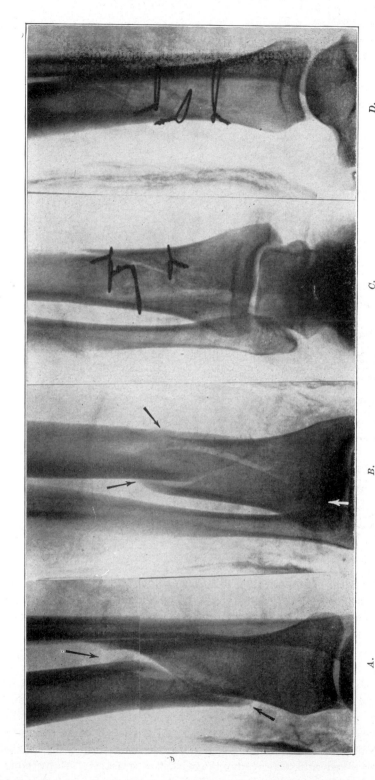

A.   *B.*   *C.*   *D.*

Fig. 1126.—Compound fracture of tibia treated by débridement and primary closure and immobilization in a plaster cast after internal fixation with wire. Sulfanilamide was implanted in the wound and primary healing occurred. One of us (J. A. K.) uses one or two non-corrosive screws for fixation in this type fracture.

the efficiency of the immobilization and we do not cut our leg plasters unless it is necessary, and it rarely is necessary. If there is considerable swelling before its application, the cast may become loose and require replacement in about a week.

The tight cast should be left on for from four to six weeks. As soon as it is hard, the patient may get up on crutches, but should refrain from bearing weight on the leg. At the end of from eight to ten weeks the cast should be removed and the stability of union tested. If union is quite firm by clinical examination and x-ray the patient may begin to exercise the leg, but should not bear weight upon it for two weeks longer. At the end of this time weight-bearing may be gradually commenced and the crutches may be discarded as the strength in the limb returns. If union is not firm when the cast is first removed, it should be reapplied and left on for two or more weeks. Due to the lack of cooperation we leave the cast on in children until we are quite sure that the leg is solid.

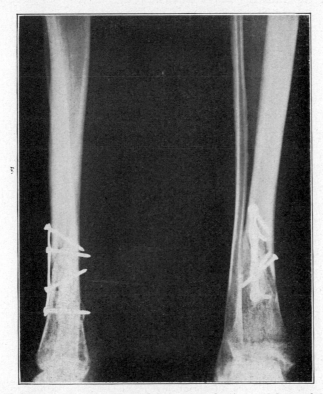

Fig. 1127.—Spiral fracture of tibia. Treated by open reduction and bone plate. (Courtesy of Dr. Joseph Lembeck.) One of us (J. A. K.) uses two screws to fix this type of fracture.

Instead of the above the Boehler skin tight plaster with walking iron may be applied and the patient may begin to bear weight on the leg as soon as the plaster is dry.

2. **Treatment of Simple Fractures of Both Bones of the Leg Which Can Be Reduced by Manipulation.**—These constitute the transverse fractures and short oblique or spiral or mildly comminuted fractures near the ends of the

bones. That is, fractures which not only can be reduced, but those in which the main fragments can be firmly locked and immobilized in a cast. Others require continuous traction or skeletal fixation after reduction.

Method of Reduction.—The patient should be anesthetized, placed on an operating table, and the materials for the application of the plaster should be at hand before the manipulation is attempted. Reduction is accomplished by means of traction with some molding of the fragments in order that the ends may be engaged. The traction is most effective if it is applied with the knee flexed from 30 to 45 degrees or more as this relaxes the tendo achillis. Some surgeons recommend cutting the tendo achillis subcutaneously. We have never found this necessary, as we have usually been able to pull these fractures down to full length if the knee is flexed. The ease of reduction varies inversely with the time that has elapsed since the fracture occurred. In fractures seen and manipulated a few hours after the injury and before shortening of the muscles takes place, reduction can, as a rule, be accomplished with surprising ease.

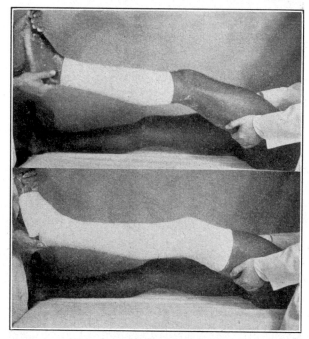

Fig. 1128.—Traction and countertraction supplied by two assistants while the surgeon molds the fragments, corrects the alignment, and applies the plaster first to the leg, then to the knee and thigh, and then to the ankle and foot. Not an efficient method for securing traction.

Traction in the Reduction of Fractures of the Leg.—In order that a fracture of both bones of the leg be reduced by manipulation and immobilized in a plaster cast, it is absolutely necessary that sufficient traction be obtained to pull the fractures down to or beyond their normal positions and that this traction be maintained while the leg is elevated for the application of the plaster-of-Paris cast.

The difficulties which many surgeons experience in the treatment of these fractures are due to the fact that they do not avail themselves of some simple mechanical support for the knee, but depend upon two assistants. The usual method is that one assistant grasps the thigh just above the knee and holds it in a position of about 45 degrees flexion, thus supplying countertraction to the leg and lifting the weight of the thigh and leg while the other assistant grasps the foot and makes manual traction on the lower fragments (Fig. 1128). The difficulty is that the assistant above who holds the thigh is in a strained position, and after a few minutes in this position he gradually gives way, the leg is gradually lowered, the knee is gradually straightened, and the traction becomes less and less efficient.

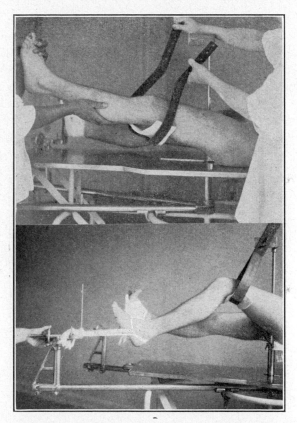

Fig. 1129.—Conwell's countertraction thigh and knee support used in fractures of the leg. This support is a band of iron one-eighth by one and one-half inches bent into a triangle and fixed to the upright attachment on the Hawley table.

All that is needed is some mechanical support under the popliteal space. This can be supplied either by a crossbar which is fixed to uprights on the side of the fracture table, or by a sling which is fixed to the upright projecting from the perineal post (Fig. 1129) or by a special gas pipe apparatus such as that devised by Boehler (Fig. 1133). The point is that the thigh should be supported by a mechanical device which will also provide countertraction. Not only does this do away with one assistant, but it also assures the surgeon that the upper fragment at least will be immobilized and all that is necessary is to have an assistant make sufficient traction on the foot to bring the fragments down into their proper positions. Lacking a mechanical support, the back of a chair may be utilized (Fig. 1135).

If the assistant who holds the foot is not sufficiently strong, a double clove hitch can be placed around the ankle with a muslin bandage and this passed around the assistant's body in order that he may use his body weight for traction. When this method is used, however, great care should be taken not to apply the plaster cast over the hitch around the ankle or extensive pressure sores may result. We have seen cases with large sloughs on the dorsum of the foot as a result of the application of a plaster-of-Paris cast over a traction bandage around the ankle.

A very efficient method is that of Boehler, who, by the use of his simple apparatus, supports the thigh and applies countertraction with a special popliteal crutch and obtains traction on the lower fragment by means of a Steinman pin through the heel and a screw traction apparatus. With Boehler's apparatus great force can be applied very gradually and maintained constantly. As a result any fracture of the leg can be pulled down to or beyond full length. The only objection is that in many instances it is not necessary to apply the Steinman pin through the heel, as quite enough traction and immobilization can be supplied by an assistant.

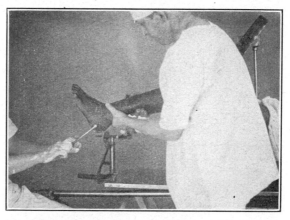

Fig. 1130.—Surgeon manipulating the fragments while an assistant applies traction by means of a pin through the os calcis.

If one of the newer traction apparatuses is available, this may be used to advantage in this type of fracture, and if there is a tendency for the fragments to slip back after the traction is released, the pins or wires may be incorporated in the cast and thus afford skeletal fixation. Where this is done, care must be taken not to pull and hold the fragments too far apart as this may cause delay in union. (Fig. 1136.)

When the traction is made, the surgeon carefully supervises the rotation of the foot until a line drawn directly downward from the patella passes between the first and second toes and corrects the alignment of the leg. He also molds the fragments by lateral pressure until approximately anatomical reduction of the tibia has been obtained and in the case of long oblique or spiral fractures attempts to engage the ends in order that the tendency to shortening be eliminated.

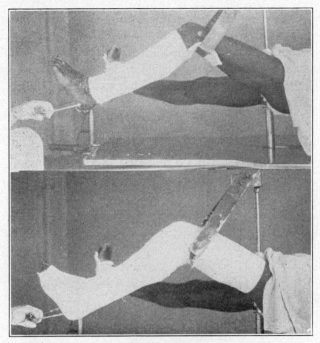

Fig. 1131.—Cast applied first to the leg, then knee, thigh, and ankle and foot.

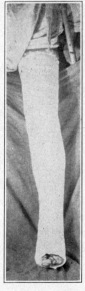

Fig. 1132.—Cast seen from front. Alignment and rotation correct.

When satisfactory reduction has been accomplished, a plaster cast is applied around the leg extending from the ankle to the knee. In beginning this plaster it is advisable to apply a posterior plaster mold to the leg and to correct the tendency of the leg to sag downward at the site of the fracture. The mold is incorporated in a cast which is applied over very little padding and extends from the ankle to the knee. The traction is maintained until this section sets. If the traction is supplied by a pin through the os calcis, the plaster can be continued down over the foot to the toes immediately. Then the cast is continued down over the foot and up over the thigh to its upper third, the assistants maintaining as much traction as possible during the application of the cast and taking especial care not to dislodge the engaged fragments. Thus the cast is applied in three sections: (1) leg; (2) foot; and (3) knee and thigh. (Figs. 1130 and 1131.)

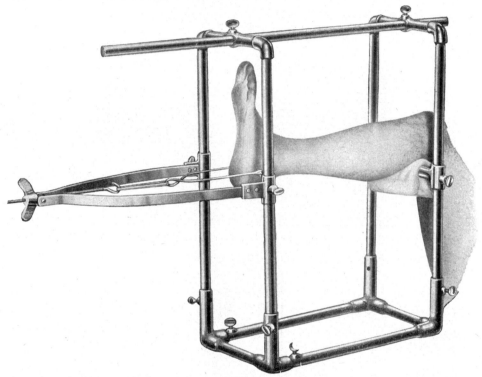

Fig. 1133.—Boehler's apparatus for the reduction of fractures of the leg. (Courtesy Zimmer Mfg. Co.)

The leg is immobilized with the knee flexed about thirty degrees. As soon as the plaster is dry the patient is put to bed with the leg elevated and the leg is kept elevated until there is no further danger of swelling. In the great majority of cases the plaster will control the swelling, but the toes should be watched carefully and if they become cold or cyanotic, the plaster should be split along one side or if necessary along both sides. We do not bivalve the plaster, however, unless it is necessary.

The patient should be kept in bed for several days or even weeks, depending upon the character of the fracture. Immediately after the reduction the position of the fragments should be checked by the x-ray, and if the position is not satisfactory, a second attempt at reduction should be made or the surgeon should remove the cast and treat the fracture by traction as described in the next section. If the fracture is stable and the reduction is satisfactory, the patient may be got up on crutches after a few days. On the other hand, in long oblique, spiral, or comminuted fractures in which there is considerable danger of displacement these patients should be kept in bed until all danger of displacement has passed. At the end of from two to four weeks the patient may be got up on crutches or in the case of feeble patients, they may be up in a chair. The plaster is left on for from eight to

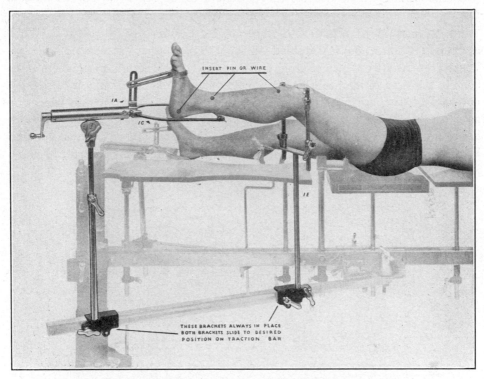

Fig. 1134.—Method of reduction by the two-pin method in fractures of both bones of the leg, using the Bell table instead of the fracture machine.

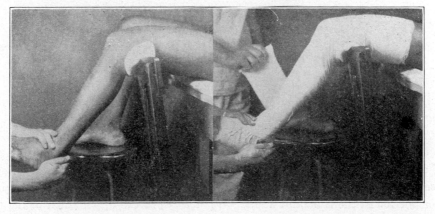

Fig. 1135.—Countertraction supplied by back of chair. (After Wilson and Cochran: *Fractures and Dislocations*, J. B. Lippincott Co., Publishers.)

ten weeks, then removed, and the stability of union is tested. If the plaster becomes loose before this time, it should be removed and reapplied. If union is not satisfactory, the plaster is replaced for four weeks longer. At the end of this time union will usually be firm enough to permit exercises of the leg with no danger of deformity, and in two weeks more, weight-bearing may be commenced and the crutches gradually discarded.

Instead of the above we now frequently use the Boehler skin tight plaster with the walking iron and let the patient bear as much weight as he comfortably can on the extremity as soon as the plaster is dry.

3. **Treatment of Simple Fractures of Both Bones of the Leg in Which Reduction Cannot Be Maintained Without Traction or Skeletal Fixation.**— These are extensively comminuted fractures in which there is not enough intact bone in the tibia to maintain length, or oblique or spiral fractures in which it is not possible to obtain stable engagement of the fragments after full length has been obtained by traction. This group also includes those fractures in which, because of swelling and lapse of time since the accident, or because of other injuries, it is not possible to perform satisfactory manipulative reduction.

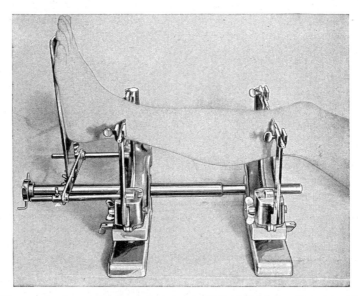

Fig. 1136.—Zimmer fracture reduction apparatus applied to the leg. (Courtesy Zimmer Manufacturing Company.)

These fractures should be treated by traction and immobilization. Immobilization can be obtained by suspending the leg in a Thomas splint which is flexed about 30 degrees at the knee and fixed to the foot of the bed. The foot of the bed should be elevated about ten inches and a frame should be placed over the bed with a trapeze in order that the patient may move himself around in bed. The most satisfactory method of applying the traction in these cases is by means of a Steinmann pin or wire through the os calcis or lower portion of the tibia and fibula. In fractures of the upper third of the tibia quite satisfactory traction can sometimes be obtained by means of adhesive

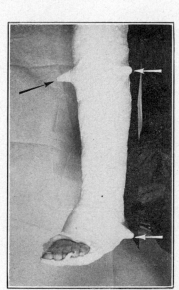

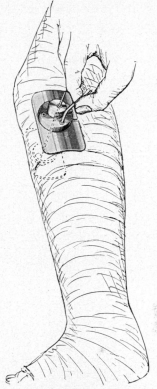

Fig. 1137.   Fig. 1138.

Fig. 1137.—Method of immobilizing the fragments by pins fixed in a plaster-of-Paris cast after reduction of fracture of both bones of the leg. The lower pin may be placed through the lower fragment of the tibia or through the os calcis, as shown in this figure.

Fig. 1138.—Zimmer button wire tightener for skeletal fixation with wires in a plaster cast. (Courtesy Zimmer Manufacturing Company.)

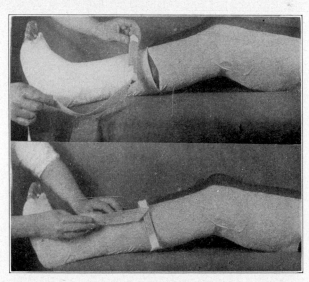

Fig. 1139.—Correction of angular deformity in any direction can be obtained by cutting plaster cast and wedging it.

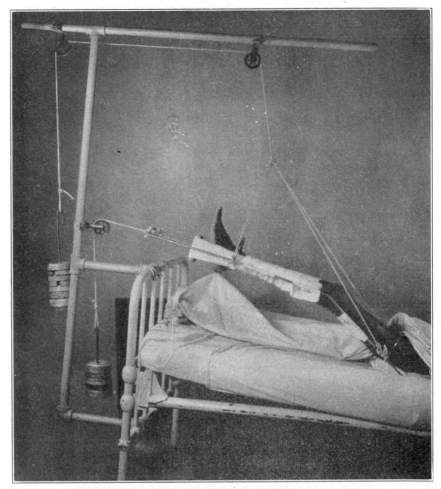

Fig. 1140.—Treatment of a high fracture of the leg by skin traction or skeletal traction, as indicated and suspension in a Hodgen splint and Conwell's one-inch iron frame attached to bed. This position and apparatus is also useful in treating fractures of the femur.

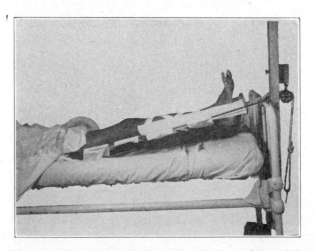

Fig. 1141.—Skin traction applied to the leg with adhesive and immobilization in a Thomas splint in the treatment of fractures of both bones of the leg. The extent of the adhesive application depends upon the site of the fracture. This type of traction is not useful in fractures of the lower third of the tibia and fibula.

applied to the skin as illustrated in Figs. 1140 and 1141. In low fractures fairly satisfactory traction can be obtained by means of some form of the Sinclair skate. The disadvantage is that the adhesive tends to slip after a few days and it needs constant attention. We usually use skeletal traction applied by means of a Kirschner wire through the lower end of the tibia.

Application of Skeletal Traction in Fractures of the Leg.—Skeletal traction may be applied by means of a wire or pin through the lower third of the tibia and fibula or through the os calcis. Personally we prefer the wire through the tibia unless the fracture involves the lower third of this bone.

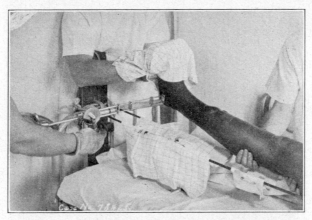

Fig. 1142.—Application of Kirschner wire through the os calcis.

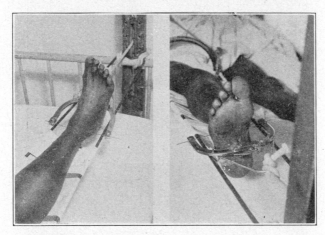

Fig. 1143.—Kirschner wire applied through lower one-fourth of tibia and fibula with DePuy bow being used. This case has a severe comminuted fracture middle one-third of the tibia and fibula.

Application of Pin or Wire Through the Os Calcis or Distal Fourth of the Tibia.—The patient is placed in a bed with fracture boards under the mattress and general or local anesthesia is administered. A Thomas splint of the correct size with the knee bent to about 45 degrees is placed over the leg. The ankle and heel in the lower portion of the leg are then cleaned with soap and water if necessary, followed by alcohol and ether and painted with strong tincture of iodine (7 per cent) (Fig. 1144). A small incision is made about one inch below and one-half inch posterior to the tip of the external malleolus, the skin being pulled up-ward while the incision is made (Fig. 1109). The pin or wire is then introduced and drilled or driven through the os calcis and out to the skin on the other side (Fig. 1145). The skin on the inner side is then pulled upward and a small in-cision is made and the pin or wire is forced through until it projects about

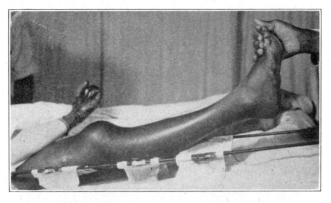

Fig. 1144.—Application of a Steinmann pin through the heel. Thomas splint is under the leg, the foot is held up by an assistant while the ankle is painted with iodine.

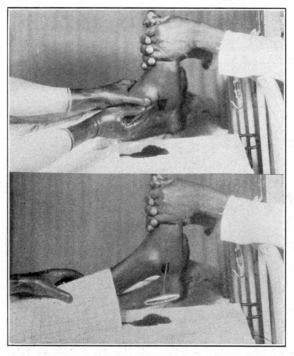

Fig. 1145.—While the skin is pulled upward a small incision is made below and posterior to the external malleolus over the center of the os calcis.

an equal distance on each side. The skin wounds are dressed with gauze, the splint is tied to the foot of the bed, the leg is suspended in the splint by slings, traction is applied to the wire or pin (Fig. 1147), and the foot of the bed is elevated about ten inches (Fig. 1148). As a rule from fifteen to twenty pounds of traction is adequate, and at the end of a few days or as soon as full length has been obtained, the weight can be decreased to from ten to twelve pounds.

We usually use a Kirschner wire drilled through the lower fourth of the tibia about an inch above the ankle joint and do not incise the skin, but push the wire through the skin.

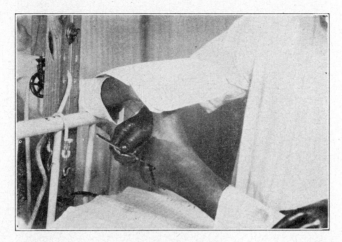

Fig. 1146.—The pin is thrust through a small incision on the inner side of the heel.

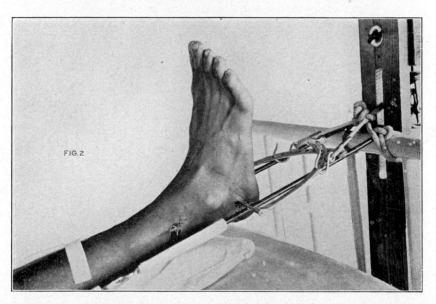

Fig. 1147.—The metal bow is applied to the pin and traction attached to the bow. The Thomas splint is fixed to the foot of the bed and the thigh and leg suspended in the splint.

Aftertreatment.—The alignment of the fragments in the anteroposterior plane is controlled by adjusting the slings over the leg and knee. Lateral alignment can be controlled by swinging the pin which is fixed in the os calcis or by pads between the leg and the side bars of the splint, or by a pressure pad such as that of Conwell, illustrated in Fig. 1149.

As soon as full length is obtained by measurement and when the alignment appears to be satisfactory, x-ray pictures are taken by portable apparatus in order to check the position of the fragments. If the position is satisfactory, the traction is continued until union is sufficiently firm to maintain length of the leg and position of the fragments after it has been immobilized

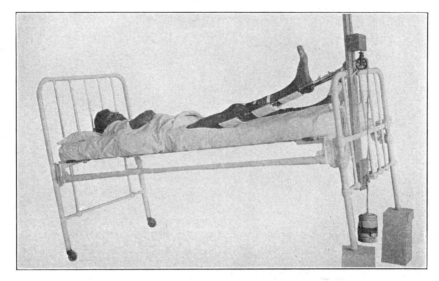

Fig. 1148.—Foot of bed is elevated ten or twelve inches.

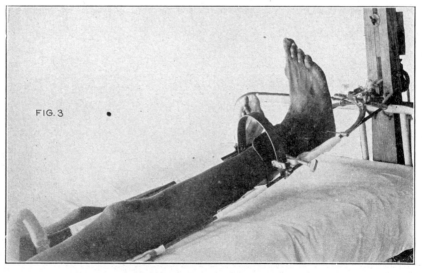

Fig. 1149.—Conwell's pressure pad for the correction of lateral deformities. To be used on the leg with care, lest pressure sores develop.

in a plaster-of-Paris cast (about three weeks). If the position is not satisfactory, an attempt should be made to correct it either by adding to the weights suspended from the pin, by changing the position of the slings or of the pressure pads, or by manual manipulation of the fragments in the splint. As soon as union has begun to take place, a plaster-of-Paris cast can be substituted for the traction, after the pin or wire has been removed.

Application of the Plaster-of-Paris Cast.—Two assistants or a mechanical rest for the knee and foot are needed to hold the leg. One assistant grasps the thigh just above the knee while the other holds the foot (Fig. 1150). With the two assistants maintaining the traction and position of the fragments, the leg

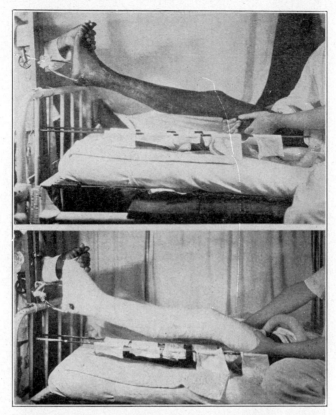

Fig. 1150.—Application of plaster-of-Paris cast after reduction and partial union have been obtained by skeletal traction, the soft structures have greatly improved, and practically a simple fracture exists.

Fig. 1151.—With the traction in place and the leg elevated by assistants, the cast is applied over the pin in the heel.

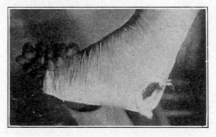

Fig. 1152.—Windows cut around the heel and pin removed.

is lifted directly upward and a circular plaster-of-Paris cast is applied around the leg from the ankle to the knee. The application of this cast is expedited if a short posterior plaster mold is first placed under the leg, as this aids in maintaining the alignment and prevents the tendency of the leg to sag at the site of the fracture. As soon as this cast has begun to harden the plaster is

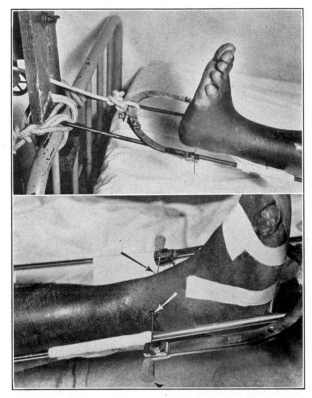

Fig. 1153.—Kirschner wire applied through os calcis and through lower end of the tibia for fractures of the leg.

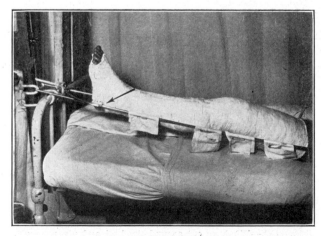

Fig. 1154.—Immobilization in a plaster cast combined with skeletal traction to the os calcis in the treatment of fractures of the leg.

continued upward around the thigh and downward around the foot and ankle to the toes, the pin being left in place and incorporated in the plaster. The plaster remains in place for from five to seven weeks or until firm union has been obtained. During this time the patient may be up on crutches.

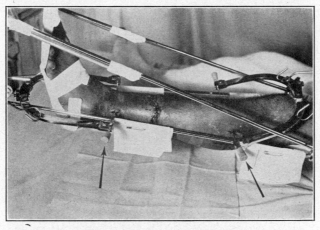

Fig. 1155.—Kirschner wires below and above the fracture site to afford traction and counter-traction in the treatment of certain fractures of the leg.

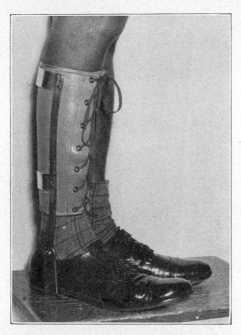

Fig. 1156.—Short, double, upright lower leg and ankle metal brace.

Traction in a Cast.—Instead of the Thomas splint we usually use a method demonstrated some years ago by H. H. Hitchcock. The traction wire is placed through the lower fourth of the tibia, the fracture is then reduced by manual traction and manipulation and a plaster cast is applied with the knee slightly flexed. The cast extends from the toes to the middle of the thigh and is well

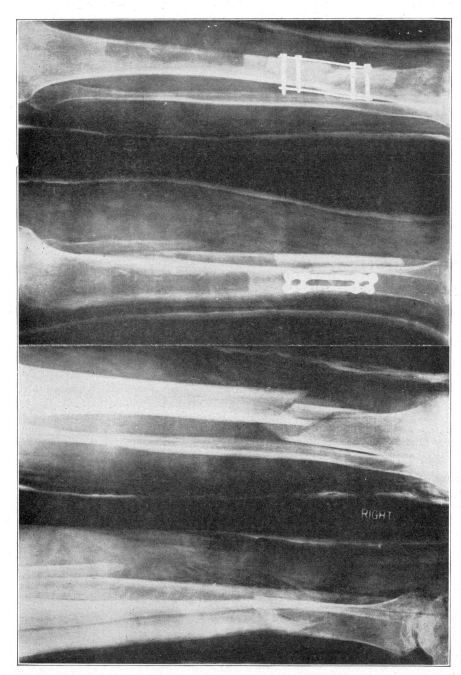

Fig. 1157.—Old fracture of the tibia with nonunion. Treated by dual plates supplemented by free grafts from same tibia.

padded around the knee to permit the cast to slip down slightly when traction is applied. A cross board may be incorporated in the cast to prevent rotation. The patient is placed in bed with the leg resting on a pillow or splint and from ten to fifteen pounds of traction is applied.

The alignment of the fragments should be checked with the portable x-ray a few days later, and if it is not satisfactory it can be corrected by cutting a circle almost around the plaster at the site of the deformity and wedging or angling it until the leg is straight and then wrapping a plaster bandage around the cut to repair the plaster.

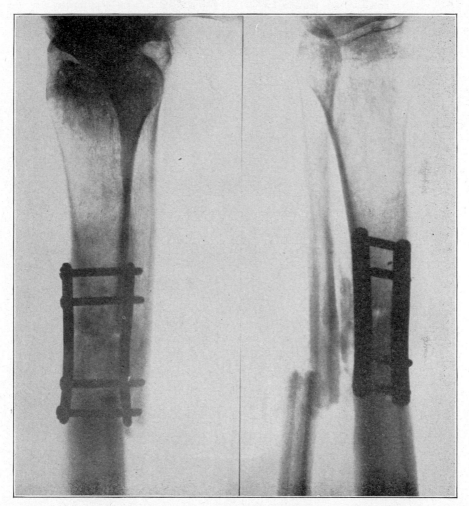

Fig. 1158.—Fracture of the tibia about three months after the accident. Treated by dual plates and an iliac graft.

The traction is continued for from four to six weeks; then it is discontinued and a new snug or skin-tight plaster is applied. This extends from the toes to the midthigh and usually is not a walking cast, but the patient may be up on crutches. In selected cases without much tendency to displacement a walking cast may be used. This is continued for from four to six weeks longer. At the

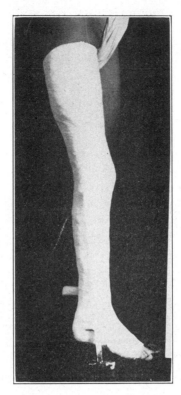

Fig. 1159.—Boehler's skin-tight plaster with weight-bearing crutch.

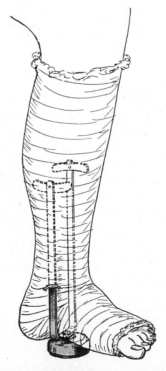

Fig. 1160—Swivel walking heel for ambulant treatment of fractures below the knee. (Courtesy Zimmer Manufacturing Company.)

end of this time it is removed, and if the leg is solid clinically, the patient may begin to use the leg.

Treatment by Skeletal Fixation.—Since the widespread use of stainless steel wire and pins for traction, this method has become deservedly popular for the treatment of difficult comminuted or oblique fractures of both bones of the leg. (Figs. 1136 and 1138.)

The method is most satisfactorily used if one of the traction machines is available. These operate by means of one or two wires or pins through each fragment and in skillful hands permit of very accurate reduction of these fractures. After the bones are in a satisfactory position, a plaster cast is applied with the pins or wires in place, and these are incorporated in the cast.

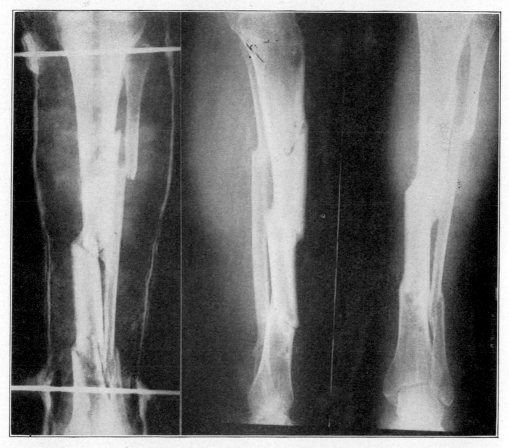

Fig. 1161.—Comminuted fractures of tibia and fibula which have been reduced and held in place with transfixation pins above and below and plaster cast. Good anatomical result. Good function and no disability.

Lacking such a machine, the pins or wires may be placed through the bones and the fracture then reduced by whatever means is available and the plaster cast applied. The pins or wires serve to immobilize the fragments and are left in situ until union is fairly firm. The patient may be up on crutches, but should not bear full weight on the extremity until the pins or wires have been removed. Then a walking plaster cast can be applied.

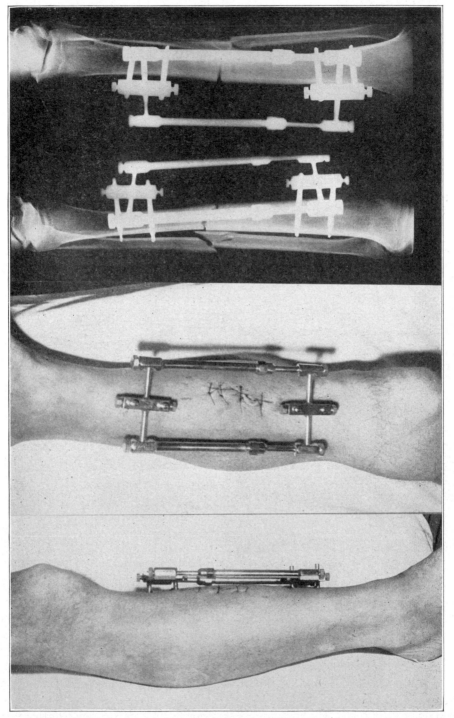

Fig. 1162.—The Haynes splint applied to a compound fracture of the leg. (Courtesy Commander H. R. Walker, United States Navy.)

Operative Reduction.—Since the introduction of stainless steel and vitallium for internal fixation and the local use of the sulfonamides in clean operations for the prevention of infection, we no longer hesitate to operate upon and internally fix the fragments, if the displacement does not yield readily to manipulation or traction. Many surgeons routinely operate upon and plate these fractures.

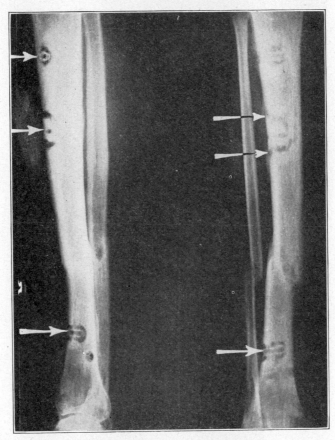

Fig. 1163.—Osteomyelitis with ring sequestra of the tibia following application of pins for treating fracture of the leg. Fractures had not healed when pins were removed, but union of tibia and fibula was accomplished with the simple application of a plaster cast without any further treatment. Patient had prolonged convalescence because of a bone infection from pins.

The operation is relatively simple, the tibia being exposed through a longitudinal incision lateral to the crest. The fracture is reduced and fixed with a noncorrosive plate or wire, the metal being placed on the lateral surface of the tibia beneath the muscle. A long oblique screw at right angles to the plate affords more rigid fixation (Murray). In oblique fractures one or more cross screws may afford ample fixation. The sulfonamide powder is then implanted in the wound, and it is then closed and treated as a simple fracture.

Aftertreatment of Fracture of the Leg.—The plaster cast is continued until the leg is clinically solid; that is, the callus is not tender, no movement or springing is noted when cross strain is placed on the leg, and there is no pain at the

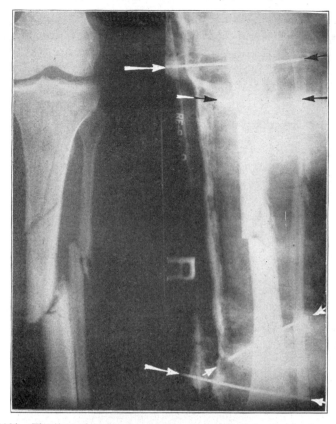

Fig. 1164.—Fixation of a fracture of the leg by multiple pins in two planes.

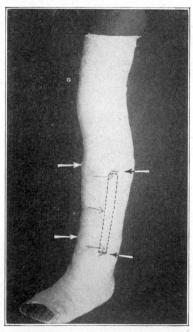

Fig. 1165.—Fixation pins incorporated in a plaster cast and length maintained by wood bars (dotted lines) between the pins and incorporated in the cast.

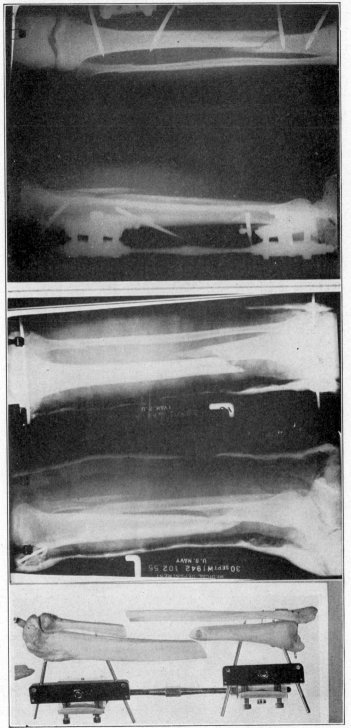

Fig. 1166.—The use of the Stader splint for fractures of the leg. (Courtesy Captain C. M. Shaar, United States Navy.)

fracture site with moderate weight-bearing. If the fracture is not solid in from eight to twelve weeks after the injury, a short skin-tight plaster is applied and in selected cases weight-bearing in a walking cast is permitted. Movement of the knee is encouraged in either case.

After the cast is removed, the patient uses crutches or a cane until the leg is strong enough to support his weight. He is given exercises to restore movement to the knee and ankle, and the foot and leg are wrapped with an elastic bandage to control the swelling. The bandage is continued for three weeks or more until the swelling is no longer troublesome.

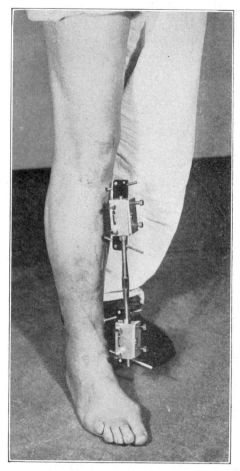

Fig. 1167.

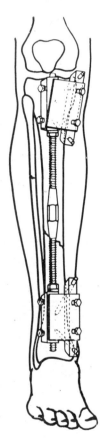

Fig. 1168.

Figs. 1167 and 1168.—Showing Stader splint in use. (Courtesy Captain C. M. Shaar, United States Navy.)

Delayed Union in Fractures of the Leg

The lower third of the tibia is one of the most frequent sites of delayed union. We may consider union delayed in fractures in which union is not present within eight or ten weeks after the injury and in which there is no evidence of callus in the roentgenogram, and in which there is evidence of an open marrow cavity. If the marrow cavity is closed by eburnated bone or if there is marked absorption of the ends of the bones, we may consider the case one of nonunion. It has been demonstrated clinically that many of these cases of delayed union will unite if the bone be stimulated by partial weight-bearing. For this reason we recommend and use in these cases weight-bearing with sufficient support to the leg to prevent the development of deformity. This support is obtained by the walking plaster (Fig. 1159). Also, we have been bringing about union in such cases by drilling the bones at the site of the fracture. We prefer opening the skin in this procedure rather than drilling through the skin. A circular cast is applied afterward.

Figs. 1166, 1167 and 1168 show the use of the Stader splint. We seldom use this splint and advise its application and use only by individuals who are familiar with and capable of applying it. Therefore, authorities who do use it state that it should be used only in certain selected cases. This same precaution applies to all external pin fixation.

CHAPTER XXVI

INJURIES IN THE REGION OF THE ANKLE

SURGICAL ANATOMY

The Lower End of the Tibia.—The tibia is moderately enlarged in its lower portion and its mesial rounded subcutaneous border is thickened and projected downward as the internal malleolus. The tip of the internal malleolus is roughened for the attachment of the internal lateral ligament of the ankle joint and its lateral or deep surface is covered with cartilage for articulation with the side of the body of the astragalus. The inferior surface is concave from before backward and articulates with the superior surface of the astragalus. Its articular cartilage is continuous with that of the deep surface of the internal malleolus. The concavity of the inferior surface is slightly deepened behind by the projection downward of the rather sharp posterior border. The anterior border is rounded and the lateral or deep border is roughened for the attachment of the inferior tibiofibular ligaments.

The Lower End of the Fibula.—The fibula is subcutaneous in its lower third and its lower extremity is enlarged and projected downward as the prominent external malleolus. The lateral surface of the external malleolus is rounded and subcutaneous, and its tip lies about a half inch below and posterior to that of the internal malleolus. Its posterior border is grooved for the peroneal tendons and its tip and anterior border are roughened for the attachment of the ligaments. Its deep or inner surface presents an articular facet for the lateral surface of the body of the astragalus.

Ossification.—The centers of ossification in the lower epiphyses of the tibia and fibula appear at about the second year and fuse with the shaft at about the eighteenth year. The epiphyseal line of the tibia runs transversely across the bone just above the attachment of the joint capsule, and the epiphysis includes the internal malleolus and the inferior articular surface. The epiphyseal line of the fibula is at a lower level, being in line with the articular surface of the tibia and the epiphysis includes the external malleolus.

The Astragalus.—This is an irregular bone which receives the body weight from the tibia and transmits it to the other tarsal bones. It consists of a body, a neck, and a head. The body is roughly quadrilateral in shape and fits into the mortise formed by the malleoli and the inferior surface of the tibia. Its superior surface is flattened from side to side and convex from before backward and this and the sides are covered by articular cartilage to articulate with the mortise of the ankle joint. The inferior surface presents articular facets for the os calcis and a central roughened area for the interosseous ligaments. The short thick neck projects downward and inward to terminate in a rounded head which articulates with the scaphoid.

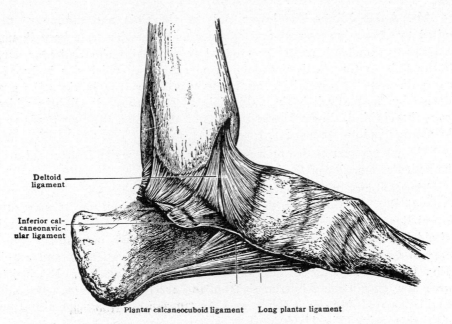

Deltoid ligament

Inferior calcaneonavicular ligament

Plantar calcaneocuboid ligament   Long plantar ligament

Fig. 1169.—Drawing of ankle joint seen from the inner aspect showing ligaments. (From Morris: *Human Anatomy*, P. Blakiston's Son & Co., Inc., Publisher.)

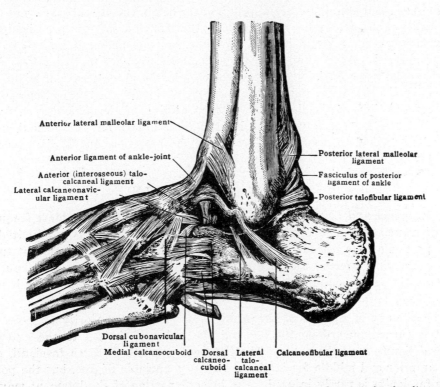

Anterior lateral malleolar ligament

Anterior ligament of ankle-joint

Anterior (interosseous) talocalcaneal ligament

Lateral calcaneonavicular ligament

Posterior lateral malleolar ligament

Fasciculus of posterior ligament of ankle

Posterior talofibular ligament

Dorsal cubonavicular ligament
Medial calcaneocuboid   Dorsal calcaneocuboid   Lateral talocalcaneal ligament   Calcaneofibular ligament

Fig. 1170.—Drawing of the ankle joint seen from the external lateral aspect showing ligaments. (Morris: *Human Anatomy*, P. Blakiston's Son & Co., Inc., Publisher.)

The Ankle Joint.—The lower ends of the tibia and fibula are firmly united by strong interosseous and anterior and posterior transverse ligaments and the two malleoli project downward from the inferior articular surface of the tibia to form a deep groove or mortise into which the body of the astragalus fits. This mortising of the body of the astragalus into the groove formed by the malleoli is the ankle joint. The groove is slightly wider in front than behind, thus a forward thrust of the leg on the foot tends to jam the astragalus into the mortise.

The joint is surrounded by a rather thin capsule which is attached around the articular margins of the involved bones.

The contours of the bones are such that the ankle joint is very strong mechanically and this strength is increased by the addition of very strong lateral ligaments which anchor the foot to the leg. The internal lateral or deltoid ligament is a heavy mass of fibers which spreads out fanlike from the internal malleolus to be attached to the os calcis, astragalus, and scaphoid (Fig. 1169). The external lateral ligament is much weaker. It consists of three diverging bands which arise from the external malleolus. The middle band is inserted into the os calcis, and the anterior and posterior are attached to the astragalus (Fig. 1170).

Movements at the Ankle.—Due to the facts that the articulating surfaces of the tibia and astragalus are approximately flat in the lateral plane and that the body of the astragalus is grasped by the malleoli, there is practically no movement at the ankle in the lateral plane, and movement is limited to the anteroposterior plane. Lateral movement of the foot on the leg takes place at the subastragaloid joint. The movements in the anteroposterior plane are hinge-like in character, the astragalus rotating in the concave articular surface of the tibia as the ligaments prevent gliding of the articular surfaces. The range of movement varies in different individuals, but the normal ankle may be expected to permit dorsiflexion of the foot to about 70 degrees and plantar flexion to about 140 degrees.

SPRAINS OF THE ANKLE

Incidence and Cause.—Sprain of the ankle is probably the most frequent of all traumatic lesions of the extremity and its occurrence is not limited to any particular age period. The most common cause is that the patient turns the ankle while bearing weight upon it. This is frequently brought about by placing the foot upon an uneven surface when walking or running, or it may occur from a fall.

Pathology of Sprains of the Ankle.—In the great majority of cases the foot is turned inward on the leg and the lesion is limited to the external lateral ligament of the ankle. The ligament consists of three fasciculi, and the anterior and middle fasciculi are torn to a variable degree, but the posterior fasciculus is rarely injured. The injured portion of the ligament may be completely torn across, or it may be avulsed from its attachment to the malleolus or to the foot, or in less severe injuries there may be only a partial tearing or stretching of the ligament. In addition to the tearing of the ligament, there is an extravasation of the blood into the surrounding tissues, more or less effusion into the joint, and a variable amount of stretching of the peroneal muscles and soft tissues on the lateral surface of the ankle.

Occasionally sprains of other joints of the foot occur. Here the pathology is the same, but the localization is at the site of the injury. This may be the anterior portion of the ankle joint, the internal lateral ligament, or the ligaments spanning any of the tarsal or tarsometatarsal joints.

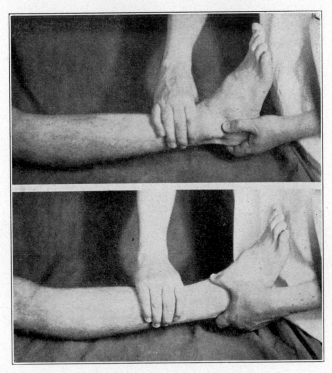

Fig. 1171.—Examination of the ankle joint. Palpation of the tip of the external malleolus and of the external lateral ligament.

Fig. 1172.—Examination of the ankle joint. Manipulation to determine presence or absence of supramalleolar fracture.

Diagnosis of Sprain of the Ankle.—The patient gives a history of an injury to the ankle, usually of the ankle turning and giving way under him or of its being injured during a fall. The injury is accompanied by severe pain which at first is felt in the outer side of the ankle and in a severe case gradually spreads to involve the entire foot, ankle, and leg. There is more or less inability to bear weight upon the foot. In a mild case the patient may be able to walk, although weight-bearing causes considerable pain. Swelling and ecchymosis appear soon after the injury and vary with the severity of the sprain. It is rather characteristic of sprains that the pain persists even when the foot is put at rest, and in a severe sprain the pain is more severe than is usually found in fractures.

On physical examination there is a variable amount of swelling which is most marked anterior to and below the external malleolus. In a severe sprain the swelling involves the entire foot and ankle and the lower half of the leg.

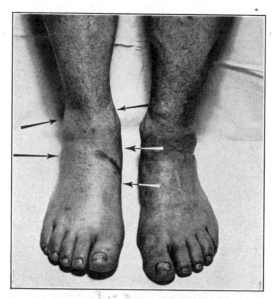

Fig. 1173.—Sprain of the right ankle. The x-ray was negative for any bone injury.

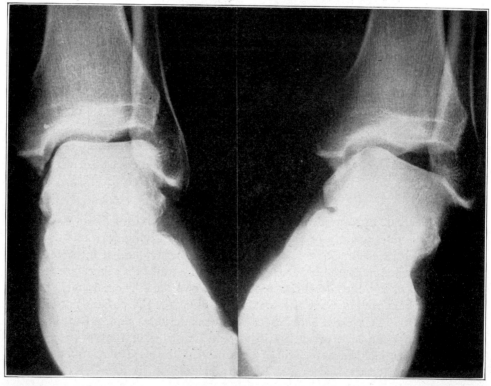

Fig. 1174.—Sprain of ankle, eleven months' duration, with continued pain. Extent of permanent ligamentous damage shown by x-ray with foot held in abduction. (Courtesy Dr. Joseph Lembeck.)

On inspection the foot is not displaced on the leg although the swelling may simulate lateral displacement. On palpation there is acute tenderness over the region of the tear in the external lateral ligament (usually anterior to and below the tip of the external malleolus) (Fig. 1171), and there may be tenderness entirely around the ankle joint and up the leg, especially along the peroneal muscles and over the external malleolus.

On manipulation all movements of the foot and ankle are possible except as limited by the swelling, but they are apt to be accompanied by pain, and adduction which puts strain on the torn ligament is especially painful.

A very helpful point in the differential diagnosis of a sprain and a fracture is that in a sprain the foot can be pressed directly upward against the articular surface of the tibia without eliciting pain, while in the presence of a fracture the maneuver usually causes pain at the site of the fracture.

In mild sprains in which the tenderness is limited to the region over the ligament below and anterior to the tip of the malleolus a diagnosis of sprain can be safely made without an x-ray picture but in moderate or severe cases the signs and symptoms of the sprain may be practically identical with those of a fracture of the external malleolus without displacement, or of a sprain fracture with avulsion of the tip of the malleolus. Consequently all cases of moderate or severe sprain, and especially those in which there is tenderness over the external malleolus, should be x-rayed in order to rule out a fracture.

Occasionally fractures of the external malleolus are not visible in the ordinary anteroposterior and lateral views and an oblique view of the external malleolus is necessary to demonstrate the fracture.

In the rare sprains of a ligament, other than the external lateral, the symptoms are similar except that tenderness is localized over the involved ligament.

Treatment of Sprains of the Ankle

The treatment depends upon the severity of the sprain and the amount of swelling present. In severe sprains the patient should be put to bed and the ankle elevated and immobilized in a pressure or hot wet dressing until the swelling has decreased.

A very simple and efficient form of pressure dressing can be improvised by covering the foot and ankle and lower third of the leg with several turns of absorbent cotton so that there is a layer of cotton from one and one-half to two inches thick around the involved region. This is then covered with a gauze bandage which is drawn tightly and is applied in such a direction that the foot is pulled into a position of eversion. The gauze bandage compresses the cotton, thus making elastic pressure on the foot and ankle, and the cotton tends to afford a considerable degree of immobilization. (Conwell then places the foot in a wire basket splint and wets the dressing with boracic acid and places the foot under a light.) If the surgeon prefers a flannel or woven elastic bandage, this may be used in place of the cotton for the temporary dressing until the swelling has largely disappeared.

The patient should remain in bed with the foot elevated three or four days or more if necessary. At the end of this time the pressure dressing should be removed, the foot washed in alcohol, and a light circular plaster cast or a stirrup and basket strapping should be applied. In mild sprains the strapping may be applied immediately and the preliminary period of rest in bed with the pressure dressing may be dispensed with. The area should be shaved and painted with tincture of benzoin or merthiolate before the adhesive is applied.

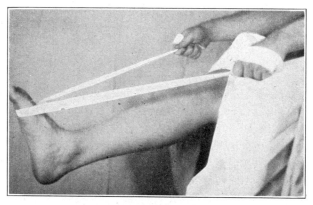

Fig. 1175.—Photograph of patient with foot supported by bandage to aid surgeon in strapping for sprain.

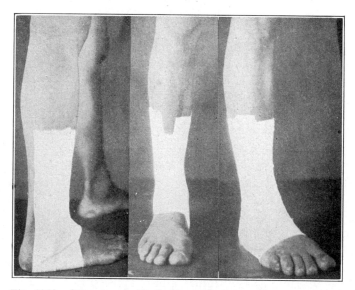

Fig. 1176.—Stirrup and shingle strapping for sprain at the ankle.

Adhesive Strapping for Sprains of the Ankle.—While the adhesive is being applied, the patient's foot should be supported and held in a position of dorsiflexion and eversion (Fig. 1175). This can be accomplished by placing the patient's heel on the surgeon's knee and by running a strip of adhesive around the ball of the foot from within outward and having the patient hold this adhesive, thus pulling the foot upward and outward from a point at about the head of the fifth metatarsal bone.

Adhesive strips about one inch wide should be at hand. These are applied as follows: the first strip is begun on the inner side of the leg about six inches above the ankle, passed down under the heel and up the other side of the leg. The second strip is begun on the inner side of the foot, carried back around the heel and pulled forward over the first strip and parallel with the sole to the lateral side of the forefoot. The third strip is placed slightly anterior to and parallel with the first (vertical) and overlapping the second (horizontal) strip. In this manner the strapping is continued forward on the foot and upward on the leg by means of alternating vertical and horizontal strips. As the vertical strips reach the front of the leg, they curve around the lower leg on either side. In this way the entire region of the ankle and lower leg and foot as far as the heads of the metatarsals is encased in a basket-like adhesive sheath. It is important that the foot be held in one position until the strapping is complete. Instead of the above a stirrup and shingle strapping may be used (Fig. 1176).

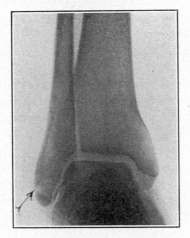

Fig. 1177.—Sprain fracture at the ankle with avulsion of the tip of the external malleolus. Treated by plaster cast (four weeks) followed by hot baths and weight-bearing one week later.

The strapping is then covered with a gauze bandage and the patient may be permitted to walk. It is advisable to elevate the outer border of the heel of the shoe from three-sixteenths to one-fourth of an inch as this tends to maintain the foot in a position of eversion and takes the strain off the torn ligament. This strapping should be worn until it becomes loose and inefficient (this is about ten days), when it should be removed and reapplied. The average sprained ankle in an adult requires from four to six weeks to heal and in severe sprains eight to ten weeks may be necessary. Support by adhesive strapping and elevation of the outer border of the heel of the shoe should be continued until healing is complete; otherwise the ankle may be permanently weak and unstable. In children sprains heal more quickly.

In the case of fracture sprains with avulsion of a portion of the external malleolus (Fig. 1177), it is advisable to immobilize the foot in eversion in a plaster-of-Paris boot over a period of about four weeks. This can be followed by the adhesive strapping and tilted heel until the patient is fully recovered (three to six weeks). If the avulsed fragment does not unite and pain persists, the fragment should be removed.

FRACTURES AND FRACTURE DISLOCATIONS IN THE REGION OF THE ANKLE

Incidence and Causation.—Fractures in the region of the ankle are rather uncommon in children, but are among the most frequent of the severe fractures in adults. The majority of the cases occur in vigorous adults who lead an outdoor life or are engaged in hazardous occupations.

Very rarely a fracture at the ankle may be the result of direct violence as in crushing injuries or the passage of the wheel of a heavy vehicle over the foot, but the great majority of these fractures are caused by indirect violence. This is usually applied by the body weight acting through the leg on the foot, as in falls from a height, getting the foot caught while the body is moving, stepping into a hole or on an uneven surface while running or walking or merely by suddenly turning, and having the ankle give way from the abnormal lateral or rotary strain.

Mechanism.—The structure of the ankle joint is such that seven different mechanisms may act on the joint to produce sprains, fractures, and dislocations in this region by indirect violence: the astragalus may be forced upward, backward, or forward on the articular surface of the tibia, or it may be inverted or everted against one of the malleoli while the other tends to be torn off by arrachement; or it may be rotated inward or outward in its mortise and thus tend to spread the malleoli apart. As upward displacement is usually combined with backward displacement, these may be considered under one group, and the same is true of inversion and internal rotation. This leaves four main groups: 1. External rotation. 2. Eversion (fibular flexion). 3. Inversion (tibial flexion). 4. Upward displacement or compression in the long axis of the leg. The details of the mechanism and pathology of each group will be discussed below.

Classification of Ankle Fractures.—The custom among physicians and surgeons is to refer to all fractures in this region as Pott's or Dupuytren's fractures and to pay little attention to the mechanism or pathology of the lesion. Of late years, however, several thoughtful students of fractures have attempted to classify ankle fractures in such a way that the reader may obtain a clear understanding of the subject. The classifications are based upon the mechanism of production or upon the pathology of the lesion.

For the purpose of treatment an anatomical classification is the most useful and we shall present one under treatment, but for a proper understanding of the various lesions, the classification of Ashhurst and Bromer* is preferable. It is as follows:

A. Fractures by External Rotation

    1. First Degree: Lower end of fibula only ("mixed oblique")   79 (26 %)
    2. Second Degree: Same plus rupture of internal lateral ligament
        or fracture of internal malleolus ("low Dupuytren")   100 (33 %)
        Viz.,
        (a) Internal lateral ligament, uncomplicated_____ 13
           Internal lateral ligament complicated by posterior
             marginal fragment of tibia_____ 13

*Ashhurst and Bromer: Arch. Surg. 4: 51-129, 1922.

(b) Internal malleolus, uncomplicated------------------ 32
Internal malleolus complicated by posterior marginal
fragment of tibia----------------------------- 42
3. Third Degree: Same plus fracture of whole lower end of tibia,
representing the internal malleolus.   5 (1.7 %)

Total Fractures by External Rotation---------------- 184 (61   %)

B. Fractures by Abduction (Fibular Flexion)

   1. First Degree: Internal malleolus only   20 (6.6 %)
   2. Second Degree: Same plus fracture of fibula (transverse, above
      or below tibiofibular joint)   41 (13.7 %)
      (a) Below inferior tibiofibular joint (no diastasis) (''bi-
         malleolar fracture'') ------------------------ 13
      (b) Above inferior tibiofibular joint (with diastasis)
         (Pott's fracture,'' ''Dupuytren type'')--------- 28
   3. Third Degree: Internal malleolus represented by whole lower
      end of tibia   2 (0.66%)

Total Fractures by Abduction------------------------ 63 (21   %)

C. Fractures by Adduction (Tibial Flexion)

   1. First Degree: External malleolus only, transverse, at or below
      level of tibial plafond   27 (9   %)
   2. Second Degree: Same plus
      (a) Internal malleolus below level of tibial plafond (''bi-
         malleolar fracture'') ------------------------ 3
      (b) Median surface of tibia up and in from joint surface 8   11 (3.6 %)
   3. Third Degree: Same, plus whole lower end of tibia (''supra-
      malleolar fracture by adduction'')----------------------   2 (0.66%)

Total Fractures by Adduction------------------------ 40 (13.3 %)

D. Fractures by Compression in Long Axis of Leg

   1. Isolated Marginal Fractures--------------------------------- 1
   2. Comminution of tibial plafond----------------------------- 3
   3. T or Y-fractures (''V-fractures of Gosselin'')-------------- 4

Total Fractures by Compression in Long Axis of Leg---- 8 (2.7 %)

E. Fractures by Direct Violence (Supramalleolar types)   5 (1.7 %)

FRACTURES AND FRACTURE DISLOCATIONS AT THE ANKLE

Mechanism and Pathology of Fractures and Fracture Dislocations at the
Ankle.—Fractures by External Rotation: When the foot is fixed on the
ground and the leg is forcibly rotated inward on the foot or when the leg is
fixed and the foot is forcibly rotated outward on the leg, the astragalus is
twisted in its mortise between the malleoli and tends to spread the malleoli
apart. With external rotation of the foot on the leg the anterior portion of
the body of the astragalus presses against the anterior border of the inner
surface of the external malleolus and forces it outward and backward. As
the inferior tibiofibular ligaments are stronger than the bone, this maneuver
tends to cause an oblique or spiral fracture of the lower end of the fibula
(Fig. 1178).

In the typical case the fracture line begins at the front of the malleolus just below the inferior tibiofibular articulation, and passes upward and backward across the joint to emerge on the posterior surface of the fibula. This is the simplest and most frequent form of ankle fracture (61 per cent in Ashhurst's series). In cases due to relatively slight violence there may be practically no displacement of the fragments and relatively little pain and disability.

Second Degree External Rotation Fractures.—If the force continues to act, the internal lateral ligament is ruptured or the internal malleolus is pulled off, and an abduction fracture of the second degree is produced. As the inner side of the ankle gives way, the astragalus is permitted to move outward and backward and carry the external malleolus with it, thus the lower fragment is displaced outward as well as rotated outward and may also be displaced backward. As a rule, however, the backward displacement is due to the outward rotation and is apparent rather than real.

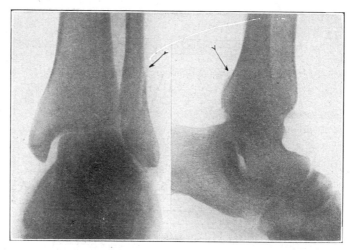

Fig. 1178.—External rotation fracture of the external malleolus with slight outward displacement of the foot. Treated by manipulative reduction under an anesthetic, followed by immobilization in a plaster-of-Paris cast for five weeks. No weight-bearing for two weeks longer. Good result.

In severe cases in which the external rotation is combined with a forward thrust of the leg on the foot, there is a chipping off of the posterior margin of the tibia, the size of the separated fragment varying from a small chip to as much as one-third of the inferior articular surface of the tibia. Very rarely there is a diastasis at the ankle joint with rupture of the tibiofibular ligaments or an avulsion of an intermediate fragment from the lateral surface of the tibia. Occasionally the fibula is broken in its upper third with or without fracture of this bone at the ankle joint.

Third Degree External Rotation Fractures.—In the third degree fractures of this type according to Ashhurst's classification, the entire lower end of the tibia is broken off; consequently, the transverse fracture through the lower portion of the tibia takes the place of the rupture of the internal lateral ligament or of the fracture of the internal malleolus. Ashhurst believes that most of the cases of separation of the lower epiphysis of the tibia are third degree external rotation fractures.

Abduction (So-Called Pott's or Dupuytren's) Fractures.—When the foot is forcibly abducted on the leg or when the leg is bent outward on the fixed foot, either by a fall on the everted foot or by a blow on the outside of the leg, the strain falls first on the internal lateral ligament of the ankle and this ligament may be ruptured and a sprain of the inner side of the ankle may result. The internal lateral ligament, however, is unusually strong and is rarely ruptured; in these abduction injuries the internal malleolus is usually fractured by arrachment (bimalleolar fracture), the fracture line tending to be roughly transverse at or just below the level of the inferior articular surface of the tibia. This is the simplest form of abduction fracture and is accompanied by little or no displacement of the detached portion of the internal malleolus.

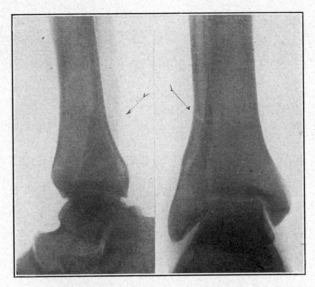

Fig. 1179.—Abduction fracture of the ankle with fracture of the fibula above the ankle and rupture of the internal lateral ligament. Treated by manipulation under an anesthetic to restore the mortise and immobilization in a plaster-of-Paris cast for six weeks. Weight-bearing two weeks later with Thomas heel. Good result.

Second Degree Abduction Fractures.—If the abducting force continues to act, the astragalus impinges upon the internal surface of the external malleolus, and this is pushed outward and upward and produces a fracture of the lower end of the fibula, which tends to be transverse and may be either above (Figs. 1179, 1180, and 1182) or below the inferior tibiofibular articulation. If the tibiofibular ligaments hold, the external malleolus is broken off transversely and the two malleoli may be displaced outward to a variable degree (bimalleolar fracture).

If the ligaments of the inferior tibiofibular joint are ruptured, there is produced a diastasis at this joint, and the fibula tends to be broken above the joint. This fracture usually occurs at the narrow portion of the fibula (surgical neck), two or three inches above the joint, and is due to the shaft

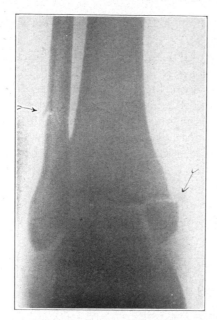
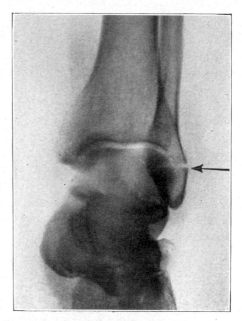

Fig. 1180.   Fig. 1181.

Fig. 1180.—Abduction fracture of the ankle with fracture of the fibula above the joint and avulsion of the inner malleolus. No manipulation was necessary. Treated by immobilization in a plaster cast for five weeks; weight-bearing two weeks later. Good result.

Fig. 1181.—A simple fracture through the external malleolus of the ankle, good position. Plaster cast with walking iron applied. Good result.

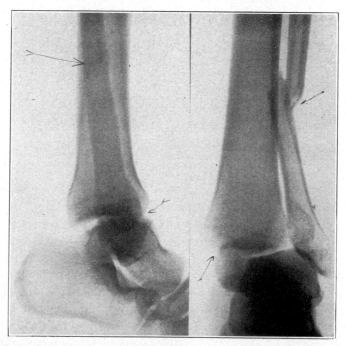

Fig. 1182.—Abduction fracture of the fibula above the ankle with avulsion of the internal malleolus and moderate outward displacement of the astragalus. Treated by manipulative reduction under an anesthetic and immobilization in a plaster-of-Paris cast for six weeks. Weight-bearing three weeks later with Thomas heel. Good result.

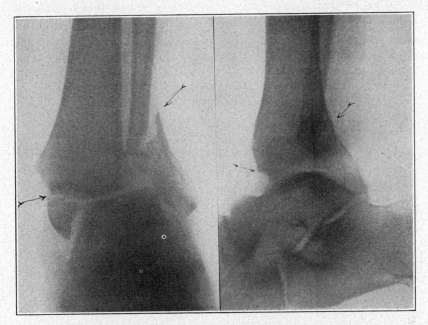

Fig. 1183.—Abduction fracture of the fibula just above the ankle with avulsion of the internal malleolus and moderate outward and posterior displacement of the astragalus. Treated by manipulative reduction under an anesthetic and immobilization in a plaster-of-Paris cast with good result.

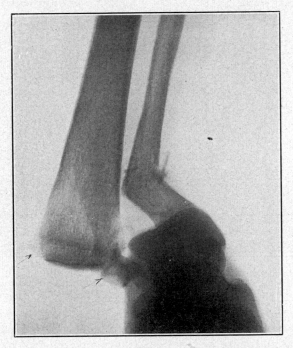

Fig. 1184.—Abduction fracture of the fibula above the ankle, avulsion of the internal malleolus, and complete lateral displacement of the astragalus on the tibia. Treated by manipulative reduction and immobilization in a plaster-of-Paris cast with good result.

of the bone being bent (or sprung) inward toward the tibia by the continuation of the upward and outward force (Fig. 1182). This is called Dupuytren's or Pott's fracture. The bending fracture of the fibula may result in comminution of the bone with separation of a wedge-shaped fragment. Either of the

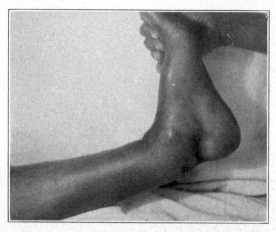

Fig. 1185.—Comminuted fracture through the lower end of the tibia and fibula with displacement. Treated by manipulative reduction and traction with a Steinman pin through the heel for three weeks followed by immobilization in a plaster-of-Paris cast for six weeks, walking in twelve weeks. Good result.

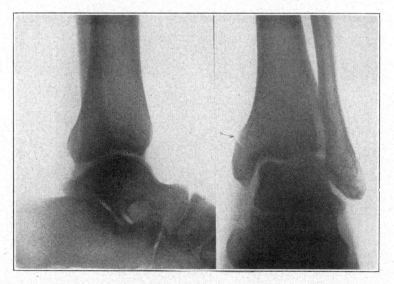

Fig. 1186.—Adduction fracture with rupture of the external lateral ligament and fracture of the internal malleolus with practically no displacement. No reduction was necessary. Treated by immobilization in a plaster-of-Paris cast for three weeks with good result. Weight-bearing six weeks following injury.

above may be complicated by a posterior marginal (Figs. 1183 and 1184) fracture of the tibia and more or less displacement of the foot or by the avulsion of an intermediate fragment from the tibia at the points of attachment of the inferior tibiofibular ligaments. In rare instances diastasis may occur without fracture of the fibula.

Third Degree Abduction Fractures.—In the third degree fractures of this type the internal malleolus is represented by the entire lower end of the tibia, and there is a transverse fracture of the lower portion of the shaft of the tibia (supramalleolar fracture).

Adduction Fractures.—When the foot is forcibly adducted on the leg, as in a fall on the adducted foot, the usual lesion is a rupture of some of the

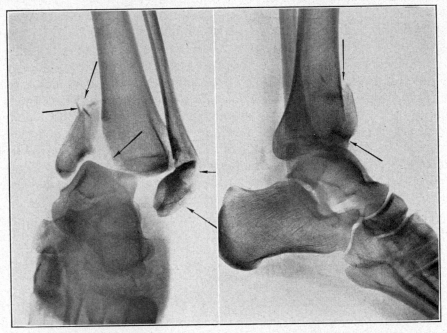

Fig. 1187.—Severe inversion fracture of both malleoli. Reduced by manipulation and immobilized in a plaster-of-Paris cast.

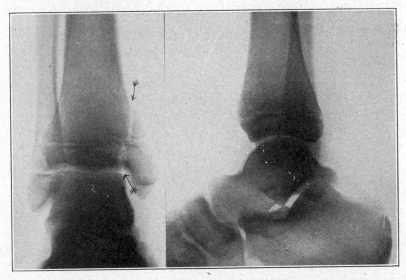

Fig. 1188.—Rare fracture of the internal malleolus through the epiphysis. No reduction was necessary. Immobilized in a plaster cast for five weeks with weight-bearing eight weeks after the injury. Good result.

fibers of the external lateral ligament or an ordinary sprain of the ankle; however, if the external lateral ligament withstands the strain and the force is sufficient, the external malleolus is torn off, the fracture being transverse and tending to lie at the level of or below the articular surface with the tibia.

Second Degree Adduction Fractures.—With a continuation of the force the body of the astragalus is forced inward and upward against the internal malleolus and this is broken off by compression (Fig. 1186). The fracture line in the internal malleolus usually begins at or below the level of the inferior articular surface of the tibia (tibial plafond) and extends obliquely upward and inward to emerge on the mesial surface of the malleolus.

In cases where much of the force is exerted from above downward, as in a fall from a height on the adducted foot, the fracture of the tibia is apt to involve the inferior articular surface, and the fracture line may begin at any point on the inferior articular surface of the tibia, or may begin at its lateral margin near the inferior tibiofibular joint and pass upward and inward to emerge on the mesial surface of the shaft, and the entire inferior articular surface may be separated from the bone and displaced upward and inward. In other instances the internal malleolus or that portion of the articular surface which is split off with it may be comminuted.

The most frequent adduction fracture is one in which the external lateral ligament is ruptured, while the fibula remains intact and the fracture is limited to that of the internal malleolus (Fig. 1186). Fracture of the posterior margin of the tibia with posterior displacement of the foot rarely occurs in these adduction fractures.

Third Degree Adduction Fractures.—In the third degree adduction fractures the tibia and fibula are broken transversely in their lower third and a supramalleolar fracture is produced.

FRACTURES BY COMPRESSION IN THE LONG AXIS OF THE LEG

These fractures are usually the result of falls from a height in which the patient lands squarely on the foot. They may be the result of a forward thrust of the foot as when the heel is caught in going downstairs, or they may be the result of forcible dorsiflexion of the foot. In the thrust fractures the posterior margin of the tibia is split off and there is a variable amount of posterior displacement of the foot. In the dorsiflexion fractures which are very rare there is a separation of a fragment from the anterior margin of the tibia which tends to be displaced upward and forward. The foot is not as a rule dislocated anteriorly. In the severe compression fractures at the ankle the lower end of the tibia may be comminuted and may be broken in a T or Y pattern and the fibula may also be broken transversely or comminuted (Fig. 1189).

Fractures From Direct Violence are usually crushing injuries and are very likely to be compound, and the bones are likely to be broken transversely (either bimalleolar fractures or supramalleolar fractures). There is not as a rule extensive displacement of the fragments.

Diagnosis of Ankle Fractures.—In severe fractures of the ankle with displacement of the foot on the leg the diagnosis of a fracture can be made at a glance (Fig. 1185), but with fractures of the external malleolus with little or no displacement, the diagnosis between a fracture and a sprain is very difficult and at times impossible without the aid of x-ray examination.

In ankle injuries it is especially important to obtain as accurate a history as possible, and to endeavor to determine the mechanism by which the injury was produced; that is, is the injury one due to external rotation, adduction, abduction, compression in the long axis of the leg, or direct violence? If the surgeon is able to determine the mechanism by which the injury was produced he can predict roughly the type of lesion present and then from his physical examination determine whether it is first, second, or third degree.

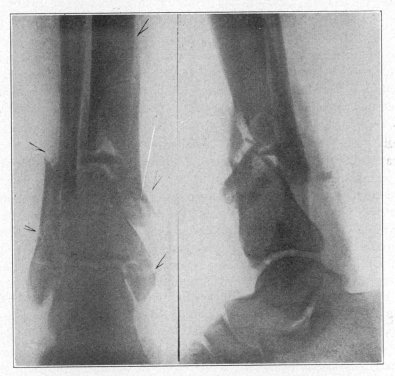

Fig. 1189.—Severe comminuted supramalleolar fracture. Treated by skeletal traction with wire through the os calcis for six weeks; then a long plaster cast.

Having obtained the history, the surgeon inspects the foot carefully and compares it with the other foot, making due allowance for swelling. The important thing to determine is whether or not the foot is displaced on the leg, and in doing this the surgeon must not be deceived by the swelling around the ankle joint, as this may simulate displacement.

If the foot occupies its normal position on the leg, the injury is either a sprain or a fracture with little or no displacement. The degree of swelling is not a safe guide in differentiating between a fracture and a sprain, as a fracture may be present with relatively little swelling, and with a severe sprain extensive swelling may be present. It should be noted especially whether or not there is a rotation deformity or a lateral or a posterior displacement of the foot. If lateral displacement is present, there is either an abduction or an external rotation fracture; and if inward displacement is present, there is an adduction fracture. Posterior displacement may be present with severe abduction or external rotation fractures or with fractures due to compression in the long axis of the leg.

The foot and ankle should be gently palpated in order to determine the points of acute tenderness. Acute tenderness below the external malleolus usually means a sprain. Acute tenderness around either malleolus usually means a fracture of that malleolus, and acute tenderness around the shafts of the bone above the malleoli usually means a fracture at the point of maximum tenderness. During the palpation it is possible to determine the position of the tips of the malleoli and thus to check the presence or absence of deformity as noted by inspection.

The foot is then manipulated, not with the idea of eliciting crepitus, as this is unnecessary and is painful, but in order to determine whether or not false motion is present, whether or not normal motion is limited, and whether or not certain movements elicit pain.

One usually begins by making direct pressure upward on the foot while the leg is fixed. In the case of a sprain, this does not elicit pain. In case of a fracture, even one of the external malleolus without displacement, it usually causes pain. Next with the leg fixed, lateral mobility is determined. This is done by grasping the heel and ankle firmly with one hand and attempting to move it outward and inward on the tibia and not by everting or inverting the foot. If lateral mobility is present there is obviously a fracture either in the lower third of the leg or of one or both malleoli. Relatively little force should be used; otherwise one may increase the displacement. Inversion and eversion of the foot are next attempted. These motions are usually painful and are not very useful in determining whether or not a fracture is present, but they are useful in determining the presence of a supramalleolar fracture, as with eversion or inversion false motion will occur at the site of the fracture above the malleoli.

Finally, the range of motion at the ankle in the anteroposterior plane is tested. If there is no posterior displacement of the foot, dorsiflexion is normal, except as limited by the swelling, but if the foot is displaced backward, dorsiflexion is limited, and limitation of dorsiflexion suggests a posterior marginal fracture with backward displacement of the foot.

The Roentgenogram in Ankle Fractures.—Due to the fact that anatomical reposition should be obtained if possible in every ankle fracture a roentgenogram should be made before the final diagnosis is complete. This is for two reasons: (1) In certain cases the surgeon is not able to determine whether a sprain or fracture is present; and (2) even with the knowledge that a fracture is present, it is not possible by physical examination to determine the details of the lesion, and these are very necessary in planning the treatment. In severe ankle fractures with displacement which are seen immediately after the injury before marked swelling has occurred, however, a rough diagnosis of the displacement and extent of the fracture can usually be made by physical examination, and as the time element is so important in these fractures, it is frequently advisable to reduce the fracture first and then obtain a roentgenogram later rather than delay treatment for several hours while waiting for one.

Prognosis in Ankle Fractures.—The prognosis in ankle fractures is very largely dependent upon whether or not anatomical reposition of the fragments is obtained and maintained over a sufficiently long period. Not only is the ankle joint a weight-bearing joint, but it is one in which the normal contours of the bones must be very accurately maintained if normal function is to be expected. Consequently, unless anatomical reposition is obtained a traumatic arthritis may develop.

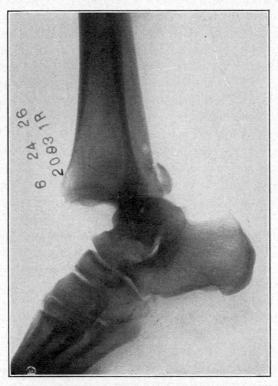

Fig. 1190.—Posterior marginal fracture of the tibia with posterior subluxation at the ankle. Treated by manipulative reduction and immobilization in a cast from midthigh to toes.

It is not enough to restore the normal alignment of the foot with the leg in both anteroposterior and lateral planes, but it is also necessary to restore the contour of the tibial plafond and to replace the malleoli in such a position that they firmly grasp the body of the astragalus. Otherwise a weak and unstable ankle will result. Nonunion is not, as a rule, to be expected. In a case of avulsion or sprain fracture of the tips of the malleoli, however, the torn off fragments sometimes fail to unite. Occasionally even with perfect anatomical reposition, the fracture lines in the articular surface may result in later degeneration of the cartilage and the development of traumatic arthritis. In the average case, however, if union is obtained with the **frag-ments** restored to their normal position, a practically normal ankle may be expected.

Treatment of Fractures and Fracture Dislocations at the Ankle.—From what has been said above, it is obvious that every fracture of the ankle in which slight displacement is present should be manipulated and an attempt made to obtain anatomical reduction. In this manipulation it is important to remember that the malleoli which are broken off tend to move with the astragalus, and that the malleoli which remain intact tend to be separated from the astragalus by a tearing of the corresponding lateral ligament. It should also be remembered that with displacement the lesion is really a frac-ture dislocation at the ankle and that the astragalus is firmly bound to and a part of the foot, and that the foot serves as a handle or lever by which the astragalus can be moved at will.

In the manipulation the object to be aimed at is the restoration of the astragalus to its normal position against the inferior articular surface of the tibia and the squeezing together of the malleoli so that they grasp the body of the astragalus in the normal manner. Also in cases in which the articular surface of the tibia is involved in the fracture it is important to restore the normal contour of this surface.

Consequently, for the purpose of treatment, it is convenient to **divide** ankle fractures into two great groups—those in which the fragments are not displaced, and those in which they are displaced. This is because the fractures in which no displacement exists need not be manipulated, but require immo-bilization, while the fractures with displacement require reduction and immo-bilization.

The second group may then be divided into supramalleolar fractures in which the ankle joint is not involved, and fractures in which the ankle joint is involved. In the supramalleolar fractures anatomical reposition is not necessary, while in fractures in which the ankle joint is involved anatomical reposition is necessary.

This second subgroup of fractures involving the ankle joint is then divided into fractures with lateral displacement, fractures with posterior displacement, fractures with mesial displacement, fractures with upward dis-placement, and anterior marginal fractures with upward displacement of the fragment. Epiphyseal separations are placed in this group because they re-quire anatomical reposition. Finally compound fractures of any type are placed in a separate group as they require special treatment. The following is the classification which we use in determining the type of treatment to be used:

Classification of Ankle Fractures Based on Treatment

1. **Fractures without displacement.** (Require immobilization only.)
   - a. Fractures of the external malleolus.
   - b. Fractures of the internal malleolus.
   - c. Fractures of both malleoli.
   - d. Fractures of the tibial plafond or margins.
   - e. Supramalleolar fractures.

2. Fractures with displacement.   (Require reduction and immobilization.)
   A. Supramalleolar fractures.   (Require functional but not anatomical reduction.)
   B. Fractures involving the ankle joint and epiphyseal separations.   (Require anatomical reduction.)
      a. Fractures with lateral displacement or rotations of the astragalus.
         1. Fractures of the external malleolus with or without rupture of the internal lateral ligament.
         2. Fractures of both malleoli.
         3. Fractures of the fibula with diastasis and rupture of the internal lateral ligament.
         4. Any of the above plus posterior marginal fracture of the tibia.
      b. Fractures with posterior displacement of the astragalus.
         1. Any of group a.   (Fractures with lateral displacement.)
         2. Isolated posterior marginal fractures.
      c. Fractures with mesial displacement of the astragalus.
         1. Fractures of the internal malleolus with rupture of the external lateral ligament.
         2. Fractures of both malleoli.
         3. Fractures of the tibial plafond.
      d. Fractures with upward displacement of the astragalus.
         1. Comminuted fractures of the tibial plafond.
         2. Fractures with marked diastasis at the inferior tibiofibular joint.
      e. Anterior marginal fractures with upward displacement of the fragment.
      f. Epiphyseal separations.
3. Compound fractures at the ankle.

Emergency Treatment of Fractures at the Ankle.—In ankle fractures even more than in most other fractures, it is important that the definitive treatment—that is to say, reduction of the displacement and immobilization of the fracture, be carried out as soon as possible after the injury and before swelling occurs and renders the reduction increasingly difficult.

However, when these fractures have to be transported to a hospital or when for some reason definitive treatment cannot be instituted immediately it is also important that some form of emergency dressing be applied to prevent movement of the foot on the leg with the resultant pain and damage to the soft tissues (Fig. 1191).   The best and most easily applied form of emergency treatment is the pillow splint as described above under the emergency treatment of fractures of the leg.   If this is not available, the ankle may be wrapped in absorbent cotton or other soft material and two lateral board splints applied.   These splints should be padded and should extend beyond the foot, but need not extend above the knee unless we are dealing with a supramalleolar fracture, when they should include the thigh.   When the splint is applied, the foot should be gently straightened and replaced in as nearly as possible its normal position on the leg.

It should be pointed out, however, that this is strictly emergency treatment, and that one of the most serious and frequent mistakes in the treatment of fractures at the ankle is for the physician to postpone the reduction and immobilization until after the swelling has subsided.   The ideal treatment is to reduce the fragment before this swelling occurs.   This will enable the surgeon to obtain a more accurate reduction, and this with immobilization of the leg tends to prevent swelling.   We regard this as so important that we believe that if a roentgenogram cannot be taken immediately a reduction should be attempted without waiting for the roentgenogram because in the case of a recent fracture before swelling has occurred a fairly accurate diagnosis can be made and the normal contours of the bones can be restored by palpation. After the reduction, the control x-ray picture can be made and if necessary the reduction can be repeated.

If extensive swelling has occurred when the fracture is first seen an x-ray picture should be taken, and the fracture should be treated immediately to the best of the surgeon's ability. The surgeon should not wait until the swelling has disappeared; this will take ten days or more. Then, if necessary, further attempts at reduction are in order.

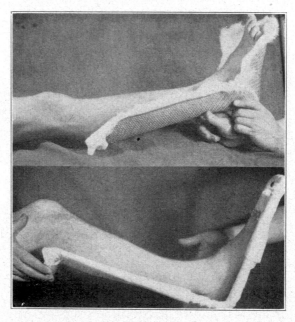

Fig. 1191.—Wire basket and Cabot posterior wire splints for the emergency treatment of fractures of the ankle. Should not be used as a permanent dressing.

Treatment of Fractures at the Ankle Without Displacement.—These fractures constitute a rather large percentage of the fractures at the ankle. They require no anesthetic and no manipulative reduction. All that is necessary is to immobilize the leg, ankle, and foot until union is firm, and this immobilization is most efficiently and conveniently obtained by means of the application of a plaster-of-Paris cast which extends from the toes to the tibial tubercle (or midthigh in supramalleolar fractures) and immobilizes the foot in line with the leg in a position of about 90 degrees dorsiflexion (Figs. 1192, 1193, and 1196).

As was stated in the classification, these fractures include fractures of either or both malleoli, of the articular surface of the tibia or of its margins, and supramalleolar fractures. In other words, they include all of the fractures around the ankle joint, any of which may occur without appreciable displacement of the fragments.

It is important, however, that the surgeon realize that the margins of error are very slight. In other words, in ankle joint fractures even with very slight displacement present, an attempt should be made to reduce the displacement and restore the normal contours of the ankle joint.

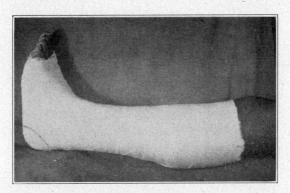

Fig. 1192.—Short plaster-of-Paris cast used only in the treatment of certain isolated fractures of the internal or external malleolus where position is good and fragments are stable. Applied with the foot at right angle to leg. Heel can be cut out if desired, but is seldom necessary.

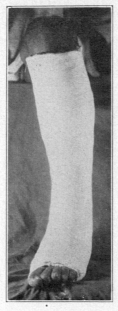

Fig. 1193.—Same as preceding seen from the front. Note slight inversion of foot. This inversion is not always necessary.

Consequently before a fracture in the region of the ankle is classed as one without displacement, anteroposterior and lateral x-ray pictures should be taken and it should be carefully noted whether or not the distance between the malleoli is broadened, whether or not the astragalus is in its normal position, whether or not the external malleolus is pushed backward, whether or not either malleolus is displaced upward, and whether or not the normal contour of the lower end of the tibia is present and whether or not

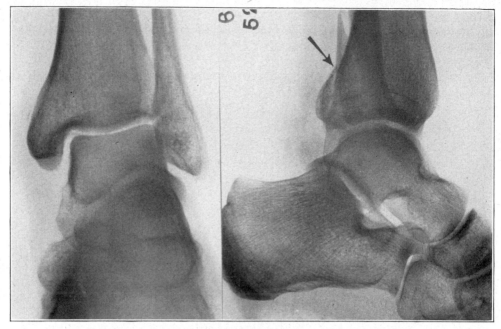

Fig. 1194.—Fracture of external malleolus and a mild fracture of posterior margin of tibia with slight diastasis. Treated by immobilization in a plaster cast for ten days; then, a new snug plaster with a walking iron attached for five weeks.

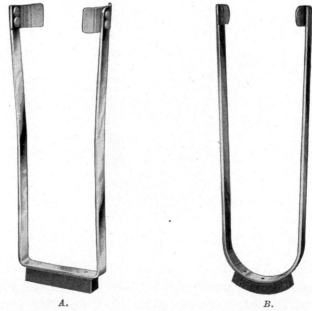

A.   *B.*

Fig. 1195.—*A,* Rubber tread walking heel; *B,* rubber tread walking heel, MacMillan style. (Courtesy Zimmer Manufacturing Co.)

diastasis of the ankle is present. If normal conditions in regard to the above-mentioned points are present, a plaster cast should be applied immediately.

Application of the Plaster.—If the fracture is seen before swelling has occurred, the plaster should be applied over very little padding. If considerable swelling has occurred, a little more padding may be permitted as it will be necessary to change the cast later. The foot should be supported by the surgeon in a position of about 90 degrees dorsiflexion at the ankle joint and in the midposition as regards adduction or abduction so that a line dropped from the center of the kneecap will pass between the first and second toes and a circular plaster-of-Paris cast should be applied. If relatively little swelling is present, a walking plaster is applied. This extends from the tibial tubercle to the toes and may be applied over a single layer of stockinet or directly to the skin. We usually use a skin-tight plaster with a thin layer of sheet cotton around the malleoli. A walking iron or felt heel is fitted to the plaster after it has set. Weight-bearing is permitted after the cast has hardened. (Fig. 1196.)

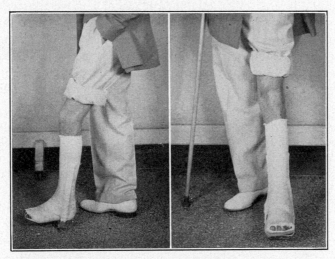

Fig. 1196.—Walking plaster cast or boot with walking iron as used in the treatment of fractures around the ankle or delayed union in the lower one-half of the tibia when weight-bearing is desired.

If the ankle is markedly swollen an ordinary padded plaster is applied and about two weeks later after the swelling has subsided this is removed and a walking plaster cast is applied.

During the first twenty-four hours after the application of the plaster the patient's toes should be watched and if he complains of great pain or if the toes become tensely swollen, cyanotic, and cold the cast should be split, preferably down the dorsum of the foot and ankle and its edges spread enough to relieve the embarrassment to the circulation. If the patient is put to bed with the foot elevated, this will rarely be necessary. No weight-bearing should be permitted in this original cast.

Aftertreatment.—The walking cast is worn for from four to six weeks after the injury, when it is removed and a stirrup strapping of adhesive is applied to the ankle and the patient begins walking in an ordinary shoe. The strapping is continued for two weeks or longer if necessary. It supports the ankle and lessens the swelling which may persist for several weeks.

Treatment of Ankle Fractures With Displacement
(Fracture Dislocations)

These fractures require manipulative reduction with anesthesia, either general or local, according to the preference of the surgeon, and this reduction should be done as soon as possible after the injury. A skillful surgeon should not hesitate to reduce such a fracture without a roentgenogram, depending upon his diagnosis as determined by physical examination and history rather than wait for a roentgenogram and permit swelling to take place.

After satisfactory reduction has been accomplished, the thigh, knee, leg, ankle and foot should be immobilized and for this no splint has yet been devised which is as satisfactory and as effective as a well fitting plaster-of-Paris cast. Some surgeons use a plaster splint such as the anteroposterior and lateral splints of Stimson or the lateral splint of Speed made of molded plaster. However, we prefer a simple circular plaster applied over very little padding and applied with the foot held in a position which maintains reduction and gives the foot as much dorsiflexion as possible. As a rule we do not markedly invert the foot but apply the cast with the foot in a position of slight inversion. The cast extends from the base of the toes to the midthigh with slight flexion at the knee.

As soon as the plaster has set, the patient is put to bed with the foot elevated, and he should remain in this position until pain and swelling disappear. Most writers advise splitting the plaster immediately, but as a matter of fact this is rarely done, even by those who advise it in their writings. The foot should be carefully watched, and if great pain, swelling, cyanosis, or coldness of the toes develops, the cast and padding should be split along the dorsal aspect and spread slightly until the circulation is restored.

This cast may be changed at the end of about three weeks, when a walking plaster may be applied or a new light plaster for simple immobilization or a bivalved plaster for physiotherapy and exercises, according to the dictates of the surgeon.

Weight-bearing is prohibited for a period of from eight to ten weeks, depending upon the severity of the fracture. At the end of this time a shoe with a stiff shank and a longitudinal arch pad is given and the fracture treated just as described above in the treatment of fractures in which no displacement has occurred.

In the reduction of these fractures in which considerable swelling has occurred, it is very helpful if the swelling around the ankle joint and malleolus be kneaded away by strong pressure and deep massage by the thumbs and knuckles of the surgeon until he can obtain a definite idea of the outline of the bones. This pushing away of the swelling and dissipating it into the surrounding tissues would seem to the uninitiated to be quite rough treatment and result in severe traumatism to the soft parts, but as a matter of fact it seems to do no harm at all and greatly facilitates accurate reduction.   One of us (H. E. C.) believes, however, that it is liable to produce emboli and does not use the deep massage.

Probably the most important single factor in the successful treatment in fractures of the ankle is for the surgeon who is responsible for the case to have the courage to tell the patient after his first attempt that the reduction has not been successful and that it will be necessary to try again and perhaps again, but not to be satisfied with an almost satisfactory reduction.   The cause of prolonged and even permanent disability in many of these fractures is due to the natural tendency of all of us to spare the patient a second or third manipulation and to be content with improvement in position rather than anatomical reposition of the fragments.

In rare instances these fractures are best treated by skeletal traction with a Steinmann pin through the heel.   Fractures demanding this type of treatment are those of the articular surface of the tibia with upward displacement which tends to recur after manipulative reduction.   These fractures can be determined by a study of the postoperative roentgenograms.

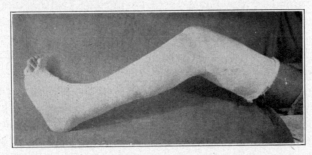

Fig. 1197.—Long plaster-of-Paris cast for severe fractures and dislocations at the ankle.

Very rarely some of these ankle fractures require open reduction.   The ones requiring open reduction are usually those in which the anterior or posterior margin of the articular surface of the tibia has been displaced upward and in which attempts at reposition by manipulation have not been successful.

The methods which we have found useful in manipulating the various types of fractures of the ankle joint will now be described, and it is to be understood that in each instance the manipulation is to be followed by the application of a plaster cast with the foot in the position which is most useful and at the same time most apt to maintain reduction.   Unless stated to the contrary this is with the foot in a position of 90 degrees dorsiflexion and in the neutral position in the anteroposterior plane—that is, at a right angle to the leg and in such a position that a line dropped from the tubercle of the tibia will pass between the first and second toes.

1. **Manipulative Reduction of Supramalleolar Fractures.**—Supramalleolar fractures are really fractures of the leg, and the manipulation is exactly the same as that described above in the treatment of fractures of the leg, except that the anatomical reposition is usually more easily obtained because the bones lie close to the surface.   Reduction is accomplished by traction and

lateral pressure or angulation, depending upon the choice of the surgeon. Traction is made with the knee flexed and the foot in slight plantar flexion in order to relax the tendo achillis. It is advantageous to have the thigh supported by a rigid mechanical support. In most of these cases manual traction will be found sufficient to pull the fracture down to full length and accomplish reduction. Reduction is satisfactory if the fragments are end on and in correct alignment as regards rotation and angulation.

It should be stated that, as in other leg fractures, anatomical reposition of the fragments is not necessary as the joint is not involved. Since the bones are quite close to the surface it is desirable and can usually be obtained without great difficulty. In long oblique or comminuted fractures in this region skeletal traction with a Steinmann pin through the heel may be necessary.

In most of these supramalleolar fractures correct alignment of the fragments can be maintained with the foot dorsiflexed 90 degrees, but occasionally this will cause posterior bowing at the site of the fracture and in these cases the surgeon should not hesitate to immobilize the foot in as much plantar flexion as is necessary to secure and maintain normal alignment as it is more important to obtain union of the bones in their normal position than to prevent structural changes in the soft parts. After the fracture is healed, the tendo achillis can be stretched, or if necessary lengthened by plastic operation. It should also be noted that in these fractures the cast should extend up to the middle of the thigh as it is necessary to immobilize the knee.

Fractures in Which the Astragalus Is Displaced Outward or Rotated Outward.—These include fractures of the external malleolus with or without rupture of the internal lateral ligaments, fractures of both malleoli, fractures of the fibula with diastasis and rupture of the internal lateral ligament, or of both lateral ligaments, and any of the above plus posterior displacement of the astragalus with or without fractures of the posterior margin of the lower end of the tibia.

In all of these injuries it is necessary to replace the astragalus in its normal position and to squeeze the malleoli together on either side of it in their normal positions. If upward displacement is present, this should first be reduced by direct traction which is most effective if it is applied with the knee flexed and the foot in moderate plantar flexion. The knee and thigh can be hung over a table or the back of a chair or over a mechanical rest, or held by an assistant in order to obtain countertraction. The surgeon should grasp the dorsum of the foot in one hand and the heel in the other and make direct traction in line with the leg (Fig. 1198).

As soon as the foot has been pulled down to its normal position on the leg, the posterior displacement, if it is present, should be corrected by pulling the foot directly upward (forward on the leg). In order to do this counterpressure is made upon the front of the lower third of the leg by an assistant or by the surgeon's left hand while his right hand pulls the foot forward on the leg. The late Sir Robert Jones placed a band or loop around the front of the leg and pulled the lower third of the leg backward (downward) with his foot in the loop, while he pulled upward on the heel with both hands. The objection to this method is that it is difficult to apply it with the knee flexed, and flexion at the knee relaxes the heel cord and renders the reduction easier.

When satisfactory reduction of the posterior displacement has occurred, the foot can be dorsiflexed to its normal range without resistance except that due to the swelling (Fig. 1199) and the amount of dorsiflexion possible for the given patient should be determined by examining the opposite normal foot and ankle. The foot should then be strongly inverted to pull the external malleolus back in place and correct the lateral displacement (Fig. 1200).

Fig. 1198.   Fig. 1199.

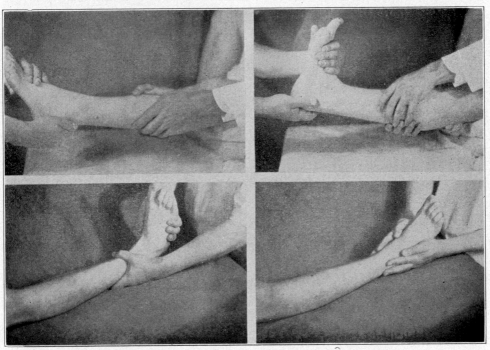

Fig. 1200.   Fig. 1201.

Fig. 1198.—Manipulative reduction of fractures and fracture dislocations at the ankle. With the foot in plantar flexion to increase the deformity, strong traction and countertraction are made to bring the foot down and then it is pulled directly forward to reduce the posterior displacement.

Fig. 1199.—The foot is then dorsiflexed while the traction and countertraction are continued.

Fig. 1200.—The foot is inverted in order to pull the external malleolus down.

Fig. 1201.—With the heels of the hands by direct pressure the malleoli are molded into their normal positions.

It is probable that during the preliminary traction when the foot has been pulled directly downward and strongly inverted most of the lateral displacement will have been reduced and that the astragalus will now be under the lower articular surface of the tibia and in its normal position. If this has not been accomplished, however, it should be pushed under by making counterpressure on the internal malleolus or on the surface of the tibia just above this with the heel of one hand while the heel of the other hand presses directly upon the external malleolus and pushes it and the foot directly inward

(Fig. 1201). If necessary this should be done while an assistant maintains traction in line with the shaft of the tibia. If both malleoli are broken, care must be taken not to displace the foot too far inward.

Finally the swelling should be pushed away from over the external malleolus by massage, and by direct pressure over the bone it should be molded into what appears to be its normal relationship. The foot should then be immobilized in a plaster cast in a position of slight inversion and dorsiflexed about 90 degrees.

In cases in which there has been posterior displacement, care should be taken to prevent a dropping back of the foot on the leg during the application of the plaster. This can sometimes be prevented by maintaining moderate tension in dorsiflexion, but in these cases the plaster should always be applied while the weight of the foot and leg is supported by grasping the forefoot and the plaster should be well molded around the heel, malleoli and tendo achillis. Another method is to apply a posterior plaster mold to the foot and leg and then incorporate this in a circular plaster cast.

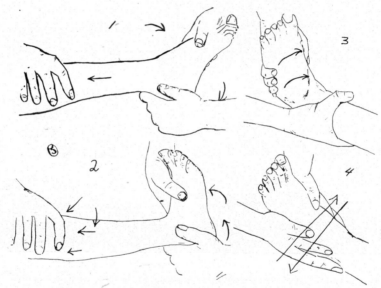

Fig. 1202.—Diagram of the four preceding figures.

The Treatment of Trimalleolar Fractures.—These are so-called Cotton fractures in which, in addition to the fractures of the malleoli, there is also a fracture of the posterior margin of the distal end of the tibia. This last involves the bearing surface of the ankle joint, and it is usual for the posterior fragment to be displaced backward and slightly upward with the foot. This posterior fragment may be small or quite large and may involve one-third or more of the articular surface. The treatment is reduction by manipulation and immobilization in a plaster cast with the foot in the neutral position.

Reduction is accomplished under general anesthesia by placing a series of large sandbags or other support under the knee and a small sandbag under the lower fourth of the leg. Traction is made in the long axis of the leg while an assistant holds the lower leg firmly against the sandbag. Then, when the foot is pulled straight, it is pulled strongly forward at right angles to the leg to reduce the posterior displacement of the foot. The malleoli are now molded into position by lateral pressure and a plaster cast is applied with the foot in the neutral position. Digital pressure behind the malleoli may help to reduce the posterior fragment of the tibia.

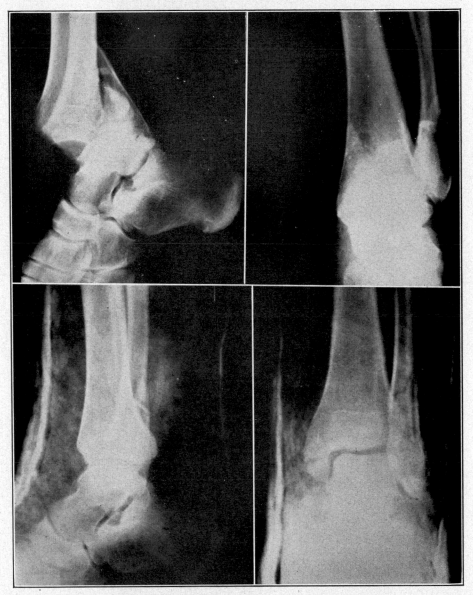

Fig. 1203.—Typical trimalleolar fracture at the ankle before and after manipulative reduction. Reduction satisfactory and open fixation of posterior fragment not necessary. Cast in this type of case should extend from midthigh to toes.

When the position is satisfactory, a plaster cast is applied over a moderate amount of padding. This cast extends up to the middle of the thigh and immobilizes the knee. During its application care is taken to hold the foot well

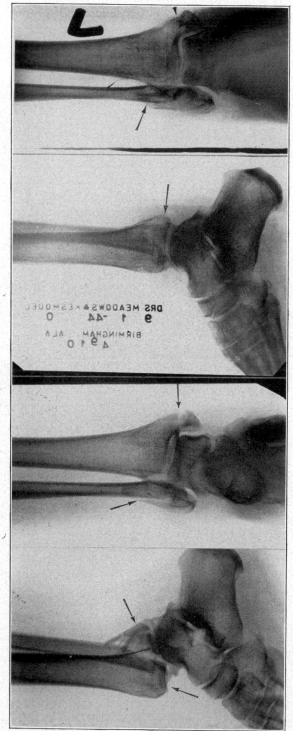

Fig. 1204.—Trimalleolar fracture of the ankle with backward displacement of the astragalus. Treated by closed reduction and circular cast. Excellent functional result without disability in six months.

forward on the leg and this is accomplished by supporting the weight of the leg by holding the foot. The cast is firmly molded around and behind the malleoli.

The cast is left on for two or three weeks and is then replaced by a short skin-tight walking cast. However, if the fracture involves more than one-fourth of the weight-bearing surface of the tibia, weight-bearing is not permitted until eight weeks after the injury.

Open Operation.—In fractures which involve more than one-fourth of the weight-bearing surface of the tibia it is important that anatomic reduction of the posterior fragment be obtained and maintained. An x-ray is taken a day or two after the reduction, and if the position is not satisfactory, an open reduction is in order.

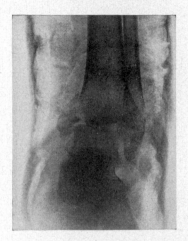 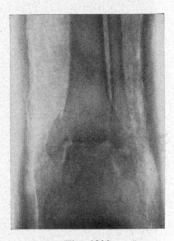

Fig. 1205.   Fig. 1206.

Fig. 1205.—Shows a bimalleolar fracture which has been inverted too much.
Fig. 1206.—Same after a second manipulation. Now in good position.

Operative Reduction.—The patient lies on his face with the lower third of the leg resting on a large sandbag and the foot hanging free. An incision about four inches long is made lateral to the tendo achillis and carried down to the bone. The loose posterior fragment is pushed down into position and fixed by two small nails or screws which should not penetrate the ankle joint. The fracture of the fibula is also exposed and accurately reduced through the same incision and, if necessary, it can be fixed internally with wire or other material. The wound is closed, and a plaster cast is applied as described above.

Internal Fixation of the Internal Malleolus.—Not infrequently in trimalleolar fractures, and also in simpler fractures of the ankle, it will be found that the fragment of the internal malleolus remains displaced distally after reduction and immobilization in a plaster cast. To fail to correct this displacement is to invite nonunion. The fracture is exposed by a short vertical incision and the fragment accurately reduced and fixed with a screw or Kirschner wire.

Manipulative Reduction of Fractures With Mesial Displacement of the Astragalus.—These include fractures of the internal malleolus with rupture of the external lateral ligament, fractures of both malleoli, and fractures of the tibial plafond.

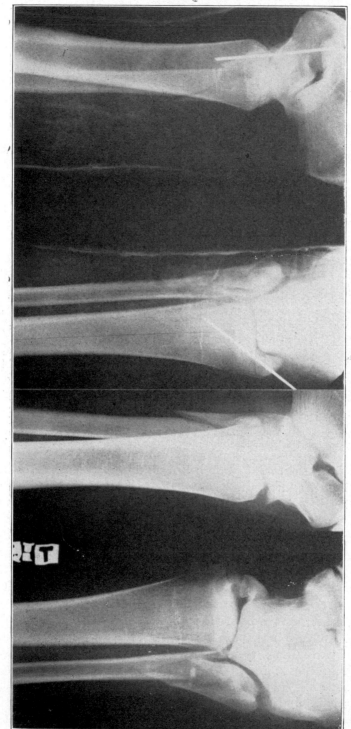

Fig. 1207.—Bimalleolar fracture treated by manipulative reduction and open reduction of internal malleolus with a Kirschner wire which projected through the skin and was removed four weeks after operation. Good functional result.

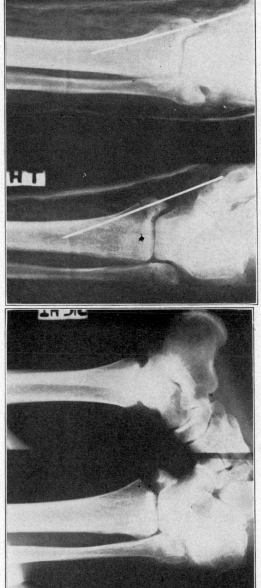

Fig. 1208.—Bimalleolar fracture with wide separation treated by open reduction and fixation with a Kirschner wire. The projecting end of the wire should be bent close to the skin. Good result.

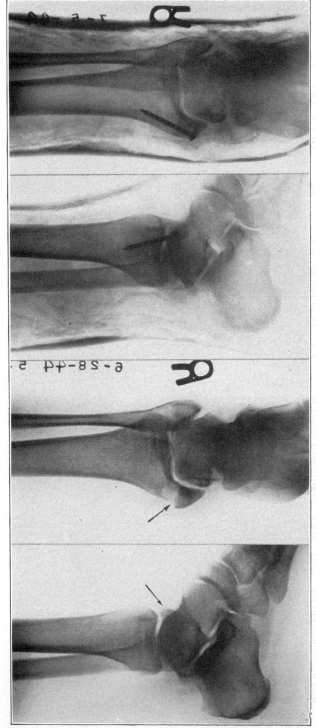

Fig. 1209.—Fracture of internal malleolus with distal displacement. Closed reduction failed and the fragment was fixed with a screw. Excellent functional result with no complications.

Reduction is accomplished as described above under fractures with lateral displacement except that the foot must be pushed outward rather than inward on the leg. Traction is first applied to pull the foot down away from the leg and this is most effectively applied with the knee flexed and supported on a rigid bar or crutch or hanging over the back of a chair or table.

When the foot has been pulled down to its normal position, it is forcibly everted and is then pushed laterally by direct pressure of the heels of the surgeon's hands on the internal malleolus, while counterpressure is made on the external malleolus and the lower third of the fibula with the heel of the other hand. In fractures of both malleoli it is important not to push the foot too far outward, but to restore the normal contour of both malleoli.

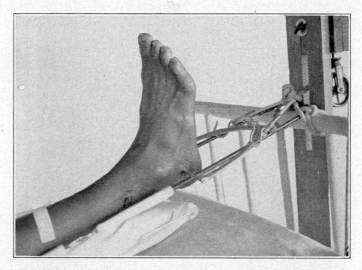

Fig. 1210.—Steinmann pin through the heel with traction as used in fractures at the ankle in which correction cannot be maintained in a plaster-of-Paris cast. The Kirschner wire is also indicated in such cases.

The most difficult fractures of this type to treat are the long oblique fractures of the tibial plafond in which the fracture line begins near the outer margin of the tibial surface and runs upward and inward to emerge on the inner surface of the shaft some inches above the joint. In these fractures the large loose fragment tends to be displaced upward and to carry the foot with it. Sometimes it is very difficult to pull this fragment down into position. The external lateral ligaments are torn, and forcible eversion of the foot does not affect the reduction. In certain instances where it is pulled down, it slips up again immediately if the traction is released. In this type of case the fracture is best treated by a wire or pin through the os calcis with sufficient traction to pull the fragment down and maintain it in normal position (Fig. 1210). This is continued two or three weeks and then a well fitting plaster cast is applied.

Fractures With Upward Displacement of the Astragalus.—These include comminuted fractures of the tibial plafond and those with marked diastasis at the inferior tibiofibular joint in which the astragalus has been pushed laterally and upward, being completely dislocated from the articular surface of the tibia.

The upward displacement is reduced by traction applied as described above with the knee flexed and the thigh supported, preferably by a rigid mechanical support. In severe cases the Boehler screw traction apparatus with the Steinmann pin through the heel may be useful. In the average case the foot can be pulled down into position by manual traction. After this has been accomplished the malleoli should be carefully molded around the astragalus by direct lateral pressure and a plaster cast applied.

If a Steinmann pin has been necessary in the reduction this should be left in place and the patient should be treated with the foot encased in the plaster and traction applied to the Steinmann pin in order to maintain reduction. If it is impossible to restore the normal contour of the articular surface of the tibia, this should be attempted by an open operation. These fractures should be given from ten to twelve weeks' freedom from weight-bearing.

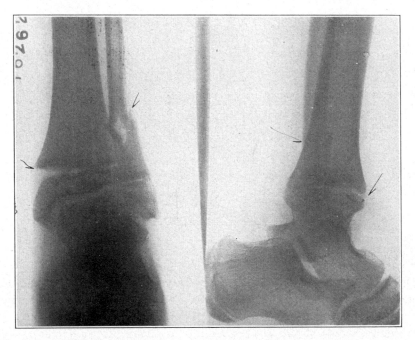

Fig. 1211.—Abduction injury with separation of the epiphysis of the tibia and fracture of the fibula with slight outward displacement. Treated by manipulative reduction under an anesthetic and immobilization in a plaster-of-Paris cast for five weeks. Weight-bearing in eight weeks. Good result.

Manipulative Reduction of Anterior Marginal Fractures With Upward Displacement of the Fragment.—An attempt should be made to pull the anterior marginal fragment down by traction and forcible plantar flexion of the foot. After it has been pulled down direct pressure should be made on the fragment in an attempt to mold it back into its normal position. Then a plaster-of-Paris cast should be applied with the foot in a position of full plantar flexion. This should be left on for three weeks. At the end of this time it can be removed and the foot gradually dorsiflexed.

In case it is not possible to obtain reduction by manipulation the fragment should be exposed by open operation, replaced in its normal position and fixed by sutures or small nails made by cutting sections from a Kirschner wire. These may be left projecting through the skin and pulled out three or four weeks later.

Diastasis at the Ankle.—Any of the above fractures may be complicated by diastasis at the ankle with broadening of the mortise which holds the astragalus. This can be recognized in the anteroposterior x-ray, and it is our experience that when it is recognized in the acute fracture, the diastasis can be corrected after the reduction by firmly pressing the malleoli together. It is reproduced by inverting or everting the foot. Consequently, the foot is then immobilized in the neutral position, and the reduction is maintained by molding the plaster around the malleoli. The tibia and fibula are firmly healed together by the time the fractures have healed.

In old cases with permanent broadening of the mortise open reduction and fixation of the fibula to the tibia are necessary.

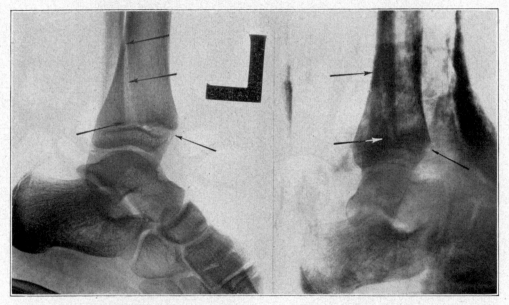

Fig. 1212.—Backward displacement of the lower epiphysis of the tibia in an adolescent with a fracture of the posterior portion of the tibia. Closed reduction. Good functional result.

Manipulative Reduction of Epiphyseal Separations at the Ankle.—In epiphyseal separations at the lower end of the tibia and fibula the epiphyses are as a rule displaced outward (Fig. 1211), but they may be displaced in any direction. (Figs. 1211 and 1214.) The reduction of these is by traction and lateral pressure just as described for supramalleolar fractures except that it is more important that approximately anatomical reposition be obtained, otherwise growth may result in the accentuation of a slight deformity. After reduction the leg and foot should be immobilized in a plaster-of-Paris cast for eight weeks.

Aftertreatment of Ankle Fractures.—In our experience most ankle fractures which require manipulative reduction are not suitable for the immediate application of a walking plaster. If they are reduced very soon after the in-

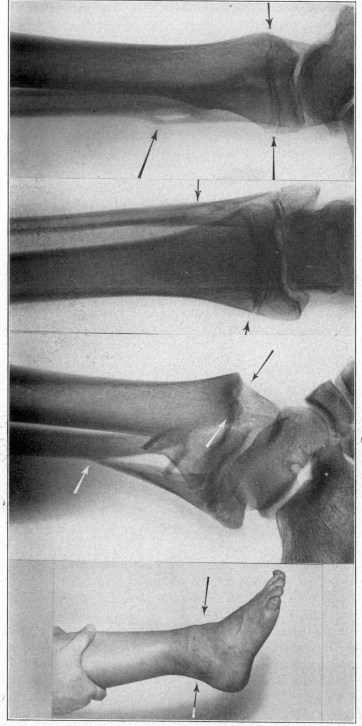

Fig. 1213.—Trimalleolar fracture of the ankle in an adolescent. Reduced by manipulation and immobilized in a cast. Excellent functional result four months following injury.

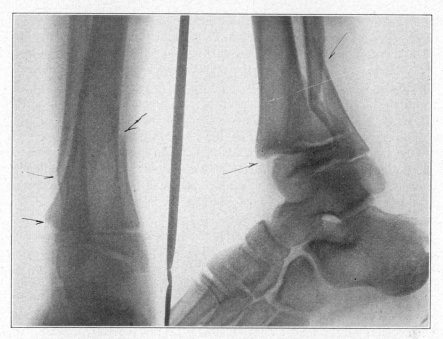

Fig. 1214.—Fracture of the fibula and separation of the epiphysis of the tibia with posterior and inward displacement. Treated by manipulative reduction under an anesthetic and immobilization in a plaster-of-Paris cast for six weeks. Weight-bearing within nine weeks. Good result.

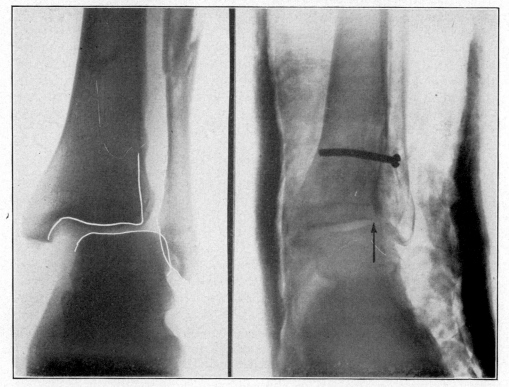

Fig. 1215.—A diastasis of the distal tibiofibular joint. Fixation with screw through the tibia and fibula. (Courtesy of Dr. R. H. Alldredge.)

jury and before extensive swelling has occurred and if the articular surface of
the tibia is not extensively involved in the fracture (more than one-fourth of
the articular surface), a walking plaster may be applied immediately and the patient may begin to bear weight on the foot as soon as the plaster has hardened.

Usually it is advisable to apply a plaster over a moderate amount of padding, and the patient may be up on crutches, but he does not bear weight on
the extremity. About two weeks later when the swelling has subsided, a skin-
tight walking plaster is applied from the tibial tubercle to the toes with the
foot in the neutral position, and this is fitted with a walking iron or felt heel,
and the patient may walk with a cane or without support. In fractures which
involve one-fourth or more of the articular surface of the tibia, we do not permit
weight-bearing until eight weeks or more after the injury and do not use a walking plaster.

The walking plaster is removed about six weeks after the injury, and the
ankle is strapped firmly with adhesive. The strapping is continued for from
two to four weeks until the bones are solidly united and an ordinary shoe is
worn.

DISLOCATIONS AT THE ANKLE

On account of the mechanical efficiency of the mortise in which the astragalus is held and of the strength of the ligaments around the joint, which
in the average individual tend to be stronger than the malleoli, true traumatic
dislocation of the ankle without fracture is an extremely rare lesion. However, occasionally such lesions do occur. The most frequent of these is the
posterior dislocation. The next is the anterior dislocation and the most rare
is the dislocation upward. A dislocation in the lateral plane without fracture
is practically impossible. The fracture dislocations have been considered in
the preceding section on fractures and fracture dislocations at the ankle. In
this section we shall consider them again very briefly along with the true
dislocations and shall merely mention the fractures which are usually present
with a given dislocation.

Posterior Dislocation at the Ankle

Since the mortise of the ankle joint is narrower behind than in front
one would expect posterior dislocations without fracture of the malleoli to be
impossible; however, they are the most frequent form of true dislocations at
the ankle. The reason is that the human foot is more frequently subjected to
trauma in a position of plantar flexion with a strong forward thrust applied
to the leg than it is to trauma in dorsiflexion. The relative frequency of posterior dislocations is also accounted for by the fact that there is no strong
tendon such as the tendo achillis in front of the ankle joint to prevent backward displacement of the foot.

These dislocations are usually accompanied by fractures of one or both
malleoli and of the posterior margin of the tibia. (Figs. 1216 and 1217.)
However, in very rare instances the ligaments may be torn and the bones
may remain intact, the malleoli being slightly spread apart as the astragalus
is forced back between them.

Diagnosis of Posterior Dislocation at the Ankle.—With a complete posterior dislocation the abnormal relation of the foot to the bones of the leg can be seen at a glance and the diagnosis should present no great difficulty. The lower ends of the tibia and fibula project beneath the skin over the front of the ankle and are both visible and palpable in this position, while the distance between the anterior border of the tibia and heel is markedly increased. If the malleoli are fractured, they are displaced backward with the foot and this point can be determined by palpating the lower ends of the bones of the leg and by palpating the displaced foot. In minor backward displacements there is inability to dorsiflex the foot on the leg, the lower end of the tibia is unusually prominent, and the forefoot appears to be definitely shortened while the lengthening of the heel can be determined by measurement.

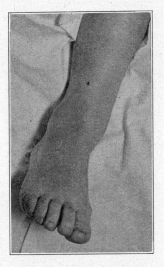

Fig. 1216.—Incomplete posterolateral dislocation at the ankle with fracture of the posterior margin of the tibia. Treated by manipulative reduction and immobilization in a plaster-of-Paris cast.

Treatment of Posterior Dislocation at the Ankle.—The treatment is immediate reduction and immobilization. Reduction should be performed under full anesthesia and is done in the manner described above in the treatment of fractures with posterior dislocation; that is, while countertraction is made on the flexed knee, traction is made on the plantar flexed foot until it is pulled down to its normal position and then it is pulled forward while counterpressure is made on the front of the lower end of the leg. After the foot has been pulled forward on the leg it should be dorsiflexed and the reduction is not to be regarded as complete until full dorsiflexion is possible.

After the reduction the leg and ankle should be immobilized in a plaster-of-Paris cast with the foot maintained in full dorsiflexion and in the neutral position as regards abduction and adduction. The plaster extends from the base of the toes to the midthigh with slight flexion at the knee. If there has been no fracture the periods of immobilization and freedom from weight-bearing are shortened and guarded active motion at the ankle joint may be begun at the end of five weeks. If there has been a fracture—and there usually has been—the treatment is exactly the same as that described above under fractures at the ankle joint. (Figs. 1218 and 1219.)

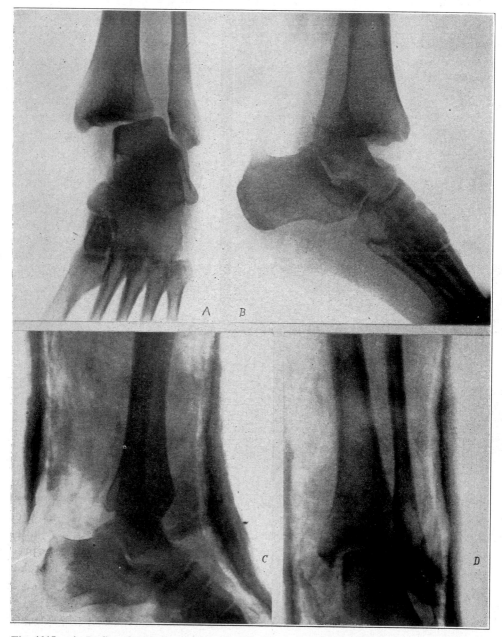

Fig. 1217.—*A, B, C,* and *D* x-ray pictures of case shown in Fig. 1216 before and after reduction.

Anterior Dislocations at the Ankle

Anterior dislocations at the ankle are very rare injuries and are almost always accompanied by a fracture of the anterior margin of the articular sur-

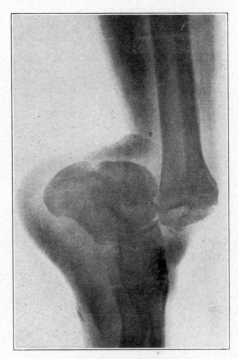

Fig. 1218.—Complete posterior dislocation at the ankle without a fracture of both malleoli. Treated by manipulative reduction and immobilization in a plaster-of-Paris cast. Good results.

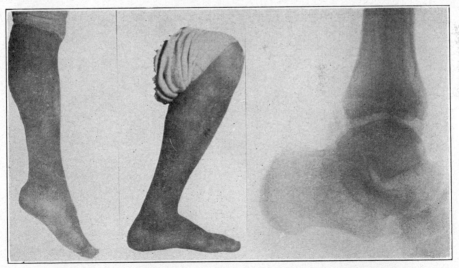

Fig. 1219.—Functional result and roentgenogram of preceding case.

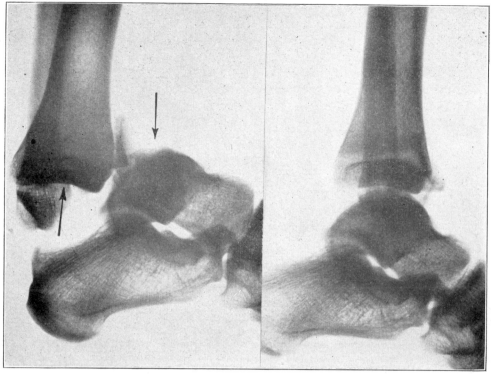

Fig. 1220.—Complete anterior dislocation of the ankle joint. Treated by closed reduction and circular cast from toes to middle third of thigh. Good functional result.

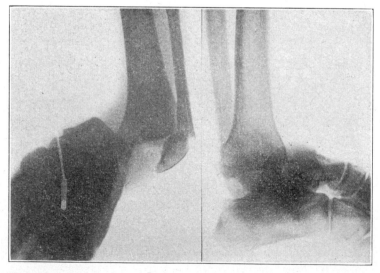

Fig. 1221.—Very unusual anterior and internal dislocation with fracture of the external malleolus. Treated by manipulative reduction and immobilization in a plaster-of-Paris cast with good result.

face of the tibia. They are the result of forcible dorsiflexion of the foot or of falls upon the heel with the foot in a position of dorsiflexion, both of which are forms of trauma to which the human foot is rarely subjected. In addition to the fracture of the anterior margin of the tibia one or both malleoli may be pulled off.

Diagnosis of Anterior Dislocations at the Ankle.—With complete anterior dislocation the diagnosis is not difficult and can usually be made at a glance, as the abnormal relation of the foot to the leg is obvious. The heel is shortened, the lower ends of the bones of the leg are prominent behind and the forefoot is lengthened while the foot is maintained in a position of dorsiflexion. Whether or not the malleoli are detached can be determined by palpating the lower ends of the bones of the leg posteriorly beneath the skin and also by palpating the malleoli in their abnormal position, as if they are fractured they tend to be displaced with the foot, but they may remain in situ (Fig. 1221). As a rule the smooth articular surface of the astragalus can be palpated in front of the lower end of the tibia.

Treatment of Anterior Dislocations at the Ankle.—The treatment is immediate reduction under anesthesia and immobilization in a plaster-of-Paris cast. In an anterior dislocation the reduction is accompanied by slightly increasing the dorsiflexion; then making traction on the foot while the knee is flexed to relax the tendo achillis. This traction disengages the astragalus, and then while counterpressure is made on the posterior surface of the lower third of the leg the foot is pushed directly backward and downward. After the reduction has been completed the foot can be plantar flexed to the normal degree and unless this is possible the reduction is incomplete.

The foot should then be immobilized in a plaster-of-Paris cast in a position of plantar flexion as this tends to maintain the reduction. The cast should extend from the base of the toes to the midthigh with slight flexion at the knee. At the end of three weeks the plaster should be removed, the foot gently dorsiflexed, and a new plaster applied with the foot in dorsiflexion. If there is no fracture, this should be bivalved and active motion begun. Weight-bearing may be begun in five weeks. If a fracture is present, the period of freedom from weight-bearing should be longer (eight to twelve weeks) as described above under fractures at the ankle.

Upward Dislocations at the Ankle

In a compression injury which causes diastasis at the inferior tibio-fibular joint the astragalus may be pushed upward between the bones of the leg (Fig. 1222). This is a rare lesion and when it occurs there is usually considerable comminution of the lower end of the tibia and also fracture of the fibula.

The lesion can be diagnosed by the abnormal broadening of the malleoli and by the approximation of the heel to one or both malleoli.

Treatment is immediate reduction under an anesthetic. The reduction is accomplished by traction directly downward in line with the tibia, while countertraction is made on the thigh with the knee flexed to relax the tendo achillis. When the foot is pulled down to such a point that the superior surface of the astragalus is below the tibial plafond, the malleoli tend to come together again. At this point, while the traction is maintained, strong lateral pressure should be exerted on the malleoli in order to squeeze them together. When the reduction is complete, the foot should be dorsiflexed and plantar flexed in order to correct any backward or anterior displacement and should then be immobilized in a plaster-of-Paris cast in a position of moderate dorsiflexion.

The aftertreatment is the same as that described above for posterior dislocation except that complete immobilization should be continued over a period of at least twelve weeks in order to permit firm healing of the inferior tibiofibular ligaments.

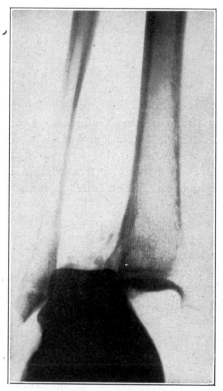

Fig. 1222.—Divergent or upward dislocation at the ankle. A severe type of ankle injury. Reduced by manipulation and immobilization in a plaster cast for eight weeks. Result fair. Ankle weak and painful. Ankle brace worn for several weeks.

Dislocations in the Lateral Plane

These are severe fracture dislocations of the abduction, external rotation, or adduction type as described previously under "Fractures at the Ankle," in which the astragalus has been displaced so far outward or inward that it is completely separated from the inferior articular surface of the tibia and tends to be moved upward. These injuries are often compound.

In these complete dislocations the diagnosis is, as a rule, easy, but considerable difficulty may be encountered in determining the extent and nature of the bone lesions. They should always be differentiated from a supramalleolar fracture, and this is not difficult as with dislocation outward or inward the end of the bone on the opposite side of the leg is usually palpable and the level at which the displacement occurs can be determined.

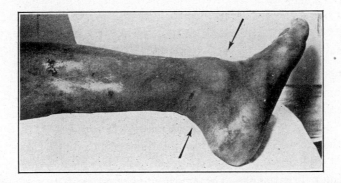

A.

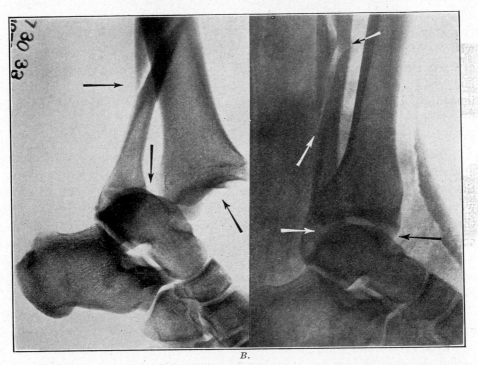

B.

Fig. 1223.—Posterior dislocation at the ankle with fractured lower third of the fibula before and after reduction.

Treatment of Dislocations in the Lateral Plane.—Treatment is immediate reduction under an anesthetic. This can be accomplished by traction on the foot while the countertraction is made on the thigh with the knee flexed. As the foot is pulled downward it should be pressed inward or outward, depending upon the character of the dislocation and should be pulled forward on the leg if necessary. It should be immobilized in a plaster-of-Paris cast in a position of dorsiflexion and this immobilization should be continued over a period of from six to ten weeks, depending upon the severity of the accompanying fracture, as described in the section on "Fractures at the Ankle." The cast should extend from the base of the toes to the midthigh with slight flexion at the knee.

COMPOUND FRACTURES AND FRACTURE DISLOCATIONS AT THE ANKLE

Incidence.—Due to the fact that the bones of the ankle are so close to the skin, compound injuries in this region are relatively frequent. In severe injuries, especially those resulting from falls from a height, the distal end of the tibia or fibula may be driven through the skin and even into the ground; as a result the wound is extensively contaminated with dirt. Likewise in injuries due to direct violence the soft parts are usually lacerated over the bone lesion.

Emergency Treatment.—The emergency treatment in compound injuries differs from that described in simple injuries of the ankle joint in that no effort should be made to reduce the fracture or dislocation immediately as this may result in the carrying of dirt into the depths of the wound. The wound should be covered with sterile gauze if this is procurable or any sort of dressing and the leg and foot should be immobilized on a pillow or a pad made of folded clothes and the patient should be rushed to the hospital for immediate definitive treatment. A tourniquet is rarely necessary as the main blood vessels are seldom torn. If there is arterial bleeding, a tourniquet should be applied.

Definitive Treatment consists of immediate operative cleansing of the wound and should be done as soon as possible after the injury. The principles are the same as those recommended in the treatment of other compound fractures with involvement of joints. On the operating table after the patient is anesthetized the wound is covered with a sterile gauze pad, and the foot and leg are scrubbed with green soap and water and shaved when necessary. The wound is then scrubbed with soap and water, and the entire leg including the wound is washed with alcohol and ether and painted with iodine or other skin antiseptic.

The leg is then draped and the wound edges are excised and any grossly contaminated or devitalized tissue is excised. Then with Dakin's solution or warm normal salt solution the wound and ankle joint are irrigated over a period of several minutes, the bones being spread apart and the ankle joint opened so that the joint is thoroughly washed out. If the ends of the bones have been driven into the dirt, the contaminated portion of the bone is excised with rongeurs, bone cutting forceps, or a chisel, as it is impossible to clean glossly contaminated bone. Loose fragments which are not contaminated and which retain their blood supply should not be removed. Powdered sulfanilamide or sulfathiazole is then implanted in the joint and in the wound. The displacement is then reduced and the wound is closed with silkworm-gut or chromic catgut (interrupted).

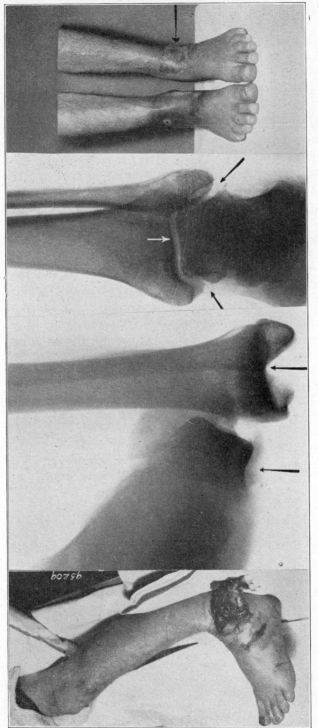

Fig. 1224.—Complete compound dislocation of the ankle joint without fracture. Treated by thorough débridement, reduction, closure of wound, and skeletal traction through the os calcis. Later plaster cast from the toes to the upper third of the thigh. Excellent results.

Often there is considerable loss of tissue and difficulty may be experienced in closing these wounds. Under these conditions a plastic skin flap may be cut by extending the incision upward from the posterior angle of the wound, thus loosening the skin and permitting it to be pulled down. Every effort should be made to cover the area of the fracture with living tissue. A small rubber tissue drain may be inserted or the skin may be sutured rather loosely, thus permitting drainage.

After the fracture has been reduced and the wound has been closed, the surgeon should choose between treatment by traction with a wire or pin through the heel and by immobilization in a plaster-of-Paris cast. In cases with severe soft tissue injury, H. E. C. treats the fracture by traction, and supports the leg in a Thomas splint in order that he may watch it carefully. At the end of about two weeks, when there is no further danger of infection, he applies a plaster cast and removes the pin. J. A. K. uses a plaster cast in practically all cases.

In cases with only moderate soft tissue injury we immobilize the fracture in a plaster-of-Paris cast which extends up to the midthigh just as is recommended above in the treatment of simple fractures. A window is cut in the plaster over the wound, it is inspected on the second or third day, and a clean dressing is applied. It is not necessary to worry about the occurrence of swelling in the plaster in these cases, as the open wound with the drainage takes care of the swelling, so that very little padding is necessary under the cast.

CHAPTER XXVII

INJURIES OF THE FOOT

SURGICAL ANATOMY

The bony framework of the foot consists of seven tarsal bones, five metatarsals and fourteen phalanges. The tarsal bones are the astragalus, os calcis, cuboid, scaphoid and three cuneiforms (Figs. 1225 and 1226). The astragalus has been described in the section on "Injuries at the Ankle." All of these bones are cancellous in structure.

The Os Calcis is a large roughly quadrilateral bone which supports the astragalus and forms the heel. It consists of a body, sustentaculum tali, and tuberosity. The body presents four surfaces and anterior and posterior extremities. The superior surface is divided into a posterior rounded nonarticular portion and an anterior articulating portion. The anterior portion presents two facets for articulation with the inferior surface of the astragalus. These are separated by a transverse groove for the attachment of an interosseous ligament. The inferior surface is rounded from side to side and slightly concave from before backward. It is roughened for the attachment of ligaments and muscles. The relatively flat lateral surface is crossed by a broad groove which extends from above downward and forward. This groove transmits the vessels, nerves, and tendons which pass from the leg to the inner side of the sole of the foot. The anterior extremity consists of a flattened articular facet for the cuboid.

The sustentaculum tali is a shelf-like process which projects from the anterior portion of the mesial surface and overhangs the groove in this surface. It presents a superior articular facet which is continuous with those on the superior surface of the body and aids in supporting the astragalus.

The Tuberosity.—The tuberosity is the enlarged rounded posterior extremity of the body of the os calcis. Its inferior portion is roughened for the attachment of the tendo achillis and its upper portion is smooth and rounded and is separated from the tendon by a bursa.

The Cuboid is a rather large bone which is roughly cuboid in shape and presents three nonarticular and three articular surfaces. The superior, lateral, and inferior surfaces are roughened for the attachment of ligaments and muscles. The posterior surface articulates with the anterior extremity of the os calcis, the anterior surface articulates with the fourth and fifth metatarsals, and the mesial surface articulates with the external cuneiform and occasionally with the scaphoid.

The Scaphoid is a disc-like bone which presents a concave posterior articular surface for the rounded head of the astragalus. Its convex anterior surface presents three facets for the cuneiform bones, and its borders are roughened for the attachment of ligaments and muscles. Its mesial border presents a prominent tubercle which forms the highest part of the anterior arch of the foot.

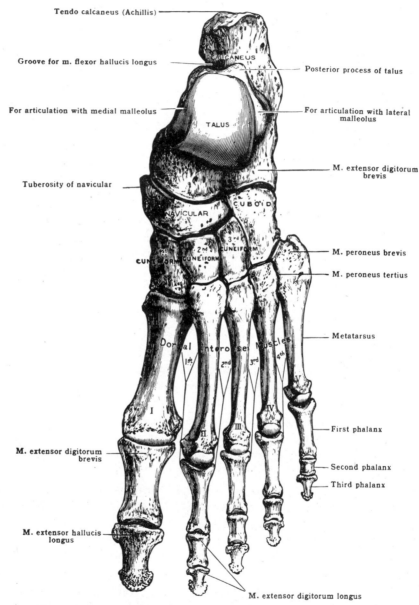

Fig. 1225.—Dorsal view of the bones of the foot in their normal positions. (From Morris: *Human Anatomy*, P. Blakiston's Son & Co., Inc., Publisher.)

The Cuneiform Bones are three wedge-shaped bones which are flattened from side to side and broader on their dorsal than on their plantar aspect. They lie side by side in front of the scaphoid, and their posterior surfaces articulate with this bone while their anterior surfaces articulate with the three inner metatarsals.

The **Metatarsal Bones** are short pipe bones each of which presents a flattened base, a cylindrical shaft, and a rounded head for articulation with the base of the first phalanx of the corresponding toe. The first metatarsal is shorter and much heavier than any of the others. The enlarged base of the fifth metatarsal presents a lateral tuberosity which projects backward and outward and overhangs the joint between this bone and the cuboid.

The **Phalanges of the Toes** resemble those of the fingers, but are shorter and those of the first toe are very thick and strong. There are two for the great toe and three for each of the other toes.

Sesamoid Bones of the Foot.—Two large sesamoid bones are constantly found beneath the first metatarsophalangeal joint and others are occasionally found under the interphalangeal joint of the great toe, or the metatarsophalangeal joint of any of the other toes, or the joint between the fifth metatarsal and the cuboid.

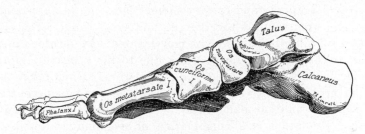

Fig. 1226.—Mesial view of the bones of the foot in their normal positions.

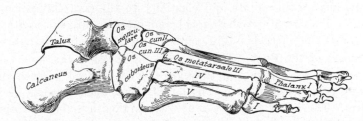

Fig. 1227.—Lateral view of the bones of the foot in their normal positions.

Ossification of the Bones of the Foot.—The os calcis develops from two centers, one for the body and one for the tuberosity. Each of the other bones of the foot develops from a single center. Those for the astragalus, body of the os calcis, and cuboid are present at birth. Ossification centers appear in the external cuneiform during the first year, in the internal cuneiform during the third year, and in the middle cuneiform and scaphoid during the fourth year.

Each metatarsal presents a single epiphysis which begins to ossify in the third year and fuses with the shaft at the sixteenth year. The epiphysis of each of the four outer metatarsals is situated at the distal end (head) of the bone while that of the first metatarsal and of each of the phalanges is situated at the proximal extremity (base).

Anomalous Bones of the Foot.—It is important to know that certain anomalous bones occur in the foot, because the presence of these may lead to an erroneous diagnosis of fracture. The os trigonum is a small bony nod-

ule sometimes present at the posterior margin of the superior articular surface of the astragalus. The os tibiale externum, or accessory tarsal scaphoid,
is a small bone which is found adjacent to the tubercle of the scaphoid at the
point where the posterior tibial muscle is inserted. It may fuse with the
scaphoid and lead to considerable enlargement of this bone and to the development of a prominence on the inner side of the foot.

Rarely sesamoids may be found on the outer border of the foot below
and lateral to the cuboid or in close proximity to the tuberosity of the fifth
metatarsal. The calcaneosecundum is a small bone which is occasionally
present near the calcaneocuboid joint.

Joints of the Foot.—The subastragaloid joint between the astragalus and
the os calcis presents anterior and posterior facets which are separated by
a dense interosseous ligament which binds the two bones together. The joint
is strengthened by the internal and external lateral ligaments of the ankle.

The astragaloscaphoid and calcaneocuboid joints lie in approximately the
same plane and are grouped together as midtarsal joint. This joint as a
whole permits of a limited amount of movement of the forefoot in all directions on the os calcis and astragalus, but due to the relative rigidity of the
lateral border of the foot and to the width of the joint when taken as a whole
this range of movement is quite limited. The movements permitted at the
midtarsal joint are plantar and dorsal flexion, adduction and abduction of
the forefoot. Pronation is a combination of eversion and abduction and
supination is a combination of inversion and adduction.

The tarsometatarsal joints add elasticity to the foot but permit of very
little motion. The metatarsophalangeal and interphalangeal joints are hinge
joints similar to the corresponding joints in the hands and fingers.

The Arches of the Foot.—The bones of the foot are fastened together by
ligaments in such a manner that they are bowed upward in both the anteroposterior and transverse planes. The longitudinal arch consists of inner and
outer pillars. The inner pillar is much the higher and has its apex at the
astragaloscaphoid joint. It includes the three inner metatarsals, the three
cuneiform bones, the scaphoid, the astragalus, and the os calcis. The outer
pillar is practically flat and consists of the two outer metatarsals, the cuboid
and the os calcis. It is thus seen that, beginning at the heads of the metatarsals, the longitudinal arch courses upward and backward to the midtarsal
region, where the two pillars fuse and course downward and backward to
terminate in the tuberosity of the os calcis. The transverse arch is confined
to the forefoot and is usually divided into anterior and posterior transverse
arches. The anterior transverse arch is rather shallow and is formed by the
heads of the metatarsal bones while the posterior transverse arch is rather
sharply and deeply curved and is formed by the anterior tarsal bones.

The Mechanism of the Foot as a Whole.—The body weight is received by
the astragalus from the lower end of the tibia and lines of force radiate
downward and backward to the heel, and downward and forward to the forefoot, being distributed through the longitudinal and transverse arches to the
weight-bearing points which are the tuberosity of the os calcis, the head of
the first metatarsal, and the outer border of the foot. The arch structure is

important in giving the foot elasticity, and it is maintained by the ligaments and muscles which bind the bones together. It is important to remember that the function of the ligaments is to check sudden strains with a tendency to displacement, but that maintenance of the normal arch structure of the foot is due to the strength of the muscles of the leg and foot. This is because ligaments, if subjected to prolonged strain, gradually become stretched and eventually yield and permit displacement. For this reason it is important that the normal muscle balance of the foot be maintained. Otherwise, deformities may be expected to occur. It should also be pointed out that as the foot is everted, the scaphoid tends to be lowered and the longitudinal arch tends to be flattened.

Movements of the Foot.—Flexion, that is dorsiflexion, and extension or plantar flexion of the foot on the leg occur at the ankle joint. The lateral movements are more complex and take place largely in the subastragaloid joint. Deviation of the foot outward in the lateral plane is called eversion or pronation, and deviation inward is called inversion or supination. These movements are usually combined with adduction and abduction which occur largely at the midtarsal joint although in the normal foot very little motion in abduction or adduction can be demonstrated. In the movement of pronation the longitudinal arch tends to be flattened.

FOOT STRAIN, FLATFOOT, OR PRONATED FOOT

In a consideration of the question of foot strain the popular notion is that the efficiency of the foot depends upon the height of the arches and is impaired when they have fallen or broken down. As a matter of fact the height of the arches has relatively little to do with the functional efficiency in the normal foot and many people with very flat feet (Figs. 1228 and 1229) go through life without foot trouble, while others who normally have a high arch may have a great deal of pain and disability in their feet, and on physical examination show relatively little flattening of the arch. In other words, feet should not be treated as flat feet but should be treated by an effort to relieve pain and disability when these occur regardless of the type of architecture which exists.

Foot strain may be divided into two types—acute and chronic. Acute foot strain is one in which a foot becomes sore, swollen, painful and unable to bear weight as a result of some sudden stretching of the ligaments. This sudden stretching of the ligaments may be an acute trauma, such as a fall from a height in which the condition is analogous to a sprain elsewhere except that the plantar ligaments are stretched or torn, or may be due to resumption of weight-bearing after the muscles have been weakened by immobilization in a plaster cast or by a considerable period of freedom of weight-bearing due to illness or confinement to bed as a result of an injury.

Chronic foot strain is one in which the feet have gradually become pronated or everted and the anterior arch is usually gradually flattened as a result of muscle imbalance, or of faulty shoes, faulty posture, or faulty habits in walking so that the ligaments have gradually become stretched, sore, and painful. In chronic foot strain the symptoms are not especially acute and the patient is able to walk, but complains of pain and disability in the foot and the pain is usually localized on the inner border at the height of the longitudinal arch at the astragaloscaphoid joint. It may radiate up the back of the leg. Many of these cases of chronic foot strain have short heel cords and dorsiflexion is limited. In other cases the symptoms are largely confined to the anterior transverse arch. This is tender and on physical examination is seen to be flattened.

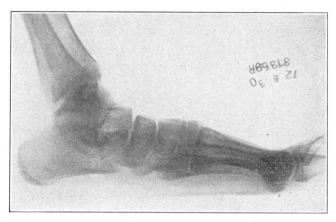

Fig. 1228.—Lateral roentgenogram of a flat or pronated foot.

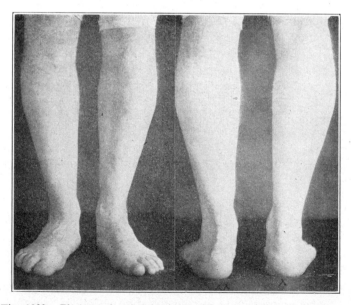

Fig. 1229.—Photographs showing pronated feet, more marked on left.

Treatment of Acute Foot Strain.—In a severe case of acute foot strain complete freedom from weight-bearing should be prescribed for a few days and the patient should be put to bed with the feet elevated. Local heat in the form of bakes or hot soaks is useful in relieving pain, although it probably has no effect upon the healing of the ligaments. As soon as the acute tenderness and swelling have disappeared the foot should be firmly strapped with adhesive applied in such a manner that the foot is held in inversion and the longitudinal and anterior arches are supported (Fig. 1230). Then the patient may be got up, wearing a shoe which has a heel sufficiently high so that when he stands on the foot the short tendo achillis does not throw the foot into pronation. The inner border of this heel should be extended forward beneath the astragaloscaphoid joint and elevated one-eighth to one-fourth of an inch, depending upon the width of the heel. In addition to this an arch support of hard felt, leather, or rubber should be placed in the shoe.

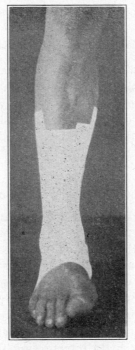

Fig. 1230.—Photograph of foot strapped in inversion in the treatment of flat foot.

As soon as the tenderness has disappeared, the patient should be given exercises which tend to strengthen the muscles that invert the foot and flex the toes. In other words the exercises should consist of inversion, dorsiflexion, and flexion of the toes, the patient being taught to pull the foot upward, turn it inward, and forcibly flex the toes from twenty-five to fifty times twice daily. They should also be taught to walk with the toes pointing straight ahead and with the weight resting upon the outer borders of the feet and to use the toes actively in walking to thrust the body forward. While standing or sitting, the patient should get in the habit of curling the toes in the shoe and pulling the arches upward and resting the weight on the outer borders of the feet. This habit, if once acquired, will gradually restore normal muscle balance and will do it more quickly and more efficiently than will any set of formal exercises. One of us (J. A. K.) instructs practically all of his foot patients to do this exercise off and on during the day and to do it two hundred times a day.

Treatment of Chronic Foot Strain.—In chronic foot strain the preliminary period of rest in bed is not indicated and it is frequently not necessary to strap the feet or give the patient arch supports. Usually all that is necessary is to prescribe a proper shoe; that is, one having a straight inner border with a heel, the inner border of which is elevated, and a stiff shank; to teach the patient to walk properly; that is, with the toes turned in and the weight resting upon the outer border of the foot; to have him acquire the habit of exercising the foot in the shoe; and to prescribe the exercises given above until the symptoms have disappeared. The efficiency of the treatment varies directly with the cooperation obtained from the patient.

FRACTURES OF THE ASTRAGALUS

Incidence and Varieties.—Fractures of the astragalus are rare injuries, but the bone is occasionally broken in falls on the feet from a height. Fracture of the astragalus may occur alone or it may occur in conjunction with fractures of the os calcis or of the ankle. According to the part of the bone which is broken these fractures may be divided into (1) fractures of the posterior process (Stieda's process), (2) fractures of the body, and (3) fractures of the neck.

1. Fractures of the Posterior Process of the Astragalus

These fractures are probably due to force transmitted upward through the heel or to forcible plantar flexion of the foot, the projecting posterior process being broken off by the impaction of the os calcis. The loose fragment is displaced backward and upward a short distance.

Diagnosis of Fractures of the Posterior Process.—Such a fracture may be suspected if after a fall on the heel or forcible plantar flexion of the foot the patient complains of pain in the region posterior to the malleoli, and if there is slight swelling and tenderness in this area with moderate pain on flexing or extending the ankle. In interpreting the roentgenogram it should be remembered that the posterior process of the astragalus may be present as the os trigonum, an anomalous bone, and that the apparent fragment may be a developmental defect and not the result of an injury.

Treatment of Fractures of the Posterior Process.—As a rule no anesthesia is necessary. The foot should be dorsiflexed and an attempt made by deep pressure on either side of the tendo achillis to push the fragment back into its normal position. Then the foot should be immobilized in a plaster-of-Paris cast in a position of dorsiflexion over a period of four weeks. At the end of this time the cast may be removed and the patient may begin to bear weight upon the foot.

2. Fractures of the Body of the Astragalus

The body of the astragalus is made up of quite dense bone and being surrounded and protected as it is by the malleoli, it is rarely broken. However, occasionally in falls on the feet from a height it is crushed between the tibial plafond and the superior surface of the os calcis. In these crushing fractures of the body there may be telescoping of the bone with disorganization of the superior and inferior articular surfaces.

Diagnosis of Fractures of the Body of the Astragalus.—The diagnosis of fracture of the body of the astragalus is difficult in the absence of positive roentgenograms and in the absence of a roentgenogram it may be impossible to differentiate it from certain fractures of the os calcis. Fracture of the astragalus may be suspected when after a fall on the feet the regions in front of and behind the malleoli are swollen and tender and when there is no puffiness of the heel such as is present in fresh fractures of the os calcis. As a rule there is not sufficient displacement or telescoping of the bone to enable one to note a shortening of the distance between the malleoli and the ground. The patient is unable to bear weight upon the leg, and movements of the ankle joint are limited and painful.

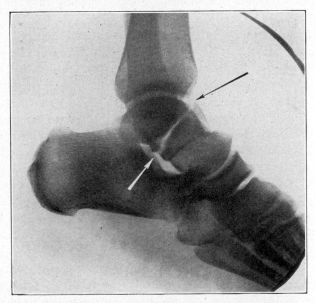

Fig. 1231.—Simple fracture through the body of the astragalus with no displacement. Treated by plaster cast. Union and good functional result.

Treatment of Fractures of the Body of the Astragalus.—Treatment of fractures of the body of the astragalus depends upon whether or not telescoping with disorganization of the articular surfaces has occurred. In cases with no displacement no anesthetic is necessary and the foot and ankle should be immobilized in a plaster-of-Paris cast with the foot held in a position of dorsiflexion and in the neutral position as regards adduction or abduction. This cast should be left on for from six to eight weeks, depending upon the age of the patient, and no weight-bearing should be permitted during this period. In certain cases a Boehler walking plaster with' an iron heel as described under fractures of the leg may be applied at the end of the second week and the patient may then begin to walk in the cast as soon as it is dry.

In fractures with displacement an attempt should be made to reduce the displacement and restore the normal contours of the articular surfaces. This demands very strong traction which is most effective if it is applied with the foot in slight plantar flexion and with the knee flexed to relax the tendo achillis. As the foot is pulled forcibly down away from the leg, the telescoping is corrected and there is a certain tendency for the fragments to slip into their normal positions. When this has been done and the impaction broken up, the foot should be gently dorsiflexed and plantar flexed through the normal range in order to restore the contour at the ankle joint, and gently inverted and everted in order to restore the contour at the subastragaloid joint.

If there is little tendency to displacement after the reduction, a posterior plaster mold incorporated in a cast or a plaster cast extending from the mid-thigh to the toes should be applied with the knee in a position of moderate flexion and the foot in dorsiflexion. The cast should be removed in six or eight weeks and exercises commenced; weight-bearing may be begun in ten or twelve weeks.

If manual manipulation fails to obtain a satisfactory reduction, the surgeon should resort to skeletal traction with a pin through the os calcis. The traction may be applied by hand or by the Hawley table with Conwell's knee-thigh countertraction apparatus or by means of the Boehler traction apparatus.

After the reduction these severe fractures should be treated in traction over a period of about three or four weeks. Traction is best applied with the Steinmann pin through the heel, and the foot may be supported in a plaster-of-Paris cast or Thomas splint. At the end of this time a well-fitting plaster-of-Paris cast is applied; weight-bearing is not permitted until ten or twelve weeks have elapsed after the fracture. If one wishes, however, a Boehler walking plaster can be applied four weeks after the injury and the patient may begin to walk on this as soon as it is hard.

3. Fractures of the Neck of the Astragalus

These are the most frequent injuries of the astragalus, but even they are quite rare fractures. They, too, are usually the result of falls upon the feet; but in addition to the crushing of the bone between the tibia and os calcis, there is a certain amount of shearing force which tends to break the neck transversely and to cause upward, and usually inward, displacement of the distal or head fragment (Figs. 1232 and 1233). In certain instances this vertical fracture through the neck lies well posterior, even into the body of the bone, and the astragalus is split vertically in the frontal plane. With this type of injury the posterior portion including most or all of the body of the bone may be displaced backward and so tilted that the fracture surface points downward against the os calcis (Figs. 1236 and 1237).

With a complete fracture of the neck or with a vertical fracture through the junction of the neck and body, it is unusual not to find displacement.

Diagnosis.—With the vertical fractures through the neck, the forefoot is usually displaced slightly upward and inward on the heel. There is marked swelling and tenderness around the front of the ankle, and it may be possible by deep palpation to detect the sharp proximal edge of the distal fragment. With posterior displacement of the body of the bone, there is marked swelling beneath the tendo achillis and the displaced bone can be palpated by deep palpation in this area. The diagnosis should be confirmed by an x-ray picture.

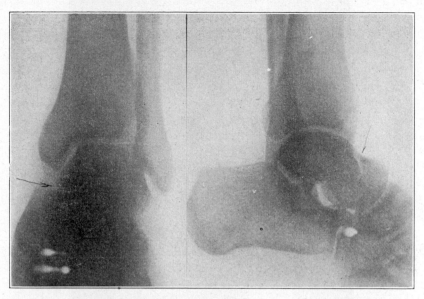

Fig. 1232.—Fracture of the neck of the astragalus with practically no displacement. No reduction indicated. Treated by immobilization in a plaster-of-Paris cast with foot at right angle to the leg. Good result.

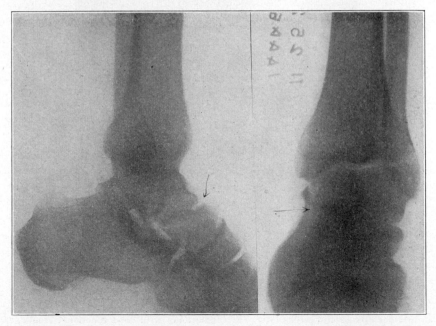

Fig. 1233.—Fracture of the posterior portion of the neck of the astragalus with slight displacement and involvement of the subastragaloid joint. Treatment: General anesthetic. Foot brought to almost a right angle to the leg, cast applied with the foot in the midposition, the cast extending from the base of the toes to the midthigh. The cast remained on for seven weeks, bivalved on fifth week. Hot baths commenced daily the sixth week. Weight-bearing in nine weeks. Good result in five months.

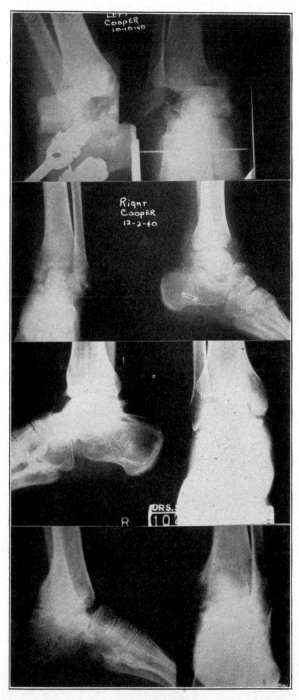

Fig. 1234.—Severe comminuted fracture dislocation of the astragalus. Closed reduction with aseptic necrosis several weeks later. Astragalectomy with good functional result. (Courtesy Drs. Schrock and Johnson.)

Treatment.—In cases with practically no displacement all that is necessary is to immobilize the foot and leg in a plaster-of-Paris cast over a period of eight weeks. At the end of this time the plaster may be removed and the patient may begin to walk, but he should wear a shoe with an arch support. In cases in which the forefoot is displaced upward and inward this can as a rule be reduced by forcible plantar flexion combined with traction and aided by direct pressure on the displaced fragment. With the thigh immobilized or supported on a mechanical support, an assistant should pull the foot downward directly away from the leg and then slowly plantar flex it and abduct it. During this maneuver the surgeon should make direct pressure with his fingers upon the displaced distal fragment. The foot should then be slowly dorsiflexed and immobilized in a plaster-of-Paris cast in a position of moderate dorsiflexion and slight inversion. Weight-bearing should not be permitted until eight weeks after the injury.

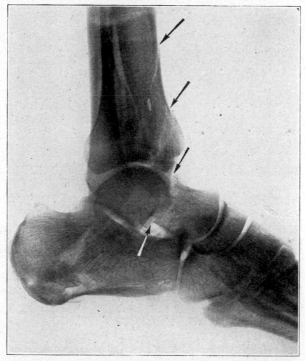

Fig. 1235.—Severe fracture involving the tibia, astragalus, and os calcis. Very little displacement is present. Treated by immobilization in a plaster-of-Paris cast for eight weeks, beginning weight-bearing at the end of ten weeks. Moderate restriction of motion at ankle but no pain.

In rare cases in which the body of the bone is displaced backward and so tilted that its fractured surface faces downward while its inferior surface faces backward, the reduction is more difficult, but is carried out in much the same manner. Strong downward traction is made on the foot with the thigh flexed and the foot in a position of plantar flexion, thus pulling the os calcis away from the tibia. This unlocks the displaced body of the astragalus which is caught between the os calcis and the tibia, and after this has been accomplished, the body can be pushed forward by direct pressure on either side

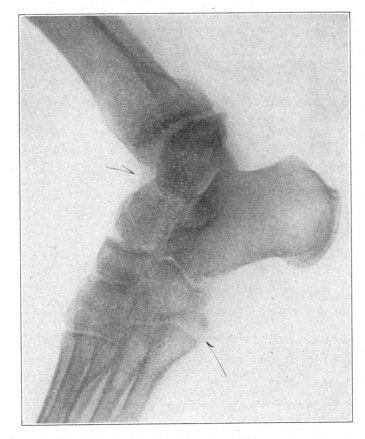

Fig. 1236.—Fracture through the neck of the astragalus with a rotation dislocation of the body of the astragalus. Closed reduction unsuccessful.

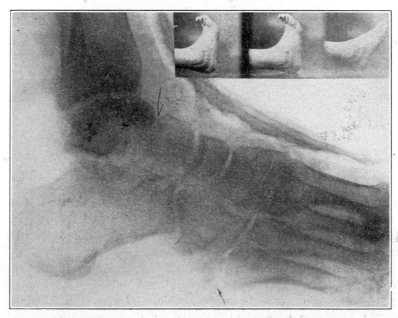

Fig. 1237.—Result obtained in preceding case by open reduction and subastragaloid arthrodesis.
(Courtesy Dr. John D. Sherrill, Birmingham, Alabama.)

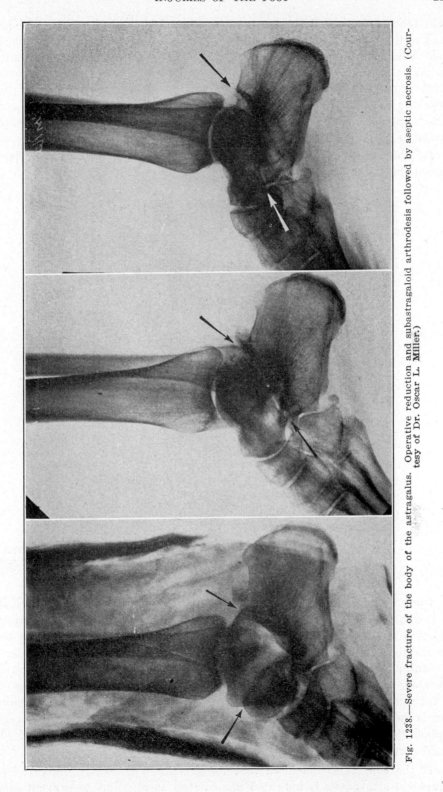

Fig. 1238.—Severe fracture of the body of the astragalus. Operative reduction and substastragaloid arthrodesis followed by aseptic necrosis. (Courtesy of Dr. Oscar L. Miller.)

of the tendo achillis and the foot can be slipped backward and slowly dorsi-flexed so that as the body is pushed forward into its socket the detached neck of the bone is brought up against it. The foot should then be immobilized in a plaster-of-Paris cast in a position of moderate plantar flexion as forcible dorsiflexion tends to redislocate the body of the bone. At the end of three weeks the cast can be removed and the foot slowly dorsiflexed and a new plaster applied. This cast should be worn for five weeks and no weight-bearing is permitted during this time without support.

In many of these fractures of the neck the Boehler walking cast can be worn at the end of two weeks after the injury.

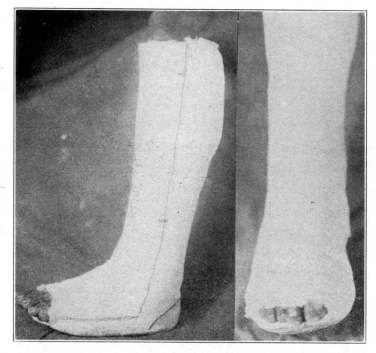

Fig. 1239.—Type of plaster cast used in the treatment of *most* fractures of the astragalus and the tarsal and metatarsal bones. The foot is at a right angle to the leg and in the neutral position. In certain severe fractures of the astragalus and os calcis the cast should extend to midthigh. With moderate flexion on the leg at the knee.

Open Reduction in Fractures of the Astragalus.—In cases in which it is not possible to reduce the displacement of the body by manipulation an open reduction should be performed immediately (Figs. 1236 and 1237). In badly comminuted fractures in which it is not possible to obtain satisfactory reduction by manipulation an open reduction is indicated, and the fragments should be accurately reduced and the articular surfaces restored. If the foot remains pain-ful for some months after the fracture has healed, an arthrodesis of the painful joint is indicated. This may be the ankle, the subastragaloid or the astragalo-scaphoid joint, or it may be necessary to fuse all of the above joints. This should give a painless foot with some limitation of movement.

If the body is so displaced that its circulation is largely destroyed pan-astragaloid arthrodesis is indicated immediately in an effort to prevent aseptic necrosis. If aseptic necrosis occurs later, the arthrodesis should be attempted, and if this fails, the astragalus should be removed and an attempt made to ankylose the tibia and the fibula to the os calcis by bone.

In some clinics an astragalectomy is preferred to the arthrodesis, but this decision must be left to the surgeon. Personally we rarely perform the operation of astragalectomy except as a means of treating sepsis with infection of this bone, and then we try to fuse the tibia and fibula to the os calcis.

FRACTURES OF THE OS CALCIS

Incidence.—The os calcis is fractured more frequently than any of the other tarsal bones and in various series these fractures comprise from 1 to 2 per cent of all fractures. During recent years considerable attention has been paid to fractures of the os calcis because most of the cases occur in laboring men and the resultant compensation and prolonged disability have forcibly impressed the importance of these injuries upon industrial surgeons. As a result considerable advancement has been made in the treatment in efforts to lessen the permanent disability and shorten the time away from work.

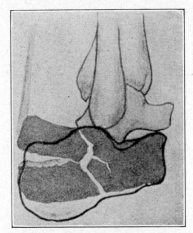

Fig. 1240.—Avulsion fracture of the tuberosity of the os calcis with comminution of the body of the bone. (Figs. 1240 to 1244 from Conn, H. R.: Ohio State M. J. 1928.)

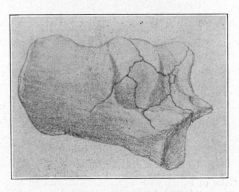

Fig. 1241.—Comminuted fracture of the body of the os calcis with involvement of the sub-astragaloid joint. (Conn.)

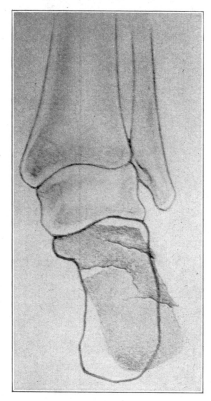

Fig. 1242.—Comminuted fracture of the os calcis with eversion of the tuberosity. (Conn.)

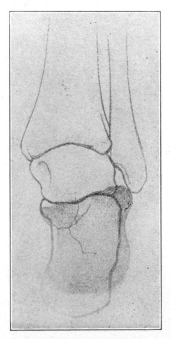

Fig. 1243.—Telescoping of the os calcis with upward displacement of fragments under the external malleolus. (Conn.)

Classification.—There are numerous classifications of these injuries. The one which we use is a slight modification of that devised by H. R. Conn.* This classification is useful, not because all fractures of the os calcis can be made to fit into the groups provided, but because it directs attention to the lesions which are the cause of disability in these injuries and which must be recognized and corrected if a useful foot is to be obtained. In fact all of the lesions enumerated in the classification may be present in a single severely crushed heel. Consequently, one injury may comprise the entire classification, but if this is true, all of the lesions must be corrected if a useful foot is to be obtained. The classification is as follows (Figs. 1240, 1241, 1242, 1243, and 1244):

1. Avulsion fractures of the tuberosity or separation of the apophysis.
2. Fractures of the medial and lateral processes of the tuberosity.
3. Isolated fractures of the sustentaculum tali.
4. Fractures of the body of the os calcis.

   a. Fracture with eversion of the tuberosity.
   b. Fractures with upward displacement of the tuberosity.
   c. Telescoping fractures with lateral mass driven up under the external malleolus.
   d. Comminuted fractures into the subastragaloid joint.
   e. Comminuted fractures of the anterior portion of the body into the calcaneocuboid joint.

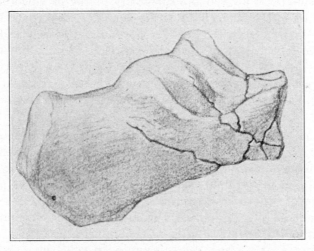

Fig. 1244.—Comminuted fracture of the anterior portion of the os calcis with relatively little disturbance of the rest of the bone. (Conn.)

1. Avulsion Fractures of the Tuberosity or Separation of the Apophysis

Cause.—These are rare injuries which are the result of sudden strain on the tendo achillis in which a portion of the tuberosity is torn off and displaced upward. They may be caused by falls upon the balls of the feet or by muscular action in jumping; they are especially apt to occur when sudden

*Conn, H. R.: Ohio State M. J., 1928.

strain is put on atrophic bone after the foot has been immobilized in plaster for a long time on account of some other lesion.

Pathology.—The avulsed fragment may vary from a small sliver of bone beneath the tendo achillis to a large mass of bone comprising the posterior portion of the tuberosity. In younger patients the apophysis may be pulled off before it has united to the rest of the bone and even in adult patients the fracture line tends to coincide rather closely with the apophyseal line. These avulsion fractures should be distinguished from those of the body of the bone in which there is also a fracture of the tuberosity with upward displacement of a separate fragment, as these latter are not true avulsion fractures, but are the result of crushing injuries.

In the true avulsion fractures the detached fragment is not the main insertion of the tendo achillis as most of this is inserted into the lower portion of the tuberosity while the separated fragment usually comprises a portion of the upper border of the posterior surface. In rare instances the entire insertion of the tendo achillis may be pulled off and displaced upward. In the average case there is relatively little displacement.

Diagnosis of Avulsion Fractures of the Os Calcis.—The history of the accident may enable the surgeon to suspect an avulsion fracture. This is especially true if the accident occurred while running or jumping or if the patient is sure that in a fall from a height he landed on the balls of his feet rather than upon the heels. On physical examination there is considerable swelling and tenderness around the tuberosity of the os calcis and posterior to the malleoli on either side of the tendo achillis, while there is practically no swelling or tenderness in the anterior portion of the foot and ankle. The patient is unable to bear weight upon the foot and has pain when he attempts to plantar flex the foot against resistance. On palpation it may be possible to feel the separated fragment in the space between the tendo achillis and the posterior surface of the tibia. The diagnosis should be confirmed by the x-ray.

Prognosis in Avulsion Fractures of the Os Calcis.—If the fragment is small, the injury is not a serious one and a normal foot may be expected after a few weeks' immobilization in a plaster-of-Paris cast. If the fragment is large and displaced upward, it must be replaced and held in position until union is obtained. Otherwise a painful heel may result. If the entire insertion of the tendo achillis is avulsed, this must be replaced and occasionally sutured in position if a normal foot is to be obtained.

Treatment of Avulsion Fractures of the Os Calcis.—The treatment is replacement of the fragment and immobilization of the foot in a position of plantar flexion in a plaster-of-Paris cast until union has occurred. Whether or not replacement is necessary must be determined by the physical examination and the roentgenogram. If the fragment is small and the displacement is slight, immobilization is all that is needed. If the fragment is rather large and so displaced that it forms a mass of bone beneath the tendo achillis, or if the insertion of the tendon is torn off, it must be replaced. This can usually be accomplished by manipulation under either local or general anesthesia.

In order to replace the fragment, the knee is flexed to relax the tendo achillis and the foot is plantar flexed to bring the main mass of bone as close as possible to the displaced fragment. Then by direct pressure of the thumbs on the displaced fragment in the space beneath the tendo achillis it should be pressed down into position. Once it is reduced, if the knee is maintained in flexion and the foot is maintained in plantar flexion, there will be relatively little tendency for displacement to occur, and a plaster cast should be applied from the midthigh to the toes and well molded around the tendo achillis and tuberosity of the os calcis in order to immobilize the fragment.

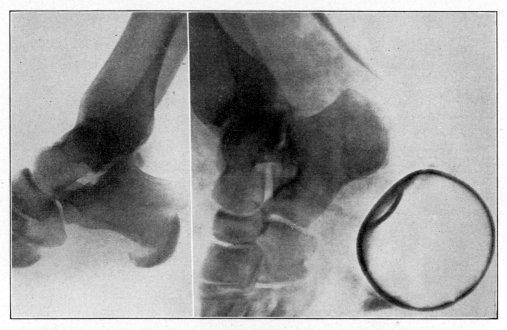

Fig. 1245.—Fracture of the tuberosity of the os calcis. Reduced by pressure from a rubber ball incorporated in the cast. (Courtesy Dr. George E. Moore.)

The original plaster should be left on for three or four weeks, depending upon the severity of the injury. At the end of this time the plaster should be bivalved and the foot very gently dorsiflexed and the knee straightened. A new plaster should be applied with the foot in as much dorsiflexion as can safely be obtained without danger of displacing the fragment; this cast need extend only to the tuberosity of the tibia. This cast should be left on for from two to four weeks, depending upon the severity of the injury, when it should then be removed and the patient may begin gradually to bear weight upon the foot. He should be given exercises to strengthen the muscles of the foot and leg.

If the fragment is large and manipulative reduction is not successful, the surgeon is justified in doing an open operation and replacing the frag-ment and fixing it in position either with a small nail or screw or by sutures. This can be done through an incision along the mesial border of the tendo achillis, and it is not necessary to cut the tendon. After the operation the foot is immobilized in slight plantar flexion.

2. Fractures of the Medial and Lateral Processes of the Tuberosity of the Os Calcis

G. E. Moore* has described a fracture of the tuberosity (Fig. 1245) in which a portion of the posterior and inferior part of the tuberosity is broken off and tends to be displaced toward the sole of the foot. The fracture is said to be due to lateral compression of the heel and is treated by immobilizing the foot and leg in a plaster cast in plantar flexion and incorporating a rather large soft rubber ball in the cast. The ball is so placed that its pressure tends to push the loose fragments back into place.

3. Fractures of the Sustentaculum Tali

These are very rare injuries which are caused by forcible inversion of the foot with the result that the sustentaculum is compressed against the inferior surface of the astragalus and either broken off or crushed into the body of the bone.

Diagnosis.—There is usually a history of a fall upon the inverted foot accompanied by sharp pain on the inner side of the foot and inability to bear weight while motions at the ankle joint are relatively free and accompanied by little pain. On physical examination there is a variable amount of swelling over the inner surface of the bone and acute tenderness just below the tip of the internal malleolus. The os calcis may appear to be slightly displaced outward and the foot tends to be held in a position of pronation. The diagnosis should, of course, be confirmed by the roentgenogram, but this is apt to be negative as the sustentaculum is difficult to show. Speed recommends a diagonal x-ray picture through the inner side of the foot in order to throw the impacted or displaced sustentaculum into profile.

Prognosis.—Unless the normal contour of the arch of the foot is restored, a flat foot will result and this may be painful over a long period.

Treatment.—If the sustentaculum is displaced, an attempt should be made to replace it. Under local or general anesthesia the foot should be inverted and plantar flexed, the head of the first metatarsal being pulled well down in the plantar direction and the forefoot pronated in order to restore the arch while direct pressure is made upward against the sustentaculum along the inner border of the foot. When satisfactory reduction has been obtained, the foot should be immobilized in a plaster-of-Paris cast in a position of plantar flexion and inversion of the heel with the forefoot pronated. The cast should extend from the toes to the tuberosities of the tibia and should be worn for six weeks. At the end of this time the cast may be removed and the patient given a shoe with the heel elevated one-eighth to one-fourth of an inch on the inner border and a hard felt arch support in the shoe.

4. Fractures of the Body of the Os Calcis

Fractures of the body of the os calcis are the most frequent of all the fractures of the tarsal bones and comprise about 90 per cent of such injuries. The great majority of the cases are due to falls upon the feet from a

*Moore, G. E.: Surg. Gynec. & Obst., 1933.

height, the mechanism of the fracture being a crushing and splitting of the os calcis by the body weight transmitted through the astragalus as the heel strikes the ground. The posterior portion of the astragalus acts as a wedge and tends to be driven into the body of the os calcis. Due to the mechanism of the injury, these fractures are not infrequently bilateral. The fractures vary from a simple crack in the bone without displacement which may be very difficult to demonstrate even with the x-ray to severe crushing injuries in which the bone is severely comminuted and distorted in its outline.

Due to the nature of the injury and to the cancellous structure of the bone, these fractures tend to be impacted when displacement of the fragments occurs. In cases of severe injury, the fracture may be compound. Most of the compound fractures of the os calcis, however, are the result of direct crushing injuries of the heel in which the soft structures are lacerated directly by the fracturing force.

As the great majority of the os calcis fractures are caused by a fall from a height, they may occur in connection with other grave injuries, such as fracture of the skull, spine, pelvis, femur, or leg, and in such cases the fracture of the os calcis may be overlooked at the time of the original examination.

Pathology of Fractures of the Body of the Os Calcis: (a) **Fractures with Eversion of the Tuberosity.**—Due to the fact that when the foot strikes the ground it is usually pronated with the tuberosity of the os calcis directed outward, backward, and downward, it tends to be carried upward, outward, and forward, permitting the sustentaculum to be displaced downward and the long arch of the foot to be flattened. There is usually an oblique fracture line through the tuberosity which communicates with vertical and transverse fractures. This main transverse line extends in a more or less horizontal direction across the posterior portion of the body and tends to be opened on its mesial aspect while the lateral surface of the bone is compressed and the tuberosity is displaced outward. As the heel is forced outward, the scaphoid becomes unusually prominent and the malleoli are brought closer to the ground than normal.

(b) **Fractures with Upward and Forward Displacement of the Tuberosity.**—As the astragalus is driven into the superior surface of the os calcis, it tends to break it in a more or less transverse direction and to force the middle of the bone downward, thus creating a relative upward displacement of the tuberosity (Figs. 1246, 1247, and 1248). This upward displacement is increased and maintained by the contraction of the tendo achillis. Due to the fact that the tuberosity of the os calcis is tilted downward and backward at an angle of about 45 degrees, force applied from beneath tends not only to drive the tuberosity upward, but also to drive it forward, thus telescoping the bone and shortening it in the long axis of the foot. In some cases the tuberosity is split in its long axis in a horizontal plane and the superior fragment is pulled upward to a greater degree than is the inferior one. This upward and forward displacement of the tuberosity is usually combined with the lateral displacement mentioned above.

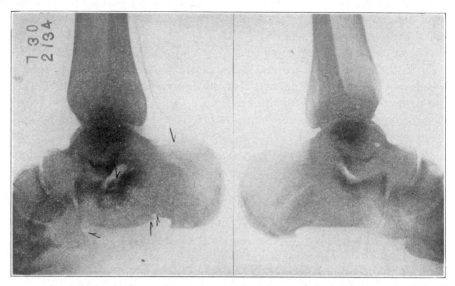

Fig. 1246.—Comminuted fracture of the os calcis with moderate upward displacement of the tuberosity. Treated by reduction on block under general anesthetic. Right angle position of foot to leg, inversion of foot at ankle. Cast extending from toes to midthigh with knee flexed 30 degrees. Good result.

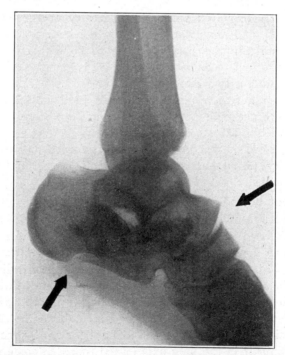

Fig. 1247.—Comminuted fracture of the os calcis with marked upward displacement and shortening of the posterior half of the bone. There is also a subluxation of the astragalo-scaphoid joint. Treated by subastragaloid arthrodesis and scaphoid-cuboid-astragaloid arthrodesis. Good result.

(c) **Telescoping Fractures with a Lateral Mass Driven Up Under the External Malleolus.**—This fracture is similar to that with eversion and is always one in which the tuberosity is displaced upward, but instead of being deviated outward without shortening, the tuberosity is forced directly upward and forward and its lateral surface is telescoped and impacted. As a result of force of the injury, some of the fragments are driven up beneath

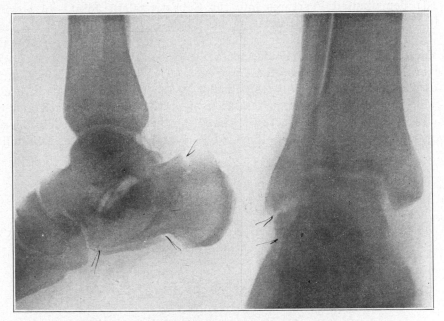

Fig. 1248.—Severely comminuted fracture of the os calcis with shortening and upward displacement. The anteroposterior view shows lateral mass of bone beneath the external malleolus. Treated by the Boehler method cast to midthigh with moderate flexion of leg at knee. Good result.

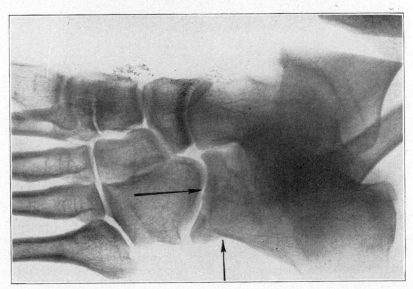

Fig. 1249.—Fracture of the anterior portion of the os calcis shown by an oblique view of the foot.

the external malleolus, especially near its posterior border (Fig. 1248). In these fractures the body of the bone is broadened and the heel is shortened, the long arch of the foot is lowered, and the tuberosity may or may not be everted. The lateral mass of bone driven up under the external malleolus encroaches upon the space occupied by the peroneal tendons and causes irritation of these tendons and of the adjacent bone.

(d) **Comminuted Fractures into the Subastragaloid Joint.**—In most of the fractures in which the fragments are displaced one or more of the fracture lines involve the articular surface of the joint between the astragalus and the os calcis and this articular surface may be severely comminuted with more or less displacement of the fragments (Fig. 1250). The comminution and displacement of fragments which make up the articular surface is of considerable importance because unless accurate reduction is obtained and the normal contour of the joint surface restored, the patient will probably develop a traumatic arthritis in the subastragaloid joint and suffer prolonged disability.

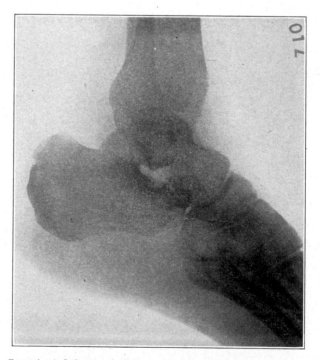

Fig. 1250.—Comminuted fracture of the os calcis in which the tuberosity is split longitudinally and in which the anterior portion is involved. The tuberosity is also displaced upward. Treated by reduction under a general anesthetic. Right angle position of foot to leg, inversion of foot at ankle. Cast from toes to midthigh with knee flexed 30 degrees. Good result.

(e) **Comminuted Fracture of the Anterior Portion of the Body of the Os Calcis.**—This is a rather rare type of compression fracture in which that portion of the bone which lies in front of the sustentaculum tali is shattered, while the posterior portion of the bone may or may not be broken. This type of fracture should be recognized because the fracture lines involve the calcaneocuboid joint, and unless accurate reduction is obtained, traumatic arthritis may supervene in this joint and result in prolonged disability.

Prognosis in Fractures of the Body of the Os Calcis.—A severe fracture of the body of the os calcis with comminution and displacement of the fragments may result in prolonged disability and necessitate operative treatment even after skillful reduction and immobilization of the fragments. The deformities which it is necessary to correct if the surgeon is to guard against pain and disability afterward are: (1) eversion and upward and forward displacement of the tuberosity; (2) excess bone behind and below the external malleolus; and (3) disorganization of the subastragaloid or calcaneocuboid joints with resultant traumatic arthritis.

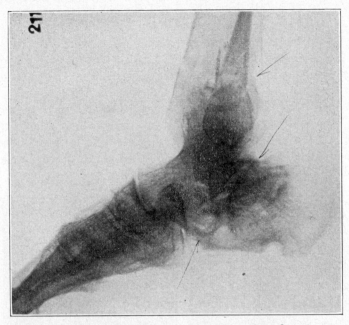

Fig. 1251.—Old fracture of the os calcis in which the displacement was not reduced. The patient has worked as a painter during the past ten years with no disability. There is a recent supramalleolar fracture.

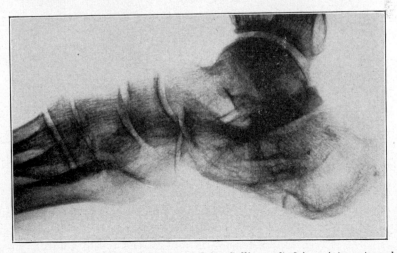

Fig. 1252.—Old fracture of the os calcis treated by Gallie graft driven into a tunnel through the posterior subastragaloid joint.

It should be mentioned, however, that inefficient reduction is not always followed by disability. We have seen many cases in which there was considerable displacement of the fragments and in which either no reduction was attempted or attempts at reduction failed, and yet these men have serviceable feet and do not have pain after prolonged walking or standing (Fig. 1251). It is for this reason that we do not recommend immediate arthrodesis of the subastragaloid and calcaneocuboid joints in cases in which the surfaces of the joints are fragmented.

Diagnosis of Fractures of the Body of the Os Calcis.—In the average case there is a history of a fall upon the feet followed by severe pain in the injured heel and inability to bear weight upon the foot. Swelling occurs soon after the accident and involves not only the entire heel, but also the middle portion of the foot and the ankle (Fig. 1253). The heel is broadened from the swelling and from the bony deformity (Fig. 1254). In addition to being swollen, the tissues on either side of the heel have a definite bluish tint. This is due to the fact that the skin is thin and the subcutaneous tissues are infiltrated with blood. The long arch of the foot is flattened due to the upward displacement of the tuberosity and the sagging of the inner border of the foot, and the malleoli are lowered on account of the upward displacement of the tuberosity.

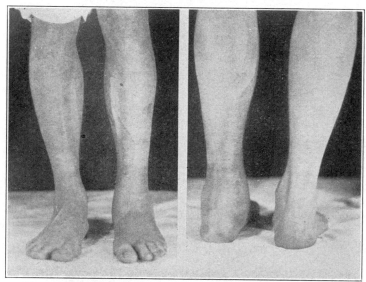

Fig. 1253.   Fig. 1254.

Fig. 1253.—Fracture of the left os calcis seen from the front. Note that the swelling involves the entire foot.

Fig. 1254.—Fracture of the os calcis seen from behind. Note the broadening of the heel and the lowering of the malleoli.

On palpation the tissues on either side of the heel have a rather characteristic elastic or semifluctuant consistency due to the fact that the subcutaneous tissues are infiltrated with blood. In spite of the swelling, motion at the ankle joint is free unless tension is put on the tendo achillis, when pain is felt in the heel, but lateral motion, which occurs at the subastragaloid joint, is limited and painful. The presence or absence of eversion and the presence or absence of excess bone behind and below the external malleolus can usually be detected by careful palpation. Lowering of the malleoli, unless it is very slight, can be detected by measuring the distance between the tips of the malleoli and the inferior surface of the heel. Likewise the heel may be definitely shortened due to the impaction and this can be determined by noting the distance between the posterior surface of the heel and the posterior border of the external malleolus. The upward and forward displacement tend to relax the tendo achillis (Hoffa's sign).

In fractures in which there is upward displacement of the tuberosity, with or without eversion, it may be assumed that fracture lines are present in the subastragaloid joint. If there is considerable acute tenderness over the anterior portion of the bone and if other evidences of fracture are present, it may be assumed that fracture lines involve the calcaneocuboid joint.

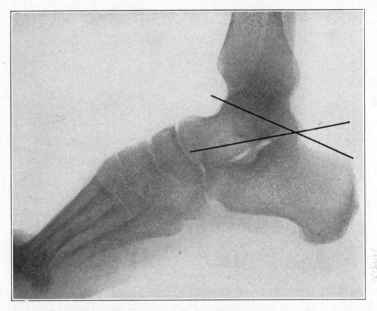

Fig. 1255.—Roentgenogram of normal foot showing Boehler's tuber joint lines. The included angle is about 40 degrees.

It should be pointed out that the diagnosis is not complete with the determination as to whether or not a fracture of the os calcis exists, but an attempt should be made to determine the extent and type of fracture and the degree of the displacement. This can be done to a certain extent by inspection and palpation, but the details of the fracture must be learned from the roentgenograms.

X-ray Examination.—The x-ray examination is important in these fractures, because it is only by this means that the surgeon is able to learn approximately with what he is dealing and thus direct his treatment in such a way that he will obtain correction of the various deformities.

Lateral roentgenograms of both heels should be taken and Boehler has pointed out that the angle of lines drawn parallel to the subastragaloid joint and to the superior surface of the tuberosity give a very important criterion by which to judge whether or not upward displacement has occurred. In the normal individual these lines should meet at an angle of about 40 degrees (Fig. 1255). With upward displacement of the tuberosity these lines tend to approach one another and be parallel, or the angulation may even be reversed. In addition to the anteroposterior and lateral views there should be a posteroanterior view which is taken obliquely through the heel with the foot dorsiflexed as much as possible, the x-ray tube being placed opposite the sole of the foot (Fig. 1256). This third view shows the lateral deviation, the presence of excess bone below the external malleolus and vertical splits through the bone (Fig. 1257).

Treatment of Fractures of the Body of the Os Calcis.—The first thing to be decided is whether or not reduction is necessary. If displacement exists it should be corrected. Consequently every fracture of the os calcis should be subjected to a careful x-ray study before treatment is instituted.

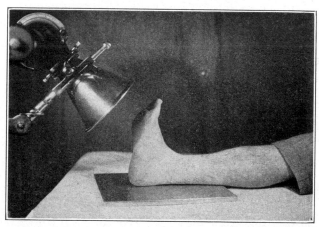

Fig. 1256.—Position of the tube and the x-ray in getting a posteroanterior view of the tuberosity of the os calcis.

Treatment of Fractures of the Body of the Os Calcis Without Displacement.—These are rather rare cases in which the fracture is limited to one or more cracks in the bone. In these cases all that is necessary is to apply a plaster-of-Paris cast over relatively little padding which extends from the toes to the midthigh. The cast is applied with a few degrees of flexion at the knee. The patient may be got up on crutches as soon as the cast is solid. This cast should be left on for four weeks. At the end of this time it may be removed and a new cast may be applied which extends from the toes to the tibial tubercle. This may be a walking cast or not, and it should be left on for four weeks or more when the patient may begin to walk with a felt arch pad in the shoe.

Prognosis in this type of fracture is a normal foot if the os calcis is protected from weight-bearing until union is firm.

Treatment of Fractures of the Body of the Os Calcis with Displacement of the Fragments.—In these injuries the displacement should be reduced if a normal foot is to be expected. As was stated in the section on pathology, the deformities which demand correction are the following:

1. Upward displacement and shortening of the posterior portion of the body of the tuberosity.
2. Lateral deviation of the tuberosity.
3. Broadening of the bone, especially with displacement of fragments in the region below and behind the external malleolus.
4. Disorganization of the subastragaloid joint.
5. Disorganization of the calcaneocuboid joint.

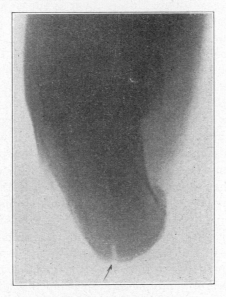

Fig. 1257.—Posteroanterior view of fracture of the os calcis showing vertical split in the tuberosity.

In order to correct these displacements, the following maneuvers are indicated: (1) the tuberosity and posterior portion of the body must be pulled downward and backward, while the center of the bone is pressed upward until the normal arch of the foot is restored; (2) if the tuberosity is deviated outward it must be pushed inward until the normal weight-bearing line of the heel is restored in the anteroposterior direction; (3) after the upward displacement and shortening and lateral deviation are corrected, the bone must be compressed laterally until it is restored to its normal diameter; (4) if the correction of the preceding deformities has not restored the contour of the articular surface, nothing short of an open operation will affect them, and this should not be considered in the primary treatment of these cases. Consequently the disorganization of the joint surfaces must be ignored for the time being and if, after union has occurred and function has been resumed, these joints are painful, arthrodesis of the involved joints should be considered.

Correction of the Upward Displacement and Shortening of the Bone.—The surgeon should decide whether or not this displacement can be corrected by manual manipulation or whether it will be necessary to introduce a pin either through or above the os calcis in order to pull the bone down and back. We do not believe that it is ever necessary to lengthen the tendo achillis in order to obtain reduction in these fresh fractures of the os calcis, since, if the manipulation is carried out with the knee in flexion, the tendo achillis will be relaxed, and if it is then immobilized with the knee flexed and the foot plantar flexed, there will be little tendency on the part of the tendon to cause displacement.

Manipulative Method of Yoerg.—Since one of us (J. A. K.) examined a large series of cases treated by Dr. O. W. Yoerg (Surgery, October, 1937) a few years ago, we have adopted this method as our routine procedure for the treatment of fractures of the body of the os calcis with displacement. His description is as follows:* (See Fig. 1263.)

"It is not necessary that the fracture be reduced immediately after the injury. In most cases swelling to some degree is present and occasionally the fracture is compounded. Several days should elapse and the patient should remain in bed with the foot elevated and with continuous applications of hot packs to relieve pain and to aid in reducing the swelling. Frequently, it becomes necessary, on account of swelling, to wait for a week or ten days, but more than two weeks should not be allowed before attempt at reduction.

"No one will deny that an impacted fracture with displacement must be disimpacted before the fragments can be replaced. If this is true in a Colles fracture it is also true in fractures of the os calcis. Impactions in fractures of the os calcis are always firm because of the severe force inflicted when the accident occurs. The amount of force required to disimpact the fracture must necessarily also be great, and the surgeon must acquire courage which will allow him to use sufficient force to break up the impaction. It must be admitted that forceful and only forceful manipulation can bring this about without open operation.

"Disimpaction can best be accomplished by placing the anesthetized patient on his affected side on a firm table, preferably a Hawley table. The injured foot is brought to the edge of the table, with the heel extending over the edge. A felt pad is placed between the foot and the table. With the left hand the surgeon firmly grasps the ankle and leg just above the ankle. The right hand grasps the heel and manipulates it laterally with sudden forceful thrusts exerted through the ball of the hand. A tremendous amount of force may be applied without danger of damage so long as a firm grip is maintained with the left hand, and only the heel itself allowed to project over the edge of the table. This thrusting force is repeated until disimpaction can be felt. Occasionally, in very firm impactions, it may be necessary to apply the compression clamp to start disimpaction and the heel can then be fully disimpacted by further manipulation.

"Disimpaction having been accomplished, we can proceed in reducing the fragments to their normal or nearly normal positions. If there is a depression of the posterior joint surface, as in the severe types, this depression must be raised into position to restore the carrying angle, or salient angle as described by Boehler. Any loss of this angle, even when no depression of the posterior

*Lancet: 59: 530, 1939.

joint surface occurs, must be corrected to normal or nearly normal. Both of
these conditions can be corrected by the same procedure, as follows:

"The patient, still on his affected side, is pulled up on the Hawley table
with the hip and knee flexed and the foot in plantar flexion. The forward

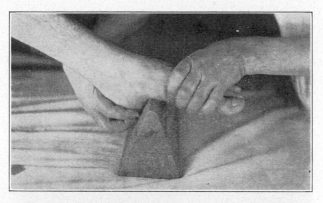

Fig. 1258.—Manipulation of the foot over a wedge in an effort to reduce the upward displacement of the posterior portion of the os calcis and restore the arch of the foot.

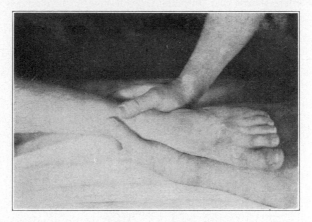

Fig. 1259.—Lateral compression of the os calcis with the heels of the hands in an effort to
restore the normal contour of the bone.

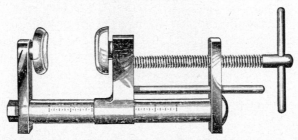

Fig. 1260.—Boehler's foot vise for correcting broadening of the os calcis. (Courtesy Zimmer
Manufacturing Co.)

portion of the foot is grasped with one hand, the heel with the other hand, and
the sole of the foot is then pulled with sudden forceful thrusts against a vertical
bar inserted in the usual slot in the middle of the table. After we have disimpacted the bones and restored the angle, the fragments are still loose and broad-

ening is still present.   An os calcis clamp is applied to squeeze the loosened
bones further into position and to overcome the broadening.   If the anterior
portion of the os calcis is fractured, the clamp must be moved forward and reapplied to overcome any spreading which may be present in this portion of the
bone.   It is well to measure the width of the uninjured heel with the calibrated
os calcis clamp and when it is applied to the injured heel to close the clamp
one-half inch more than on the well heel.

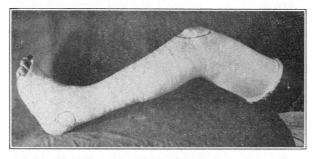

Fig. 1261.—Plaster-of-Paris cast extending from the toes to the midthigh with the knee in
a position of moderate flexion to relax the posterior leg muscles used in the treatment of fractures of the os calcis.

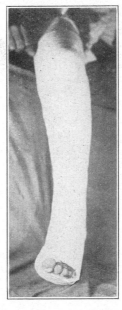

Fig. 1262.—Same as preceding seen from front. Note that the foot is in slight inversion.
Fractures of the os calcis are the only fractures of the tarsal bones which are treated with the
foot in inversion.

"Roentgenograms should then be made and if reduction is satisfactory,
the patient is turned on his back and a moderately padded boot cast is applied.
The knee is held flexed, and the foot in full plantar flexion. The patient is pulled
down on the table with the leg extending at right angles at the knee over the
edge of the table. The surgeon sitting on a low stool molds the cast well under
the malleoli and over the back of the heel, keeping firm traction over the back

of the heel and with the sole of the foot resting on the surgeon's flexed knee to build up an arch in the drying cast. The knee is flexed and the foot is in full plantar flexion in all of the procedures.

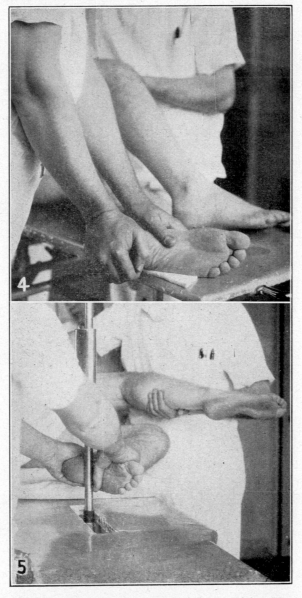

Fig. 1263.—Manipulative reduction of fractures of the os calcis. Above, the impaction is being broken up over the edge of the table and below the arch is being restored by hammering the arch of the foot against the post of the fracture table. (Courtesy of Dr. O. W. Yoerg, Minneapolis.)

"The patient is allowed to be up on crutches in a few days and is discharged from the hospital, but is not allowed weight-bearing. One month after reduction, the cast is removed, as union is then sufficiently firm so that a cast is no longer necessary, but not firm enough for weight-bearing. The patient is instructed to move the foot actively and passively, and to use vigorous massage and manipulation for one month. At the end of this month, or two months after reduction, union is firm enough for weight-bearing. The patient is instructed to walk on the foot, using his crutches, but is encouraged to discard support as soon as possible. He continues his massage and manipulation and is taught to rise on his toes frequently to strengthen the plantar and calf muscles.

"Massage and persistent use of the foot play an important part in early recovery. It is only by early mobilization that we can expect return of muscular and joint function. The patient is encouraged to return to work as soon as possible as only in regular prescribed work will recovery be hastened. We all know that unemployment breeds laziness and that it is easier to sit than to walk when some soreness exists in a foot."

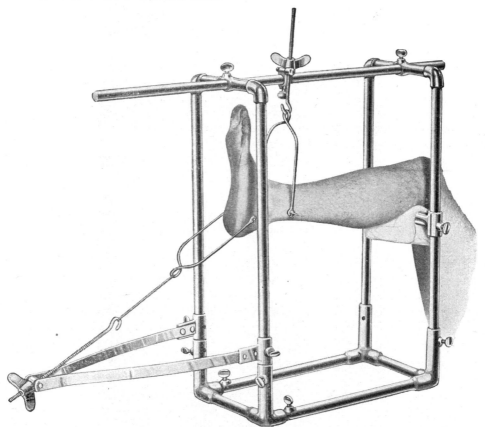

Fig. 1264.—Boehler's apparatus as used in the reduction of fractures of the os calcis. (Courtesy Zimmer Mfg. Co.)

Boehler's Method of Reduction of Fractures of the Os Calcis.—In order to obtain traction on the os calcis in line with the long axis of the bone, Boehler[*] has recently devised and published an original method in which two steel pins or drills are used in conjunction with his screw traction apparatus for the leg. (Fig. 1264.) It aims at correction of the axial deviation, flattening, shortening, and broadening of the bone. The correction is maintained by

[*]Boehler: J. Bone and Joint Surg. 13: 75-89, 1931.

two pins which are incorporated in a plaster cast. The reduction is performed from six to ten days after the injury, when much of the swelling has disappeared.

Under general or spinal anesthesia, the swelling is removed by pressure massage, and the impaction is broken up by placing the sole over a wooden wedge and forcing the foot into strong plantar flexion (Fig. 1258). If this is not successful, the tuberosity is gripped in the os calcis vise and moved to and fro.

The points where the pins are to be inserted are marked on the moistened skin with silver nitrate and appear as white spots when the tincture of iodine is applied. The skin of the leg and foot is painted with strong tincture of iodine and "one pin is placed through the tibia four fingerbreadths above the ankle joint; the other pin is placed parallel to the former, through the posterior upper corner of the tuberosity of the os calcis, the pins being driven through with hammer or drill. The skin wounds are covered with the nicked sponges moistened with balsam of peru. Before the pin is driven through the posterior upper corner of the os calcis, it is necessary to place the foot in maximum dorsiflexion in order to relax the skin, which easily tears unless this precaution is taken. Both pins are now engaged in the freely turning wire stirrups. The free movement of the latter is essential since subsequent traction is to occur in two directions. If on the other hand the stirrup loop were tight against the pin, a traction in different directions would only be possible by turning the pin in the bone; this would be conducive to drill-hole infection.

"Now the limb is placed upon the screw extension apparatus with the knee in flexion. The pin placed above the ankle joint is suspended on its stirrup so as to make the leg horizontal. The right-angle flexion of the knee relaxes the tendo achillis. The pin through the os calcis is attached to the hook of the screw extension apparatus after interposition of a spring balance. Then traction is applied—first in the long axis of the leg to the amount of fifteen to twenty kilograms, in order to pull the tuberosity of the os calcis downward and to restore the tuber-joint angle; the forefoot at the same time being placed in pronation and maximum plantar flexion. The screw is then lowered, and traction of from fifteen to twenty kilograms is made in the direction of the axis of the os calcis, in order to overcome the shortening of the bone and the axial deviation in the transverse plane, the forefoot again being plantar flexed and pronated. The screw and stirrup are again raised, and horizontal traction of from ten to twelve kilograms in the axis of the leg is applied. By means of this longitudinal traction in the axis of the os calcis and the subsequent traction in the axis of the tibia, as well as by means of the plantar flexion and pronation of the forefoot, the axial kinking, the shortening, and also a part of the broadening of the os calcis are corrected. The astragalus is lifted off the os calcis and the joint space between the two bones is again restored.

"In order to correct the remaining broadening, the screw vise (Fig. 1260) is applied under constant longitudinal traction in such a manner as to place the straight pad on the outside, the concave on the inside below the sustentaculum tali; then the vise is screwed together until a distance of from 35 to

50 millimeters is obtained. The proper distance for each case is determined by applying the vise first tightly to the sound heel and by reading off the breadth of the os calcis. On the affected side the compression is then carried to five millimeters beyond the normal amount. The vise is released rapidly so as to avoid pressure necrosis of the skin. Under continued traction lateral and axial x-rays are made to determine whether the tuber-joint angle has been restored and whether the broadening and the adduction deviation have disappeared. The tuber-joint angle should be somewhat overcorrected, amounting to from 35 to 40 degrees.

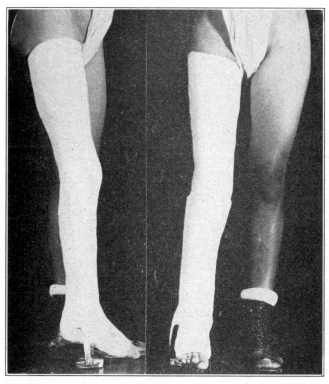

Fig. 1265.—Boehler's walking cast used in the convalescent treatment of fractures of the os calcis. In most cases it is only necessary to extend the cast up to the upper one-third of the leg.

"To retain the good position of the fragments, an unpadded plaster splint is applied, under continuous longitudinal traction from the tip of the toes to the popliteal space. On the dorsal side the toes are left exposed. The splint is nicked on both sides at the heel and also about the pins to avoid wrinkles. This splint is then fastened with three circular plaster bandages, which must be placed loosely on both sides of the heel in order that they may not be too tight over the depressions caused by the pressure of the pads. Care must be taken to insure good modelling; there should be no pressure on either side of the tendo achillis. The forefoot must be held constantly in plantar flexion and pronation, and, at the same time, the great toe is held in dorsiflexion.

"After a few minutes, when the plaster has hardened, the traction is released, the stirrups are removed, and the limb is placed upon a Braun's splint.

The two pins now hold the fragments immovably in the plaster cast. For the next forty-eight hours the circulation of the toes must be watched very closely and if the toes are swollen, bluish, or cold, the plaster dressing must be split immediately; this, however, occurs but rarely. Formerly both pins were removed immediately after completed reduction; but this did not prove advisable, because the tuberosity of the os calcis was displaced upward by the pull of the tendo achillis, and the tuber-joint angle became diminished or even disappeared.

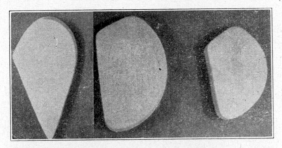

Fig. 1266.—Types of hard felt pads used in making arch supports in the convalescent treatment of fractures of the tarsal bones. These are shaved down to conform to the arch.

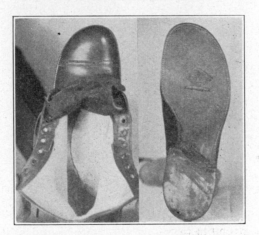

Fig. 1267.—Felt pad in the shoe glued to the inner sole, and Thomas heel on shoe. Another excellent support is one made of sponge rubber, which can be cut out and glued in the shoe the same as the felt.

"Should the skin break during reduction, the pins must be removed to avoid infection; in this case it is better to eliminate at once the pull of the tendon, by achillotenotomy. If signs of inflammation appear, the pins must be removed at once; otherwise they remain in place for from three to five weeks according to the degree of fragmentation. At this time the pins are removed and a new plaster cast with walking stirrup is applied (Fig. 1265). This remains until from nine to fourteen weeks after injury. If this is removed too soon, the soft callus may yield to pressure, and new axial kinks of the bone may occur. A zinc glue dressing is applied for the after-treatment to avoid subsequent swelling and flatfoot plates of strong material with lateral flange are used.

"Complete functional ability of the foot is observed after from four to eight months, varying with the age of the patient and the degree of comminution of the bone."

We have used this method with the variation that we use a well-padded plaster cast immediately after the reduction and incorporate the pins in this cast. At the end of this time we remove the cast and pins and apply a new cast either over very little padding, or a Boehler unpadded walking plaster is applied and worn for from four to eight weeks. Conn's method* reduces the displacements by means of a special traction apparatus and then incorporates his pins in a well-padded cast and four weeks later performs a triple arthrodesis as mentioned below under treatment of old fractures of the os calcis. He adopts this procedure because in his hands the Boehler method has often failed to give painless feet and he reports excellent results in seventeen out of nineteen acute fractures treated by reduction followed by triple arthrodesis.

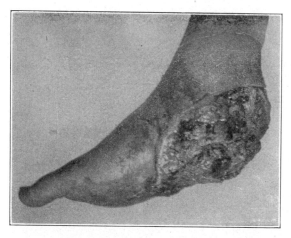

Fig. 1268.—Photograph of severe compound fracture of the os calcis with loss of substance. Treated by Dakin's solution followed by skin graft. Useful foot was obtained.

Cotton's Method of Impaction.—The Cotton method which is rather popular in this country attempts to reduce the upward and posterior displacement by direct manual traction and then to maintain the reduction by lateral impaction. Reduction is accomplished by pulling the heel downward and backward or by manipulating the foot over a wedge as described above. Then the foot is laid on a sandbag with the inner side down, a pad of felt is placed over the lateral surface of the os calcis, a rounded piece of wood is placed over this, and with a mallet the os calcis is impacted laterally. This method is excellent, if it is possible to reduce the upward and backward displacement. If this cannot be done the lateral impaction does not affect it. However, even when the upward and lateral displacement cannot be reduced the lateral impaction tends to get rid of the broadening of the heel and of the fragments which are displaced posteriorly and below the external malleolus. After the impaction the foot and leg are immobilized in a plaster-of-Paris cast for ten

*Conn, H. R.: J. Bone & Joint Surg., 1935.

weeks. At the end of this time the cast is removed and the patient may begin to exercise the foot and bear weight in a shoe with an arch support and a Thomas heel.

Treatment of Old Fractures of the Os Calcis.—In a certain percentage of the old fractures of the os calcis in which reduction has not been obtained or in which there has been disorganization of the subastragaloid or calcaneo-cuboid joints, there is pain with weight-bearing and prolonged disability. In some of these cases the symptoms can be relieved by arch supports or by a shoe with a Thomas heel, but in the majority of them operative intervention is necessary if the patient is to have a useful and painless foot. Before the operation is undertaken, careful x-ray and physical examination should be made in an effort to determine the cause of the pain. In the great majority of cases the pain and disability are due to traumatic arthritis in the subas-tragaloid joint. The next most frequent cause of trouble is the presence of excess bone behind and beneath the external malleolus. The third cause is traumatic arthritis in the calcaneocuboid joint. Rare causes of disability are upward displacement of the heel with resultant flattening of the arch of the foot and the presence of spurs or loose fragments of bones on the plantar surface of the heel causing points of painful pressure.

After the cause of disability has been determined, the surgeon should plan his operation in such a way that this will be relieved. Frequently there is trouble in the subastragaloid joint and in the calcaneocuboid joint, and also there is excess bone behind the external malleolus. In these cases it is necessary to correct all three conditions and this can be done at one operation. Through a lateral incision below the external malleolus the excess bone on the lateral surface of the os calcis is removed with a chisel and some of the underlying bone is removed. The object is to get rid of enough bone.

Then the subastragaloid joint is excised, and in the excision the joint sur-faces are so modeled that the os calcis will be restored to its normal line of weight-bearing; that is, in many instances the os calcis will be found to be tilted outward and it will be necessary to remove a wedge from the inner side of the joint. Some surgeons prefer to make a separate incision on the inner side of the ankle and thus obtain a better and an easier access to the region of the sustentaculum tali.

The lateral incision is then extended forward on the lateral border of the foot crossing the calcaneocuboid joint, and the cartilage from this joint should be excised.

After these two joints have been excised, it is frequently found that the foot cannot be placed in its normal position and that it is necessary to shorten the neck of the astragalus. This may be done by excising the astragalo-scaphoid joint through a lateral or mesial incision and removing a portion of the head of the astragalus and thus shortening it. We usually do the triple arthrodesis operation, excising the subastragaloid, calcaneocuboid, and as-tragaloscaphoid joints, thus ankylosing the astragalus, os calcis, cuboid, and scaphoid to one another. This permits free motion at the ankle and stabilizes the heel in the lateral plane and gives the patient a firm, stable and painless foot.

The rare instances with loose fragments or spurs in the plantar surface of the heel are usually cured by removing the offending bone. The upward displacement of the tuberosity and the posterior portion of the body can be corrected by an oblique osteotomy through the body. The separated tuberosity is then pulled downward and backward and fixed in place by a screw or nail. This is an extensive and difficult operation and is rarely necessary.

After any of these operations the foot should be immobilized in a plaster-of-Paris cast for eight weeks. At the end of this time the cast can be removed and the patient may begin to bear weight in a shoe with a Thomas heel and an arch support (Figs. 1266 and 1267).

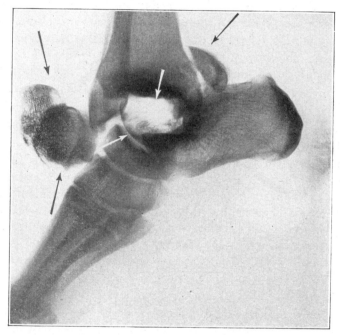

Fig. 1269.—Severe compound comminuted fracture dislocation of astragalus. Astragalectomy was performed. Fairly good function.

TOTAL DISLOCATION OF THE ASTRAGALUS

Dislocation of the astragalus is a very rare injury which may result from a fall from a height in which the patient lands on the foot and as a result of leverage combined with compression, the astragalus is torn loose from most, if not all, of its ligamentous attachments and is forced out of its socket and comes to rest in the subcutaneous tissues around the ankle while the malleoli settle down on the superior surface of the os calcis. The lesion is often compound and may be complicated by a fracture of the astragalus or of the malleoli or of some of the other bones of the foot. The bone may be displaced forward and outward or inward or backward.

Diagnosis of Total Dislocation of the Astragalus.—There is great swelling and complete disability, but despite the swelling, the mass of the displaced astragalus can usually be seen and can always be palpated beneath the skin in its abnormal position. The malleoli may or may not be intact, the os calcis is usually intact and the malleoli are lowered on the os calcis. The foot may be displaced backward or forward on the leg. The diagnosis should be confirmed by the x-ray.

Prognosis in Total Dislocation of the Astragalus.—If the dislocation is successfully reduced soon after the accident, a practically normal foot and ankle may be expected. If the dislocation is not reduced soon after the accident, there may be sloughing of the tense skin over the displaced bone and infection may supervene and amputation be necessary.

Treatment of Total Dislocation of the Astragalus.—Treatment is immediate reduction which should be accomplished by manipulation if possible. In order to accomplish reduction it is necessary to pull the os calcis down away from the malleoli so that the astragalus may be replaced in its normal bed. Consequently the first maneuver in reduction is to apply strong traction to the foot while countertraction is applied to the leg with the knee flexed. When the os calcis has been pulled down and while this traction is maintained by an assistant or by a screw traction apparatus with a pin through the os calcis, the surgeon endeavors by direct pressure to force the astragalus back into its normal position. If this is not possible, an open reduction is indicated and should be done immediately.

At the operation the astragalus should be replaced in its normal position, the wound closed, and the foot immobilized in a plaster-of-Paris cast extending from the toes to the middle of the thigh. Immobilization should be continued for four weeks. At the end of this time the cast may be removed, the patient may begin to exercise the foot and gradually restore motion at the ankle. At the end of two or three weeks more, the patient may begin to bear weight upon the foot in a shoe with a Thomas heel and an arch support. If the wound becomes infected, astragalectomy may be necessary.

SUBASTRAGALOID DISLOCATION

Subastragaloid dislocations are rare injuries which may result from falls or severe torsion injuries of the foot, such as usually result in fractures and fracture dislocations at the ankle. The astragalus remains in the mortise of the ankle joint while the foot is torn loose at the subastragaloid and astragalo-scaphoid joints and is displaced upon the astragalus. The displacement may be forward, backward, inward, or outward, the direction being dependent upon the force causing the injury. It may be complete or incomplete.

Prognosis.—The prognosis is good if the dislocation is reduced soon after the injury.

Diagnosis.—There is marked swelling and complete disability, the foot is fixed in an abnormal position on the leg, and the circulation of the foot may be impeded. The malleoli are intact and motion at the ankle joint is possible but painful. Palpation of the os calcis will usually enable the surgeon to determine the direction and degree of the displacement. When the foot is displaced backward the head of the astragalus is palpable in front of the ankle, and the forefoot is shortened. When it is displaced forward there is a prominence beneath the tendo achillis, and the heel is shortened. The lateral displacement can be determined by noting the alignment of the foot with the leg. The diagnosis should be confirmed by the x-ray when possible, but the surgeon should not delay reduction in order to obtain an x-ray picture.

Treatment.—Treatment is immediate reduction. This is especially true if there is circulatory impairment. Reduction can as a rule be accomplished by manipulation and with relatively little difficulty. Traction is made on the foot by an assistant while countertraction on the leg with the knee flexed is made by another assistant or by a mechanical rest. Then, with direct pressure with the hands, when the bones have been pulled apart, the surgeon should mold the foot or ankle so that normal relationship will be restored, moving it forward or backward as necessary.

After reduction the foot, ankle and leg are immobilized in a plaster-of-Paris cast or posterior plaster mold incorporated in a cast for six weeks. At the end of this time the cast is removed and the patient may begin to exercise the foot and ankle, and three weeks later he may begin to bear weight in a shoe with an ankle support and a Thomas heel.

DISLOCATION AT THE MIDTARSAL JOINT

The midtarsal joint includes the astragaloscaphoid joint on the mesial side of the foot and the calcaneocuboid joint on the lateral side of the foot and separates the anterior from the posterior tarsal bones. Dislocation at the midtarsal joint is a rare lesion, but it may occur in severe crushing or torsion injuries of the foot or in falls from a height and may be either incomplete or complete. In the incomplete type the anterior tarsal bones and forefoot may be displaced in any direction. In the total type the anterior tarsal bones and the forefoot are usually displaced downward, but may be displaced in any direction just as in the incomplete type. The injury may be compound and associated with multiple fractures of the foot and may result in amputation.

Diagnosis of Dislocation at the Midtarsal Joint.—The malleoli and ankle regions are intact, but the entire foot and ankle are markedly swollen and in the complete type the forefoot is grossly displaced and the foot is shortened. With complete dislocation even with great swelling, it is possible to palpate the head of the astragalus and the proximal borders of the displaced anterior tarsal bones in their abnormal positions. Motions at the ankle are not greatly disturbed, but the forefoot is fixed in an abnormal position on the posterior tarsal bones. The diagnosis should be confirmed by the x-ray.

Treatment of Dislocation at the Midtarsal Joint.—Treatment is immediate reduction by manipulation under an anesthetic. The swelling should be massaged away in order that the contours of the bones may be palpable, then with the ankle immobilized by an assistant, another assistant makes strong traction directly forward on the forefoot and the surgeon endeavors by direct pressure with the heels of his hands to force the anterior tarsal bones back into their normal position. If this is not possible, open reduction should be resorted to. When satisfactory reduction has been obtained, the foot should be immobilized in a plaster-of-Paris cast, and the patient put in bed

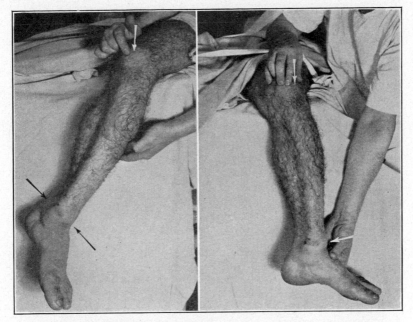

A.

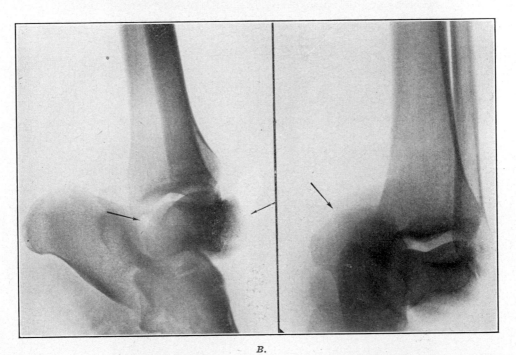

B.

Fig. 1270 *A* and *B*.—Posterior and mesial dislocation at the subastragaloid joint. Reduced by manipulation.

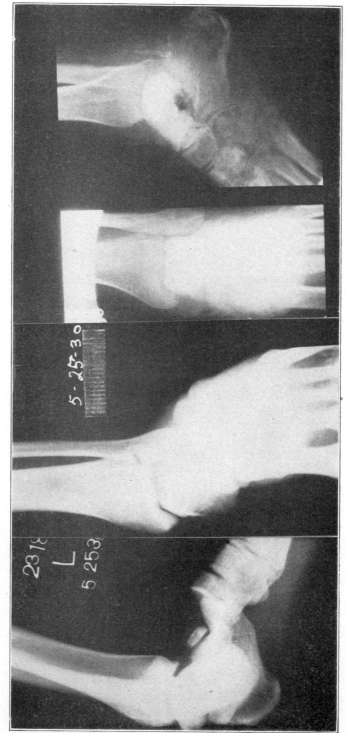

Fig. 1271.—Subastragalar and astragaloscaphoid dislocation of the left ankle with a chip fracture of the head of the astragalus. Aseptic necrosis of the body of the astragalus necessitated astragalectomy. Good result. (Courtesy Drs. Schrock, Johnson, and Waters.)

with the foot elevated. Frequently an incomplete reduction is followed by partial ankylosis with a stiff and painful foot. Consequently postoperative roentgenograms should be made as soon as the cast is dry. If the position is satisfactory, the cast should remain on for eight weeks. At the end of this time, the patient may be permitted to walk, but should wear a shoe with a Thomas heel and an arch support of hard felt. If persistent pain results, the painful joints should be arthrodesed.

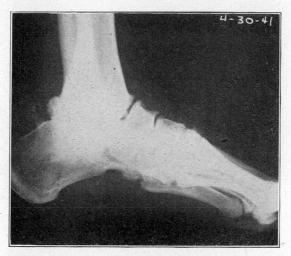

Fig. 1272.—Roentgenogram of case shown in Fig. 1271 eleven years later.

FRACTURES OF THE ANTERIOR TARSAL BONES

Fractures of the Scaphoid

The scaphoid may be fractured alone (Fig. 1273) or as a complication of other fractures of the foot and ankle. The usual mechanism is one in which force transmitted upward from the forefoot through the cuneiform bones compresses the scaphoid between these bones and the head of the astragalus. Consequently the scaphoid may be broken in falls upon the balls of the feet, in forcible dorsiflexion of the foot, or in torsion injuries of the foot. The fracture line tends to be vertical across the body of the bone or the tuberosity may be broken off or the bone may be comminuted. The mesial fragment tends to be displaced inward or forward (upward) and may be palpable as a prominence on the anterior border of the foot. In other instances the bone is crushed from below upward and is compressed.

Diagnosis of Fractures of the Scaphoid.—When the injury occurs in conjunction with fractures at the ankle, the injury to the scaphoid is apt to be overlooked unless it is seen in the x-ray plates. In an isolated injury of the scaphoid the diagnosis can usually be made from the physical examination. There is a history of an acute injury followed by pain and swelling in the region over the scaphoid and inability to bear weight upon the foot. The foot tends to be held in a position of eversion and attempts to invert or dorsiflex it cause pain at the site of the tenderness. If the fragments are displaced,

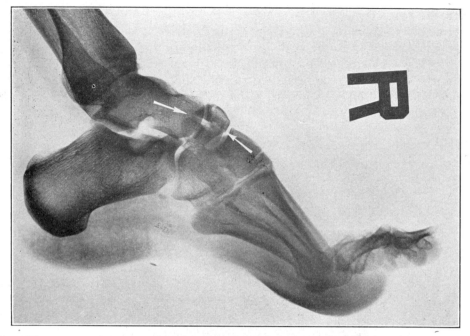

Fig. 1273.—Fracture of the scaphoid. No reduction necessary. Immobilized in a plaster-of-Paris cast.

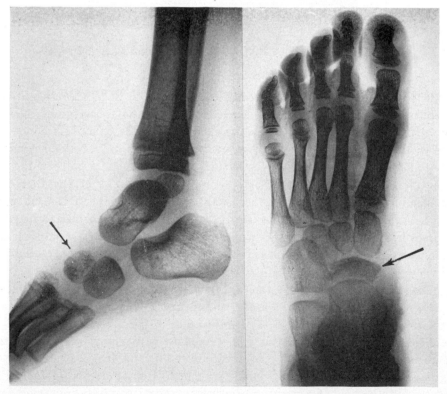

Fig. 1274.—A. Showing Köhler's disease in its early stage. B. Showing same case several months later. Treatment in this case usually demands prolonged fixation in a cast with limited weight-bearing.

it may be possible to palpate the displaced fragment in the subcutaneous tissues over the scaphoid. The diagnosis should be confirmed by x-ray, and the presence of an accessory scaphoid should be ruled out.

In children the surgeon should be on the watch for Köhler's disease. This is an osteitis of the scaphoid with symptoms simulating those of a fracture. The treatment is conservative: prolonged rest (two to four months) in a plaster cast with freedom from weight-bearing or strapping to relieve symptoms.

Treatment of Fractures of the Scaphoid.—If there is no displacement of the fragments, the foot and ankle should be immobilized in a plaster boot extending from the toes to the tibial tubercle, the foot being immobilized in a position of slight plantar flexion and in the neutral position as regards inversion and eversion. This plaster is worn for from four to six weeks. At the end of this time it may be discontinued and the patient may be permitted to wear a shoe with a Thomas heel which is elevated one-fourth of an inch on its inner border and which contains a hard felt or sponge rubber arch support.

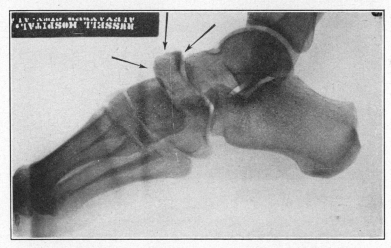

Fig. 1275.—Anterior subluxation of the carpal scaphoid. Open reduction was necessary followed by immobilization in a plaster-of-Paris cast.

If there is displacement an attempt should be made to reduce the displacement and restore the normal contours of the bone. This is especially important as the scaphoid enters into the formation of two weight-bearing joints. Reduction can usually be accomplished by having an assistant fix the heel while another assistant makes strong traction on the forefoot and at the same time everts it and plantar flexes it, thus widening the space between the cuneiforms and the head of the astragalus. While the traction is maintained, the surgeon should, by means of his thumbs, endeavor to press the displaced fragments back into their normal position. If the fracture is several days old, it may be necessary to place a piece of saddler's felt over the bone and drive the displaced fragments back with a mallet. When reduction has been accomplished, the traction should be released while the surgeon maintains pressure on the fragments, and if displacement does not recur, the foot should be immobilized in a plaster-of-Paris cast as described above.

If dislocation does occur when the traction is released, the foot should be immobilized in eversion and plantar flexion over a period of three weeks. This position will usually maintain reduction. At the end of three weeks this plaster is removed, the foot gently brought into the midposition and into as much dorsiflexion as possible, and a new plaster applied. This is worn from two to three weeks, when it is removed and the patient given a shoe as described above.

In old cases in which reduction has not been accomplished and in which a painful flatfoot has developed, an arthrodesing operation of either the astragaloscaphoid joint or of the joint between the scaphoid and the cuneiform bones should be performed, and the foot corrected under an anesthetic and immobilized in the correct position.

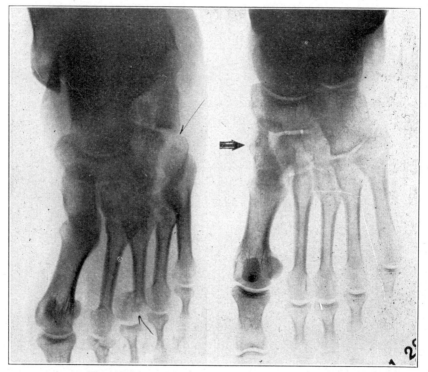

Fig. 1276.   Fig. 1277.

Fig. 1276.—Crush fracture of the cuboid, third and fourth metatarsals and the os calcis. Treated by immobilization in a plaster cast for six weeks, weight-bearing on felt pad in nine weeks. Good result in twelve weeks.

Fig. 1277.—Old fracture of the internal cuneiform not diagnosed or treated. Poor result with necrosis of the bone. Cast was then applied; no weight-bearing for three months. Good result.

Fractures of the Cuboid and Cuneiform Bones

Occasionally one or more of these bones are fractured by direct violence in severely crushed feet (Figs. 1276 and 1277). In other instances they are fractured in the severe torsion injuries in which there is displacement either at the midtarsal or at the tarsometatarsal joint.

Diagnosis.—Due to the position of the bones, the diagnosis is usually dependent upon the x-ray pictures which should always be obtained in these severely crushed feet, even though no deformity be present. The diagnosis may be suspected by the presence of swelling and localized tenderness over the site of the fracture.

Treatment.—As a rule there is practically no displacement of the fragments. If the fracture is a part of some major injury to the foot, this should be treated and the fractures of the cuboid and cuneiforms may be ignored.

In isolated fractures of these bones all that is necessary is to immobilize the foot in a plaster-of-Paris cast in a neutral position over a period of from four to five weeks. At the end of this time the cast may be removed, the foot strapped firmly with adhesive, and the patient may begin walking in a shoe with a Thomas heel and a hard felt arch support.

DISLOCATION AT THE TARSOMETATARSAL JOINTS

These injuries are fairly common and vary greatly in their pathology. The entire group of metatarsals may be dislocated en masse upon the tarsal bones and the displacement may be lateral or upward or downward (Figs. 1278, 1279, 1280, and 1281). In other instances a single metatarsal is dislocated

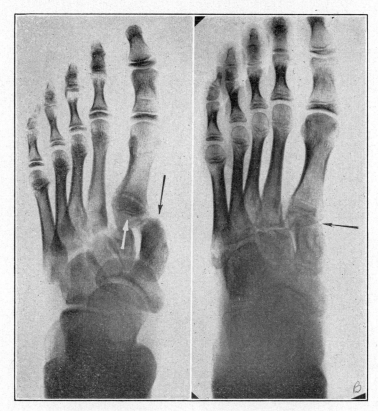

Fig. 1278.—Dislocation at the tarsometatarsal joint. Open reduction was necessary. Immobilized in a plaster-of-Paris cast. Good result.

and here the displacement is usually upward, but it may be downward or lateral, or two or more of the metatarsals may be dislocated upward, downward or laterally. The most frequent tarsometatarsal dislocations are those of the first and the fifth metatarsals. The dislocation may be the result of falls on the ball of the foot, or of direct crushing injuries or of torsion injuries and is not as a rule associated with fractures.

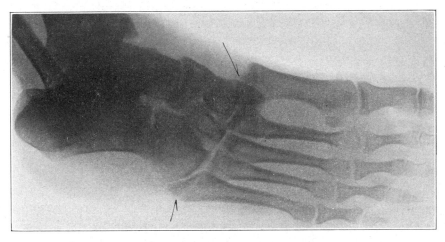

Fig. 1279.—Dislocation of the first metatarsal with fracture of the second metatarsal shaft and base of the fifth metatarsal. Reduction with cast applied for seven weeks. Weight-bearing in nine weeks. Good result in twelve weeks.

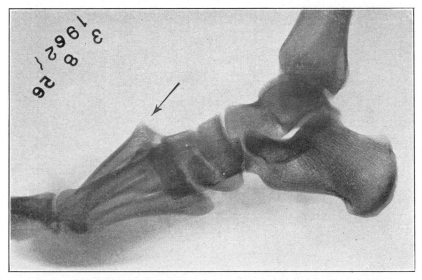

Fig. 1280.—Dorsal dislocation of the second metatarsal. Reduced by open operation and immobilized in a plaster cast.

Diagnosis.—Following the accident there is marked swelling of the entire forefoot and this swelling may involve the ankle and extend up the leg. It may be so great as to obscure the deformity. Ordinarily, however, the deformity is visible, especially in dorsal dislocations where the thick base of the dislocated metatarsal produces a marked prominence on the dorsum of the foot. The extensor tendons are drawn tightly over this prominence. In lateral dislocations the deformity is usually visible as well as palpable. Motions at the ankle are free, but abduction and adduction are painful and limited. The diagnosis should be confirmed by the x-ray, as it is not as a rule possible by physical examination alone to get an exact idea of the total damage.

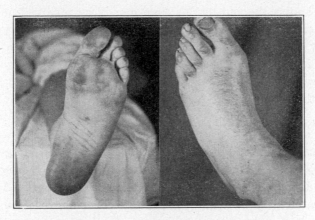

Fig. 1281.—Dislocation of the first metatarsal with fracture of the second and third. Treated by manipulative reduction and plaster cast for seven weeks. Weight-bearing with felt pad in nine weeks. No improvement. Metal arch, no improvement. Arthrodesis at the first, second, third, and fourth tarsometatarsal joints was performed with good result in ten weeks.

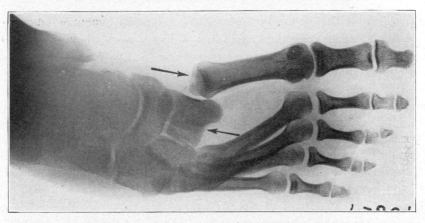

Fig. 1282.—Roentgenogram of preceding case.

Treatment of Dislocation at the Tarsometatarsal Joint.—The treatment is immediate reduction. If the patient is seen soon after the injury, this can usually be accomplished with relatively little difficulty by traction and direct pressure. One assistant should immobilize the heel while another makes strong traction on the toes. It is advisable to place a loop of bandage around the toe in order to secure a firm grip for traction. If the metatarsals are displaced en masse a bandage can be looped around the forefoot just behind the metatarsal heads. When the dislocated bone or bones have been pulled down by an assistant, the surgeon should, by direct pressure with his hands on the base of the metatarsal bones, force them back into their normal positions. In order to be fairly certain that accurate reduction has been obtained, the swelling over the bases of the bones should be pressed away by deep massage in order that the contour of the dorsum of the foot may be restored.

When satisfactory reduction has been obtained, the foot should be immobilized in a plaster-of-Paris cast with the instep well molded and the patient put to bed with the foot elevated. The plaster should be worn for four or five weeks and at the end of this time it may be removed and the patient may begin to exercise the foot. Motion at the tarsometatarsal joint, however, is of relatively little importance and there is no indication for a lot of physiotherapy in order to obtain motion. After another week the patient may be given a shoe with a Thomas heel and a hard felt arch pad and begin to bear weight upon the foot. The reduction should, of course, be controlled by an x-ray picture, and if satisfactory reduction has not been obtained by the manipulation, an open reduction should be performed as it is very important that the bones be accurately replaced if a painless functioning foot is to be obtained. This can be done through a dorsal incision and it may be necessary to suture the displaced bone into place with chromic catgut. After the open reduction, treatment is the same as that described above after reduction by manipulation.

FRACTURES OF THE METATARSAL BONES

Fractures of the metatarsal bones are relatively common and are frequently the cause of prolonged disability, either because they are overlooked at the preliminary examination or are unsuccessfully treated. Most of the cases occur in laboring men and are the result of direct crushing injuries such as the dropping of a heavy object on the foot or of the foot being run over by an automobile. The fractures may involve one bone alone, may be multiple (Fig. 1283), or may be comminuted (Fig. 1284). In a considerable percentage of the cases there is little or no displacement. In other instances there is complete displacement with shortening of the bone and as a rule the proximal end of the distal fragment is displaced downward into the sole of the foot.

Diagnosis of Fractures of the Metatarsal Bones.—The diagnosis is difficult because after the injury there is swelling and pain involving the entire forefoot (Fig. 1288) and the bones lie so close to one another that palpation of an individual bone is difficult. If there is gross displacement, especially of the first or fifth metatarsal bone, the diagnosis can usually be made by palpation and by the demonstration of false motion when the distal fragment is grasped between the thumb and fingers and pushed upward or downward or moved in flexion and extension while the proximal end is immobilized by the other hand (Fig. 1289). In the case of the second, third, and fourth, relatively little false motion can be demonstrated. It may be possible, however, to demonstrate crepitus by gently flexing and extending the involved toe.

A very important point in the diagnosis is the production of either false motion or of distinct pain by making axial pressure in the line of the shaft of

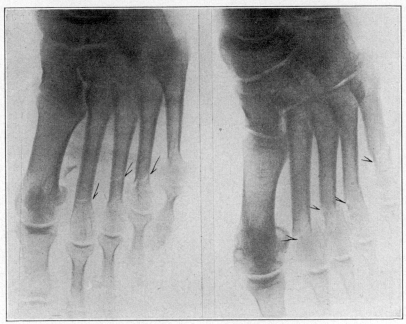

A.   B.

Fig. 1283.—*A*, Transverse fracture of the second, third, and fourth metatarsals with practically no displacement. Treated by immobilization in a plaster-of-Paris cast for six weeks. Weight-bearing in eight weeks with felt pad in instep of shoe. Good result.

B, Transverse fractures of the distal thirds of the four lateral metatarsals with slight displacement. Treated by immobilization in a plaster-of-Paris cast for eight weeks. Weight-bearing in ten weeks. Felt pad in instep of shoe. Good result.

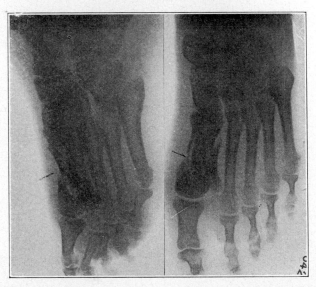

Fig. 1284.—Comminuted fracture of the first metatarsal. Treated by closed manipulative reduction and immobilization in plaster-of-Paris cast for six weeks. Walking in nine weeks with sponge rubber arch support. Good result.

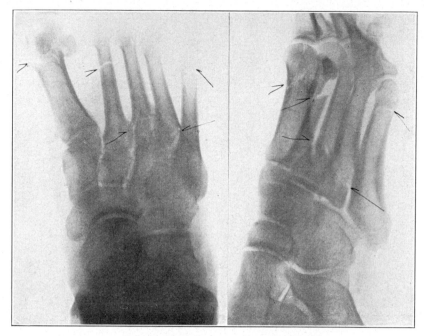

Fig. 1285.—Multiple fractures of the metatarsal bones with slight displacement. Treated by closed manipulative reduction of the fracture near the head of the first metatarsal and prolonged immobilization for eight weeks and freedom from weight-bearing for ten weeks. Felt arch pad. Good result.

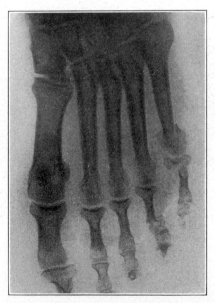

Fig. 1286.—Subcapital fracture of the fifth metatarsal and of the fourth and fifth toes. Treated by manipulative reduction and immobilization in plaster-of-Paris cast for three weeks with weight-bearing in six and one-half weeks. Good result.

each bone in turn. In order to do this the foot is held with one hand and the moderately flexed toe is grasped between the finger and thumb of the other and the toe is pressed up against the head of the metatarsal, or the toe can be hyperextended and direct pressure made on the head of the metatarsal.

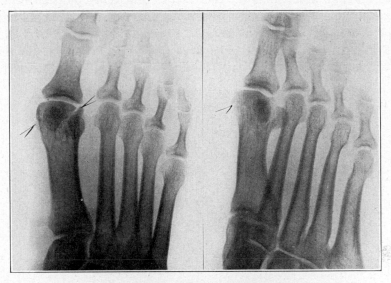

Fig. 1287.—Impacted fracture of the head of the first metatarsal. This type often leads to traumatic arthritis. Treated by reduction and by immobilization in a plaster-of-Paris cast for three weeks, then daily hot baths with freedom from weight-bearing for seven weeks. Good result.

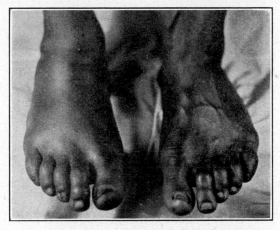

Fig. 1288.—Multiple fractures of the metatarsals. Note the swelling of the forefoot and of the toes.

If there is a fracture, even without displacement, these maneuvers will produce pain at the site of the fracture. The difficulty is that occasionally in severe contusions or sprains in the region of the tarsometatarsal joint this manipulation produces pain and leads to the false diagnosis of a fracture. Consequently the diagnosis of fracture of a metatarsal bone should be confirmed by the x-ray.

Treatment of Fractures of the Metatarsal Bones.—These fractures should be treated seriously; unless accurate reduction and firm union in the correct position are obtained, prolonged disability may result.

Fractures Without Displacement.—In fractures without displacement the indications are to immobilize the foot in the functional position in a plaster-of-Paris cast until firm union has occurred. The plaster cast should include the toes and extend to the tubercle of the tibia, and it should be well molded under the arch in order that this be preserved (Fig. 1292). If the first metatarsal has been fractured, the immobilization should be continued over a

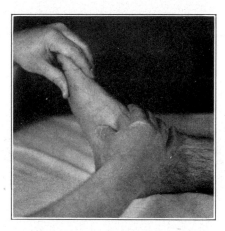

Fig. 1289.—Examination of the forefoot and method of manipulating in suspected fracture of the metatarsals.

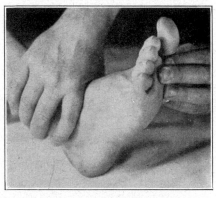

Fig. 1290.—Examination of the forefoot making pressure over the head of the metatarsal. If the fracture is present this maneuver usually elicits pain.

period of from five to six weeks. The shaft of the other metatarsal may be expected to heal in four or five weeks. If one desires, a Boehler walking plaster with an iron heel may be used as soon as the swelling has disappeared and the patient may walk on the foot. The prolonged immobilization is to be preferred to the treatment by physiotherapy, massage, and attempts to maintain motion at the ankle joint, as these efforts may lead to the production of exuberant callus with resultant pain on weight-bearing (Fig. 1293). Early motion and weight-bearing are usually to be avoided in these cases.

After the cast has been removed, the patient may begin to walk in a shoe with a Thomas heel (Figs. 1267 and 1268) and a rather large hard felt or sponge rubber arch support which extends down well under the shafts of the metatarsals to a point just behind the heads, or a metatarsal bar and anterior arch

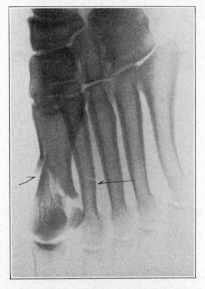

Fig. 1291.—Fracture of the first and second metatarsals with rotation of the distal fragment of the first. Treated by closed manipulative reduction and immobilization in a plaster cast for eight weeks with weight-bearing in ten weeks. Good result.

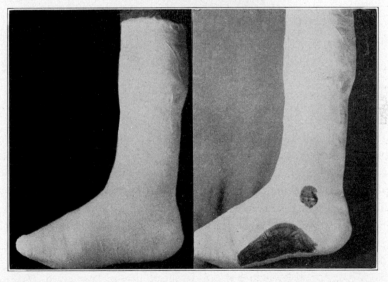

Fig. 1292.—Type of cast used in the treatment of fractures of the metatarsal bones. On the right the cast is marked over the area where it is molded in to restore the arch of the foot.

pad (Fig. 1294). This is very important as the callus should be protected from strain, otherwise it may bend when weight-bearing is resumed and prolonged disability result.

Fractures of the Metatarsal Bones With Displacement must be reduced, and the reduction must be practically anatomical. Reduction can usually be accomplished by manipulation in the following manner: While an assistant immobilizes the foot, another makes traction on the involved toe by means of a loop of bandage around the toe, and the surgeon, by direct pressure, molds the fragments back into normal position.

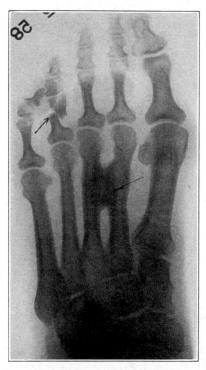

Fig. 1293.—Synostosis between the first and second metatarsal shafts following a fracture. There is also a fracture of the fourth toe with nonunion, but no symptoms. Synostosis caused considerable pain and was removed by operation. Good result.

If the fracture is a long oblique or comminuted one, and if the surgeon does not find it possible to obtain and maintain reduction, the fracture should be treated by traction. This can be applied in a manner similar to the banjo splint used for traction of the metacarpals of the hands. A plaster-of-Paris cast is placed upon the foot, which immobilizes the foot in the neutral position with moderate plantar flexion. A wire loop extending out over the toes is incorporated in the plaster, traction is applied to the toes and fastened to the loop by elastic rubber bands. Due to the shortness of the toes this traction should be either skeletal traction or through the pulp of the toe by rustless steel wire, a pin, or silkworm-gut, as directed under fractures of the fingers. Traction is maintained for three weeks, and at the end of this time union will usually be solid enough to permit removal of the traction and the application of the plaster cast. The immobilization should be continued for three or four weeks more when the cast may be removed and the patient fitted with a shoe with a Thomas heel and an arch support as described under fractures without displacement. The Davis metatarsal splint may be used instead of the banjo splint, but is less efficient.

In case accurate reduction cannot be obtained by conservative methods, the surgeon should not hesitate to operate upon these patients and perform an open reduction, as prolonged disability may follow with relatively slight displacement.

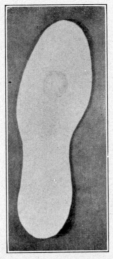

Fig. 1294.—Soft felt insole with a hard anterior arch pad sometimes used in the convalescent treatment of fractures of the metatarsals, especially with anterior arch involvement.

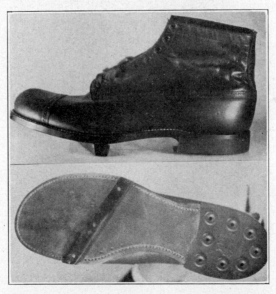

Fig. 1295.—Leather bar nailed to the sole used in the convalescent treatment of fractures of the toes and sometimes in fractures of the heads of the metatarsals. The top of the shoe frequently has to be cut away over the toes.

Fractures of the Base of the Fifth Metatarsal Bone

The fifth metatarsal differs from the others in that it may be fractured across the base or across the tuberosity by indirect violence either in inver-

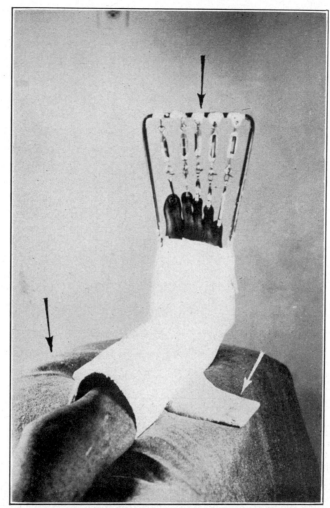

Fig. 1296.—Banjo splint and plaster cast used in maintaining traction of the toes for fractures of the phalanges or metatarsals where traction is necessary. Courtesy Dr. Charles Colquitt, Bessemer, Ala.

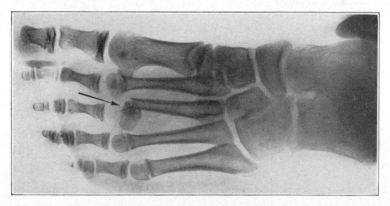

Fig. 1297.—Fracture of the distal end of 2nd and 3rd metatarsals. Treated by open reduction and fixation with chromic catgut. Cast applied. Good result.

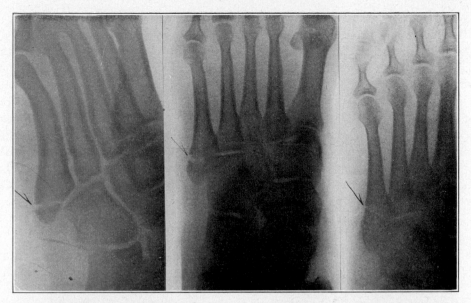

Fig. 1298.—Three cases of inversion fracture of the base of the fifth metatarsal. Treated by immobilization in a plaster-of-Paris cast for four weeks. Weight-bearing was begun at the end of seven weeks. Good result in each. This type of fracture is not infrequently received by women due to a sudden twisting of the foot usually caused by high heels.

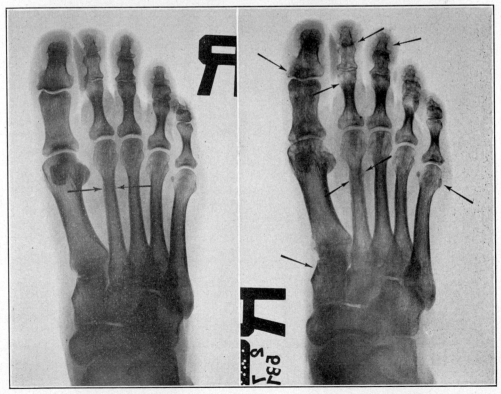

Fig. 1299.—March fracture of the distal third of the shaft of the second metatarsal bone. Treated by immobilization in a plaster-of-Paris cast. There is considerable atrophy as shown in the print on the right, but union with relatively little callus has occurred.

sion of the foot or possibly by a pull of the peroneus brevis muscle which is attached to the tuberosity. The fracture line may pass through the tip of the tuberosity, through the base of the tuberosity, or through the proximal end of the bone (Fig. 1298). The fracture usually occurs when force acts upon the supinated foot in plantar flexion.

Diagnosis.—If one is able to obtain an accurate history of the position of the foot at the time when the trauma acted, the diagnosis should be suspected, especially if the patient felt something give way or snap while the foot was inverted and plantar flexed. There is local pain and swelling with tenderness over the site of the fracture and pain on weight-bearing. The diagnosis should be confirmed by the x-ray. False motion cannot as a rule be demonstrated.

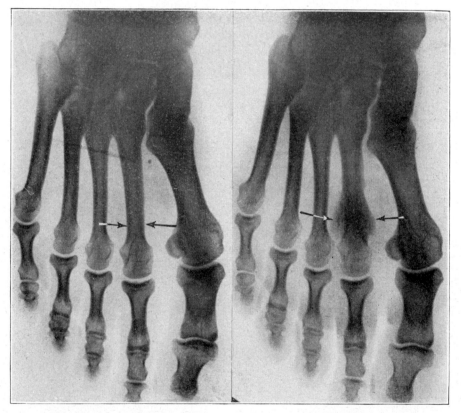

Fig. 1300.—A march fracture in which the first x-ray was negative. The excessive callus resulted from failure to protect the foot with a metatarsal bar and restrict activity but caused no permanent disability.

Treatment.—There is rarely ever sufficient displacement to make reduction necessary. The foot should be immobilized in a plaster-of-Paris cast which extends up to the tibial tubercle and this should be left on for four weeks. At the end of this time the cast should be removed and an x-ray picture taken. If there are no signs of union, the plaster should be reapplied and immobilization continued for four weeks longer. If union has not occurred at the end of the eighth week, the patient should be permitted to try to walk with the foot firmly strapped. If pain persists, the loose fragment should be excised. The delayed union and failure to unite which frequently occur in fractures of the fifth metatarsal have been explained by the poor blood supply to the proximal end of the fifth metatarsal. For this reason these fractures should be considered seriously, as they may result in prolonged disability.

March Fracture.—A rather unusual metatarsal fracture is one which occurs without unusual trauma and is consequently called march fracture. The fracture occurs as a simple transverse fracture of the distal half of the shaft of one of the three middle metatarsals, and there is little tendency to displacement, but unless the arch of the foot is supported by a metatarsal bar, it tends to produce excess callus and may remain painful for a long time.

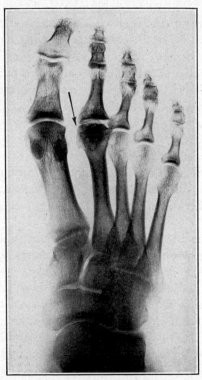

Fig. 1301.—Infraction of the head of the second metatarsal bone (Freiberg's disease). Treated by excision of the metatarsal head.

The patient notices a moderate pain in the anterior portion of the foot and local tenderness and swelling lead the surgeon to suspect a fracture which is then shown in the x-ray.

The fracture may be treated by a walking plaster well molded under the arch of the foot but this is rarely necessary. Rest for a few days until the acute pain subsides and then restricted activity in a shoe fitted with a metatarsal bar afford relief and the fracture may be expected to heal without complications and result in no disability.

Infraction of the Second Metatarsal Head.—Painful enlargement of the head of the second metatarsal was described by Freiberg as a clinical entity.

It is probable that in some instances no injury other than that due to walking is required, as some patients can recall no injury.

The patient complains of pain in the anterior arch and on palpation the head of the second metatarsal is found to be thickened and tender. There is a callus under the ball of the foot and movement of the joint causes pain. The x-rays shows the metatarsal head enlarged with the extremity flattened, and the base of the first phalanx of the toe may be deformed. The joint may contain loose bodies.

Treatment.—A metatarsal bar and a relatively loose shoe may afford relief. In severe cases one of us (J. A. K.) has removed the metatarsal head and the base of the phalanx of the toe with satisfactory results.

FRACTURES OF THE TOES

Most of the fractures of the toes are due to direct violence as in a weight falling upon the foot, and for this reason many of them are compound even though the shoe be not broken. Occasionally the proximal phalanx is broken indirectly as when a patient kicks an object while barefooted. In the fractures due to direct violence the phalanges may be comminuted or split longitudinally. This is especially true of the distal phalanx.

In fractures due to indirect violence, the fracture line tends to be transverse or oblique.

Diagnosis.—Due to the fact that the bones are superficial and can be easily grasped with the fingers, the diagnosis can in most cases be made without difficulty. Crepitus and deformity are present, and false motion can be demonstrated. If there is any doubt the diagnosis should be confirmed by x-ray.

Treatment.—Treatment is reduction and immobilization. If the toe is simply crushed and the phalanges are split or comminuted without displacement of the fragments no reduction is necessary. Occasionally in oblique fractures the reduction is difficult to maintain without traction. In the average case either no reduction is necessary or the displacement can be corrected by direct traction on the end of the toe, and the fracture when reduced will tend to remain reduced. In these cases all that is necessary is to immobilize the toe by strapping it to a small wooden splint made from a tongue depressor (Fig. 1304). The patient should be kept off the feet for a few days, and the splint should be worn for from two to three weeks. At the end of this time union will be fairly firm and the toe can be immobilized by strapping with adhesive.

One of us (J. A. K.) treats most of these fractures of the toes by immobilizing the toe with an adhesive dressing which is not disturbed for three or four weeks. The patient is given a large or cut-out shoe with a metatarsal bar and may return to work in a few days.

Treatment by Traction.—If reduction is not possible or if it is not possible to maintain reduction after it has been accomplished, these fractures may be treated by traction. This is most successfully applied in the manner described for the treatment of fractures of the metatarsals by traction; that is, the foot is encased in a plaster boot and a wire loop which extends out beyond the toes is incorporated in this boot. Traction by adhesive may be

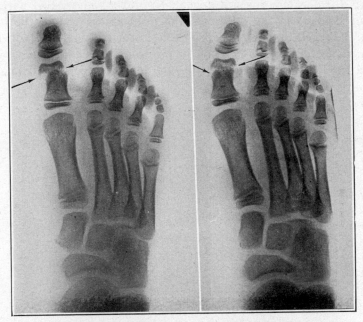

Fig. 1302.—Fracture of the first phalanx of the great toe in a child. Treated by manipulative reduction under local anesthesia and immobilization in a plaster-of-Paris splint with good result.

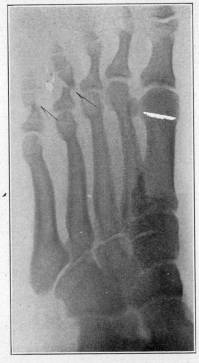

Fig. 1303.—Transverse fractures of the first phalanges of the fourth and fifth toes. Treated by manipulative reduction and immobilization in a molded plaster splint for ten days. Weight-bearing in twelve days with shoe with leather bar. Good result.

tried, but if it does not succeed a small loop of stainless steel wire or of silk-worm gut should be passed through the pulp at the end of the toe and this should be fastened to a wire loop by an elastic rubber band which is drawn taut enough to hold the fragments in position. A small wooden spreader is placed in the loop just in front of the toe in order to prevent it cutting into the skin.

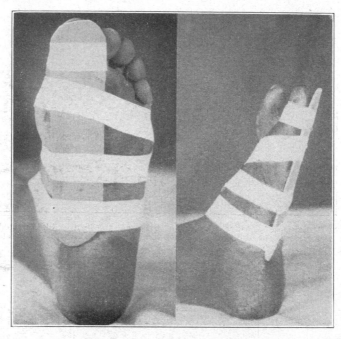

Fig. 1304.—Plantar wooden splint applied to the toe for immobilization. No padding has been used in order to show detail. This splint is practical only in mild cases.

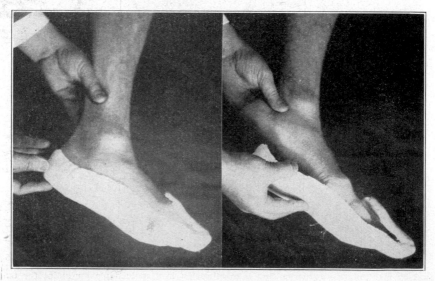

Fig. 1305.—Molded plaster slipper used in the immobilization of moderately traumatized toes. Useful also where frequent baths to toes are necessary. This dressing is also excellent in fractures of the sesamoids.

DISLOCATION AT THE METATARSOPHALANGEAL JOINTS

These are rare injuries which may be due to falls, stubbing the toe, or to direct violence such as occurs when a heavy weight falls upon the foot. The majority of cases occur in the great toe joint and a considerable percentage of these are compound dislocations.

Diagnosis.—The diagnosis can usually be made without difficulty as the toe is maintained in an abnormal position on the head of the metatarsal (Fig. 1306).

Fig. 1306.   Fig. 1307.

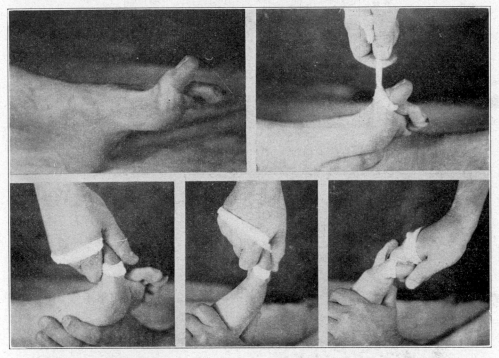

Fig. 1308.   Fig. 1309.   Fig. 1310.

Fig. 1306.—Dislocation at the first metatarsophalangeal joint.
Fig. 1307.—Manipulative reduction of the preceding posterior dislocation.
Fig. 1308.—Hyperextending the toes and bringing the base forward.
Fig. 1309.—Traction downward with countertraction to the foot.
Fig. 1310.—Flexion and traction of the toe to complete the reduction.

Treatment.—Treatment is reduction by manipulation. The manipulation is rendered more efficient if a bandage is looped around the toe and used to make traction. As the dislocation is usually on the dorsal aspect of the head of the metatarsal, traction should be made in a direction upward and forward with one hand while the thumb of the other hand presses the proximal end of the phalanx distally and then downward over the head of the metatarsal (Figs. 1306-1310).

In the case of the big toe it may be necessary first to hyperextend the dislocated toe and thus unlock the flexor tendons from the head of the metatarsal. Then the hyperextended toe is pushed directly downward over the metatarsal head. After reduction has been accomplished, there is, as a rule, little tendency for the dislocation to recur. The toe, however, should be immobilized for from one to two weeks on a small wooden splint made of a tongue depressor which is padded with cotton and strapped to the plantar surface of the foot with adhesive. A normal foot may be expected. In severe cases a plaster boot (Fig. 1311) or traction on a banjo splint may be necessary.

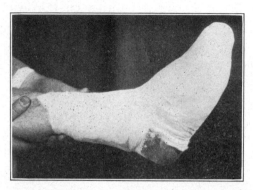

Fig. 1311.—Type of plaster used in the immobilization of simple fractures of the toe. This cast should be bivalved if necessary.

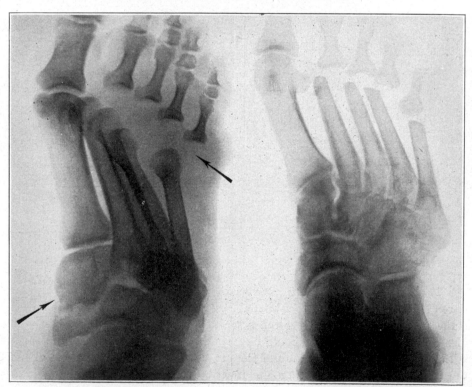

Fig. 1312.   Fig. 1313.

Fig. 1312.—Severe dislocation of the outer four toes and fracture of the scaphoid. Manipulative reduction was not possible. Treated by resection of the heads of the metatarsals. (Courtesy of John D. Sherrill, Birmingham, Alabama.)

Fig. 1313.—Same as preceding after resection of the metatarsal heads. Excellent functional result. Note the excellent results of the fractured scaphoid.

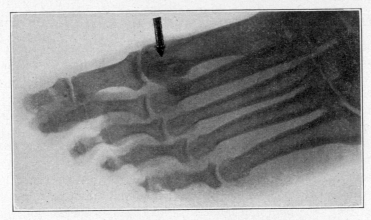

Fig. 1314.—Fracture of the sesamoid. Immobilized in a cast for two weeks with weight-bearing in three weeks. Moderate pain for eight weeks. Felt pad with hole used with relief. Good result in ten weeks. No union resulted.

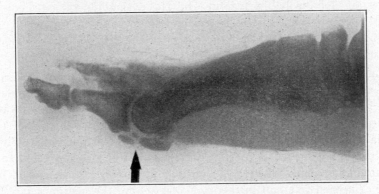

Fig. 1315.—Tripartate sesamoid. Note that the edges of the bone are smooth and that they do not coincide.

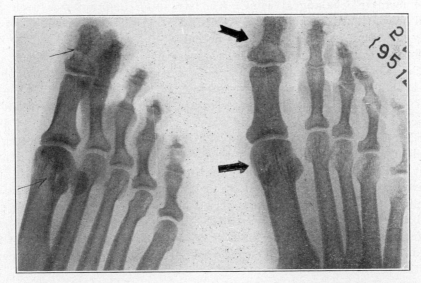

Fig. 1316.—Fracture of the mesial sesamoid of the great toe with transverse fracture of the distal phalanx. This sesamoid was removed when cast failed to cure.

FRACTURES OF THE SESAMOIDS OF THE GREAT TOE

Normally two relatively large sesamoid bones lie in the tendons of the flexor brevis hallucis muscle just beneath the head of the first metatarsal. These sesamoids are imbedded in a sheet of dense fibrous tissue and the superior surfaces are smooth for articulation with the inferior surface of the metatarsal. They may be injured by direct violence as when a weight falls upon the joint, or by a fall upon the feet when they are crushed between the head of the metatarsal and ground, or by jumping, or by forcible hyperextension of the great toe.

Diagnosis.—The injury is often overlooked because the only localizing signs are pain and tenderness over the sesamoids and pain on hyperextension of the great toe. The pain and tenderness may lead to considerable prolonged disability as they are especially pronounced with weight-bearing. The diagnosis should be confirmed by the x-ray (Fig. 1314). In examining the roentgenogram for probable fracture of the sesamoid, the surgeon should rule out bipartate sesamoids which are sometimes present (Fig. 1315). These can be ruled out by the fact that the edges of the fragments are smooth and rounded, while those in a fresh fracture are usually irregular.

Treatment of Fractures of the Sesamoids: Acute Cases.—If the patient is seen soon after the injury, an attempt should be made to obtain union of the fractured bone. In order to do this, the entire foot, ankle, and toe must be immobilized in a plaster-of-Paris cast which extends from the tip of the toes to the tibial tubercle and should be applied with the great toe moderately flexed. This plaster should be worn for three weeks. At the end of this time, the plaster should be removed, and the patient given an anterior arch support consisting of a hard felt pad in the shoe just behind the metatarsals. He may begin to walk while the toe is strapped with adhesive in order to limit motion at the metatarsophalangeal joint. The strapping and anterior arch pads should be continued for about four weeks. At the end of this time union may or may not occur, but there should be no pain.

Chronic Cases.—Many of these cases are not seen by the surgeon until some time after the accident, and in these cases it is not advisable to immobilize the foot in a plaster-of-Paris cast, as there is little chance of obtaining union by this method of treatment. On the other hand, many of these cases can be relieved by conservative treatment which consists of the application of a pad of hard felt just posterior to the heads of the metatarsals, the pad being cut in such a manner that it relieves the sesamoid from pressure incident to weight-bearing. At the same time, the great toe should be strapped with adhesive in order to limit motion at the metatarsophalangeal joint. If this does not relieve the symptoms within a period of two weeks, the offending sesamoid bone should be excised (Fig. 1316). This can be done through a small plantar incision, or in case the internal sesamoid is broken, the incision may be made along the mesial border of the sole. A normal foot may be expected after the operation.